PDR®

for Nutritional Supplements™

THOMSON REUTERS

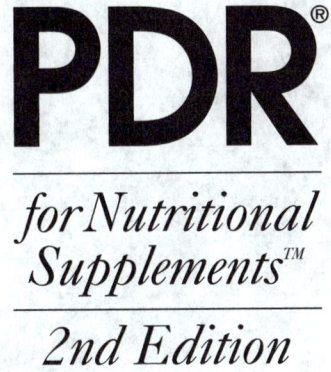

PDR®
for Nutritional Supplements™
2nd Edition

Sheldon Saul Hendler, PhD, MD, FACP, FACN, FAIC with David Rorvik, MS

Senior Director, Editorial & Publishing: Bette LaGow
Manager, Clinical Services: Nermin Shenouda, PharmD
Manager, Editorial Services: Lori Murray
Lead Project Editor: Kathleen Engel
Drug Information Specialists: Anila Patel, PharmD;
 Christine Sunwoo, PharmD; Greg Tallis, RPh
Project Editor: Sabina Borza
Associate Editor: Jennifer Reed
Manager, Art Department: Livio Udina
Electronic Publishing Designers: Deana DiVizio, Carrie Spinelli Faeth

Senior Director, Client Services: Stephanie Struble
Project Manager: Christina Klinger
Manager, Production Purchasing: Thomas Westburgh
Index Supervisor: Noel Deloughery
Index Editor: Allison O'Hare

PHYSICIANS' DESK REFERENCE
Executive Vice President, PDR: Thomas Rice
Vice President, Product Management: Cy Caine
Vice President, Publishing & Operations: Valerie Berger
Vice President, Clinical Relations: Mukesh Mehta, RPh
Vice President, Strategy & Business Development: Ray Zoeller
Vice President, Finance: Donna Santarpia
Vice President, Manufacturing: Brian Holland
Senior Director, Copy Sales: Bill Gaffney
Senior Product Manager: Richard Buchwald

Officers of Thomson Reuters (Healthcare): *President & Chief Executive Officer:* Mike Boswood; *Senior Vice President & Chief Technology Officer:* Frank Licata; *Chief Strategy Officer:* Courtney Morris; *Executive Vice President, Payer Decision Support:* Jon Newpol; *Executive Vice President, Management Decision Support:* Terry Cameron; *Executive Vice President, Marketing & Innovation:* Doug Schneider; *Senior Vice President, Finance:* Phil Buckingham; *Executive Vice President, PDR:* Thomas Rice; *Executive Vice President, Clinical Decision Support:* Thomas Hegelund; *General Counsel:* Darren Pocsik; *Senior Vice President, Human Resources:* Robin Hembree

ISBN: 978-1-56363-710-0   Printed in the United States

Contents

Foreword

The new *PDR® for Nutritional Supplements*™, *2nd Edition* takes an already excellent book to an even higher level. I was surprised at the amount of research in nutritional medicine that has taken place since the first edition was published in 2001. For many of the supplements, there were at least 10 times the number of references than were available for the first edition. The information found in this new research has been incorporated into the extensive revisions of the monographs.

In one way or another, just about everyone is exposed to supplementary nutrition, whether in the form of nutritional and dietary supplements; food fortification (eg, vitamins A and D in milk, iodine in iodized salt, and more); or functional foods (those that encompass potentially healthful products, including any modified food or food ingredient that may provide a health benefit beyond the traditional nutrients it contains, such as cholesterol-lowering phytosterols in spreads, salad dressings and snack bars, or fermented foods containing blood pressure-lowering peptides). Six out of 10 Americans use supplements on a regular basis. However, many medical practitioners are still not conversant with these supplements and many of those who use supplements are unclear as to why they are doing so.

In the rapidly evolving field of nutritional medicine, designing a safe and effective supplement regimen can be a daunting task. One must weigh the claims, the research and its quality, as well as possible side effects and drug, food, herb, supplement and disease interactions, among other things. The *PDR for Nutritional Supplements, 2nd Edition* is a source that consumers, physicians and health professionals in general can turn to for well-considered, trustworthy and relevant information about nutritional remedies.

The *PDR for Nutritional Supplements, 2nd Edition* is fortunate to have the guidance of one of the world's most respected authorities in biochemistry and clinical nutrition, Dr. Sheldon Saul Hendler, whom I met over 35 years ago when he was a Postdoctoral Fellow at the Salk Institute. As the Editor-in-Chief of the international *Journal of Medicinal Food* and the author of scores of peer-reviewed papers and patents, he brings unmatched experience, insight and judgment to this frequently controversial field.

In addition to the extensively revised existing monographs of the first edition, there are 30 new entries in this second edition. I was particularly interested in the monographs on fisetin, baicalein and the curcuminoids, since some of the major research on these substances is being performed by Drs. David Schubert and Pamela Maher, both of the Salk Institute. There is fascinating reading in the entries on vitamins C, D, and E, citrulline, and carnosine, among many others. Overall, it is very well written and a good read.

PDR for Nutritional Supplements, 2nd Edition should be a basic book for everyone's personal library. It will be for mine.

Roger Guillemin, M.D., Ph.D.
Interim President, Salk Institute
Distinguished Professor, Salk Institute
Nobel Laureate in Physiology and Medicine

How to Use This Book

Drawing on over 60 years' experience in the dissemination of pharmaceutical information, *Physicians' Desk Reference*® is proud to offer *PDR*® *for Nutritional Supplements*™, *2nd Edition*. This newly updated guide provides a comprehensive overview of the spectrum of current nutritional products.

In all, you'll find over 230 monographs—including 30 monographs new to this edition—designed to arm you with the information you need to make educated, health-promoting supplement decisions. In addition to supplying a summary of clinical research, the monographs address the practical issues encountered during routine use, from proper dosage to crucial precautions. Each profile includes up to nine sections. Here's a closer look at what they contain:

Description: A detailed discussion of the nature of the substance and its place in human biochemistry, along with its chemical structure, when available.

Actions and Pharmacology: An overview of the nutrient's best-documented actions, the proposed or verified mechanisms through which it exerts its effects, and its pharmacokinetics.

Indications and Usage: The specific therapeutic uses proposed for the supplement, ranging from the accepted indications to more speculative possibilities.

Research Summary: This section enumerates the leading claims made for the substance and evaluates the merits of each. Included are the most significant findings, both pro and con, drawn from retrospective reviews, meta-analyses, and controlled clinical trials.

Contraindications, Precautions, Adverse Reactions: The important safety considerations to remember when evaluating the supplement for personal use or, for healthcare professionals, when recommending the supplement and while monitoring the patient's progress.

Interactions: Listed here are the drugs, herbs, foods, and supplements with which the substance may interact.

Overdosage: The potential for overdose and list of the warning signs of overdose (if any are known).

Dosage and Administration: Typical dosage recommendations for the supplement, together with special measures to be taken during administration.

■ **Literature:** Relevant citations from the clinical literature.

To help you quickly locate information, the monographs have been indexed by supplement name, nutritional category, indications, side effects, and adjunctive uses. You'll also find all the interactions cited in the text listed by the supplement and the interacting substance. Here's an overview of what each index provides:

■ **Supplement Name Index:** Lists nutrients by all the names most frequently employed in the literature. Names that serve as monograph titles are highlighted by bold type. Alternative names and associated forms are cross-referenced to the appropriate monograph.

■ **Category Index:** Monographs are listed by type, such as glycosupplements, hormones, and probiotics.

■ **Indications Index:** Directs you to the nutrients customarily used for a particular therapeutic or preventative purpose. For ease of comparison with prescription and over-the-counter medications, the index employs the same headings found in the Indications Index of the *PDR Guide to Drug Interactions, Side Effects, and Indications.*

■ **Side Effects Index:** Supplements are grouped by potential adverse reactions cited in the text. Like the Indications Index, this index employs nomenclature used in the *PDR Guide to Drug Interactions, Side Effects, and Indications.*

■ **Interactions Guide:** Lists problem combinations by both the name of the nutrient and the name of the interacting agent. Drug, herb, and food interactions are included. A description of the interaction's potential effect appears in each entry.

■ **Companion Drug Index:** This section suggests nutritional supplements that may be used, in conjunction with prescription drug therapy, to reverse drug-induced side effects, relieve symptoms of the illness itself, or treat sequelae of the initial disease. Supplements are listed alphabetically under each condition.

At the end of the book, you'll find five tables designed for quick comparisons of combination supplement products. They include:

■ Calcium Combination Products

- Iron Combination Products
- Multivitamin Products
- Multivitamin and Mineral Products
- Vitamin B Complex Products

PDR for Nutritional Supplements, 2nd Edition, is the result of one of the most thorough and inclusive examinations of the literature ever undertaken. Nevertheless, it's important to remember that the book summarizes and synthesizes key data from the underlying reports, and of necessity includes neither every published report nor every recorded fact. As in all scientific investigation, conclusions regarding the effectiveness of the supplements discussed in this compendium are based on the preponderance of current evidence and cannot be considered firm or final.

The publisher does not warrant that any substance will unfailingly and uniformly exhibit the properties ascribed to it by researchers in the field. Additionally, the products discussed in this book are marketed under the provisions of the Dietary Supplement and Health Education Act of 1994, which prohibits their sale for the diagnosis, treatment, cure, or prevention of any disease. The monographs in this reference discuss scientific findings regarding the substance itself and should not be construed as recommending any specific preparation. Enumeration of specific products within a monograph implies no claim or warranty of their efficacy for any purpose, by either the manufacturer or the publisher. Furthermore, it should be understood that, just as omission of a product does not signify rejection, inclusion of a product does not imply endorsement, and that the publisher is not advocating the use of any product or substance described herein. Please remember, too, that the potency and the purity of nutritional supplements are subject to substantial variation. Dosage ranges set forth in the monographs must therefore be employed only as general guidelines.

Likewise, safety information found in the monographs applies only to the substance itself, and does not account for the effects of adulterants and variations in the manufacturing process. In addition, the publisher does not guarantee that every possible hazard, adverse effect, contraindication, precaution, or consequence of overdose is included in the summaries presented here. The publisher has performed no independent verification of the data reported herein, and expressly disclaims responsibility for any error, whether inherent in the underlying literature or resulting from erroneous translation, transcription, or typography.

Whether you are a healthcare professional or a health-conscious individual wanting to learn more about the latest nutritional discovery to hit the nightly news, we hope that *PDR for Nutritional Supplements, 2nd Edition*, provides you with the guidance you need to make informed, health-promoting choices.

Supplement Name Index

This index lists nutrients by the names most frequently employed in the literature. Names that serve as monograph titles appear in bold type. Alternative names and associated forms are cross-referenced to the appropriate monograph.

Category Index

In this index, monographs are organized by type of nutrient. United States Adopted Names (USAN) and commonly used acronyms follow the supplement names when applicable. To locate supplements advocated for a specific medical problem or purpose, please consult the Indications Index.

Indications Index

Entries in this index are organized by specific complaint, enabling you to quickly review the nutritional measures appropriate to a given situation. United States Adopted Names (USAN) and commonly used acronyms follow the supplement names when applicable. For ease of comparison with prescription and over-the-counter medications, the index employs the same headings found in the Indications Index of the PDR Guide to Drug Interactions, Side Effects, and Indications.

Side Effects Index

Presented here is an alphabetical list of every potential side effect cited in the book. Under each side effect is a list of the monographs in which it appears. United States Adopted Names (USAN) and commonly used acronyms follow the supplement names when applicable. For ease of comparison with prescription and over-the-counter medications, the index employs the same headings found in the Side Effects Index of the PDR Guide to Drug Interactions, Side Effects, and Indications.

Interactions Guide

This section catalogs potentially adverse interactions between nutritional supplements and drugs, herbs, alcohol, food, tobacco, and other nutrients. Under each bold-face entry, you'll find a list of potentially interactive substances. A description of the interaction's effect follows each item in the list. All interactions are indexed under each element in the combination.

5-HT1 RECEPTOR AGONISTS

5-Hydroxytryptophan
(5-HTP may increase risk of side effects)

L-Tryptophan
(Concurrent use of L-tryptophan with a 5-HT1 agonist may increase the risk of adverse reactions)

Myo-Inositol
(May have additive effects with Myo-Inositol)

5-HYDROXYTRYPTOPHAN

5-HT1 Receptor Agonists
(5-HTP may increase risk of side effects)

Carbidopa
(Increases 5-HTP levels in the brain)

Cyproheptadine Hydrochloride
(5-HTP may decrease effects)

Hypericum
(5-HTP may potentiate antidepressant effects and increase risk of side effects)

Hypericum Perforatum
(5-HTP may potentiate antidepressant effects and increase risk of side effects)

Methyldopa
(Inhibits 5-HTP metabolism to serotonin)

Methysergide Maleate
(5-HTP may decrease effects)

Monoamine Oxidase Inhibitors
(5-HTP may increase risk of side effects)

Phenoxybenzamine Hydrochloride
(Inhibits 5-HTP metabolism to serotonin)

SSRIs
(5-HTP may potentiate antidepressant effects and increase risk of side effects)

Serotoninergic Agents
(5-HTP may potentiate antidepressant effects and increase risk of side effects)

Vitamin B6
(May enhance 5-HTP conversion to serotonin)

7-OXO-DEHYDROEPIANDROSTERONE

Warfarin Sodium
(7-Oxo-DHEA may have an effect on platelet membrane fluidity. Therefore those taking warfarin should exercise caution in the use of 7-Oxo-DHEA)

ACE INHIBITORS

Capsiate and Capasicin
(Those with chronic cough syndromes, including chronic cough due to the use of angiotensin-converting enzyme (ACE) inhibitors, may notice an increase in coughing when using capsinoids. To date, this has not been reported, but since capsinoids as well as capsaicin are agonists for the ligand-gated cation channel TRPV1, it is something to watch out for)

Potassium
(Increased serum Potassium due to inhibition of aldosterone production)

ABCIXIMAB

Alpha-Tocopherol Polyethylene Glycol Succinate (TPGS)
(High doses of TPGS may enhance the effects of abciximab)

Gamma-Tocopherol
(Increased effects of abciximab)

Nattokinase (Subtilisin NAT)
(The use of nattokinase along with parenteral antiplatelet drugs (GPIIB/IIA inhibitors such as abciximab) may cause serious adverse events, especially excessive bleeding. Administration of nattokinase is contraindicated in those with bleeding disorders and should be avoided in those receiving antiplatelet agents)

Vitamin E
(High doses of vitamin E may potentiate the effects of antiplatelet drugs)

Vitamin E Phosphate
(Vitamin E phosphate may potentiate the effects of antiplatelet drugs (eg, abciximab))

ACARBOSE

Inositol Nicotinate
(High dose nicotinic acid may
antagonize effects)

Niacin
(High dose nicotinic acid may
antagonize effects requiring dose
adjustment)

Supplemental Enzymes
(Decreased efficacy of acarbose
when taken with amylase,
pancreatin, and pancrelipase)

ACETAMINOPHEN

L-Methionine
(L-Methionine may decrease
hepatic toxicity with overdosage)

Molybdenum
(High dose molybdate may inhibit
acetaminophen metabolism)

ACETYL-L-CARNITINE

Didanosine
(May lead to decreased acetyl-L-
carnitine levels)

Pivalic Acid-Containing Antibiotics
(May lead to L-carnitine
deficiencies)

Stavudine
(May lead to decreased acetyl-L-
carnitine levels)

Valproic Acid
(May lead to L-carnitine
deficiencies)

Zalcitabine
(May lead to decreased acetyl-L-
carnitine levels)

ACETYLCYSTEINE

Carbamazepine
(NAC may reduce serum levels of
carbamazepine)

Nitrates and Nitrites
(May cause headaches when taken
with NAC)

ACITRETIN

Vitamin A
(May produce additive toxicity
effects)

ACTIVATED CHARCOAL

Drugs, unspecified
(Avoid using Activated Charcoal
within two hours of taking these
products)

Food, unspecified
(Avoid using Activated Charcoal
within two hours of taking these
products)

Herbal Medicines, unspecified
(Avoid using Activated Charcoal
within two hours of taking these
products)

Nutritional Supplement
(Avoid using Activated Charcoal
within two hours of taking these
products)

ALCOHOL

Gamma-Hydroxybutyrate
(GHB)
(May be life-threatening with
GHB)

Niacin
(May increase nicotinic acid-
induced flushing)

Vitamin B6
(Chronic and excessive use may
cause vitamin B6 deficiency)

ALL-TRANS-RETINOIC ACID

Vitamin A
(May produce additive toxicity
effects)

ALLIUM SATIVUM

Alpha-Tocopherol
Polyethylene Glycol
Succinate (TPGS)
(Some herbs, such as garlic and
ginkgo, possess antithrombotic
activity. High does of TPGS, used
concomitantly with these herbs,
may enhance antithrombotic
activity)

Borage Oil
(Interactions may occur with
Borage Oil)

Eicosapentaenoic Acid (EPA)
(May interact with EPA. Such
reactions might be manifested by
increased susceptibility to
bruising, nosebleeds, hemoptysis,
hematemesis, hematuria, and blood
in the stool. Most who take the
EPA supplements do not suffer
from these problems and if they
occur, they are rare. If they do

occur, the EPA dose should be
lowered or discontinued)

Evening Primrose Oil
(EPO may increase bleeding
tendencies)

Fish Oil
(May interact with fish oil. Such
interactions might be manifested
by increased susceptibility to
bruising, nosebleeds, hemoptysis,
hematemesis, hematuria, and blood
in the stool. Most who take fish
oil supplements do not suffer
from these problems and if they
occur, they are rare. If they do
occur, the fish oil dose should be
lowered or discontinued)

Flaxseed Oil
(Interactions may occur between
alpha-linoleic acid and its
metabolites with such herbs as
garlic (allium sativum). Such
interactions might be manifested
by nosebleeds and easy bruising)

Gamma-Tocopherol
(Enhanced antithrombotic activity
of garlic)

Nattokinase (Subtilisin NAT)
(Co-administration of nattokinase
with garlic (allium sativa) may
lead to increased bleeding
tendencies manifested by increased
susceptibility to bruising,
nosebleeds, hematemesis,
hematuria, and blood in the stool)

Perilla Oil
(Increased antithrombotic effects
with Perilla Oil)

Tocotrienols
(May enhance antithrombotic
activity)

Vitamin E
(Some herbs, including garlic and
ginkgo, possess antithrombotic
activity. High doses of vitamin E
used at the same time as these
herbs may enhance their
antithrombotic activity)

ALPHA ADRENERGIC BLOCKERS

Inositol Nicotinate
(High dose nicotinic acid may
potentiate hypotensive effects)

Niacin
(High dose nicotinic acid may potentiate hypotensive effects and may cause postural hypotension)

ALPHA CAROTENE

Beta-Sitosterol
(May lower serum levels of alpha- and beta-carotene)

Phytostanols
(Phytostanols may interfere with absorption and lower serum levels)

Phytosterols
(Phytosterols may interfere with absorption and lower serum levels)

ALPHA GALACTOSIDASE ENZYME

Prebiotics
(Decreased effectiveness of the soy oligosaccharides)

ALPHA TOCOPHEROL ACETATE

Coenzyme Q10 (CoQ10)
(Elevation in CoQ10 levels in mitochondria by dietary supplementation is linked to a corresponding rise in alpha-tocopherol content)

Gamma-Tocopherol
(Decreased plasma Gamma-Tocopherol levels)

Iron
(Iron may cause oxidation of the tocopherols)

ALPHA-LIPOIC ACID

Antidiabetic Drugs, unspecified
(Alpha-lipoic acid may lower blood glucose levels. Those with diabetes on antidiabetic medication should have their blood glucose monitored and antidiabetic drug dose adjusted appropriately, if necessary, to avoid possible hypoglycemia)

Insulin
(Alpha-lipoic acid may lower blood glucose levels. Those with diabetes on antidiabetic medication should have their blood glucose monitored and antidiabetic drug dose adjusted appropriately, if necessary, to avoid possible hypoglycemia)

ALPHA-TOCOPHEROL POLYETHYLENE GLYCOL SUCCINATE (TPGS)

Abciximab
(High doses of TPGS may enhance the effects of abciximab)

Allium sativum
(Some herbs, such as garlic and ginkgo, possess antithrombotic activity. High does of TPGS, used concomitantly with these herbs, may enhance antithrombotic activity)

Amprenavir
(TPGS is used as an absorption and bioavailability enhancer for amprenavir)

Antiplatelet Drugs
(High doses of TPGS may enhance the effects of antiplatelet drugs)

Aspirin
(High doses of TPGS may enhance the effects of aspirin)

Coenzyme Q-10
(TPGS may increase the absorption of coenzyme Q-10)

Cyclosporine
(TPGS may increase absorption of cyclosporine)

Dipyridamole
(High doses of TPGS may enhance the effects of dipyridamole)

Eptifibatide
(High doses of TPGS may enhance the effects of eptifibatide)

Flavonoids
(TPGS may increase the absorption of flavonoids)

Ginkgo biloba
(Some herbs, such as garlic and ginkgo, possess antithrombotic activity. High does of TPGS, used concomitantly with these herbs, may enhance antithrombotic activity)

Lipophilic drugs, unspecified
(TPGS may increase absorption of lipophilic drugs)

Polyphenols
(TPGS may increase the absorption of polyphenols)

Selenium
(May function synergistically with d-alpha-tocopherol)

Ticlopidine Hydrochloride
(High doses of TPGS may enhance the effects of ticlopidine)

Tocotrienols
(TPGS may increase the absorption of all forms of vitamin E (gamma-tocopherol, tocotrienols))

Vitamin A
(TPGS may increase the absorption of vitamin A)

Vitamin C
(May help maintain d-alpha-tocopherol in its reduced (antioxidant) form)

Vitamin D
(TPGS may increase the absorption of vitamin D)

Vitamin E
(TPGS may increase the absorption of all forms of vitamin E (gamma-tocopherol, tocotrienols))

Vitamin K
(TPGS may increase the absorption of vitamin K)

Warfarin Sodium
(High doses (greater than 500 mg) of TPGS may enhance the anticoagulant response of warfarin. Monitor INRs and adjust dose of warfarin if necessary)

ALPHA-LACTALBUMIN

L-Tryptophan
(May increase the brain availability of L-tryptophan)

ALPRAZOLAM

DHEA
(May increase DHEA levels)

ALUMINUM HYDROXIDE

Vanadium
(May decrease absorption of vanadium)

ALUMINUM-CONTAINING COMPOUNDS, UNSPECIFIED

Ascorbyl Palmitate
(Large dose Vitamin C may increase urinary Aluminum excretion)

Silicon
(Silicon may inhibit aluminum absorption)

Vitamin C
(Large doses of vitamin C used at the same time as aluminum-containing antacids has been reported to increase urinary aluminum excretion, suggesting increased aluminum absorption from these antacids)

AMILORIDE HYDROCHLORIDE

Potassium
(Concomitant potassium-sparing diuretic and Potassium supplements can produce severe hyperkalemia)

AMINOBENZOIC ACID

(*See under* Para-Aminobenzoic Acid (PABA))

AMINOGLUTETHIMIDE

Chrysin
(Chrysin may have additive effects)

AMINOGLYCOSIDES

Sesame Seed Lignans
(Antibiotics may decrease the production of the mammalian lignans enterolactone (ENT) and enterodiol (END) from sesame seed lignans)

AMIODARONE HYDROCHLORIDE

Arnica
(Increased risk of prolonged QT interval when given with Arnica)

Luteolin
(Luteolin has been found to inhibit the metabolism of the sedative drug midazolam by human liver microsomes and cytochrome P450 3A4 (CYP3A4) and CYP3A5. Midazolam is a probe substrate for CYP3A4 and CYP3A5 enzymes. CYP3A4 is located in the intestine and liver, and its inhibition leads to delayed absorption and reduced first pass metabolism in the liver, resulting in higher plasma levels of the drug. However, given this finding, those using midazolam or other drugs metabolized by CYP3A4, including amiodarone, should exercise caution in the use of luteolin-containing dairy supplements)

Vitamin B6
(Concomitant vitamin B6 may enhance amiodarone-induced photosensitivity reactions)

Vitamin E
(Alpha-tocopherol may ameliorate some of the adverse side effects of amiodarone)

AMITRIPTYLINE HYDROCHLORIDE

Arnica
(Increased risk of prolonged QT interval when given with Arnica)

AMOXICILLIN

Bromelain
(Bromelain may increase amoxicillin levels)

AMPRENAVIR

Alpha-Tocopherol Polyethylene Glycol Succinate (TPGS)
(TPGS is used as an absorption and bioavailability enhancer for amprenavir)

ANASTROZOLE

Chrysin
(Chrysin may have additive effects)

ANDROSTENEDIOL

DHEA
(May increase adverse effects of DHEA)

ANDROSTENEDIONE

DHEA
(May increase adverse effects of DHEA)

ANTACIDS, ALUMINUM-CONTAINING

Fluoride
(Decreased absorption of Fluoride)

Iron
(May decrease absorption of iron)

Phosphorus
(Decreased absorption of Phosphorus)

ANTACIDS, MAGNESIUM-CONTAINING

Manganese
(May decrease absorption of manganese)

ANTACIDS, NON-ABSORBABLE

Lactulose
(May increase Lactulose effects)

ANTACIDS, UNSPECIFIED

Indole-3-Carbinol
(Block the conversion of Indole-3-Carbinol to DIM and ICZ)

ANTHRACYCLINE ANTIBIOTICS AND THEIR DERIVATIVES

Sesame Seed Lignans
(Antibiotics may decrease the production of the mammalian lignans enterolactone (ENT) and enterodiol (END) from sesame seed lignans)

ANTIBIOTICS, BROAD SPECTRUM, UNSPECIFIED

Vitamin K
(Broad spectrum antibiotics may sterilize the bowel and decrease the vitamin K contribution to the body by the intestinal microflora)

ANTIBIOTICS, UNSPECIFIED

Biotin
(May decrease Biotin absorption)

Equol
(Antibiotics may decrease equol formation)

Flaxseed Lignans
(Antibiotics may decrease the production of enterodiol (END) and enterolactone (ENL) from secoisolariciresinol diglucoside (SDG))

Spruce Lignans (7-Hydroxymatairesinol)
(Antibiotics may decrease the production of enterolactone (ENL) from 7-hydroxymatairesinol (HMR))

Vitamin B12
(The use of antibiotics may alter the intestinal microflora and may decrease the possible contribution of vitamin B12 by certain inhabitants of the microflora to the body's requirement for the vitamin. This may particularly be a problem for vegetarians)

ANTICHOLINESTERASE DRUGS
Huperzine A
(Additive effects and increased adverse effects with Huperzine A)

ANTICOAGULANT DRUGS, UNSPECIFIED
Borage Oil
(Increased anticoagulant and antiplatelet effects when taken with Borage Oil)
Bromelain
(Bromelain may enhance anticoagulant effects)
Supplemental Enzymes
(Enhanced anticoagulant activity when taken with Bromelain)
Tiratricol (TRIAC)
(May increase hypoprothrombinemic effect)

ANTICONVULSANTS
Gamma-Hydroxybutyrate (GHB)
(May be life-threatening with GHB)
Vitamin E
(Anticonvulsants may lower plasma vitamin E levels)

ANTIDEPRESSANT MEDICATIONS, UNSPECIFIED
Melatonin
(May increase sedation and adverse effects with Melatonin)

ANTIDIABETIC DRUGS, UNSPECIFIED
Alpha-Lipoic Acid
(Alpha-lipoic acid may lower blood glucose levels. Those with diabetes on antidiabetic medication should have their blood glucose monitored and antidiabetic drug dose adjusted appropriately, if necessary, to avoid possible hypoglycemia)

Coenzyme Q10 (CoQ10)
(May need dosing adjustments)
D-Ribose
(D-Ribose may cause hypoglycemia)
Glucosamine
(Glucosamine may increase insulin resistance and affect glucose tolerance)

ANTIHISTAMINES
Gamma-Hydroxybutyrate (GHB)
(May be life-threatening with GHB)
L-Histidine
(L-Histidine might decrease the efficacy of)
Melatonin
(May increase sedation and adverse effects with Melatonin)

ANTIPLATELET DRUGS
Alpha-Tocopherol Polyethylene Glycol Succinate (TPGS)
(High doses of TPGS may enhance the effects of antiplatelet drugs)
Borage Oil
(Increased anticoagulant and antiplatelet effects when taken with Borage Oil)
Curcuminoids
(Curcuminoids may enhance the antiplatelet effect)
Gamma-Tocopherol
(Increased effects of antiplatelet drugs)
Green Tea Catechins
(Enhanced effect with green tea catechins)
Myco-Polysaccharides
(Ganoderma may enhance antiplatelet effects)
Tocotrienols
(Tocotrienol may potentiate antiplatelet effects)
Vitamin E
(High doses of vitamin E may potentiate the effects of antiplatelet drugs)

ANTITHROMBOTIC AGENTS
Bromelain
(Bromelain may enhance antithrombotic effects)
Supplemental Enzymes
(Enhanced antithrombotic activity when taken with Bromelain)

ANTITHYROID AGENTS
Iodine
(May potentiate the hypothyroid effect of iodides)

ARGATROBAN
Nattokinase (Subtilisin NAT)
(The use of nattokinase along with direct thrombin inhibitors (eg, argatroban) may cause serious adverse events, especially excessive bleeding.)

ARGININE
(See under L-Arginine)

ARGININE HYDROCHLORIDE
Xylitol
(Arginine-containing mints have been found to have anticariogenic activity secondary to their ability to buffer the acid produced by cariogenic bacteria. The combination of xylitol and arginine-containing mints may give better anticariogenic effects than the use of either alone)

ARGININE BASE
Xylitol
(Arginine-containing mints have been found to have anticariogenic activity secondary to their ability to buffer the acid produced by cariogenic bacteria. The combination of xylitol and arginine-containing mints may give better anticariogenic effects than the use of either alone)

ARNICA
Amiodarone Hydrochloride
(Increased risk of prolonged QT interval when given with Arnica)
Amitriptyline Hydrochloride
(Increased risk of prolonged QT interval when given with Arnica)

Chlorpromazine
(Increased risk of prolonged QT interval when given with Arnica)

Desipramine Hydrochloride
(Increased risk of prolonged QT interval when given with Arnica)

Disopyramide
(Increased risk of prolonged QT interval when given with Arnica)

Doxepin Hydrochloride
(Increased risk of prolonged QT interval when given with Arnica)

Doxorubicin Hydrochloride
(Increased cardiotoxicity with Arnica)

Haloperidol
(Increased risk of prolonged QT interval when given with Arnica)

Pentamidine Isethionate
(Increased risk of prolonged QT interval when given with Arnica)

Procainamide
(Increased risk of prolonged QT interval when given with Arnica)

Prochlorperazine
(Increased risk of prolonged QT interval when given with Arnica)

Quinidine
(Increased risk of prolonged QT interval when given with Arnica)

Sotalol Hydrochloride
(Increased risk of prolonged QT interval when given with Arnica)

AROMATASE INHIBITORS

Chrysin
(Chrysin may have additive effects)

ARSENIC TRIOXIDE

Vitamin C
(Ascorbic acid has been found to enhance arsenic trioxide-induced cytotoxicity in multiple myeloma cells. It has also been found to overcome drug resistance in myeloma and to significantly increase the anti-myeloma effects of both arsenic trioxide and melphalan in cell culture models and in animal models)

ASCORBATE

Chromium
(May increase absorption of chromium)

ASCORBIC ACID

(*See under* Vitamin C)

L-Cysteine
(May inhibit the oxidation of L-Cysteine)

ASCORBYL PALMITATE

Aluminum-containing Compounds, unspecified
(Large dose Vitamin C may increase urinary Aluminum excretion)

Aspirin
(May decrease Vitamin C absorption and large aspirin doses may cause Vitamin C deficiency)

Carbamazepine
(Grapefruit flavonoids may increase bioavailability due to cytochrome P-450 3A4 inhibition)

Cisplatin
(Vitamin C may potentiate antineoplastic activity)

Copper
(High dose Vitamin C may decrease absorption)

Cyclosporine
(Grapefruit flavonoids may increase bioavailability due to cytochrome P-450 3A4 inhibition)

Doxorubicin Hydrochloride
(Vitamin C may potentiate antineoplastic activity)

Estrogen
(Vitamin C may enhance inhibition of LDL formation)

Felodipine
(Grapefruit flavonoids may increase bioavailability due to cytochrome P-450 3A4 inhibition)

Flavonoids
(Vitamin C may have synergistic effects)

Glutathione
(Vitamin C may maintain reduced Glutathione levels)

Iron Supplements
(Vitamin C may cause iron overload)

Lovastatin
(Grapefruit flavonoids may increase bioavailability due to cytochrome P-450 3A4 inhibition)

Nisoldipine
(Grapefruit flavonoids may increase bioavailability due to cytochrome P-450 3A4 inhibition)

Paclitaxel
(Vitamin C may potentiate antineoplastic activity)

Saquinavir
(Grapefruit flavonoids may increase bioavailability due to cytochrome P-450 3A4 inhibition)

Simvastatin
(Grapefruit flavonoids may increase bioavailability due to cytochrome P-450 3A4 inhibition)

ASPIRIN

Alpha-Tocopherol Polyethylene Glycol Succinate (TPGS)
(High doses of TPGS may enhance the effects of aspirin)

Ascorbyl Palmitate
(May decrease Vitamin C absorption and large aspirin doses may cause Vitamin C deficiency)

Borage Oil
(Increased anticoagulant and antiplatelet effects when taken with Borage Oil)

Curcuminoids
(Curcuminoids may enhance the antiplatelet effect)

Eicosapentaenoic Acid (EPA)
(May interact with EPA. Such reactions might be manifested by increased susceptibility to bruising, nosebleeds, hemoptysis, hematemesis, hematuria, and blood in the stool. Most who take the EPA supplements do not suffer from these problems and if they occur, they are rare. If they do occur, the EPA dose should be lowered or discontinued)

Evening Primrose Oil
(EPO may increase bleeding
tendencies)
Fish Oil
(May interact with fish oil. Such
interactions might be manifested
by increased susceptibility to
bruising, nosebleeds, hemoptysis,
hematemesis, hematuria, and blood
in the stool. Most who take fish
oil supplements do not suffer
from these problems and if they
occur, they are rare. If they do
occur, the fish oil dose should be
lowered or discontinued)
Flaxseed Oil
(Interactions may occur between
flaxseed oil and its metabolites
and warfarin, aspirin, and
NSAIDs. Such interactions, if they
were to occur, might be
manifested by nosebleeds and
increased susceptibility to
bruising. If this does occur,
consideration should be given to
lowering or stopping intake)
Gamma-Tocopherol
(Increased effects of aspirin)
Green Tea Catechins
(Enhanced effect with green tea
catechins)
Hemp Seed Oil
(Increased bleeding and
susceptibility to bruising)
Inositol Nicotinate
(May decrease high dose nicotinic
acid flushing effects)
Melatonin
(May decrease Melatonin levels)
Nattokinase (Subtilisin NAT)
(The use of nattokinase along
with antiplatelet drugs (eg,
aspirin) may cause serious adverse
events, especially excessive
bleeding. Administration of
nattokinase is contraindicated in
those with bleeding disorders and
should be avoided in those
receiving antiplatelet agents)
Niacin
(May decrease high dose nicotinic
acid flushing effects)

Perilla Oil
(Increased antithrombotic effects
with Perilla Oil)
Policosanol
(Policosanol showed a synergism
with the antithrombotic properties
of aspirin in different
experimental models)
Vitamin C
(Chronic use of high dose aspirin
may lead to impaired vitamin C
status)
Vitamin E
(High doses of vitamin E may
potentiate the effects of
antiplatelet drugs)
Vitamin E Phosphate
(Vitamin E phosphate may
potentiate the effects of
antiplatelet drugs (eg, aspirin))
Vitamin K
(Salicylates in large doses may
inhibit vitamin K epoxide
reductase resulting in vitamin K
deficiency)

ASPIRIN BUFFERED
Curcuminoids
(Curcuminoids may enhance the
antiplatelet effect)
Eicosapentaenoic Acid (EPA)
(May interact with EPA. Such
reactions might be manifested by
increased susceptibility to
bruising, nosebleeds, hemoptysis,
hematemesis, hematuria, and blood
in the stool. Most who take the
EPA supplements do not suffer
from these problems and if they
occur, they are rare. If they do
occur, the EPA dose should be
lowered or discontinued)
Fish Oil
(May interact with fish oil. Such
interactions might be manifested
by increased susceptibility to
bruising, nosebleeds, hemoptysis,
hematemesis, hematuria, and blood
in the stool. Most who take fish
oil supplements do not suffer
from these problems and if they
occur, they are rare. If they do

occur, the fish oil dose should be
lowered or discontinued)
Green Tea Catechins
(Enhanced effect with green tea
catechins)
Nattokinase (Subtilisin NAT)
(The use of nattokinase along
with antiplatelet drugs (eg,
aspirin) may cause serious adverse
events, especially excessive
bleeding. Administration of
nattokinase is contraindicated in
those with bleeding disorders and
should be avoided in those
receiving antiplatelet agents)
Policosanol
(Policosanol showed a synergism
with the antithrombotic properties
of aspirin in different
experimental models)
Vitamin E Phosphate
(Vitamin E phosphate may
potentiate the effects of
antiplatelet drugs (eg, aspirin))

ASPIRIN, ENTERIC COATED
Curcuminoids
(Curcuminoids may enhance the
antiplatelet effect)
Eicosapentaenoic Acid (EPA)
(May interact with EPA. Such
reactions might be manifested by
increased susceptibility to
bruising, nosebleeds, hemoptysis,
hematemesis, hematuria, and blood
in the stool. Most who take the
EPA supplements do not suffer
from these problems and if they
occur, they are rare. If they do
occur, the EPA dose should be
lowered or discontinued)
Fish Oil
(May interact with fish oil. Such
interactions might be manifested
by increased susceptibility to
bruising, nosebleeds, hemoptysis,
hematemesis, hematuria, and blood
in the stool. Most who take fish
oil supplements do not suffer
from these problems and if they
occur, they are rare. If they do

occur, the fish oil dose should be lowered or discontinued)

Green Tea Catechins
(Enhanced effect with green tea catechins)

Nattokinase (Subtilisin NAT)
(The use of nattokinase along with antiplatelet drugs (eg, aspirin) may cause serious adverse events, especially excessive bleeding. Administration of nattokinase is contraindicated in those with bleeding disorders and should be avoided in those receiving antiplatelet agents)

Policosanol
(Policosanol showed a synergism with the antithrombotic properties of aspirin in different experimental models)

Vitamin E Phosphate
(Vitamin E phosphate may potentiate the effects of antiplatelet drugs (eg, aspirin))

ASTAXANTHIN

Beta-Carotene
(Concomitant intake of beta-carotene and astaxanthin may increase the absorption of astaxanthin)

Cholestyramine
(Concomitant intake of cholestyramine and astaxanthin may decrease the absorption of astaxanthin)

Cod Liver Oil
(Dietary oils such as olive oil and fish oils may enhance the absorption of astaxanthin. Corn oil is less likely to enhance astaxanthin absorption)

Colestipol
(Concomitant intake of colestipol and astaxanthin may decrease the absorption of astaxanthin)

Colestipol Hydrochloride
(Concomitant intake of colestipol and astaxanthin may decrease the absorption of astaxanthin)

Fish Oils
(Dietary oils such as olive oil and fish oils may enhance the

absorption of astaxanthin. Corn oil is less likely to enhance astaxanthin absorption)

Medium-Chain Triglycerides
(Concomitant intake of medium-chain triglycerides and lycopene may decrease the absorption of astaxanthin)

Mineral Oil
(Concomitant intake of mineral oil and astaxanthin may reduce the absorption of astaxanthin)

Oils, dietary
(Dietary oils such as olive oil and fish oils may enhance the absorption of astaxanthin. Corn oil is less likely to enhance astaxanthin absorption)

Olestra
(Olestra may reduce the absorption of astaxanthin)

Orlistat
(Orlistat may decrease the absorption of astaxanthin)

Pectin
(Concomitant intake of pectin and astaxanthin may decrease the absorption of astaxanthin)

Salmon Oil
(Dietary oils such as olive oil and fish oils may enhance the absorption of astaxanthin. Corn oil is less likely to enhance astaxanthin absorption)

Shark Liver Oil
(Dietary oils such as olive oil and fish oils may enhance the absorption of astaxanthin. Corn oil is less likely to enhance astaxanthin absorption)

Vitamin E
(Concomitant intake of vitamin E and astaxanthin may decrease astaxanthin absorption)

AZOLE ANTIFUNGALS

Red Yeast Rice
(Increased risk of myopathy)

Sesame Seed Lignans
(Antibiotics may decrease the production of the mammalian lignans enterolactone (ENT) and

enterodiol (END) from sesame seed lignans)

BACLOFEN

Glycine
(Glycine may increase effect of)

BACTERIOSTATIC ANTIBIOTICS

Sesame Seed Lignans
(Antibiotics may decrease the production of the mammalian lignans enterolactone (ENT) and enterodiol (END) from sesame seed lignans)

BAICALEIN

Beta Blockers
(Baicalein and beta-lactams have shown synergistic activity against MRSA (methicillin-resistant Staphylococcus aureus) in vitro)

Gentamicin
(Baicalein and gentamicin have shown synergistic activity against vancomycin-resistant Enterococcus in vitro)

Gentamicin Sulfate
(Baicalein and gentamicin have shown synergistic activity against vancomycin-resistant Enterococcus in vitro)

Tetracyclines, unspecified
(Baicalein and tetracycline have shown synergistic activity against MRSA (methicillin-resistant Staphylococcus aureus) in vitro)

BENTONITE

Drugs, unspecified
(Bentonite may adsorb certain drugs)

Food, unspecified
(Bentonite may adsorb certain food components)

Herbal Medicines, unspecified
(Bentonite may adsorb certain herb components)

Nutritional Supplement
(Bentonite may adsorb certain nutritional supplements)

BENZODIAZEPINES

Gamma-Hydroxybutyrate
(GHB)
(May be life-threatening with GHB)

Melatonin
(May increase sedation and adverse effects with Melatonin)

BERRIES

Sesame Seed Lignans
(An extract of Schisandra chinensis berry when combined with sesamin was found to decrease blood viscosity and improve blood fluidity in a human clinical study)

BETA BLOCKERS

Baicalein
(Baicalein and beta-lactams have shown synergistic activity against MRSA (methicillin-resistant Staphylococcus aureus) in vitro)

Chromium
(Elevated HDL cholesterol levels after two months of chromium use)

Melatonin
(May lead to decreased Melatonin levels)

BETA-ALANINE

Creatine Phosphate
(Creatine and beta-alanine may increase skeletal creatine phosphate and carnosine and may work synergistically to delay fatigue and increase exercise performance, especially in trained athletes)

BETA-CAROTENE

Astaxanthin
(Concomitant intake of beta-carotene and astaxanthin may increase the absorption of astaxanthin)

Beta-Sitosterol
(May lower serum levels of alpha- and beta-carotene)

Cholestyramine
(May decrease the absorption of beta-carotene)

Colestipol
(May decrease the absorption of beta-carotene)

Fucoxanthin
(Concomitant intake of beta-carotene and fucoxanthin may increase the absorption of fucoxanthin)

Iron
(May enhance absorption of iron)

Lutein
(May decrease the absorption of beta-carotene)

Lutein and Zeaxanthin
(Decreased absorption of Lutein and Zeaxanthin)

Lycopene
(Increased absorption of Lycopene)

Mineral Oil
(May decrease the absorption of beta-carotene)

Olestra
(May decrease the absorption of beta-carotene)

Orlistat
(May decrease the absorption of beta-carotene)

Pectin
(May decrease the absorption of beta-carotene)

Phytostanols
(Phytostanols may interfere with absorption and lower serum levels)

Phytosterols
(Phytosterols may interfere with absorption and lower serum levels)

Piperine
(Piperine may enhance the absorption)

Sodium Alginates and other Phyco-Polysaccharides
(Decreased absorption of Beta Carotene)

Vitamin E
(Some studies have suggested that oral supplements of beta-carotene may cause a decrease in serum levels of alpha-tocopherol. However, more recent and much larger and longer studies have demonstrated that supplementation with beta-carotene does not alter serum concentrations of vitamin E)

BETA-SITOSTEROL

Alpha Carotene
(May lower serum levels of alpha- and beta-carotene)

Beta-Carotene
(May lower serum levels of alpha- and beta-carotene)

Lycopene
(May lower serum levels of lycopene)

Vitamin E
(May lower serum levels of vitamin E)

BETA-LACTAM ANTIBIOTICS

Sesame Seed Lignans
(Antibiotics may decrease the production of the mammalian lignans enterolactone (ENT) and enterodiol (END) from sesame seed lignans)

BETAINE AND BETAINE HYDROCHLORIDE

Folic Acid
(May be synergistic in lowering serum homocysteine levels)

BETHANECHOL CHLORIDE

Huperzine A
(Additive effects and increased adverse effects with Huperzine A)

BEVERAGES, CAFFEINE-CONTAINING

Creatine
(May interfere with effects of Creatine)

Zinc
(Concomitant intake of coffee, caffeinated beverages, or caffeine and zinc may depress the absorption of zinc)

BEVERAGES, HOT

Inositol Nicotinate
(May increase nicotinic acid-induced flushing)

Niacin
(May increase nicotinic acid-induced flushing)

BEVERAGES, SULFITES

Thiamin
(May inactivate Thiamin)

BEXAROTENE

Vitamin A
(May produce additive toxicity effects)

BIOTIN

Antibiotics, unspecified
(May decrease Biotin absorption)
Carbamazepine
(May decrease Biotin levels)
Pantothenic Acid
(May decrease Biotin absorption)
Phenobarbital
(May decrease Biotin levels)
Phenytoin
(May decrease Biotin levels)
Primidone
(May decrease Biotin levels)

BISPHOSPHONATES

Bone Meal
(Decreased absorption of
Bisphosphonate)
Calcium
(May decrease absorption of
bisphosphonate)
Ipriflavone
(Additive effects with Ipriflavone)
Iron
(May decrease absorption of
bisphosphonate)
Magnesium
(May decrease absorption of
bisphosphonates)
Zinc
(Concomitant intake of a
bisphosphonate and zinc may
decrease the absorption of both
the bisphosphonate and zinc)

BIVALIRUDIN

Nattokinase (Subtilisin NAT)
(The use of nattokinase along
with direct thrombin inhibitors
(eg, bivalirudin) may cause
serious adverse events, especially
excessive bleeding)

BONE MEAL

Bisphosphonates
(Decreased absorption of the
Bisphosphonate)
Calcitriol
(Increased absorption of Calcium)
Dietary Fiber
(Decreased absorption of Calcium)
Fructo-oligosaccharides
(Increased absorption of Calcium)

Histamine H2-receptor antagonists
(Decreased absorption of Calcium)
Inositol
(Decreased absorption of Calcium)
Inulin
(Increased absorption of Calcium)
Levothyroxine Sodium
(Decreased levothyroxine
absorption and increased serum
thyrotropin levels)
Oxalic Acid
(Decreased absorption of Calcium)
Proton Pump Inhibitor
(Decreased absorption of Calcium)
Quinolones
(Decreased absorption of
quinolones)
Sodium Alginate
(Decreased absorption of Calcium)
Tetracyclines, unspecified
(Decreased absorption of
tetracyclines)
Vitamin D
(Increased absorption of Calcium)

BORAGE OIL

Allium sativum
(Interactions may occur with
Borage Oil)
Anticoagulant drugs, unspecified
(Increased anticoagulant and
antiplatelet effects when taken
with Borage Oil)
Antiplatelet Drugs
(Increased anticoagulant and
antiplatelet effects when taken
with Borage Oil)
Aspirin
(Increased anticoagulant and
antiplatelet effects when taken
with Borage Oil)
Chlorpromazine
(May cause seizures when taken
with Borage Oil)
Fish Oils
(Increased antithrombotic activity
with Borage oil)
Ginkgo biloba
(Interactions may occur with
Borage Oil)

Nonsteroidal Anti-Inflammatory
Drugs
(Increased anticoagulant and
antiplatelet effects when taken
with Borage Oil)
Phenothiazines
(May cause seizures when taken
with Borage Oil)
Warfarin Sodium
(Increased anticoagulant and
antiplatelet effects when taken
with Borage Oil)

BORON

Ipriflavone
(Additive effects with Ipriflavone)
Magnesium
(May increase magnesium levels)

BREWER'S YEAST

Monoamine Oxidase Inhibitors
(May cause hypertension with
Brewer's Yeast)
Pargyline Hydrochloride
(May cause hypertension with
Brewer's Yeast)
Phenelzine Sulfate
(May cause hypertension with
Brewer's Yeast)
Tranylcypromine Sulfate
(May cause hypertension with
Brewer's Yeast)

BROMELAIN

Amoxicillin
(Bromelain may increase
amoxicillin levels)
Anticoagulant drugs, unspecified
(Bromelain may enhance
anticoagulant effects)
Antithrombotic Agents
(Bromelain may enhance
antithrombotic effects)
Tetracyclines, unspecified
(Bromelain may increase
tetracycline levels)

BROMELAINS

(*See also under* Bromelain)
Curcuminoids
(May enhance absorption of
curcuminoids)
Quercetin
(Increase absorption of Quercetin)

BUMETANIDE

Thiamin
  (Chronic use may cause Thiamin deficiency)

C-GLUOSYLFLAVONES

Iodine
  (Inhibit thyroid peroxidase activity)

CAFFEINE

Green Tea Catechins
  (Synergistic effect with green tea catechins in enhancing thermogenesis)

Zinc
  (Concomitant intake of coffee, caffeinated beverages, or caffeine and zinc may depress the absorption of zinc)

CALCITONIN, UNSPECIFIED

Gelatin Hydrolysates
  (Gelatin Hydrosylates may enhance the osteoporosis treatment effects)

Hydrolyzed Collagen
  (Enhanced effect (in the treatment of osteoporosis) with hydrolyzed collagen)

Ipriflavone
  (Additive effects with Ipriflavone)

CALCITRIOL

Bone Meal
  (Increased absorption of Calcium)

Calcium
  (May increase absorption of calcium)

CALCIUM

Bisphosphonates
  (May decrease absorption of bisphosphonate)

Calcitriol
  (May increase absorption of calcium)

Dietary Fiber
  (May decrease absorption of calcium)

Fluoride
  (Decreased absorption of Fluoride)

Fructo-oligosaccharides
  (May increase absorption of calcium)

Histamine H2-receptor antagonists
  (May decrease absorption of calcium)

Inositol
  (May decrease absorption of calcium)

Inositol Hexaphosphate
  (May form chelates with Inositol Hexaphosphate)

Inulin
  (May increase absorption of calcium)

Ipriflavone
  (Additive effects with Ipriflavone)

Iron
  (May decrease absorption of iron)

L-Lysine
  (L-lysine may increase Calcium absorption)

Lactulose
  (Lactulose may enhance colonic absorption of dietary and supplemental Calcium)

Levothyroxine Sodium
  (May decrease levothyroxine absorption and increase serum thyrotropin levels)

Magnesium
  (May decrease absorption of magnesium)

Manganese
  (May decrease absorption of manganese)

Medium-Chain Triglycerides
  (MCT may facilitate the absorption of Calcium)

Oxalic Acid
  (May decrease absorption of calcium)

Pectin
  (Decreased absorption of Calcium)

Phytic Acid
  (May decrease absorption of calcium)

Prebiotics
  (Enhanced absorption of Calcium)

Proton Pump Inhibitor
  (May decrease absorption of calcium)

Psyllium
  (Decreased absorption of Calcium)

Quinolones
  (May decrease absorption of quinolones)

Sodium Alginate
  (May decrease absorption of calcium)

Sodium Alginates and other Phyco-Polysaccharides
  (Decreased absorption of Calcium)

Soy Protein
  (May reduce availability of calcium)

Synbiotics
  (Enhanced colonic absorption of Calcium)

Tetracyclines, unspecified
  (May decrease absorption of tetracyclines)

Thyroxine
  (May decrease thyroxine absorption)

Transgalacto-Oligosaccharides
  (Enhanced colonic absorption of Calcium)

Vitamin B12
  (May reverse metformin-induced decrease of vitamin B12 absorption)

Vitamin D
  (May increase absorption of calcium. Concomitant intake of calcium and vitamin D may be more effective than no therapy or calcium alone in corticosteroid-induced osteoporosis)

Zinc
  (Concomitant intake of calcium and zinc may depress zinc absorption in postmenopausal women)

CALCIUM CHANNEL BLOCKERS, UNSPECIFIED

Inositol Nicotinate
  (High dose nicotinic acid may potentiate hypotensive effects)

Niacin
  (High dose nicotinic acid may potentiate hypotensive effects)

CALCIUM PANTOTHENATE

(*See under* Pantothenic Acid)

CALCIUM SALTS

L-Lysine
(L-lysine may increase Calcium absorption)

CAPSIATE AND CAPASICIN

ACE Inhibitors
(Those with chronic cough syndromes, including chronic cough due to the use of angiotensin-converting enzyme (ACE) inhibitors, may notice an increase in coughing when using capsinoids. To date, this has not been reported, but since capsinoids as well as capsaicin are agonists for the ligand-gated cation channel TRPV1, it is something to watch out for)

CARBAMAZEPINE

Acetylcysteine
(NAC may reduce serum levels of carbamazepine)

Ascorbyl Palmitate
(Grapefruit flavonoids may increase bioavailability due to cytochrome P-450 3A4 inhibition)

Biotin
(May decrease Biotin levels)

Folate
(May decrease folate levels and increase homocysteine levels; high dose folic acid may decrease serum levels)

Nicotinamide
(Nicotinamide may decrease carbamazepine clearance)

Psyllium
(Reduced absorption of carbamazepine)

Vitamin B6
(Chronic use may decrease plasma pyridoxal 5'-phosphate levels)

Vitamin C
(Grapefruit flavonoids may increase bioavailability due to cytochrome P-450 3A4 inhibition)

Vitamin E
(Anticonvulsants may lower plasma vitamin E levels)

CARBIDOPA

5-Hydroxytryptophan
(Increases 5-HTP levels in the brain)

Octacosanol
(Worsened dyskinesias in Parkinson's disease)

CARBOHYDRATES

L-Tryptophan
(May increase the brain availability of L-tryptophan)

CAROTENOIDS

Chitosan
(Might bind to Chitosan)

Medium-Chain Triglycerides
(MCT may facilitate the absorption of carotenoids)

CEFAMANDOLE NAFATE

Vitamin K
(Can cause vitamin K deficiency and hypoprothrombinemia)

CEFAZOLIN SODIUM

Vitamin K
(Can cause vitamin K deficiency and hypoprothrombinemia)

CEFMENOXIME

Vitamin K
(Can cause vitamin K deficiency and hypoprothrombinemia)

CEFOPERAZONE SODIUM

Vitamin K
(Can cause vitamin K deficiency and hypoprothrombinemia)

CEFOTETAN

Vitamin K
(Can cause vitamin K deficiency and hypoprothrombinemia)

CHEMOTHERAPEUTIC AGENTS

Vitamin C
(May diminish the efficacy of some chemotherapeutic agents)

CHITOSAN

Carotenoids
(Might bind to Chitosan)

Chondroitin Sulfate
(May decrease absorption of chondroitin sulfate)

Diet, lipid
(Might bind to Chitosan)

Flavonoids
(Might bind to Chitosan)

Lipophilic drugs, unspecified
(Might bind to Chitosan)

Vitamin A
(Might bind to Chitosan)

Vitamin C
(May enhance the benefits of Chitosan)

Vitamin D
(Might bind to Chitosan)

Vitamin E
(Might bind to Chitosan)

Vitamin K
(Might bind to Chitosan)

Zinc
(Might bind to Chitosan)

CHLORELLA

Warfarin Sodium
(Chlorella may interfere with effects)

CHLORIDE

Vanadium
(May decrease absorption of vanadium)

CHLORPROMAZINE

Arnica
(Increased risk of prolonged QT interval when given with Arnica)

Borage Oil
(May cause seizures when taken with Borage Oil)

Riboflavin (Vitamin B2)
(May inhibit riboflavin conversion to FMN and FAD)

CHOLECALCIFEROL

(*See under* Vitamin D)

CHOLESTYRAMINE

Astaxanthin
(Concomitant intake of cholestyramine and astaxanthin may decrease the absorption of astaxanthin)

Beta-Carotene
(May decrease the absorption of beta-carotene)

Folate
(May decrease folic acid absorption)

Fucoxanthin
(Concomitant intake of cholestyramine and fucoxanthin may decrease the absorption of fucoxanthin)

Gamma-Tocopherol
(Decreased Gamma-Tocopherol absorption)

Inositol Nicotinate
(May reduce nicotinic acid absorption and may have synergistic antihyperlipidemic effects)

Lutein and Zeaxanthin
(Decreased absorption of Lutein and Zeaxanthin)

Lycopene
(Decreased absorption of Lycopene)

Niacin
(May reduce nicotinic acid absorption and may have synergistic antihyperlipidemic effects)

Psyllium
(Enhanced cholesterol-lowering action)

Riboflavin (Vitamin B2)
(May decrease absorption of riboflavin)

Tocotrienols
(May decrease Tocotrienol absorption)

Vitamin A
(May decrease vitamin A absorption)

Vitamin B12
(May decrease enterohepatic reabsorption of vitamin B12)

Vitamin D
(Concomitant intake of cholestyramine and vitamin D may reduce the absorption of vitamin D)

Vitamin E
(May decrease vitamin E absorption)

Vitamin K
(May reduce vitamin K absorption)

CHOLINE

Homocysteine
(Increased metabolism with Choline, Vitamin B6, Vitamin B12 and Folic Acid)

Huperzine A
(Additive effects and increased adverse effects with Huperzine A)

L-Carnitine
(May lead to increased L-Carnitine retention)

Methotrexate Sodium
(May decrease Choline metabolites)

CHOLINERGIC AGENTS

Huperzine A
(Additive effects and increased adverse effects with Huperzine A)

CHONDROITIN SULFATE

Chitosan
(May decrease absorption of chondroitin sulfate)

CHROMIUM

Ascorbate
(May increase absorption of chromium)

Beta Blockers
(Elevated HDL cholesterol levels after two months of chromium use)

Phytic Acid
(May decrease absorption of chromium)

Sodium Alginates and other Phyco-Polysaccharides
(Decreased absorption of Chromium)

Vanadium
(May decrease absorption of vanadium)

CHRYSIN

Aminoglutethimide
(Chrysin may have additive effects)

Anastrozole
(Chrysin may have additive effects)

Aromatase Inhibitors
(Chrysin may have additive effects)

CISPLATIN

Ascorbyl Palmitate
(Vitamin C may potentiate antineoplastic activity)

Luteolin
(Luteolin was shown to sensitize the anticancer effect of cisplatin (cisdiamminediachloroplatinum))

Quercetin
(May cause genotoxicity in normal tissues when taken with Quercetin)

Vitamin C
(Vitamin C may potentiate the antineoplastic activity of cisplatin. It may also help ameliorate the nephrotoxic effect of cisplatin)

CLINDAMYCIN HYDROCHLORIDE

Pectin
(Decreased absorption of clindamycin)

CLOPIDOGREL BISULFATE

Curcuminoids
(Curcuminoids may enhance the antiplatelet effect)

Gamma-Tocopherol
(Increased effects of clopidogrel)

Green Tea Catechins
(Enhanced effect with green tea catechins)

Nattokinase (Subtilisin NAT)
(The use of nattokinase along with antiplatelet drugs (eg, clopidogrel) may cause serious adverse events, especially excessive bleeding. Administration of nattokinase is contraindicated in those with bleeding disorders and should be avoided in those receiving antiplatelet agents)

Vitamin E
(High doses of vitamin E may potentiate the effects of antiplatelet drugs)

Vitamin E Phosphate
(Vitamin E phosphate may potentiate the effects of antiplatelet drugs (eg, clopidogrel))

COD LIVER OIL

Astaxanthin
(Dietary oils such as olive oil and fish oils may enhance the absorption of astaxanthin. Corn oil is less likely to enhance astaxanthin absorption)

Fucoxanthin
(Dietary oils, such as fish oils and olive oils, may enhance the absorption of fucoxanthin)

COENZYME Q10 (COQ10)

Alpha Tocopherol Acetate
(Elevation in CoQ10 levels in mitochondria by dietary supplementation is linked to a corresponding rise in alpha-tocopherol content)

Alpha-Tocopherol Polyethylene Glycol Succinate (TPGS)
(TPGS may increase the absorption of coenzyme Q-10)

Antidiabetic Drugs, unspecified
(May need dosing adjustments)

Corticosteroids
(May need dosing adjustment)

Doxorubicin Hydrochloride
(May ameliorate the cardiotoxicity of doxorubicin)

Doxorubicin Hydrochloride Liposome
(May ameliorate the cardiotoxicity of doxorubicin)

Lovastatin
(Decreases CoQ10 levels)

Piperine, found in black pepper
(May enhance absorption and increase plasma levels of CoQ10)

Pravastatin Sodium
(Decreases CoQ10 levels)

Propranolol Hydrochloride
(May inhibit some CoQ10-dependent enzymes)

Simvastatin
(Decreases CoQ10 levels)

Tocopherol Acetate
(Elevation in CoQ10 levels in mitochondria by dietary supplementation is linked to a corresponding rise in alpha-tocopherol content)

Tocopherols
(Elevation in CoQ10 levels in mitochondria by dietary supplementation is linked to a corresponding rise in alpha-tocopherol content)

Warfarin Sodium
(May decrease the effectiveness of warfarin)

COLCHICINE

Folate
(May decrease folate levels)

Vitamin B12
(May decrease absorption of vitamin B12)

COLESTIPOL

Astaxanthin
(Concomitant intake of colestipol and astaxanthin may decrease the absorption of astaxanthin)

Beta-Carotene
(May decrease the absorption of beta-carotene)

Folate
(May decrease folic acid absorption)

Fucoxanthin
(Concomitant intake of colestipol and fucoxanthin may decrease the absorption of fucoxanthin)

Gamma-Tocopherol
(Decreased Gamma-Tocopherol absorption)

Inositol Nicotinate
(May reduce nicotinic acid absorption and may have synergistic antihyperlipidemic effects)

Lutein and Zeaxanthin
(Decreased absorption of Lutein and Zeaxanthin)

Niacin
(May reduce nicotinic acid absorption and may have synergistic antihyperlipidemic effects)

Tocotrienols
(May decrease Tocotrienol absorption)

Vitamin A
(May decrease vitamin A absorption)

Vitamin B12
(May decrease enterohepatic reabsorption of vitamin B12)

Vitamin D
(Concomitant intake of colestipol and vitamin D may reduce the absorption of vitamin D)

Vitamin E
(May decrease vitamin E absorption)

Vitamin K
(May reduce vitamin K absorption)

COLESTIPOL HYDROCHLORIDE

Astaxanthin
(Concomitant intake of colestipol and astaxanthin may decrease the absorption of astaxanthin)

Fucoxanthin
(Concomitant intake of colestipol and fucoxanthin may decrease the absorption of fucoxanthin)

Lycopene
(Decreased absorption of Lycopene)

Riboflavin (Vitamin B2)
(May decrease absorption of riboflavin)

COPPER

Ascorbyl Palmitate
(High dose Vitamin C may decrease absorption)

Diet high in fructose
(Decreased copper levels)

Inositol Hexaphosphate
(May form chelates with Inositol Hexaphosphate)

Iron
(May decrease copper levels in tissues)

Molybdenum
(High dose of molybdenum may antagonize dietary copper absorption and high dose copper may antagonize molybdenum absorption)

Pectin
(Decreased absorption of Copper)

Penicillamine
(Decreased absorption of copper and penicillamine)
Phytic Acid
(Decreased absorption of copper)
Psyllium
(Decreased absorption of Copper)
Soy Protein
(May reduce availability of copper)
Vitamin C
(One study showed that high doses of vitamin C negatively affected copper status in men. Other studies have shown no such effects)
Zinc
(Concomitant intake of copper and zinc may depress the absorption of copper. Intake of large doses of zinc can negatively affect the copper status of the body)

CORTICOSTEROIDS
Coenzyme Q10 (CoQ10)
(May need dosing adjustment)

CREATINE
Beverages, caffeine-containing
(May interfere with effects of Creatine)

CREATINE PHOSPHATE
Beta-Alanine
(Creatine and beta-alanine may increase skeletal creatine phosphate and carnosine and may work synergistically to delay fatigue and increase exercise performance, especially in trained athletes)

CURCUMIN
Piperine
(Piperine may enhance the absorption)

CURCUMINOIDS
Antiplatelet Drugs
(Curcuminoids may enhance the antiplatelet effect)
Aspirin
(Curcuminoids may enhance the antiplatelet effect)

Aspirin Buffered
(Curcuminoids may enhance the antiplatelet effect)
Aspirin, Enteric Coated
(Curcuminoids may enhance the antiplatelet effect)
Bromelains
(May enhance absorption of curcuminoids)
Clopidogrel Bisulfate
(Curcuminoids may enhance the antiplatelet effect)
Dipyridamole
(Curcuminoids may enhance the antiplatelet effect)
Nutritional Supplement
(Bromelain and piperine may enhance the absorption of curcuminoids)
Piperine, found in black pepper
(May enhance absorption of curcuminoids)
Ticlopidine Hydrochloride
(Curcuminoids may enhance the antiplatelet effect)
Warfarin Sodium
(Curcuminoids may enhance the anticoagulant effect)

CYANOCOBALAMIN
(*See under* Vitamin B12)

CYCLOSERINE
Vitamin B6
(May result in vitamin B6 deficiency)

CYCLOSPORINE
Alpha-Tocopherol
Polyethylene Glycol Succinate (TPGS)
(TPGS may increase absorption of cyclosporine)
Ascorbyl Palmitate
(Grapefruit flavonoids may increase bioavailability due to cytochrome P-450 3A4 inhibition)
L-Arginine
(L-Arginine may counteract antinaturetic effects)
Red Yeast Rice
(Increased risk of myopathy)

Vitamin C
(Grapefruit flavonoids may increase bioavailability due to cytochrome P-450 3A4 inhibition)
Vitamin E
(Based on cell culture studies, alpha-tocopherol may help to ameliorate the renal side effects of cyclosporine)

CYPROHEPTADINE HYDROCHLORIDE
5-Hydroxytryptophan
(5-HTP may decrease effects)

CYSTEINE
Iron
(May increase absorption of iron)

CYSTEINE-CONTAINING PROTEINS
Zinc
(Foods rich in cysteine-containing proteins (eg, animal muscle tissue) may increase the absorption of zinc if ingested concomitantly)

CYTOCHROME P450 1A2 SUBSTRATES (SELECTED)
Gamma-Oryzanol
(Gamma-oryzanol was found to have no more than a slight inhibitory effect on cytochrome P450 activities in human liver microsomes, indicating that gamma-oryzanol would not be expected to cause clinically significant interactions with cytochrome P450-metabolized drugs)
Xanthohumol
(Xanthohumol inhibits cytochrome p450, and although there are no known reports of any interactions with drugs and xanthohumol, those using drugs that are metabolized via the cytochrome p450 system, for example, the statin atorvastatin, should be cautious in the use of xanthohumol supplements)

CYTOCHROME P450 2C8 SUBSTRATES (SELECTED)
Gamma-Oryzanol
(Gamma-oryzanol was found to have no more than a slight inhibitory effect on cytochrome

P450 activities in human liver microsomes, indicating that gamma-oryzanol would not be expected to cause clinically significant interactions with cytochrome P450-metabolized drugs)

Xanthohumol

(Xanthohumol inhibits cytochrome p450, and although there are no known reports of any interactions with drugs and xanthohumol, those using drugs that are metabolized via the cytochrome p450 system, for example, the statin atorvastatin, should be cautious in the use of xanthohumol supplements)

CYTOCHROME P450 2C9 SUBSTRATES (SELECTED)

Gamma-Oryzanol

(Gamma-oryzanol was found to have no more than a slight inhibitory effect on cytochrome P450 activities in human liver microsomes, indicating that gamma-oryzanol would not be expected to cause clinically significant interactions with cytochrome P450-metabolized drugs)

Xanthohumol

(Xanthohumol inhibits cytochrome p450, and although there are no known reports of any interactions with drugs and xanthohumol, those using drugs that are metabolized via the cytochrome p450 system, for example, the statin atorvastatin, should be cautious in the use of xanthohumol supplements)

CYTOCHROME P450 2C18 SUBSTRATES (SELECTED)

Gamma-Oryzanol

(Gamma-oryzanol was found to have no more than a slight inhibitory effect on cytochrome P450 activities in human liver microsomes, indicating that gamma-oryzanol would not be

expected to cause clinically significant interactions with cytochrome P450-metabolized drugs)

Xanthohumol

(Xanthohumol inhibits cytochrome p450, and although there are no known reports of any interactions with drugs and xanthohumol, those using drugs that are metabolized via the cytochrome p450 system, for example, the statin atorvastatin, should be cautious in the use of xanthohumol supplements)

CYTOCHROME P450 2C19 SUBSTRATES (SELECTED)

Gamma-Oryzanol

(Gamma-oryzanol was found to have no more than a slight inhibitory effect on cytochrome P450 activities in human liver microsomes, indicating that gamma-oryzanol would not be expected to cause clinically significant interactions with cytochrome P450-metabolized drugs)

Xanthohumol

(Xanthohumol inhibits cytochrome p450, and although there are no known reports of any interactions with drugs and xanthohumol, those using drugs that are metabolized via the cytochrome p450 system, for example, the statin atorvastatin, should be cautious in the use of xanthohumol supplements)

CYTOCHROME P450 2D6 SUBSTRATES (SELECTED)

Gamma-Oryzanol

(Gamma-oryzanol was found to have no more than a slight inhibitory effect on cytochrome P450 activities in human liver microsomes, indicating that gamma-oryzanol would not be expected to cause clinically significant interactions with

cytochrome P450-metabolized drugs)

Xanthohumol

(Xanthohumol inhibits cytochrome p450, and although there are no known reports of any interactions with drugs and xanthohumol, those using drugs that are metabolized via the cytochrome p450 system, for example, the statin atorvastatin, should be cautious in the use of xanthohumol supplements)

CYTOCHROME P450 3A SUBSTRATES (SELECTED)

Gamma-Oryzanol

(Gamma-oryzanol was found to have no more than a slight inhibitory effect on cytochrome P450 activities in human liver microsomes, indicating that gamma-oryzanol would not be expected to cause clinically significant interactions with cytochrome P450-metabolized drugs)

Xanthohumol

(Xanthohumol inhibits cytochrome p450, and although there are no known reports of any interactions with drugs and xanthohumol, those using drugs that are metabolized via the cytochrome p450 system, for example, the statin atorvastatin, should be cautious in the use of xanthohumol supplements)

CYTOCHROME P450 3A4 SUBSTRATES (SELECTED)

DHEA

(DHEA inhibits CYP3A4 in vitro and could increase serum concentrations of drugs metabolized by this isoenzyme)

Gamma-Oryzanol

(Gamma-oryzanol was found to have no more than a slight inhibitory effect on cytochrome P450 activities in human liver microsomes, indicating that gamma-oryzanol would not be expected to cause clinically significant interactions with cytochrome P450-metabolized drugs)

Luteolin
(Luteolin has been found to inhibit the metabolism of the sedative drug midazolam by human liver microsomes and cytochrome P450 3A4 (CYP3A4) and CYP3A5. Midazolam is a probe substrate for CYP3A4 and CYP3A5 enzymes. CYP3A4 is located in the intestine and liver, and its inhibition leads to delayed absorption and reduced first pass metabolism in the liver, resulting in higher plasma levels of the drug. However, given this finding, those using midazolam or other drugs metabolized by CYP3A4, including statins - atorvastatin, lovastatin and simvastatin - as well as amiodarone, buspirone, cisapride, etoposide, quinidine and sildenafil, tadalafil, vardenafil and others, should exercise caution in the use of luteolin-containing dairy supplements)

Xanthohumol
(Xanthohumol inhibits cytochrome p450, and although there are no known reports of any interactions with drugs and xanthohumol, those using drugs that are metabolized via the cytochrome p450 system, for example, the statin atorvastatin, should be cautious in the use of xanthohumol supplements)

D-GLUCARATE

Fluorouracil
(Synergistic antitumor activity)
Retinoids
(Synergistic chemopreventive effects)

D-RIBOSE

Antidiabetic Drugs, unspecified
(D-Ribose may cause hypoglycemia)

DHEA

Alprazolam
(May increase DHEA levels)
Androstenediol
(May increase adverse effects of DHEA)
Androstenedione
(May increase adverse effects of DHEA)
Cytochrome p450 3a4 substrates (selected)
(DHEA inhibits CYP3A4 in vitro and could increase serum concentrations of drugs metabolized by this isoenzyme)
Danazol
(May decrease DHEA levels)
Dexamethasone
(May decrease DHEA levels)
Diltiazem Hydrochloride
(May increase DHEA levels)
Insulin
(May decrease DHEA levels)
Morphine Sulfate
(May decrease DHEA levels)
Testosterone
(May increase adverse effects of DHEA)

DL-PHENYLALANINE

Monoamine Oxidase Inhibitors
(May cause hypertension with Brewer's Yeast)
Neuroleptics
(L-Phenylalanine may potentiate tardive dyskinesia side effects)
Pargyline Hydrochloride
(May cause hypertension with Brewer's Yeast)
Phenelzine Sulfate
(May cause hypertension with Brewer's Yeast)
Selegiline Hydrochloride
(May have synergistic antidepressant activity)
Tranylcypromine Sulfate
(May cause hypertension with Brewer's Yeast)

DAIDZEIN

Ethanol
(Daidzein/daidzin may increase the bioavailability of ingested ethanol)

DAIRY PRODUCTS

Fluoride
(Decreased absorption of Fluoride)

DALTEPARIN SODIUM

Nattokinase (Subtilisin NAT)
(The use of nattokinase along with parenteral anticoagulants (eg, low molecular weight heparins) may cause serious adverse events, especially excessive bleeding. Administration of nattokinase is contraindicated in those with bleeding disorders and should be avoided in those receiving anticoagulant agents)

DANAZOL

DHEA
(May decrease DHEA levels)

DANTROLENE SODIUM

Glycine
(Glycine may increase effect of)

DAPSONE

Piperine
(Piperine may inhibit metabolism)

DEGLYCYRRHIZINATED LICORICE (DGL)

Nitrofurantoin
(Increased excretion rate of nitrofurantoin)

DESIPRAMINE HYDROCHLORIDE

Arnica
(Increased risk of prolonged QT interval when given with Arnica)

DEXAMETHASONE

DHEA
(May decrease DHEA levels)

DEXTROAMPHETAMINE

Pycnogenol
(May be synergistic with Pycnogenol for attention deficit-hyperactivity disorder management)

DIAZEPAM

Glycine
(Glycine may increase effect of)

DIDANOSINE

Acetyl-L-Carnitine
(May lead to decreased acetyl-L-carnitine levels)

L-Carnitine
(May produce L-Carnitine
deficiencies)
Riboflavin (Vitamin B2)
(Riboflavin may reverse
nucleoside analogue-induced lactic
acidosis in mild riboflavin
deficiencies)

DIET HIGH IN FRUCTOSE
Copper
(Decreased copper levels)

DIET HIGH IN PROTEIN
Inositol Hexaphosphate
(May form chelates with Inositol
Hexaphosphate)

DIET, LIPID
Chitosan
(Might bind to Chitosan)

DIETARY FIBER
Bone Meal
(Decreased absorption of Calcium)
Calcium
(May decrease absorption of
calcium)
Vitamin E
(Dietary fiber supplementation
may decrease the antioxidative
effect of a supplement containing
alpha-tocopherol and carotenoids)

DIGOXIN
Pectin
(Decreased absorption of digoxin)
Psyllium
(Reduced absorption of digoxin)

DILTIAZEM HYDROCHLORIDE
DHEA
(May increase DHEA levels)

DIMETHYL SULFOXIDE (DMSO)
Sulindac
(May decrease the effects of
DMSO and increase side effects)

DIPYRIDAMOLE
Alpha-Tocopherol
Polyethylene Glycol
Succinate (TPGS)
(High doses of TPGS may
enhance the effects of
dipyridamole)

Curcuminoids
(Curcuminoids may enhance the
antiplatelet effect)
Gamma-Tocopherol
(Increased effects of dipyridamole)
Green Tea Catechins
(Enhanced effect with green tea
catechins)
Nattokinase (Subtilisin NAT)
(The use of nattokinase along
with antiplatelet drugs (eg,
dipyridamole) may cause serious
adverse events, especially
excessive bleeding. Administration
of nattokinase is contraindicated
in those with bleeding disorders
and should be avoided in those
receiving antiplatelet agents)
Vitamin E
(High doses of vitamin E may
potentiate the effects of
antiplatelet drugs)
Vitamin E Phosphate
(Vitamin E phosphate may
potentiate the effects of
antiplatelet drugs (eg,
dipyridamole))

DISOPYRAMIDE
Arnica
(Increased risk of prolonged QT
interval when given with Arnica)

DOCOSAHEXAENOIC ACID (DHA)
Gamma-Oryzanol
(Administration of the omega-3
long chain polyunsaturated acids
DHA (docosahexaenoic acid) and
EPA (eicosapentaenoic acid) along
with gamma-oryzanol may
produce a synergistic effect in
lipid lowering)
Warfarin Sodium
(Because DHA my have
antithrombotic activity, caution
should be exercised with
concomitant warfarin therapy)

DONEPEZIL HYDROCHLORIDE
Huperzine A
(Additive effects and increased
adverse effects with Huperzine A)

DOXEPIN HYDROCHLORIDE
Arnica
(Increased risk of prolonged QT
interval when given with Arnica)

DOXORUBICIN HYDROCHLORIDE
Arnica
(Increased cardiotoxicity with
Arnica)
Ascorbyl Palmitate
(Vitamin C may potentiate
antineoplastic activity)
Coenzyme Q10 (CoQ10)
(May ameliorate the cardiotoxicity
of doxorubicin)
L-Theanine
(L-Theanine may enhance
antitumor effects and decrease
adverse effects)
Luteolin
(Luteolin was found to reverse
tumor resistance to doxorubicin in
human and murine breast cancer
cells under hypoxic conditions)
Riboflavin (Vitamin B2)
(May inhibit riboflavin conversion
to FMN and FAD)
Vitamin C
(Vitamin C may potentiate the
antineoplastic activity of
doxorubicin. It may also help
ameliorate the cardiotoxic effect
of doxorubicin)

DOXORUBICIN HYDROCHLORIDE LIPOSOME
Coenzyme Q10 (CoQ10)
(May ameliorate the cardiotoxicity
of doxorubicin)
Luteolin
(Luteolin was found to reverse
tumor resistance to doxorubicin in
human and murine breast cancer
cells under hypoxic conditions)

DOXYCYCLINE
Sesame Seed Lignans
(Antibiotics may decrease the
production of the mammalian
lignans enterolactone (ENT) and
enterodiol (END) from sesame
seed lignans)

DRUGS, UNSPECIFIED

Activated Charcoal
(Avoid using Activated Charcoal within two hours of taking these products)

Bentonite
(Bentonite may adsorb certain drugs)

Piperine
(Piperine may inhibit metabolism)

EICOSAPENTAENOIC ACID (EPA)

Allium sativum
(May interact with EPA. Such reactions might be manifested by increased susceptibility to bruising, nosebleeds, hemoptysis, hematemesis, hematuria, and blood in the stool. Most who take the EPA supplements do not suffer from these problems and if they occur, they are rare. If they do occur, the EPA dose should be lowered or discontinued)

Aspirin
(May interact with EPA. Such reactions might be manifested by increased susceptibility to bruising, nosebleeds, hemoptysis, hematemesis, hematuria, and blood in the stool. Most who take the EPA supplements do not suffer from these problems and if they occur, they are rare. If they do occur, the EPA dose should be lowered or discontinued)

Aspirin Buffered
(May interact with EPA. Such reactions might be manifested by increased susceptibility to bruising, nosebleeds, hemoptysis, hematemesis, hematuria, and blood in the stool. Most who take the EPA supplements do not suffer from these problems and if they occur, they are rare. If they do occur, the EPA dose should be lowered or discontinued)

Aspirin, Enteric Coated
(May interact with EPA. Such reactions might be manifested by increased susceptibility to

bruising, nosebleeds, hemoptysis, hematemesis, hematuria, and blood in the stool. Most who take the EPA supplements do not suffer from these problems and if they occur, they are rare. If they do occur, the EPA dose should be lowered or discontinued)

Gamma-Oryzanol
(Administration of the omega-3 long chain polyunsaturated acids DHA (docosahexaenoic acid) and EPA (eicosapentaenoic acid) along with gamma-oryzanol may produce a synergistic effect in lipid lowering)

Garlic Extract
(May interact with EPA. Such reactions might be manifested by increased susceptibility to bruising, nosebleeds, hemoptysis, hematemesis, hematuria, and blood in the stool. Most who take the EPA supplements do not suffer from these problems and if they occur, they are rare. If they do occur, the EPA dose should be lowered or discontinued)

Garlic Oil
(May interact with EPA. Such reactions might be manifested by increased susceptibility to bruising, nosebleeds, hemoptysis, hematemesis, hematuria, and blood in the stool. Most who take the EPA supplements do not suffer from these problems and if they occur, they are rare. If they do occur, the EPA dose should be lowered or discontinued)

Ginkgo biloba
(May interact with EPA. Such reactions might be manifested by increased susceptibility to bruising, nosebleeds, hemoptysis, hematemesis, hematuria, and blood in the stool. Most who take the EPA supplements do not suffer from these problems and if they occur, they are rare. If they do

occur, the EPA dose should be lowered or discontinued)

Nonsteroidal Anti-Inflammatory Drugs
(May interact with EPA. Such reactions might be manifested by increased susceptibility to bruising, nosebleeds, hemoptysis, hematemesis, hematuria, and blood in the stool. Most who take the EPA supplements do not suffer from these problems and if they occur, they are rare. If they do occur, the EPA dose should be lowered or discontinued)

Warfarin Sodium
(Because of the possible antithrombotic activity of EPA, caution should be exercised with concomitant warfarin therapy)

ENOXAPARIN

Nattokinase (Subtilisin NAT)
(The use of nattokinase along with parenteral anticoagulants (eg, low molecular weight heparins) may cause serious adverse events, especially excessive bleeding. Administration of nattokinase is contraindicated in those with bleeding disorders and should be avoided in those receiving anticoagulant agents)

EPTIFIBATIDE

Alpha-Tocopherol Polyethylene Glycol Succinate (TPGS)
(High doses of TPGS may enhance the effects of eptifibatide)

Gamma-Tocopherol
(Increased effects of eptifibatide)

Nattokinase (Subtilisin NAT)
(The use of nattokinase along with parenteral antiplatelet drugs (GPIIB/IIA inhibitors such as eptifibatide) may cause serious adverse events, especially excessive bleeding. Administration of nattokinase is contraindicated in those with bleeding disorders and should be avoided in those receiving antiplatelet agents)

Vitamin E
(High doses of vitamin E may potentiate the effects of antiplatelet drugs)

Vitamin E Phosphate
(Vitamin E phosphate may potentiate the effects of antiplatelet drugs (eg, eptifibatide))

EQUOL

Antibiotics, unspecified
(Antibiotics may decrease equol formation)

Fructo-oligosaccharides
(May promote the formation of equol)

Green Tea Extract
(May promote the formation of equol)

Starch
(May promote the formation of equol)

ERYTHROMYCIN

Sesame Seed Lignans
(Antibiotics may decrease the production of the mammalian lignans enterolactone (ENT) and enterodiol (END) from sesame seed lignans)

ESTROGEN

Ascorbyl Palmitate
(Vitamin C may enhance inhibition of LDL formation)

Ipriflavone
(Additive effects with Ipriflavone)

Vitamin C
(Ascorbic acid may enhance 17 beta-estradiol inhibition of oxidized LDL formation)

ETHACRYNIC ACID

Thiamin
(Chronic use may cause Thiamin deficiency)

ETHAMBUTOL HYDROCHLORIDE

Piperine
(Piperine may inhibit metabolism)

ETHANOL

Daidzein
(Daidzein/daidzin may increase the bioavailability of ingested ethanol)

Inositol Nicotinate
(May increase nicotinic acid-induced flushing)

Niacin
(May increase nicotinic acid-induced flushing)

ETHIONAMIDE

Vitamin B6
(May increase vitamin B6 requirements)

ETHYL ALCOHOL

Niacin
(May increase nicotinic acid-induced flushing)

ETHYLENEDIAMINETETRAACETIC ACID

Vanadium
(May decrease absorption of vanadium)

ETRETINATE

Vitamin A
(May produce additive toxicity effects)

EVENING PRIMROSE OIL

Allium sativum
(EPO may increase bleeding tendencies)

Aspirin
(EPO may increase bleeding tendencies)

Fish Oils
(EPO may increase bleeding tendencies)

Ginkgo biloba
(EPO may increase bleeding tendencies)

Nonsteroidal Anti-Inflammatory Drugs
(EPO may increase bleeding tendencies)

Phenothiazines
(EPO lowers seizure threshold)

Warfarin Sodium
(EPO may increase bleeding tendencies)

EZETIMIBE

Gamma-Oryzanol
(Ezetimibe may inhibit the uptake of the phytosterols into the enterocytes of the small intestine)

Vitamin E
(May inhibit the intestinal absorption of alpha-tocopherol)

FAT SUBSTITUTE

Gamma-Tocopherol
(Inhibits absorption of Gamma-Tocopherol)

Lutein and Zeaxanthin
(Decreased absorption of Lutein and Zeaxanthin)

Lycopene
(Reduced absorption of Lycopene)

Tocotrienols
(May inhibit Tocotrienol absorption)

Vitamin A
(May inhibit vitamin A absorption)

Vitamin D
(Olestra inhibits the absorption of vitamin D as well as the other fat-soluble vitamins A, E, and K)

Vitamin E
(Olestra inhibits the absorption of vitamin E, as well as the other fat-soluble vitamins, A, D, and K, carotenoids and flavonoids)

Vitamin K
(Inhibits absorption of vitamin K as well as the other fat-soluble vitamins A, D, and E)

FATTY ACIDS

Medium-Chain Triglycerides
(MCT may facilitate the absorption of fatty acids)

FATTY ACIDS, POLYUNSATURATED

Vitamin E
(Supplementary PUFAs may increase vitamin E requirements. High polyunsaturated fatty acid intakes should be accompanied by increased vitamin E intakes to prevent their oxidation)

FELODIPINE

Ascorbyl Palmitate
(Grapefruit flavonoids may increase bioavailability due to cytochrome P-450 3A4 inhibition)

Vitamin C
(Grapefruit flavonoids may increase bioavailability due to cytochrome P-450 3A4 inhibition)

FERROUS FUMARATE

Vanadium

(May decrease absorption of vanadium)

FERROUS GLUCONATE

Vanadium

(May decrease absorption of vanadium)

FERROUS SULFATE

Vanadium

(May decrease absorption of vanadium)

FIBER

Vitamin E

(Dietary fiber supplementation may decrease the antioxidative effect of a supplement containing alpha-tocopherol and carotenoids)

FIBRATES

Red Yeast Rice

(Increased risk of myopathy)

FISH OIL

Allium sativum

(May interact with fish oil. Such interactions might be manifested by increased susceptibility to bruising, nosebleeds, hemoptysis, hematemesis, hematuria, and blood in the stool. Most who take fish oil supplements do not suffer from these problems and if they occur, they are rare. If they do occur, the fish oil dose should be lowered or discontinued)

Aspirin

(May interact with fish oil. Such interactions might be manifested by increased susceptibility to bruising, nosebleeds, hemoptysis, hematemesis, hematuria, and blood in the stool. Most who take fish oil supplements do not suffer from these problems and if they occur, they are rare. If they do occur, the fish oil dose should be lowered or discontinued)

Aspirin Buffered

(May interact with fish oil. Such interactions might be manifested by increased susceptibility to

bruising, nosebleeds, hemoptysis, hematemesis, hematuria, and blood in the stool. Most who take fish oil supplements do not suffer from these problems and if they occur, they are rare. If they do occur, the fish oil dose should be lowered or discontinued)

Aspirin, Enteric Coated

(May interact with fish oil. Such interactions might be manifested by increased susceptibility to bruising, nosebleeds, hemoptysis, hematemesis, hematuria, and blood in the stool. Most who take fish oil supplements do not suffer from these problems and if they occur, they are rare. If they do occur, the fish oil dose should be lowered or discontinued)

Garlic Extract

(May interact with fish oil. Such interactions might be manifested by increased susceptibility to bruising, nosebleeds, hemoptysis, hematemesis, hematuria, and blood in the stool. Most who take fish oil supplements do not suffer from these problems and if they occur, they are rare. If they do occur, the fish oil dose should be lowered or discontinued)

Garlic Oil

(May interact with fish oil. Such interactions might be manifested by increased susceptibility to bruising, nosebleeds, hemoptysis, hematemesis, hematuria, and blood in the stool. Most who take fish oil supplements do not suffer from these problems and if they occur, they are rare. If they do occur, the fish oil dose should be lowered or discontinued)

Ginkgo biloba

(May interact with fish oil. Such interactions might be manifested by increased susceptibility to bruising, nosebleeds, hemoptysis, hematemesis, hematuria, and blood in the stool. Most who take fish

oil supplements do not suffer from these problems and if they occur, they are rare. If they do occur, the fish oil dose should be lowered or discontinued)

Nonsteroidal Anti-Inflammatory Drugs

(May interact with fish oil. Such interactions might be manifested by increased susceptibility to bruising, nosebleeds, hemoptysis, hematemesis, hematuria, and blood in the stool. Most who take fish oil supplements do not suffer from these problems and if they occur, they are rare. If they do occur, the fish oil dose should be lowered or discontinued)

Warfarin Sodium

(Because of the possible antithrombotic effect of fish oil supplements, caution should be exercised with concomitant warfarin therapy)

FISH OILS

Astaxanthin

(Dietary oils such as olive oil and fish oils may enhance the absorption of astaxanthin. Corn oil is less likely to enhance astaxanthin absorption)

Borage Oil

(Increased antithrombotic activity with Borage oil)

Evening Primrose Oil

(EPO may increase bleeding tendencies)

Flaxseed Oil

(Interactions may occur if flaxseed oil is used with other nutritional supplements, such as fish oils, which have antithrombotic activity)

Fucoxanthin

(Dietary oils, such as fish oils and olive oils, may enhance the absorption of fucoxanthin)

Gamma-Oryzanol

(Administration of the omega-3 long chain polyunsaturated acids DHA (docosahexaenoic acid) and

EPA (eicosapentaenoic acid) along with gamma-oryzanol may produce a synergistic effect in lipid lowering)

Nattokinase (Subtilisin NAT)
(Co-administration of nattokinase with fish oil may lead to increased bleeding tendencies manifested by increased susceptibility to bruising, nosebleeds, hematemesis, hematuria, and blood in the stool)

Vitamin E Phosphate
(Fish oils possess antiplatelet activity. Vitamin E phosphate may potentiate the antiplatelet activity of fish oils)

FLAVONOIDS

Alpha-Tocopherol Polyethylene Glycol Succinate (TPGS)
(TPGS may increase the absorption of flavonoids)

Ascorbyl Palmitate
(Vitamin C may have synergistic effects)

Chitosan
(Might bind to Chitosan)

Gamma-Tocopherol
(Helps to maintain levels of reduced Gamma-Tocopherol)

Medium-Chain Triglycerides
(MCT may facilitate the absorption of flavonoids)

Vitamin C
(Vitamin C may act synergistically with various flavonoids)

FLAXSEED LIGNANS

Antibiotics, unspecified
(Antibiotics may decrease the production of enterodiol (END) and enterolactone (ENL) from secoisolariciresinol diglucoside (SDG))

FLAXSEED OIL

Allium sativum
(Interactions may occur between alpha-linoleic acid and its metabolites with such herbs as garlic (allium sativum). Such

interactions might be manifested by nosebleeds and easy bruising)

Aspirin
(Interactions may occur between flaxseed oil and its metabolites and warfarin, aspirin, and NSAIDs. Such interactions, if they were to occur, might be manifested by nosebleeds and increased susceptibility to bruising. If this does occur, consideration should be given to lowering or stopping intake)

Fish Oils
(Interactions may occur if flaxseed oil is used with other nutritional supplements, such as fish oils, which have antithrombotic activity)

Nonsteroidal Anti-Inflammatory Drugs
(Interactions may occur between flaxseed oil and its metabolites and warfarin, aspirin, and NSAIDs. Such interactions, if they were to occur, might be manifested by nosebleeds and increased susceptibility to bruising. If this does occur, consideration should be given to lowering or stopping intake)

Warfarin Sodium
(Interactions may occur between flaxseed oil and its metabolites and warfarin, aspirin, and NSAIDs. Such interactions, if they were to occur, might be manifested by nosebleeds and increased susceptibility to bruising. If this does occur, consideration should be given to lowering or stopping intake)

FLUORIDE

Antacids, aluminum-containing
(Decreased absorption of Fluoride)

Calcium
(Decreased absorption of Fluoride)

Dairy products
(Decreased absorption of Fluoride)

FLUORINE & FLUORIDE PREPARATIONS

Ipriflavone
(Additive effects with Ipriflavone)

Xylitol
(The combination of xylitol and the use of fluoride toothpastes may give better anticariogenic effects than the use of either alone)

FLUOROQUINOLONE ANTIBIOTICS

Sesame Seed Lignans
(Antibiotics may decrease the production of the mammalian lignans enterolactone (ENT) and enterodiol (END) from sesame seed lignans)

FLUOROURACIL

D-Glucarate
(Synergistic antitumor activity)

FLUOXETINE HYDROCHLORIDE

Folate
(Folic acid may enhance antidepressant effects)

Melatonin
(Psychotic episode reported with Melatonin)

FLUVOXAMINE MALEATE

Melatonin
(Increases the bioavailability of oral Melatonin)

FOLATE

Carbamazepine
(May decrease folate levels and increase homocysteine levels; High dose folic acid may decrease serum levels)

Cholestyramine
(May decrease folic acid absorption)

Colchicine
(May decrease folate levels)

Colestipol
(May decrease folic acid absorption)

Fluoxetine Hydrochloride
(Folic acid may enhance antidepressant effects)

Food, unspecified
(Decrease in folic acid availability)

Fosphenytoin
(May decrease folate levels and increase homocysteine levels; high

dose folic acid may decrease
serum levels)

Lithium
(Folic acid may increase efficacy)

Lometrexol
(Folic acid may be synergistic and
decrease adverse effects)

Metformin
(Long-term use of metformin has
been associated with elevated
homocysteine levels which are
reduced with folic acid
administration)

Methotrexate
(Folic acid may reduce toxic side
effects)

Nonsteroidal Anti-Inflammatory
Drugs
(Large doses may exert antifolate
activity)

Phenobarbital
(May decrease folate levels and
increase homocysteine levels;
High dose folic acid may decrease
serum levels)

Phenytoin
(May decrease folate levels and
increase homocysteine levels;
High dose folic acid may decrease
serum levels)

Primidone
(May decrease folate levels and
increase homocysteine levels;
High dose folic acid may decrease
serum levels)

Pyrimethamine
(Folic acid may decrease
antiparasitic effects)

Sulfasalazine
(May decrease folic acid
absorption)

Valproic Acid
(May decrease folate levels and
increase homocysteine; High dose
folic acid may decrease serum
levels)

Vitamin B6
(May be synergistic in lowering
serum homocysteine levels)

Vitamin B12
(May be synergistic in lowering
serum homocysteine levels)

Zinc
(Folic acid may decrease zinc
absorption)

FOLIC ACID

(*See also under* Folate)

Betaine and Betaine
Hydrochloride
(May be synergistic in lowering
serum homocysteine levels)

Vitamin B12
(Synergistic with vitamin B12 to
lower homocysteine levels)

FOOD, HOT

Inositol Nicotinate
(May increase nicotinic acid-
induced flushing)

Niacin
(May increase nicotinic acid-
induced flushing)

FOOD, SULFITES

Thiamin
(May inactivate Thiamin)

FOOD, UNSPECIFIED

Activated Charcoal
(Avoid using Activated Charcoal
within two hours of taking these
products)

Bentonite
(Bentonite may adsorb certain
food components)

Folate
(Decrease in folic acid
availability)

Thiamin
(Antithiamin factors in food
inactivate Thiamin)

FOSPHENYTOIN

Folate
(May decrease folate levels and
increase homocysteine levels;
High dose folic acid may decrease
serum levels)

Vitamin B6
(Vitamin B6 may lower plasma
phenytoin levels)

FRUCTO-OLIGOSACCHARIDES

Bone Meal
(Increased absorption of Calcium)

Calcium
(May increase absorption of
calcium)

Equol
(May promote the formation of
equol)

Magnesium
(May increase absorption of
magnesium)

FUCOXANTHIN

Beta-Carotene
(Concomitant intake of beta-
carotene and fucoxanthin may
increase the absorption of
fucoxanthin)

Cholestyramine
(Concomitant intake of
cholestyramine and fucoxanthin
may decrease the absorption of
fucoxanthin)

Cod Liver Oil
(Dietary oils, such as fish oils and
olive oils, may enhance the
absorption of fucoxanthin)

Colestipol
(Concomitant intake of colestipol
and fucoxanthin may decrease the
absorption of fucoxanthin)

Colestipol Hydrochloride
(Concomitant intake of colestipol
and fucoxanthin may decrease the
absorption of fucoxanthin)

Fish Oils
(Dietary oils, such as fish oils and
olive oils, may enhance the
absorption of fucoxanthin)

Medium-Chain Triglycerides
(Concomitant intake of medium-
chain triglycerides and fucoxanthin
may enhance the absorption of
fucoxanthin)

Mineral Oil
(Concomitant intake of mineral oil
and fucoxanthin may decrease the
absorption of fucoxanthin)

Oils, dietary
(Dietary oils, such as fish oils and
olive oils, may enhance the
absorption of fucoxanthin)

Oils, unspecified
(Dietary oils, such as fish oils and
olive oils, may enhance the
absorption of fucoxanthin)

Olestra

(Olestra may reduce the absorption of fucoxanthin)

Orlistat

(Orlistat may decrease the absorption of fucoxanthin)

Pectin

(Concomitant intake of pectin and fucoxanthin may decrease the absorption of fucoxanthin)

Salmon Oil

(Dietary oils, such as fish oils and olive oils, may enhance the absorption of fucoxanthin)

Shark Liver Oil

(Dietary oils, such as fish oils and olive oils, may enhance the absorption of fucoxanthin)

Vitamin A

(Concomitant intake of beta-carotene and fucoxanthin may increase the absorption of fucoxanthin)

FUROSEMIDE

Thiamin

(Chronic use may cause Thiamin deficiency)

GAMMA-HYDROXYBUTYRATE (GHB)

Alcohol

(May be life-threatening with GHB)

Anticonvulsants

(May be life-threatening with GHB)

Antihistamines

(May be life-threatening with GHB)

Benzodiazepines

(May be life-threatening with GHB)

Opiates

(May be life-threatening with GHB)

Protease Inhibitors

(May be life-threatening with GHB)

Skeletal Muscle Relaxants

(May be life-threatening with GHB)

Tranquilizers

(May be life-threatening with GHB)

GAMMA-ORYZANOL

Cytochrome p450 1a2 substrates (selected)

(Gamma-oryzanol was found to have no more than a slight inhibitory effect on cytochrome P450 activities in human liver microsomes, indicating that gamma-oryzanol would not be expected to cause clinically significant interactions with cytochrome P450-metabolized drugs)

Cytochrome p450 2c8 substrates (selected)

(Gamma-oryzanol was found to have no more than a slight inhibitory effect on cytochrome P450 activities in human liver microsomes, indicating that gamma-oryzanol would not be expected to cause clinically significant interactions with cytochrome P450-metabolized drugs)

Cytochrome p450 2c9 substrates (selected)

(Gamma-oryzanol was found to have no more than a slight inhibitory effect on cytochrome P450 activities in human liver microsomes, indicating that gamma-oryzanol would not be expected to cause clinically significant interactions with cytochrome P450-metabolized drugs)

Cytochrome p450 2c18 substrates (selected)

(Gamma-oryzanol was found to have no more than a slight inhibitory effect on cytochrome P450 activities in human liver microsomes, indicating that gamma-oryzanol would not be expected to cause clinically significant interactions with

cytochrome P450-metabolized drugs)

Cytochrome p450 2c19 substrates (selected)

(Gamma-oryzanol was found to have no more than a slight inhibitory effect on cytochrome P450 activities in human liver microsomes, indicating that gamma-oryzanol would not be expected to cause clinically significant interactions with cytochrome P450-metabolized drugs)

Cytochrome p450 2d6 substrates (selected)

(Gamma-oryzanol was found to have no more than a slight inhibitory effect on cytochrome P450 activities in human liver microsomes, indicating that gamma-oryzanol would not be expected to cause clinically significant interactions with cytochrome P450-metabolized drugs)

Cytochrome p450 3a substrates (selected)

(Gamma-oryzanol was found to have no more than a slight inhibitory effect on cytochrome P450 activities in human liver microsomes, indicating that gamma-oryzanol would not be expected to cause clinically significant interactions with cytochrome P450-metabolized drugs)

Cytochrome p450 3a4 substrates (selected)

(Gamma-oryzanol was found to have no more than a slight inhibitory effect on cytochrome P450 activities in human liver microsomes, indicating that gamma-oryzanol would not be expected to cause clinically significant interactions with cytochrome P450-metabolized drugs)

Docosahexaenoic Acid (DHA)
(Administration of the omega-3 long chain polyunsaturated acids DHA (docosahexaenoic acid) and EPA (eicosapentaenoic acid) along with gamma-oryzanol may produce a synergistic effect in lipid lowering)

Eicosapentaenoic Acid (EPA)
(Administration of the omega-3 long chain polyunsaturated acids DHA (docosahexaenoic acid) and EPA (eicosapentaenoic acid) along with gamma-oryzanol may produce a synergistic effect in lipid lowering)

Ezetimibe
(Ezetimibe may inhibit the uptake of the phytosterols into the enterocytes of the small intestine)

Fish Oils
(Administration of the omega-3 long chain polyunsaturated acids DHA (docosahexaenoic acid) and EPA (eicosapentaenoic acid) along with gamma-oryzanol may produce a synergistic effect in lipid lowering)

HMG-CoA Reductase Inhibitors
(Administration of an HMG-CoA reductase inhibitor (a 'statin') along with gamma-oryzanol may have an additive effect on the lowering of total and LDL-cholesterol)

GAMMA-TOCOPHEROL

Abciximab
(Increased effects of abciximab)

Allium sativum
(Enhanced antithrombotic activity of garlic)

Alpha Tocopherol Acetate
(Decreased plasma Gamma-Tocopherol levels)

Antiplatelet Drugs
(Increased effects of antiplatelet drugs)

Aspirin
(Increased effects of aspirin)

Cholestyramine
(Decreased Gamma-Tocopherol absorption)

Clopidogrel Bisulfate
(Increased effects of clopidogrel)

Colestipol
(Decreased Gamma-Tocopherol absorption)

Dipyridamole
(Increased effects of dipyridamole)

Eptifibatide
(Increased effects of eptifibatide)

Fat Substitute
(Inhibits absorption of Gamma-Tocopherol)

Flavonoids
(Helps to maintain levels of reduced Gamma-Tocopherol)

Ginkgo biloba
(Enhanced antithrombotic activity of gingko biloba)

Iron
(The ferrous form of iron can oxidize Gamma-Tocopherol to its pro-oxidant form)

Isoniazid
(Decreased Gamma-Tocopherol absorption)

Medium-Chain Triglycerides
(Enhanced Gamma-Tocopherol absorption)

Mineral Oil
(Decreased Gamma-Tocopherol absorption)

Neomycin
(Impaired utilization of Gamma-Tocopherol)

Ox Bile, Desiccated
(Increased Gamma-Tocopherol absorption)

Phytostanols
(Decreased plasma Gamma-Tocopherol levels)

Phytosterols
(Decreased plasma Gamma-Tocopherol levels)

Plant Phenolic Compounds
(Helps to maintain levels of reduced Gamma-Tocopherol)

Selenium
(Synergistic effect with Gamma-Tocopherol)

Sesame Seed Lignans
(A single dose of the sesame seed lignans sesamin and sesamolin

(136 mg) was found to reduce the urinary excretion of co-administered gamma-tocopherol in a human study)

Sucralfate
(Interferes with Gamma-Tocopherol absorption)

Ticlopidine Hydrochloride
(Increased effects of ticlopidine)

Tirofiban Hydrochloride
(Increased effects of tirofiban)

Vitamin C
(Helps to maintain Gamma-Tocopherol in its reduced (antioxidant) form)

Warfarin Sodium
(Enhanced anticoagulant response of warfarin)

GANGLIONIC BLOCKING AGENTS

Inositol Nicotinate
(Nicotinic acid may potentiate effects)

Niacin
(Nicotinic acid may potentiate effects, resulting in postural hypotension)

GARLIC EXTRACT

Eicosapentaenoic Acid (EPA)
(May interact with EPA. Such reactions might be manifested by increased susceptibility to bruising, nosebleeds, hemoptysis, hematemesis, hematuria, and blood in the stool. Most who take the EPA supplements do not suffer from these problems and if they occur, they are rare. If they do occur, the EPA dose should be lowered or discontinued)

Fish Oil
(May interact with fish oil. Such interactions might be manifested by increased susceptibility to bruising, nosebleeds, hemoptysis, hematemesis, hematuria, and blood in the stool. Most who take fish oil supplements do not suffer from these problems and if they occur, they are rare. If they do occur, the fish oil dose should be lowered or discontinued)

GARLIC OIL

Eicosapentaenoic Acid (EPA)
(May interact with EPA. Such reactions might be manifested by increased susceptibility to bruising, nosebleeds, hemoptysis, hematemesis, hematuria, and blood in the stool. Most who take the EPA supplements do not suffer from these problems and if they occur, they are rare. If they do occur, the EPA dose should be lowered or discontinued)

Fish Oil
(May interact with fish oil. Such interactions might be manifested by increased susceptibility to bruising, nosebleeds, hemoptysis, hematemesis, hematuria, and blood in the stool. Most who take fish oil supplements do not suffer from these problems and if they occur, they are rare. If they do occur, the fish oil dose should be lowered or discontinued)

GELATIN

(*See under* Gelatin Hydrolysates)

GELATIN HYDROLYSATES

Calcitonin, unspecified
(Gelatin Hydrosylates may enhance the osteoporosis treatment effects)

GEMFIBROZIL

Inositol Nicotinate
(High dose nicotinic acid may have synergistic antihyperlipidemic effects)

Niacin
(High dose nicotinic acid may have synergistic antihyperlipidemic effects)

Red Yeast Rice
(Increased risk of myopathy)

GENISTEIN

Letrozole
(Genistein may negate the inhibitor effect of letrozole)

Tamoxifen Citrate
(Genistein may negate the inhibitory effect of tamoxifen)

GENTAMICIN

Baicalein
(Baicalein and gentamicin have shown synergistic activity against vancomycin-resistant Enterococcus in vitro)

L-Methionine
(Methionine may protect against ototoxicity)

GENTAMICIN SULFATE

Baicalein
(Baicalein and gentamicin have shown synergistic activity against vancomycin-resistant Enterococcus in vitro)

GINKGO BILOBA

Alpha-Tocopherol Polyethylene Glycol Succinate (TPGS)
(Some herbs, such as garlic and ginkgo, possess antithrombotic activity. High does of TPGS, used concomitantly with these herbs, may enhance antithrombotic activity)

Borage Oil
(Interactions may occur with Borage Oil)

Eicosapentaenoic Acid (EPA)
(May interact with EPA. Such reactions might be manifested by increased susceptibility to bruising, nosebleeds, hemoptysis, hematemesis, hematuria, and blood in the stool. Most who take the EPA supplements do not suffer from these problems and if they occur, they are rare. If they do occur, the EPA dose should be lowered or discontinued)

Evening Primrose Oil
(EPO may increase bleeding tendencies)

Fish Oil
(May interact with fish oil. Such interactions might be manifested by increased susceptibility to bruising, nosebleeds, hemoptysis, hematemesis, hematuria, and blood in the stool. Most who take fish oil supplements do not suffer from these problems and if they occur, they are rare. If they do occur, the fish oil dose should be lowered or discontinued)

Gamma-Tocopherol
(Enhanced antithrombotic activity of gingko biloba)

Nattokinase (Subtilisin NAT)
(Co-administration of nattokinase with Ginkgo (Ginkgo biloba) may lead to increased bleeding tendencies manifested by increased susceptibility to bruising, nosebleeds, hematemesis, hematuria, and blood in the stool)

Perilla Oil
(Increased antithrombotic effects with Perilla Oil)

Tocotrienols
(May enhance antithrombotic activity)

Vitamin E
(Some herbs, including garlic and ginkgo, possess antithrombotic activity. High doses of vitamin E used at the same time as these herbs may enhance their antithrombotic activity)

GINSENG

Nattokinase (Subtilisin NAT)
(Co-administration of nattokinase with ginseng or curcuminoids may lead to increased bleeding tendencies manifested by increased susceptibility to bruising, nosebleeds, hematemesis, hematuria, and blood in the stool)

GLUCOMANNAN

Vitamin A
(Decreased absorption of fat-soluble vitamins)

Vitamin D
(Decreased absorption of fat-soluble vitamins)

Vitamin E
(Decreased absorption of fat-soluble vitamins)

Vitamin K
(Decreased absorption of fat-soluble vitamins)

GLUCOSAMINE

Antidiabetic Drugs, unspecified
  (Glucosamine may increase insulin resistance and affect glucose tolerance)
Hypoglycemic Drugs
  (Glucosamine may increase insulin resistance and affect glucose tolerance)
Insulin
  (Glucosamine may increase insulin resistance and affect glucose tolerance)

GLUTAMINE PEPTIDES

Human Growth Hormone
  (L-Glutamine may enhance nutrient absorption with short bowel syndrome)
Indomethacin
  (L-Glutamine may inhibit intestinal permeability caused by indomethacin)
Methotrexate Sodium
  (May decrease L-Glutamine effects)
Paclitaxel
  (L-Glutamine may prevent paclitaxel adverse reactions)

GLUTATHIONE

Ascorbyl Palmitate
  (Vitamin C may maintain reduced Glutathione levels)
Vitamin C
  (Vitamin C may maintain reduced Glutathione levels in cells)

GLYCINE

Baclofen
  (Glycine may increase effect of)
Dantrolene Sodium
  (Glycine may increase effect of)
Diazepam
  (Glycine may increase effect of)
L-Methionine
  (L-Methionine may decrease Glycine levels with low-protein diet)
Tizanidine Hydrochloride
  (Glycine may increase effect of)

GOITROGENS

Iodine
  (May compete with iodide and cause hypothyroidism)

GRAPEFRUIT JUICE

Red Yeast Rice
  (Increased risk of myopathy)

GREEN TEA CATECHINS

Antiplatelet Drugs
  (Enhanced effect with green tea catechins)
Aspirin
  (Enhanced effect with green tea catechins)
Aspirin Buffered
  (Enhanced effect with green tea catechins)
Aspirin, Enteric Coated
  (Enhanced effect with green tea catechins)
Caffeine
  (Synergistic effect with green tea catechins in enhancing thermogenesis)
Clopidogrel Bisulfate
  (Enhanced effect with green tea catechins)
Dipyridamole
  (Enhanced effect with green tea catechins)
Ticlopidine Hydrochloride
  (Enhanced effect with green tea catechins)

GREEN TEA EXTRACT

Equol
  (May promote the formation of equol)
Iron
  (May decrease absorption of iron)

GUAIAC

Iron
  (High false positive occult blood with iron supplements)

HMG-COA REDUCTASE INHIBITORS

Gamma-Oryzanol
  (Administration of an HMG-CoA reductase inhibitor (a 'statin') along with gamma-oryzanol may have an additive effect on the lowering of total and LDL-cholesterol)
Inositol Nicotinate
  (May produce rhabdomyolysis and may have synergistic antihyperlipidemic effects)

Niacin
  (May produce rhabdomyolysis and may have synergistic antihyperlipidemic effects; monitor carefully)
Pantethine
  (May have additive lipid-modulatory effects)
Phytostanols
  (Phytostanol supplementation may be additive to the cholesterol-lowering effects of the statins)
Red Yeast Rice
  (Increased risk of adverse reactions)
Tocotrienols
  (Tocotrienols may have synergistic cholesterol-lowering effects)

HALOPERIDOL

Arnica
  (Increased risk of prolonged QT interval when given with Arnica)

HEMP SEED OIL

Aspirin
  (Increased bleeding and susceptibility to bruising)
Nonsteroidal Anti-Inflammatory Drugs
  (Increased bleeding and susceptibility to bruising)
Warfarin Sodium
  (Increased bleeding and susceptibility to bruising)

HEPARIN

Nattokinase (Subtilisin NAT)
  (The use of nattokinase along with parenteral anticoagulants (eg, unfractionated heparin) may cause serious adverse events, especially excessive bleeding. Administration of nattokinase is contraindicated in those with bleeding disorders and should be avoided in those receiving anticoagulant agents)
Vitamin E Phosphate
  (Vitamin E phosphate may potentiate the effects of anticoagulant drugs (eg, heparin))

HEPARIN CALCIUM

Nattokinase (Subtilisin NAT)
  (The use of nattokinase along with parenteral anticoagulants (eg,

unfractionated heparin) may cause serious adverse events, especially excessive bleeding. Administration of nattokinase is contraindicated in those with bleeding disorders and should be avoided in those receiving anticoagulant agents)

Vitamin E Phosphate
(Vitamin E phosphate may potentiate the effects of anticoagulant drugs (eg, heparin))

HEPARIN SODIUM

Nattokinase (Subtilisin NAT)
(The use of nattokinase along with parenteral anticoagulants (eg, unfractionated heparin) may cause serious adverse events, especially excessive bleeding. Administration of nattokinase is contraindicated in those with bleeding disorders and should be avoided in those receiving anticoagulant agents)

Vitamin E Phosphate
(Vitamin E phosphate may potentiate the effects of anticoagulant drugs (eg, heparin))

HERBAL MEDICINES, UNSPECIFIED

Activated Charcoal
(Avoid using Activated Charcoal within two hours of taking these products)

Bentonite
(Bentonite may adsorb certain herb components)

HERBALS, MULTIPLE

Vitamin E Phosphate
(Some herbal products, including garlic, ginkgo, ginseng and curcuminoids, possess antithrombotic activity. Concomitant use of vitamin E phosphate with these herbals may enhance their antithrombotic activity)

HISTAMINE H2-RECEPTOR ANTAGONISTS

Bone Meal
(Decreased absorption of Calcium)

Calcium
(May decrease absorption of calcium)

Indole-3-Carbinol
(Block the conversion of Indole-3-Carbinol to DIM and ICZ)

Iron
(May decrease absorption of carbonyl iron)

L-Histidine
(L-Histidine might decrease the efficacy of)

Vitamin B12
(Chronic use of H2-blockers may result in decreased absorption of vitamin B12 naturally found in food sources. They are unlikely to affect the absorption of supplemental vitamin B12)

Zinc L-Carnosine
(The combination of an H2 blocker and zinc L-carnosine may be more effective than when each agent is used alone)

HOMOCYSTEINE

Choline
(Increased metabolism with Choline, Vitamin B6, Vitamin B12 and Folic Acid)

HUMAN GROWTH HORMONE

Glutamine Peptides
(L-Glutamine may enhance nutrient absorption with short bowel syndrome)

L-Glutamine
(L-Glutamine may enhance nutrient absorption with short bowel syndrome)

HUPERZINE A

Anticholinesterase drugs
(Additive effects and increased adverse effects with Huperzine A)

Bethanechol Chloride
(Additive effects and increased adverse effects with Huperzine A)

Choline
(Additive effects and increased adverse effects with Huperzine A)

Cholinergic Agents
(Additive effects and increased adverse effects with Huperzine A)

Donepezil Hydrochloride
(Additive effects and increased adverse effects with Huperzine A)

Phosphatidylcholine
(Additive effects and increased adverse effects with Huperzine A)

Physostigmine Salicylate
(Additive effects and increased adverse effects with Huperzine A)

Tacrine Hydrochloride
(Additive effects and increased adverse effects with Huperzine A)

HYDRALAZINE

Vitamin B6
(May increase vitamin B6 requirements)

HYDROLYZED COLLAGEN

Calcitonin, unspecified
(Enhanced effect (in the treatment of osteoporosis) with hydrolyzed collagen)

HYPERICUM

5-Hydroxytryptophan
(5-HTP may potentiate antidepressant effects and increase risk of side effects)

Myo-Inositol
(May have additive effects with Myo-Inositol)

HYPERICUM PERFORATUM

5-Hydroxytryptophan
(5-HTP may potentiate antidepressant effects and increase risk of side effects)

HYPOGLYCEMIC DRUGS

Glucosamine
(Glucosamine may increase insulin resistance and affect glucose tolerance)

IBUPROFEN

L-Arginine
(L-Arginine may increase absorption)

IDARUBICIN HYDROCHLORIDE

L-Theanine
(L-Theanine may enhance antitumor effects and decrease adverse effects)

INDINAVIR SULFATE

Vitamin D
(The HIV protease inhibitors ritonavir, indinavir, and nelfinavir

may impair vitamin D
bioactivation to 1, 25-
dihydroxyvitamin D)

INDOLE-3-CARBINOL
Antacids, unspecified
(Block the conversion of Indole-3-
Carbinol to DIM and ICZ)
Histamine H2-receptor antagonists
(Block the conversion of Indole-3-
Carbinol to DIM and ICZ)
Proton Pump Inhibitor
(Block the conversion of Indole-3
Carbinol to DIM and ICZ)
Tamoxifen Citrate
(May be synergistic with Indole-3-
Carbinol in protecting against
breast cancer)

INDOMETHACIN
Glutamine Peptides
(L-Glutamine may inhibit
intestinal permeability caused by
indomethacin)
L-Glutamine
(L-Glutamine may inhibit
intestinal permeability caused by
indomethacin)

INOSITOL
Bone Meal
(Decreased absorption of Calcium)
Calcium
(May decrease absorption of
calcium)
Iron
(May decrease absorption of iron)
Magnesium
(May decrease absorption of
magnesium)
Zinc
(Concomitant intake of inositol
hexaphosphate and zinc may
depress the absorption of zinc)

INOSITOL HEXAPHOSPHATE
Calcium
(May form chelates with Inositol
Hexaphosphate)
Copper
(May form chelates with Inositol
Hexaphosphate)
Diet high in protein
(May form chelates with Inositol
Hexaphosphate)

Iron
(May form chelates with Inositol
Hexaphosphate)
Magnesium
(May form chelates with Inositol
Hexaphosphate)
Manganese
(May form chelates with Inositol
Hexaphosphate)
Zinc
(May form chelates with Inositol
Hexaphosphate)

INOSITOL NIACINATE
(*See under* Inositol Nicotinate)

INOSITOL NICOTINATE
Acarbose
(High dose nicotinic acid may
antagonize effects)
Alpha Adrenergic Blockers
(High dose nicotinic acid may
potentiate hypotensive effects)
Aspirin
(May decrease high dose nicotinic
acid flushing effects)
Beverages, hot
(May increase nicotinic acid-
induced flushing)
Calcium Channel Blockers,
Unspecified
(High dose nicotinic acid may
potentiate hypotensive effects)
Cholestyramine
(May reduce nicotinic acid
absorption and may have
synergistic antihyperlipidemic
effects)
Colestipol
(May reduce nicotinic acid
absorption and may have
synergistic antihyperlipidemic
effects)
Ethanol
(May increase nicotinic acid-
induced flushing)
Food, hot
(May increase nicotinic acid-
induced flushing)
Ganglionic Blocking Agents
(Nicotinic acid may potentiate
effects)

Gemfibrozil
(High dose nicotinic acid may
have synergistic antihyperlipidemic
effects)
HMG-CoA Reductase Inhibitors
(May produce rhabdomyolysis and
may have synergistic
antihyperlipidemic effects)
Metformin
(High dose nicotinic acid may
antagonize effects)
Miglitol
(High dose nicotinic acid may
antagonize effects)
Nicotine
(Transdermal nicotine may
enhance nicotinic acid flushing
reaction)
Nitrates and Nitrites
(High dose nicotinic acid may
potentiate hypotensive effects)
Nonsteroidal Anti-Inflammatory
Drugs
(May decrease high dose nicotinic
acid flushing effects)
Pioglitazone Hydrochloride
(High dose nicotinic acid may
antagonize effects)
Repaglinide
(High dose nicotinic acid may
antagonize effects)
Rosiglitazone Maleate
(High dose nicotinic acid may
antagonize effects)
Sulfonylureas
(High dose nicotinic acid may
antagonize effects)
Warfarin Sodium
(Nicotinic acid may enhance
anticoagulant effects)

INSULIN
Alpha-Lipoic Acid
(Alpha-lipoic acid may lower
blood glucose levels. Those with
diabetes on antidiabetic medication
should have their blood glucose
monitored and antidiabetic drug
dose adjusted appropriately, if
necessary, to avoid possible
hypoglycemia)

DHEA
(May decrease DHEA levels)
Glucosamine
(Glucosamine may increase insulin resistance and affect glucose tolerance)

INTERLEUKEN-2
Melatonin
(Possible augmentation of the antitumor effect by Melatonin)

INULIN
(*See also under* Inulins)
Bone Meal
(Increased absorption of Calcium)
Calcium
(May increase absorption of calcium)
Magnesium
(May increase absorption of magnesium)

INULINS
Calcium
(Inulins may enhance colonic absorption of dietary and supplemental Calcium)
Magnesium
(Inulins may enhance colonic absorption of dietary and supplemental Magnesium)
Probiotics
(Inulins may increase beneficial effects of Probiotics)

IODINE
Antithyroid Agents
(May potentiate the hypothyroid effect of iodides)
C-Gluosylflavones
(Inhibit thyroid peroxidase activity)
Goitrogens
(May compete with iodide and cause hypothyroidism)
Lithium
(Potassium iodide and lithium may result in hypothyroidism)
Selenium
(Synergistic activity in the treatment of Kashin-Beck disease, and osteoarthropathy)

Soybean Preparations
(Inhibit thyroid peroxidase)
Warfarin Sodium
(Potassium iodide may decrease the anticoagulant effectiveness of warfarin)

IODINE PREPARATIONS
Selenium
(May have synergistic activity in the treatment of Kashin-Beck disease)

IPRIFLAVONE
Bisphosphonates
(Additive effects with Ipriflavone)
Boron
(Additive effects with Ipriflavone)
Calcitonin, unspecified
(Additive effects with Ipriflavone)
Calcium
(Additive effects with Ipriflavone)
Estrogen
(Additive effects with Ipriflavone)
Fluorine & Fluoride Preparations
(Additive effects with Ipriflavone)
Nifedipine
(Increased serum levels with Ipriflavone)
Selective Estrogen Receptor Modulators
(Additive effects with Ipriflavone)
Theophylline
(Metabolism and elimination may be inhibited by Ipriflavone)
Tolbutamide
(Increased serum levels with Ipriflavone)
Vitamin D
(Additive effects with Ipriflavone)
Vitamin K
(Additive effects with Ipriflavone)

IRON
Alpha Tocopherol Acetate
(Iron may cause oxidation of the tocopherols)
Antacids, aluminum-containing
(May decrease absorption of iron)
Beta-Carotene
(May enhance absorption of iron)
Bisphosphonates
(May decrease absorption of bisphosphonate)

Calcium
(May decrease absorption of iron)
Copper
(May decrease copper levels in tissues)
Cysteine
(May increase absorption of iron)
Gamma-Tocopherol
(The ferrous form of iron can oxidize Gamma-Tocopherol to its pro-oxidant form)
Green Tea Extract
(May decrease absorption of iron)
Guaiac
(High false positive occult blood with iron supplements)
Histamine H2-receptor antagonists
(May decrease absorption of carbonyl iron)
Inositol
(May decrease absorption of iron)
Inositol Hexaphosphate
(May form chelates with Inositol Hexaphosphate)
L-Cysteine
(May increase absorption of iron)
Levodopa
(May decrease absorption of levodopa)
Levothyroxine Sodium
(May decrease absorption of levothyroxine)
Magnesium
(May decrease absorption of iron)
Manganese
(May reduce absorption of manganese)
N-Acetyl-L-Cysteine (NAC)
(May increase absorption of iron)
Oxalic Acid
(May decrease absorption of iron)
Pectin
(Decreased absorption of Iron)
Penicillamine
(May decrease absorption of penicillamine)
Phytic Acid
(May decrease absorption of iron)
Proton Pump Inhibitor
(May decrease absorption of carbonyl iron)

Psyllium
  (Decreased absorption of Iron)
Quinolones
  (May decrease absorption of both
  quinolone and iron)
Soy Protein
  (May reduce availability of iron)
Tannins
  (May decrease absorption of iron)
Tetracyclines, unspecified
  (May decrease absorption of both
  tetracycline and iron)
Tocopherols
  (Iron may cause oxidation of
  tocotrienols)
Tocotrienols
  (Iron may cause oxidation of the
  tocotrienols. May decrease
  Tocotrienol absorption)
Vanadium
  (May decrease absorption of iron)
Vitamin C
  (May enhance absorption of iron)
Vitamin E
  (Most iron supplements contain
  the ferrous form of iron. This
  cation can oxidize unesterified
  vitamin E to its pro-oxidant form
  if taken concomitantly. This does
  not occur with esterified vitamin
  E (alpha-tocopherol acetate and
  succinate))
Zinc
  (Concomitant intake of iron and
  zinc may depress the absorption
  of both iron and zinc)

IRON SUPPLEMENTS
Ascorbyl Palmitate
  (Vitamin C may cause iron
  overload)
Liver Hydrolysate/Desiccated
  Liver
  (Liver Hydrolysate and Desiccated
  Liver may have additive effects)
Vitamin C
  (Vitamin C used concomitantly
  with nonheme iron supplements
  may increase the uptake of iron)

ISONIAZID
Gamma-Tocopherol
  (Decreased Gamma-Tocopherol
  absorption)

Melatonin
  (Possible enhanced effect with
  Melatonin)
Piperine
  (Piperine may inhibit metabolism)
Tocotrienols
  (May decrease Tocotrienol
  absorption)
Vitamin B6
  (May result in vitamin B6
  deficiency)
Vitamin E
  (May decrease vitamin E
  absorption)

ISOTRETINOIN
Vitamin A
  (May produce additive toxicity
  effects)

KETOCONAZOLE
Vitamin D
  (Ketoconazole may inhibit the
  biosynthesis and catabolism of 1,
  25-dihydroxyvitamin D)

L-ARGININE
Cyclosporine
  (L-Arginine may counteract
  antinaturetic effects)
Ibuprofen
  (L-Arginine may increase
  absorption)
Nitrates, organic
  (L-Arginine may potentiate
  effects)
Sildenafil Citrate
  (L-Arginine may potentiate
  effects)
Xylitol
  (Arginine-containing mints have
  been found to have anticariogenic
  activity secondary to their ability
  to buffer the acid produced by
  cariogenic bacteria. The
  combination of xylitol and
  arginine-containing mints may
  give better anticariogenic effects
  than the use of either alone)
Yohimbine Hydrochloride
  (L-Arginine may potentiate
  effects)

L-CARNITINE
Choline
  (May lead to increased L-
  Carnitine retention)
Didanosine
  (May produce L-Carnitine
  deficiencies)
Stavudine
  (May produce L-Carnitine
  deficiencies)
Valproic Acid
  (May produce L-Carnitine
  deficiencies)
Zalcitabine
  (May produce L-Carnitine
  deficiencies)

L-CYSTEINE
Ascorbic Acid
  (May inhibit the oxidation of L-
  Cysteine)
Iron
  (May increase absorption of iron)
Zinc
  (Concomitant intake of L-cysteine
  and zinc may enhance the
  absorption of zinc)

L-GLUTAMINE
Human Growth Hormone
  (L-Glutamine may enhance
  nutrient absorption with short
  bowel syndrome)
Indomethacin
  (L-Glutamine may inhibit
  intestinal permeability caused by
  indomethacin)
Methotrexate Sodium
  (May decrease L-Glutamine
  effects)
Paclitaxel
  (L-Glutamine may prevent
  paclitaxel adverse reactions)

L-HISTIDINE
Antihistamines
  (L-Histidine might decrease the
  efficacy of)
Histamine H2-receptor antagonists
  (L-Histidine might decrease the
  efficacy of)
Medroxyprogesterone Acetate
  (L-Histidine may enhance the
  antineoplastic effect)

Zinc
(Concomitant intake of L-histidine and zinc may enhance the absorption of zinc)

L-LYSINE

Calcium
(L-lysine may increase Calcium absorption)
Calcium Salts
(L-lysine may increase Calcium absorption)

L-METHIONINE

Acetaminophen
(L-Methionine may decrease hepatic toxicity with overdosage)
Gentamicin
(Methionine may protect against ototoxicity)
Glycine
(L-Methionine may decrease Glycine levels with low-protein diet)
Methotrexate
(L-Methionine may decrease hepatic toxicity with overdosage)
Zinc
(Concomitant intake of L-methionine and zinc may enhance the absorption of zinc)

L-PHENYLALANINE

Neuroleptics
(L-Phenylalanine may potentiate tardive dyskinesia adverse effects)
Pargyline Hydrochloride
(L-Phenylalanine may cause hypertension)
Phenelzine Sulfate
(L-Phenylalanine may cause hypertension)
Selegiline Hydrochloride
(L-Phenylalanine may have synergistic antidepressant effects)
Tranylcypromine Sulfate
(L-Phenylalanine may cause hypertension)

L-THEANINE

Doxorubicin Hydrochloride
(L-Theanine may enhance antitumor effects and decrease adverse effects)

Idarubicin Hydrochloride
(L-Theanine may enhance antitumor effects and decrease adverse effects)

L-TRYPTOPHAN

5-HT1 Receptor Agonists
(Concurrent use of L-tryptophan with a 5-HT1 agonist may increase the risk of adverse reactions)
Alpha-lactalbumin
(May increase the brain availability of L-tryptophan)
Carbohydrates
(May increase the brain availability of L-tryptophan)
Lithium
(Clinical observations suggest the possibility that the combination of L-tryptophan and lithium may reduce the need for the higher, more toxic doses of lithium necessary to control bipolar affective disorders)
MAO Inhibitors
(Concurrent use of L-tryptophan with an MAOI (type A) may increase risk of adverse reactions)
SSRIs
(Concurrent use of L-tryptophan with an SSRI may potentiate the antidepressant effect of the SSRI and may also increase the risk of adverse reactions)
Whey Protein Isolate
(May increase the brain availability of L-tryptophan)
Whey protein
(May increase the brain availability of L-tryptophan)

L-TYROSINE

Pargyline Hydrochloride
(L-Phenylalanine may cause hypertension)
Phenelzine Sulfate
(L-Phenylalanine may cause hypertension)
Tranylcypromine Sulfate
(L-Phenylalanine may cause hypertension)

LACTULOSE

Antacids, non-absorbable
(May increase Lactulose effects)
Calcium
(Lactulose may enhance colonic absorption of dietary and supplemental Calcium)
Magnesium
(Lactulose may enhance colonic absorption of dietary and supplemental Magnesium)
Probiotics
(Probiotics may increase Lactulose beneficial effects)

LAMIVUDINE

Riboflavin (Vitamin B2)
(Riboflavin may reverse nucleoside analogue-induced lactic acidosis in mild riboflavin deficiencies)

LATAMOXEF

Vitamin K
(Can cause vitamin K deficiency and hypothrombinemia)

LAXATIVES, MAGNESIUM-CONTAINING

Manganese
(May decrease absorption of manganese)

LEPIRUDIN

Nattokinase (Subtilisin NAT)
(The use of nattokinase along with direct thrombin inhibitors (eg, lepirudin) may cause serious adverse events, especially excessive bleeding.)

LETROZOLE

Genistein
(Genistein may negate the inhibitor effect of letrozole)

LEVODOPA

Iron
(May decrease absorption of levodopa)
Octacosanol
(Worsened dyskinesias in Parkinson's disease)
Vitamin B6
(Vitamin B6 may reverse therapeutic effects of levodopa if not given with carbidopa)

LEVOTHYROXINE SODIUM

Bone Meal
  (Decreased levothyroxine
  absorption and increased serum
  thyrotropin levels)
Calcium
  (May decrease levothyroxine
  absorption and increase serum
  thyrotropin levels)
Iron
  (May decrease absorption of
  levothyroxine)

LIPOPHILIC DRUGS, UNSPECIFIED

Alpha-Tocopherol
  Polyethylene Glycol
  Succinate (TPGS)
  (TPGS may increase absorption of
  lipophilic drugs)
Chitosan
  (Might bind to Chitosan)
Medium-Chain Triglycerides
  (MCT may facilitate the
  absorption of lipophilic drugs)

LIPOPHILIC SUBSTANCES, UNSPECIFIED

Medium-Chain Triglycerides
  (MCT may facilitate the
  absorption of lipophilic
  substances)

LITHIUM

Folate
  (Folic acid may increase efficacy)
Iodine
  (Potassium iodide and lithium may
  result in hypothyroidism)
L-Tryptophan
  (Clinical observations suggest the
  possibility that the combination of
  L-tryptophan and lithium may
  reduce the need for the higher,
  more toxic doses of lithium
  necessary to control bipolar
  affective disorders)
Psyllium
  (Reduced absorption of Lithium)

LIVER HYDROLYSATE/DESICCATED LIVER

Iron Supplements
  (Liver Hydrolysate and Desiccated
  Liver may have additive effects)

LOMETREXOL

Folate
  (Folic acid may be synergistic and
  decrease adverse effects)

LOVASTATIN

Ascorbyl Palmitate
  (Grapefruit flavonoids may
  increase bioavailability due to
  cytochrome P-450 3A4 inhibition)
Coenzyme Q10 (CoQ10)
  (Decreases CoQ10 levels)
Pectin
  (Decreased absorption of
  lovastatin)
Vitamin C
  (Grapefruit flavonoids may
  increase bioavailability due to
  cytochrome P-450 3A4 inhibition)

LUTEIN

Beta-Carotene
  (May decrease the absorption of
  beta-carotene)
Pectin
  (Decreased absorption of Lutein)
Sodium Alginates and other
  Phyco-Polysaccharides
  (Decreased absorption of Lutein)

LUTEIN AND ZEAXANTHIN

Beta-Carotene
  (Decreased absorption of Lutein
  and Zeaxanthin)
Cholestyramine
  (Decreased absorption of Lutein
  and Zeaxanthin)
Colestipol
  (Decreased absorption of Lutein
  and Zeaxanthin)
Fat Substitute
  (Decreased absorption of Lutein
  and Zeaxanthin)
Medium-Chain Triglycerides
  (Enhanced absorption of Lutein
  and Zeaxanthin)
Mineral Oil
  (Decreased absorption of Lutein
  and Zeaxanthin)
Oils, dietary
  (Increased absorption of Lutein
  and Zeaxanthin)
Pectin
  (Decreased absorption of Lutein
  and Zeaxanthin)

LUTEOLIN

Amiodarone Hydrochloride
  (Luteolin has been found to
  inhibit the metabolism of the
  sedative drug midazolam by
  human liver microsomes and
  cytochrome P450 3A4 (CYP3A4)
  and CYP3A5. Midazolam is a
  probe substrate for CYP3A4 and
  CYP3A5 enzymes. CYP3A4 is
  located in the intestine and liver,
  and its inhibition leads to delayed
  absorption and reduced first pass
  metabolism in the liver, resulting
  in higher plasma levels of the
  drug. However, given this finding,
  those using midazolam or other
  drugs metabolized by CYP3A4,
  including amiodarone, should
  exercise caution in the use of
  luteolin-containing dairy
  supplements)
Cisplatin
  (Luteolin was shown to sensitize
  the anticancer effect of cisplatin
  (cisdiamminediachloroplatinum))
Cytochrome p450 3a4 substrates
(selected)
  (Luteolin has been found to
  inhibit the metabolism of the
  sedative drug midazolam by
  human liver microsomes and
  cytochrome P450 3A4 (CYP3A4)
  and CYP3A5. Midazolam is a
  probe substrate for CYP3A4 and
  CYP3A5 enzymes. CYP3A4 is
  located in the intestine and liver,
  and its inhibition leads to delayed
  absorption and reduced first pass
  metabolism in the liver, resulting
  in higher plasma levels of the
  drug. However, given this finding,
  those using midazolam or other
  drugs metabolized by CYP3A4,
  including statins - atorvastatin,
  lovastatin and simvastatin - as
  well as amiodarone, buspirone,
  cisapride, etoposide, quinidine and
  sildenafil, tadalafil, vardenafil and
  others, should exercise caution in
  the use of luteolin-containing
  dairy supplements)
Doxorubicin Hydrochloride
  (Luteolin was found to reverse
  tumor resistance to doxorubicin in

human and murine breast cancer
cells under hypoxic conditions)
Doxorubicin Hydrochloride
Liposome
(Luteolin was found to reverse
tumor resistance to doxorubicin in
human and murine breast cancer
cells under hypoxic conditions)
PDE5 inhibitors
(Luteolin has been found to
inhibit the metabolism of the
sedative drug midazolam by
human liver microsomes and
cytochrome P450 3A4 (CYP3A4)
and CYP3A5. Midazolam is a
probe substrate for CYP3A4 and
CYP3A5 enzymes. CYP3A4 is
located in the intestine and liver,
and its inhibition leads to delayed
absorption and reduced first pass
metabolism in the liver, resulting
in higher plasma levels of the
drug. However, given this finding,
those using midazolam or other
drugs metabolized by CYP3A4,
including statins - atorvastatin,
lovastatin and simvastatin - as
well as amiodarone, buspirone,
cisapride, etoposide, quinidine and
sildenafil, tadalafil, vardenafil and
others, should exercise caution in
the use of luteolin-containing
dairy supplements)

LYCOPENE

Beta-Carotene
(Increased absorption of
Lycopene)
Beta-Sitosterol
(May lower serum levels of
lycopene)
Cholestyramine
(Decreased absorption of
Lycopene)
Colestipol Hydrochloride
(Decreased absorption of
Lycopene)
Fat Substitute
(Reduced absorption of Lycopene)
Medium-Chain Triglycerides
(Enhanced absorption of
Lycopene)

Mineral Oil
(Reduced absorption of Lycopene)
Oils, dietary
(Enhanced absorption of
Lycopene)
Pectin
(Decreased absorption of
Lycopene)
Pectin
(Decreased absorption of
Lycopene)
Phytostanols
(Phytostanols may interfere with
absorption and lower serum
levels)
Phytosterols
(Phytosterols may interfere with
absorption and lower serum
levels)
Sodium Alginates and other
Phyco-Polysaccharides
(Decreased absorption of
Lycopene)

LYSINE

(See under L-Lysine)

MACROLIDE ANTIBIOTICS

Red Yeast Rice
(Increased risk of myopathy)
Sesame Seed Lignans
(Antibiotics may decrease the
production of the mammalian
lignans enterolactone (ENT) and
enterodiol (END) from sesame
seed lignans)

MAGNESIUM

Bisphosphonates
(May decrease absorption of
bisphosphonates)
Boron
(May increase magnesium levels)
Calcium
(May decrease absorption of
magnesium)
Fructo-oligosaccharides
(May increase absorption of
magnesium)
Inositol
(May decrease absorption of
magnesium)

Inositol Hexaphosphate
(May form chelates with Inositol
Hexaphosphate)
Inulin
(May increase absorption of
magnesium)
Iron
(May decrease absorption of iron)
Lactulose
(Lactulose may enhance colonic
absorption of dietary and
supplemental Magnesium)
Manganese
(May decrease absorption of
manganese)
Medium-Chain Triglycerides
(MCT may facilitate the
absorption of Magnesium)
Oxalic Acid
(May decrease absorption of
magnesium)
Pectin
(Decreased absorption of
Magnesium)
Phosphate Salts
(May decrease absorption of
phosphate and magnesium)
Phytic Acid
(May decrease absorption of
magnesium)
Prebiotics
(Enhanced absorption of
Magnesium)
Psyllium
(Decreased absorption of
Magnesium)
Quinolones
(May decrease absorption of
quinolones)
Sodium Alginate
(May decrease absorption of
magnesium)
Sodium Alginates and other
Phyco-Polysaccharides
(Decreased absorption of
Magnesium)
Soy Protein
(May reduce availability of
magnesium)
Synbiotics
(Enhanced colonic absorption of
Magnesium)

Tetracyclines, unspecified
(May decrease absorption of tetracycline)

Transgalacto-Oligosaccharides
(Enhanced colonic absorption of Magnesium)

MANGANESE

Antacids, magnesium-containing
(May decrease absorption of manganese)

Calcium
(May decrease absorption of manganese)

Inositol Hexaphosphate
(May form chelates with Inositol Hexaphosphate)

Iron
(May reduce absorption of manganese)

Laxatives, magnesium-containing
(May decrease absorption of manganese)

Magnesium
(May decrease absorption of manganese)

Oxalic Acid
(May decrease absorption of manganese)

Phytic Acid
(May decrease absorption of manganese)

Sodium Alginates and other Phyco-Polysaccharides
(Decreased absorption of Manganese)

Soy Protein
(May reduce availability of manganese)

Tetracyclines, unspecified
(May reduce absorption of manganese)

MEDIUM-CHAIN TRIGLYCERIDES

Astaxanthin
(Concomitant intake of medium-chain triglycerides and lycopene may decrease the absorption of astaxanthin)

Calcium
(MCT may facilitate the absorption of Calcium)

Carotenoids
(MCT may facilitate the absorption of carotenoids)

Fatty Acids
(MCT may facilitate the absorption of fatty acids)

Flavonoids
(MCT may facilitate the absorption of flavonoids)

Fucoxanthin
(Concomitant intake of medium-chain triglycerides and fucoxanthin may enhance the absorption of fucoxanthin)

Gamma-Tocopherol
(Enhanced Gamma-Tocopherol absorption)

Lipophilic drugs, unspecified
(MCT may facilitate the absorption of lipophilic drugs)

Lipophilic substances, unspecified
(MCT may facilitate the absorption of lipophilic substances)

Lutein and Zeaxanthin
(Enhanced absorption of Lutein and Zeaxanthin)

Lycopene
(Enhanced absorption of Lycopene)

Magnesium
(MCT may facilitate the absorption of Magnesium)

Tocotrienols
(May increase Tocotrienol absorption)

Vitamin A
(MCT may facilitate the absorption of Vitamin A)

Vitamin D
(MCT may facilitate the absorption of Vitamin D)

Vitamin E
(MCT may facilitate the absorption of Vitamin E)

Vitamin K
(MCT may facilitate the absorption of Vitamin K)

MEDROXYPROGESTERONE ACETATE

L-Histidine
(L-Histidine may enhance the antineoplastic effect)

MELATONIN

Antidepressant Medications, unspecified
(May increase sedation and adverse effects with Melatonin)

Antihistamines
(May increase sedation and adverse effects with Melatonin)

Aspirin
(May decrease Melatonin levels)

Benzodiazepines
(May increase sedation and adverse effects with Melatonin)

Beta Blockers
(May lead to decreased Melatonin levels)

Fluoxetine Hydrochloride
(Psychotic episode reported with Melatonin)

Fluvoxamine Maleate
(Increases the bioavailability of oral Melatonin)

Interleuken-2
(Possible augmentation of the antitumor effect by Melatonin)

Isoniazid
(Possible enhanced effect with Melatonin)

Nonsteroidal Anti-Inflammatory Drugs
(May decrease Melatonin levels)

Progestins
(Concomitant Melatonin may cause additive effect in inhibiting ovarian function)

MELPHALAN

Vitamin C
(Ascorbic acid has been found to enhance arsenic trioxide-induced cytotoxicity in multiple myeloma cells. It has also been found to overcome drug resistance in myeloma and to significantly increase the anti-myeloma effects of both arsenic trioxide and melphalan in cell culture models and in animal models)

MELPHALAN HYDROCHLORIDE

Vitamin C
(Ascorbic acid has been found to enhance arsenic trioxide-induced

cytotoxicity in multiple myeloma cells. It has also been found to overcome drug resistance in myeloma and to significantly increase the anti-myeloma effects of both arsenic trioxide and melphalan in cell culture models and in animal models)

METFORMIN

Folate

(Long-term use of metformin has been associated with elevated homocysteine levels which are reduced with folic acid administration)

Inositol Nicotinate

(High dose nicotinic acid may antagonize effects)

Niacin

(High dose nicotinic acid may antagonize effects requiring dose adjustment)

Vitamin B12

(May decrease absorption of vitamin B12)

METHIONINE

(*See under* L-Methionine)

METHOTREXATE

Folate

(Folic acid may reduce toxic side effects)

L-Methionine

(L-Methionine may decrease hepatic toxicity with overdosage)

METHOTREXATE SODIUM

Choline

(May decrease Choline metabolites)

Glutamine Peptides

(May decrease L-Glutamine effects)

L-Glutamine

(May decrease L-Glutamine effects)

METHYLDOPA

5-Hydroxytryptophan

(Inhibits 5-HTP metabolism to serotonin)

METHYSERGIDE MALEATE

5-Hydroxytryptophan

(5-HTP may decrease effects)

METOCLOPRAMIDE HYDROCHLORIDE

Riboflavin (Vitamin B2)

(May decrease absorption of riboflavin)

MIGLITOL

Inositol Nicotinate

(High dose nicotinic acid may antagonize effects)

Niacin

(High dose nicotinic acid may antagonize effects requiring dose adjustment)

MINERAL OIL

Astaxanthin

(Concomitant intake of mineral oil and astaxanthin may reduce the absorption of astaxanthin)

Beta-Carotene

(May decrease the absorption of beta-carotene)

Fucoxanthin

(Concomitant intake of mineral oil and fucoxanthin may decrease the absorption of fucoxanthin)

Gamma-Tocopherol

(Decreased Gamma-Tocopherol absorption)

Lutein and Zeaxanthin

(Decreased absorption of Lutein and Zeaxanthin)

Lycopene

(Reduced absorption of Lycopene)

Tocotrienols

(May decrease Tocotrienol absorption)

Vitamin A

(May decrease vitamin A absorption)

Vitamin D

(Concomitant use of mineral oil and vitamin D may reduce the absorption of vitamin D)

Vitamin E

(May decrease vitamin E absorption)

Vitamin K

(May reduce vitamin K absorption)

MOLYBDENUM

Acetaminophen

(High dose molybdate may inhibit acetaminophen metabolism)

Copper

(High dose of molybdenum may antagonize dietary copper absorption and high dose copper may antagonize molybdenum absorption)

MONOAMINE OXIDASE INHIBITORS (MAO INHIBITORS)

5-Hydroxytryptophan

(5-HTP may increase risk of side effects)

Brewer's Yeast

(May cause hypertension with Brewer's Yeast)

DL-Phenylalanine

(May cause hypertension with Brewer's Yeast)

L-Tryptophan

(Concurrent use of L-tryptophan with an MAOI (type A) may increase the risk of adverse reactions)

MORPHINE SULFATE

DHEA

(May decrease DHEA levels)

MYCO-POLYSACCHARIDES

Antiplatelet Drugs

(Ganoderma may enhance antiplatelet effects)

MYO-INOSITOL

5-HT1 Receptor Agonists

(May have additive effects with Myo-Inositol)

Hypericum

(May have additive effects with Myo-Inositol)

Selective Serotonin Reuptake Inhibitors

(May have additive effects with Myo-Inositol)

N-ACETYL-L-CYSTEINE (NAC)

Iron

(May increase absorption of iron)

Zinc

(Concomitant intake of NAC and zinc may enhance the absorption of zinc)

NATTOKINASE (SUBTILISIN NAT)

Abciximab

(The use of nattokinase along with parenteral antiplatelet drugs (GPIIB/IIA inhibitors such as abciximab) may cause serious adverse events, especially excessive bleeding. Administration of nattokinase is contraindicated in those with bleeding disorders and should be avoided in those receiving antiplatelet agents)

Allium sativum

(Co-administration of nattokinase with garlic (allium sativa) may lead to increased bleeding tendencies manifested by increased susceptibility to bruising, nosebleeds, hematemesis, hematuria, and blood in the stool)

Argatroban

(The use of nattokinase along with direct thrombin inhibitors (eg, argatroban) may cause serious adverse events, especially excessive bleeding.)

Aspirin

(The use of nattokinase along with antiplatelet drugs (eg, aspirin) may cause serious adverse events, especially excessive bleeding. Administration of nattokinase is contraindicated in those with bleeding disorders and should be avoided in those receiving antiplatelet agents)

Aspirin Buffered

(The use of nattokinase along with antiplatelet drugs (eg, aspirin) may cause serious adverse events, especially excessive bleeding. Administration of nattokinase is contraindicated in those with bleeding disorders and should be avoided in those receiving antiplatelet agents)

Aspirin, Enteric Coated

(The use of nattokinase along with antiplatelet drugs (eg, aspirin) may cause serious adverse events, especially excessive

bleeding. Administration of nattokinase is contraindicated in those with bleeding disorders and should be avoided in those receiving antiplatelet agents)

Bivalirudin

(The use of nattokinase along with direct thrombin inhibitors (eg, bivalirudin) may cause serious adverse events, especially excessive bleeding.)

Clopidogrel Bisulfate

(The use of nattokinase along with antiplatelet drugs (eg, clopidogrel) may cause serious adverse events, especially excessive bleeding. Administration of nattokinase is contraindicated in those with bleeding disorders and should be avoided in those receiving antiplatelet agents)

Dalteparin Sodium

(The use of nattokinase along with parenteral anticoagulants (eg, low molecular weight heparins) may cause serious adverse events, especially excessive bleeding. Administration of nattokinase is contraindicated in those with bleeding disorders and should be avoided in those receiving anticoagulant agents)

Dipyridamole

(The use of nattokinase along with antiplatelet drugs (eg, dipyridamole) may cause serious adverse events, especially excessive bleeding. Administration of nattokinase is contraindicated in those with bleeding disorders and should be avoided in those receiving antiplatelet agents)

Enoxaparan

(The use of nattokinase along with parenteral anticoagulants (eg, low molecular weight heparins) may cause serious adverse events, especially excessive bleeding. Administration of nattokinase is contraindicated in those with bleeding disorders and should be

avoided in those receiving anticoagulant agents)

Eptifibatide

(The use of nattokinase along with parenteral antiplatelet drugs (GPIIB/IIA inhibitors such as eptifibatide) may cause serious adverse events, especially excessive bleeding. Administration of nattokinase is contraindicated in those with bleeding disorders and should be avoided in those receiving antiplatelet agents)

Fish Oils

(Co-administration of nattokinase with fish oil may lead to increased bleeding tendencies manifested by increased susceptibility to bruising, nosebleeds, hematemesis, hematuria, and blood in the stool)

Ginkgo biloba

(Co-administration of nattokinase with Ginkgo (Ginkgo biloba) may lead to increased bleeding tendencies manifested by increased susceptibility to bruising, nosebleeds, hematemesis, hematuria, and blood in the stool)

Ginseng

(Co-administration of nattokinase with ginseng or curcuminoids may lead to increased bleeding tendencies manifested by increased susceptibility to bruising, nosebleeds, hematemesis, hematuria, and blood in the stool)

Heparin

(The use of nattokinase along with parenteral anticoagulants (eg, unfractionated heparin) may cause serious adverse events, especially excessive bleeding. Administration of nattokinase is contraindicated in those with bleeding disorders and should be avoided in those receiving anticoagulant agents)

Heparin Calcium

(The use of nattokinase along with parenteral anticoagulants (eg, unfractionated heparin) may cause serious adverse events, especially excessive bleeding. Administration of nattokinase is contraindicated in those with bleeding disorders and should be avoided in those receiving anticoagulant agents)

Heparin Sodium
(The use of nattokinase along with parenteral anticoagulants (eg, unfractionated heparin) may cause serious adverse events, especially excessive bleeding. Administration of nattokinase is contraindicated in those with bleeding disorders and should be avoided in those receiving anticoagulant agents)

Lepirudin
(The use of nattokinase along with direct thrombin inhibitors (eg, lepirudin) may cause serious adverse events, especially excessive bleeding.)

Ticlopidine Hydrochloride
(The use of nattokinase along with antiplatelet drugs (eg, ticlopidine) may cause serious adverse events, especially excessive bleeding. Administration of nattokinase is contraindicated in those with bleeding disorders and should be avoided in those receiving antiplatelet agents)

Tinzaparin Sodium
(The use of nattokinase along with parenteral anticoagulants (eg, low molecular weight heparins) may cause serious adverse events, especially excessive bleeding. Administration of nattokinase is contraindicated in those with bleeding disorders and should be avoided in those receiving anticoagulant agents)

Tirofiban Hydrochloride
(The use of nattokinase along with parenteral antiplatelet drugs (GPIIB/IIA inhibitors such as tirofiban hydrochloride) may cause serious adverse events, especially excessive bleeding. Administration of nattokinase is contraindicated

in those with bleeding disorders and should be avoided in those receiving antiplatelet agents)

Warfarin Sodium
(The use of nattokinase along with oral anticoagulants (eg, warfarin) may cause serious adverse events, especially excessive bleeding. Nattokinase is contraindicated in patients taking the anticoagulant warfarin. Administration of nattokinase is contraindicated in those with bleeding disorders and in those taking the anticoagulant warfarin)

NEFAZODONE HYDROCHLORIDE
Red Yeast Rice
(Increased risk of myopathy)

NELFINAVIR MESYLATE
Vitamin D
(The HIV protease inhibitors ritonavir, indinavir, and nelfinavir may impair vitamin D bioactivation to 1, 25-dihydroxyvitamin D)

NEOMYCIN
Gamma-Tocopherol
(Impaired utilization of Gamma-Tocopherol)
Tocotrienols
(May decrease Tocotrienol effects)
Vitamin E
(May impair utilization of vitamin E)

NEUROLEPTICS
DL-Phenylalanine
(L-Phenylalanine may potentiate tardive dyskinesia side effects)
L-Phenylalanine
(L-Phenylalanine may potentiate tardive dyskinesia adverse effects)

NIACIN
Acarbose
(High dose nicotinic acid may antagonize effects requiring dose adjustment)
Alcohol
(May increase nicotinic acid-induced flushing)

Alpha Adrenergic Blockers
(High dose nicotinic acid may potentiate hypotensive effects and may cause postural hypotension)
Aspirin
(May decrease high dose nicotinic acid flushing effects)
Beverages, hot
(May increase nicotinic acid-induced flushing)
Calcium Channel Blockers, Unspecified
(High dose nicotinic acid may potentiate hypotensive effects)
Cholestyramine
(May reduce nicotinic acid absorption and may have synergistic antihyperlipidemic effects)
Colestipol
(May reduce nicotinic acid absorption and may have synergistic antihyperlipidemic effects)
Ethanol
(May increase nicotinic acid-induced flushing)
Ethyl Alcohol
(May increase nicotinic acid-induced flushing)
Food, hot
(May increase nicotinic acid-induced flushing)
Ganglionic Blocking Agents
(Nicotinic acid may potentiate effects, resulting in postural hypotension)
Gemfibrozil
(High dose nicotinic acid may have synergistic antihyperlipidemic effects)
HMG-CoA Reductase Inhibitors
(May produce rhabdomyolysis and may have synergistic antihyperlipidemic effects; monitor carefully)
Metformin
(High dose nicotinic acid may antagonize effects requiring dose adjustment)

Miglitol
(High dose nicotinic acid may antagonize effects requiring dose adjustment)
Nicotine
(Transdermal nicotine may enhance nicotinic acid-induced flushing)
Nitrates and Nitrites
(High dose nicotinic acid may potentiate hypotensive effects)
Nonsteroidal Anti-Inflammatory Drugs
(May decrease high dose nicotinic acid-induced flushing)
Pioglitazone Hydrochloride
(High dose nicotinic acid may antagonize effects which may require dose adjustment)
Repaglinide
(High dose nicotinic acid may antagonize effects which may require dose adjustment)
Rosiglitazone Maleate
(High dose nicotinic acid may antagonize effects which may require dose adjustment)
Sulfonylureas
(High dose nicotinic acid may antagonize effects which may require dose adjustment)
Warfarin Sodium
(Nicotinic acid may enhance anticoagulant effects; monitor closely)

NIACINAMIDE
(*See under* Nicotinamide)

NICOTINAMIDE
Carbamazepine
(Nicotinamide may decrease carbamazepine clearance)

NICOTINE
Inositol Nicotinate
(Transdermal nicotine may enhance nicotinic acid flushing reaction)
Niacin
(Transdermal nicotine may enhance nicotinic acid-induced flushing)

NICOTINIC ACID
Pantethine
(May have additive lipid-modulatory effects)
Red Yeast Rice
(Increased risk of myopathy)

NIFEDIPINE
Ipriflavone
(Increased serum levels with Ipriflavone)

NISOLDIPINE
Ascorbyl Palmitate
(Grapefruit flavonoids may increase bioavailability due to cytochrome P-450 3A4 inhibition)
Vitamin C
(Grapefruit flavonoids may increase bioavailability due to cytochrome P-450 3A4 inhibition)

NITRATES AND NITRITES
Acetylcysteine
(May cause headaches when taken with NAC)
Inositol Nicotinate
(High dose nicotinic acid may potentiate hypotensive effects)
Niacin
(High dose nicotinic acid may potentiate hypotensive effects)

NITRATES, ORGANIC
L-Arginine
(L-Arginine may potentiate effects)

NITROFURANTOIN
Deglycyrrhizinated Licorice (DGL)
(Increased excretion rate of nitrofurantoin)

NITROUS OXIDE
Vitamin B12
(Inhalation of the anesthetic agent nitrous oxide can produce a functional vitamin B12 deficiency)

NONSTEROIDAL ANTI-INFLAMMATORY DRUGS (NSAIDS)
Borage Oil
(Increased anticoagulant and antiplatelet effects when taken with Borage Oil)

Eicosapentaenoic Acid (EPA)
(May interact with EPA. Such reactions might be manifested by increased susceptibility to bruising, nosebleeds, hemoptysis, hematemesis, hematuria, and blood in the stool. Most who take the EPA supplements do not suffer from these problems and if they occur, they are rare. If they do occur, the EPA dose should be lowered or discontinued)
Evening Primrose Oil
(EPO may increase bleeding tendencies)
Fish Oil
(May interact with fish oil. Such interactions might be manifested by increased susceptibility to bruising, nosebleeds, hemoptysis, hematemesis, hematuria, and blood in the stool. Most who take fish oil supplements do not suffer from these problems and if they occur, they are rare. If they do occur, the fish oil dose should be lowered or discontinued)
Flaxseed Oil
(Interactions may occur between flaxseed oil and its metabolites and warfarin, aspirin, and NSAIDs. Such interactions, if they were to occur, might be manifested by nosebleeds and increased susceptibility to bruising. If this does occur, consideration should be given to lowering or stopping intake)
Folate
(Large doses may exert antifolate activity)
Hemp Seed Oil
(Increased bleeding and susceptibility to bruising)
Inositol Nicotinate
(May decrease high dose nicotinic acid flushing effects)
Melatonin
(May decrease Melatonin levels)
Niacin
(May decrease high dose nicotinic acid-induced flushing)

Perilla Oil
(Increased antithrombotic effects with Perilla Oil)

NUTRITIONAL SUPPLEMENT

Activated Charcoal
(Avoid using Activated Charcoal within two hours of taking these products)

Bentonite
(Bentonite may adsorb certain nutritional supplements)

Curcuminoids
(Bromelain and piperine may enhance the absorption of curcuminoids)

OCTACOSANOL

Carbidopa
(Worsened dyskinesias in Parkinson's disease)

Levodopa
(Worsened dyskinesias in Parkinson's disease)

OILS, DIETARY

Astaxanthin
(Dietary oils such as olive oil and fish oils may enhance the absorption of astaxanthin. Corn oil is less likely to enhance astaxanthin absorption)

Fucoxanthin
(Dietary oils, such as fish oils and olive oils, may enhance the absorption of fucoxanthin)

Lutein and Zeaxanthin
(Increased absorption of Lutein and Zeaxanthin)

Lycopene
(Enhanced absorption of Lycopene)

OILS, UNSPECIFIED

Fucoxanthin
(Dietary oils, such as fish oils and olive oils, may enhance the absorption of fucoxanthin)

OLESTRA

Astaxanthin
(Olestra may reduce the absorption of astaxanthin)

Beta-Carotene
(May decrease the absorption of beta-carotene)

Fucoxanthin
(Olestra may reduce the absorption of fucoxanthin)

Vitamin D
(Olestra inhibits the absorption of vitamin D as well as the other fat-soluble vitamins A, E, and K)

Vitamin E
(Olestra inhibits the absorption of vitamin E, as well as the other fat-soluble vitamins, A, D, and K, carotenoids and flavonoids)

Vitamin K
(Inhibits absorption of vitamin K as well as the other fat-soluble vitamins A, D, and E)

OLEUROPEIN AND OLEUROPEIN AGLYCONE

Trastuzumab
(Oleuropein aglycone was reported to reverse acquired autoresistance to trastuzumab in human epidermal growth factor receptor-2 (HER-2)-overexpressing breast cancer)

OPIATES

Gamma-Hydroxybutyrate (GHB)
(May be life-threatening with GHB)

ORAL CONTRACEPTIVES

Riboflavin (Vitamin B2)
(May decrease serum levels of riboflavin)

Vitamin A
(May increase serum retinol)

Vitamin B6
(May increase vitamin B6 requirements)

ORLISTAT

Astaxanthin
(Orlistat may decrease the absorption of astaxanthin)

Beta-Carotene
(May decrease the absorption of beta-carotene)

Fucoxanthin
(Orlistat may decrease the absorption of fucoxanthin)

Tocotrienols
(May inhibit Tocotrienol absorption)

Vitamin A
(May decrease vitamin A absorption)

Vitamin D
(Orlistat may decrease the absorption of vitamin D)

Vitamin E
(Inhibits vitamin E absorption)

Vitamin K
(May reduce vitamin K absorption)

OX BILE, DESICCATED

Gamma-Tocopherol
(Increased Gamma-Tocopherol absorption)

Tocotrienols
(May increase Tocotrienol absorption)

Vitamin E
(Dessicated ox bile may increase absorption of vitamin E)

OXALIC ACID

Bone Meal
(Decreased absorption of Calcium)

Calcium
(May decrease absorption of calcium)

Iron
(May decrease absorption of iron)

Magnesium
(May decrease absorption of magnesium)

Manganese
(May decrease absorption of manganese)

Zinc
(Concomitant intake of zinc with foods rich in oxalic acid (eg, spinach, sweet potatoes, rhubarb, beans) may depress the absorption of zinc)

PDE5 INHIBITORS

Luteolin
(Luteolin has been found to inhibit the metabolism of the sedative drug midazolam by human liver microsomes and cytochrome P450 3A4 (CYP3A4)

and CYP3A5. Midazolam is a probe substrate for CYP3A4 and CYP3A5 enzymes. CYP3A4 is located in the intestine and liver, and its inhibition leads to delayed absorption and reduced first pass metabolism in the liver, resulting in higher plasma levels of the drug. However, given this finding, those using midazolam or other drugs metabolized by CYP3A4, including statins - atorvastatin, lovastatin and simvastatin - as well as amiodarone, buspirone, cisapride, etoposide, quinidine and sildenafil, tadalafil, vardenafil and others, should exercise caution in the use of luteolin-containing dairy supplements)

PACLITAXEL
Ascorbyl Palmitate
(Vitamin C may potentiate antineoplastic activity)
Glutamine Peptides
(L-Glutamine may prevent paclitaxel adverse reactions)
L-Glutamine
(L-Glutamine may prevent paclitaxel adverse reactions)
Vitamin C
(Vitamin C may potentiate the antineoplastic activity of paclitaxel)

PANTETHINE
HMG-CoA Reductase Inhibitors
(May have additive lipid-modulatory effects)
Nicotinic Acid
(May have additive lipid-modulatory effects)

PANTOTHENIC ACID
Biotin
(May decrease Biotin absorption)

PAPAIN
Quercetin
(Increase absorption of Quercetin)

PARA-AMINOBENZOIC ACID (PABA)
Sulfonamides
(Decreased effectiveness)

PARA-AMINOSALICYLIC ACID
Vitamin B12
(Chronic use of the anti-tuberculosis drug may decrease the absorption of vitamin B12)

PARGYLINE HYDROCHLORIDE
Brewer's Yeast
(May cause hypertension with Brewer's Yeast)
DL-Phenylalanine
(May cause hypertension with Brewer's Yeast)
L-Phenylalanine
(L-Phenylalanine may cause hypertension)
L-Tyrosine
(L-Phenylalanine may cause hypertension)

PECTIN
Astaxanthin
(Concomitant intake of pectin and astaxanthin may decrease the absorption of astaxanthin)
Beta-Carotene
(May decrease the absorption of beta-carotene)
Calcium
(Decreased absorption of Calcium)
Clindamycin Hydrochloride
(Decreased absorption of clindamycin)
Copper
(Decreased absorption of Copper)
Digoxin
(Decreased absorption of digoxin)
Fucoxanthin
(Concomitant intake of pectin and fucoxanthin may decrease the absorption of fucoxanthin)
Iron
(Decreased absorption of Iron)
Lovastatin
(Decreased absorption of lovastatin)
Lutein
(Decreased absorption of Lutein)
Lutein and Zeaxanthin
(Decreased absorption of Lutein and Zeaxanthin)

Lycopene
(Decreased absorption of Lycopene)
Magnesium
(Decreased absorption of Magnesium)
Tetracycline Hydrochloride
(Decreased absorption of tetracycline)
Zinc
(Decreased absorption of Zinc)

PENICILLAMINE
Copper
(Decreased absorption of copper and penicillamine)
Iron
(May decrease absorption of penicillamine)
Vitamin B6
(May result in vitamin B6 deficiency)
Zinc
(Concomitant administration of penicillamine and zinc may depress absorption of zinc)

PENICILLINS
Sesame Seed Lignans
(Antibiotics may decrease the production of the mammalian lignans enterolactone (ENT) and enterodiol (END) from sesame seed lignans)

PENTAMIDINE ISETHIONATE
Arnica
(Increased risk of prolonged QT interval when given with Arnica)

PERILLA OIL
Allium sativum
(Increased antithrombotic effects with Perilla Oil)
Aspirin
(Increased antithrombotic effects with Perilla Oil)
Ginkgo biloba
(Increased antithrombotic effects with Perilla Oil)
Nonsteroidal Anti-Inflammatory Drugs
(Increased antithrombotic effects with Perilla Oil)

PHENELZINE SULFATE

Brewer's Yeast
(May cause hypertension with Brewer's Yeast)

DL-Phenylalanine
(May cause hypertension with Brewer's Yeast)

L-Phenylalanine
(L-Phenylalanine may cause hypertension)

L-Tyrosine
(L-Phenylalanine may cause hypertension)

Vitamin B6
(May result in vitamin B6 deficiency)

PHENOBARBITAL

Biotin
(May decrease Biotin levels)

Folate
(May decrease folate levels and increase homocysteine levels; High dose folic acid may decrease serum levels)

Vitamin B6
(Vitamin B6 may lower phenobarbital plasma levels)

Vitamin D
(Phenobarbital may reduce the plasma levels of 25-hydroxyvitamin D by inhibiting vitamin D 25-hydroxylase activity in the liver)

Vitamin E
(Anticonvulsants may lower plasma vitamin E levels)

PHENOTHIAZINES

Borage Oil
(May cause seizures when taken with Borage Oil)

Evening Primrose Oil
(EPO lowers seizure threshold)

PHENOXYBENZAMINE HYDROCHLORIDE

5-Hydroxytryptophan
(Inhibits 5-HTP metabolism to serotonin)

PHENYLALANINE

(*See under* DL-Phenylalanine; L-Phenylalanine)

PHENYTOIN

Biotin
(May decrease Biotin levels)

Folate
(May decrease folate levels and increase homocysteine levels; High dose folic acid may decrease serum levels)

Piperine
(Piperine may inhibit metabolism)

Vitamin B6
(Vitamin B6 may lower phenytoin plasma levels)

Vitamin D
(Phenytoin may reduce the plasma levels of 25-hydroxyvitamin D by inhibiting vitamin D 25-hydroxylase activity in the liver)

Vitamin E
(Anticonvulsants may lower plasma vitamin E levels)

PHOSPHATE SALTS

Magnesium
(May decrease absorption of phosphate and magnesium)

Zinc
(Concomitant intake of zinc and phosphate salts may decrease the absorption of zinc)

PHOSPHATIDYLCHOLINE

Huperzine A
(Additive effects and increased adverse effects with Huperzine A)

PHOSPHORUS

Antacids, aluminum-containing
(Decreased absorption of Phosphorus)

Zinc
(Decreased absorption of Zinc)

PHYSOSTIGMINE SALICYLATE

Huperzine A
(Additive effects and increased adverse effects with Huperzine A)

PHYTIC ACID

Calcium
(May decrease absorption of calcium)

Chromium
(May decrease absorption of chromium)

Copper
(Decreased absorption of copper)

Iron
(May decrease absorption of iron)

Magnesium
(May decrease absorption of magnesium)

Manganese
(May decrease absorption of manganese)

Zinc
(Concomitant intake of zinc with foods rich in phytic acid (eg, unleavened bread, raw beans, seeds, nuts, grains, soy isolates) may depress the absorption of zinc)

PHYTONADIONE

(*See under* Vitamin K)

PHYTOSTANOLS

Alpha Carotene
(Phytostanols may interfere with absorption and lower serum levels)

Beta-Carotene
(Phytostanols may interfere with absorption and lower serum levels)

Gamma-Tocopherol
(Decreased plasma Gamma-Tocopherol levels)

HMG-CoA Reductase Inhibitors
(Phytostanol supplementation may be additive to the cholesterol-lowering effects of the statins)

Lycopene
(Phytostanols may interfere with absorption and lower serum levels)

Tocotrienols
(May decrease Tocotrienol levels)

Vitamin E
(Phytostanols may interfere with absorption and lower serum levels)

PHYTOSTEROLS

Alpha Carotene
(Phytosterols may interfere with absorption and lower serum levels)

Beta-Carotene
(Phytosterols may interfere with absorption and lower serum levels)
Gamma-Tocopherol
(Decreased plasma Gamma-Tocopherol levels)
Lycopene
(Phytosterols may interfere with absorption and lower serum levels)
Tocotrienols
(May decrease Tocotrienol levels)
Vitamin E
(Phytosterols may interfere with absorption and lower serum levels)

PIOGLITAZONE HYDROCHLORIDE
Inositol Nicotinate
(High dose nicotinic acid may antagonize effects)
Niacin
(High dose nicotinic acid may antagonize effects which may require dose adjustment)

PIPERINE
Beta-Carotene
(Piperine may enhance the absorption)
Coenzyme Q-10
(Piperine may enhance the absorption)
Curcumin
(Piperine may enhance the absorption)
Dapsone
(Piperine may inhibit metabolism)
Drugs, unspecified
(Piperine may inhibit metabolism)
Ethambutol Hydrochloride
(Piperine may inhibit metabolism)
Isoniazid
(Piperine may inhibit metabolism)
Phenytoin
(Piperine may inhibit metabolism)
Propranolol
(Piperine may inhibit metabolism)
Pyrazinamide
(Piperine may inhibit metabolism)
Rifampicin
(Piperine may inhibit metabolism)

Selenium
(Piperine may enhance the absorption)
Sulfadiazine
(Piperine may inhibit metabolism)
Theophylline
(Piperine may inhibit metabolism)
Vitamin B6
(Piperine may enhance the absorption)
Vitamin C
(Piperine may enhance the absorption)

PIPERINE, FOUND IN BLACK PEPPER
Coenzyme Q10 (CoQ10)
(May increase plasma levels of CoQ10)
Curcuminoids
(May enhance absorption of curcuminoids)

PIVALIC ACID-CONTAINING ANTIBIOTICS
Acetyl-L-Carnitine
(May lead to L-carnitine deficiencies)

PLANT PHENOLIC COMPOUNDS
Gamma-Tocopherol
(Helps to maintain levels of reduced Gamma-Tocopherol)
Vitamin E
(These substances may participate in redox cycling reactions and help maintain levels of reduced vitamin E)

POLICOSANOL
Aspirin
(Policosanol showed a synergism with the antithrombotic properties of aspirin in different experimental models)
Aspirin Buffered
(Policosanol showed a synergism with the antithrombotic properties of aspirin in different experimental models)
Aspirin, Enteric Coated
(Policosanol showed a synergism with the antithrombotic properties of aspirin in different experimental models)

POLYPHENOLS
Alpha-Tocopherol Polyethylene Glycol Succinate (TPGS)
(TPGS may increase the absorption of polyphenols)

POTASSIUM
ACE Inhibitors
(Increased serum Potassium due to inhibition of aldosterone production)
Amiloride Hydrochloride
(Concomitant potassium-sparing diuretic and Potassium supplements can produce severe hyperkalemia)
Spironolactone
(Concomitant potassium-sparing diuretic and Potassium supplements can produce severe hyperkalemia)
Triamterene
(Concomitant potassium-sparing diuretic and Potassium supplements can produce severe hyperkalemia)

POTASSIUM CHLORIDE
Vitamin B12
(May decrease absorption of dietary vitamin B12)

PRAVASTATIN SODIUM
Coenzyme Q10 (CoQ10)
(Decreases CoQ10 levels)

PREBIOTICS
Alpha Galactosidase Enzyme
(Decreased effectiveness of the soy oligosaccharides)
Calcium
(Enhanced absorption of Calcium)
Magnesium
(Enhanced absorption of Magnesium)
Probiotics
(Enhanced effectiveness of the Probiotics)
Probiotics
(Synergistic effects with Prebiotics)

PRIMIDONE

Biotin
(May decrease Biotin levels)
Folate
(May decrease folate levels and increase homocysteine levels; High dose folic acid may decrease serum levels)

PROBENECID

Riboflavin (Vitamin B2)
(May inhibit absorption of riboflavin)

PROBIOTICS

Inulins
(Inulins may increase beneficial effects of Probiotics)
Lactulose
(Probiotics may increase Lactulose beneficial effects)
Prebiotics
(Enhanced effectiveness of the Probiotics)
Transgalacto-Oligosaccharides
(Enhanced beneficial effects of TOS)

PROCAINAMIDE

Arnica
(Increased risk of prolonged QT interval when given with Arnica)

PROCHLORPERAZINE

Arnica
(Increased risk of prolonged QT interval when given with Arnica)

PROGESTINS

Melatonin
(Concomitant Melatonin may cause additive effect in inhibiting ovarian function)

PROPANTHELINE BROMIDE

Riboflavin (Vitamin B2)
(May enhance absorption of riboflavin)

PROPRANOLOL

Piperine
(Piperine may inhibit metabolism)
Vitamin C
(Ascorbic acid may affect both the absorption process and the first-pass metabolism of propranolol. Heart rate has been found to decrease less when propranolol was administered with ascorbic acid, when compared to controls. The interaction has little biological importance)

PROPRANOLOL HYDROCHLORIDE

Coenzyme Q10 (CoQ10)
(May inhibit some CoQ10-dependent enzymes)
Vitamin C
(Ascorbic acid may affect both the absorption process and the first-pass metabolism of propranolol. Heart rate has been found to decrease less when propranolol was administered with ascorbic acid, when compared to controls. The interaction has little biological importance)

PROTEASE INHIBITORS

Gamma-Hydroxybutyrate (GHB)
(May be life-threatening with GHB)
Red Yeast Rice
(Increased risk of myopathy)

PROTON PUMP INHIBITORS

Bone Meal
(Decreased absorption of Calcium)
Calcium
(May decrease absorption of calcium)
Indole-3-Carbinol
(Block the conversion of Indole-3 Carbinol to DIM and ICZ)
Iron
(May decrease absorption of carbonyl iron)
Vitamin B12
(Chronic use of proton pump inhibitors may result in decreased absorption of vitamin B12 found naturally in food sources. They are unlikely to affect the absorption of supplemental vitamin B12)

PSYLLIUM

Calcium
(Decreased absorption of Calcium)
Carbamazepine
(Reduced absorption of carbamazepine)
Cholestyramine
(Enhanced cholesterol-lowering action)
Copper
(Decreased absorption of Copper)
Digoxin
(Reduced absorption of digoxin)
Iron
(Decreased absorption of Iron)
Lithium
(Reduced absorption of Lithium)
Magnesium
(Decreased absorption of Magnesium)
Warfarin Sodium
(Reduced absorption of warfarin sodium)
Zinc
(Decreased absorption of Zinc)

PSYLLIUM HUSK

(*See under* Psyllium)

PYCNOGENOL

Dextroamphetamine
(May be synergistic with Pycnogenol for attention deficit-hyperactivity disorder management)

PYRAZINAMIDE

Piperine
(Piperine may inhibit metabolism)

PYRIDOXINE HYDROCHLORIDE

(*See under* Vitamin B6)

PYRIMETHAMINE

Folate
(Folic acid may decrease antiparasitic effects)

QUERCETIN

Bromelains
(Increase absorption of Quercetin)
Cisplatin
(May cause genotoxicity in normal tissues when taken with Quercetin)
Papain
(Increase absorption of Quercetin)

Quinolones
  (Competitively inhibited by
  Quercetin)

QUINACRINE HYDROCHLORIDE
Riboflavin (Vitamin B2)
  (May inhibit riboflavin conversion
  to FMN and FAD)

QUINIDINE
Arnica
  (Increased risk of prolonged QT
  interval when given with Arnica)

QUINOLONES
Bone Meal
  (Decreased absorption of
  quinolones)
Calcium
  (May decrease absorption of
  quinolones)
Iron
  (May decrease absorption of both
  quinolone and iron)
Magnesium
  (May decrease absorption of
  quinolones)
Quercetin
  (Competitively inhibited by
  Quercetin)
Rutin
  (Inhibition of activity due to
  Rutin)
Zinc
  (Concomitant intake of a
  quinolone and zinc may decrease
  the absorption of both the
  quinolone and zinc)

RED YEAST RICE
Azole Antifungals
  (Increased risk of myopathy)
Cyclosporine
  (Increased risk of myopathy)
Fibrates
  (Increased risk of myopathy)
Gemfibrozil
  (Increased risk of myopathy)
Grapefruit Juice
  (Increased risk of myopathy)
HMG-CoA Reductase Inhibitors
  (Increased risk of adverse
  reactions)

Macrolide Antibiotics
  (Increased risk of myopathy)
Nefazodone Hydrochloride
  (Increased risk of myopathy)
Nicotinic Acid
  (Increased risk of myopathy)
Protease Inhibitors
  (Increased risk of myopathy)
Warfarin Sodium
  (Increase in the INR as well as
  bleeding)

REPAGLINIDE
Inositol Nicotinate
  (High dose nicotinic acid may
  antagonize effects)
Niacin
  (High dose nicotinic acid may
  antagonize effects which may
  require dose adjustment)

RETINOIDS
D-Glucarate
  (Synergistic chemopreventive
  effects)

RIBOFLAVIN (VITAMIN B2)
Chlorpromazine
  (May inhibit riboflavin conversion
  to FMN and FAD)
Cholestyramine
  (May decrease absorption of
  riboflavin)
Colestipol Hydrochloride
  (May decrease absorption of
  riboflavin)
Didanosine
  (Riboflavin may reverse
  nucleoside analogue-induced lactic
  acidosis in mild riboflavin
  deficiencies)
Doxorubicin Hydrochloride
  (May inhibit riboflavin conversion
  to FMN and FAD)
Lamivudine
  (Riboflavin may reverse
  nucleoside analogue-induced lactic
  acidosis in mild riboflavin
  deficiencies)
Metoclopramide Hydrochloride
  (May decrease absorption of
  riboflavin)

Oral Contraceptives
  (May decrease serum levels of
  riboflavin)
Probenecid
  (May inhibit absorption of
  riboflavin)
Propantheline Bromide
  (May enhance absorption of
  riboflavin)
Quinacrine Hydrochloride
  (May inhibit riboflavin conversion
  to FMN and FAD)
Stavudine
  (Riboflavin may reverse
  nucleoside analogue-induced lactic
  acidosis in mild riboflavin
  deficiencies)
Tricyclic Antidepressants
  (May inhibit riboflavin conversion
  to FMN and FAD)
Zidovudine
  (Riboflavin may reverse
  nucleoside analogue-induced lactic
  acidosis in mild riboflavin
  deficiencies)

RIFAMPICIN
Piperine
  (Piperine may inhibit metabolism)

RITONAVIR
Vitamin D
  (The HIV protease inhibitors
  ritonavir, indinavir, and nelfinavir
  may impair vitamin D
  bioactivation to 1, 25-
  dihydroxyvitamin D)

ROSIGLITAZONE MALEATE
Inositol Nicotinate
  (High dose nicotinic acid may
  antagonize effects)
Niacin
  (High dose nicotinic acid may
  antagonize effects which may
  require dose adjustment)

RUTIN
Quinolones
  (Inhibition of activity due to
  Rutin)
Vitamin C
  (Prevention of Vitamin C
  oxidation, enhanced and/or

inhibition of absorption with
flavonoids)

SALICYLATES

Vitamin K
(Salicylates in large doses may
inhibit vitamin K epoxide
reductase resulting in vitamin K
deficiency)

SALMON OIL

Astaxanthin
(Dietary oils such as olive oil and
fish oils may enhance the
absorption of astaxanthin. Corn oil
is less likely to enhance
astaxanthin absorption)

Fucoxanthin
(Dietary oils, such as fish oils and
olive oils, may enhance the
absorption of fucoxanthin)

SAQUINAVIR

Ascorbyl Palmitate
(Grapefruit flavonoids may
increase bioavailability due to
cytochrome P-450 3A4 inhibition)

Vitamin C
(Grapefruit flavonoids may
increase bioavailability due to
cytochrome P-450 3A4 inhibition)

**SELECTIVE ESTROGEN RECEPTOR
MODULATORS**

Ipriflavone
(Additive effects with Ipriflavone)

**SELECTIVE SEROTONIN REUPTAKE
INHIBITORS (SSRIS)**

5-Hydroxytryptophan
(5-HTP may potentiate
antidepressant effects and increase
risk of side effects)

L-Tryptophan
(Concurrent use of L-tryptophan
with an SSRI may potentiate the
antidepressant effect of the SSRI
and may also increase the risk of
adverse reactions)

Myo-Inositol
(May have additive effects with
Myo-Inositol)

SELEGILINE HYDROCHLORIDE

DL-Phenylalanine
(May have synergistic
antidepressant activity)

L-Phenylalanine
(L-Phenylalanine may have
synergistic antidepressant effects)

SELENIUM

Alpha-Tocopherol
Polyethylene Glycol
Succinate (TPGS)
(May function synergistically with
d-alpha-tocopherol)

Gamma-Tocopherol
(Synergistic effect with Gamma-
Tocopherol)

Iodine
(Synergistic activity in the
treatment of Kashin-Beck disease,
and osteoarthropathy)

Iodine Preparations
(May have synergistic activity in
the treatment of Kashin-Beck
disease)

Piperine
(Piperine may enhance the
absorption)

Vitamin C
(May decrease absorption of
selenium. The protective effect of
selenite in tumorgenesis may be
nullified by vitamin C)

Vitamin E
(Selenium may function
synergistically with vitamin E)

SEROTONINERGIC AGENTS

5-Hydroxytryptophan
(5-HTP may potentiate
antidepressant effects and increase
risk of side effects)

SESAME SEED LIGNANS

Aminoglycosides
(Antibiotics may decrease the
production of the mammalian
lignans enterolactone (ENT) and
enterodiol (END) from sesame
seed lignans)

Anthracycline antibiotics and their
derivatives
(Antibiotics may decrease the
production of the mammalian
lignans enterolactone (ENT) and
enterodiol (END) from sesame
seed lignans)

Azole Antifungals
(Antibiotics may decrease the
production of the mammalian
lignans enterolactone (ENT) and
enterodiol (END) from sesame
seed lignans)

Bacteriostatic antibiotics
(Antibiotics may decrease the
production of the mammalian
lignans enterolactone (ENT) and
enterodiol (END) from sesame
seed lignans)

Berries
(An extract of Schisandra
chinensis berry when combined
with sesamin was found to
decrease blood viscosity and
improve blood fluidity in a human
clinical study)

Beta-lactams antibiotics
(Antibiotics may decrease the
production of the mammalian
lignans enterolactone (ENT) and
enterodiol (END) from sesame
seed lignans)

Doxycycline
(Antibiotics may decrease the
production of the mammalian
lignans enterolactone (ENT) and
enterodiol (END) from sesame
seed lignans)

Erythromycin
(Antibiotics may decrease the
production of the mammalian
lignans enterolactone (ENT) and
enterodiol (END) from sesame
seed lignans)

Fluoroquinolone antibiotics
(Antibiotics may decrease the
production of the mammalian
lignans enterolactone (ENT) and
enterodiol (END) from sesame
seed lignans)

Gamma-tocopherol
(A single dose of the sesame seed
lignans sesamin and sesamolin
(136 mg) was found to reduce the
urinary excretion of co-
administered gamma-tocopherol in
a human study)

Macrolide Antibiotics
(Antibiotics may decrease the production of the mammalian lignans enterolactone (ENT) and enterodiol (END) from sesame seed lignans)

Penicillins
(Antibiotics may decrease the production of the mammalian lignans enterolactone (ENT) and enterodiol (END) from sesame seed lignans)

Tetracyclines
(Antibiotics may decrease the production of the mammalian lignans enterolactone (ENT) and enterodiol (END) from sesame seed lignans)

Tocopherols
(A single dose of the sesame seed lignans sesamin and sesamolin (136 mg) was found to reduce the urinary excretion of co-administered gamma-tocopherol in a human study)

SHARK LIVER OIL

Astaxanthin
(Dietary oils such as olive oil and fish oils may enhance the absorption of astaxanthin. Corn oil is less likely to enhance astaxanthin absorption)

Fucoxanthin
(Dietary oils, such as fish oils and olive oils, may enhance the absorption of fucoxanthin)

SILDENAFIL CITRATE

L-Arginine
(L-Arginine may potentiate effects)

SILICON

Aluminum-containing Compounds, unspecified
(Silicon may inhibit aluminum absorption)

SIMVASTATIN

Ascorbyl Palmitate
(Grapefruit flavonoids may increase bioavailability due to cytochrome P-450 3A4 inhibition)

Coenzyme Q10 (CoQ10)
(Decreases CoQ10 levels)

Vitamin C
(Grapefruit flavonoids may increase bioavailability due to cytochrome P-450 3A4 inhibition)

SKELETAL MUSCLE RELAXANTS

Gamma-Hydroxybutyrate (GHB)
(May be life-threatening with GHB)

SODIUM ALGINATE

Bone Meal
(Decreased absorption of Calcium)

Calcium
(May decrease absorption of calcium)

Magnesium
(May decrease absorption of magnesium)

SODIUM ALGINATES AND OTHER PHYCO-POLYSACCHARIDES

Beta-Carotene
(Decreased absorption of Beta Carotene)

Calcium
(Decreased absorption of Calcium)

Chromium
(Decreased absorption of Chromium)

Lutein
(Decreased absorption of Lutein)

Lycopene
(Decreased absorption of Lycopene)

Magnesium
(Decreased absorption of Magnesium)

Manganese
(Decreased absorption of Manganese)

Zinc
(Decreased absorption of Zinc)

SODIUM FLUORIDE

Xylitol
(The combination of xylitol and the use of fluoride toothpastes may give better anticariogenic effects than the use of either alone)

SOTALOL HYDROCHLORIDE

Arnica
(Increased risk of prolonged QT interval when given with Arnica)

SOY PROTEIN

Calcium
(May reduce availability of calcium)

Copper
(May reduce availability of copper)

Iron
(May reduce availability of iron)

Magnesium
(May reduce availability of magnesium)

Manganese
(May reduce availability of manganese)

Zinc
(May reduce availability of zinc)

SOY-CONTAINING DIETARY SUPPLEMENTS

Supplemental Enzymes
(Decreased prebiotic activity of Soy products when taken with alpha-galactosidase)

SOYBEAN PREPARATIONS

Iodine
(Inhibit thyroid peroxidase)

SPIRONOLACTONE

Potassium
(Concomitant potassium-sparing diuretic and Potassium supplements can produce severe hyperkalemia)

SPRUCE LIGNANS (7-HYDROXYMATAIRESINOL)

Antibiotics, unspecified
(Antibiotics may decrease the production of enterolactone (ENL) from 7-hydroxymatairesinol (HMR))

SQUALENE

Vitamin K
(May reduce vitamin K absorption)

STARCH

Equol
(May promote the formation of equol)

STAVUDINE

Acetyl-L-Carnitine
(May lead to decreased acetyl-L-carnitine levels)

L-Carnitine
(May produce L-Carnitine deficiencies)

Riboflavin (Vitamin B2)
(Riboflavin may reverse nucleoside analogue-induced lactic acidosis in mild riboflavin deficiencies)

SUCRALFATE

Gamma-Tocopherol
(Interferes with Gamma-Tocopherol absorption)

Tocotrienols
(May inhibit Tocotrienol absorption)

Vitamin E
(Interferes with vitamin E absorption)

Zinc L-Carnosine
(The combination of cytoprotectant sucralfate and zinc L-carnosine may be more effective than when each agent is used alone)

SULFADIAZINE

Piperine
(Piperine may inhibit metabolism)

SULFASALAZINE

Folate
(May decrease folic acid absorption)

SULFONAMIDES

Para-Aminobenzoic Acid (PABA)
(Decreased effectiveness)

SULFONYLUREAS

Inositol Nicotinate
(High dose nicotinic acid may antagonize effects)

Niacin
(High dose nicotinic acid may antagonize effects which may require dose adjustment)

SULFUR HEXAFLUORIDE

Xylitol
(The combination of xylitol and the use of fluoride toothpastes may give better anticariogenic effects than the use of either alone)

SULINDAC

Dimethyl Sulfoxide (DMSO)
(May decrease the effects of DMSO and increase side effects)

SUPPLEMENTAL ENZYMES

Acarbose
(Decreased efficacy of acarbose when taken with amylase, pancreatin, and pancrelipase)

Anticoagulant drugs, unspecified
(Enhanced anticoagulant activity when taken with Bromelain)

Antithrombotic Agents
(Enhanced antithrombotic activity when taken with Bromelain)

Soy-containing dietary supplements
(Decreased prebiotic activity of Soy products when taken with alpha-galactosidase)

SYMPATHOMIMETIC AGENTS

Tiratricol (TRIAC)
(Possible increased risk of coronary insufficiency in patients with coronary artery disease)

SYNBIOTICS

Calcium
(Enhanced colonic absorption of Calcium)

Magnesium
(Enhanced colonic absorption of Magnesium)

TACRINE HYDROCHLORIDE

Huperzine A
(Additive effects and increased adverse effects with Huperzine A)

TAMOXIFEN CITRATE

Genistein
(Genistein may negate the inhibitory effect of tamoxifen)

Indole-3-Carbinol
(May be synergistic with Indole-3-Carbinol in protecting against breast cancer)

Tangeretin
(Tangeretin was found to neutralize the tumor-suppressing effect of tamoxifen)

TANGERETIN

Tamoxifen Citrate
(Tangeretin was found to neutralize the tumor-suppressing effect of tamoxifen)

TANNINS

Iron
(May decrease absorption of iron)

Thiamin
(May inactivate Thiamin)

Zinc
(Concomitant intake of tea (tannins) and zinc may cause decreased absorption of zinc)

TESTOSTERONE

DHEA
(May increase adverse effects of DHEA)

TETRACYCLINE HYDROCHLORIDE

Pectin
(Decreased absorption of tetracycline)

TETRACYCLINES

Sesame Seed Lignans
(Antibiotics may decrease the production of the mammalian lignans enterolactone (ENT) and enterodiol (END) from sesame seed lignans)

Zinc
(Concomitant intake of a tetracycline and zinc may decrease the absorption of both the tetracycline and zinc)

TETRACYCLINES, UNSPECIFIED

Baicalein
(Baicalein and tetracycline have shown synergistic activity against MRSA (methicillin-resistant Staphylococcus aureus) in vitro)

Bone Meal
(Decreased absorption of tetracyclines)

Bromelain
(Bromelain may increase tetracycline levels)

Calcium
(May decrease absorption of tetracyclines)

Iron
  (May decrease absorption of both
  tetracycline and iron)
Magnesium
  (May decrease absorption of
  tetracycline)
Manganese
  (May reduce absorption of
  manganese)

THEOPHYLLINE
Ipriflavone
  (Metabolism and elimination may
  be inhibited by Ipriflavone)
Piperine
  (Piperine may inhibit metabolism)
Vitamin B6
  (Vitamin B6 may increase risk of
  theophylline-induced seizures)

THIAMIN
Beverages, sulfites
  (May inactivate Thiamin)
Bumetanide
  (Chronic use may cause Thiamin
  deficiency)
Ethacrynic Acid
  (Chronic use may cause Thiamin
  deficiency)
Food, sulfites
  (May inactivate Thiamin)
Food, unspecified
  (Antithiamin factors in food
  inactivate Thiamin)
Furosemide
  (Chronic use may cause Thiamin
  deficiency)
Tannins
  (May inactivate Thiamin)

THIAZIDES
Vitamin D
  (Concomitant use of thiazides and
  pharmacologic doses of vitamin D
  may cause hypercalcemia in some)

THYROID PREPARATIONS
Tiratricol (TRIAC)
  (May produce additive effects
  with tiratricol)

THYROXINE
Calcium
  (May decrease thyroxine
  absorption)

TICLOPIDINE HYDROCHLORIDE
Alpha-Tocopherol
  Polyethylene Glycol
  Succinate (TPGS)
  (High doses of TPGS may
  enhance the effects of ticlopidine)
Curcuminoids
  (Curcuminoids may enhance the
  antiplatelet effect)
Gamma-Tocopherol
  (Increased effects of ticlopidine)
Green Tea Catechins
  (Enhanced effect with green tea
  catechins)
Nattokinase (Subtilisin NAT)
  (The use of nattokinase along
  with antiplatelet drugs (eg,
  ticlopidine) may cause serious
  adverse events, especially
  excessive bleeding. Administration
  of nattokinase is contraindicated
  in those with bleeding disorders
  and should be avoided in those
  receiving antiplatelet agents)
Vitamin E
  (High doses of vitamin E may
  potentiate the effects of
  antiplatelet drugs)
Vitamin E Phosphate
  (Vitamin E phosphate may
  potentiate the effects of
  antiplatelet drugs (eg, ticlopidine))

TINZAPARIN SODIUM
Nattokinase (Subtilisin NAT)
  (The use of nattokinase along
  with parenteral anticoagulants (eg,
  low molecular weight heparins)
  may cause serious adverse events,
  especially excessive bleeding.
  Administration of nattokinase is
  contraindicated in those with
  bleeding disorders and should be
  avoided in those receiving
  anticoagulant agents)

TIRATRICOL (TRIAC)
Anticoagulant drugs, unspecified
  (May increase
  hypoprothrombinemic effect)
Sympathomimetic Agents
  (Possible increased risk of
  coronary insufficiency in patients
  with coronary artery disease)

Thyroid Preparations
  (May produce additive effects
  with tiratricol)
Warfarin Sodium
  (May increase
  hypoprothrombinemic effect)

TIROFIBAN HYDROCHLORIDE
Gamma-Tocopherol
  (Increased effects of tirofiban)
Nattokinase (Subtilisin NAT)
  (The use of nattokinase along
  with parenteral antiplatelet drugs
  (GPIIB/IIA inhibitors such as
  tirofiban hydrochloride) may cause
  serious adverse events, especially
  excessive bleeding. Administration
  of nattokinase is contraindicated
  in those with bleeding disorders
  and should be avoided in those
  receiving antiplatelet agents)
Vitamin E
  (High doses of vitamin E may
  potentiate the effects of
  antiplatelet drugs)
Vitamin E Phosphate
  (Vitamin E phosphate may
  potentiate the effects of
  antiplatelet drugs (eg, tirofiban))

TIZANIDINE HYDROCHLORIDE
Glycine
  (Glycine may increase effect of)

TOCOPHEROL ACETATE
Coenzyme Q10 (CoQ10)
  (Elevation in CoQ10 levels in
  mitochondria by dietary
  supplementation is linked to a
  corresponding rise in alpha-
  tocopherol content)

TOCOPHEROLS
Coenzyme Q10 (CoQ10)
  (Elevation in CoQ10 levels in
  mitochondria by dietary
  supplementation is linked to a
  corresponding rise in alpha-
  tocopherol content)
Iron
  (Iron may cause oxidation of the
  tocopherols)
Sesame Seed Lignans
  (A single dose of the sesame seed
  lignans sesamin and sesamolin

(136 mg) was found to reduce the urinary excretion of co-administered gamma-tocopherol in a human study)

TOCOTRIENOLS

Allium sativum
(May enhance antithrombotic activity)

Alpha-Tocopherol Polyethylene Glycol Succinate (TPGS)
(TPGS may increase the absorption of all forms of vitamin E (gamma-tocopherol, tocotrienols))

Antiplatelet Drugs
(Tocotrienol may potentiate antiplatelet effects)

Cholestyramine
(May decrease Tocotrienol absorption)

Colestipol
(May decrease Tocotrienol absorption)

Fat Substitute
(May inhibit Tocotrienol absorption)

Ginkgo biloba
(May enhance antithrombotic activity)

HMG-CoA Reductase Inhibitors
(Tocotrienols may have synergistic cholesterol-lowering effects)

Iron
(Iron may cause oxidation of tocotrienols)

Iron
(May decrease Tocotrienol absorption)

Isoniazid
(May decrease Tocotrienol absorption)

Medium-Chain Triglycerides
(May increase Tocotrienol absorption)

Mineral Oil
(May decrease Tocotrienol absorption)

Neomycin
(May decrease Tocotrienol effects)

Orlistat
(May inhibit Tocotrienol absorption)

Ox Bile, Desiccated
(May increase Tocotrienol absorption)

Phytostanols
(May decrease Tocotrienol levels)

Phytosterols
(May decrease Tocotrienol levels)

Sucralfate
(May inhibit Tocotrienol absorption)

Warfarin Sodium
(Large dose Tocotrienols may enhance anticoagulant effects)

TOLBUTAMIDE

Ipriflavone
(Increased serum levels with Ipriflavone)

TRANQUILIZERS

Gamma-Hydroxybutyrate (GHB)
(May be life-threatening with GHB)

TRANSGALACTO-OLIGOSACCHARIDES

Calcium
(Enhanced colonic absorption of Calcium)

Magnesium
(Enhanced colonic absorption of Magnesium)

Probiotics
(Enhanced beneficial effects of TOS)

TRANYLCYPROMINE SULFATE

Brewer's Yeast
(May cause hypertension with Brewer's Yeast)

DL-Phenylalanine
(May cause hypertension with Brewer's Yeast)

L-Phenylalanine
(L-Phenylalanine may cause hypertension)

L-Tyrosine
(L-Phenylalanine may cause hypertension)

TRASTUZUMAB

Oleuropein and Oleuropein Aglycone
(Oleuropein aglycone was reported to reverse acquired autoresistance to trastuzumab in human epidermal growth factor receptor-2 (HER-2)-overexpressing breast cancer)

TRIAMTERENE

Potassium
(Concomitant potassium-sparing diuretic and Potassium supplements can produce severe hyperkalemia)

TRICYCLIC ANTIDEPRESSANTS

Riboflavin (Vitamin B2)
(May inhibit riboflavin conversion to FMN and FAD)

TYROSINE

(See under L-Tyrosine)

VALPROIC ACID

Acetyl-L-Carnitine
(May lead to L-carnitine deficiencies)

Folate
(May decrease folate levels and increase homocysteine; high dose folic acid may decrease serum levels)

L-Carnitine
(May produce L-Carnitine deficiencies)

Vitamin B6
(Chronic use may decrease plasma pyridoxal 5'-phosphate)

VANADIUM

Aluminum Hydroxide
(May decrease absorption of vanadium)

Chloride
(May decrease absorption of vanadium)

Chromium
(May decrease absorption of vanadium)

Ethylenediaminetetraacetic Acid
(May decrease absorption of vanadium)

Ferrous Fumarate
(May decrease absorption of vanadium)

Ferrous Gluconate
(May decrease absorption of vanadium)

Ferrous Sulfate
(May decrease absorption of vanadium)

Iron
(May decrease absorption of iron)

VINPOCETINE

Warfarin Sodium
(Slight changes in prothrombin time noted when used concomitantly; regular monitoring of INR is advised)

VITAMIN A

Acitretin
(May produce additive toxicity effects)

All-trans-retinoic Acid
(May produce additive toxicity effects)

Alpha-Tocopherol Polyethylene Glycol Succinate (TPGS)
(TPGS may increase the absorption of vitamin A)

Bexarotene
(May produce additive toxicity effects)

Chitosan
(Might bind to Chitosan)

Cholestyramine
(May decrease vitamin A absorption)

Colestipol
(May decrease vitamin A absorption)

Etretinate
(May produce additive toxicity effects)

Fat Substitute
(May inhibit vitamin A absorption)

Fucoxanthin
(Concomitant intake of beta-carotene and fucoxanthin may increase the absorption of fucoxanthin)

Glucomannan
(Decreased absorption of fat-soluble vitamins)

Isotretinoin
(May produce additive toxicity effects)

Medium-Chain Triglycerides
(MCT may facilitate the absorption of Vitamin A)

Mineral Oil
(May decrease vitamin A absorption)

Oral Contraceptives
(May increase serum retinol)

Orlistat
(May decrease vitamin A absorption)

Vitamin K
(Large doses of vitamin A may decrease absorption of vitamin K)

VITAMIN B6

5-Hydroxytryptophan
(May enhance 5-HTP conversion to serotonin)

Alcohol
(Chronic and excessive use may cause vitamin B6 deficiency)

Amiodarone Hydrochloride
(Concomitant vitamin B6 may enhance amiodarone-induced photosensitivity reactions)

Carbamazepine
(Chronic use may decrease plasma pyridoxal 5'-phosphate levels)

Cycloserine
(May result in vitamin B6 deficiency)

Ethionamide
(May increase vitamin B6 requirements)

Folate
(May be synergistic in lowering serum homocysteine levels)

Fosphenytoin
(Vitamin B6 may lower plasma phenytoin levels)

Hydralazine
(May increase vitamin B6 requirements)

Isoniazid
(May result in vitamin B6 deficiency)

Levodopa
(Vitamin B6 may reverse therapeutic effects of levodopa if not given with carbidopa)

Oral Contraceptives
(May increase vitamin B6 requirements)

Penicillamine
(May result in vitamin B6 deficiency)

Phenelzine Sulfate
(May result in vitamin B6 deficiency)

Phenobarbital
(Vitamin B6 may lower phenobarbital plasma levels)

Phenytoin
(Vitamin B6 may lower phenytoin plasma levels)

Piperine
(Piperine may enhance the absorption)

Theophylline
(Vitamin B6 may increase risk of theophylline-induced seizures)

Valproic Acid
(Chronic use may decrease plasma pyridoxal 5'-phosphate)

Vitamin B12
(Synergistic with vitamin B12 to lower homocysteine levels)

VITAMIN B12

Antibiotics, unspecified
(The use of antibiotics may alter the intestinal microflora and may decrease the possible contribution of vitamin B12 by certain inhabitants of the microflora to the body's requirement for the vitamin. This may particularly be a problem for vegetarians)

Calcium
(May reverse metformin-induced decrease of vitamin B12 absorption)

Cholestyramine
(May decrease enterohepatic reabsorption of vitamin B12)

Colchicine
(May decrease absorption of vitamin B12)

Colestipol
(May decrease enterohepatic reabsorption of vitamin B12)

Folate
(May be synergistic in lowering serum homocysteine levels)

Folic Acid
(Synergistic with vitamin B12 to lower homocysteine levels)

Histamine H2-receptor antagonists
(Chronic use of H2-blockers may result in decreased absorption of vitamin B12 naturally found in food sources. They are unlikely to affect the absorption of supplemental vitamin B12)

Metformin
(May decrease absorption of vitamin B12)

Nitrous Oxide
(Inhalation of the anesthetic agent nitrous oxide can produce a functional vitamin B12 deficiency)

Para-Aminosalicylic Acid
(Chronic use of the anti-tuberculosis drug may decrease the absorption of vitamin B12)

Potassium Chloride
(May decrease absorption of dietary vitamin B12)

Proton Pump Inhibitor
(Chronic use of proton pump inhibitors may result in decreased absorption of vitamin B12 found naturally in food sources. They are unlikely to affect the absorption of supplemental vitamin B12)

Vitamin B6
(Synergistic with vitamin B12 to lower homocysteine levels)

VITAMIN C

Alpha-Tocopherol Polyethylene Glycol Succinate (TPGS)
(May help maintain d-alpha-tocopherol in its reduced (antioxidant) form)

Aluminum-containing Compounds, unspecified
(Large doses of vitamin C used at the same time as aluminum-containing antacids has been reported to increase urinary aluminum excretion, suggesting increased aluminum absorption from these antacids)

Arsenic Trioxide
(Ascorbic acid has been found to enhance arsenic trioxide-induced cytotoxicity in multiple myeloma cells. It has also been found to overcome drug resistance in myeloma and to significantly increase the anti-myeloma effects of both arsenic trioxide and melphalan in cell culture models and in animal models)

Aspirin
(Chronic use of high dose aspirin may lead to impaired vitamin C status)

Carbamazepine
(Grapefruit flavonoids may increase bioavailability due to cytochrome P-450 3A4 inhibition)

Chemotherapeutic agents
(May diminish the efficacy of some chemotherapeutic agents)

Chitosan
(May enhance the benefits of Chitosan)

Cisplatin
(Vitamin C may potentiate the antineoplastic activity of cisplatin. It may also help ameliorate the nephrotoxic effect of cisplatin)

Copper
(One study showed that high doses of vitamin C negatively affected copper status in men. Other studies have shown no such effects)

Cyclosporine
(Grapefruit flavonoids may increase bioavailability due to cytochrome P-450 3A4 inhibition)

Doxorubicin Hydrochloride
(Vitamin C may potentiate the antineoplastic activity of doxorubicin. It may also help ameliorate the cardiotoxic effect of doxorubicin)

Estrogen
(Ascorbic acid may enhance 17 beta-estradiol inhibition of oxidized LDL formation)

Felodipine
(Grapefruit flavonoids may increase bioavailability due to cytochrome P-450 3A4 inhibition)

Flavonoids
(Vitamin C may act synergistically with various flavonoids)

Gamma-Tocopherol
(Helps to maintain Gamma-Tocopherol in its reduced (antioxidant) form)

Glutathione
(Vitamin C may maintain reduced Glutathione levels in cells)

Iron
(May enhance absorption of iron)

Iron Supplements
(Vitamin C used concomitantly with nonheme iron supplements may increase the uptake of iron)

Lovastatin
(Grapefruit flavonoids may increase bioavailability due to cytochrome P-450 3A4 inhibition)

Melphalan
(Ascorbic acid has been found to enhance arsenic trioxide-induced cytotoxicity in multiple myeloma cells. It has also been found to overcome drug resistance in myeloma and to significantly increase the anti-myeloma effects of both arsenic trioxide and melphalan in cell culture models and in animal models)

Melphalan Hydrochloride
(Ascorbic acid has been found to enhance arsenic trioxide-induced cytotoxicity in multiple myeloma cells. It has also been found to overcome drug resistance in myeloma and to significantly increase the anti-myeloma effects of both arsenic trioxide and melphalan in cell culture models and in animal models)

Nisoldipine
(Grapefruit flavonoids may increase bioavailability due to cytochrome P-450 3A4 inhibition)

Paclitaxel
  (Vitamin C may potentiate the
  antineoplastic activity of
  paclitaxel)
Piperine
  (Piperine may enhance the
  absorption)
Propranolol
  (Ascorbic acid may affect both
  the absorption process and the
  first-pass metabolism of
  propranolol. Heart rate has been
  found to decrease less when
  propranolol was administered with
  ascorbic acid, when compared to
  controls. The interaction has little
  biological importance)
Propranolol Hydrochloride
  (Ascorbic acid may affect both
  the absorption process and the
  first-pass metabolism of
  propranolol. Heart rate has been
  found to decrease less when
  propranolol was administered with
  ascorbic acid, when compared to
  controls. The interaction has little
  biological importance)
Rutin
  (Prevention of Vitamin C
  oxidation, enhanced and/or
  inhibition of absorption with
  flavonoids)
Saquinavir
  (Grapefruit flavonoids may
  increase bioavailability due to
  cytochrome P-450 3A4 inhibition)
Selenium
  (May decrease absorption of
  selenium. The protective effect of
  selenite in tumorgenesis may be
  nullified by vitamin C)
Simvastatin
  (Grapefruit flavonoids may
  increase bioavailability due to
  cytochrome P-450 3A4 inhibition)
Vitamin E
  (Vitamin C may regenerate or
  spare d-aplha-tocopherol)

VITAMIN D
Alpha-Tocopherol
  Polyethylene Glycol
  Succinate (TPGS)
  (TPGS may increase the
  absorption of vitamin D)
Bone Meal
  (Increased absorption of Calcium)
Calcium
  (Concomitant intake of calcium
  and vitamin D may be more
  effective than no therapy or
  calcium alone in corticosteroid-
  induced osteoporosis)
Chitosan
  (Might bind to Chitosan)
Cholestyramine
  (Concomitant intake of
  cholestyramine and vitamin D
  may reduce the absorption of
  vitamin D)
Colestipol
  (Concomitant intake of colestipol
  and vitamin D may reduce the
  absorption of vitamin D)
Fat Substitute
  (Olestra inhibits the absorption of
  vitamin D as well as the other
  fat-soluble vitamins A, E, and K)
Glucomannan
  (Decreased absorption of fat-
  soluble vitamins)
Indinavir Sulfate
  (The HIV protease inhibitors
  ritonavir, indinavir, and nelfinavir
  may impair vitamin D
  bioactivation to 1, 25-
  dihydroxyvitamin D)
Ipriflavone
  (Additive effects with Ipriflavone)
Ketoconazole
  (Ketoconazole may inhibit the
  biosynthesis and catabolism of 1,
  25-dihydroxyvitamin D)
Medium-Chain Triglycerides
  (MCT may facilitate the
  absorption of Vitamin D)
Mineral Oil
  (Concomitant use of mineral oil
  and vitamin D may reduce the
  absorption of vitamin D)

Nelfinavir Mesylate
  (The HIV protease inhibitors
  ritonavir, indinavir, and nelfinavir
  may impair vitamin D
  bioactivation to 1, 25-
  dihydroxyvitamin D)
Olestra
  (Olestra inhibits the absorption of
  vitamin D as well as the other
  fat-soluble vitamins A, E, and K)
Orlistat
  (Orlistat may decrease the
  absorption of vitamin D)
Phenobarbital
  (Phenobarbital may reduce the
  plasma levels of 25-
  hydroxyvitamin D by inhibiting
  vitamin D 25-hydroxylase activity
  in the liver)
Phenytoin
  (Phenytoin may reduce the plasma
  levels of 25-hydroxyvitamin D by
  inhibiting vitamin D 25-
  hydroxylase activity in the liver)
Ritonavir
  (The HIV protease inhibitors
  ritonavir, indinavir, and nelfinavir
  may impair vitamin D
  bioactivation to 1, 25-
  dihydroxyvitamin D)
Thiazides
  (Concomitant use of thiazides and
  pharmacologic doses of vitamin D
  may cause hypercalcemia in some)

VITAMIN E
Abciximab
  (High doses of vitamin E may
  potentiate the effects of
  antiplatelet drugs)
Allium sativum
  (Some herbs, including garlic and
  ginkgo, possess antithrombotic
  activity. High doses of vitamin E
  used at the same time as these
  herbs may enhance their
  antithrombotic activity)
Alpha-Tocopherol
  Polyethylene Glycol
  Succinate (TPGS)
  (TPGS may increase the
  absorption of all forms of vitamin

E (gamma-tocopherol, tocotrienols))

Amiodarone Hydrochloride
(Alpha-tocopherol may ameliorate some of the adverse side effects of amiodarone)

Anticonvulsants
(Anticonvulsants may lower plasma vitamin E levels)

Antiplatelet Drugs
(High doses of vitamin E may potentiate the effects of antiplatelet drugs)

Aspirin
(High doses of vitamin E may potentiate the effects of antiplatelet drugs)

Astaxanthin
(Concomitant intake of vitamin E and astaxanthin may decrease astaxanthin absorption)

Beta-Carotene
(Some studies have suggested that oral supplements of beta-carotene may cause a decrease in serum levels of alpha-tocopherol. However, more recent and much larger and longer studies have demonstrated that supplementation with beta-carotene does not alter serum concentrations of vitamin E)

Beta-Sitosterol
(May lower serum levels of vitamin E)

Carbamazepine
(Anticonvulsants may lower plasma vitamin E levels)

Chitosan
(Might bind to Chitosan)

Cholestyramine
(May decrease vitamin E absorption)

Clopidogrel Bisulfate
(High doses of vitamin E may potentiate the effects of antiplatelet drugs)

Colestipol
(May decrease vitamin E absorption)

Cyclosporine
(Based on cell culture studies, alpha-tocopherol may help to ameliorate the renal side effects of cyclosporine)

Dietary Fiber
(Dietary fiber supplementation may decrease the antioxidative effect of a supplement containing alpha-tocopherol and carotenoids)

Dipyridamole
(High doses of vitamin E may potentiate the effects of antiplatelet drugs)

Eptifibatide
(High doses of vitamin E may potentiate the effects of antiplatelet drugs)

Ezetimibe
(May inhibit the intestinal absorption of alpha-tocopherol)

Fat Substitute
(Olestra inhibits the absorption of vitamin E, as well as the other fat-soluble vitamins, A, D, and K, carotenoids and flavonoids)

Fatty Acids, polyunsaturated
(Supplementary PUFAs may increase vitamin E requirements. High polyunsaturated fatty acid intakes should be accompanied by increased vitamin E intakes to prevent their oxidation)

Fiber
(Dietary fiber supplementation may decrease the antioxidative effect of a supplement containing alpha-tocopherol and carotenoids)

Ginkgo biloba
(Some herbs, including garlic and ginkgo, possess antithrombotic activity. High doses of vitamin E used at the same time as these herbs may enhance their antithrombotic activity)

Glucomannan
(Decreased absorption of fat-soluble vitamins)

Iron
(Most iron supplements contain the ferrous form of iron. This

cation can oxidize unesterified vitamin E to its pro-oxidant form if taken concomitantly. This does not occur with esterified vitamin E (alpha-tocopherol acetate and succinate))

Isoniazid
(May decrease vitamin E absorption)

Medium-Chain Triglycerides
(MCT may facilitate the absorption of Vitamin E)

Mineral Oil
(May decrease vitamin E absorption)

Neomycin
(May impair utilization of vitamin E)

Olestra
(Olestra inhibits the absorption of vitamin E, as well as the other fat-soluble vitamins, A, D, and K, carotenoids and flavonoids)

Orlistat
(Inhibits vitamin E absorption)

Ox Bile, Desiccated
(Dessicated ox bile may increase absorption of vitamin E)

Phenobarbital
(Anticonvulsants may lower plasma vitamin E levels)

Phenytoin
(Anticonvulsants may lower plasma vitamin E levels)

Phytostanols
(Phytostanols may interfere with absorption and lower serum levels)

Phytosterols
(Phytosterols may interfere with absorption and lower serum levels)

Plant Phenolic Compounds
(These substances may participate in redox cycling reactions and help maintain levels of reduced vitamin E)

Selenium
(Selenium may function synergistically with vitamin E)

Sucralfate
(Interferes with vitamin E absorption)
Ticlopidine Hydrochloride
(High doses of vitamin E may potentiate the effects of antiplatelet drugs)
Tirofiban Hydrochloride
(High doses of vitamin E may potentiate the effects of antiplatelet drugs)
Vitamin C
(Vitamin C may regenerate or spare d-aplha-tocopherol)
Vitamin K
(Intake of very large doses of vitamin E may result in vitamin K deficiency)
Warfarin Sodium
(Vitamin E may enhance anticoagulant response. Monitor INRs and adjust dose of warfarin appropriately if necessary)
Zidovudine
(Vitamin E may ameliorate myelosuppressive side effects of zidovudine)

VITAMIN E PHOSPHATE

Abciximab
(Vitamin E phosphate may potentiate the effects of antiplatelet drugs (eg, abciximab))
Aspirin
(Vitamin E phosphate may potentiate the effects of antiplatelet drugs (eg, aspirin))
Aspirin Buffered
(Vitamin E phosphate may potentiate the effects of antiplatelet drugs (eg, aspirin))
Aspirin, Enteric Coated
(Vitamin E phosphate may potentiate the effects of antiplatelet drugs (eg, aspirin))
Clopidogrel Bisulfate
(Vitamin E phosphate may potentiate the effects of antiplatelet drugs (eg, clopidogrel))
Dipyridamole
(Vitamin E phosphate may potentiate the effects of

antiplatelet drugs (eg, dipyridamole))
Eptifibatide
(Vitamin E phosphate may potentiate the effects of antiplatelet drugs (eg, eptifibatide))
Fish Oils
(Fish oils possess antiplatelet activity. Vitamin E phosphate may potentiate the antiplatelet activity of fish oils)
Heparin
(Vitamin E phosphate may potentiate the effects of anticoagulant drugs (eg, heparin))
Heparin Calcium
(Vitamin E phosphate may potentiate the effects of anticoagulant drugs (eg, heparin))
Heparin Sodium
(Vitamin E phosphate may potentiate the effects of anticoagulant drugs (eg, heparin))
Herbals, Multiple
(Some herbal products, including garlic, ginkgo, ginseng and curcuminoids, possess antithrombotic activity. Concomitant use of vitamin E phosphate with these herbals may enhance their antithrombotic activity)
Ticlopidine Hydrochloride
(Vitamin E phosphate may potentiate the effects of antiplatelet drugs (eg, ticlopidine))
Tirofiban Hydrochloride
(Vitamin E phosphate may potentiate the effects of antiplatelet drugs (eg, tirofiban))
Warfarin Sodium
(Vitamin E phosphate may potentiate the effects of anticoagulant drugs (eg, warfarin))

VITAMIN K

Alpha-Tocopherol Polyethylene Glycol Succinate (TPGS)
(TPGS may increase the absorption of vitamin K)

Antibiotics, broad spectrum, unspecified
(Broad spectrum antibiotics may sterilize the bowel and decrease the vitamin K contribution to the body by the intestinal microflora)
Aspirin
(Salicylates in large doses may inhibit vitamin K epoxide reductase resulting in vitamin K deficiency)
Cefamandole Nafate
(Can cause vitamin K deficiency and hypoprothrombinemia)
Cefazolin Sodium
(Can cause vitamin K deficiency and hypoprothrombinemia)
Cefmenoxime
(Can cause vitamin K deficiency and hypoprothrombinemia)
Cefoperazone Sodium
(Can cause vitamin K deficiency and hypoprothrombinemia)
Cefotetan
(Can cause vitamin K deficiency and hypoprothrombinemia)
Chitosan
(Might bind to Chitosan)
Cholestyramine
(May reduce vitamin K absorption)
Colestipol
(May reduce vitamin K absorption)
Fat Substitute
(Inhibits absorption of vitamin K as well as the other fat-soluble vitamins A, D, and E)
Glucomannan
(Decreased absorption of fat-soluble vitamins)
Ipriflavone
(Additive effects with Ipriflavone)
Latamoxef
(Can cause vitamin K deficiency and hypothrombinemia)
Medium-Chain Triglycerides
(MCT may facilitate the absorption of Vitamin K)
Mineral Oil
(May reduce vitamin K absorption)

Olestra
(Inhibits absorption of vitamin K as well as the other fat-soluble vitamins A, D, and E)

Orlistat
(May reduce vitamin K absorption)

Salicylates
(Salicylates in large doses may inhibit vitamin K epoxide reductase resulting in vitamin K deficiency)

Squalene
(May reduce vitamin K absorption)

Vitamin A
(Large doses of vitamin A may decrease absorption of vitamin K)

Vitamin E
(Intake of very large doses of vitamin E may result in vitamin K deficiency)

Warfarin Sodium
(Vitamin K can antagonize effects of warfarin)

VITAMINS WITH FLUORIDE

Xylitol
(The combination of xylitol and the use of fluoride toothpastes may give better anticariogenic effects than the use of either alone)

WARFARIN SODIUM

7-Oxo-Dehydroepiandrosterone
(7-Oxo-DHEA may have an effect on platelet membrane fluidity. Therefore those taking warfarin should exercise caution in the use of 7-Oxo-DHEA)

Alpha-Tocopherol Polyethylene Glycol Succinate (TPGS)
(High doses (greater than 500 mg) of TPGS may enhance the anticoagulant response of warfarin. Monitor INRs and adjust dose of warfarin if necessary)

Borage Oil
(Increased anticoagulant and antiplatelet effects when taken with Borage Oil)

Chlorella
(Chlorella may interfere with effects)

Coenzyme Q10 (CoQ10)
(May decrease the effectiveness of warfarin)

Curcuminoids
(Curcuminoids may enhance the anticoagulant effect)

Docosahexaenoic Acid (DHA)
(Because DHA my have antithrombotic activity, caution should be exercised with concomitant warfarin therapy)

Eicosapentaenoic Acid (EPA)
(Because of the possible antithrombotic activity of EPA, caution should be exercised with concomitant warfarin therapy)

Evening Primrose Oil
(EPO may increase bleeding tendencies)

Fish Oil
(Because of the possible antithrombotic effect of fish oil supplements, caution should be exercised with concomitant warfarin therapy)

Flaxseed Oil
(Interactions may occur between flaxseed oil and its metabolites and warfarin, aspirin, and NSAIDs. Such interactions, if they were to occur, might be manifested by nosebleeds and increased susceptibility to bruising. If this does occur, consideration should be given to lowering or stopping intake)

Gamma-Tocopherol
(Enhanced anticoagulant response of warfarin)

Hemp Seed Oil
(Increased bleeding and susceptibility to bruising)

Inositol Nicotinate
(Nicotinic acid may enhance anticoagulant effects)

Iodine
(Potassium iodide may decrease the anticoagulant effectiveness of warfarin)

Nattokinase (Subtilisin NAT)
(The use of nattokinase along with oral anticoagulants (eg, warfarin) may cause serious adverse events, especially excessive bleeding. Nattokinase is contraindicated in patients taking the anticoagulant warfarin. Administration of nattokinase is contraindicated in those with bleeding disorders and in those taking the anticoagulant warfarin)

Niacin
(Nicotinic acid may enhance anticoagulant effects; monitor closely)

Psyllium
(Reduced absorption of warfarin sodium)

Red Yeast Rice
(Increase in the INR as well as bleeding)

Tiratricol (TRIAC)
(May increase hypoprothrombinemic effect)

Tocotrienols
(Large dose Tocotrienols may enhance anticoagulant effects)

Vinpocetine
(Slight changes in prothrombin time noted when used concomitantly; regular monitoring of INR is advised)

Vitamin E
(Vitamin E may enhance anticoagulant response. Monitor INRs and adjust dose of warfarin appropriately if necessary)

Vitamin E Phosphate
(Vitamin E phosphate may potentiate the effects of anticoagulant drugs (eg, warfarin))

Vitamin K
(Vitamin K can antagonize effects of warfarin)

Wheat Grass/Barley Grass
(Wheat Grass supplements may affect the INR)

WHEAT GRASS/BARLEY GRASS

Warfarin Sodium
(Wheat Grass supplements may affect the INR)

WHEY PROTEIN ISOLATE

L-Tryptophan
(May increase the brain availability of L-tryptophan)

WHEY PROTEIN

L-Tryptophan
(May increase the brain availability of L-tryptophan)

XANTHOHUMOL

Cytochrome p450 1a2 substrates (selected)
(Xanthohumol inhibits cytochrome p450, and although there are no known reports of any interactions with drugs and xanthohumol, those using drugs that are metabolized via the cytochrome p450 system, for example, the statin atorvastatin, should be cautious in the use of xanthohumol supplements)

Cytochrome p450 2c8 substrates (selected)
(Xanthohumol inhibits cytochrome p450, and although there are no known reports of any interactions with drugs and xanthohumol, those using drugs that are metabolized via the cytochrome p450 system, for example, the statin atorvastatin, should be cautious in the use of xanthohumol supplements)

Cytochrome p450 2c9 substrates (selected)
(Xanthohumol inhibits cytochrome p450, and although there are no known reports of any interactions with drugs and xanthohumol, those using drugs that are metabolized via the cytochrome p450 system, for example, the statin atorvastatin, should be cautious in the use of xanthohumol supplements)

Cytochrome p450 2c18 substrates (selected)
(Xanthohumol inhibits cytochrome p450, and although there are no known reports of any interactions with drugs and xanthohumol,

those using drugs that are metabolized via the cytochrome p450 system, for example, the statin atorvastatin, should be cautious in the use of xanthohumol supplements)

Cytochrome p450 2c19 substrates (selected)
(Xanthohumol inhibits cytochrome p450, and although there are no known reports of any interactions with drugs and xanthohumol, those using drugs that are metabolized via the cytochrome p450 system, for example, the statin atorvastatin, should be cautious in the use of xanthohumol supplements)

Cytochrome p450 2d6 substrates (selected)
(Xanthohumol inhibits cytochrome p450, and although there are no known reports of any interactions with drugs and xanthohumol, those using drugs that are metabolized via the cytochrome p450 system, for example, the statin atorvastatin, should be cautious in the use of xanthohumol supplements)

Cytochrome p450 3a substrates (selected)
(Xanthohumol inhibits cytochrome p450, and although there are no known reports of any interactions with drugs and xanthohumol, those using drugs that are metabolized via the cytochrome p450 system, for example, the statin atorvastatin, should be cautious in the use of xanthohumol supplements)

Cytochrome p450 3a4 substrates (selected)
(Xanthohumol inhibits cytochrome p450, and although there are no known reports of any interactions with drugs and xanthohumol, those using drugs that are metabolized via the cytochrome p450 system, for example, the

statin atorvastatin, should be cautious in the use of xanthohumol supplements)

XYLITOL

Arginine Hydrochloride
(Arginine-containing mints have been found to have anticariogenic activity secondary to their ability to buffer the acid produced by cariogenic bacteria. The combination of xylitol and arginine-containing mints may give better anticariogenic effects than the use of either alone)

Arginine base
(Arginine-containing mints have been found to have anticariogenic activity secondary to their ability to buffer the acid produced by cariogenic bacteria. The combination of xylitol and arginine-containing mints may give better anticariogenic effects than the use of either alone)

Fluorine & Fluoride Preparations
(The combination of xylitol and the use of fluoride toothpastes may give better anticariogenic effects than the use of either alone)

L-Arginine
(Arginine-containing mints have been found to have anticariogenic activity secondary to their ability to buffer the acid produced by cariogenic bacteria. The combination of xylitol and arginine-containing mints may give better anticariogenic effects than the use of either alone)

Sodium Fluoride
(The combination of xylitol and the use of fluoride toothpastes may give better anticariogenic effects than the use of either alone)

Sulfur Hexafluoride
(The combination of xylitol and the use of fluoride toothpastes may give better anticariogenic

effects than the use of either alone)

Vitamins with Fluoride
(The combination of xylitol and the use of fluoride toothpastes may give better anticariogenic effects than the use of either alone)

YOHIMBINE HYDROCHLORIDE

L-Arginine
(L-Arginine may potentiate effects)

ZALCITABINE

Acetyl-L-Carnitine
(May lead to decreased acetyl-L-carnitine levels)

L-Carnitine
(May produce L-Carnitine deficiencies)

ZIDOVUDINE

Riboflavin (Vitamin B2)
(Riboflavin may reverse nucleoside analogue-induced lactic acidosis in mild riboflavin deficiencies)

Vitamin E
(Vitamin E may ameliorate myelosuppressive side effects of zidovudine)

ZINC

Beverages, caffeine-containing
(Concomitant intake of coffee, caffeinated beverages, or caffeine and zinc may depress the absorption of zinc)

Bisphosphonates
(Concomitant intake of a bisphosphonate and zinc may decrease the absorption of both the bisphosphonate and zinc)

Caffeine
(Concomitant intake of coffee, caffeinated beverages, or caffeine and zinc may depress the absorption of zinc)

Calcium
(Concomitant intake of calcium and zinc may depress zinc absorption in postmenopausal women)

Chitosan
(Might bind to Chitosan)

Copper
(Concomitant intake of copper and zinc may depress the absorption of copper. Intake of large doses of zinc can negatively affect the copper status of the body)

Cysteine-Containing Proteins
(Foods rich in cysteine-containing proteins (eg, animal muscle tissue) may increase the absorption of zinc if ingested concomitantly)

Folate
(Folic acid may decrease zinc absorption)

Inositol
(Concomitant intake of inositol hexaphosphate and zinc may depress the absorption of zinc)

Inositol Hexaphosphate
(May form chelates with Inositol Hexaphosphate)

Iron
(Concomitant intake of iron and zinc may depress the absorption of both iron and zinc)

L-Cysteine
(Concomitant intake of L-cysteine and zinc may enhance the absorption of zinc)

L-Histidine
(Concomitant intake of L-histidine and zinc may enhance the absorption of zinc)

L-Methionine
(Concomitant intake of L-methionine and zinc may enhance the absorption of zinc)

N-Acetyl-L-Cysteine (NAC)
(Concomitant intake of NAC and zinc may enhance the absorption of zinc)

Oxalic Acid
(Concomitant intake of zinc with foods rich in oxalic acid (eg, spinach, sweet potatoes, rhubarb, beans) may depress the absorption of zinc)

Pectin
(Decreased absorption of Zinc)

Penicillamine
(Concomitant administration of penicillamine and zinc may depress absorption of zinc)

Phosphate Salts
(Concomitant intake of zinc and phosphate salts may decrease the absorption of zinc)

Phosphorus
(Decreased absorption of Zinc)

Phytic Acid
(Concomitant intake of zinc with foods rich in phytic acid (eg, unleavened bread, raw beans, seeds, nuts, grains, soy isolates) may depress the absorption of zinc)

Psyllium
(Decreased absorption of Zinc)

Quinolones
(Concomitant intake of a quinolone and zinc may decrease the absorption of both the quinolone and zinc)

Sodium Alginates and other Phyco-Polysaccharides
(Decreased absorption of Zinc)

Soy Protein
(May reduce availability of zinc)

Tannins
(Concomitant intake of tea (tannins) and zinc may cause decreased absorption of zinc)

Tetracyclines
(Concomitant intake of a tetracycline and zinc may decrease the absorption of both the tetracycline and zinc)

ZINC L-CARNOSINE

Histamine H2-receptor antagonists
(The combination of an H2 blocker and zinc L-carnosine may be more effective than when each agent is used alone)

Sucralfate
(The combination of cytoprotectant sucralfate and zinc L-carnosine may be more effective than when each agent is used alone)

Companion Drug Index

This index suggests nutritional supplements that may be used, in conjunction with prescription drug therapy, to reverse drug-induced side effects, relieve symptoms of the illness itself, or treat sequelae of the initial disease. Supplements, together with their associated brands, are listed alphabetically under each condition. Italic page numbers refer to combination-product tables.

ACNE MEDICAMENTOSA

May result from the use of azathioprine, dantrolene sodium, ethionamide, haloperidol, isoniazid, lithium carbonate, lithium citrate, oral contraceptives containing norethindrone or norgestrel, phenytoin, thyroid hormones or trimethadione. The following products may be recommended:

NOBILETIN 455
VITAMIN A 627

ALCOHOLISM, HYPOCALCEMIA SECONDARY TO

Alcoholism may be treated with disulfiram or naltrexone hydrochloride. The following products may be recommended for relief of hypocalcemia:

CALCIUM 109
CALCIUM COMBINATION PRODUCTS . 743

ALCOHOLISM, HYPOMAGNESEMIA SECONDARY TO

Alcoholism may be treated with disulfiram or naltrexone hydrochloride. The following products may be recommended for relief of hypomagnesemia:

MAGNESIUM 404

ALCOHOLISM, VITAMINS AND MINERALS DEFICIENCY SECONDARY TO

Alcoholism may be treated with disulfiram or naltrexone

hydrochloride. The following products may be recommended for relief of vitamins and minerals deficiency:

ALPHA-TOCOPHERYL NICOTINATE . . . 31
ALPHA-TOCOPHEROL POLYETHYLENE
GLYCOL SUCCINATE (TPGS) 29
MULTIVITAMIN PRODUCTS 750
MULTIVITAMIN AND MINERAL
PRODUCTS 758
RIBOFLAVIN (VITAMIN B2) 547
SPIRULINA 589
THIAMIN 609
VITAMIN A 627
VITAMIN B COMPLEX PRODUCTS . . . 785
VITAMIN B6 634
VITAMIN B12 644
VITAMIN C 654
VITAMIN D 669
VITAMIN E 682
VITAMIN E PHOSPHATE 703
VITAMIN K 708

ANCYLOSTOMIASIS, IRON-DEFICIENCY ANEMIA SECONDARY TO

Ancylostomiasis may be treated with mebendazole or thiabendazole. The following products may be recommended for relief of iron-deficiency anemia:

IRON 324
IRON COMBINATION PRODUCTS 746

ANEMIA, IRON-DEFICIENCY

May result from the use of chronic salicylate therapy or nonsteroidal anti-inflammatory drugs. The

following products may be recommended:

IRON 324
IRON COMBINATION PRODUCTS 746

ANGINA, UNSTABLE

May be treated with beta blockers, calcium channel blockers or nitrates. The following products may be recommended for relief of symptoms:

8-PRENYLNARINGENIN 7
ACETYLCYSTEINE 16
ALPHA-LIPOIC ACID 25
ASTAXANTHIN 42
BAICALEIN 50
COCOA FLAVONOIDS 149
COENZYME Q10 (COQ10) 151
COPPER 161
CURCUMINOIDS 167
DAIDZEIN 175
DOCOSAHEXAENOIC ACID (DHA) . . . 190
EICOSAPENTAENOIC ACID (EPA) . . . 195
EQUOL 198
FISH OIL 208
FLAXSEED LIGNANS 214
FLAXSEED OIL 218
FOLATE 225
GAMMA-ORYZANOL 249
GENISTEIN 258
GLYCITEIN 282
GREEN TEA CATECHINS 285
HYDROXYTYROSOL 303
L-CITRULLINE 344
L-THEANINE 365

ARTHRITIS

May be treated with biologicals, corticosteroids or nonsteroidal anti-inflammatory drugs. The following products may be recommended for relief of symptoms:

BRONCHITIS, CHRONIC, ACUTE EXACERBATION OF

May be treated with cefdinir, cefixime, cefpodoxime proxetil, cefprozil, ceftibuten dihydrate, cefuroxime axetil, cilastatin sodium, clarithromycin, imipenem, quinolones or sulfamethoxazole-trimethoprim. The following products may be recommended for relief of symptoms:

BURN INFECTIONS, SEVERE, NUTRIENTS DEFICIENCY SECONDARY TO

Severe burn infections may be treated with anti-infectives. The following products may be recommended for relief of nutrient deficiency:

CANCER, NUTRIENTS DEFICIENCY SECONDARY TO

Cancer may be treated with chemotherapeutic agents. The following products may be recommended for relief of nutrient deficiency:

CONGESTIVE HEART FAILURE, NUTRIENTS DEFICIENCY SECONDARY TO

Congestive heart failure may be treated with ace inhibitors, angiotensin II receptor antagonists, beta blockers, cardiac glycosides or diuretics. The following products may be recommended for relief of nutrient deficiency:

CONSTIPATION

May result from the use of ace inhibitors, anticholinergics, anticonvulsants, antidepressants, beta blockers, bile acid sequestrants, butyrophenones, calcium and aluminum-containing antacids, calcium channel blockers, ganglionic blockers, hematinics, monoamine oxidase inhibitors, narcotic analgesics, nonsteroidal anti-inflammatory drugs or phenothiazines and statins. The

following products may be recommended:

CYSTIC FIBROSIS, NUTRIENTS DEFICIENCY SECONDARY TO

Cystic fibrosis may be treated with dornase alfa. The following products may be recommended for relief of nutrient deficiency:

DENTAL CARIES

May be treated with fluoride preparations or vitamin and fluoride supplements. The following products may be recommended for relief of symptoms:

DIABETES MELLITUS, CONSTIPATION SECONDARY TO

Diabetes mellitus may be treated with insulins or oral hypoglycemic agents. The following products may be recommended for relief of constipation:

DIABETES MELLITUS, POORLY CONTROLLED, VITAMINS AND MINERALS DEFICIENCY SECONDARY TO

Diabetes mellitus may be treated with insulins or oral hypoglycemic agents. The following products may be recommended for relief of vitamin and mineral deficiency:

DIARRHEA

May result from the use of acarbose, ace inhibitors, alprazolam, antibiotics, beta blockers, cardiac glycosides, chemotherapeutic agents, colchicine, diuretics, divalproex sodium, ethosuximide, fluoxetine hydrochloride, hydralazine hydrochloride, levodopa, lithium carbonate, lithium citrate, magnesium-containing antacids, mesna, metformin hydrochloride, misoprostol, nonsteroidal anti-inflammatory drugs, olsalazine sodium, pancrelipase, potassium supplements, procainamide hydrochloride, reserpine, succimer, ticlopidine hydrochloride or valproic acid. The following products may be recommended:

DIARRHEA, INFECTIOUS

May be treated with ciprofloxacin, sulfamethoxazole-trimethoprim or vancomycin hydrochloride. The following products may be recommended for relief of symptoms:

FLUSHING EPISODES

May result from the use of lipid lowering doses of niacin. The following products may be recommended:

GASTRITIS, IRON-DEFICIENCY SECONDARY TO

Gastritis may be treated with histamine H2 receptor antagonists, proton pump inhibitors or sucralfate. The following products may be recommended for relief of iron deficiency:

GASTROESOPHAGEAL REFLUX DISEASE

May be treated with histamine H2 receptor antagonists, proton pump inhibitors or sucralfate. The following products may be recommended for relief of symptoms:

HUMAN IMMUNODEFICIENCY VIRUS (HIV) INFECTIONS, NUTRIENTS DEFICIENCY SECONDARY TO

HIV infections may be treated with fusion inhibitors, hiv and integrase strand transfer inhibitors, non-nucleoside reverse transcriptase inhibitors, nucleoside reverse transcriptase inhibitors or protease inhibitors. The following products may be recommended for relief of nutrient deficiency:

HYPERPARATHYROIDISM, NUTRIENTS DEFICIENCY SECONDARY TO

Hyperparathyroidism may be treated with propylthiouracil. The following products may be recommended for relief of nutrient deficiency:

HYPERTHYROIDISM, NUTRIENTS DEFICIENCY SECONDARY TO

Hyperthyroidism may be treated with methimazole or propylthiouracil. The following products may be recommended for relief of nutrient deficiency:

HYPOKALEMIA

May result from the use of aldesleukin, amphotericin B, carboplatin, corticosteroids, diuretics, foscarnet sodium, mycophenolate mofetil, pamidronate disodium, tacrolimus or thiazides. The following products may be recommended:

HYPOMAGNESEMIA

May result from the use of aldesleukin, aminoglycosides, amphotericin B, caroboplatin, cisplatin, cyclosporine, diuretics, foscarnet, pamidronate, sargramostim or tacrolimus. The following products may be recommended:

HYPOPARATHYROIDISM

May be treated with vitamin d sterols. The following products may be recommended for relief of symptoms:

HYPOTHYROIDISM, CONSTIPATION SECONDARY TO

Hypothyroidism may be treated with

thyroid hormones. The following products may be recommended for relief of constipation:

INFECTIONS, BACTERIAL, UPPER RESPIRATORY TRACT

May be treated with amoxicillin-clavulanate, cephalosporins, doxycycline, erythromycin, macrolide antibiotics, minocycline hydrochloride or penicillins. The following products may be recommended for relief of symptoms:

INFECTIONS, SKIN AND SKIN STRUCTURE

May be treated with aminoglycosides, amoxicillin, amoxicillin-clavulanate, cephalosporins, daptomycin, doxycycline, erythromycin, linezolid, macrolide antibiotics, penicillins, quinolones or tigecycline. The following products may be recommended for relief of symptoms:

IRRITABLE BOWEL SYNDROME

May be treated with 5-HT3 receptor antagonists, anticholinergic and combinations, dicyclomine hydrochloride or hyoscyamine

sulfate. The following products may be recommended for relief of symptoms:

ISCHEMIC HEART DISEASE

May be treated with beta blockers, calcium channel blockers, isosorbide dinitrate, isosorbide mononitrate or nitroglycerin. The following products may be recommended for relief of symptoms:

MYOCARDIAL INFARCTION, ACUTE

May be treated with ace inhibitors, anticoagulants, beta blockers, nitroglycerin or thrombolytic agents. The following products may be recommended for relief of symptoms:

NECATORIASIS, IRON-DEFICIENCY ANEMIA SECONDARY TO

Necatoriasis may be treated with mebendazole or thiabendazole. The following products may be recommended for relief of iron-deficiency anemia:

OSTEOPOROSIS

May be treated with biphosphonates, calcitonin or estrogens. The following products may be recommended for relief of symptoms:

OSTEOPOROSIS, SECONDARY

May result from the use of carbamazepine, chemotherapeutic agents, heparin, methotrexate sodium, phenytoin, prolonged glucocorticoid therapy or thyroid hormones. The following products may be recommended:

OTITIS MEDIA, ACUTE

May be treated with amoxicillin, amoxicillin-clavulanate, cephalosporins, erythromycin-sulfisoxazole, macrolide antibiotics or sulfamethoxazole-trimethoprim. The following products may be recommended for relief of symptoms:

PANCREATIC INSUFFICIENCY, NUTRIENTS DEFICIENCY SECONDARY TO

Pancreatic insufficiency may be treated with pancrelipase. The following products may be recommended for relief of nutrients deficiency:

PARKINSON'S DISEASE, CONSTIPATION SECONDARY TO

Parkinson's disease may be treated with carbidopa, centrally active anticholinergic agents, COMT inhibitors, dopaminergic agents, levodopa or selective inhibitor of MAO type B. The following products may be recommended for relief of constipation:

PEPTIC ULCER DISEASE

May be treated with histamine H2 receptor antagonists, proton pump inhibitors or sucralfate. The following products may be recommended for relief of symptoms:

PEPTIC ULCER DISEASE, IRON DEFICIENCY SECONDARY TO

Peptic ulcer disease may be treated with histamine H2 receptor antagonists, proton pump inhibitors or sucralfate. The following products may be recommended for relief of iron deficiency:

PHARYNGITIS

May be treated with cephalosporins, macrolide antibiotics or penicillins. The following products may be recommended for relief of symptoms:

RENAL OSTEODYSTROPHY, HYPOCALCEMIA SECONDARY TO

Renal osteodystrophy may be treated with vitamin d sterols. The following products may be recommended for relief of hypocalcemia:

SINUSITIS

May be treated with amoxicillin, amoxicillin-clavulanate, cefprozil, cefuroxime axetil or clarithromycin. The following products may be recommended for relief of symptoms:

SKIN IRRITATION

May result from the use of transdermal drug delivery systems. The following products may be recommended:

TUBERCULOSIS, NUTRIENTS DEFICIENCY SECONDARY TO

Tuberculosis may be treated with capreomycin sulfate, ethambutol hydrochloride, ethionamide, isoniazid, pyrazinamide, rifampin or streptomycin sulfate. The following products may be recommended for relief of nutrient deficiency:

VAGINOSIS, BACTERIAL

May be treated with metronidazole or sulfabenzamide/sulfacetamide/sulfathiozole. The following products may be recommended for relief of symptoms:

VULVOVAGINITIS, CANDIDAL

May result from the use of estrogen-containing oral contraceptives, immunosuppressants or recent broad-spectrum antibiotic therapy. The following products may be recommended:

Supplement Monographs

5-Hydroxytryptophan (5-HTP)

DESCRIPTION

5-Hydroxytryptophan is the immediate precursor in the biosynthesis of the neurotransmitter 5-hydroxytryptamine (5-HT or serotonin). 5-HT itself is derived biochemically from the essential protein amino acid L-tryptophan (see L-Tryptophan).

5-HTP, along with carbidopa, is used in Europe as a pharmaceutical agent for the treatment of depression. It has also been used in the treatment of Gilles de la Tourette syndrome and for the treatment of the self-mutilation symptoms of Lesch-Nyhan syndrome. 5-HTP is an orphan drug in the U.S. for the treatment of postanoxic intention myoclonus, a rare complication of CPR (cardiopulmonary resuscitation). It is used in this disorder in combination with carbidopa.

Until November 1989, L-tryptophan was a popular nutritional supplement in the U.S. In November 1989, the FDA recalled supplementary L-tryptophan because of several reports associating the amino acid with some severe side effects. These side effects were part of a syndrome called the eosinophilia-myalgia syndrome (EMS). The cause of the syndrome was thought to be due to a contaminant in L-tryptophan that was produced from a genetically modified microorganism (GMO), and not from the L-tryptophan itself. The hunt for possible toxicants and contaminants in the suspected L-tryptophan supplements that could be identified as causing EMS immediately began, but although some suspects were identified, none were positively identified that could have caused EMS.

In 1991, the FDA banned L-tryptophan supplements from sale in the U.S. In 2001, the FDA loosened the restriction on the marketing of L-tryptophan supplements, but did ban its importation except under certain circumstances. As of May 2, 2005, the FDA completely cancelled the import ban alert for L-tryptophan. Soon thereafter, L-tryptophan supplements began again appearing on the nutritional supplement marketplace, including in health food stores, compounding pharmacies and over the Internet, where they continue to be found.

5-HTP was intended to fill the gap created by the removal of L-tryptophan from the nutritional supplement marketplace. Because of its chemical and biochemical relationship to L-tryptophan, 5-HTP has been under vigilance by government, academia, industry and consumers for its safety. As of August 1998, the FDA reported that 10 cases of EMS possibly associated with 5-HTP had been documented worldwide, none resulting in death. No new cases of EMS have since been reported.

However, 5-HTP suffers from another problem. High doses of 5-HTP are metabolized peripherally to 5-hydroxytryptamine (5-HT or serotonin) and this can result in elevated serum levels of serotonin, with consequent adverse reactions related to the elevated levels (see Adverse Reactions). In Europe, where 5-HTP is used for the treatment of depression, it is used in combination with carbidopa, which inhibits the peripheral conversion of 5-HTP to serotonin. This is similar to the situation with the use of levodopa in the treatment of Parkinson's disease. For levodopa to be effective in this disorder, its peripheral conversion to dopamine must be prevented. This is the reason why L-dopa is combined with carbidopa and both are used in the treatment of Parkinson's disease. Carbidopa inhibits this conversion.

5-Hydroxytryptophan or 5-HTP is also known as L-5-HTP, L-5-hydroxytryptophan, oxitriptan and L-2-amino-3-(5-hydroxy-1-H-indol-3-yl)propionic acid. Its molecular formula is $C_{11}H_{12}N_2O_3$ and its molecular weight is 220.23 daltons. The structural formula of 5-hydroxytryptophan is:

5-Hydroxytryptophan

A major commercial source of 5-HTP is the African plant *Griffonia simplicifolia*, a relative of carob. Small amounts of 5-HTP, as well as serotonin, are found in food sources, including bananas, tomatoes, plums, avocados, eggplant, walnuts and pineapples.

ACTIONS AND PHARMACOLOGY

ACTIONS

5-HTP may have antidepressant activity. It has putative analgesic and bariatric actions. 5-HTP may also have antioxidant activity.

MECHANISM OF ACTION

The mechanism of the possible antidepressant activity of 5-HTP is accounted for by its conversion to the neurotransmitter serotonin which plays a central role in the affective state. Antidepressants may work by either binding to one or more of the family of serotonin 5-HT receptors (5-HT$_1$ -5-HT$_7$) or by inhibiting the reuptake of serotonin. The tricyclic antidepressants may work, in part, by binding to the serotonin 5-HT$_6$ receptor, a member of the G protein superfamily, which is positively coupled to an adenylate cyclase second-messenger system. The selective serotonin reuptake inhibitors (SSRIs) selectively inhibit the reuptake of serotonin. 5-HTP most likely binds to one or more of the 5-HT receptors, although which one(s) is not known for sure.

There is some evidence that 5-HTP has some analgesic activity in those with fibromyalgia, and, in one study, 5-HTP was found to have some beneficial effect in those with chronic tension headache. The possible analgesic effect of 5-HTP may be accounted for, in part, by its conversion to serotonin. 5-HTP has also been found to increase plasma beta-endorphin and platelet met-enkephalin levels, which may signify a reinforcing effect upon an endogenous analgesic effect.

The mechanism of the putative bariatric action of 5-HTP is not well understood. Serotonin is known to regulate feeding behavior and decrease food intake in humans and rodents. One study suggests that this effect may be mediated via leptin. Serum leptin levels in mice were found to increase following systemic injection of 5-HTP. Leptin, an adipocyte-derived protein product of the ob(obesity) gene, is a multifunctional polypeptide associated with the development of obesity-related disorders in humans.

The hydroxyl radical is one of the most potent, and destructive, of all of the reactive oxygen species (ROS). 5-HTP was reported to be a more potent *in vitro* hydroxyl radical scavenger than either vitamin C or melatonin.

PHARMACOKINETICS

A significant amount of an ingested dose of 5-HTP is decarboxylated in the small intestine to 5-hydroxytryptamine (5-HT or serotonin). Carbidopa, if administered with 5-HTP, inhibits this decarboxylation which is catalyzed by a vitamin B_6-dependent decarboxylase. Peripheral decarboxylation of 5-HTP occurs to a much lesser extent in those with low vitamin B_6 status, and most likely to a greater extent in those who take concurrent vitamin B_6 supplements of doses 5 milligrams or greater.

The efficiency of absorption of 5-HTP, as well as its decarboxylation product serotonin, is approximately 47 to 84%. Absorption of 5-HTP occurs by an active transport process. 5-HTP is transported by the portal circulation to the liver where approximately 25% of an administered dose is metabolized via vitamin B_6-dependent L-aromatic amino acid decarboxylase to 5-HT. 5-HT is subsequently metabolized to 5-hydroxyindole acetaldehyde which is rapidly metabolized to 5-hydroxyindoleacetic acid (5-HIAA). 5-HTP that is not metabolized in the liver is transported by the general circulation to the various tissues of the body, including the brain. 5-HTP readily crosses the blood-brain barrier, and is converted to serotonin in brain cells. 5-HIAA is the principal renal excretion product of 5-HTP.

5-HTP has shown some usefulness in some conditions characterized, in part, by serotonin deficits, principally depression. It has also been shown to be useful in some individuals with obesity, insomnia, fibromyalgia and chronic tension headache.

Scattered studies have shown that supplemental 5-HTP has significant antidepressant effects in some. In one double-blind, multi-center study, 5-HTP was said to have antidepressant effects slightly better than the SSRI fluvoxamine. Other studies have been more equivocal. One study indicated that 5-HTP is not effective in those whose depression is not responsive to serotonin reuptake inhibitors (SSRIs). More rigorous, longer term studies are needed.

In a double-blind, placebo-controlled crossover study of 19 obese female subjects given 5-HTP (8 milligrams per kilogram of body weight daily) for five weeks, significant weight loss (about 5 percent) was recorded in 5-HTP treated subjects, compared with controls. No dietary prescriptions were prescribed during the course of this study.

These findings were confirmed in a second double-blind, placebo-controlled, randomized study conducted over a longer period of time—two consecutive six-week periods.

In a more recent double-blind study, subjects with non-insulin dependent diabetes were randomized to receive either placebo or 750 milligrams of 5-HTP daily for two weeks without dietary restrictions. Significant weight loss was achieved in the 5-HTP group. A 5-HTP-inhibiting effect on carbohydrate intake was noted.

There is preliminary, dated (1977) evidence that 5-HTP can be of benefit in those described as "mildly insomniac."

Evidence that 5-HTP might be helpful in fibromyalgia is also preliminary but more recent. In a 90-day open trial, 50 patients with primary fibromyalgia were reported to achieve significant improvement in all clinical variables measured, including tender points, anxiety, quality of sleep and fatigue.

There is evidence in some animal work, as well as some *in vitro* work, that 5-HTP is radioprotective. Combined with a thiol compound, 5-HTP protected peripheral blood and sperm cells.

In a recently reported randomized, double-blind, placebo-controlled trial, subjects who took 300 milligrams daily of 5-HTP were found to have a significant decrease in their use of analgesics for chronic tension-type headache, and also a significant decrease in the number of days with headaches following the conclusion of the trial.

CONTRAINDICATIONS, PRECAUTIONS, ADVERSE REACTIONS

CONTRAINDICATIONS

5-HTP is contraindicated in those hypersensitive to any component of a 5-HTP-containing product. It is also contraindicated in those with carcinoid tumors, and during or within 2 weeks after discontinuing MAOIs (type A), including isocarboxazid, phenelzine sulfate and tranylcypromine.

PRECAUTIONS

Those who are interested in the use of 5-HTP for any health condition should first discuss its use with his or her physician.

Large doses of 5-HTP can trigger excess serotonin formation in tissues other than the target organ and may cause significant adverse reactions.

5-HTP should not be used concurrently with any antidepressant, including selective serotonin reuptake inhibitors (SSRIs), tricyclic antidepressants or monoamine oxidase inhibitors (MAOIs). Concurrent use of 5-HTP with an antidepressant may increase the risk of adverse reactions.

5-HTP should not be used concurrently with serotonin 5-HT$_1$ receptor agonists, including naratriptan, sumatriptan and zolmitriptan. Such use may increase the risk of adverse reactions.

5-HTP should be avoided by those with ischemic heart disease (history of myocardial infarction, angina pectoris, documented silent ischemia), coronary artery spasm (eg, Prinzmetal's angina), uncontrolled hypertension and any other significant cardiovascular disease.

5-HTP should be avoided by pregnant women and nursing mothers.

ADVERSE REACTIONS

As of August 1998, the FDA reported that 10 cases of eosinophilia myalgia syndrome (EMS) possibly associated with 5-HTP had been documented worldwide, none resulting in death. No new cases of EMS have since been reported. (See Description above.) A scleroderma-like skin condition has been reported in some taking a combination of 5-HTP and carbidopa.

Reported side effects, include nausea, diarrhea, loss of appetite, vomiting and difficult breathing. Neurological side effects, including dilation of the pupils, abnormally sensitive reflexes, loss of muscle coordination and blurring of vision, have been reported in those taking large doses of 5-HTP. Cardiac dysrhythmias have also been reported.

Large doses of 5-HTP may significantly increase serum levels of serotonin, and theoretically, this may result in the serotonin syndrome. Symptoms and signs of the serotonin syndrome include confusion, agitation, diaphoresis, diarrhea, tachycardia, myoclonus and hyperreflexia. In addition, hypertension, coma/unresponsiveness, seizures, and death may occur if the syndrome is not promptly recognized and treated. There are no reports of the serotonin syndrome occurring with use of 5-HTP in humans. However, it conceivably could occur and the combination of 5-HTP with another serotonergic agent can increase the risk of it occurring. As a side note, there are 21 cases of 5-HTP toxicosis reported in dogs. Accidental ingestion of 5-HTP by dogs resulted in a serotonin-like syndrome. Three of the dogs died.

Although a full-blown serotonin syndrome is unlikely in those using 5-HTP, symptoms associated with elevated serum levels of serotonin may occur. For example, a recent report described a 56-year-old woman who presented to the clinic with a 12-week history of diarrhea (6-8 loose stools daily). The only abnormal finding in her initial workup was a severely elevated 5-hydroxyindole acetic acid (5-HIAA) level in a 24-hour urine collection. (5-HIAA is a metabolite of serotonin and is the test used to determine if the patient has abnormally high levels of serotonin.) A medical oncologist suggested that the patient might have carcinoid syndrome. He told the patient that her elevated 5-HIAA level was consistent with a disseminated carcinoid malignancy, which was really bad news, and he ordered further tests. However, during an appointment to sign a consent for endoscopy, she reported that for the past 18 months she had been taking 5-HTP, 100 mg daily. She was asked to stop taking the supplement. A 24-hour urine collection was repeated two weeks later and was found to be within normal limits. Her diarrhea also improved. That was really good news.

INTERACTIONS

DRUGS

5-HT antagonists (methysergide, cyproheptadine): 5-HTP may decrease the effectiveness of methysergide and cyproheptadine.

5-HT$_1$ receptor agonists (naratriptan, sumatriptan, zolmitriptan): Concurrent use of 5-HTP with a 5-HT$_1$ agonist may increase the risk of adverse reactions.

Carbidopa: Carbidopa suppresses peripheral 5-HTP metabolism, allowing greater amounts of 5-HTP to reach the brain.

Methyldopa: Methyldopa inhibits the enzymatic conversion of 5-HTP to serotonin.

Monoamine oxidase inhibitors (MAOIs; isocarboxazid, phenelzine sulfate, tranylcypromine): Concurrent use of 5-HTP with an MAOI (type A) may increase the risk of adverse reactions.

Phenoxybenzamine: Phenoxybenzamine inhibits the conversion of 5-HTP to serotonin.

Selective serotonin reuptake inhibitors (SSRIs; citalopram, fluvoxamine maleate, fluoxetine, paroxetine, sertraline, venlafaxine): Concurrent use of 5-HTP with a SSRI may potentiate the antidepressant effect of the SSRI and may also increase the risk of adverse reactions.

NUTRITIONAL SUPPLEMENTS

Vitamin B_6: Concurrent intake of 5-HTP and doses of vitamin B_6 5 milligrams or greater, may enhance the peripheral decarboxylation of 5-HTP to serotonin.

HERBS

Saint John's wort: Theoretically, concurrent use of 5-HTP and Saint John's wort may both potentiate the possible antidepressant activity of the herbal product and increase the risk of adverse reactions.

OVERDOSAGE

There are no reports of overdosage in humans. There are reports of overdosage and subsequent serotonin-like syndrome in dogs. Some of these overdosages resulted in death to the animals.

DOSAGE AND ADMINISTRATION

Those who wish to try 5-HTP should discuss dosage with his or her physician. Doses should generally not exceed those recommended on the label.

In Europe, a combination of 5-HTP with carbidopa is available, and this combination appears to have a safer profile. However, those who wish to use this combination product must do so only under medical supervision and prescription. It has been found that doses of 100 milligrams to 2 grams daily are required to observe any desired effect. These doses, without concomitant carbidopa, can cause adverse events (see Precautions).

LITERATURE

Boiardi A, Picotti GB, Di Giulio AM, et al. Platelet met-enkephalin immunoreactivity and 5-hydroxytryptamine concentrations in migraine patients: effects of 5-hydroxytryptophan, amitriptyline and chlorimipramine treatment. *Cephalalgia.* 1984;4:81-84.

Byerley WF, Judd LL, Reimherr FW, et al. 5-Hydroxytryptophan: a review of its antidepressant efficacy and adverse effects. *J Clin Psychopharmacol.* 1987;7:127-137.

Cangiano C, Ceci F, Cascino A, et al. Eating behavior and adherence to dietary prescriptions in obese adult subjects treated with 5-hydroxytryptophan. *Am J Clin Nutr.* 1992;56:863-867.

Cangiano C, Laviano A, Del Ben M, et al. Effects of oral5-hydroxytryptophan on energy intake and macronutrient selection in non-insulin dependent diabetes mellitus. *Int J Obes Relat Metab Disord.* 1998;22:648-654.

Caruso I, Sarzi Puttini P, Cazzola M, et al. Double-blind study of 5-hydroxytryptophan versus placebo in the treatment of primary fibromyalgia syndrome. *J Int Med Res.* 1990;18:201-209.

Ceci F, Cangiano C, Cairella M, et al. The effects of oral 5-hydroxytryptophan administration on feeding behavior in obese adult female subjects. *J Neural Transm.* 1989;76:109-117.

Das YT, Bagchi M, Bagchi D, et al. Safety of 5-hydroxy-L-tryptophan. *Toxicol Lett.* 2004;150(1):111-122.

Genazzani AR, Sandrini G, Facchinetti F, et al. Effects of L-5HTP with and without carbidopa on plasma beta-endorphin and pain perception. Possible implications in migraine prophylaxis. *Cephalalgia.* 1986;6:241-245.

Gwaltney-Brant SM, Albertsen JC, Khan SA. 5-Hydroxy-trytophan toxicosis in dogs: 21 cases (1989-1999). *J Am Vet Med Assoc.* 2000;216:1937-1940.

Imeri L, Mancia M, Bianchi S, et al. 5-Hydroxytryptophan, but not L-tryptophan, alters sleep and brain temperature in rats. *Neuroscience.* 2000;95:445-452.

Keithahn C, Lerchl A. 5-hydroxytryptophan is a more potent in vitro hydroxyl radical scavenger than melatonin or vitamin C. *J Pineal Res.* 2005;38(1):62-66.

Klarskov K, Johnson KL, Benson LM, et al. Eosinophilia-myalgia syndrome case-associated contaminants in commercially available 5-hydroxytryptophan. *Adv Exp Med Biol.* 1999;467:461-468.

Lowe SL, Yeo KP, Teng L, et al. L-5-Hydroxytryptophan augments the neuroendocrine response to a SSRI. *Psychoneuroendocrinology.* 2006;31(4):473-484.

Michelson D, Page SW, Casey R, et al. An eosinophilia-myalgia syndrome related disorder associated with exposure to L-5-hydroxytryptophan. *J Rheumatol.* 1994;21:2261-2265.

Morrow JD, Vikraman S, Imeri L, et al. Effects of serotonergic activation by 5-hydroxytryptophan on sleep and body temperature of C57BL/6J and interleukin-6-deficient mice are dose and time related. *Sleep.* 2008;31(1):21-33.

Nicoladi M, Sicuteri F. L-5-hydroxytryptophan can prevent nociceptive disorders in man. *Adv Exp Med Biol.* 1999;467:177-182.

Preshaw RM, Leavitt D, Hoag G. The dietary supplement 5-hydroxytryptophan and urinary 5-hydroxyindole acetic acid. *CMAJ.* 2008;178(8):993.

Puttini PS, Caruso I. Primary fibromyalgia syndrome and 5-hydroxy-L-tryptophan: a 90-day open study. *J Int Med Res.* 1992;20:182-189.

Ribeiro CA. L-5-Hydroxytryptophan in the prophylaxis of chronic tension-type headache: a double-blind, randomized, placebo-controlled study. For the Portuguese Head Study. *Headache.* 2000;40:451-456.

Shaw K, Turner J, Del Mar C. Are tryptophan and 5-hydroxytryptophan effective treatments for depression? A meta-analysis. *Aust N Z J Psychiatry.* 2002;36(4):488-91.

Shaw K, Turner J, Del Mar C. Tryptophan and 5-hydroxytryptophan for depression. *Cochrane Database Syst Rev.* 2002;(1):CD003198.

Smarius LJ, Jacobs GE, Hoeberechts-Lefrandt DH, et al. Pharmacology of rising oral doses of 5-hydroxytryptophan with carbidopa. *J Psychopharmacol.* 2008;22(4):426-433.

Sternberg EM, Van Woert MH, Young SN, et al. Development of a scleroderma-like illness during therapy with L-5-hydroxy-tryptophan and carbidopa. *N Engl J Med.* 1980;303:782-787.

U. S. Food and Drug Administration, Center for Food Safety and Applied Nutrition, Office of Nutritional Products, Labeling, and Dietary Supplements. February 2001. Information Paper on L-tryptophan and 5-hydroxy-L-tryptophan. http://www.cfsan.fda.gov/~dms/ds-tryp1.html. Date accessed: September 23, 2008.

Williamson BL, Klarskov K, Tolminson AJ, et al. Problems with over-the-counter 5-hydroxy-L-tryptophan. *Nat Med.* 1998;4:983.

Yamada J, Ujikawa M, Sugimoto Y. Serum leptin levels after central and systemic injection of a serotonin precursor, 5-hydroxytryptophan, in mice. *Eur J Pharmacol.* 2000;406:159-162.

Zhou SY, Goshgarian HG. 5-Hydroxytryptophan-induced respiratory recovery after cervical spinal cord hemisection in rats. *J Appl Physiol.* 2000;89:1528-1536.

7-Oxo-Dehydroepiandrosterone (7-Oxo-DHEA)

DESCRIPTION

7-Oxo-Dehydroepiandrosterone, abbreviated as 7-oxo-DHEA, is a natural substance produced in the adrenal glands, gonads and brain. 7-Oxo-DHEA is a metabolite of the steroid hormone DHEA (see DHEA). DHEA and its metabolite dehydroepiandrosterone-3-sulfate, or DHEAS, are the major secretory steroidal products of the adrenal glands and the most abundant steroids in human blood. DHEA has been found to promote leanness in some obese animals, and, in mostly animal studies, has been found to decrease serum cholesterol, to decrease blood glucose in diabetic mice, to enhance immune function, to possess anticancer activity and to improve memory in old mice. DHEA is believed by some to have great importance in human physiology. However, to date, its exact role in human physiology remains unknown. 7-Oxo-DHEA has been studied to better understand, among other things, the biological role of DHEA. A major biochemical difference between 7-oxo-DHEA and DHEA is that DHEA is metabolized to the sex hormones (androgens and estrogens) while 7-oxo-DHEA does not appear to be metabolized to these hormones.

7-Oxo-DHEA is being studied for its possible cognition-enhancing and thermogenic activities. Steroids that are made in the brain are referred to as neurosteroids; steroids that may have thermogenic activity are referred to as ergosteroids. 7-Oxo-DHEA is also known as 3beta-hydroxyandrost-5-ene-7,17-dione,delta5-androstene-3beta-ol-7,17-dione and 7-keto-DHEA. The structural formula is:

7-Oxo-Dehydroepiandrosterone

7-Oxo-DHEA is marketed as a nutritional supplement. The form of 7-oxo-DHEA most commonly marketed is the 3-acetyl ester of 7-oxo-DHEA, also known as 3-acetyl-7-oxo-DHEA.

ACTIONS AND PHARMACOLOGY

ACTIONS

Supplemental 7-oxo-DHEA has putative cognition-enhancing, thermogenic and immunomodulatory activities.

MECHANISM OF ACTION

7-Oxo-DHEA was found to reverse scopolamine-induced cholinergic dysfunction in mice. It is speculated that 7-oxo-DHEA's effect on memory is via allosteric inhibition of the $GABA_A$ receptor. In fact, studies have shown that DHEAS is a potent allosteric inhibitor of the $GABA_A$ receptor. DHEAS has been found to rapidly reduce $GABA_A$-gated chloride and voltage-gated calcium currents, thereby increasing the general excitability of the hippocampus.

DHEA has been found to promote leanness in genetically obese and normal experimental animals without altering food intake. The amount of DHEA necessary to elicit this response is much larger than is required to obtain responses to hormones, and it was thought that this effect was probably mediated by a metabolite of DHEA. The DHEA metabolite 7-oxo-DHEA was found to be much more effective than DHEA at promoting leanness in experimental animals. 7-Oxo-DHEA appears to promote leanness via a thermogenic effect. 7-Oxo-DHEA has been demonstrated to enhance the activities in rats of the two thermogenic enzymes, liver mitochondrial *sn*-glycerol 3-phosphate dehydrogenase and cytosolic malic enzyme. It is thought that the induction of these enzymes may account for the thermogenic effect of 7-oxo-DHEA in animal models. 7-Keto-DHEA was shown to be significantly more potent than DHEA per se in the induction of these thermogenic enzymes.

7-Oxo-DHEA has been reported to augment interleukin 2 (IL-2) production by human lymphocytes *in vitro*. The mechanism of this effect is unknown.

PHARMACOKINETICS

There is little on the pharmacokinetics of 7-oxo-DHEA in humans. Preliminary studies indicate that it is absorbed following ingestion. However, the efficiency of its absorption, as well as its distribution, metabolism and excretion, needs to be elucidated. 7-Oxo-DHEA is not converted to DHEA, nor does it appear to be converted to the sex hormones testosterone and estrogens; DHEA, on the other hand, is.

INDICATIONS AND USAGE

Claims for 7-oxo-DHEA include metabolic enhancements that help promote weight loss and increase lean body mass, favorable effects on immunity, improved memory and various anti-aging effects. These claims are largely extravagant extrapolations from animal and *in vitro* studies and from very preliminary human studies. Some claim that 7-oxo-DHEA is superior to DHEA itself because 7-oxo-DHEA appears not to be converted to sex hormones (see DHEA).

RESEARCH SUMMARY

In a recent animal study, 7-oxo-DHEA was tested for its possible ability to reverse chemically induced memory abolition in young mice and for its effects on memory in old mice. Significant positive effects were reported in both test groups, compared with controls. A single dose of 7-oxo-DHEA reportedly completely reversed scopolamine-induced memory impairment in the young mice. And, in the old mice, single doses resulted in significant memory retention, as measured by water maze training, through a four-week test period. Memory retention was not improved in controls or in those animals given DHEA itself.

Several experimental studies have suggested that 7-oxo-DHEA might enhance thermogenesis. Some researchers have concluded that it is a more effective inducer of thermogenic enzymes than its parent steroid, DHEA. In large doses, DHEA has been shown to induce weight loss in genetically obese and in some normal animals without affecting food intake, but similar effects in humans have not been reliably confirmed. Similarly, there is little evidence that 7-oxo-DHEA significantly decreases weight or increases lean muscle mass in humans.

There are some data indicating that 7-oxo-DHEA might favorably impact some immune activities, such as stimulation of interleukin-2 and increased production of CD-4 and CD-8 cells *in vitro*.

CONTRAINDICATIONS, PRECAUTIONS, ADVERSE REACTIONS

CONTRAINDICATIONS

7-Oxo-DHEA is contraindicated in those hypersensitive to any component of a 7-oxo-DHEA-containing product.

PRECAUTIONS

7-Oxo-DHEA supplementation should be avoided by pregnant women and nursing mothers.

Those who wish to try 7-oxo-DHEA for any health reason should first discuss its use with his or her physician.

INTERACTIONS

DRUGS

7-Oxo-DHEA may have an effect on platelet membrane fluidity. Therefore, those taking the anticoagulant warfarin (Coumadin) should exercise caution in the use of 7-oxo-DHEA.

NUTRITIONAL SUPPLEMENTS

None known.

HERBS

None known.

FOODS

None known.

ADVERSE REACTIONS

Vivid dreams have been reported in some taking 7-oxo-DHEA. Vivid dreams occur during REM (rapid eye movement) sleep, seem very real and are easier to remember.

OVERDOSAGE

No reports.

DOSAGE AND ADMINISTRATION

7-Oxo-DHEA is available in the dietary supplement marketplace. It is marketed as the 3-acetyl ester of 7-oxo-DHEA. Typical dosage is 25 milligrams per day. Doses higher than those stated on the label should be avoided.

LITERATURE

Bobyleva V, Bellei M, Kneer N, et al. The effects of the ergosteroid 7-oxo-dehydroepiandrosterone on mitochondrial membrane potential: possible relationship to thermogenesis. *Arch Biochem Biophys*. 1997;341:122-128.

Hampl R, Hill M, Bílek R, et al. Relationship of dehydroepiandrosterone and its 7-hydroxylated metabolites to thyroid parameters and sex hormone-binding globulin (SHBG) in healthy subjects. *Clin Chem Lab Med*. 2003;41(8):1081-1086.

Hampl R, Lapčík O, Hill M, et al. 7-Hydroxydehydroepiandrosterone—a natural antiglucocorticoid and a candidate for steroid replacement therapy? *Physiol Res*. 2000;49 Suppl 1:S107-112.

Ihler G, Chami-Stemmann H. 7-oxo-DHEA and Raynaud's phenomenon. *Med Hypotheses*. 2003;60(3):391-397.

Lardy H, Partridge B, Kneer N, et al. Ergosteroids: induction of thermogenic enzymes in liver of rats treated with steroids derived from dehydroepiandrosterone. *Proc Natl Acad Sci USA*. 1995;92:6617-6619.

Rose KA, Stapleton G, Dott K, et al. Cyp7b, a novel brain cytochrome P450, catalyzes the synthesis of neurosteroids 7alpha-hydroxy dehydroepiandrosterone and 7alpha-hydroxypregnenolone. *Proc Natl Acad Sci USA*. 1997;94:4925-4930.

Shi J, Schulze S, Lardy HA. The effect of 7-oxo-DHEA acetate on memory in young and old C57BL/6 mice. *Steroids*. 2000;65:124-129.

Zenk JL, Frestedt JL, Kuskowski MA. HUM5007, a novel combination of thermogenic compounds, and 3-acetyl-7-oxo-dehydroepiandrosterone: each increases the resting metabolic rate of overweight adults. *J Nutr Biochem*. 2007;18(9):629-634.

8-Prenylnaringenin (8-PN)

DESCRIPTION

Beer is a fermented aqueous drink based on starch and flavored with hops. Hops provide the characteristic bitterness of the beer and contribute to its aroma and foam stability.

The hop plant (*Humulus lupulus* L.) is a dioecious plant, meaning that there are separate male and female hop plants. Only the female produces the flowers, or, more specifically, the strobiles that are used for brewing or for potential medicinal purposes.

The term 'hop' refers to the plant, and the term 'hops' refers to the flower cones ("hop cones" or "hops") of the hop plant. However, both terms are commonly used interchangeably. The flowers in a female hop plant are arranged in characteristic clusters on stems. The flower cluster is called an inflorescence. The female inflorescences are rich in polyphenolic compounds and acyl phloroglucides that are widely used to preserve beer and give beer its characteristic flavor and aroma.

The hop cones are green, are built like pine cones and vary in size. At the base of the leaves (bracts, also called scales) of the cones are collections of small, yellow spheres called the lupulin glands. The lupulin glands are little sacs of bitter and aromatic acids and oils. In the lupulin glands can be found the alpha-acids and their derivatives, including the iso-alpha-acids and the rho-iso-alpha acids, the beta acids, xanthohumol and 8-PN, among several other compounds. The iso-alpha-acids, including isohumulone, mainly account for the bitter taste of beer. The oils in the hops are mainly responsible for the aroma of beer.

In addition to their roles in beer, there has been great interest in studying the hop phytochemicals for possible medicinal uses. Two of the phytochemicals found in hops that have been receiving much of the attention are the flavonoid, 8-PN, for its phytoestrogenic activity, and the prenylated chalcone, xanthohumol (see Xanthohumol), for its possible broad-spectrum chemopreventive and anticancer activities. Recently, the iso-alpha acids have also been receiving attention for their possible anti-inflammatory activities.

8-PN is a prenylated flavonoid found in the lupulin glands of the female inflorescence. It is secreted as part of the hop resin (lupulin) by glandular trichomes found on the adaxial surfaces of cone bracts.

The estrogenic effects of hops have been recognized for a long time. The frequent menstrual disturbances observed in female hop-pickers during the early days of hop cone harvesting, when hops were picked by hand, suggested a potential hormonal activity of the hops. An old folk legend held that female hop-pickers, who normally lived a distance from hop gardens, regularly began to menstruate two days after arriving to pick hops. In Germany, brewery sludge baths containing about 30% hops extracts ("hop baths") were traditionally used for the treatment of gynecological disorders. Hop baths and hops extracts were reported to be effective in reducing hot flashes in menopausal women. In 1953, Koch and Heim, in a short communication, reported that hops contained the equivalent of 20 to 300 micrograms of the female hormone 17beta-estradiol. This was the first scientific confirmation that hops possess estrogenic activity. In 1999, 8-PN, the major estrogenic substance in hops, was isolated and characterized. It has been found to be the most potent plant-derived estrogen (phytoestrogen) to date.

8-PN's empirical formula is $C_{20}H_{20}O_5$, and its molecular weight is 340.37. It is described chemically as (2*S*)-5,7-dihydroxy-2-(4-hydroxyphenyl)-8-(3-methylbut-2-enyl)chroman-4-one. It is also known as prenylnaringenin. Its abbreviation is 8-PN. 8-PN exists as the enantiomers 2*S*(–)8-PN and 2*R*(+)8-PN, and as a racemic mixture containing both enantiomers. An enantiomer is one of two stereoisomers that are nonsuperimposable, complete mirror images of each other. The 2*S*(–)8-PN enantiomer has slightly more potent estrogenic activity than the 2*R*(+)8-PN enantiomer. Both enantiomers are found in hops. 8-PN is classified as a prenylated flavonoid, a prenylflavonoid, a prenylated flavanone, a prenylflavanone, and as a polyphenol. It belongs to the flavanone subclass of flavonoids. In addition to hops, 8-PN is also found in A*naxagorea luzonensis* A. Gray, a tree indigenous to Thailand, the extracts of which are used in traditional Thai medicine for the treatment of a number of diseases. In fact, 8-PN was first identified as a phytoestrogen in the heartwood of the tree. The concentration of 8-PN in most beers is below 30 micrograms per liter. Some beers, particularly strong ales, have been reported to contain concentrations of up to 250 micrograms (0.24 milligrams) or higher per liter. Beer is the major dietary source of 8-PN.

8-PN is represented by the following chemical structure.

8-prenylnaringenin

ACTIONS AND PHARMACOLOGY

ACTIONS

8-prenylnaringenin (8-PN) has estrogenic activity. It may also have anticancer and antiangiogenic activities.

MECHANISM OF ACTION

Antiangiogenesio activity: 8-PN was shown to inhibit angiogenesis induced by basic fibroblast growth factor (bFGF), vascular endothelial growth factor (VEGF) or the synergistic effect of the two cytokines in combination. The effect was seen with bovine microvascular endothelial cells derived from the adrenal cortex and with endothelial cells from the bovine thoracic aorta. Given this finding, 8-PN could have therapeutic applications for diseases in which angiogenesis is an important component—for example, certain cancers. The exact mechanism of the antiangiogenic action of 8-PN is unclear.

Anticancer activity: 8-PN was found to inhibit estrogen receptor alpha mediated cell growth and induce apoptosis in MCF-7 human breast cancer cells.

8-PN showed a biphasic action on cell growth. At concentrations below 10 micromolar (microM), 8-PCN showed estrogenic properties, increasing cell growth in estrogen receptor-positive MCF-7 human breast cancer cells, while high concentrations of 8-PN inhibited proliferation and induced apoptosis in hormone responsive cells. The exact mechanism of this action is unclear.

Treatment of the prostate cancer cell lines PC-3 and DU145 with 8-PN was demonstrated to induce a caspase-independent form of cell death. Caspases are essential in cells for apoptosis or programmed cell death. The mechanism of action of this anticancer effect is not clear. However, vacuoles were noted in some of the cells, suggesting the induction of autophagy and consequent cell death. Autophagy is a type of programmed cell death, which is characterized by the accumulation of autophage vacuoles and the absence of caspase activation. Autophagy is a cell survival mechanism during nutrient starvation that supplies vital components until conditions improve. Autophagy has also been found to be a novel tumor suppression mechanism.

Estrogenic activity: Studies with racemic 8-PN and its enantiomers 2S(−)8-PN and 2R(+)8-PN have revealed that 8-PN is the first ER_{alpha} (estrogen receptor alpha) selective phytoestrogen with a two- to threefold higher affinity for the ER_{alpha} than for the ER_{beta} (estrogen receptor beta). 8-PN is the most potent plant-derived ER_{alpha} agonist to date. It is 10-fold more potent than coumestrol and 100-fold more potent than genistein, but 70 times weaker than 17beta-estradiol.

Studies have revealed a greater than 3.6-fold higher estrogenic activity of 8-PN at ER_{alpha} than at ER_{beta}. This is in contrast to other phytoestrogens, including genistein and coumestrol, which are primarily ER_{beta} agonists. 8-PN is a pure estrogen receptor agonist *in vitro*. Its estrogenic activity is comparable to that of estrone. Estrone is one of the three major estrogens and is much less potent than 17beta-estradiol, the primary estrogen. Although 8-PN demonstrated only 70 times weaker ER_{alpha} agonist activity than 17beta-estradiol in an *in vitro* or test tube study, an *in vivo* study showed the estrogenic activity of 8-PN in reproductive tissue to be about 20,000-fold weaker when compared to that of beta-estradiol. The 2S(−)8-PN enantiomer shows moderately higher estrogenic activity *in vitro* and *in vivo* than the 2R(+)8-PN enantiomer.

Studies on the *in vivo* pharmacological profile of 8-PN were performed using three different techniques: the short-term uterus growth test in juvenile rats, the 4-week bone mineral density (BMD) model in adult ovariectomized rats and the ERE-luc (estrogen response elements luciferase) transgenic mouse model. The ERE-luc transgenic mice carry a luciferase gene that is driven by two estrogen response elements. The model appears to report reliably on the activity of liganded and unliganded estrogen receptors induced by endogenous and exogenous stimuli.

Data obtained in the BMD study in adult ovariectomized rats demonstrated that 8-PN completely protected the rats from bone loss induced by ovariectomy without stimulating the uterus and the endometrium to the extent seen for a 17beta-estradiol dose that was necessary for the same bone-protective effect. It was estimated that 8-PN had a 10-fold higher sensitivity for bone tissue compared with 17beta-estradiol. Whereas 17beta-estradiol maximally stimulated uterus growth and epithelial height, the effect of 8-PN on uterus growth and epithelial height was marginal and not different from that found in ovariectomized control animals. 8-PN was also found to have a pronounced bone tissue-specific estrogenic effect in the transgenic ERE-luc mouse model.

Given the above findings, 8-PN can be termed a natural selective estrogen receptor modulator, or SERM. A substance that demonstrates low stimulatory effects on the uterus at bone tissue-effective doses makes 8-PN a serious candidate for HRT (hormone replacement therapy). However, before it can be recommended for HRT, large scale human clinical trials, including long-term safety studies, are clearly needed and clearly warranted.

At menopause, the ovaries stop releasing eggs and a severe decline in serum 17beta-estradiol levels occurs. Low estradiol levels typically result in symptoms such as hot flashes (vasomotor symptoms), vulvar and vaginal atrophy and dryness, mood disturbances and loss of libido. It also can result in degenerative processes such as osteoporosis and cardiovascular disease. This situation once prompted many women to start HRT in order to treat and prevent these problems. Since estrogens alone stimulate endometrial proliferation, which may result in cancer, estrogens were given in combination with progestins. In 2002, a report from the Women's Health Initiative (WHI) study published in the *Journal of the American Medical Association* (*JAMA*) cast doubt on the beneficial effects of HRT. Results from the WHI study showed a higher incidence in cardiovascular disease complications, such as heart attacks and strokes, and a higher incidence of breast cancers in those postmenopausal women who were using HRT in the form of conjugated estrogens plus medroxyprogesterone. The report rekindled an interest in alternatives to classical HRT, such as plant estrogens (phytoestrogens). 8-PN is the most potent phytoestrogen known, but not much is known about its safety. The following study examined morphologic changes induced by oral long-term treatment with 8-PN in the uterus, vagina and mammary gland of castrated rats.

Rats were ovariectomized and fed for three months with soy-free chow containing either 17beta-estradiol or 8-PN, both given in two doses (a low dose and a high dose). The uteri of the rats treated with both 17beta-estradiol doses and the high 8-PN dose were found to have increased weight and showed histologic estrogen-induced features. High-dose 8-PN induced epithelial polyploidy formation unique to this group. Compared to the atrophic controls, both 17beta-estradiol doses and the high 8-PN dose induced hyperplastic epithelia in the vagina. The high doses of both 17beta-estradiol and 8PN caused secretion in the mammary gland, whereas proliferation and progesterone receptor expression were stimulated by both 17beta estradiol doses and the high 8-PN dose. 8-PN, at least at a high dose, did not come out with a clean bill of health from this study.

Further animal toxicity and human toxicity studies are needed and warranted.

PHARMACOKINETICS

A human pharmacokinetic (PK) study of 8-PN was performed in healthy postmenopausal women. The study was performed using a randomized, double-blind, placebo-controlled, dose-escalation design with three groups of eight women. In each group, six subjects received 8-PN and two subjects received placebo. 8-PN was given orally in doses of 50, 250 or 750 milligrams (mg).

All treatments were well tolerated. Serum concentrations of 8-PN demonstrated rapid enteral absorption of the prenylflavonoid, and secondary peaks were suggestive of a pronounced presystemic elimination with subsequent marked enterohepatic recirculation. Comparatively little phase 1 metabolism was recorded. Conjugation to beta-glucuronides or sulfates seemed to constitute the main metabolic pathway. Approximately 30% of the dose was recovered in the urine and feces, either as unchanged or as conjugated metabolites, over the 48-hour observation period. 8-PN elimination seemed to be a combination of hepatic conjugation, hepatic elimination and renal excretion of conjugates. Secondary peaks hindered the calculation of the disposition half-life of 8-PN. However, the rapid decrease in serum concentration after the peaks suggested a short elimination phase with a half-life of one to three hours. The 750 mg dose decreased serum luteinizing hormone (LH) concentrations. The decrease in serum LH concentrations found after the highest dose demonstrated the ability of 8-PN to cross the blood-brain barrier and interact with the hypothalamo-pituitary axis, which is regarded as a prerequisite for the successful treatment of menopausal symptoms. Follicle-stimulating hormone (FSH) serum concentrations were not significantly influenced by 8-PN at any of the doses tested.

Further human studies on the PK of 8-PN in humans are warranted, as is investigation of 8-PN and its biological effects following multiple doses.

The PK of 8-PN in rats and dogs is characterized by a low oral bioavailability caused by extensive presystemic elimination after complete enteral absorption. 8-PN is almost completely excreted via the bile in unchanged form and in urine in the form of conjugates.

In vitro studies of intestinal permeability and hepatic and intestinal metabolism of 8-PN have been performed using monolayers of the human intestinal epithelial cancer line Caco-2 (a cell model of intestinal absorption and intestinal metabolism) and human hepatocytes (a cell model of hepatic metabolism). 8-PN showed good intestinal absorption via passive diffusion. Both glucuronide and sulfate conjugates of 8-PN were detected in the Caco-2 cell incubations. The 4′-O-glucuronide was the predominant Caco-2 metabolite, followed by the 7-O-sulfate and the 4′-O-sulfate. Both phase 1 and phase 2 metabolites of 8-PN were formed by human hepatocytes. The 7-O-glucuronide was the most abundant hepatocyte metabolite, and no sulfate conjugates were detected.

INDICATIONS AND USAGE

The flavonoid 8-prenylnaringenin (8-PN) found in hops is the most potent known phytoestrogen and thus has been proposed as an alternative to hormone therapy for the treatment of perimenopausal symptoms. The safety and efficacy of its use in menopausal and post-menopausal women has not been established. Claims that it is an effective "breast enhancer" are unsubstantiated. It may have some cardioprotective and anticancer potential.

RESEARCH SUMMARY

Because there is some evidence that standard estrogen/progestin therapy for the treatment and prevention of perimenopausal symptoms (such as "hot flushes") may place some women at higher risk of some cancers, heart attack and stroke, "natural" alternative treatments have focused on such phytoestrogenic substances as 8-PN. Both *in vitro* and *in vivo* studies leave no doubt that 8-PN is a potent estrogen receptor agonist in estrogen-responsive cells. Its estrogenic activity exceeds that of other phytoestrogenic agents such as genistein (see Genistein) and daidzein (see Daidzein). When given in drinking water to ovariectomized mice, the substance induced estrogenic stimulation of the vaginal epithelium with doses that were calculated to be 500-fold greater than that present in any beer. Another group of researchers reported that 8-PN is 100 times more potent than genistein. And though considerably weaker than the principal endogenous mammalian estrogen—estradiol—it is still potent enough that one group of authors concluded that it has "remarkable" potential for the treatment of conditions characterized by estrogen deficiency. In an animal model of menopausal hot flushes, 8-PN modulated vasomotor response in a way that lowered skin temperature, suggesting that the flavonoid might, indeed, be useful for ameliorating or preventing hot flushes.

Other experiments, however, have raised safety issues. Some data suggest that 8-PN, in doses sufficient to be effective in preventing/treating perimenopausal symptoms, would act on the hypothalamo-pituitary-uterine axis in some of the same negative ways that estrogen therapies do. Thus, the authors of one study concluded that, just as in standard HRT, progestins might have to be co-administered with 8-PN in order to reduce/prevent endometrial overstimulation. That would, of course, negate one of the putative advantages of this "natural" alternative therapy. In the first oral long-term treatment with 8-PN, changes were observed in the uteri, vaginas and mammary glands of ovariectomized rats that raised additional doubts about the safety of this substance.

Again, many of the same unfavorable sequelae of standard HRT were observed. In addition, what was described as a novel lesion was observed in the endometria of some of the 8-PN-dosed animals, a lesion not hitherto seen in animals treated with estradiol. Its significance is unknown. In view of this and prior findings that 8-PN can stimulate growth of human breast cancer cells, these researchers concluded that the clinical use of this substance could have adverse effects. More research is clearly needed before 8-PN can be said to be either safe or efficacious in the prevention and treatment of perimenopausal symptoms.

On the other hand, some *in vitro* studies have shown that 8-PN has antiproliferative effects on some human breast and colon cancer cell lines. It has also induced cell death in a prostate cancer cell line and, in still other studies, has inhibited angiogenesis, which could make it useful in treating vascularized forms of cancer and other angiogenesis-associated diseases. Whether it is potent enough, in this context, to have any impact in a clinical setting is unknown. Again, much more research is needed to determine the efficacy and safety of this substance as a potential anticancer agent.

Dosing ovariectomized rats for three months with 8-PN had effects on lipids that were said to be more favorable than those achieved with estradiol benzoate. However, the 8-PN had no effect on triglycerides or on HDL-cholesterol. The researchers discerned a role for it in the prevention of cardiovascular disease associated with estrogen deficiency. That use, however, is clearly premature, pending clinical safety and efficacy trials.

Finally, it has been claimed that 8-PN, and other constituents of hops, can enhance breast size in women. Thus, these constituents have been added to some "breast-enhancement pills" currently being marketed. There is no evidence that these substances are either safe or efficacious.

CONTRAINDICATIONS, PRECAUTIONS, ADVERSE REACTIONS

CONTRAINDICATIONS

8-PN-containing dietary supplements are contraindicated in those hypersensitive to any component of an 8-PN-containing product.

PRECAUTIONS

Those who wish to use an 8-PN-containing dietary supplement for a health condition should first discuss this with his or her physician.

Pregnant females and nursing mothers should avoid the use of 8-PN-containing dietary supplements. Women with breast, uterine or ovarian cancer should avoid the use of 8-PN.

ADVERSE REACTIONS

No reports.

INTERACTIONS

DRUGS

None known.

NUTRITIONAL SUPPLEMENTS

None known.

HERBS

None known.

OVERDOSAGE

There are no reports of overdosage.

DOSAGE AND ADMINISTRATION

The optimal dosage of 8-PN for any health condition is unknown.

A number of 8-PN-containing dietary supplements are available which are marketed for breast enhancement. Because of the lack of long-term safety studies, these supplements are not recommended for use.

Beer is the major dietary source of 8-PN. The concentration of 8-PN in most beers is below 30 micrograms per liter. Some beers, particularly strong ales, have been reported to contain concentrations of up to 250 micrograms (0.24 milligrams) or higher per liter. Beer itself contains isoxanthohumol, a mild phytoestrogen which can be metabolized to 8-PN via the intestinal microflora. This could increase the exposure to 8-PN from beer by up to 4 mg per liter.

LITERATURE

Böttner M, Christoffel J, Wuttke W. Effects of long-term treatment with 8-PN and oral estradiol on the GH-IGF-1 axis and lipid metabolism in rats. *J Endocrinol.* 2008;198:395-401.

Bowe J, Li XF, Kinsey-Jones J, et al. The hop phytoestrogen, 8-PN, reverses the ovariectomy-induced rise in skin temperature in an animal model of menopausal hot flushes. *J Endocrinol.* 2006;191(2):399-405.

Brunelli E, Minassi A, Appendino G, et al. 8-PN, inhibits estrogen receptor-alpha mediated cell growth and induces apoptosis in MCF-7 breast cancer cells. *J Steroid Biochem Mol Biol.* 2007;107(3-5):140-148.

Christoffel J, Rimoldi G, Wuttke W. Effects of 8-PN on the hypothalamo-pituitary-uterine axis in rats after 3-month treatment. *J Endocrinol.* 2006;188(3):397-405.

Delmulle L, Berghe TV, Keukeleire DD, et al. Treatment of PC-3 and DU145 prostate cancer cells by prenylflavonoids from hop (Humulus lupulus L.) induces a caspase-independent form of cell death. *Phytother Res.* 2008;22(2):197-203.

Diel P, Thomae RB, Caldarelli A, et al. Regulation of gene expression by 8-PN in uterus and liver of Wistar rats. *Planta Med.* 2004;70(1):39-44.

Milligan S, Kalita J, Pocock V, et al. Oestrogenic activity of the hop phyto-oestrogen, 8-PN. *Reproduction.* 2002;123(2):235-242.

Milligan SR, Kalita JC, Pocock V, et al. The endocrine activities of 8-PN and related hop (*Humulus lupulus* L.) flavonoids. *J Clin Endocrinol Metab.* 2000;85(12):4912-4915.

Nikolic D, Li Y, Chadwick LR, et al. In vitro studies of intestinal permeability and hepatic and intestinal metabolism of 8-PN, a potent phytoestrogen from hops (Humulus lupulus L.). *Pharm Res.* 2006;23(5):864-872.

Nikolic D, Li Y, Chadwick LR, et al. Metabolism of 8-PN, a potent phytoestrogen from hops (Humulus lupulus), by human liver microsomes. *Drug Metab Dispos.* 2004;32(2):272-279.

Pepper MS, Hazel SJ, Hümpel M, et al. 8-PN, a novel phytoestrogen, inhibits angiogenesis in vitro and in vivo. *J Cell Physiol.* 2004;199(1):98-107.

Rad M, Hümpel M, Schaefer O, et al. Pharmacokinetics and systemic endocrine effects of the phyto-oestrogen 8-PN after single oral doses to postmenopausal women. *Br J Clin Pharmacol.* 2006;62(3):288-296.

Rimoldi G, Christoffel J, Wuttke W. Morphologic changes induced by oral long-term treatment with 8-PN in the uterus, vagina, and mammary gland of castrated rats. *Menopause.* 2006;13(4):669-677.

Roelens F, Heldring N, Dhooge W, et al. Subtle side-chain modifications of the hop phytoestrogen 8-PN result in distinct agonist/antagonist activity profiles for estrogen receptors alpha and beta. *J Med Chem.* 2006;49(25):7357-7365.

Rong H, Boterberg T, Maubach J, et al. 8-PN, the phytoestrogen in hops and beer, upregulates the function of the E-cadherin/catenin complex in human mammary carcinoma cells. *Eur J Cell Biol.* 2001;80(9):580-585.

Schaefer O, Hümpel M, Fritzemeier KH, et al. 8-PN is a potent ERalpha selective phytoestrogen present in hops and beer. *J Steroid Biochem Mol Biol.* 2003;84(2-3):359-360.

Sehmisch S, Hammer F, Christoffel J, et al. Comparison of the phytohormones genistein, resveratrol and 8-PN as agents for preventing osteoporosis. *Planta Med.* 2008;74(8):794-801.

Zierau O, Hauswald S, Schwab P, et al. Two major metabolites of 8-PN are estrogenic in vitro. *J Steroid Biochem Mol Biol.* 2004;92(1-2):107-110.

19-Norandrostenedione

It is illegal to use or possess 19-Norandrostenedione except if enrolled in FDA-allowed clinical trials or if prescribed by a qualified physician.

DESCRIPTION

Following the passage of the Dietary Supplement Health and Education Act (DSHEA) of 1994, a number of putative anabolic substances, including 19-norandrostenedione, began to be marketed as dietary supplements. In March 2004, Senators Joseph Biden and Orrin Hatch co-authored and introduced a bill known as the Anabolic Steroid Control Act of 2004. The Act revised the term "anabolic steroid" to mean any drug or hormonal substance chemically and pharmacologically related to testosterone (other than estrogens, progestins, corticosteroids, and dehydroepiandrosterone [DHEA]). The list attached to the bill contained 59 specific substances, 26 of which were added to the existing 1990 list of steroids that are classified as schedule III controlled substances. The two isomers of 19-norandrostenedione—19-nor-4-androstene-3, 17-dione and 19-nor-5-androstene-3, 17-dione—were included in the list. The bill passed the Senate by unanimous consent on October 6, 2004, passed the House of Representatives two days later and was signed by President George W. Bush on October 22, 2004. It went into effect on January 20, 2005.

19-norandrostenedione refers to two steroid isomers that had been marketed as dietary supplements and mainly used by body builders. The difference between the two 19-norandrostenedione isomers is in the position of the double bond in the cyclopentanoperhydrophenanthrene ring structure. The delta4 isomer has a double bond between carbons 4 and 5; the delta5 isomer has a double bond between carbons 5 and 6.

The delta4 isomer is also known as 19-nor-4-androstene-3, 17-dione. The delta5 isomer is also known as 19-nor-5-androstene-3, 17-dione. The delta4 isomer is sometimes referred to as 19-nor and is the more popular of the two substances. The term "nor" refers to the absence of a 19 methyl group on the steroid ring structure. 19-norandrostenedione is synthesized in the adrenal gland and gonads from androstenedione. It is metabolized by the aromatase complex to estrone. The delta4, as well as delta5, 19-norandrostenedione may also be metabolized by the enzyme 17 beta-hydroxy steroid dehydrogenase to 19-nortestosterone, also known as nandrolone. In this monograph, 19-norandrostenedione will generally be used in the singular to refer to both the delta4 and delta5 isomers.

ACTIONS AND PHARMACOLOGY

ACTIONS

Supplemental 19-norandrostenedione is a putative anabolic substance.

MECHANISM OF ACTION

19-norandrostenedione may be metabolized to 19-nortestosterone in both men and women. 19-Norandrostenedione, also known as nandrolone, is the basic substance of some very popular injectable anabolic steroids. 19-Norandrostenedione is not metabolized to testosterone. Whether increases in 19-nortestosterone levels that may be produced by taking oral 19-norandrostenedione would be sustained long enough to show increase in nitrogen retention and muscle strength and mass is unknown.

PHARMACOKINETICS

There is scant human pharmacokinetic data on 19-norandrostenedione. Absorption appears variable, but some absorption does occur. Following ingestion of 19-norandrostenedione, metabolites, including 19-norandrosterone and 19-noretiocholanolone, appear in the urine. 19-norandrostenedione and 19-noretiocholanolone are detectable in the urine for seven to 10 days after a single 50-mg oral dose. Specific metabolites of 19-nor-5-androstene-3, 17-dione are 19-nor-dehydroandrosterone and 19-nordehydroepiandrosterone. In the later stages of excretion, higher levels of 19-noretiocholanolone relative to 19-norandrosterone indicate intake of 19-nor delta5 steroids.

INDICATIONS AND USAGE

The claim that supplemental 19-norandrostenedione has anabolic effects is unsubstantiated. The use of this substance may pose serious health risks in some.

RESEARCH SUMMARY

There is no research showing that either oral or injectable 19-norandrostenedione has significant anabolic effects.

CONTRAINDICATIONS, PRECAUTIONS, ADVERSE REACTIONS

CONTRAINDICATIONS

19-norandrostenedione is contraindicated in those with prostate, breast, ovarian and uterine cancer and those at risk for these cancers. 19-norandrostenedione is also contraindicated in those who are hypersensitive to any component of a 19-norandrostenedione-containing preparation.

PRECAUTIONS

19-norandrostenedione is illegal to use or possess except if enrolled in an FDA-allowed clinical trial or if prescribed by a qualified physician.

ADVERSE REACTIONS

No data are available on the long-term safety of taking supplemental 19-norandrostenedione. Adverse effects of exogenous testosterone in men include acne, testicular atrophy, gynecomastia, behavioral changes and possibly an increased risk of prostate cancer. Adverse effects of exogenous testosterone in women include hirsutism, deepening of the voice, acne, clitoral hypertrophy, amenorrhea, male-pattern baldness and coarsening of the skin. In adolescents, exogenous testosterone can lead to early closing of bone growth plates and decreased adult height. Other adverse effects of testosterone include hepatic failure and increased platelet aggregation.

Many, if not all, of the above adverse reactions may occur with long-term use of 19-norandrostenedione.

INTERACTIONS

No drug, nutritional supplement, food or herb interactions have yet been reported.

OVERDOSAGE

No reports of overdosage.

DOSAGE AND ADMINISTRATION

19-norandrostenedione is illegal to use or possess except if enrolled in an FDA-allowed clinical trial or if prescribed by a qualified physician.

LITERATURE

Anabolic Steroid Control Act of 2004. http://frwebgate.access. gpo.gov/cgi-bin/getdoc.cgi?dbname=108_cong_public_ laws&docid=f:publ358.108.pdf. Accessed September 22, 2008.

Uralets VP, Gillette PA. Over-the-counter anabolic steroids 4-androsten-3, 17-dione; 4-androsten-3beta, 17beta-diol; and 19-nor-4-androstene-3, 17-dione: excretion studies in men. *J Anal Toxicol.* 1999;23:357-366.

Uralets VP, Gillette PA. Over-the-counter delta5 anabolic steroids 5-androsten-3, 17-dione, 5-androsten-3beta, 17 beta-diol; dehydroxyepiandrosterone; and 19-nor-5-androstene-3, 17-dione: excretion studies in men. *J Anal Toxicol.* 2000;24:188-193.

Acetyl-L-Carnitine

DESCRIPTION

Acetyl-L-Carnitine is the acetyl ester of L-carnitine. It occurs naturally in animal products. Chemically, acetyl-L-carnitine is known as beta-acetoxy-gamma-N, N, N-trimethylamino-butyrate and is represented by the following chemical structure:

$$(CH_3)_3\overset{+}{N}\text{---}CH_2\text{-}CH\text{---}CH_2\text{-}COO^-$$
$$| $$
$$O$$
$$\text{CCH}_3$$
$$||$$
$$O$$

Acetyl-L-Carnitine

Acetyl-L-carnitine is also known as acetyl-carnitine, L-acetycarnitine, acetylcarnitine, acetyl levocarnitine, N-acetyl-L-carnitine, ALC and ALCAR.

Acetyl-L-carnitine is a delivery form for both L-carnitine and acetyl groups.

ACTIONS AND PHARMACOLOGY

ACTIONS

Supplemental acetyl-L-carnitine may have neuroprotective activity. In addition, it, like L-carnitine, may have cardioprotective activity and may beneficially affect cardiac function. It may enhance sperm motility. Acetyl-L-carnitine may also have cytoprotective, antioxidant and anti-apoptotic activity.

MECHANISM OF ACTION

Acetyl-L-carnitine is a delivery form for L-carnitine and acetyl groups. The functions of L-carnitine include transport of long-chain fatty acids across the mitochondrial membranes into the mitochondria (wherein their metabolism produces bioenergy) and transport of small-chain and medium-chain fatty acids out of the mitochondria in order to, among other things, maintain normal coenzyme A levels in these organelles. It may also have antioxidant activity.

The acetyl component of acetyl-L-carnitine provides for the formation of the neurotransmitter acetylcholine. Abnormal acetylcholine metabolism in the brain, leading to acetylcholine deficits in certain brain regions, is thought to be associated with age-related dementias, including Alzheimer's disease.

Acetyl-L-carnitine has been found to decrease glycation of lens proteins *in vitro*. It is thought to do so by acetylating certain lens proteins called crystallins. In so doing it protects them from glycation-mediated damage.

Many biochemical changes occur during the aging process. These include decreased cardiolipin synthesis in the heart and impaired mitochondrial function. Cardiolipin is a key phospholipid necessary for mitochondrial transport processes in the heart. Mitochondria are vital for the production of cellular energy. Experiments in aged rats have shown that acetyl-L-carnitine supplementation leads to improved mitochondrial function and increased cardiolipin production.

Acetyl-L-carnitine serves as a readily accessible energy pool for use in both activation of respiration and motility in human spermatozoa.

PHARMACOKINETICS

The pharmacokinetics of acetyl-L-carnitine is similar to L-Carnitine (see L-carnitine). There is speculation that it is better absorbed than L-carnitine, but this has not yet been established.

INDICATIONS AND USAGE

Acetyl-L-carnitine has recently demonstrated some efficacy as a possible neuroprotective agent and may be indicated for use in strokes, Alzheimer's disease, Down's syndrome and for the management of various neuropathies. It may also have anti-aging properties. Research regarding acetyl-L-carnitine's possible beneficial effect on sperm motility is early-stage but promising. One group of researchers suggested that acetyl-L-carnitine might be useful in the treatment of HIV lipoatrophy, although evidence for this is presently lacking.

RESEARCH SUMMARY

Several studies have now demonstrated some positive effects of acetyl-L-carnitine supplementation in Alzheimer's patients especially with regard to tasks involving attention and concentration. In a double-blind, parallel design, placebo-controlled pilot study of 30 patients whose mild-to-moderate dementias were believed to be symptoms of Alzheimer's disease, there were significant, positive results as measured by some of the neuropsychological tests used in the study.

In another early double-blind, placebo-controlled study of 130 patients with clinical diagnoses of Alzheimer's disease, a slower rate of deterioration was observed in 13 of 14 outcome measures at the end of this one-year study. Some of these measures reached statistical significance, including measures of logical intelligence, long-term verbal memory and selective attention.

More recent studies continue to show beneficial effects in Alzheimer's disease. Younger patients seem to benefit most.

It has been suggested that cognitive function may be improved in subjects with Alzheimer's disease by acetyl-L-carnitine's hypothesized ability to inhibit apoptosis of cerebral nerve cells.

Significant improvement in visual memory and attention in Down's syndrome subjects treated with acetyl-L-carnitine has also been reported. These researchers hypothesized that acetyl-L-carnitine's positive actions in both Alzheimer's disease and Down's syndrome result from its direct and indirect cholinomimetic effects.

There is also preliminary evidence that acetyl-L-carnitine can slow mental decline in the elderly who are not afflicted with dementias.

Neuroprotective effects of acetyl-L-carnitine have been reported after stroke in both animal models and in humans. Cerebral blood flow reportedly improves in acetyl-L-carnitine treated subjects with cerebrovascular disease.

Peripheral nerve function has been improved with the use of acetyl-L-carnitine in experimental diabetes. There is also early clinical evidence that acetyl-L-carnitine may be helpful in various peripheral neuropathies, and it has been suggested that this supplement might be helpful in alleviating the neurotoxicity associated with the nucleoside analogues used in the treatment of AIDS. This latter hypothesis has yet to be tested.

There is some evidence in animal work that acetyl-L-carnitine might have anti-aging effects. Mitochondrial function and ambulatory activity were assessed in a study of old rats fed acetyl-L-carnitine. Ambulatory activity was significantly increased in the old rats, and an examination of liver cells in the treated animals showed a significant reversal of age-associated decline of mitochondrial membrane potential. Cardiolipin, which declines with age, was significantly restored.

Recently, there has been some further work with lipoic acid, in combination with acetyl-L-carnitine, related to aging. In one study, feeding acetyl-L-carnitine and alpha-lipoic acid to old rats was said to significantly improve metabolic function while decreasing oxidative stress. In another study, this same combination was reported to maintain myocardial function in aging rats. Beagle dogs between 7.6 and 8.8 years of age that were administered a twice-daily supplement of these agents over a two-month period reportedly made fewer errors in two learning tests, compared with controls. The researchers concluded that they believe long-term supplementation could slow cognitive decline in these animals. Whether these findings might have clinical relevance is unknown.

One group of researchers hypothesized that acetyl-L-carnitine might be useful in the treatment of HIV lipoatrophy, a syndrome that features both fat accumulation and wasting, sometimes accompanied by metabolic derangement of glucose and lipids. The researchers proposed a pilot study to test this hypothesis. As yet, there are no results to support or refute the idea.

Finally, acetyl-L-carnitine has been reported to increase sperm motility *in vitro*, and in one human trial, 4 grams daily of this substance given to 20 oligoasthenospermic men produced increased progressive sperm motility, which was associated with a greater number of pregnancies.

CONTRAINDICATIONS, PRECAUTIONS, ADVERSE REACTIONS

CONTRAINDICATIONS

Known hypersensitivity to an acetyl-L-carnitine-containing product.

PRECAUTIONS

Because of lack of long-term safety studies, acetyl-L-carnitine is not advised for pregnant women or nursing mothers. Those with seizure disorders should only use acetyl-L-carnitine under medical advisement and supervision.

ADVERSE REACTIONS

Mild gastrointestinal symptoms may occur in those taking acetyl-L-carnitine supplements. These include nausea, vomiting, abdominal cramps and diarrhea.

Increased agitation has been reported in some with Alzheimer's disease when taking oral acetyl-L-carnitine. In those with seizure disorders, an increase in seizure frequency and/or severity has been reported in some taking this substance. The incidence of this in this population is low.

INTERACTIONS

Therapy with the nucleoside analogues didanosine (ddI), zalcitabine (ddC) and stavudine (d4T) may lead to decreased acetyl-L-carnitine levels.

Therapy with valproic acid and the pivalic acid-containing antibiotics may lead to secondary L-carnitine deficiencies (see L-carnitine).

OVERDOSAGE

There are no reports of overdosage.

DOSAGE AND ADMINISTRATION

Typical doses of supplemental acetyl-L-carnitine are 500 milligrams to 2 grams daily in divided doses.

LITERATURE

Aliev G, Liu J, Shenk JC, et al. Neuronal mitochondrial amelioration by feeding acetyl-L-carnitine and lipoic acid to aged rats. *J Cell Mol Med.* Epub: 2008 Mar 28.

Brooks JO 3rd, Yesavage JA, Carta A, et al. Acetyl-L-carnitine slows decline in younger patients with Alzheimer's disease: a reanalysis of a double-blind, placebo-controlled trial using the trilinear approach. *Int Psychogeriatr.* 1998;10:193-203.

Chiechio S, Copani A, Gereau RW 4th, et al. Acetyl-L-carnitine in neuropathic pain: experimental data. *CNS Drugs.* 2007;21 Suppl 1:31-80;discussion 45-60.

Chiechio S, Copani A, Nicoletti F, et al. L-acetylcarnitine: a proposed therapeutic agent for painful peripheral neuropathies. *Curr Neuropharmacol.* 2006;4(3):233-237.

Chuang WW, Lin WW, Lamb DJ, et al. Effect of acetylcarnitine on sperm motility. *J Urol.* 2000; 163(4 Suppl):Abstract1324.

Day L, Shikuma C, Gerschenson M. Acetyl-L-carnitine for the treatment of HIV lipoatrophy. *Ann NY Acad Sci.* 2004;1033:139-146.

De Grandis D. Acetyl-L-carnitine for the treatment of chemotherapy-induced peripheral neuropathy: a short review. *CNS Drugs.* 2007;21 Suppl 1:39-43; discussion 45-60.

Famularo G, Morreti S, Marcellini S, et al. Acetyl-carnitine deficiency in AIDS patients with neurotoxicity on treatment with antiretroviral nucleoside analogues. *AIDS.* 1997;11:185-190.

Gorini A, D'Angelo A, Villa RF. Action of L-acetylcarnitine on different cerebral mitochondrial populations from cerebral cortex. *Neurochem Res.* 1998;23:1485-1491.

Hagen TM, Ingersoll RT, Wehr CM, et al. Acetyl-L-carnitine fed to old rats partially restores mitochondrial function and ambulatory activity. *Proc Natl Acad Sci USA.* 1998;95:9562-9566.

Hagen TM, Liu J, Lykkesfeldt J, et al. Feeding acetyl-L-carnitine and lipoic acid to old rats significantly improves

metabolic function while decreasing oxidative stress. *Proc Natl Acad Sci U S A.* 2002;99(4):1870-1875.

Hagen TM, Wehr CM, Ames BN. Mitochondrial decay in aging. Reversal through supplementation of acetyl-L-carnitine and N-tert-butyl-alpha-phenyl-nitrone. *Ann NY Acad Sci.* 1998;854:214-223.

Hudson S, Tabet N. Acetyl-L-carnitine for dementia. *Cochrane Database Syst Rev.* 2003;(2):CD003158.

Lolic MM, Fiskum G, Rosenthal RE. Neuroprotective effects of acetyl-L-carnitine after stroke in rats. *Ann Emerg Med.* 1997;29:758-765.

Milgram NW, Araujo JA, Hagen TM, et al. Acetyl-L-carnitine and alpha-lipoic acid supplementation of aged beagle dogs improves learning in two landmark discrimination tests. *FASEB J.* 2007;21(13):3756-3762.

Moncada ML, Vicari E, Cimino C, et al. Effect of acetylcarnitine treatment in oligoasthenospermic patients. *Acta Eur Fertil.* 1992:23:221-224.

Onofrj M, Fulgente T, Melchiadona D, et al. L-acetylcarnitine as a new therapeutic approach for peripheral neuropathies with pain. *Int J Clin Pharmacol Res.* 1995;15:9-15.

Pettegrew JW, Klunke WE, Panchalingam K. Clinical and biochemical effects of acetyl-L-carnitine in Alzheimer's disease. *Neurobiol Aging.* 1995;16:1-4.

Pettegrew JW, Levine J, McClure RJ. Acetyl-L-carnitine physical-chemical, metabolic, and therapeutic properties: relevance for its mode of action in Alzheimer's disease and geriatric depression. *Mol Psychiatry.* 2000;5(6):616-632.

Piovesan P, Quatrini G, Pacifici L, et al. Acetyl-L-carnitine restores choline acetyltransferase activity in the hippocampus of rats with partial unilateral fimbria-fornix transection. *Int J Dev Neurosci.* 1995;13:13-19.

Rebouche CJ. Kinetics, pharmacokinetics, and regulation of L-carnitine and acetyl-L-carnitine metabolism. *Ann N Y Acad Sci.* 2004;1033:30-41.

Salvioli G, Neri M. L-acetylcarnitine treatment of mental decline in the elderly. *Drugs Exp Clin Res.* 1994;20:169-176.

Sano M, Bell K, Cote L, et al. Double-blind parallel pilot study of acetyl levocarnitine in patients with Alzheimer's disease. *Arch Neurol.* 1992;49:1137-1141.

Sima AA. Acetyl-L-carnitine in diabetic polyneuropathy: experimental and clinical data. *CNS Drugs.* 2007;21 Suppl 1:13-23; discussion 45-60.

Thal LJ, Carta A, Clarke WR, et al. A one year multicenter placebo-controlled study of acetyl-L-carnitine in patients with Alzheimer's disease. *Neurology.* 1996;47:705-711.

White HL, Scates PW. Acetyl-L-carnitine as a precursor of acetylcholine. *Neurochem Res.* 1990;15:597-601.

Youle M. Acetyl-L-carnitine in HIV-associated antiretroviral toxic neuropathy. *CNS Drugs.* 2007;21 Suppl 1:25-30; discussion 45-46.

Zhou X, Liu F, Zhai S. Effect of L-carnitine and/or L-acetyl-carnitine in nutrition treatment for male infertility: a systematic review. *Asia Pac J Clin Nutr*. 2007;16 Suppl 1:383-390.

Acetylcysteine

DESCRIPTION

Acetylcysteine, or N-acetylcysteine, commonly abbreviated as NAC, is the N-acetyl derivative of the protein amino acid L-cysteine (see L-Cysteine). NAC is available as a nutritional supplement and as a drug. It is given orally or by slow intravenous infusion in the treatment of acetaminophen (known as paracetamol in Europe) overdose. NAC is also used in the treatment of respiratory disorders, such as acute and chronic bronchitis associated with the production of excessive or viscous mucus. For such respiratory disorders, it is delivered as an inhalant.

NAC is a delivery form of L-cysteine. L-cysteine is hygroscopic and slowly decomposes and oxidizes. NAC is more stable than L-cysteine, and it may be better absorbed. NAC, in addition to being known as N-acetylcysteine, is known as acetylcysteine and N-acetyl-L-cysteine. It is represented by the following chemical structure:

$$HS-CH_2-CH \begin{cases} COOH \\ NH-\underset{\underset{O}{\parallel}}{C}-CH_3 \end{cases}$$

N-acetyl-L-cysteine

ACTIONS AND PHARMACOLOGY

ACTIONS

NAC is a reducing agent and has antioxidant activity. It is also a mucolytic and a hepatoprotectant, and it may have anti-apoptotic activity.

MECHANISM OF ACTION

NAC's efficacy in the treatment of acetaminophen overdose is due mainly to its ability to regenerate liver stores of glutathione. NAC is a delivery form of L-cysteine, which serves as a major precursor to the antioxidant glutathione. An overdose of acetaminophen leads to its metabolism to large quantities of N-acetyl-benzoquinoneimine or NABQI in the liver. NABQI depletes hepatic glutathione stores, placing an enormous oxidative stress on the liver, which can lead to hepatic failure and be life-threatening.

NAC's mucolytic activity is believed to be due to its ability to reduce disulfide bonds in mucoproteins found in mucus, liquefying this viscous substance.

The hepatoprotectant activity of NAC is also due to its ability to serve as a precursor to glutathione. A major role of glutathione is the maintenance of a normal redox state of the liver. A normal redox state is vital to normal hepatic function.

There is some evidence that NAC may have anti-apoptotic activity, particularly in pancreatic beta-cells and nerve cells. This research is still preliminary, but it is believed that the possible anti-apoptotic effect of NAC is due to its antioxidant activity. Specifically, it is thought that NAC, in its role as a precursor to L-cysteine and glutathione, may protect cell membranes against lipid peroxidation and protein oxidation.

PHARMACOKINETICS

NAC is rapidly absorbed from the gastrointestinal tract and transported to the liver via the portal circulation, where it undergoes extensive first-pass metabolism. Peak plasma concentrations are observed approximately 0.5 to 1 hour following oral administration of doses of 200 to 600 milligrams. NAC is metabolized to N-acetylcysteine, N,N'-diacetylcysteine, N, N-diacetylcystine and L-cysteine, among other metabolites. L-cysteine itself is metabolized to glutathione, protein, taurine and sulfate. NAC has low bioavailability, probably because of its extensive first-pass metabolism in the liver. The terminal half-life of total NAC is approximately 6.25 hours after ingestion.

INDICATIONS AND USAGE

Broad claims are made for NAC. There is some support for claims that it is hepatoprotective, that it is of benefit in some with early adult respiratory distress syndrome and chronic obstructive pulmonary disease and that it might help protect against cardiovascular disease. There is also some preliminary suggestion that it might have some usefulness in the treatment of diabetes, some cancers and some immune disorders. A recent study suggests that NAC might have some favorable impact on age-related memory loss. Its benefit in reversing tolerance to nitrates in patients with coronary artery disease remains controversial. However, NAC may benefit some individuals who have noise-induced hearing loss.

RESEARCH SUMMARY

High-dose NAC has been used successfully as an antidote for acetaminophen poisoning and *Amanita phalloides* intoxication. In one series of 11 patients with *Amanita phalloides* poisoning, a detoxifying regimen that included NAC produced successful recovery in all but one subject without need of liver transplantation. Fulminant hepatic failure induced by acetaminophen overdose has similarly been significantly ameliorated by NAC treatment. It is believed that NAC accomplishes these benefits by preventing hepatic necrosis through replenishment of glutathione and, possibly, through enhanced oxygen delivery and consumption.

Given that acetaminophen overdose is the most common cause of calls to poison control centers in the United States, NAC's contribution is quite significant in this context. It has been suggested that NAC might also be useful in some infectious liver disorders, such as hepatitis C. As of yet, there is no evidence of efficacy in those diseases.

Several studies have indicated that NAC might be helpful in treating chronic obstructive pulmonary disease (COPD). In an open, controlled multicenter study of 169 patients with moderate-to-severe COPD, subjects were randomized to receive standard treatment plus 600 milligrams of NAC once daily or standard therapy alone for a six-month period. Exacerbations of COPD were reduced 41% in the NAC-treated group, compared with the standard therapy-only group. There was also a significant reduction in number of sick days among the NAC-treated. Another study found benefit from NAC and rutin in protecting the lungs of patients, with early adult respiratory distress syndrome ARDS. However, not all with ARDS benefit from NAC.

NAC has improved myocardial contraction in an animal model of myocardial ischemia. It has also been shown to inhibit platelet aggregation; and it has lowered lipoprotein (a) levels to a degree not previously achieved by either drugs or diet, according to some researchers. Additionally, some recent clinical studies have demonstrated that intravenous infusion of NAC during thrombolysis is associated with decreased size of infarct and increased rescue of left ventricular function.

One group of researchers concluded: "Short-and long-term studies indicated that also on patients with unstable angina pectoris and threat of infarct, the intravenous or oral administration of N-acetylcysteine in association with nitroglycerin is highly effective in decreasing the risk of worsening, mainly by preventing the occurrence of acute myocardial infarction."

Animal model work has produced preliminary evidence that NAC, apparently more than either vitamins C or E, or both, can be of some benefit in insulin-dependent diabetes mellitus. NAC reportedly inhibits pancreatic beta-cell apoptosis without affecting the rate of beta-cell proliferation. NAC has also been shown to moderately decrease blood glucose levels and to retain glucose-stimulated insulin secretion.

There is some interest in NAC as a possible anti-cancer agent. There is some preliminary work indicating that it might be helpful in the early stages of some cancers. It is hypothesized to be a logical chemopreventive agent in some cancers based on its properties and some experimental data demonstrating, among other things, extracellular inhibition of mutagenic agents, protection of DNA and nuclear enzymes, and dampening of reactive oxygen species.

One group of researchers, however, claims to have found some evidence of NAC-induced DNA damage in a human leukemia cell line and has cautioned that NAC "may have the dual function of carcinogenic and anti-carcinogenic potentials." More research is needed.

NAC's therapeutic role, if any, in the treatment of immune disorders is similarly undecided. NAC has been shown to inhibit factors that are believed to stimulate HIV; this inhibition has been attributed to NAC-induced increases in intracellular thiol levels. These *in vitro* findings have not yet been demonstrated in clinical trials.

Recently, NAC was administered to eight patients with steroid-resistant acute graft-versus-host disease. Prompt significant response was seen in six of these subjects, four complete and two partial responses. More studies are needed.

A recent study of aged mice found some evidence that NAC can help prevent apoptotic death of neuronal cells and help protect against oxidative damage in synaptic mitochondria. NAC-supplemented mice were compared with unsupplemented mice fed standard food pellets. After 23 weeks, there was significant correction of some memory deficits in the aged mice receiving NAC, compared with those on the standard diet. And there were significant reductions in lipid peroxide and protein carbonyl levels in the synaptic mitochondria of the NAC-supplemented mice.

While some studies suggest that NAC can reverse tolerance to nitrates in patients with coronary artery disease, other studies have failed to demonstrate any benefit. On the other hand, NAC might help prevent/ameliorate noise-induced hearing loss, which is a growing problem; it is estimated that 600 million people worldwide are exposed to noise hazards occupationally, including 50 million in the United States. NAC has shown benefit in some, but not all, animal models of acute acoustic trauma. The military is reportedly investigating the use of NAC as a possible treatment agent to be administered shortly after acute acoustic trauma. Some preliminary clinical trials (typically using 900 mg of NAC, sometimes prior to exposure to loud noise such as occurs in a discotheque or on a shooting range) have produced mildly promising but inconclusive results. The rationale for trying NAC in this context relates to its antioxidant and cell-death inhibiting properties, experimentally found to be useful in protecting against noise-induced cochlear injury. More-rigorous trials are needed and warranted.

CONTRAINDICATIONS, PRECAUTIONS, ADVERSE REACTIONS

CONTRAINDICATIONS

Known hypersensitivity to an NAC-containing product.

PRECAUTIONS

Supplemental NAC should be avoided by nursing mothers and should only be used by pregnant women if prescribed by a physician.

N-acetylcysteine clearance is reduced in those with chronic liver disease as well as in pre-term newborns.

NAC may be harmful if administered early in the treatment of critically ill patients.

NAC may intensify headaches in those taking nitrates for the treatment of angina.

Although the incidence of cystine renal stones is low, they do occur. Those who do form renal stones, particularly cystine stones, should avoid NAC supplements.

NAC and its sulfhydryl metabolites, like other sulfhydryl-containing substances, could produce a false-positive result in the nitroprusside test for ketone bodies used in diabetes.

NAC should be used with caution in those with a history of peptic ulcer disease, since mucolytic agents may disrupt the gastric mucosal barrier.

ADVERSE REACTIONS

Adverse reactions reported with oral NAC include nausea, vomiting, diarrhea, headache (especially when used along with nitrates) and rashes. There are rare reports of renal stone formation.

Adverse reactions reported with intravenous NAC include bronchospasm, nausea, vomiting, stomatitis, rhinorrhea, headache, tinnitus, urticaria, rashes, chills and fever. There are rare reports of anaphylactic reactions. The most common symptoms of those experiencing anaphylactoid reactions are rash, pruritus, flushing, nausea, vomiting, angioedema, tachycardia, bronchospasm, hypotension, hypertension and ECG change. The anaphylactoid reactions are pseudo-allergic rather than immunologic.

INTERACTIONS

Nitrates: Use of supplemental NAC along with nitrates may cause headaches.

Carbamazepine: Use of supplemental NAC along with carbamazepine may cause reduced serum levels of carbamazepine.

No interactions with nutritional supplements, food or herbs are known.

OVERDOSAGE

There are no reports of overdosage with oral, supplemental NAC. There are reports of overdosage when using intravenous NAC for treatment of acetaminophen poisoning. Symptoms of overdosage are similar to those of anaphylaxis (rash, pruritis, flushing, nausea, vomiting, angioedema, tachycardia, bronchospasm, hypotension, hypertension, ECG abnormalities) but have been more severe. Hypotension appears to be a major symptom of overdosage. Other symptoms include respiratory depression, hemolysis, DIC (disseminated intravascular coagulation) and renal failure. It is unclear whether some of these symptoms may have been due to acetaminophen poisoning. Death has occurred in three patients receiving an overdosage of NAC while being treated for acetaminophen poisoning. The role of NAC in these deaths was unclear in two of the patients.

DOSAGE AND ADMINISTRATION

Use of NAC for mucus liquefaction in severe broncho-pulmonary disease or acetaminophen overdosage should be dosed according to instructions in the package insert.

Supplemental intake ranges from 600 milligrams once to three times daily. Those who supplement with NAC should drink 6 to 8 glasses of water daily in order to prevent cystine renal stones. Cystine renal stones are rare but do occur.

LITERATURE

Ahola T, Fellman V, Laaksonen R, et al. Pharmacokinetics of intravenous N-acetylcysteine in pre-term new-born infants. *Eur J Clin Pharmacol.* 1999;55:645-650.

Ardissino D, Melini PA, Savonitto S, et al. Effect of transdermal nitroglycerin or N-acetylcysteine, or both, in the long-term treatment of unstable angina pectoris. *J Am Coll Cardiol.* 1997;29:941-947.

Bielefeld EC, Kopke RD, Jackson RL, et al. Noise protection with N-acetyl-l-cysteine (NAC) using a variety of noise exposures, NAC doses, and routes of administration. *Acta Otolaryngol.* 2007;127(9):914-919.

Bongers V, de Jong J, Steen I, et al. Antioxidant-related parameters in patients treated for cancer chemoprevention with N-acetylcysteine. *Europ J Cancer.* 1995;31A:921-923.

Colombo AA, Alessandrino EP, Bernasconi P, et al. N-acetylcysteine in the treatment of steroid-resistant acute graft-versus-host-disease: preliminary results. Gruppo Italiano Trapianto di Midollo Osseo (GITMO) *Transplantation.* 1999;68:1414-1416.

Dawson AH, et al. Adverse reactions to N-acetylcysteine during treatment for paracetamol poisoning. *Med J Aust.* 1989;150:329-331.

De Flora S, Grassi C, Carati L. Attenuation of influence-like symptomatology and improvement of cell-mediated immunity with long-term N-acetylcysteine treatment. *Eur RespirJ.* 1997;10:1535-1541.

DeVries N, De Flora S. N-acetyl-L-cysteine. *J Cell Biochem.* 1993;Supp 17F:270-277.

Gavish D, Breslow JL. Lipoprotein (a) reduction by N-acetylcysteine. *Lancet.* 1991;337:203-204.

Hamernik RP, Qiu W, Davis B. The effectiveness of N-acetyl-L-cysteine (L-NAC) in the prevention of severe noise-induced hearing loss. *Hear Res.* 2008;239(1-2):99-106.

Harrison PM, Wendon JA, Gimson AES, et al. Improvement by acetylcysteine of hemodynamics and oxygen transport in fulminant hepatic failure. *N Engl J Med.* 1991;324:1852-1857.

Heard KJ. Acetylcysteine for acetaminophen poisoning. *N Engl J Med.* 2008;359(3):285-292.

Ho E, Chen G, Bray TM. Supplementation of N-acetylcysteine inhibits NFkappaB activation and protects against alloxan-induced diabetes in CD-1 mice. *FASEB J.* 1999;13:1845-1854.

Hogan JC, Lewis MJ, Henderson AH. Chronic administration of N-acetylcysteine fails to prevent nitrate tolerance in patients with stable angina pectoris. *Br J Clin Pharmacol.* 1990;30:573-577.

Hogan JC, Lewis MJ, Henderson AH. N-acetylcysteine fails to attenuate haemodynamic tolerance to glyceryl trinitrate in healthy volunteers. *Br J Clin Pharmacol.* 1989;28:421-426.

Holdiness MR. Clinical pharmacokinetics of N-acetylcysteine. *Clinical Pharmacokinet.* 1991;20:123-134.

Horowitz JD, Henry CA, Syrjanen ML, et al. Nitroglycerine/N-acetylcysteine in the management of unstable angina pectoris. *Eur Heart J.* 1988;9 Suppl A:95-100.

Iversen HK. N-acetylcysteine enhances nitroglycerin-induced headache and cranial arterial response. *Clin Pharmacol Ther.* 1992;52:125-133.

Jones AL, Jarvie DR, Simpson D, et al. Pharmacokinetics of N-acetylcysteine are altered in patients with chronic liver disease. *Aliment Pharmacol Ther.* 1997;11:787-791.

Kelebic T, Kinter A, Poli G, et al. Suppression of human immunodeficiency virus expression in chronically infected monocyte cells by glutathione, glutathione ester, and N-acetylcysteine. *Proc Natl Accd Sci.* 1991;88:986-990.

Kopke RD, Jackson RL, Coleman JK, et al. NAC for noise: from the bench top to the clinic. *Hear Res.* 2007;226(1-2):114-125.

Lorito G, Giordano P, Petruccelli J, et al. Different strategies in treating noiseinduced hearing loss with N-acetylcysteine. *Med Sci Monit.* 2008;14(8):BR159-164.

Lorito G, Giordano P, Prosser S, et al. Noise-induced hearing loss: a study on the pharmacological protection in the Sprague Dawley rat with N-acetyl-cysteine. *Acta Otorhinolaryngol Ital.* 2006;26(3):133-139.

Louwerse ES, Weverling GJ, Bossuyt PM, et al. Randomized double-blind controlled trial of acetylcysteine in amyotrophic lateral sclerosis. *Arch Neurol.* 1995;52:559-564.

Mani TGK, et al. Adverse reactions to acetylcysteine and effects of overdose. *Br Med J.* 1984;289:217-219.

Marchetti G, Lodola E, Licciardello L, et al. Use of N-acetylcysteine in the management of coronary artery diseases. *Cardiologia.* 1999;44:633-637.

Martinez M, Hernandez AI, Martinez N. N-acetylcysteine delays age-associated memory impairment in mice: role in synaptic mitochondric. *Brain Res.* 2000;855:100-106.

Molnar Z, Schearer E, Lowe D. N-acetylcysteine treatment to prevent the progression of multisystem organ failure: a prospective, randomized placebo-controlled study. *Crit Care Med.* 1999;27:1100-1104.

Montanini S, Sinardi D, Pratico C, et al. Use of acetylcysteine as the life-saving antidote in Amanita phalloides (death cap) poisoning. Case report on 11 patients. *Arzneimittel-forschung.* 1999;49:1044-1047.

Oikawa S, Yamada K, Yamashita N, et al. N-acetylcysteine, a cancer chemopreventive agent, causes oxidative damage to cellular and isolated DNA. *Carcinogenesis.* 1999;20:1485-1490.

Ortolani O, Conti A, De Gaudio AR, et al. Protective effects of N-acetylcysteine and rutin on the lipid peroxidation of the lung epithelium during the adult respiratory distress syndrome. *Shock.* 2000;13:14-18.

Pela R, Calcagni AM, Subiaco S, et al. N-acetylcysteine reduces the exacerbation rate in patients with moderate to severe COPD. *Respiration.* 1999;66:495-500.

Roederer M, Staal FJT, Raju PA, et al. Cytoline-stimulated human immunodeficiency virus replication is inhibited by N-acetyl-L-cysteine. *Proc Natl Accd Sci.* 1990;87:4884-4888.

Sala R, Moriggi E, Corvasce G, et al. Protection by N-acetylcysteine against pulmonary endothelial cell damage induced by oxidant damage. *Eur Respir J.* 1993;6:440-446.

Unverferth DV, Jagadeesh JM, Unverferth BJ, et al. Attempt to prevent doxorubicin-induced acute human myocardial morphologic damage with acetylcysteine. *J Natl Canc Inst.* 1983;71:917-920.

Activated Charcoal

DESCRIPTION

Activated charcoal is a type of amorphous carbon prepared by destructive distillation of such materials as wood, vegetables and coconut shells, materials that have much higher surface areas than charcoal itself. It is a fine, black powder of largely pure carbon. The large surface area of activated charcoal confers a great adsorptive capacity to this material. It is this great adsorptive capacity that is the basis for its many industrial as well as medical uses. There are different types of activated charcoal with different adsorption characteristics. The adsorptive characteristics are determined by the configuration of the surface of activated charcoal.

Activated charcoal is widely used in the treatment of acute poisoning (overdose) with such substances as acetaminophen, salicylates, barbiturates and tricyclic antidepressants. Activated charcoal strongly adsorbs aromatic substances such as the above, reducing their absorption from the gastrointestinal tract. Most inorganic poisons are not significantly adsorbed by activated charcoal. A major industrial use of activated charcoal is as a decolorizer. For example, it is used in the late stages of sugar refining to produce white sugar. Activated charcoal is commonly used in air and water filters.

Activated charcoal, in addition to some other substances, has been used in Russia for the treatment of a number of disorders and diseases, including hyperlipidemia, liver, biliary tract and renal diseases. The practice is known as enterosorption and carbon sorption therapy, when activated charcoal is the principle therapeutic component. Oral activated charcoal is known to lower cholesterol levels.

Activated charcoal is also known as active carbon, activated carbon, adsorbent charcoal, carbo activatus, carbo medicinalis, carbon active, carbon attivo, decolorizing charcoal, activkohle (German) and medicinal charcoal.

ACTIONS AND PHARMACOLOGY

ACTIONS
Activated charcoal is a gastrointestinal adsorbent. It may also have hypocholesterolemic activity.

MECHANISM OF ACTION
The large surface area of activated charcoal confers a great adsorptive capacity to this material. The adsorptive capacity of this substance differs for various chemical entities. Activated charcoal is most effective in adsorbing aromatic or benzenoid-type substances. Less well adsorbed are non-aromatic (non-benzenoid) substances, such as the various fatty acids and fatty alcohols. Inorganic substances are poorly adsorbed by activated charcoal. Aromatic substances, such as acetaminophen, salicylates, barbiturates and tricyclic antidepressants, are very strongly adsorbed by activated charcoal, and that is why activated charcoal is commonly used in the management of overdosage of these substances. Adsorption of these drugs reduces their absorption from the gastrointestinal tract.

The mechanism of the hypocholesterolemic effect of activated charcoal is not entirely clear. It is thought that the cholesterol-lowering effect of activated charcoal is caused by its interference with the enterohepatic circulation of bile acids.

PHARMACOKINETICS
Activated charcoal is not absorbed via the gastrointestinal tract, and all ingested activated charcoal is excreted in the feces.

INDICATIONS AND USAGE

Results have been mixed in studies using charcoal in patients with gas complaints. There is some evidence that activated charcoal can favorably affect lipids and that it might be helpful in alleviating symptoms associated with cholestasis of pregnancy. Activated charcoal looks promising for the treatment of uremic pruritis, as well as for congenital erythropoietic porphyria.

RESEARCH SUMMARY

There are inconsistent results in studies related to activated charcoal's efficacy in reducing intestinal gas and symptoms related thereto. In one double-blind study, the substance significantly reduced bloating and abdominal cramps associated with gaseousness. Some other studies have confirmed this effect, and some others have not, discrepancies that may be related to dosing and sampled populations. One researcher reported that activated charcoal effectively adsorbs intestinal gas in healthy subjects but that it "has not been properly investigated in patients with gas complaints."

Oral activated charcoal has significantly lowered plasma total cholesterol and LDL-cholesterol in both animals and humans. It has also raised HDL-cholesterol in some studies. In one crossover study of seven subjects ingesting 4, 8, 16 or 32 grams per day of activated charcoal, serum total and LDL-cholesterol were decreased (maximum 29% and 41% respectively) and the ratio of HDL/LDL-cholesterol was increased (maximum 121%) by activated charcoal in a dose-dependent pattern.

Ten additional subjects with severe hypercholesterolemia took daily, in random order, for three weeks, 16 grams of activated charcoal, 16 grams of cholestyramine or 8 grams of activated charcoal plus 8 grams of cholestyramine. Activated charcoal reduced total and LDL-cholesterol concentrations 23% and 29%, respectively; cholestyramine reduced them 32% and 39%; in combination, they reduced them 30% and 38%. The ratio of HDL/LDL-cholesterol increased from 0.13 to 0.23 with activated charcoal, to 0.29 with cholestyramine and to 0.25 with the combination. Cholestyramine increased serum triglycerides, but activated charcoal did not. Research is ongoing.

Given that elevated serum bile acid levels are thought to play a role in cholestasis of pregnancy, activated charcoal was administered to women with this condition to see if it could decrease these levels. The women were given 50 grams of the substance three times a day for eight days. By day eight, serum total bile acid concentrations were significantly reduced. Outcome of pregnancy was good. This preliminary study needs followup to see whether activated charcoal might be an option in the treatment of entrahepatic cholestasis of pregnancy.

Activated charcoal given as an oral dose of 6 grams provided symptomatic relief in nearly 50% of patients with uremic pruritis, a poorly understood symptom of uremia. The studies have, however, been limited. More research is needed.

Finally, activated charcoal was more effective in reducing plasma porphyrin levels than oral cholestyramine in a patient with congenital erythropoietic porphyria or Gunther's disease. Again, more research is needed.

CONTRAINDICATIONS, PRECAUTIONS, ADVERSE REACTIONS

CONTRAINDICATIONS

Activated charcoal is contraindicated in those whose gastrointestinal tract is not anatomically intact.

PRECAUTIONS

Activated charcoal adsorbs a wide range of drugs and nutrients. Those using activated charcoal should avoid using it within two hours of drug, food, nutritional supplement or herb intake or within two hours before their intake.

ADVERSE REACTIONS

Black stools (from the activated charcoal) occur frequently. Other reported adverse reactions include nausea, vomiting, blackening of the teeth and mouth, abdominal discomfort, diarrhea (more frequent) and constipation (less frequent).

There are occasional reports of drug failure in those who use activated charcoal concomitantly with a drug.

INTERACTIONS

Activated charcoal adsorbs a wide range of drugs and nutrients. Therefore, those using activated charcoal should avoid using it within two hours of drug, food, nutritional supplement or herb intake or within two hours before their intake.

OVERDOSAGE

None reported.

DOSAGE AND ADMINISTRATION

Those who use activated charcoal as an antflatulant typically use 500 to 1000 milligrams as needed. Those who use activated charcoal for its possible cholesterol-lowering effect take 5 to 8 grams two to three times daily. Those who use activated charcoal combine it with plenty of water and must not use it within two hours before or after ingesting any drug, food, nutritional supplement or herb.

LITERATURE

Friedman EA, Saltzman MJ, Delano BG, Bayer MM. Reduction in hyperlipidemia in hemodialysis patients treated with charcoal and oxidized starch (oxystarch). *Am J Clin Nutr.* 1978; 31:1903-1914.

Giovannetti S, Barsotti G, Cupisti A, et al. Oral activated charcoal in patients with uremic pruritis. *Nephron.* 1995; 70:193-196.

Kaaja RJ, Kontula KK, Raiho A, Laatikainen T. Treatment of cholestasis of pregnancy with peroral activated charcoal. A preliminary study. *Scand J Gastroenterol.* 1994; 29:178-181.

Korkushko OV, Bogatskaia LN, Novikova SN, et al. [Use of enterosorption for correction of dyslipoproteinemias in patients with ischemic heart disease in geriatric patients]. [Article in Russian]. *Klin Med (Mosk).* 1991; 69:51-53.

Kuusisto P, Vapaatalo H, Manninen V, et al. Effect of activated charcoal on hypercholesterolaemia. *Lancet.* 1986; 2(8503):366-367.

Neuvonen PJ, Kuusisto P, Manninen V, et al. The mechanism of the hypocholesterolaemic effect of activated charcoal. *Eur J Clin Invest.* 1989; 19:251-254.

Neuvonen PJ, Kuusisto P, Vapaatalo H, Manninen V. Activated charcoal in the treatment of hypercholesterolaemia: dose-response relationships and comparison with cholestyramine. *Eur J Clin Pharmacol.* 1989; 37:225-230

Nikolaev VG. Peroral application of synthetic activated charcoal in USSR. *Biomater Artif Cells Artif Organs.* 1990; 18:555-568.

Pimstone NR, Gandhi SN, Mukerji SK. Therapeutic efficacy of oral charcoal in congenital erythropoietic porphyria. *N Engl J Med.* 1987; 316:390-393.

Robertson KE, Mueller BA. Uremic pruritis. *Am J Health Syst Pharm.* 1996; 53:2159-2170.

Suarez FL, Furne J. Springfield J, Levitt MD. Failure of activated charcoal to reduce the release of gases produced by the colonic flora. *Am J Gastroenterol.* 1999; 94:208-212.

Windrum P, Hull DR, Morris TCM. Herb-drug interactions. *Lancet.* 2000; 355:1019-1020.

Alkoxyglycerols

DESCRIPTION

Alkoxyglycerols are ether-linked glycerols derived from shark liver oil. They include such substances as batyl alcohol, chimyl alcohol and selachyl alcohol. They are also known as alkylglycerols, ether lipids and dietary ether lipids. The terms alkoxyglycerols and shark liver oil are frequently used interchangeably. Alkoxyglycerols are found naturally in shark liver oil in the form of fatty acid esters. These fatty acid esters are called 1-O-alkyl-2,3-diacyl-sn-glycerols and are represented by the following chemical structure:

$$H_2C\!-\!OH$$
$$HO\!-\!CH$$
$$H_2C\!-\!OR$$

Alkoxyglycerol

ACTIONS AND PHARMACOLOGY

ACTIONS

Alkoxyglycerols have putative antiproliferative and immuno-modulatory activities.

MECHANISM OF ACTION

The mechanism of the putative antiproliferative and immunomodulatory actions of alkoxyglycerols is not known. Speculative mechanisms include protein kinase C inhibition, macrophage activation and natural killer cell activation.

PHARMACOKINETICS

Ether glycerols, when absorbed, may be incorporated into plasmalogens and alkylacyl glycerophospholipids. Little is available on the specific pharmacokinetics of the shark oil alkoxyglycerols in humans.

INDICATIONS AND USAGE

Support for claims that the alkoxyglycerols are indicated for the prevention and treatment of any cancer or for the treatment of wounds and inflammatory conditions in humans is limited and unsystematic. There is little support for claims that they are immune-enhancing in humans.

RESEARCH SUMMARY

This shark-liver oil derivative has been touted as an effective anti-cancer treatment. Unfortunately, there is little evidence to support this claim, at least for humans. There is scant evidence it inhibits tumor growth or reduces cancer mortality in humans. It should in no way be relied upon in the treatment of any form of cancer. Similarly, there is little evidence to support claims that this substance is useful for treating wounds and inflammatory conditions. Neither has it been demonstrated in appropriate human clinical studies that it has immune-enhancing effects. There are some *in vitro* and animal studies reporting antiproliferative and immunomodulatory effects for these substances, and perhaps alkoxyglycerols may eventually have a role to play in adjuvant management of certain types of cancer. However, this would need to be established by well-designed, double-blind, placebo-controlled trials, which have not yet been done.

CONTRAINDICATIONS, PRECAUTIONS, ADVERSE REACTIONS

CONTRAINDICATIONS

Known hypersensitivity to an alkoxyglycerol-containing product.

PRECAUTIONS

Those with cancer who are interested in alkoxyglycerols should discuss their use with their physicians. Under no circumstance should they be relied upon as principle elements in the management of their disease. Pregnant women and nursing mothers should avoid alkoxyglycerol supplements.

ADVERSE REACTIONS

Mild gastrointestinal symptoms, including diarrhea, have been reported.

DOSAGE AND ADMINISTRATION

There are no typical doses. Those who use shark liver oil products are cautioned that some preparations may contain high amounts of vitamins A and D.

LITERATURE

Brohult A, Brohult J, Brohult S, Joelsson I. Reduced mortality in cancer patients after administration of alkoxyglycerols. *Acta Obstet Gynecol Scand.* 1986; 65:779-785.

Das AK, Holmes RD, Wilson GN, Hajra AK. Dietary ether lipid incorporation into tissue plasmologens of humans and rodents. *Lipids.* 1992; 27:401-405.

Hallgren B, Niklasson A, Stallberg G, Thorin H. On the occurrence of 1-O-(2-methoxyalkyl)glycerols and 1-O-phytanylglycerol in marine animals. *Acta Chem Scand B.* 1974; 28:1035-1040.

Hasle H, Rose C. [Shark liver oil (alkoxyglycerol) and cancer treatment]. [Article in Danish]. *Ugesk Laeger.* 1991; 153:343-346.

Oh SY, Jadhav LS. Effects of dietary alkoxyglycerols in lactating rats on immune responses in pups. *Pediatr Res.* 1994; 36:300-305.

Alpha-Amylase Inhibitor (Phaseolamin)

DESCRIPTION

The enzyme pancreatic alpha-amylase plays a major role in the digestion of the starch. Starch is comprised of two polysaccharides—amylose and amylopectin. Amylose is comprised of long unbranched chains of D-glucose units bound in alpha (1>4) linkages. Amylopectin is a highly branched structure, also made up of D-glucose units. The backbone glycosidic linkages are alpha (1>4), as in amylose, but the branch points have alpha (1>6) glycosidic linkages. Pancreatic alpha-amylase hydrolyzes alpha (1>4) linkages randomly to produce maltotriose, oligosaccharides, maltose and some D-glucose. Alpha-amylase cannot hydrolyze alpha (1>6) linkages, which occur at the branch points of amylopectin, consequently forming a highly branched core called limit dextrin. A debranching enzyme—alpha (1>6) glycosidase—hydrolyzes the alpha (1>6) linkages at the branch points producing D-glucose. The brush border of the cells lining the lumen of the small intestine contains enzymes that covert oligosaccharides and disaccharides to D-glucose. Alpha-glucosidases convert maltose and maltotriose to D-glucose. D-glucose is then the major end product of the digestion of starch.

The regulation of plasma glucose levels and of glucose metabolism is one of the most important homeostatic mechanisms in the body. In a normal situation, some of the D-glucose formed from starch digestion is stored as glycogen in the liver and some is metabolized to produce biological energy. This occurs when an appropriate amount of non-resistant insulin is secreted in response to the glucose formed via digestion. Under conditions of insulin resistance, postprandial serum glucose is abnormally elevated and less glucose goes into the production of glycogen and into the pathways that produce biological energy, among other metabolic events. A way of rectifying this abnormal situation would be to decrease the amount of D-glucose produced from carbohydrate digestion, slowing down its absorption and consequently diminishing postprandial excursions of insulin and D-glucose. One way of doing that might be to inhibit the enzyme pancreatic alpha-amylase.

Alpha-amylase inhibitors are found in many plants and are abundant in cereals and legumes. A major impetus for research and discovery of these inhibitors is their potential as bioinsecticides. Three different isoforms of an alpha-amylase inhibitor are found in the common bean *Phaseolus vulgaris*. These isoforms are designated alphaAI-1, alphaAI-2 and alphaAI-3.

AlphaAI-1 was purified and analyzed in the mid 1970s and found to be a glycoprotein having a molecular weight of 45 kDa (kilo Daltons) to 50 kDa. This glycoprotein was named phaseolamin in recognition of its origin. Later, it was determined that this glycoprotein had a molecular weight of 56.7 kDa, that it was composed of two kinds of glycopeptide structures, alpha and beta, and that it had a tetrameric structure, $alpha_2beta_2$.

AlphaAI-1 inhibits animal alpha-amylase and forms the basis of a dietary supplement that was introduced into the dietary supplement marketplace in the early 1980s. It was called a "starch blocker," with claims that it would lower plasma glucose levels and also help in weight reduction. However, even though it was demonstrated in some animal studies to have a serum glucose-lowering effect, and even though alpha-amylase inhibition seemed like a good bet for an agent that would result in a decreased release of glucose and insulin, phaseolamin did not appear to work in humans and almost disappeared from the marketplace. However, phaseolamin had a rebirth in the early 2000s that coincided with an increased interest in low-carbohydrate diets for weight management.

ACTIONS AND PHARMACOLOGY

ACTIONS

Alpha-amylase inhibitor (phaseolamin) has possible hypoglycemic activity and possible anorexigenic activity.

MECHANISM OF ACTION

Phaseolamin has demonstrated alpha-amylase activity, *in vitro,* and in animal studies. Further, inhibition of pancreatic alpha-amylase might be expected to demonstrate less of an increase in plasma glucose and plasma insulin levels following a meal, and possibly even a modest weight reduction effect. Parallels might be drawn between a pancreatic alpha-amylase inhibitor and two drugs that inhibit a related enzyme (alpha-glucosidase) in the digestion of starch—acarbose (a maltotetrose derivative) and miglitol (N-hydroxyethyl-1-deoxynojirimycin, a monosaccharide-like substance). Both of these drugs reduce fasting and postprandial serum glucose levels and have a modest effect on weight reduction. The possible mechanism of action of these substances is unclear, but may be due to energy loss from increased colonic fermentation of oligosaccharides and maltose and/or may be due to adiponectin elevation caused by these drugs, among other possibilities. Gastrointestinal side effects, including flatulence, abdominal cramping, borborygms, bloating, diarrhea and nausea, are common in those who use acarbose or miglitol and have to do with undigested carbohydrates entering the large intestine and undergoing fermentation to short-chain fatty acids and the gases methane and hydrogen. Interestingly, these adverse effects have rarely been reported in those using phaseolamin, suggesting the possibility that very little or no inhibition of alpha-amylase is taking place *in vivo*. These gastrointestinal symptoms would very likely occur if undigested starch were to enter the large intestine to be fermented by its bacterial microflora. In this way, the undigested starch would be acting like resistant starch (see Resistant Starch).

Assuming that the inhibition of alpha-amylase does have a weight reduction effect, the mechanism of action of this effect is unclear. It is known that a reduction in postprandial insulin secretion, by preventing rebound hypoglycemia, can have a favorable effect on appetite control. There are other possibilities and it is conceivable that this might occur via yet unknown mechanisms.

The phaseolamin marketed in the 1980s as a "starch blocker" to control hyperglycemia and obesity showed little or no effect on plasma glucose levels or on weight. It was thought that was because the preparations at the time were very crude, had many impurities and little of the alpha-amylase inhibitor. The "new" alpha-amylase inhibitor is said to have no impurities and to have much higher alpha-amylase activity.

Much research and evidence-based clinical trials are needed in order to determine if the new, reformulated phaseolamin has a role in postprandial glucose control and weight management.

PHARMACOKINETICS

Little is known about the pharmacokinetics of phaseolamin. Most importantly, research is needed on the stability of phaseolamin in the stomach and small intestine.

INDICATIONS AND USAGE

There is some evidence that alpha-amylase inhibitor, a so-called "starch blocker" derived from the common white kidney bean (*Phaseolus vulgaris*), may have hypoglycemic and anorexigenic actions and might thus be of benefit in the prevention and treatment of diabetes and obesity. A suggestion that this substance might be protective against colorectal cancer is, at this point, based entirely upon a theoretical mode of action that remains to be demonstrated.

RESEARCH SUMMARY

So-called starch blockers have been marketed for some time as antiobesity and antidiabetic agents. The claim has been that these starch blockers interfere with the breakdown of complex carbohydrate, reducing or prolonging its digestibility and thus reducing carbohydrate absorption, as well as reducing postprandial glucose and insulin levels. There are *in vitro* as well as *in vivo* animal and human data to support this hypothesis, but studies have yielded mixed results over the years. The inconsistency of these results has been attributed by one recent reviewer of the relevant literature to inefficient extraction methods that resulted in products with impurities and low alpha-amylase inhibiting activity. Newer, improved extraction techniques have resulted in purer, more potent products.

Various rat studies using kidney beans or alpha-amylase inhibitor have demonstrated reduced food intake and subsequent modest weight loss. There is some evidence that prolonged administration of the inhibitor is necessary in order to get any meaningful results. Clinical studies have been few, have again reported mixed results and, when positive, have mostly reported what the authors of a review article called "subtle weight loss." It appears that more research is needed in order to establish that alpha-amylase inhibitor has consistent, significant appetite-suppressing/weight-reducing effects.

Rats have exhibited reduced postprandial glucose levels when given amylase inhibitor with or before starch-containing meals. Reductions have also been observed in some human subjects similarly treated. Decreased serum insulin levels have been found in both normal and diabetic rats fed amylase inhibitor. There is sufficient preliminary data to warrant further study of the possible beneficial effects of alpha-amylase inhibitor in diabetes.

The suggestion that alpha-amylase inhibitor might have some protective effects against colon cancer is purely hypothetical but may be worthy of further investigation.

CONTRAINDICATIONS, PRECAUTIONS, ADVERSE REACTIONS

CONTRAINDICATIONS

Products containing alpha-amylase (phaseolamin) should not be used by anyone who is allergic to any component of a phaseolamin-containing product.

PRECAUTIONS

Those with type 2 diabetes who wish to try phaseolamin should do so only with a physician's approval and supervision.

Pregnant women and nursing mothers should avoid the use of phaseolamin.

ADVERSE REACTIONS

If phaseolamin does inhibit pancreatic alpha-amylase, the following gastrointestinal adverse events may be expected: flatulence, abdominal cramping, borborygms, bloating, diarrhea and nausea.

INTERACTIONS

DRUGS

None known.

FOODS

No known interactions.

DIETARY SUPPLEMENTS

No known interactions.

OVERDOSAGE

No reports.

DOSAGE AND ADMINISTRATION

Phaseolamin is available in 500mg and 600mg capsules. Those who use phaseolamin take two pills either once a day in the morning before meals, or two pills before or with each meal.

LITERATURE

Carlson GL, Li BU, Bass P, et al. A bean alpha-amylase inhibitor formulation (starch blocker) is ineffective in man. *Science.* 1983;219(4583):393-395.

Celleno L, Tolaini MV, D'Amore A, et al. A Dietary supplement containing standardized Phaseolus vulgaris extract influences body composition of overweight men and women. *Int J Med Sci.* 2007;4(1):45-52.

Chokshi D. Toxicity studies of Blockal, a dietary supplement containing Phase 2 Starch Neutralizer (Phase 2), a standardized extract of the common white kidney bean (Phaseolus vulgaris). *Int J Toxicol.* 2006;25(5):361-371.

Draeger KE, Vértesy L, Grigoleit HG. Starch blockers. *Lancet.* 1983;1(8320):354-355.

Garrow JS, Scott PF, Heels S, et al. A study of 'starch blockers' in man using 13C-enriched starch as a tracer. *Hum Nutr Clin Nutr.* 1983;37(4):301-305.

Guzman-Partida AM, Jatomea-Fino O, Robles-Burgueño MR, et al. Characterization of alpha-amylase inhibitor from Palo Fierro seeds. *Plant Physiol Biochem.* 2007;45(9):711-715.

Lee SC, Gepts PL, Whitaker JR. Protein structures of common bean (Phaseolus vulgaris) alpha-amylase inhibitors. *J Agric Food Chem.* 2002;50(22):6618-6627.

Marshall JJ, Lauda CM. Purification and properties of phaseolamin, an inhibitor of alpha-amylase, from the kidney bean, Phaseolus vulgaris. *J Biol Chem.* 1975;250(20):8030-8037.

Nakaguchi T, Arakawa T, Philo JS, et al. Structural characterization of an alpha-amylase inhibitor from a wild common bean (Phaseolus vulgaris): insight into the common structural features of leguminous alpha-amylase inhibitors. *J Biochem.* 1997;121(2):350-354.

Obiro WC, Zhang T, Jiang B. The nutraceutical role of the Phaseolus vulgaris alpha-amylase inhibitor. *Br J Nutr.* 2008;100(1):1-12.

Tormo MA, Gil-Exojo I, Romero de Tejada A, et al. Hypoglycaemic and anorexigenic activities of an alpha-amylase inhibitor from white kidney beans (*Phaseolus vulgaris*) in Wistar rats. *Br J Nutr.* 2004;92(5):785-790.

Udani J, Hardy M, Madsen DC. Blocking carbohydrate absorption and weight loss: a clinical trial using Phase 2 brand proprietary fractionated white bean extract. *Altern Med Rev.* 2004;9(1):63-69.

Valencia-Jiménez A, Arboleda Valencia JW, Grossi-De-Sá MF. Activity of alpha-amylase inhibitors from Phaseolus coccineus on digestive alpha-amylases of the coffee berry borer. *J Agric Food Chem.* 2008;56(7):2315-2320.

Zhang XQ, Yang MY, Ma Y, et al. Isolation and activity of an alpha-amylase inhibitor from white kidney beans. *Yao Xue Xue Bao.* 2007;42(12):1282-7.

Alpha-Lipoic Acid

DESCRIPTION

Alpha-lipoic acid, also known as thioctic acid, is a disulfide compound that is a cofactor in vital energy-producing reactions in the body. It is also a potent biological antioxidant. Alpha-lipoic acid was once thought to be a vitamin for animals and humans. It is made endogenously in humans—the details of its synthesis are still not fully understood—and so it is not an essential nutrient. There are, however, certain situations, for example, diabetic polyneuropathy, where alpha-lipoic acid might have conditional essentiality. And recent research indicates that the antioxidant roles of alpha-lipoic acid may confer several health benefits. Alpha-lipoic acid is found widely in plant and animal sources.

Most of the metabolic reactions in which alpha-lipoic acid participates occur in mitochondria. These include the oxidation of pyruvic acid (as pyruvate) by the pyruvate dehydrogenase enzyme complex and the oxidation of alpha-ketoglutarate by the alpha-ketoglutarate dehydrogenase enzyme complex. It is also a cofactor for the oxidation of branched-chain amino acids (leucine, isoleucine and valine) via the branched-chain alpha-keto acid dehydrogenase enzyme complex.

Alpha-lipoic acid is approved in Germany as a drug for the treatment of polyneuropathies, such as diabetic and alcoholic polyneuropathies, and liver disease.

Alpha-lipoic acid contains a chiral center and consists of two enantiomers, the natural R- or D- enantiomer and the S- or L- enantiomer. Commercial preparations of alpha-lipoic acid consist of the racemic mixture, i.e. a 50/50 mixture of the R- and E-enantiomers. It is represented by the following chemical structure:

Alpha-Lipoic acid

Alpha-lipoic acid has a variety of names. In addition to being known as alpha-lipoic acid and thioctic acid, it is also known as lipoic acid, 1,2-dithiolane-3-pentanoic acid; 1,2-ditholane-3-valeric acid; 6,8-thiotic acid; 5-[3-C1,2-dithiolanyl)]-pentanoic acid; delta-[3-(1,2-dithiacyclopentyl)] pentanoic acid; acetate replacing factor and pyruvate oxidation factor. Alpha-lipoic acid is water-insoluble.

Although the details of its synthesis have yet to be worked out, alpha-lipoic acid is synthesized in mitochondria; octanoic acid and L-cysteine (for its sulfur) are precursors in its synthesis.

ACTIONS AND PHARMACOLOGY

ACTIONS

Alpha-lipoic acid has biological antioxidant activity, antioxidant recycling activity and activity in enhancing biological energy production.

MECHANISM OF ACTION

Alpha-lipoic acid and its reduced metabolite, dihydrolipoic acid (DHLA), form a redox couple and may scavenge a wide range of reactive oxygen species. Both alpha-lipoic acid and DHLA can scavenge hydroxyl radicals, the nitric oxide radical, peroxynitrite, hydrogen peroxide and hypochlorite. Alpha-lipoic acid, but not DHLA, may scavenge singlet oxygen, and DHLA, but not alpha-lipoic acid, may scavenge superoxide and peroxyl reactive oxygen species.

Alpha-lipoic acid has been found to decrease urinary isoprostanes, O-LDL and plasma protein carbonyls, markers of oxidative stress. Further, alpha-lipoic acid and its redox couple DHLA have been found to have antioxidant activity in aqueous, as well as in lipophilic regions, and in extracellular and intracellular environments. Finally, with regard to alpha-lipoic acid's antioxidant activity, alpha-lipoic acid appears to participate in the recycling of other important biologic antioxidants, such as vitamins E and C, ubiquinone and glutathione.

Exogenous alpha-lipoic acid has been shown to increase ATP production and aortic blood flow during reoxygenation after hypoxia in a working heart model. It is thought that this is due to its role in the oxidation of pyruvate and alpha-ketoglutarate in the mitochondria, ultimately enhancing energy production. This activity, and possibly its antioxidant activity, may account for its possible benefit in diabetic polyneuropathy.

PHARMACOKINETICS

Most pharmacokinetic studies have been performed in animals. Alpha-lipoic acid is absorbed from the small intestine and distributed to the liver via the portal circulation and to various tissues in the body via the systemic circulation. The natural R-enantiomer is more readily absorbed than the L-enantiomer and is the more active form. Alpha-lipoic acid readily crosses the blood-brain barrier. It is found, after its distribution to the various body tissues, intracellularly, intramitochondrialy and extracellularly.

Alpha-lipoic acid is metabolized to its reduced form, dihydrolipoic acid (DHLA), by mitochondrial lipoamide dehydrogenase. DHLA, together with lipoic acid, form a redox couple. It is also metabolized to lipoamide, which functions as the lipoic acid cofactor in the multienzyme complexes that catalyze the oxidative decarboxylations of pyruvate and alpha-ketoglutarate. Alpha-lipoic acid may be metabolized to dithiol octanoic acid, which can undergo catabolism.

INDICATIONS AND USAGE

Lipoic acid shows evidence of being effective in the treatment of diabetic neuropathy and may be useful in treating some other aspects of diabetes. It may help prevent the oxidation of LDL cholesterol and may be protective, generally, against oxidative stress and, specifically, against atherosclerosis, ischemia-reperfusion injury and various radiologic and chemical toxins. It may also be useful in some inborn metabolic disorders. There is less evidence that it might be helpful in some neurodegenerative conditions. There is preliminary evidence that it might have some

immune-modulating effects. It has been suggested that lipoic acid may slow aging of the brain and that it may be an anti-aging substance, in general. Alpha-lipoic acid is not effective in alleviating burning mouth syndrome.

RESEARCH SUMMARY

Lipoic acid is an approved treatment for diabetic neuropathy in Germany. Numerous studies in both animals and humans have produced promising results with lipoic acid in this neuropathy. In animal models and culture studies, lipoic acid has demonstrated antioxidant properties that help reduce or eliminate a sequence of events that include reduced endon-eural blood flow and oxygen tension, which are pre-requisites of neuropathy. In addition, some of these studies have revealed favorable lipoic acid effects that appear to be independent of its antioxidant properties, including increased glucose uptake, promotion of new neurite growth and chelation of transition metals thought to play a role in diabetic neuropathy.

In some animal experiments, lipoic acid, administered for up to three months, significantly reversed the increase in nerve vascular resistance and the decrease in nerve blood flow in diabetic rats. Nerve conduction velocity was entirely restored in some nerve groups after three months of treatment.

Human clinical trials have been similarly encouraging. In one of these studies, subjects received 200 milligrams of intravenous lipoic acid daily. After 21 days, significant pain reduction was achieved in most subjects.

In a larger, multi-center, double-blind, randomized, placebo-controlled study of 328 patients with type 2 diabetes, significant improvements were recorded in several clinical measures of diabetic polyneuropathy, including pain, numbness, paresthesia and burning sensations. These results were evident after three weeks of intravenous lipoic acid given five times weekly in doses of 600 and 1200 milligrams.

Nerve conduction velocity has not been shown to improve in the short-term human studies conducted so far. One group of researchers has suggested that proof of neurophysiological improvement in these neuropathies may emerge from long-term lipoic acid supplementation studies, as has been the case in some animal model studies. "A period of several years," they have observed, "is required to slow progress of diabetic neuropathy due to normalization of blood glucose levels."

A recent study again demonstrated that lipoic acid may improve symptomatic diabetic polyneuropathy. Pain symptoms were significantly reduced in subjects receiving 600 mg of lipoic acid daily over a five-week period. There is evidence, too, that lipoic acid may help prevent or slow the development of the atherosclerosis for which diabetics are at higher risk. It may do this, in part, through a gene-regulatory mechanism that helps prevent endothelial cell activity that has been implicated in the progression of atherosclerosis.

With respect to atherosclerosis, in general, lipoic acid's antioxidant and metabolic effects appear to offer some protection, as demonstrated in various animal models. Recently, researchers demonstrated, in a 16-week randomized trial, that lipoic acid, in oral doses of 600 milligrams daily for eight weeks, significantly inhibits the oxidation of LDL-cholesterol in healthy human subjects. The supplements also significantly reduced levels of F-2 isoprostanes, markers of oxidative stress. In this study, lipoic acid proved to be superior to vitamin E in decreasing levels of plasma protein carbonyls. Protein oxidation and LDL-cholesterol oxidation are implicated in heart disease.

Various animal studies have suggested that lipoic acid can prevent or reduce cell and tissue damage in heart attacks and stroke. There is extensive animal work showing that lipoic acid can exert significant protective effects against ischemia-reperfusion injury.

Lipoic acid is believed to work in this context, at least in part, through its antioxidant properties and its reported ability to increase cellular levels of glutathione that are typically depleted by the reactive oxygen species formation that characterizes ischemia-reperfusion. More research is needed to further elucidate these mechanisms and determine whether these results will apply in humans.

Animal work is also suggestive of some modest benefit from lipoic acid in the treatment of various neurodegenerative disorders, including Parkinson's disease, Alzheimer's disease, amyotrophic lateral sclerosis and Huntington's disease. In one human study, a dose of 600 mg of lipoic acid was administered daily to 43 patients with Alzheimer's disease over an observation period of up to 48 months. No significant improvement was seen in these patients in this open label study, although the authors indicated there might have been slower progression of disease among those with mild dementia. There is some very preliminary evidence from a cellular model of Parkinson's disease that a combination of lipoic acid and acetyl-L-carnitine might exert some positive effects in that disease. More research is needed and warranted.

There is some evidence that children afflicted with inborn errors of pyruvate metabolism may derive some benefit from lipoic acid treatment. Those with Wilson's disease, a genetic disorder characterized by disturbed copper metabolism, may be helped by lipoic acid as well. The supplement has also proved useful in conferring some protection against cadmium poisoning and hexane inhalation. It has also been used in some liver toxicities, such as *Amanita phalloides* mushroom poisoning.

Lipoic acid's role in immunity is not well understood. There are reports that it can augment antibody response in some animal models of immunosuppression. This research warrants follow-up.

Lipoic acid was judged to have favorable effects in a pilot study testing its use in subjects with multiple sclerosis (MS). This study determined that lipoic acid supplementation can inhibit a class of activated T cell-produced proteases implicated in MS. This preliminary study needs follow-up and expansion.

Claims that lipoic acid slows aging of the brain and is an anti-aging substance generally seem to be related to its potent antioxidant properties. Direct proof of anti-aging is lacking, but there is some animal work suggestive of some possible anti-aging effects.

Rats were fed a lipoic-acid supplemented diet to see whether the substance can reverse age-related declines in metabolism and mitochondrial function. Unsupplemented aged rats (24 to 26 months) exhibited ambulatory activity, said to be a general measure of metabolic activity, that was threefold lower than that of young controls. But this decline was significantly reversed in similarly aged rats supplemented with lipoic acid for two weeks.

Hepatocytes from untreated aged rats, compared with hepatocytes of young controls (three to five months), had significantly lower oxygen consumption and mitochondrial membrane potential. But in supplemented aged rats, hepatocytes, by the same measures, were comparable to those of the young controls.

Lipoic acid supplementation was reported to completely reverse age-related declines in hepatocyte ascorbic acid and glutathione levels. There was additional evidence of decreased oxidative damage in the lipoic-acid supplemented aged rats. The researchers concluded: "Little is known about whether lipoic acid may be an effective anti-aging supplement ... in humans. Our present findings using rats would suggest that lipoic acid supplementation may be a safe and effective means to improve general metabolic activity and increase antioxidant status, affording increased protection against external oxidative and xenobiotic insults with age."

Recently, there has been some further work with lipoic acid, in combination with acetyl-L-carnitine, related to aging. In one study, feeding acetyl-L-carnitine and lipoic acid to old rats was said to significantly improve metabolic function while decreasing oxidative stress. In another study, this same combination was reported to maintain myocardial function in aging rats. Beagle dogs between 7.6 and 8.8 years of age that were administered a twice-daily supplement of these agents over a two-month period reportedly made fewer errors in two learning tests, compared with controls. The researchers concluded that they believe long-term supplementation could slow cognitive decline in these animals. Whether these findings might have clinical relevance is unknown.

Finally, a recent double-blind, randomized, placebo-controlled study found that lipoic acid is of no benefit in burning mouth syndrome, a chronic facial pain syndrome suffered primarily by middle-aged/elderly women with hormonal changes or, some believe, psychological disorders.

CONTRAINDICATIONS, PRECAUTIONS, ADVERSE REACTIONS

CONTRAINDICATIONS

Known hypersensitivity to an alpha-lipoic acid-containing product.

PRECAUTIONS

Because of lack of long-term safety data, alpha-lipoic acid should be avoided by pregnant women and nursing mothers.

Those with diabetes and problems with glucose intolerance are cautioned that supplemental alpha-lipoic acid may lower blood glucose levels. Blood glucose should be monitored and antidiabetic drug dose adjusted, if necessary, to avoid possible hypoglycemia.

ADVERSE REACTIONS

To date, alpha-lipoic acid in doses up to 600 milligrams daily has been well tolerated.

INTERACTIONS

Supplemental alpha-lipoic acid may lower blood glucose levels. Those with diabetes on antidiabetic medication should have their blood glucose monitored and antidiabetic drug dose appropriately adjusted, if necessary, to avoid possible hypoglycemia.

OVERDOSAGE

There are no reports of alpha-lipoic acid overdosage.

DOSAGE AND ADMINISTRATION

Alpha-lipoic acid is mainly available as a racemic mixture of R- and S-enantiomers, as well as R-alpha-lipoic acid. Some studies showing significant antioxidant effects have used doses of the racemic mixture of 600 milligrams daily.

Alpha-lipoic acid is available in Germany as a drug to treat polyneuropathy, such as diabetic polyneuropathy, and liver disorders. It is available for oral and parenteral use. Those with diabetic neuropathy use 300 milligrams daily of the oral preparation, taken in divided doses.

LITERATURE

Aliev G, Liu J, Shenk JC, et al. Neuronal mitochondrial amelioration by feeding acetyl-L-carnitine and lipoic acid to aged rats. *J Cell Mol Med.* Epub: 2008 Mar 28.

Ames BN. Delaying the mitochondrial decay of aging. *Ann N Y Acad Sci.* 2004;1019:406-411.

Bast A, Haenen GR. Lipoic acid: a multifunctional antioxidant. *Biofactors.* 2003;17(1-4):207-213.

Bilska A, Wodek L. Lipoic acid—the drug of the future? *Pharmacol Rep.* 2005;57(5):570-577.

Carbone M, Pentenero M, Carrozzo M, et al. Lack of efficacy of alpha-lipoic acid in burning mouth syndrome: A double-blind, randomized, placebo-controlled study. *Eur J Pain.* Epub: 2008 Jul 31.

Doggrell SA. Alpha-lipoic acid, an anti-obesity agent? *Expert Opin Investig Drugs.* 2004;13(12):1641-1643.

Hagen TM, Ingersoll RT, Lykkesfeldt J, et al. (R)-alpha-lipoic acid-supplemented old rats have improved mitochondrial function, decreased oxidative damage, and increased metabolic rate. *FASEB J. 1999;*13:411-418.

Hagen TM, Liu J, Lykkesfeldt J, et al. Feeding acetyl-L-carnitine and lipoic acid to old rats significantly improves metabolic function while decreasing oxidative stress. *Proc Natl Acad Sci U S A.* 2002;99(4):1870-1875.

Hagen TM, Moreau R, Suh JH, et al. Mitochondrial decay in the aging rat heart: evidence for improvement by dietary supplementation with acetyl-L-carnitine and/or lipoic acid. *Ann N Y Acad Sci.* 2002;959:491-507.

Lykkesfeldt J, Hagen TM, Vinarsky V, et al. Age-associated decline in ascorbic and concentration, recycling and biosynthesis in rat hepatocytes-reversal with (R)-alpha-lipoic acid supplementation. *FASEB J.* 1998;12:1183-1189.

Maczurek A, Hager K, Kenklies M, et al. Lipoic acid as an anti-inflammatory and neuroprotective treatment for Alzheimer's disease. *Adv Drug Deliv Rev.* Epub: 2008 Jul 4.

Marangon K, Devaraj S, Tirosh O, et al. Comparison of the effect of alpha-lipoic acid and alpha-tocopherol supplementation on measures of oxidative stress. *Free Rad Biol Med.* 1999;27:1114-1121.

Milgram NW, Araujo JA, Hagen TM, et al. Acetyl-L-carnitine and alpha-lipoic acid supplementation of aged beagle dogs improves learning in two landmark discrimination tests. *FASEB J.* 2007;21(13):3756-3762.

Moreira PI, Harris PL, Zhu X, et al. Lipoic acid and N-acetyl cysteine decrease mitochondrial-related oxidative stress in Alzheimer disease patient fibroblasts. *J Alzheimers Dis.* 2007;12(2):195-206.

Natrej CV, Gandhi VM, Melon KKG. Lipoic acid and diabetes: effect of dihydrolipoic acid administration in diabetic rats and rabbits. *J Biosci* 1984;6:37-46.

Nickander KK, McPhee BR, Low PA, et al. Alpha-lipoic acid: antioxidant potency against lipid peroxidation of neural tissues in vitro and implications for diabetic neuropathy. *Free Rad Biol Med.* 1996;21:631-639.

Novotny L, Rauko P, Cojocel C. alpha-Lipoic acid: the potential for use in cancer therapy. *Neoplasma.* 2008;55(2):81-86.

Ohmori H, Yamauchi T, Yamamoto I. Augmentation of the antibody response by lipoic acid in mice II. Restoration of the antibody response in immunosuppressed mice. *Japan J Pharmacol* 1986;42:275-280.

Packer L, Tritschler HJ, Wessel K. Neuroprotection by the metabolic antioxidant alpha-lipoic acid. *Free Rad Biol Med.* 1997;22:359-378.

Packer L, Witt EH, Tritschler, et al. Alpha-lipoic as a biological antioxidant. *Free Rad Biol Med.* 1995;19:227-250.

Reed LJ. The chemistry and function of lipoic acids. *Adv Enzymol.* 1957;18:319-347.

Sachse G, Willms B. Efficacy of throctic acid in the therapy of peripheral diabetic neuropathy. *Horm Metab Res Suppl.* 1980;9:105-107.

Salinthone S, Yadav V, Bourdette DN, et al. Lipoic acid: a novel therapeutic approach for multiple sclerosis and other chronic inflammatory diseases of the CNS. *Endocr Metab Immune Disord Drug Targets.* 2008 Jun;8(2):132-142.

Sauer J, Tabet N, Howard R. Alpha lipoic acid for dementia. *Cochrane Database Syst Rev.* 2004;(1):CD004244.

Smith AR, Shenvi SV, Widlansky M, et al. Lipoic acid as a potential therapy for chronic diseases associated with oxidative stress. *Curr Med Chem.* 2004;11(9):1135-1146.

Tang J, Wingerchuk DM, Crum BA, et al. Alpha-lipoic acid may improve symptomatic diabetic polyneuropathy. *Neurologist.* 2007;13(3):164-167.

Tirosh O, Sen CK, Roy S, et al. Neuroprotective effects of alpha-lipoic acid and its positively charged amide analogue. *Free Rad Biol Med.* 1999;26:1418-1426.

Wagh SS, Natraj CV, Menon KKG. Mode of action of lipoic acid in diabetes. *J Biosci.* 1987;11:59-74.

Wollin SD, Jones PJ. Alpha-lipoic acid and cardiovascular disease. *J Nutr.* 2003;133(11):3327-3330.

Yadav V, Marracci G, Lovera J, et al. Lipoic acid in multiple sclerosis: a pilot study. *Mult Scler.* 2005;11(2):159-165.

Ziegler D, Hanefeld M, Ruhnau KJ, et al. Treatment of symptomatic diabetic peripheral neuropathy with the antioxidant alpha-lipoic acid. A three-week multicentre randomized controlled trial (ALADIN study). *Diabetologia.* 1995;38:1425-1433.

Zimmer G, Beikler TK, Schneider M, et al. Dose/response curves of lipoic acid R- and S- forms in the working rat heart during reoxygenation: superiority of the R-entantiomer in the enhancement of aortic flow. *J Mol Cell Cardiol.* 1995;27:1895-1903.

Zhang H, Jia H, Liu J, et al. Combined R-alpha-lipoic acid and acetyl-L-carnitine exerts efficient preventative effects in a cellular model of Parkinson's disease. *J Cell Mol Med.* Epub: 2008 Jun 20.

Alpha-Tocopherol Polyethylene Glycol Succinate (TPGS)

DESCRIPTION

D-alpha-tocopheryl polyethylene glycol succinate, abbreviated as TPGS, is a water-soluble derivative of d-alpha-tocopheryl succinate. TPGS is used as a water-soluble delivery form of vitamin E for those with fat malabsorption syndromes, such as chronic childhood cholestasis. It is also used as an absorption and bioavailability enhancer for certain water-insoluble drugs (e.g. the HIV protease inhibitor amprenavir) and fat-soluble vitamins such as vitamin D.

TPGS is synthesized by esterifying d-alpha tocopheryl succinate with polyethylene glycol (PEG) 1000 (the molecular weight of PEG 1000 is approximately 1,000 daltons). It is a pale yellow, waxy solid substance that is amphipathic and hydrophilic. Its molecular weight is approximately 1,513 daltons. D-alpha-tocopherol comprises 26% of TPGS. TPGS is also known as d-alpha-tocopheryl polyethylene glycol 1000 succinate and d-alpha-tocopheryl PEG 1000 succinate. Since there are eight stereoisomers of alpha-tocopherol, the designation d-alpha-tocopherol, although commonly used, is chemically incorrect. Correct chemical names for TPGS include *RRR*-alpha-tocopheryl polyethylene glycol 1000 succinate, 2R, 4′R, 8′R-alpha-tocopheryl polyethylene glycol 1000 succinate and 2, 5, 7, 8-tertramethyl-2-(4′,8′,12′-trimethyltridecyl)-6-chromanyl polyethylene glycol 1000 succinate.

ACTIONS AND PHARMACOLOGY

ACTIONS

TPGS is a water-soluble delivery form of d-alpha-tocopherol. See Vitamin E for actions of this vitamin. TPGS may also enhance the absorption and bioavailability of certain drugs and nutritional substances. It has applications as an emulsifier, a drug solublizer, an absorption enhancer, a vehicle for lipid-based drug delivery and as a source of natural vitamin E (*RRR*-alpha-tocopherol).

MECHANISM OF ACTION

In contrast to other forms of vitamin E, which require emulsification and micelle formation by bile salts for their absorption, TPGS, because of its amphipathic nature (has both hydrophilic and lipophilic ends), forms its own micelles and thus does not require bile salts to do so. This makes it an excellent alpha-tocopherol substance for those who have problems secreting bile salts into the intestine (e.g., those with chronic childhood cholestasis).

TPGS may enhance the absorption of lipophilic drugs if formulated together with them. For this reason, the HIV protease inhibitor amprenavir is formulated with TPGS. Further, the enhancement of the oral bioavailability of some drugs when co-administered with TPGS may, in part, be due to inhibition of P-glycoprotein (P-gp) in the intestine. P-glycoprotein, a member of the ATP-binding cassette family of transporters, is the multidrug resistance transporter and is involved in the mediation of multidrug resistance.

PHARMACOKINETICS

The pharmacokinetics of TPGS is not completely known. TPGS is more efficiently absorbed from the lumen of the small intestine following ingestion than other forms of vitamin E. As mentioned above, TPGS forms micelles in the small intestine and does not require bile salts to do so. The mechanism of it's absorption into enterocytes remains unclear. A few possibilities exist. TPGS is hydrolyzed within the lumen of the small intestine to form d-alpha-tocopherol; it is hydrolyzed by lipase on the surface of the enterocytes to form d-alpha-tocopherol; or the entire TPGS micelle is taken up by the enterocytes and it is hydrolyzed within them to d-alpha-tocopherol. Whichever the case, d-alpha-tocopherol is secreted by the enterocytes into the lymphatics and is processed in a similar manner to other forms of vitamin E. (See Vitamin E.)

INDICATIONS AND USAGE

TPGS is indicated in some with chronic cholestatic liver disease of infancy and childhood. It may be helpful in some other forms of liver disease and in fat-soluble vitamin deficiency generally. It is useful in treating vitamin E malabsorption in short-bowel syndrome. It may protect the liver against some toxins. When co-administered it enhances the absorbability of some pharmaceutical drugs. It has been suggested that it might be helpful in treating some of the malabsorption problems associated with Crohn's disease, HIV disease, ulcerative colitis, cystic fibrosis and others, but this hypothesis has not been adequately tested.

RESEARCH SUMMARY

There is considerable research supporting the use of TPGS in chronic childhood cholestasis and in some forms of liver disease characterized by significantly reduced bile acid secretion into the intestine. In a multicenter study, children with chronic cholestasis unresponsive to other forms of vitamin E were given TPGS supplements. All of the children experienced normalization of vitamin E status. Improvements were noted in the neurological function, which had deteriorated prior to the study's onset, in 25 of the subjects. Neurological function stabilized in 27 others and worsened in only two of the subjects; functions were measured after a mean of 2.5 years of TPGS therapy.

In addition, TPGS has been used with some preliminary success to help overcome the difficulty those with cholesta-sis have in absorbing other fat-soluble vitamins (A, D, K). Through admixture and co-administration of these other fat-soluble vitamins in TPGS preparations, absorption has reportedly been enhanced.

Similarly, co-administration of some poorly absorbed drugs with TPGS has enhanced the absorption of those drugs even in healthy volunteers. TPGS, used in this context, increases the absorbability of the HIV protease inhibitor amprenavir. TPGS has improved the absorbability of cyclosporin in children receiving liver transplants. It is useful in combating vitamin E malabsorption in short-bowel syndrome. It has also demonstrated hepatoprotective effects against carbon tetrachloride in animal studies.

CONTRAINDICATIONS, PRECAUTIONS, ADVERSE REACTIONS

CONTRAINDICATIONS

TPGS is contraindicated in those with known hypersensitivity to the substance.

PRECAUTIONS

Typically, TPGS is prescribed and monitored by a physician. Those on warfarin need to be aware that high doses of TPGS (greater than 500 milligrams daily, equivalent to 130 milligrams of d-alpha-tocopherol) may enhance the anticoagulant effect of warfarin, and therefore they should have their INRs carefully monitored and their warfarin doses appropriately adjusted if indicated. Those with vitamin K deficiencies should be aware that high doses of TPGS may have anticoagulant activity. TPGS should be used with caution in those with lesions with a propensity to bleed (e.g., bleeding peptic ulcers), those with a history of hemorrhagic stroke and those with inherited bleeding disorders (e.g., hemophilia).

High-dose TPGS should be stopped about one month before surgical procedures, unless one's physician advises otherwise.

Those on the HIV protease inhibitor amprenavir need to be aware that, if they are taking the recommended daily adult dose of this drug, they are receiving 1,168 milligrams (1,744 IUs) daily of d-alpha-tocopherol. Vitamin E supplements higher than RDA amounts should only be taken by those taking amprenavir if directed to do so by one's physician.

ADVERSE REACTIONS

No adverse reactions have been reported.

INTERACTIONS

DRUGS

Amprenavir: TPGS is used as an absorption and bioavailability enhancer for the HIV protease inhibitor amprenavir.

Antiplatelet drugs, such as aspirin, dipyridamole, eptifibatide, clopidogrel, ticlopidine, tirofiban and abciximab: High doses of TPGS may enhance the effects of these antiplatelet drugs.

Cyclosporine and other lipophilic drugs: TPGS may increase absorption if taken concomitantly.

Warfarin: High dose (greater than 500 milligram daily) of TPGS may enhance the anticoagulant response of warfarin. Monitor INRs and appropriately adjust dose of warfare if necessary.

NUTRITIONAL SUPPLEMENTS

Flavonoids, polyphenols, CoQ$_{10}$: TPGS may increase the absorption of these supplements if taken concomitantly.

Selenium: may function synergistically with d-alpha-tocopherol.

Vitamin C: may help maintain d-alpha-tocopherol in its reduced (antioxidant) form.

Vitamin A, D and K: TPGS may increase the absorption of vitamins A, D and K if taken concomitantly. It may also increase the absorption of all forms of vitamin E (gamma-tocopherol, tocotrienols) if taken concomitantly.

HERBS

Some herbs, such as garlic and ginkgo, possess antithrombotic activity. High doses of TPGS used concomitantly with these herbs may enhance antithrombotic activity.

OVERDOSAGE

No reports of TPGS overdosage appear in the literature.

DOSAGE AND ADMINISTRATION

TPGS is typically used for the treatment of vitamin E deficiency states due to fat malabsorption, such as chronic childhood cholestasis. Doses used for this condition range from 10 to 17 milligrams (as d-alpha-tocopherol) per kilogram daily. Doses of up to 670 milligrams (as d-alpha-tocopherol) daily for up to three years have been used in the treatment of vitamin E deficiency secondary to short-bowel syndrome. Use of TPGS in these disorders, as well as other disorders of fat malabsorption, such as cystic fibrosis, requires medical supervision. It is unclear if TPGS offers any advantages, as a vitamin E supplement, to those without vitamin E deficiencies.

LITERATURE

Dintaman JM, Silverman JA. Inhibition of P-glycoprotein by d-alpha-tocopheryl polyethylene glycol 1000 succinate (TPGS). *Pharm Res.* 1999;16:1550-1556.

Socha P, Koletzko B, Pawlowska J, et al. Treatment of cholestatic children with water-soluble vitamin E (alpha-tocopheryl polyethylene glycol succinate): effects on serum vitamin E, lipid peroxides, and polyunsaturated fatty acids. *J Pediatr Gastroenterol Nutr.* 1997;24:189-193.

Sokol RJ, Butler-Simon N, Conner C, et al. Multicenter trial of d-alpha-tocopheryl polyethylene glycol 1000 succinate for treatment of vitamin E deficiency in children with chronic cholestasis. *Gastroenterology.* 1993;104:1727-1735.

Traber MG, Shiano TD, Steephen AC, et al. Efficacy of water-soluble vitamin E in the treatment of vitamin E malabsorption in short-bowel syndrome. *Am J Clin Nutr.* 1994;59:1270-1274.

Traber MG, Thellman CA, Rindler MJ, et al. Uptake of intact TPGS (d-alpha-tocopheryl polyethylene glycol 1000 succinate) a water-miscible form of vitamin E by human cells in vitro. *Am J Clin Nutr.* 1998;48:605-611.

Alpha-Tocopheryl Nicotinate

DESCRIPTION

Alpha-tocopheryl nicotinate is a synthetic ester formed from d1-alpha-tocopherol and nicotinic acid. It is a delivery form of nicotinic acid and is used in Europe and Japan for the treatment of hyperlipidemia. It is marketed in the United States as a nutritional supplement, usually in a combination formula.

Alpha-tocopheryl nicotinate is also known as vitamin E nicotinate and tocopheryl nicotinate.

ACTIONS AND PHARMACOLOGY

ACTIONS

Alpha-tocopheryl nicotinate may have triglyceride- and cholesterol-lowering activity in some.

MECHANISM OF ACTION

See the monograph on nicotin (nicotinic acid) for mechanism of action information.

PHARMACOKINETICS

There is little information on the pharmacokinetics of alpha-tocopheryl nicotinate. Absorption from the lumen of the small intestine is dependent on the presence or the absence of food. Absorption is much higher with food. Alpha-tocopheryl nicotinate appears to be transported by the lymphatics to the systemic circulation. It is taken up by the liver where it is hydrolyzed to d1-tocopherol and nicotinic acid.

See the Vitamin E and Niacin (Nicotinic Acid) monographs for information on these metabolites of alpha-tocoperyl nicotinate.

INDICATIONS AND USAGE

Alpha-tocopheryl nicotinate has shown some experimental antiarrhythmic activity and is used in Europe and Japan as a lipid-lowering agent.

RESEARCH SUMMARY

Alpha-tocopheryl nicotinate demonstrated an ability to significantly inhibit experimentally induced antiarrhythmic activity in isolated animal atria, as well as *in vivo* in an animal model. Of three substances tested (the other two were dodecanoic acid and alpha-tocopherol), alpha-tocopheryl nicotinate showed the greatest inhibiting activity.

Alpha-tocopheryl nicotinate is a delivery form of nicotinic acid which does possess hypocholesterolemic and hypotriglyceridemic activities. However, there is no evidence that it is superior to nicotinic acid itself in this regard (see Niacin [Nicotinic Acid]). Further, the doses typically used are unlikely to have hypolipidemic activity in most people.

CONTRAINDICATIONS, PRECAUTIONS, ADVERSE REACTIONS

See Niacin. (Nicotinic Acid).

OVERDOSAGE

The literature does not contain reports of alpha-tocopheryl nicotinate overdosage.

DOSAGE AND ADMINISTRATION

Typical dosing is 100 to 200 milligrams three times a day. This dose is equivalent to about 120 to 240 milligrams of d-alpha-tocopherol daily and about 60 to 120 milligrams of nicotinic acid daily.

LITERATURE

Aigner O, Schlick W. [Effect of tocopherol nicotinate on serum lipids]. [Article in German]. *Int J Clin Pharmacol.* 1974; 10:216-219.

Hasegawa J, Tomono Y, Fujita T, et al. The effect of food on the absorption of alpha-tocopheryl nicotinate in beagle dogs and human volunteers. *Int J Clin Pharmacol Ther Toxicol.* 1981; 19:216-219.

Iino K, Abe K, Kariya S, et al. A controlled double-blind study of dl-alpha-tocopheryl nicotinate (Juvela-Nicotinate) for treatment of symptoms in hypertension and cerebral arteriosclerosis. *Jpn Heart J.* 1977; 18:277-283.

Noma A, Maseda S, Okuno M, et al. Reduction of serum lipoprotein(a) levels in hyperlipidaemic patients with alpha-tocopheryl nicotinate. *Atherosclerosis.* 1990; 84:213-217.

Suzuki N, Nakamura T. Metabolism of the nicotinic acid moiety of dl-alpha tocopheryl nicotinate. *J Nutr Sci Vitaminol.* 1983; 29:93-103.

Androstenediol

It is illegal to use or possess Androstenediol except if enrolled in an FDA-allowed clinical trial or if prescribed by a qualified physician.

DESCRIPTION

Following the passage of the Dietary Supplement Health and Education Act (DSHEA) of 1994, a number of putative anabolic substances, including androstenediol, began to be marketed as dietary supplements. In March 2004, Senators Joseph Biden and Orrin Hatch co-authored and introduced a bill known as the Anabolic Steroid Control Act of 2004. The Act revised the term "anabolic steroid" to mean any drug or hormonal substance chemically and pharmacologically related to testosterone (other than estrogens, progestins, corticosteroids, and dehydroepiandrosterone [DHEA]). The list attached to the bill contained 59 specific substances, 26 of which were added to the existing 1990 list of steroids that are classified as schedule III controlled substances. The two isomers of androstenediol—delta4-androstenediol and delta5-androstenediol—were included in the list. The bill passed the Senate by unanimous consent on October 6, 2004, passed the House of Representatives two days later and was signed by President George W. Bush on October 22, 2004. It went into effect on January 20, 2005.

Androstenediol refers to two steroid isomers that had been marketed as dietary supplements and mainly used by body builders. The two androstenediol isomers are delta4-androstenediol and delta5-androstenediol. The difference between the two isomers is in the position of the double bond in the cyclopentanoperhydrophenanthrene ring structure. Delta4-androstenediol has a double bond between carbons 4 and 5; delta5-androstenediol has a double bond between carbons 5 and 6.

Delta4-androstenediol is also known as 4-androstene-3beta, 17beta-diol and (3beta, 17beta)-androst-4-ene-3,17-diol. Delta5-androstenediol is also known as 5-androstene-3beta, 17beta-diol, androst-5-ene-3beta,17beta-diol, (3beta, 17beta)-androst-5-ene-3, 17-diol and Adiol. The molecular formula of both delta4-androstenediol and delta5-androstenediol is $C_{19}H_{30}O_2$, and the molecular weight of these substances is 290.45 daltons.

Delta4-androstenediol and delta5-androstenediol are synthesized in the adrenal gland and gonads from dehydroepiandrosterone (DHEA) via the enzyme 17beta-hydroxysteroid dehydrogenase. They are metabolized to testosterone via the enzyme 3beta-hydroxysteroid dehydrogenase. Delta5-androstenediol is similar in structure to methandriol. Androstenediol is represented by the following structural formula:

Androstenediol

ACTIONS AND PHARMACOLOGY

ACTIONS

Supplemental delta4- and delta5-androstenediol have putative anabolic activity. Delta5-androstenediol may have immunomodulatory and radioprotective activities.

MECHANISM OF ACTION

Supplemental delta4- and delta5-androstenediol may be metabolized to testosterone in both men and women. Whether increases in testosterone levels that may be produced by taking oral delta4- or delta5-androstenediol would be sustained long enough to show increases in nitrogen retention and muscle strength and mass is unknown. Delta5-androstenediol is similar in structure to methandriol, a one-time popular injectable anabolic steroid.

5-Androstenediol has been demonstrated to enhance survival in mice and monkeys exposed to whole body gamma-ionizing radiation. It has been shown to stimulate hematopoiesis, suggesting that the steroid may act on hematopoietic progenitor cells. 5-Androstenediol was found to exert survival-enhancing effects on irradiated human hematopoietic progenitor cells via induction, stabilization, and activation of nuclear factor-kappaB (NF-kappaB), which resulted in increased secretion of the hematopoietic growth factor, granulocyte-colony stimulating factor (G-CSF).

Delta5-androstenediol has been demonstrated to enhance the immune response against infection in mice. It is thought that this is due, in part, to delta5-androstenediol's possible role in counter-regulating the immunosuppressive effects of glucocorticoids. That is, delta5-androstenediol may have antiglucocorticoid activity.

PHARMACOKINETICS

There are scant human pharmacokinetic data on the androstenediol isomers. Absorption is variable following ingestion, but some absorption does occur. First-pass metabolism appears to render much of an oral dose of delta4-androstenediol into the inactive metabolites androsterone and etiocholanolone. Androsterone and etiocholanolone are found in the urine after ingestion of delta4-androstenediol and delta5-

androstenediol. Both delta4- and delta5-androstenediol may be metabolized to testosterone.

INDICATIONS AND USAGE

The claim that oral androstenediol has anabolic effects is unsubstantiated. There is preliminary evidence that androstenediol may have some immunomodulating and radioprotective effects. Use of androstenediol may pose health hazards in some.

RESEARCH SUMMARY

Androstenediol significantly protected mice from lethal bacterial infections (*Enterococcus faecalis* and *Pseudomonas veruginosa*) in one recent experiment. There was no evidence of direct antibacterial activity; rather, the researchers believed that the steroids exerted a neuroendocrine regulation of antibacterial immune resistance.

Subsequently, androstenediol was reported to augment antiviral immune response in another animal study, again through immuno-endocrine regulation. The antiglucocorticoid activity of androstenediol was credited with reducing bacterial counts and prolonging survival in a mouse model of pulmonary tuberculosis. Research is ongoing.

The radioprotective effect of 5-androstenediol against ionizing radiation exposure should be further explored, considering, among other things, that exposure to nuclear radiation in the form of a "dirty" bomb is no longer unthinkable, and an agent that might protect against radiation damage of the bone marrow would be an important countermeasure.

CONTRAINDICATIONS, PRECAUTIONS, ADVERSE REACTIONS

CONTRAINDICATIONS

Delta4-androstenediol and delta5-androstenediol are contraindicated in those with prostate, breast, ovarian and uterine cancer and in those at risk for these cancers. Delta4-androstenediol and delta5-androstenediol are also contraindicated in those who are hypersensitive to any component of a delta4- or delta5-androstenediol-containing product.

PRECAUTIONS

Androstenediol is illegal to use or possess except if enrolled in an FDA-allowed clinical trial or if prescribed by a qualified physician.

ADVERSE REACTIONS

No data are available on the long-term safety of supplemental 4delta- or 5delta-androstenediol. Adverse effects of exogenous testosterone—to which androstenediol may be metabolized—in men, include acne, testicular atrophy, gynecomastia, behavioral changes and possibly an increased risk of prostate cancer. Adverse effects of exogenous testosterone in women include hirsutism, deepening of the voice, acne, clitoral hypertrophy, amenorrhea, male-pattern baldness and coarsening of the skin. In adolescents, exogenous testosterone can lead to early closing of bone growth plates and decreased adult height. Other adverse effects of testosterone include hepatic failure and increased platelet aggregation.

INTERACTIONS

No drug, nutritional supplement, food or herb interactions have been reported.

OVERDOSAGE

No reports of overdosage.

DOSAGE AND ADMINISTRATION

Androstenediol is illegal to use or possess except if enrolled in an FDA-allowed clinical trial or if prescribed by a qualified physician.

LITERATURE

Anabolic Steroid Control Act of 2004. http://frwebgate.access. gpo.gov/cgi-bin/getdoc.cgi?dbname=108_cong_public_ laws&docid=f:publ358.108.pdf. Accessed September 22, 2008.

Ben-Nathan D, Padgett DA, Loria RM. Androstenediol and dehydroepiandrosterone protect mice against lethal bacterial infections and lipopolysaccharide toxicity. *J Med Microbiol.* 1999;48:425-431.

Earnest CP, Olson MA, Broeder CE, et al. In vivo 4-androstene-3,17-dione and 4-androstene-3beta, 17beta-diol supplementation in young men. *Eur J Appl Physiol.* 2000;81:229-232.

Hernandez-Pando R, De La Luz Streber M, Orozco H, et al. The effects of androstenediol and dehydroepiandrosterone on the course and cytokine profile of tuberculosis in BALB/c mice. *Immunology.* 1998;95:234-241.

Miyamoto H, Yeh S, Lardy H, et al. Delta5-androstenediol is a natural hormone with androgenic activity in human prostate cancer cells. *Proc Natl Acad Sci USA.* 1998;95:11083-11088.

Padgett DA, Loria RM, Sheridan JF. Endocrine regulation of the immune response to influenza virus infection with a metabolite of DHEA-androstenediol. *J Neuroimmunol.* 1997;78:203-211.

Padgett DA, Sheridan JF. Androstenediol (AED) prevents neuroendocrine-mediated suppression of the immune response to an influenza viral infection. *J Neuroimmunol.* 1999;98:121-129.

Singh VK, Grace MB, Jacobsen KO, et al. Administration of 5-androstenediol to mice: pharmacokinetics and cytokine gene expression. *Exp Mol Pathol.* 2008;84(2):178-188.

Uralets VP, Gillette PA. Over-the-counter delta5 anabolic steroids 5-androsten-3, 17-dione; 5-androstene-3beta, 17beta-diol; dehydroepiandrosterone; and 19-nor-5-androstene-3, 17-dione: excretion studies in men. *J Anal Toxicol.* 2000;24:188-193.

Whitnall MH, Elliott TB, Harding RA, et al. Androstenediol stimulates myelopoiesis and enhances resistance to infection in gamma-irradiated mice. *Int J Immunopharmacol.* 2000;22(1):1-14.

Whitnall MH, Elliott TB, Landauer MR, et al. Protection against gamma-irradiation with 5-androstenediol. *Mil Med.* 2002;167(2 Suppl):64-65.

Whitnall MH, Inal CE, Jackson WE 3rd, et al. In vivo radioprotection by 5-androstenediol: stimulation of the innate immune system. *Radiat Res.* 2001;156(3):283-293.

Whitnall MH, Villa V, Seed TM, et al. Molecular specificity of 5-androstenediol as a systemic radioprotectant in mice. *Immunopharmacol Immunotoxicol.* 2005;27(1):15-32.

Xiao M, Inal CE, Parekh VI, et al. 5-Androstenediol promotes survival of gamma-irradiated human hematopoietic progenitors through induction of nuclear factor-kappaB activation and granulocyte colony-stimulating factor expression. *Mol Pharmacol.* 2007;72(2):370-379.

Androstenedione

It is illegal to use or possess Androstenedione except if enrolled in an FDA-allowed clinical trial or if prescribed by a qualified physician.

DESCRIPTION

Following the passage of the Dietary Supplement Health and Education Act (DSHEA) of 1994, a number of putative anabolic substances, including androstenedione, began to be marketed as dietary supplements. In March 2004, Senators Joseph Biden and Orrin Hatch introduced a bill into the US Senate that they co-authored and that is known as the Anabolic Steroid Control Act of 2004. The act revised the term 'anabolic steroid' to mean any drug or hormonal substance, chemically and pharmacologically related to testosterone (other than estrogens, progestins, corticosteroids, and dehydroepiandrosterone [DHEA]). The list attached to the bill contained 59 specific substances, 26 of which were added to the existing 1990 list of steroids that are classified as schedule III controlled substances. Androstenedione was included in the list. The bill passed the Senate by unanimous consent on October 6, 2004, passed the House of Representatives on October 8, 2004, was signed by President George W. Bush on October 22, 2004 and went into effect on January 20, 2005.

Androstenedione, a steroid hormone, is a natural substance made in the adrenal gland and the gonads. It is also found in small amounts in some plants. Androstenedione, commonly known as "andro," became popular because of its use by the baseball player Mark McGwire. McGwire stopped using androstenedione in May, 1999.

Androstenedione is synthesized in the adrenal gland and gonads from dehydroepiandrosterone. It is metabolized by the enzyme 17 beta-hydroxy steroid dehydrogenase to testosterone, and by the aromatase enzyme complex to estrone. Estrone is metabolized to estradiol.

Androstenedione is also known as 4-androstenedione and chemically as 4-androstene-3,17-dione. The chemical structure is:

Androstenedione
(4-Androstene-3,17-dione)

ACTIONS AND PHARMACOLOGY

ACTIONS

Androstenedione is a putative anabolic substance.

MECHANISM OF ACTION

Androstenedione is metabolized to testosterone in both men and women. Supraphysiologic doses of testosterone have been reported to increase nitrogen retention and increase muscle mass and strength. Women taking 100-milligram oral doses of androstenedione have had significant increases in serum testosterone. The results with men have been variable. One study reported that an androstenedione dose of 300 milligrams daily led to significant elevation of serum testosterone. The elevation was not seen, in the same study, in those receiving daily doses of 100 milligrams. Another study reported that neither 100- nor 300-milligram daily doses of androstenedione led to significant increases in serum testosterone. In any case, whether increases in testosterone levels that may be produced by taking oral androstenedione would be sustained long enough to show increases in nitrogen retention and muscle strength and mass is unknown.

PHARMACOKINETICS

There is scant pharmacokinetic data on orally administered androstenedione. Absorption appears variable, but some absorption does occur. Androstenedione is distributed to various tissues of the body and is metabolized to testosterone and estrone. The amount of testosterone produced per given dose of androstenedione appears to vary. Typically, a greater increase in serum testosterone is found in women compared to men, following intake of oral androstenedione.

INDICATIONS AND USAGE

It has been claimed that supplemental androstenedione can significantly increase blood testosterone levels and build muscle. Recent research is conflicting with respect to the testosterone effect, but is unified in suggesting that prolonged use of this steroid could result in serious health risks.

RESEARCH SUMMARY

A very small 1962 study is often cited by those who claim that androstenedione can significantly boost serum testosterone. Marketers often neglect to mention, however, that this study involved only two subjects—both women.

In 1999, for the first time, androstenedione was tested in healthy young men. This was a well-designed, double-blind, placebo-controlled study. The 30 subjects, aged 19 to 29, all had normal testosterone levels and were not taking nutritional supplements or anabolic steroids at baseline. Nor were they, at the outset, engaged in resistance training. Subjects were randomized to receive 300 milligrams of androstenedione daily or placebo and, concurrently, entered an eight-week program of whole-body resistance training.

The researchers found that androstenedione exerted no effect on serum free and total testosterone levels. Nor was there any difference in lean body mass between those taking the steroid and those receiving placebo.

On the other hand, the researchers reported that serum estradiol and estrone levels increased significantly in those taking androstenedione, and serum HDL-cholesterol levels dropped by 12 percent in those receiving the steroid. The researchers expressed concern over these findings, noting that there is considerable research suggesting that increased estrogen levels may be associated with increased risk of gynecomastia, cardiovascular disease, breast cancer (in women) and pancreatic cancer (in men). Increased levels of androstenedione itself have been associated in some, but not all, studies with increased risk of prostate and pancreatic cancers.

The reduction in HDL-cholesterol seen in this study did not reach the level that is regarded as a risk factor for cardiovascular disease. Nonetheless, the researchers regarded the observed reduction as clinically relevant, and others have observed that the higher doses used by many bodybuilders and athletes over longer periods of time could result in significant cardiovascular risk.

The dose of androstenedione used in this study exceeds the 100 to 200 milligram dose typically recommended by manufacturers of this supplement. But many athletes are reported to be taking far higher doses, often 500 to 1200 milligrams daily.

Two more recent studies, one using 100 milligrams of androstenedione for five days and the other (a randomized placebo-controlled, double-blind study) also using 100 milligrams daily over a 12-week period, similarly found no increase in testosterone levels and no anabolic effect in healthy males.

Another study, however, did find increased testosterone levels in those taking 300 milligrams of androstenedione daily. This study did not measure athletic performance. It also found that the steroid in these doses significantly increased estradiol levels. More research is needed to resolve the testosterone issue.

Some have suggested that more research is also needed to determine whether androstenedione may have some usefulness in those with low and declining testosterone levels, such as some women and older men. There is some evidence that supplementation with the steroid in doses under 300 milligrams a day might increase serum testosterone levels in those who are hypotestosterogenic.

CONTRAINDICATIONS, PRECAUTIONS, ADVERSE REACTIONS

CONTRAINDICATIONS

Androstenedione is contraindicated in those with prostate, breast and uterine cancer.

PRECAUTIONS

Androstenedione is illegal to use or possess except if enrolled in an FDA-allowed clinical trial or if prescribed by a qualified physician.

ADVERSE REACTIONS

No data are available on the long-term safety of taking supplemental androstenedione. Adverse effects of exogenous testosterone in men include acne, testicular atrophy, gynecomastia, behavioral changes and possibly an increased risk of prostate cancer. Adverse effects of exogenous testosterone in women include hirsutism, deepening of the voice, acne, clitoral hypertrophy, amenorrhea, male-pattern baldness and coarsening of the skin. In adolescents, exogenous testosterone can lead to early closing of bone growth plates and decreased adult height. Other adverse effects of testosterone include hepatic failure and increased platelet aggregation.

Oral androstenedione has been found to decrease HDL-cholesterol levels, which may increase risk of cardiovascular disease.

OVERDOSAGE

There are no reports of overdosage.

DOSAGE AND ADMINISTRATION

Androstenedione is illegal to use or possess except if enrolled in an FDA-allowed clinical trial or if prescribed by a qualified physician.

LITERATURE

Anabolic Steroid Control Act of 2004. Available at: http://frwebgate.access.gpo.gov/cgi-bin/getdoc.cgi?dbname=108cong publiclaws&docid=f:publ358.108.pdf. Accessed August 23, 2008

King DS, Sharp RL, Vukovich MD, et al. Effect of oral androstenedione on serum testosterone and adaptations to resistance training in young men. A randomized controlled trial. *J Am Med Assoc*. 1999; 281:2020-2028.

Leder BZ, Longcope C, Catlin DH, et al. Oral androstenedione administration and serum testosterone concentrations in young men. *J Am Med Assoc*. 2000; 283:779-782.

Rasmussen BB, Volpi E, Gore DC, Wolfe RR. Androstenedione does not stimulate protein metabolism anabolism in young healthy men. *J Clin Endocrin Metab*. 2000; 85:55-59.

Wallace MB, Lim J, Cutler A, Bucci L. Effects of dehydroepiandrosterone vs. androstenedione supplementation in men. *Med Sci Sports Exerc*. 1999; 31:1788-1792.

Yesalis III CE. Medical, legal, and social implications of androstenedione use. *J Am Med Assoc*. 1999; 281:2043-2044.

Arginine Pyroglutamate

DESCRIPTION

Arginine pyroglutamate is the L-arginine salt of pyroglutamic acid. It is also known as pirglutargine and arginine pidolate. It is represented by the following chemical structure:

Arginine pyroglutamate

Arginine pyroglutamate is a delivery form of pyroglutamate. Pyroglutamate is formed in the body by the cyclization of the amino acid glutamic acid and is found naturally in plant and animal products, including the brain. Pyroglutamate is also known as 2-oxo-pyrrolidone carboxylic acid or PCA and 5-oxoproline. Pyroglutamate is an intermediate of the gamma-glutamyl cycle of glutathione synthesis and degradation.

Arginine pyroglutamate, which is comprised of the amino acid L-arginine and the imino acid pyroglutamate, is a water-soluble substance.

ACTIONS AND PHARMACOLOGY

ACTIONS

Arginine pyroglutamate is reputed to have cognition-enhancing activity. The activity is attributed to pyroglutamate.

MECHANISM OF ACTION

Since the action of arginine pyroglutamate is unclear, its mechanism of action is entirely speculative. However, pyroglutamate is structurally related to the drug piracetam, and more is known about piracetam's activity. Piracetam belongs to a class of drugs known as nootropics. The term "nootropic," from the Greek, means "acting on the mind." Piracetam, like pyroglutamate, is a pyrrolidone. Piracetam and related nootropics facilitate learning and memory in animal models, although human studies give mixed results except perhaps in dyslexia.

The effects of piracetam are thought to be mediated through effects on membrane fluidity in the brain. Further, some pyrrolidone-nootropic agents appear to interact with metabotropic glutamate receptors. It is not known whether pyroglutamate has any of these activities.

PHARMACOKINETICS

Little is known in detail about the pharmacokinetics of arginine pyroglutamate. Arginine pyroglutamate gets absorbed across the small intestine and is transported by the portal circulation to the liver, where both L-arginine and pyroglutamate enter into various metabolic pathways. Some pyroglutamate appears to pass into the brain.

INDICATIONS AND USAGE

Arginine pyroglutamate may help improve cognition (e.g. verbal memory) in the aged, though more research is required to confirm this.

RESEARCH SUMMARY

The primary claim made for this arginine salt of pyroglutamic acid relates to cognitive enhancement. It is asserted by some that this substance can help overcome memory defects induced by alcohol abuse and in those with some forms of dementia. Some use the supplement in Italy to treat alcoholism, senility and mental retardation. While such sweeping use is unwarranted based on current findings, there are data that suggest a cognitive-enhancing role for arginine pyroglutamate, though how significant a role is far from established. Some animal studies show that the substance has positive effects in cortical and cholinergic mechanisms and that it has cognition-enhancing properties. And in one double-blind study of aged human subjects, verbal memory was said to be improved in those taking arginine pyroglutamate compared with controls who received placebo.

CONTRAINDICATIONS, PRECAUTIONS, ADVERSE REACTIONS

CONTRAINDICATIONS

Known hypersensitivity to an arginine pyroglutamate-containing product.

PRECAUTIONS

Children, pregnant women and nursing mothers should avoid taking arginine pyroglutamate supplements.

ADVERSE REACTIONS

Arginine pyroglutamate is generally well tolerated. Minor gastrointestinal complaints have been noted.

OVERDOSAGE

There are no known reports of overdosage.

DOSAGE AND ADMINISTRATION

The usual recommended dose is 500 to 1000 milligrams daily. A 500 milligram dose delivers about 150 milligrams of L-arginine and about 350 milligrams of pyroglutamate.

LITERATURE

Barone D, Spignal G. Investigations on the binding properties of the nootropic agent pyroglutamic acid. *Drugs Exp Clin Res.* 1990; 16:85-99.

Drago F, Valerio C, D'Agata V, et al. Pyroglutamic acid improves learning and memory capacities in old rats. *Funct Neurol.* 1988; 3:137-143.

Moos WH, Hershenson FM. Potential therapeutic strategies for senile cognitive disorders. *Drug News Perspect.* 1989; 2:397-409.

Provenzano PM, Brucato A, Gianguzza S, et al. Chemistry and pharmacology of arginine pyroglutamate. Analysis of its effects on the CNS. *Arzneimittelforschung.* 1977; 27:1553-1557.

Sinforiani E, Trucco M, Cavalline A, et al. Reversibility of cognitive disorders among chronic alcoholics in phases of withdrawal. Effect of arginine pyroglutamate. *Minerva Psichiatr.* 1985; 26:339-346.

Spignoli G, Magnani M, Giovannini MG, Pepeu G. Effect of pyroglutamic acid stereoisomers on ECS and scopalamine-induced memory disruption and brain acetylcholine levels in the rat. *Pharmacol Res Commun.* 1987; 19:901-912.

Arnica

DESCRIPTION

Arnica is perhaps best known as a homeopathic remedy for muscle strain and soreness. Arnica, also known as leopard's bane, mountain tobacco, mountain daisy and wolf's bane, is made from the dried flowers and sometimes roots of a few members of the daisy (*Asteraceae/Compositae*) family. These members include *Arnica montana L.,* the major source of arnica in Europe, *Arnica chamissonis* ssp foliosa, *Arnica fulgens* Pursh, *arnica soraria* Greene, *Arnica cordifolia* Hook and *Arnica latifolia* Bong. The dried flowers of another member of the daisy family, *Heterotheca inuloides,* also called arnica, are used in Mexico as a folk remedy.

In the United States, arnica is listed by the FDA as an unsafe herb and is only allowed for food use in alcoholic beverages, where it serves as a flavoring agent. Arnica contains some highly poisonous compounds, such as helenalin, and is considered unsafe for oral use. In addition to the sesquiterpenoid lactone helenalin, arnica contains carbohydrates, such as inulin; amines, such as betaine and choline; coumarins; flavonoids, such as quercetin, kaempferol, isorhamnetin and luteolin; thymol; caffeic acid; phytosterols; and other sesquiterpenoid lactones, such as 11alpha, 13-dihydrohelenalin and chamissonolid. Arnica from the Mexican medicinal plant *Heterotheca inuloides* also contains the sesquiterpenoids 7-hydroxy-3, 4-dihydrocadalin and 7-hydroxycadalin.

Arnica is available in homeopathic preparations, in herbal tinctures and in topical products. Externally applied tinctures of arnica are commonly used in countries such as Germany to treat contusions, sprains, hematomas, rheumatic disorders and superficial inflammations of the skin.

ACTIONS AND PHARMACOLOGY

ACTIONS
Arnica has putative analgesic and anti-inflammatory activities.

MECHANISM OF ACTION
The sesquiterpenoid lactone helenalin and, to lesser degrees, the sesquiterpenoid lactones 11alpha, 13-dihydrohelenalin and chamissonolid are reported to inhibit the activation of the transcription factor NF-kappa B by directly modifying this factor. Activation of NF-kappa B leads to inflammatory activity. This could account, at least in part, for the possible anti-inflammatory and analgesic actions of topical arnica preparations. There is no credible research supporting anti-inflammatory and/or analgesic activity for ingested arnica.

The sesquiterpenoids isolated from *Heterotheca inuloides*—7-hydroxy-3, 4-dihydrocadalin and 7-hydroxycadalin—have been reported to have activity against Gram-positive bacteria, including methicillin-resistant *Staphylococcus aureus* (MRSA). The mechanism of this antibacterial activity is unknown. Similarly unknown is how the antibacterial activities of the compounds relate to any possible action of Mexican arnica. In fact, one study reported only slight *in vitro* activity of arnica against oral pathogens.

PHARMACOKINETICS
There are no reports on the pharmacokinetics of arnica.

INDICATIONS AND USAGE
Claims that oral arnica is helpful in relieving pain and stiffness of muscle soreness and useful, generally, in tissue trauma are not supported by credible research.

RESEARCH SUMMARY
A recent review of all placebo-controlled studies related to the clinical efficacy of oral arnica found that the homeopathic remedy is no more efficacious than placebo.

A placebo-controlled study examining the possible ameliorative effect of oral arnica on the tissue trauma following removal of impacted wisdom teeth found more pain and swelling in the arnica-treated group than in the placebo group. A double-blind, placebo-controlled, randomized trial of its use in treating pain and infection after total hysterectomy found no significant difference between it and placebo. In another double-blind, placebo-controlled study, arnica-treated participants in a marathon race were no different than controls in terms of post-race cell damage and restitution time. There was some positive effect in the arnica group with respect to muscle stiffness. A subsequent study of long-distance runners, however, found arnica ineffective in reducing muscle soreness.

There is some positive evidence that arnica has some anti-inflammatory activity when applied externally. On the other hand, arnica is also reported to cause contact allergies in some.

CONTRAINDICATIONS, PRECAUTIONS, ADVERSE REACTIONS

CONTRAINDICATIONS
Oral use of arnica is considered unsafe. Topical use of arnica on broken skin and open wounds is also considered unsafe.

Arnica is contraindicated in those who are allergic to it or who have known allergies or hypersensitivity to other members of the daisy family, such as chamomile and marigolds. It is contraindicated in pregnant women and nursing mothers.

PRECAUTIONS
Sesquiterpenoid lactones in arnica, such as helenalin, are intensely poisonous and cardiotoxic. Therefore, oral use of arnica is considered unsafe, as is topical use of arnica on broken skin and open wounds. Those with hypertension, cardiac arrythmias, and those taking drugs known to cause a prolonged QT interval or drugs known to be potentially cardiotoxic, should be extremely cautious about the use of arnica (see Interactions).

ADVERSE REACTIONS
Ingested arnica may cause nausea, vomiting, abdominal pain, diarrhea, coma and death. Those allergic or hypersensitive to arnica or to other members of the daisy family can develop rhinitis, conjunctivitis, urticaria, bronchospasm, asthmatic attacks and anaphylaxis.

Topical arnica can cause contact dermatitis manifested as pruritis and erythema.

INTERACTIONS

DRUGS
Arnica may potentiate the adverse effects of drugs known to cause a prolonged QT interval. Such drugs include quinidine, procainamide, disopyramide, sotalol, amiodarone, chlorpromazine, prochlorperazine, haloperidol, pentamidine, amitryptyline, desipramine and doxepim.

Arnica may potentiate the cardiotoxicity of such drugs as doxorubicin.

OVERDOSAGE

Overdosage can cause cardiac arrhythmias, coma and death.

DOSAGE AND ADMINISTRATION

No recommended dose.

Arnica is available in homeopathic preparations, herbal tinctures and topical ointments, gels and creams. Arnica is listed in the Homeopathic Pharmacopeia of the United States (HPUS).

LITERATURE

Ernst E, Pittler MH. Efficacy of homeopathic arnica: a systematic review of placebo-controlled clinical trials. *Arch Surg.* 1998; 133:1187-1190.

Hart O, Mullee MA, Lewith G, Miller J. Double-blind, placebo-controlled, randomized clinical trial of homeopathic arnica C30 for pain and infection after total abdominal hysterectomy. *J R Soc Med.* 1997; 90:73-78.

Hausen BM. [Arnica allergy.] [Article in German.] *Hautartz.* 1980; 31:10-17.

Lyss G, Knorre A, Schmidt TJ, et al. The anti-inflammatory sesquiterpene lactone helenalin inhibits the transcription factor NF-kappa B by directly targeting p65. *J Bio Chem.* 1998; 273:33508-33516.

Lyss G, Schmidt TJ, Merfort I, Pahl HL. Helenalin, an anti-inflammatory sesquiterpene lactone from arnica, selectively inhibits transcription factor NF-kappa B. *Biol Chem.* 1997; 378:951-961

Schroder H, Losche W, Strobach H, et al. Helenalin and 11alpha, 13-dihydrohelenalin, two constituents from *Arnica montana* L., inhibit human platelet function via thiol-dependent pathways. *Thromb Res.* 1990; 57:839-845.

Tveiten D, Bruseth S, Borchgrevink CF, Lohne K. [Effect of Arnica D 30 during hard physical exertion. A double-blind trial during the Oslo Marathon 1990]. [Article in Norwegian]. *Tidsskr Nor Laegeforen.* 1991; 111:3630-3631.

Vickers AJ, Fisher P, Smith C, et al Homeopathic Arnica 30X is ineffective for muscle soreness after long-distance running: a randomized, double-blind, placebo-controlled trial. *Clin J Pain.* 1998; 14:227-231.

Arsenic

DESCRIPTION

Arsenic is a metalloid with atomic number 33 and symbol As. It occurs in many ores and is widely distributed in nature, being present in minute quantities in the soil, the sea and in living matter, such as the human body. Arsenic occurs mainly in the trivalent and pentavalent states as compounds of arsenite and arsenate. Arsenic-containing ribofuranosides (arsenosugars) have been identified in living matter. Methyl-containing arsenic compounds, such as arsenocholine and arsenobetaine, are also found in living organisms.

Arsenic is presently not considered an essential nutrient for humans. However, arsenic deficiency states have been reported in some animals. Goats, miniature pigs and rats fed low-arsenic diets were reported to have depressed growth, impaired fertility and increased perinatal mortality. In addition, goats fed arsenic-deficient diets have been found to have depressed triglyceride concentrations and an increased death rate during lactation. Lactating goats on low-arsenic diets suffer myocardial damage, which is associated with injury to the mitochondria.

Worldwide, the daily dietary intake of arsenic ranges from 12 to 60 micrograms. In the United States, the average daily dietary intake of arsenic is approximately 30 micrograms. This figure excludes any contribution from shellfish. Major sources of dietary arsenic are fish, grain and cereal products.

Arsenic is best known as a deadly poison. To a large degree this reputation derived from a 1944 film classic, *Arsenic and Old Lace.* In the movie, two spinsters, as acts of charity, murder lonely old men with their homemade elderberry wine laced with arsenic. Less known is the fact that the wine was also laced with strychnine and cyanide. The fact is that the manifestations of arsenic poisoning, except in very high doses, are typically not acute. However, arsenic can be toxic and is a known carcinogen and teratogen, and high dietary intake of arsenic is a serious public health problem in certain parts of the world, such as Bengal and Bangladesh.

Arsenic has a special role in medical history. Paul Ehrlich, considered the father of modern chemotherapy, discovered the first treatment for syphilis, which he called 606 (salvarsan), an arsenic-containing compound. The trivalent arsenical melarsoprol is used in the treatment of protozoal diseases. And, in the 1930s, arsenic trioxide was found to be effective in the treatment of chronic myelogenous leukemia (CML). Arsenic preparations are widely used in homeopathy. In the 1990s, intravenous arsenic trioxide was found to induce complete remission in patients with acute promyelocytic leukemia (APL), apparently by upregulating apoptosis. Randomized clinical trials led to FDA approval of arsenic trioxide in September 2000 for refractory or relapsed APL. Presently, there are a number of ongoing studies with arsenic trioxide as possible treatment for multiple myeloma, astrocytoma and other malignancies. Interestingly, vitamin C appears to work synergistically with arsenic trioxide in inducing apoptosis in multiple myeloma cells. Vitamin C acts as a prooxidant, not an antioxidant, in this case (see Vitamin C).

ACTIONS AND PHARMACOLOGY

ACTIONS

The actions of dietary arsenic are unknown. Pharmaceutical arsenic appears to induce apoptosis in a number of cancer cells.

PHARMACOKINETICS

Water-soluble arsenic acids and their salts are more rapidly absorbed from the gastrointestinal tract than poorly soluble arsenicals such as arsenic trioxide. Following absorption, arsenic is stored mainly in the liver, kidneys, heart and lungs, with smaller amounts in the muscle and nervous tissue. A couple of weeks following ingestion, arsenic is deposited in the hair and nails, and remains fixed to the keratin for years. Arsenic is also deposited in the bones and teeth.

In the liver, pentavalent arsenic is reduced to some degree to the more toxic trivalent form, and trivalent arsenic is slowly and extensively oxidized to pentavalent arsenic. Both pentavalent and trivalent arsenic are methylated with S-adenosylmethione to relatively non-toxic derivatives. These metabolites of arsenic are excreted in the urine mainly as dimethylarsinic acid and smaller amounts of monomethylarsinic acid and inorganic arsenic compounds. Approximately 50% of ingested arsenic is eliminated within three to five days. Small amounts may continue to be excreted for several weeks following a single dose. Small amounts of arsenic are excreted in the feces, sweat, lungs and skin. Arsenic is excreted in breast milk and readily crosses the placenta.

INDICATIONS AND USAGE

There are no indications for the use of supplemental arsenic. Homeopathic claims made for the use of arsenicum album are not supported by credible research. Arsenic trioxide as a drug is beneficial in the treatment of acute promyelocytic leukemia and possibly some other cancers.

RESEARCH SUMMARY

Complete remission in up to 90% of patients with acute promyelocytic leukemia, including some resistant to standard treatments, has been demonstrated. Clinical, randomized, controlled studies are ongoing, investigating the potential use of arsenic trioxide in acute promyelocytic leukemia and in various other tumors. Arsenic trioxide, however, is not a dietary supplement, and physicians should caution patients who hear about these studies not to take arsenic supplements.

CONTRAINDICATIONS, PRECAUTIONS, ADVERSE REACTIONS

CONTRAINDICATIONS

Supplemental arsenic is contraindicated for everyone.

PRECAUTIONS

Supplemental arsenic is not recommended for anyone. Arsenic trioxide is presently in clinical trials for the treatment of various cancers and is an approved drug for the treatment of acute promyelocytic leukemia. Under no circumstance should cancer patients self-medicate with arsenic trioxide or any other form of arsenic.

ADVERSE REACTIONS

Toxicity from dietary intake of arsenic—up to 60 micrograms daily—is relatively low. Intakes of higher amounts of arsenic on a chronic basis may cause hyperkeratosis, especially of the palms and soles, skin pigmentation, eczematous or follicular dermatitis, edema (especially of the eyelids), alopecia, muscle-aching and weakness, stomatitis, excessive salivation, anemia, leukopenia, thrombocytopenia, jaundice, cirrhosis, ascites, peripheral neuropathy, paresthesias, proteinuria, hematuria and anuria. Chronic-high arsenic ingestion has been associated with various cancers, such as basal cell carcinoma and bladder, liver and lung cancers. The nail changes associated with arsenic toxicity are known as Mees' lines or transverse striate leukonychia.

Ingested arsenic salts cause oral irritation and a sensation of burning in the mouth and throat.

OVERDOSAGE

Intake of 70 to 300 milligrams of arsenic trioxide may be fatal. Death typically occurs between 12 to 48 hours but can occur within one hour. Those who survive arsenic trioxide poisoning may develop encephalopathy or severe peripheral neuropathies. Toxicity of inorganic arsenic increases with greater solubility. Trivalent compounds (e.g., arsenic trioxide) are more toxic than pentavalent compounds. Some organic arsenic compounds, such as arsenobetaine, are significantly less toxic. Symptoms of acute poisoning usually occur within one hour of ingestion but may be delayed for up to 12 hours, particularly in the presence of food. The principle toxic effects are hemorrhagic gastro-enteritis, profound dehydration, cardiac arrhythmias, convulsions, muscle cramps, shock and death.

DOSAGE AND ADMINISTRATION

No recommended dosage of supplemental arsenic.

There were not sufficient data to set dietary reference intakes (DRIs), including tolerable upper intake levels (UL) for arsenic.

Small amounts of arsenic may be found in colloidal or liquid minerals. Arsenic is also found in several homeopathic remedies, including arsenicum album (arsenic trioxide), arsenicum bromatum, arsenicum vodatum, arsenicum metallicum and arsenicum sulfuratum flavum-arsenic trisulph.

LITERATURE

Hei TM, Liu SX, Waldren C. Mutagenicity of arsenic in mammalian cells: role of reactive oxygen species. *Proc Natl Acad Sci.* 1998;95:8103-8107.

Hertz-Picciotto I, Arrighi HM, Hu SW. Does arsenic exposure increase the risk for circulatory disease? *Am J Epidemiol.* 2000;151:174-181.

Institute of Medicine, Food and Nutrition Board. Dietary Reference Intakes for vitamin A, vitamin K, arsenic, boron, chromium, copper, iodine, iron, manganese, molybdenum, nickel, silicon, vanadium, and zinc. Washington, DC: National Academy Press, 2001.

Lehmann S, Paul C. Arsenic efficient in acute promyelocytic leukemia. [Article in Swedish.] *Lakartidningen.* 1999;96:5626-5628.

Mazunder DN, Das Gupta J, Santra A, et al. Chronic arsenic toxicity in west Bengal—the worst calamity in the world. *J Indian Med Assoc.* 1998;96:4-7,18.

Nielsen FH. Ultratrace minerals. In: Shils ME, Olson JA, Shike M, Ross AC, eds. *Modern Nutrition in Health and Disease.* 9th ed. Baltimore, MD: Williams and Wilkins; 1999;283-303.

Pergantis SA, Wangkarn S, Francesconi KA, et al. Identification of arsenosugars at the picogram level using nanoelectrospray quadropole-time-of-flight mass spectrometry. *Anal Chem.* 2000;72:357-366.

Shen ZY, Shen J, Cai WJ, et al. The alteration of mitochondria is an early event of arsenic trioxide induced apoptosis in esophageal carcinoma cells. *Int J Mol Med.* 2000;5:155-158.

Soignet SL, Maslak PM, Wang Z-G, et al. Complete remission after treatment of acute promyelocytic leukemia with arsenic trioxide. *N Engl J Med.* 1998;339:1341-1348.

Ascorbyl Palmitate

DESCRIPTION

Ascorbyl palmitate is a synthetic ester comprised of the 16-carbon chain saturated fatty acid palmitic acid and L-ascorbic acid. The ester linkage is at the 6 carbon of ascorbic acid. It is used as an antioxidant in foods, pharmaceuticals and cosmetics, and is also used as a preservative for the natural oils, oleates, fragrances, colors, vitamins and other edible oils and waxes which are used in pharmaceuticals, cosmetics and foods.

Ascorbyl palmitate is a white or yellowish powder having a slight odor. It is very slightly soluble in water and in vegetable oils. Ascorbic acid comprises 42.5% of the weight of ascorbyl palmitate. Its molecular weight is 414.54 daltons and its empirical formula is $C_{22}H_{38}O_7$. Ascorbyl palmitate is also known as vitamin C palmitate, L-ascorbyl-6-palmitate and 3-oxo-L-gulofuranolactone 6-palmitate.

Ascorbyl palmitate is marketed as a nutritional supplement and claimed by some to be a superior delivery form of vitamin C. Since ascorbyl palmitate is a fat-soluble derivative of ascorbic acid, theoretically it can concentrate into the lipid domains of biological systems and protect cell membranes and low density lipoproteins (LDL) against oxidation.

ACTIONS AND PHARMACOLOGY

ACTIONS

Ascorbyl palmitate is a delivery form of ascorbic acid. Refer to the vitamin C monograph for the action of ascorbic acid.

MECHANISM OF ACTION

If ascorbyl palmitate is absorbed intact, it may be expected to be a better antioxidant in the lipid domains of the cell membranes and in LDL than is ascorbic acid. It may also be expected to be a more efficient partner with d-alpha-tocopherol than is ascorbic acid with regard to sparing vitamin E, as well as regenerating it from its radical form. However, to date, little is known of the pharmacokinetics of ascorbyl palmitate. Refer to the vitamin C monograph for details on the mechanism of action of ascorbic acid.

PHARMACOKINETICS

As mentioned above, little is known of the pharmacokinetics of ascorbyl palmitate. For details on the pharmacokinetics of ascorbic acid, refer to the vitamin C monograph.

INDICATIONS AND USAGE

Ascorbyl palmitate has indications similar to those of vitamin C. (See Vitamin C.) There is one report suggesting that it might be more effective than other forms of vitamin C in protecting against lipid peroxide-induced endothelial injury.

RESEARCH SUMMARY

There is one preliminary *in vitro* study suggesting that ascorbyl palmitate can protect cultured human umbilical vein endothelial cells from the cytotoxicity of linoleic acid hydroperoxide in circumstances where ascorbic acid itself failed to perform the same protective function. At this early state, however, there is no reason to recommend preferential use of ascorbyl palmitate. See the monograph for vitamin C for the research summary of ascorbic acid.

CONTRAINDICATIONS, PRECAUTIONS, ADVERSE REACTIONS

See Vitamin C.

INTERACTIONS

See Vitamin C.

DOSAGE AND ADMINISTRATION

Multiply ascorbyl palmitate dose by 0.425 to derive the amount of ascorbic acid in the preparation. For recommended dosage and administration, refer to the vitamin C monograph.

LITERATURE

Kaneko T, Kaji K, Matsuo M. Protective effects of lipophilic derivatives of ascorbic acid on lipid peroxide-induced endothelial injury. *Arch Biochem Biophys.* 1993; 304:176-180.

Perricone N, Nagy K, Horvath F, et al. The hydroxyl free radical reactions of ascorbyl palmitate as measured in various in vitro models. *Biochem Biophys Res Commun.* 1999; 262:661-665.

Refer to the vitamin C monograph to review further literature references for ascorbic acid.

Astaxanthin

DESCRIPTION

Astaxanthin is a member of the carotenoid family, specifically, the xanthophyll subfamily of the carotenoids, oxygenated derivatives of carotenoids (oxycarotenoids) whose biosynthesis involves steps with beta-carotene (see Beta-carotene) and/or lycopene (see Lycopene). Astaxanthin is related to beta-carotene, but in contrast to beta-carotene, astaxanthin does not possess provitamin A activity. Astaxanthin, like other carotenoids, is a fat-soluble pigment.

Pure astaxanthin has a reddish-orange color. However, astaxanthin is usually found in nature bound to proteins, and the color of these complexes can be red, red/pink, green, brown or sometimes even bluish. In fact, it is astaxanthin that is responsible for the red/pink color of salmon flesh, which is perceived by consumers as one of the most important quality criteria of the fish. The color of trout, red sea bream, shrimp and lobster, as well as such birds as flamingo and quail, is also due to astaxanthin. The carotenoprotein complexes found in crustaceans provide a bluish-brown coloring. When the complexes are denatured by heat, astaxanthin is exposed and develops the typical reddish-orange color expected by consumers. None of the above fish, crustaceans or birds synthesizes its own astaxanthin. They obtain the carotenoid from consumption of certain microalgae, zooplankton and insects, or from supplemented feeds containing synthetic astaxanthin. (Farmed fish typically feed on synthetic astaxanthin.) Astaxanthin generally enters the human food chain via these fish and crustaceans.

The richest natural sources of astaxanthin are the green microalgae *Haematoccus pluvialis* and the red yeast *Phaffia rhodozyma,* with *H. pluvialis* being the richest source. Both of these organisms do biosynthesize their own astaxanthin. Astaxanthin accumulation by *H. pluvialis* is a phenomenon known as "blood rain and blood snow." Green microalgae from the *Scenedesmus* species and the *Chlorococcum* species can also biosynthesize astaxanthin, as can the green microalgae *Chlorella zofingiensis* and the marine bacteria *Agrobacterium aurantiacum.* Astaxanthin functions as a light-harvesting pigment for the microalgae, partnering with chlorophyll in the photosynthetic process. In addition, astaxanthin serves to protect these organisms against the toxic effects of oxygen and ultraviolet radiation. Astaxanthin may also be protective to humans against certain disorders, such as cataracts, macular degeneration, diabetic kidney disease and others.

Astaxanthin is chemically described as 6-hydroxy-3-[(1E,3E,5E,7E,9E,11E,13E,15E,17E)-18-(4-hydroxy-2,6,6-trimethyl-3-oxo-1-cyclohexenyl)-3,7,12,16-tetramethyloctadeca-1,3,5,7,9,11,13,15,17-nonaenyl]-2,4,4-trimethylcyclohex-2-en-1-one. It is also called 3,3'-dihydroxy-beta,beta-carotene-4,4'-dione. Astaxanthin's CAS (Chemical Abstract Services) registry number is 472-61-7, its molecular weight is 596.84 and its empirical formula is $C_{40}H_{52}O_4$. Astaxanthin is represented by the following chemical structure.

Astaxanthin

Astaxanthin has two chiral carbon atom centers (a chiral center is one that does not possess a center of symmetry and is nonsuperimposable on its mirror image), which are at the 3 and 3' positions of the ionone rings. (See accompanying figure; the chiral carbon atoms are the ones attached to the hydroxyl or OH groups.) The two chiral centers can exist either as R or S forms (R for right-handed and S for left-handed), thus there is a total of three stereoisomers (3R, 3'R), (3R, 3'S or meso) and (3S, 3'S). Astaxanthin possesses several double bonds in the chain of conjugated double bonds comprising the polyenic part of the molecule. Each double bond of the polyenic chain may exist in one of two configurations; as geometric isomers cis (Z) or trans (E). Significantly, the thermodynamically most stable form of the molecule is all-E or all-trans astaxanthin. Several geometric isomers of astaxanthin exist—isomers that differ in which atoms in the polyenic structure are Z (cis) or E (trans). The most important moiety of the astaxanthin molecule is the polyenic chain. The 13 conjugated double bonds of the astaxanthin C40 molecule, in contrast to the seven in the C40 beta carotene structure, gives astaxanthin significantly greater antioxidant capacity, and its long chain conjugated polyene structure makes it highly reactive to singlet oxygen and reactive oxygen and reactive nitrogen species.

Astaxanthin exists in several different forms, which can be classified according to stereoisomers (R and S), geometric isomers (E or trans and Z or cis) and free or esterified forms. All of these forms are found in various natural sources. Astaxanthin found in the red yeast *Phaffia rhodozyma* is in the free, unesterified form containing the 3R, 3'R stereoisomer, while astaxanthin found in microalgae *Haematoccus pluvialis* is present mainly as di- or mono-fatty acid esters, and the steroisomeric form 3*S*, 3'*S* predominates.

Synthetic astaxanthin contains a steroisomeric mixture comprised of 25% of the 3*S*,3'*S* form, 25% of the 3*R*, 3'*R* form and 50% of 3*R*,3'*S*. The *all-E* (*all-trans*) structure is the major geometric isomer in synthetic astaxanthin.

ACTIONS AND PHARMACOLOGY

ACTIONS

Astaxanthin has antioxidant activity and possible antiatherogenic, anticancer, antihypertensive/neuroprotective, anti-inflammatory/ophthalmoprotective, antioxidant/opthalmoprotective and renoprotective activities.

Antiatherogenic activity: The oxidation of LDL (low-density lipoprotein) plays a major role in the atherogenic process. Macrophages bind intra-luminal LDL via receptors known as scavenger receptors, which recognize LDL only after it has been oxidized. Uptake of oxidized-LDL renders the macrophages less mobile and promotes the accumulation of lipid-laden foam cells in the intima of the blood vessels.

Astaxanthin has been shown to inhibit the oxidation of LDL. Astaxanthin was reported to reduce LDL oxidation *in vitro* and *ex vivo,* and a daily dose of 3.6 mg of the carotenoid for two consecutive weeks demonstrated that astaxanthin could protect LDL-cholesterol against induced-oxidation in an *in vitro* test.

However, prospective clinical trials are needed and warranted to determine the efficacy of astaxanthin in protecting against atherosclerosis and to determine acceptable daily intakes of the carotenoid.

Anticancer activity: Astaxanthin was reported to inhibit mouse urinary bladder carcinogenesis induced by N-butyl-N(4-hydroxybutyl)nitrosamine (OH-BBN), to suppress azoxymethane (AOM)-induced rat colon carcinogenesis and to inhibit oral carcinogenesis in rats induced by 4-nitroquinoline 1-oxide (4NQO).

Astaxanthin was shown to suppress tumor growth in mice inoculated with methylcholanthene-induced fibrosarcoma cells. Further, astaxanthin stimulated the cytotoxic T lymphocyte immune response against the fibrosarcoma tumor antigen.

Mastocytoma cells (mast cell tumor cells) were inoculated into mice, followed by the mice being subjected to oxidative stress. The oxidative stress promoted hepatic metastasis. Oral administration of astaxanthin attenuated the promotion of hepatic metastasis induced by oxidative stress. The mode of action of astaxanthin in this case was ascribed to the carotenoid's inhibition of lipid peroxidation of the cytotoxic T lymphocytes.

Antihypertensive and neuroprotective activities: Astaxanthin was found to significantly lower blood pressure—mean blood pressure, systolic blood pressure and diastolic blood pressure—in the spontaneous hypertensive rat (SHR) model. It also delayed the incidence of stroke in the SHR-stroke prone (SHR-SP) model.

In addition, astaxanthin showed significant neuroprotective effects in ischemic mice by preventing the ischemia-induced impairment of spatial memory in these mice. Pretreatment of the mice with astaxanthin significantly shortened the latency of escaping onto the platform in the Morris water maze learning performance test. All of these findings suggested that astaxanthin may attenuate the development of hypertension and may help to protect the brain against stroke and ischemic insults.

The mechanism of action of the blood pressure-lowering effect of astaxanthin is unclear. It possibly has something to do with the antioxidant effects of the carotenoid. The peptide angiotensin II (Ang II) produced in the renin angiotensin system (RAS) pathway possesses vasoconstrictor activity. Vasoconstriction is caused when Ang II binds to its receptor, Ang IIR. Ang IIR not only signals vasoconstriction but may also activate the enzyme NADPH (nicotinamide adenine dinucleotide phosphate reduced) oxidase. NADPH oxidase produces superoxide anions. Endothelial nitric oxide (NO) is the major factor in the regulation of arteriolar tone. Vasoconstriction and elevated blood pressure occur when the endothelial bioavailability of NO decreases. Superoxide anions from the NADPH oxidase reaction can react with endothelial NO to produce the potent reactive nitrogen species peroxynitrite. When that occurs, the endothelial bioavailability of NO decreases, the blood vessels constrict and blood pressure increases. Astaxanthin is a superoxide anion scavenger and as such can prevent the formation of peroxynitrite and prevent blood pressure elevation.

More research, and most of all clinical trials, are needed and warranted to determine the mechanism of astaxanthin's blood pressure-lowering effect and to determine if the carotenoid has any role in the treatment and prevention of hypertension as well as in neuroprotection.

Anti-inflammatory/ophthalmoprotective activity: The uvea, also called the uveal layer or uveal tract, is the pigmented middle layer of the three concentric layers that comprise the eye. Uveitis or inflammation of the uvea is responsible for about ten percent of the blindness in the United States. From two-thirds to 90% of uveitis cases are anterior in location and are often referred to as iritis (inflammation of the iris and anterior chamber).

Endotoxin-induced uveitis (EIU) (induced by lipopolysaccharide [LPS]) is an acute anterior segment intraocular inflammation. EIU was induced in male Lewis rats by footpad injections of LPS. Immediately following the injections, astaxanthin in varying doses was injected intravenously. Aqueous humor was collected from six to 24 hours after the LPS injections, and the number of infiltrating cells in the anterior chamber was counted. In addition, the concentration of proteins, nitric oxide (NO), tumor necrosis factor (TNF)-alpha and prostaglandin E2 (PGE2) were assayed. Astaxanthin suppressed the development of EIU in a dose-dependent fashion. The rats injected with astaxanthin demonstrated a significant decrease in the number of cells infiltrating the anterior chamber and also demonstrated lower concentrations of protein, NO, TNF-alpha and PGE2 in the aqueous humor. The results of this study suggested that astaxanthin reduced the LPS-induced ocular inflammation by downregulating proinflammatory factors and by inhibiting the nuclear factor (NF)-kappaB signaling pathway.

Age-related macular degeneration (ARMD or AMD) is the leading cause of central vision loss (blindness) in the United States, for those over the age of 50, and its prevalence increases with age. In ARMD, the macula area of the retina, the center of the inner lining of the eye, undergoes atrophy and, in some cases, bleeding. ARMD is classified as either wet or neovascular, or dry or non-neovascular. About 10 percent of those with ARMD have the wet form. New blood vessels form to improve the blood supply to the retina. However, the new vessels are delicate and easily break, causing bleeding and damage to the surrounding tissue.

The choroid is the vascular layer of the eye lying between the retina and the sclera. Choroidal neovascularization (CNV) is the creation of new blood vessels in the choroid layer of the eye. This occurs in wet ARMD. Several proinflammatory-related molecules have been implicated in the pathogenesis of choroidal neovascularization and ARMD.

The cellular and molecular mechanisms underlying choroidal neovascularization are not completely understood. CNV in ARMD develops in the context of oxidative stress and inflammation. Vascular endothelial growth factor (VEGF) is critical for promoting CNV. CNV is also associated with the influx of inflammatory cells, including macrophages, which are the source of VEGF. CNV tissues express a number of inflammation-related molecules, including intercellular adhesion molecule (ICAM)-1, monocyte chemotactic protein (MCP)-1, interleukin (IL)-6, vascular endothelial growth factor (VEGF), VEGF receptor (VEGFR)-1 and VEGFR-2.

CNV was induced in mice by laser photocoagulation. The mice were treated with intraperitoneal injections of astaxanthin for three days prior to photocoagulation and treatments were continued daily until the end of the study. The CNV response was analyzed by volumetric measurements one week after the laser injury. The retinal pigment epithelium (RPE)-choroid complex levels of IkappaB-alpha, (ICAM)-1, (MCP)-1, (IL)-6, VEGF, VEGFR-1, and VEGFR-2 were examined by Western blotting or ELISA, and astaxanthin was applied to capillary endothelial cells, macrophages and retinal pigmented epithelial (RPE) cells to analyze the activation of nuclear factor (NF)-kappaB and the expression of inflammatory molecules.

The astaxanthin/CNV study revealed a number of findings on the anti-inflammatory activities of astaxanthin on choroidal neovascularization (CNV): Treatment with astaxanthin led to significant suppression of CNV; the cellular and molecular mechanisms of astaxanthin included inhibitory effects on macrophage infiltration into CNV and inhibition of inflammation-related molecules in the RPE-choroid complex, as well as in cultured macrophages, RPE cells and microvascular endothelial cells; and astaxanthin treatment led to inhibition of NF-kappaB activation *in vitro* and *in vivo*. Astaxanthin inhibited the activation of NF-kappaB via its suppression of IkappaB-alpha degradation and its suppression of p65 nuclear translocation. IkappaB-alpha controls the activity of NF-kappaB by inhibiting its DNA binding activity. p65 is involved in the degradation of IkappaB-alpha. The major conclusion emerging from this study was that the data suggested the importance of astaxanthin's capability to inhibit NF-kappaB activation.

Antioxidant activity: Astaxanthin is the most important defense in the microalgae *Haematoccus pluvialis* against exposure to ultraviolet (UV) light. The microalgae encounter a great quantity of ultraviolet B (UVB) radiation. Exposure to UVB leads to the generation of reactive oxygen species (ROS). Oxidative stress results from the disruption of the cellular homeostasis of ROS production via the excitation of O_2 to form singlet oxygen (the ground state of molecular oxygen is triplet oxygen) and the transfer of one, two or three electrons to form superoxide anions, hydrogen peroxide and hydroxyl radicals, respectively. The ROS generated lead to oxidative destruction of the cell compartments via oxidative damage of membrane lipids, nucleic acids, carbohydrates and proteins. Oxidative damage to membrane lipids results in lipid peroxidation, which can be measured by levels of malondialdehyde and conjugate dienes; DNA damage can be assayed by levels of 8-hydroxydeoxyguanosine (8OHdG), levels of RNA damage by 8-hydroxyguanosine (8OHG) and protein damage by levels of protein-bound carbonyls.

Astaxanthin has demonstrated its ability to quench singlet oxygen, to scavenge hydroxyl radicals, superoxide anions, hydrogen peroxide and to inhibit lipid peroxidation, protein oxidation and nucleic acid oxidation. Interestingly, although the *all-trans* (*all-E*) form of astaxanthin appears to be the most thermodynamically stable form of the carotenoid, *cis* (*Z*) astaxanthin, and especially 9-*cis* (*Z*) astaxanthin, was found to exhibit higher antioxidant activity *in vitro* when compared to the *all-trans* (*E*) isomer. This was assayed by stable radical DPPH (1,1-diphenyl-2-picrylhydrazyl) radical scavenging activity, by rat microsome and rabbit erythrocyte lipid peroxidation inhibitory activity, by inhibition of ROS generation in human neuroblastoma SH-SY5Y cells and by inhibition of collagen II degradation induced by lipid hydroperoxides.

Inorganic mercury, which is still used in certain types of batteries and in fluorescent light bulbs, can cause renal problems, including acute renal failure if absorbed into the body. Inorganic mercury has a nonuniform distribution following absorption, being accumulated mainly in kidneys. The major mode of inorganic mercury nephrotoxicity is via oxidative damage and changes in the activities of the antioxidant enzymes superoxide dismutase, glutathione peroxidase and catalase. Astaxanthin was administered to rats, following which the rats were injected with mercuric chloride. The rats were sacrificed 12 hours after the mercuric chloride injections, and it was found that astaxanthin prevented increases in lipid and protein oxidation, attenuated histopathological changes caused by the inorganic mercury and prevented changes in the antioxidant enzymes.

Ethanol is known to induce ulcerative gastric lesions in some who are excessive drinkers. It is thought that these lesions are caused by oxidative stress. Astaxanthin was shown to be protective against these lesions in ethanol-induced gastric mucosal injury in rats. Astaxanthin inhibited lipid peroxidation and also increased the activities of radical scavenging enzymes—superoxide dismutase, catalase and glutathione peroxidase. Histologically, the acute gastric mucosal lesions induced by ethanol nearly disappeared after treatment with astaxanthin.

The nonsteroidal anti-inflammatory drug (NSAID) naproxen has also been known to induce ulcerative gastric lesions thought to be due to lipid peroxides and free radicals induced by the drug. Administration of astaxanthin showed a significant protection against naproxen-induced gastric antral ulceration in rats. As in the ethanol study, it inhibited elevation of lipid peroxides in the gastric mucosa and resulted in a significant increase in superoxide dismutase, catalase and glutathione peroxidase. Histologically, the acute gastric mucosal lesions induced by naproxen nearly disappeared after treatment with astaxanthin.

Antioxidant/Ophthalmoprotective activity: Astaxanthin has been reported to protect against oxidative stress- and calcium-induced lens protein degradation.

Lens opacification, or cataracts, develop for a variety of reasons, including ultraviolet exposure, diseases such as diabetes, and as a normal process of aging. Nuclear cataracts are the most common type of age-related cataracts. Crystallins are proteins comprising the human lens, which are found damaged in cataracts. It is thought that the common link between possible causes of cataracts and damaged lens crystallins is oxidative stress.

Porcine lens was subjected to calcium-ion activated protease (calpain), or to crystallin oxidative damage mediated by iron-activated hydroxyl radicals produced via the Fenton reaction. Astaxanthin was found to protect the porcine lens from oxidative damage in both situations. Astaxanthin provided better protection than the endogenous antioxidant reduced glutathione in terms of suppressing calcium-induced turbidity of lens proteins.

Renoprotective activity: Oxidative stress is implicated as an important mechanism by which diabetes causes nephropathy. The effect of astaxanthin on diabetic nephropathy in female db/db mice, a rodent model of type 2 diabetes, when compared with a control group not receiving the carotenoid, showed significant inhibition in the increase of urinary 8-hydroxydeoxyguanosine (8-OHdG), a marker of DNA oxidative damage, and significant amelioration in the progression and acceleration of diabetic nephropathy.

The mesangial cell occupies a central position in the renal glomerulus. It has characteristics of a modified smooth muscle cell, but it is also capable of a number of other functions. Mesangial cells not only surround vascular endothelium in the glomerulus and produce the extracellular matrix to support surrounding cells, but they also produce cytokines that interact with vascular endothelial cells or inflammatory cells. In addition, the overproduction of mesangial matrix is an important event in the pathogenesis of diabetic nephropathy. In a follow-up study by the above group that reported that astaxanthin prevented the onset of diabetic nephropathy using an animal model of type 2 diabetes, the researchers investigated the protective mechanism of astaxanthin on the progression of diabetic nephropathy using an *in vitro* model of hyperglycemia, focusing on mesangial cells.

Normal human mesangial cells (NHMCs) were cultured in medium containing normal or high concentrations of D-glucose. The following were evaluated in the presence or in the absence of astaxanthin: reactive oxygen species (ROS) production, nuclear factor kappaB (NF-kappaB) and activator protein-1 (AP-1) activation, and monocyte chemoattractant protein-1 (MCP-1). High glucose exposure induced significant ROS production in the mitochondria of the mesangial cells, which resulted in the activation of transcription factors and expression and production of cytokines that play important roles in mesangial expansion, an important event in the pathogenesis of diabetic nephropathy.

Astaxanthin significantly suppressed the high glucose-induced ROS production. Astaxanthin also accumulated in the mitochondria of the mesangial cells and reduced the production of ROS-modified proteins in the mitochondria. The mechanism of action of this activity is not completely understood, however, it may have to do with astaxanthin's prevention of diabetic nephropathy via a ROS scavenging effect in the mitochondria of the mesangial cells.

PHARMACOKINETICS

There is much unknown about the pharmacokinetics (PK) of astaxanthin, in particular its distribution and its metabolism. There is some evidence from animal studies that suggests that astaxanthin can penetrate the blood-brain barrier.

From a small human trial, astaxanthin appears to be similar to the PK of some other carotenoids, especially the oxycarotenoids. The following describes the PK of astaxanthin as best we know it at this time.

Astaxanthin is available in nutritional supplements dissolved in various oils or as an oleoresin. In foods, including salmon, trout, shrimp and lobster, astaxanthin exists as part of a matrix within these foods. The efficiency of absorption of astaxanthin from foods is less than it is from nutritional supplements. Cooking the foods does help release astaxanthin and astaxanthin esters from the matrix.

In the lumen of the small intestine, astaxanthin from supplements or food is either solubilized in the lipid core of micelles (formed from bile salts and dietary fat) or forms clathrate complexes with conjugated bile salts. Micelles and clathrate complexes deliver astaxanthin to the enterocytes. Esterases liberate unesterified astaxanthin from astaxanthin esters.

Astaxanthin is released from the enterocytes into the lymphatics in the form of chylomicrons. Astaxanthin is transported by the lymphatics to the general circulation via the thoracic duct. In the circulation, lipoprotein lipase hydrolyzes much of the triglycerides in the chylomicrons, resulting in the formation of chylomicron remnants. Chylomicron remnants retain apolipoproteins E and B48 on their surfaces and are mainly taken up by hepatocytes and to lesser degrees by other tissues. Within hepatocytes, astaxanthin is incorporated into lipoproteins. Astaxanthin is released into the circulation from the hepatocytes in the form of very-low-density lipoproteins (VLDL) and low-density lipoproteins (LDL). In the plasma, VLDL is converted by lipoprotein lipase to LDL. In the small human study mentioned above, astaxanthin was transported in the plasma

predominantly as VLDL and less so as LDL and HDL. It was also found that a selective process increased the relative proportion of astaxanthin Z or *cis* isomers to astaxanthin *all-E* or all-*trans* isomers during uptake into the circulatory system.

INDICATIONS AND USAGE

Recent research suggests that astaxanthin, a red-orange carotenoid pigment found in some marine animals and vegetables, as well as in some birds, is a potent antioxidant and anti-inflammatory with cardioprotective, neuroprotective, antidiabetic, anticancer, antiasthmatic, oculoprotective, nephroprotective, gastroprotective, immunoprotective effects. There is some additional preliminary evidence that it may have some physical endurance-enhancing effects and may be helpful in treating male infertility. Among the richest sources of this carotenoid are the green microalgae *Haematoccus pluvialis* and the red yeast *Phaffia rhodozyma*.

RESEARCH SUMMARY

Numerous studies attest to the anti-inflammatory and antioxidative properties of astaxanthin. The pigment's ability to neutralize reactive oxygen species was credited, in part, with protecting rats from naproxen-induced and ethanol-induced gastric antral ulcerations in a dose-dependent manner. In another rat study, kidney function was reportedly protected against mercuric chloride-induced oxidative stress—via the carotenoid's ability to prevent lipid and protein oxidation. In an *in vitro* study, pretreatment of human lens epithelial cells with a xanthophyll complex-containing astaxanthin provided significant protection against lipid peroxidation and stress signaling induced by ultraviolet B light. In a double-blind study of visual display terminal workers, the carotenoid improved accommodation amplitude. In various studies of astaxanthin on ocular health, the carotenoid has provided more protection than such other antioxidants as glutathione (in a study that measured suppression of calcium-induced turbidity of lens proteins) and alpha-tocopherol (in terms of protection against UVB insult). Astaxanthin's anti-inflammatory properties have also been credited with helping it to protect the eye. In a rat model, it suppressed endotoxin-induced uveitis by inhibiting the nuclear factor-kappaB signaling pathway and downregulating proinflammatory factors. Its potential for reducing inflammation of the eye warrants further research, especially with regard to the possibility that it may have a beneficial role in protecting against age-related macular degeneration (see Anti-inflammatory/ophthalmoprotective activity).

In other work, further exploring astaxanthin's immunomodulating, anti-inflammatory effects, the carotenoid alone, as well as in combination with ginkgolide B, suppressed T cell activation at a level comparable to two commonly used antihistamines, cetirizine dihydrochloride and azelastine, suggesting that it might have a role as an antiasthmatic. (This study involved peripheral blood mononuclear cells derived from asthma patients.) There is some preliminary animal and human data suggesting that astaxanthin might reduce gastric inflammation in those with functional dyspepsia. Further research is needed to determine whether the carotenoid will have any clinical significance in treating or preventing these inflammatory disorders.

Astaxanthin's antioxidative properties have also shown some ability to inhibit cancer in very preliminary studies *in vitro*. Hepatic metastasis experimentally induced was inhibited in a mouse model, reportedly through inhibition of stress-induced lipid peroxidation. Far more research will be needed to establish that the carotenoid can play any role as an effective anticancer agent.

Again, astaxanthin's antioxidative and anti-inflammatory capacities are given credit for its ability to combat cardiovascular and diabetic risk factors, including hypertension, obesity, hyperlipidemia and insulin resistance. In a rat model of the metabolic syndrome, encompassing these risk factors, astaxanthin significantly reduced arterial blood pressure and fasting blood glucose levels, while improving insulin sensitivity. Among other positive effects noted were a significant increase in HDL cholesterol and significant decrease in plasma triglycerides and non-esterified fatty acids. Improved adiponectin level was seen. A decrease in the size of fat cells was also observed. Astaxanthin's ability to protect LDL from oxidation has been observed in both animals and humans. A derivative of the carotenoid, astaxanthin disuccinate disodium salt, has exhibited up to 70% protection against ischemic damage in an animal reperfusion-ischemic damage model. The same derivative significantly reduced infarct size in a rat model of ischemia-reperfusion and did so in a dose-dependent manner. The derivative has reduced rethrombosis after vascular thrombotic occlusion in a canine model. Whether these effects can be reproduced clinically remains to be seen. More research is needed and warranted to further investigate the potential for this potent antioxidant in the prevention and treatment of cardiovascular disease and diabetes.

Neuroprotective effects have also been reported. The carotenoid might help protect against post-ischemic damage to brain tissue in stroke victims primarily through its antioxidative actions. There is only very preliminary non-clinical data in support of this idea but it deserves further investigation. Similarly, a mouse study indicating that an astaxanthin-enriched algal powder added to diet might enhance memory performance needs more rigorous follow-up.

In terms of a possible exercise-enhancement effect, exercise-induced damage to mouse skeletal muscle and heart was reportedly attenuated by administration of the pigment. In another study using mice, swimming endurance was said to be enhanced by astaxanthin supplementation. The effect was attributed to an increase in utilization of fatty acids as an energy source. More research is needed before any meaningful conclusions can be reached.

Data suggest that diets rich in antioxidant-delivering foods, including the carotenoids, may be associated with enhanced male reproductive health, specifically greater sperm number and motility. In a randomized, double-blind study, 30 men with established infertility (and fertile wives) received either 16 mg of astaxanthin or placebo daily for a period of three months. By several measures, including, most significantly, pregnancy rates, the carotenoid was effective. As the researchers noted, however, this intriguing result needs to be confirmed in a larger trial before the carotenoid can be recommended as a useful treatment in infertile men.

CONTRAINDICATIONS, PRECAUTIONS, ADVERSE REACTIONS
CONTRAINDICATIONS
Astaxanthin is contraindicated in those hypersensitive to any component of an astaxanthin-containing supplement.

PRECAUTIONS
Pregnant women and nursing mothers should avoid astaxanthin-containing supplements.

ADVERSE REACTIONS
No reports.

INTERACTIONS
DRUGS
Cholestyramine: Concomitant intake of cholestyramine and astaxanthin may decrease the absorption of astaxanthin.

Colestipol: Concomitant intake of colestipol and astaxanthin may decrease the absorption of astaxanthin.

Mineral oil: Concomitant intake of mineral oil and astaxanthin may reduce the absorption of astaxanthin.

Orlistat: Orlistat (Xenical, Alli) may decrease the absorption of astaxanthin.

NUTRITIONAL SUPPLEMENTS
Beta-carotene: Concomitant intake of beta-carotene and astaxanthin may increase the absorption of astaxanthin.

Medium-chain triglycerides: Concomitant intake of medium-chain triglycerides and lycopene may enhance the absorption of astaxanthin.

Pectin: Concomitant intake of pectin and astaxanthin may decrease the absorption of astaxanthin.

Vitamin E: Concomitant intake of vitamin E and astaxanthin may decrease astaxanthin absorption.

FOODS

Oils: Dietary oils, such as olive oil and fish oils, may enhance the absorption of astaxanthin. Corn oil is less likely to enhance astaxanthin absorption.

Olestra: Olestra may reduce the absorption of astaxanthin.

HERBS

No known interactions.

OVERDOSAGE

No reports.

DOSAGE AND ADMINISTRATION

Astaxanthin supplements are available as gel capsules containing up to 5mg of astaxanthin per capsule. It is also available as an oleoresin.

The optimal doses of astaxanthin for support of health conditions are not known.

A 1997 study conducted by the FDA assessed the amounts of astaxanthin in a variety of wild salmon species.

The following lists the astaxanthin contents of some wild salmon species:

Species	Astaxanthin range	Astaxanthin average
Sockeye salmon	30-58 mg/kg	40.4 mg/kg
Coho salmon	9-28 mg/kg	12.8 mg/kg
Pink salmon	3-7 mg/kg	5.4 mg/kg
Chum salmon	1-8 mg/kg	5.6 mg/kg
Chinook king salmon	1-22 mg/kg	8.9 mg/kg
Atlantic salmon	5-7 mg/kg	5.3mg/kg

The average astaxanthin concentration in the salmon ranges from 5 to 40 ppm (5 mg/kg to 40mg/kg) of flesh. A supplement delivering 2 mg of astaxanthin per day is equivalent to about 400 grams of Atlantic salmon daily. Pregnant women, nursing mothers and children are advised to eat no more than two cans of salmon or one salmon steak per week because of possible risk of mercury exposure. Salmon is considered to be a low-mercury fish.

LITERATURE

Abadie-Guedes R, Santos SD, Cahú TB, et al. Dose-Dependent Effects of Astaxanthin on Cortical Spreading Depression in Chronically Ethanol-Treated Adult Rats. *Alcohol Clin Exp Res.* 2008;32(8):1417-1421.

Andersen LP, Holck S, Kupcinskas L, et al. Gastric inflammatory markers and interleukins in patients with functional dyspepsia treated with astaxanthin. *FEMS Immunol Med Microbiol.* 2007;50(2):244-248.

Anderson ML. A preliminary investigation of the enzymatic inhibition of 5alpha-reduction and growth of prostatic carcinoma cell line LNCap-FGC by natural astaxanthin and Saw Palmetto lipid extract in vitro. *J Herb Pharmacother.* 2005;5(1):17-26.

Aoi W, Naito Y, Sakuma K, et al. Astaxanthin limits exercise-induced skeletal and cardiac muscle damage in mice. *Antioxid Redox Signal.* 2003;5(1):139-144.

Aoi W, Naito Y, Takanami Y, et al. Astaxanthin improves muscle lipid metabolism in exercise via inhibitory effect of oxidative CPT I modification. *Biochem Biophys Res Commun.* 2008;366(4):892-897.

Augusti PR, Conterato GM, Somacal S, et al. Effect of astaxanthin on kidney function impairment and oxidative stress induced by mercuric chloride in rats. *Food Chem Toxicol.* 2008;46(1):212-219.

Bennedsen M, Wang X, Willén R, et al. Treatment of H. pylori infected mice with antioxidant astaxanthin reduces gastric inflammation, bacterial load and modulates cytokine release by splenocytes. *Immunol Lett.*1999;70(3):185-189.

Bloomer RJ. The role of nutritional supplements in the prevention and treatment of resistance exercise-induced skeletal muscle injury. *Sports Med.* 2007;37(6):519-32.

Bloomer RJ, Fry A, Schilling B, et al. Astaxanthin supplementation does not attenuate muscle injury following eccentric exercise in resistance-trained men. *Int J Sport Nutr Exerc Metab.* 2005;15(4):401-412.

Briviba K, Bornemann R, Lemmer U. Visualization of astaxanthin localization in HT29 human colon adenocarcinoma cells by combined confocal resonance Raman and fluorescence microspectroscopy. *Mol Nutr Food Res.* 2006;50(11):991-995.

Cardounel AJ, Dumitrescu C, Zweier JL, et al. Direct superoxide anion scavenging by a disodium disuccinate astaxanthin derivative: Relative efficacy of individual stereoisomers versus the statistical mixture of stereoisomers by electron paramagnetic resonance imaging. *Biochem Biophys Res Commun.* 2003;307(3):704-712.

Comhaire FH, El Garem Y, Mahmoud A, et al. Combined conventional/antioxidant 'Astaxanthin' treatment for male infertility: a double blind, randomized trial. *Asian J Androl.* 2005;7(3):257-262.

Cremades O, Parrado J, Jover M, et al. Nutritional treatment of cancer cachexia in rats. Use of a diet formulated with a crayfish enzymatic extract. *Eur J Nutr.* 2007;46(6):347-353.

Daubrawa F, Sies H, Stahl W. Astaxanthin diminishes gap junctional intercellular communication in primary human fibroblasts. *J Nutr.* 2005;135(11):2507-2511.

Gross GJ, Hazen SL, Lockwood SF. Seven day oral supplementation with Cardax (disodium disuccinate astaxanthin) provides significant cardioprotection and reduces oxidative stress in rats. *Mol Cell Biochem.* 2006;283(1-2):23-30.

Gross GJ, Lockwood SF. Acute and chronic administration of disodium disuccinate astaxanthin (Cardax) produces marked cardioprotection in dog hearts. *Mol Cell Biochem*. 2005;272(1-2):221-227.

Gross GJ, Lockwood SF. Cardioprotection and myocardial salvage by a disodium disuccinate astaxanthin derivative (Cardax). *Life Sci*. 2004;75(2):215-224.

Hansen KB, Tauson AH, Inborr J. Effect of supplementation with the antioxidant astaxanthin on reproduction, pre-weaning growth performance of kits and daily milk intake in mink. *J Reprod Fertil Suppl*. 2001;57:331-334.

Higuera-Ciapara I, Félix-Valenzuela L, Goycoolea FM. Astaxanthin: a review of its chemistry and applications. *Crit Rev Food Sci Nutr*. 2006;46(2):185-196.

Hussein G, Goto H, Oda S, et al. Antihypertensive potential and mechanism of action of astaxanthin: III. Antioxidant and histopathological effects in spontaneously hypertensive rats. *Biol Pharm Bull*. 2006;29(4):684-688.

Hussein G, Nakagawa T, Goto H, et al. Astaxanthin ameliorates features of metabolic syndrome in SHR/NDmcr-cp. *Life Sci*. 2007;80(6):522-529.

Hussein G, Nakamura M, Zhao Q, et al. Antihypertensive and neuroprotective effects of astaxanthin in experimental animals. *Biol Pharm Bull*. 2005;28(1):47-52.

Hussein G, Sankawa U, Goto H, et al. Astaxanthin, a carotenoid with potential in human health and nutrition. *J Nat Prod*. 2006;69(3):443-449.

Ikeuchi M, Koyama T, Takahashi J, et al. Effects of astaxanthin in obese mice fed a high-fat diet. *Biosci Biotechnol Biochem*. 2007;71(4):893-899.

Ikeuchi M, Koyama T, Takahashi J, et al. Effects of astaxanthin supplementation on exercise-induced fatigue in mice. *Biol Pharm Bull*. 2006;29(10):2106-2110.

Izumi-Nagai K, Nagai N, Ohgami K, et al. Inhibition of choroidal neovascularization with an anti-inflammatory carotenoid astaxanthin. *Invest Ophthalmol Vis Sci*. 2008;49(4):1679-1685.

Iwamoto T, Hosoda K, Hirano R, et al. Inhibition of low-density lipoprotein oxidation by astaxanthin. *J Atheroscler Thromb*. 2000;7(4):216-222.

Jacobsson LS, Yuan XM, Ziedén B, et al. Effects of alpha-tocopherol and astaxanthin on LDL oxidation and atherosclerosis in WHHL rabbits. *Atherosclerosis*. 2004;173(2):231-237.

Jyonouchi H, Sun S, Iijima K, et al. Antitumor activity of astaxanthin and its mode of action. *Nutr Cancer*. 2000;36(1):59-65.

Kang JO, Kim SJ, Kim H. Effect of astaxanthin on the hepatotoxicity, lipid peroxidation and antioxidative enzymes in the liver of CCl4-treated rats. *Methods Find Exp Clin Pharmacol*. 2001;23(2):79-84.

Karppi J, Rissanen TH, Nyyssönen K, et al. Effects of astaxanthin supplementation on lipid peroxidation. *Int J Vitam Nutr Res*. 2007;77(1):3-11.

Kim JH, Choi SK, Choi SY, et al. Suppressive effect of astaxanthin isolated from the Xanthophyllomyces dendrorhous mutant on ethanol-induced gastric mucosal injury in rats. *Biosci Biotechnol Biochem*. 2005;69(7):1300-1305.

Kim JH, Kim YS, Song GG, et al. Protective effect of astaxanthin on naproxen-induced gastric antral ulceration in rats. *Eur J Pharmacol*. 2005;514(1):53-59.

Kistler A, Liechti H, Pichard L, et al. Metabolism and CYP-inducer properties of astaxanthin in man and primary human hepatocytes. *Arch Toxicol*. 2002;75(11-12):665-675.

Kupcinskas L, Lafolie P, Lignell A, et al. Efficacy of the natural antioxidant astaxanthin in the treatment of functional dyspepsia in patients with or without Helicobacter pylori infection: A prospective, randomized, double blind, and placebo-controlled study. *Phytomedicine*. 2008;15(6-7):391-399.

Kurashige M, Okimasu E, Inoue M, et al. Inhibition of oxidative injury of biological membranes by astaxanthin. *Physiol Chem Phys Med NMR*. 1990;22(1):27-38.

Kurihara H, Koda H, Asami S, et al. Contribution of the antioxidative property of astaxanthin to its protective effect on the promotion of cancer metastasis in mice treated with restraint stress. *Life Sci*. 2002;70(21):2509-2520.

Lauver DA, Driscoll EM, Lucchesi BR. Disodium disuccinate astaxanthin prevents carotid artery rethrombosis and ex vivo platelet activation. *Pharmacology*. 2008;82(1):67-73.

Lee SJ, Bai SK, Lee KS, et al. Astaxanthin inhibits nitric oxide production and inflammatory gene expression by suppressing I(kappa)B kinase-dependent NF-kappaB activation. *Mol Cells*. 2003;16(1):97-105.

Li W, Hellsten A, Jacobsson LS, et al. Alpha-tocopherol and astaxanthin decrease macrophage infiltration, apoptosis and vulnerability in atheroma of hyperlipidaemic rabbits. *J Mol Cell Cardiol*. 2004;37(5):969-978.

Liu X, Osawa T. Cis astaxanthin and especially 9-cis astaxanthin exhibits a higher antioxidant activity in vitro compared to the all-trans isomer. *Biochem Biophys Res Commun*. 2007;357(1):187-193.

Lockwood SF, Gross GJ. Disodium disuccinate astaxanthin (Cardax): antioxidant and anti-inflammatory cardioprotection. *Cardiovasc Drug Rev*. 2005;23(3):199-216.

Lockwood SF, Penn MS, Hazen SL, et al. The effects of oral Cardax (disodium disuccinate astaxanthin) on multiple independent oxidative stress markers in a mouse peritoneal inflammation model: influence on 5-lipoxygenase in vitro and in vivo. *Life Sci*. 2006;79(2):162-174.

Mahmoud FF, Haines DD, Abul HT, et al. In vitro effects of astaxanthin combined with ginkgolide B on T lymphocyte activation in peripheral blood mononuclear cells from asthmatic subjects. *J Pharmacol Sci*. 2004;94(2):129-136.

Manabe E, Handa O, Naito Y, et al. Astaxanthin protects mesangial cells from hyperglycemia-induced oxidative signaling. *J Cell Biochem*. 2008;103(6):1925-1937.

Mercke Odeberg J, Lignell A, Pettersson A, et al. Oral bioavailability of the antioxidant astaxanthin in humans is enhanced by incorporation of lipid based formulations. *Eur J Pharm Sci.* 2003;19(4):299-304.

Naguib YM. Antioxidant activities of astaxanthin and related carotenoids. *J Agric Food Chem.* 2000;48(4):1150-1154.

Naito Y, Uchiyama K, Mizushima K, et al. Microarray profiling of gene expression patterns in glomerular cells of astaxanthin-treated diabetic mice: a nutrigenomic approach. *Int J Mol Med.* 2006;18(4):685-695.

Nishikawa Y, Minenaka Y, Ichimura M, et al. Effects of astaxanthin and vitamin C on the prevention of gastric ulcerations in stressed rats. *J Nutr Sci Vitaminol* (Tokyo). 2005;51(3):135-141.

Obajimi O, Black KD, Glen I, et al. Antioxidant modulation of oxidant-stimulated uptake and release of arachidonic acid in eicosapentaenoic acid-supplemented human lymphoma U937 cells. *Prostaglandins Leukot Essent Fatty Acids.* 2007;76(2):65-71.

Ohgami K, Shiratori K, Kotake S, et al. Effects of astaxanthin on lipopolysaccharide-induced inflammation in vitro and in vivo. *Invest Ophthalmol Vis Sci.* 2003;44(6):2694-2701.

Palozza P, Barone E, Mancuso C, et al. The protective role of carotenoids against 7-keto-cholesterol formation in solution. *Mol Cell Biochem.* 2008;309(1-2):61-68.

Parisi V, Tedeschi M, Gallinaro G, et al.; CARMIS Study Group. Carotenoids and antioxidants in age-related maculopathy Italian study: multifocal electroretinogram modifications after 1 year. *Ophthalmology.* 2008;115(2):324-333.

Pashkow FJ, Watumull DG, Campbell CL. Astaxanthin: a novel potential treatment for oxidative stress and inflammation in cardiovascular disease. *Am J Cardiol.* 2008;101(10A):58D-68D.

Petri D, Lundebye AK. Tissue distribution of astaxanthin in rats following exposure to graded levels in the feed. *Comp Biochem Physiol C Toxicol Pharmacol.* 2007;145(2):202-209.

Santocono M, Zurria M, Berrettini M, et al. Lutein, zeaxanthin and astaxanthin protect against DNA damage in SK-N-SH human neuroblastoma cells induced by reactive nitrogen species. *J Photochem Photobiol B.* 2007;88(1):1-10.

Suzuki Y, Ohgami K, Shiratori K, et al. Suppressive effects of astaxanthin against rat endotoxin-induced uveitis by inhibiting the NF-kappaB signaling pathway. *Exp Eye Res.* 2006;82(2):275-278.

Tripathi DN, Jena GB. Astaxanthin inhibits cytotoxic and genotoxic effects of cyclophosphamide in mice germ cells. *Toxicology.* 2008;248(2-3):96-103.

Turujman SA, Wamer WG, Wei RR, et al. Rapid liquid chromatographic method to distinguish wild salmon from aquacultured salmon fed synthetic astaxanthin. *J AOAC Int.*1997;80(3):622-632.

Uchiyama K, Naito Y, Hasegawa G, et al. Astaxanthin protects beta-cells against glucose toxicity in diabetic db/db mice. *Redox Rep.* 2002;7(5):290-293.

Wu TH, Liao JH, Hou WC, et al. Astaxanthin protects against oxidative stress and calcium-induced porcine lens protein degradation. *J Agric Food Chem.* 2006;54(6):2418-2423.

Zhang X, Pan L, Wei X, et al. Impact of astaxanthin-enriched algal powder of Haematococcus pluvialis on memory improvement in BALB/c mice. *Environ Geochem Health.* 2007;29(6):483-489.

Baicalein

DESCRIPTION

Baicalein is a polyphenolic substance and a member of the flavone subclass of flavonoids. Its conjugate, baicalein-7-glucuronide, also called baicalin, is found naturally, mainly in the roots of the Baical skullcap (*Scutellaria baicalensis* Georgi). It is also found in the leaves of the commonly used herb thyme (*Thymus vulgaris*), the mad-dog skullcap (*Scutellaria lateriflora* L.) and the midnight horror or broken bones plant (*Oroxylum indicum*).

Baicalein has a long and interesting history in traditional Chinese medicine (TCM) and also in Kampo medicine, traditional Japanese medicine. According to the *Pharmacopoeia of the People's Republic of China*, the dried root of *Scutellaria baicalensis* Georgi, Radix *Scutellariae*, (Huang-qin [golden root] in Chinese and Ogon in Japanese), which is rich in baicalin, 'has the following actions: "To remove *damp-heat*, to quench *fire* and counteract toxicity, to arrest bleeding, and to prevent abortion." Its indications, again quoting from the *Pharmacopoeia*, are: "Discomfort in the chest, nausea and vomiting... febrile diseases caused by *damp-heat* or *summer heat*; feeling of stuffiness in the abdomen, acute dysentery or jaundice caused by *damp heat*; cough due to heat in the lung; high fever with dire thirst; spitting of blood and nosebleeds due to *heat* in blood; carbuncles and sores; threatened abortion." The recommended dose of Huangqin is three to nine grams daily, or approximately 120 mg to 360 mg of baicalin.

Baicalin is a major constituent of a number of drugs used in traditional Asian medicines, including the TCM formulas Xiao-Chai-Hu-Tang and Yin-Zi-Huang, used for liver disorders; Qing-Fe-Tang and Huangqin-Tang, used for respiratory concerns; and Huang-Lian-Jie-Du-Tang, used to treat fever and infection; in addition to Saiboku-To and Sho-Saiko-To, used in Japan for the treatment of asthma and liver disorders, respectively. Tablets are available in China containing 250 mg of baicalin; doses of up to 250 mg taken three times a day are often recommended for liver conditions. Baicalin-containing drugs are mainly used for conditions due to 'damp-heat, summer-heat or fire,' which can be translated as infection and inflammation. These flavonoids have been used for many years in China to treat antibacterial and antiviral infections, including upper respiratory infections and viral hepatitis, and as antipyretics and anti-inflammatories.

Baicalein has intrigued the Chinese for centuries and seems to be intriguing modern scientists as well. Research is ongoing as to the anti-inflammatory activity of baicalein, as well as its possible neuroprotective, anticancer and angiogenic activities. There is hope that it may even play a role in the management of Alzheimer's disease some day.

Baicalein is chemically described as 5,6,7-trihydroxy-2-phenyl-4H-1-benzopyran-4-one. It is also called 5,6,7-trihydroxyflavone and noroxylin. Its CAS registry number is 401-67-8. Its empirical formula is $C_{15}H_{10}O_5$ and its molecular weight is 270.64. Baicalin is also known as baicalein-7-glucuronide and its empirical formula is $C_{21}H_{18}O_{11}$.

All flavonoids possess a basic 15-carbon skeleton that can be represented as C_6-C_3-C_6 (see figure). The common structure is that of a diphenylpropane molecule, consisting of two aromatic rings linked through the three carbons. Flavones possess a carbonyl group on position 4 of the C ring. Baicalein (trihydroxyflavone) possesses hydroxyl groups on positions 5, 6 and 7 of the A ring, making the A ring a pyrogallol moiety. The chemical structures below are described within this monograph.

Baicalein

Flavone Skeleton

Flavonoid Skeleton

ACTIONS AND PHARMACOLOGY

ACTIONS

Baicalein has antioxidant activity and possible angiogenic, anticancer, anxiolytic, anti-inflammatory and neuroprotective activities.

MECHANISM OF ACTION

Angiogenic activity: The first reaction by many to the term 'angiogenesis' is a negative one. The reason for that is that 'angiogenesis' is usually heard in connection with cancer. And, indeed, when it comes to cancer, angiogenesis is not desirable. The sprouting of new blood vessels is a major way for cancer cells to be nourished. Thus, antiangiogenic therapies would be desirable in the context of cancer. However, in the context of myocardial or limb ischemia, the sprouting of new blood vessels would be a way of preventing tissue from dying. For years, most of the research effort in angiogenesis has been concentrated on the role of angiogenic factors, such as vascular endothelial growth factor (VEGF) in tumors. Only recently has interest been growing in the study of angiogenic factors in ischemic diseases.

Angiogenesis is a dynamic process in which angiogenic signals are controlled by local release of vascular growth factors. Oxygen homeostasis is one of the major homeostatic mechanisms in the body. Hypoxia-inducible factor (HIF)-1 is a major transcription factor that functions as a master regulator of oxygen homeostasis. HIF-1 plays essential roles in cellular and systemic pathophysiology. HIF-1 is an alpha/beta heterodimer comprised of two subunits—HIF-1alpha and HIF-1beta. While both HIF-1alpha and HIF-1beta are constitutively expressed, HIF-1alpha, but not HIF-1beta, is degraded during normal oxygen conditions via the ubiquitin-proteasome system (basically, HIF-1alpha gets "chewed up" by this system). HIF-1alpha expression and HIF-1 transcriptional activity increase exponentially as cellular oxygen concentration is decreased. Over 60 target genes, including those for VEGF, are transactivated by HIF-1.

Ischemia is a stimulus for production of angiogenic cytokines which activate local vascular cells and mobilize angiogenic cells to the circulation. These responses are impaired in elderly persons with peripheral vascular disease (PVD) and other ischemic diseases. During the aging process, HIF-1 becomes less functional, thus impairing the expression of angiogenic cytokines and the mobilization of angiogenic cells. If HIF-1 could be activated, that might counteract these pathological effects of aging. However, it might also do this for malignant cells.

It is known that the enzymes HIF-1alpha-specific prolyl-4-hydroxylases (PHDs) prime the ubiquitin-proteasome degradation of HIF-1alpha. If the PHDs could be inhibited, then the HIF pathway could be upregulated. In a screen searching for small molecules that could inhibit the PHDs, it was demonstrated that baicalein inhibited HIF-1alpha-specific prolyl-4-hydroxylase-2 (PHD2), which was found to abolish asparaginyl hydroxylation of HIF-1alpha. Further, baicalein was found to suppress ubiquitination of HIF-1alpha, which works together with the inhibition of the HIF-specific hydroxylases to increase the HIF-1alpha concentration. Increasing the HIP-1alpha concentration leads to induction of HIF-1-mediated reporter gene activity and targets gene transcription in tissue culture cells, where it induces HIF-independent activation of other genes. All of these findings came out of *in vitro* studies. Significantly, baicalein was demonstrated to promote new blood vessel formation *in vivo* in the chick chorioallantoic membrane model. At the second week of the study, baicalein strongly elicited an angiogenic response, forming new capillaries from the existing vascular network. This was similar to the vascular endothelial growth factor (VEGF)-treated positive control. The eggs that were treated with dimethysulfoxide (DMSO) alone showed no significant growth of new blood vessels.

Continued research in this important area is necessary and warranted. Among other things, the exact mechanisms by which baicalein modulates the HIF-1 pathway and modulates angiogenesis *in vivo* require elucidation. And most important, conditions need to be worked out to optimize the activity for the ischemic situation without stimulating a cancer situation, as well as to optimize antiangiogenic conditions for a cancer situation without negatively affecting an ischemic situation. Baicalein might turn out to be the model molecule on which to build towards the discovery and development of a more ideal drug that will be able to counteract the aging effects in angiogenesis for the treatment of such serious diseases as peripheral vascular disease.

Anticancer activity: Baicalein was found to inhibit proliferation of LNCaP and JCA-1 human prostate cancer cells associated with apparent accumulation of cells in the G1 phase of the cell cycle and induction of apoptosis. Baicalein and baicalin were demonstrated to inhibit proliferation in DU-145 and PC3 human prostate cells and to inhibit the growth of human umbilical vein endothelial cells, associated with a decreased number of sprouts formed by the endothelial cell aggregates. The latter finding suggests that baicalein and baicalin may cause inhibition of proliferation via an antiangiogenic mechanism. In an *in vivo* mouse study, baicalein was also found to reduce the volume of prostate tumors.

In studies of human pancreatic cancer cells and human pancreatic xenografts, it was found that baicalein inhibited growth of the cancer cells and induced apoptosis. It was thought that theses activities could be accounted for by the known inhibition of 12-LOX (lipoxygenase) by baicalein. 5-LOX and 12-LOX have been found to be elevated in human pancreatic cancer cells. Baicalein was also found to induce apoptosis in human breast cancer cells and human lung non-small carcinoma H460 cells, again thought to be due to inhibition of 12-LOX by the flavonoid.

Anti-inflammatory activity: Many of the activities of baicalein discussed in this monograph may be attributed to the possible anti-inflammatory activities of baicalein. Perhaps baicalein's single most important anti-inflammatory activity is its ability to inhibit 12-lipoxygenase (12-LOX) or 12/15 LOX. Lipoxygenases comprise a heterogeneous family of enzymes that catalyze the stereospecific dioxygenation of polyunsaturated fatty acids to their corresponding hydroperoxy derivatives. In mammals, including humans, lipoxygenases are categorized with respect to their positional specificity of arachidonic acid oxygenation into 5-LOX, 8-LOX, 12-LOX and 15-LOX. 15-LOX is also known as 12/15-LOX in mice. The LOX enzymes induce structural and pathological processes, including inflammation, carcinogenesis and atherogenesis. The LOX enzymes and their pathways are the subject of much recent investigation. Importantly, accumulating research suggests diverse and opposing roles for the various LOX pathways.

Baicalein appears to possess other types of anti-inflammatory activities as well.

Human mast cells have been implicated in acute and chronic inflammatory responses. They are multifunctional cells that are involved in a number of inflammatory and immune reactions. Mast cells are most well-known, however, for their involvement in the allergic response.

Human mast cells (HMCs)-1 were stimulated either with the inflammatory cytokine mediators interleukin (IL)-1beta or tumor necrosis factor (TNF)-alpha in the absence or presence of baicalein. It was found that the flavonoid-inhibited production of IL-6, IL-8 and monocyte chemotactic protein (MCP)-1 in IL-1beta-activated HMCs-1 and also inhibited the production of these inflammatory mediators in HMCs-1 when activated by TNF-alpha. The cytokine gene expression was mildly decreased in IL-1beta-activated HMCs-1, but markedly decreased in TNF-alpha-activated HMCs-1. It was concluded that baicalein inhibited the production of the inflammatory cytokines via inhibition of activation of the major proinflammatory transcription factor, nuclear factor (NF)-kappaB.

Antioxidant activity: Both baicalein and its conjugate baicalin-7-glucuronide are polyphenols and, like other polyphenols, possess antioxidant activities. Several factors influence the antioxidant capacity of flavonoids, including the number and the position of the hydroxyl groups, the saturation status of the heterocyclic C ring and the extent and nature of the substituents. For baicalein (see figure), there are three hydroxyl groups in the A ring and a 2,3-double bond in conjugation with a 4-oxo group in the C ring, a structure that would be predicted to have good reactive oxygen and reactive nitrogen scavenging activity. It would also be predicted that baicalin, which essentially has one phenolic hydroxyl group out of play, may not have antioxidant activity as potent as baicalein. In addition to having reactive oxygen and reactive scavenging activity, the possible cytoprotective effects of flavonoids are probably determined by their lipid solubility. Baicalein is much more lipid soluble than is baicalin and, therefore, is expected to have greater cytoprotective activity than baicalin.

Both baicalein and baicalin can scavenge the reactive oxygen species superoxide anions and hydroxyl radicals. Baicalein has been demonstrated to inhibit microsomal lipid peroxidation, and a mixture containing both baicalein and baicalin has been shown to protect against hydrogen peroxide-induced oxidative stress in the human neuroblastoma cell line, HS-SY5Y.

Peroxynitrite ($ONOO^-$) is one of the most reactive of reactive oxygen and reactive nitrogen species that cells and tissues may encounter. It can react with a number of major biological molecules, including nucleic acids, lipids and proteins, which can significantly influence cellular function; peroxynitrite may be involved in the pathogenesis of a number of diseases. Baicalein has been demonstrated to scavenge peroxynitrite anions and also to protect SIN-1 (3-morpholinosydnonimine, a radical generator)-treated LLC-PK_1 cells (pig kidney epithelial cells) against peroxynitrite-induced toxicity.

Lipopolysaccharide (LPS), the outer membrane component of gram-negative bacterial cell walls, is the major trigger of gram-negative sepsis and septic shock, a life-threatening condition and the most common cause of death in intensive care units. Baicalein was reported to have a protective effect against endotoxic shock in rats *in vitro* and *in vivo*. In the study, rats were injected with LPS, which caused sepsis, hypotension, tachycardia, circulatory failure and vascular dysfunction in the animals. Treatment with baicalein significantly attenuated the hemodynamic changes and inhibited the elevation of tumor necrosis factor (TNF)-alpha, decreased the levels of inducible nitric oxide synthase (iNOS) and the overproduction of NO and superoxide anions caused by the LPS, and reduced the infiltration of neutrophils into the liver and the lungs. The protective effect of baicalein was thought to be derived, in large part, from the reactive oxygen and reactive nitrogen species scavenging activity of the flavonoid.

Anxiolytic activity: Baicalin-containing teas have had a long history of use for their supposed "nerve calming" activity. There is now some evidence that may support this use.

The Vogel lick-shock conflict test is an instrument that has become a standard test for fast screening of the potential anxiolytic properties of drugs. In this procedure, the drinking behavior is punished by mild electrical shocks, leading to a significant reduction of water consumption in deprived animals. Drinking responses are then reestablished by drugs with anxiolytic properties.

The $GABA_A$ receptor is one of two ligand-gated ion channels responsible for mediating the effects of the neurotransmitter GABA (gamma-aminobutyric acid). The $GABA_A$ receptor is the major inhibitory neurotransmitter in the brain. The $GABA_A$ receptor is also the molecular target of the benzodiazepine class of minor tranquilizer, anxiolytic drugs, including diazepam. Baicalein was demonstrated, in an *in vitro* study, to interact with the benzodiazepine binding site of $GABA_A$ receptors in mouse cerebral cortex preparations. In an *in vivo* study, both baicalein and baicalin significantly increased the number of shocks accepted by mice in the Vogel test, as did a positive control. The anxiolytic-like effect of baicalein or baicalin was antagonized by co-administration with a benzodiazepine receptor antagonist. The conclusion drawn from this study was that the anxiolytic-like effect of baicalein or baicalin was probably mediated via their interaction with and activation of the benzodiazepine binding site of the $GABA_A$ receptors.

Neuroprotectant activity: Baicalein was reported to improve clinical rating scores following multiple small clot embolic strokes in rabbits. Importantly, it was found that baicalein, even if administered at extended times following the embolic strokes, could still produce significant neuroprotection and behavioral improvement. Prior to this *in vivo* study, the researchers demonstrated that baicalein effectively attenuated cell death *in vitro* using a cultured HT22 mouse hippocampal cell line in combination with iodoacetic acid, a known irreversible inhibitor of glycolysis that results in free radical production, lipid peroxidation and cell death. The exact mechanism by which baicalein leads to neuroprotection is unclear. Baicalein is an inhibitor of 12-lipoxygenase (12-LOX), also known as 12/15 lipoxygenase (12/15-LOX) in mice, and that inhibition may account, in part, for baicalein's neuroprotective activity. Baicalein is also an antioxidant and that activity may also play a role in its neuroprotective action.

It has been shown that a decrease in reduced glutathione (GSH) in nerve cells leads to the activation of constitutively expressed 12-LOX. The loss of GSH and activation of 12-LOX are steps in many different forms of toxin-induced nerve damage and death, including those that are caused by protein misfolding.

In another study by a different group of researchers, a mouse model of transient middle cerebral artery occlusion was used to test the neuroprotective effects of baicalein. In this model, 12/15-LOX is increased in the peri-infarct area surrounding the primary infarction, predominantly in neurons. Baicalein protected the mice against transient local ischemia. A similar degree of protection was seen in 12/15-LOX knockout mice when compared with wild-type mice. However, the 12/15-LOX knockout mice were not further protected when administered baicalein. In this case, it appeared that inhibition of 12/15-LOX by baicalein played the major role in its neuroprotective activity; its antioxidant capabilities appeared to play a much smaller role.

In another study, baicalein was demonstrated in rats to improve cognitive deficits induced by chronic cerebral hypoperfusion. In a rat model of chronic cerebral hypoperfusion induced by permanent, bilateral common carotid artery occlusion (two-vessel occlusion, or 2VO), baicalein improved 2VO-induced deficits and neuropathological changes. The mechanism of baicalein's neuroprotective effects was thought to have something to do with its antioxidant action.

The pathobiochemistry of Alzheimer's disease includes, as major features, protein folding and aggregation due to the accumulation of abnormally folded amyloid beta (Abeta) peptide in the brains of those with this disease. Abeta is a peptide that is an abnormal proteolytic byproduct (via the enzyme beta-secretase) of the transmembrane protein amyloid precursor protein (APP). Abeta monomers at sufficiently high concentrations undergo conformational changes to form beta sheet-rich tertiary structures that aggregate to form amyloid fibrils, which deposit outside neurons in dense formation. These dense formations are known as senile or neuritic plaques.

Amyloid beta peptide has been reported to increase reactive oxygen and reactive nitrogen species and lipid peroxidation in PC12 nerve cells. PC12 cells are derived from a transplantable rat pheochromocytoma. Baicalein and baicalin have been shown to reduce the cytotoxicity of Abeta peptide, thought possibly to be due to oxidative stress reduction and/ or inhibition of 12/15-LOX. Another study reported that baicalein aggregates inhibit amyloid polymerization.

Several observations suggest that baicalein inhibits nerve cell death caused by misfolded and toxic peptides and proteins, as well as by oxidative stress. Baicalein has been reported to inhibit the formation of toxic fibrils of Abeta peptide, both in cell-free systems and in nerve cell lines. Baicalein has also been reported to prevent the polymerization of alpha-synuclein. Alpha-synuclein is a protein with unknown function

that is primarily found in nerve tissue. Alpha-synuclein is often found in the amyloid plaques of Alzheimer's disease, where it is known as the non-Abeta component of the plaque.

Much more research is necessary and clearly warranted on the possible anti-Alzheimer's disease activity of baicalein. Baicalein may also have activity in other amyloid diseases, and there are several of them. Finally, baicalein may be a chemical model for the development of more effective molecules for the treatment of various diseases and disorders, including Alzheimer's disease.

PHARMACOKINETICS

Most of the pharmacokinetic (PK) studies of baicalein and baicalin (baicalein-7-glucuronide) have been performed in experimental animals, mainly rats. Absorption and metabolic studies have been performed in Caco-2 cells, a human adenocarcinoma of the colon cell line. Baicalein has demonstrated an extensive first pass metabolism related to glucuronidation or sulfation, but mainly to glucuronidation, in rats following oral administration. Baicalein is absorbed from the small intestine via passive diffusion and it is thought that it undergoes extensive phase II metabolism within the enterocytes. Baicalein was shown to be rapidly metabolized via UDP-glucuronyl transferases and sulfotransferases following its absorption by passive absorption in the Caco-2 cell model. Following glucuronidation and sulfation of baicalein to baicalein-7-glucuronide and baicalein-6-O-sulfate in the Caco-2 cells, the conjugated flavonoids are carried out of the cells via a transporter.

Animal studies have shown that baicalein-7-glucuronide is the predominant form of baicalein in the general circulation following oral administration.

After oral administration of one gram of baicalin to human subjects, urine was collected and the following three metabolites were found: baicalein-6-O-beta-glucopyranuronoside, 6-O-methyl-baicailin-7-O-beta-glucopyranuronoside and baicalin.

Baicalin itself is poorly absorbed from the rat gut. However, when baicalin was administered orally to rats, it was detected in the plasma for 24 hours after administration, but the aglycone baicalein was not detected. Baicalin reaching the colon after oral administration is probably metabolized by bacterial enzymes to baicalein. Baicalein is then absorbed by the colonic enterocytes, converted back to baicalin and then transported from the cells to the circulatory system, which distributes the baicalin to various cells and tissues of the body.

INDICATIONS AND USAGE

In vitro and animal data suggest that baicalein, a polyphenolic flavonoid compound, derived from such natural sources as "skullcap" (*Scutellaria baicalensis* Georgi), has antimicrobial, cardioprotective, neuroprotective, anticancer, antianxiety, anti-inflammatory and antioxidant effects.

RESEARCH SUMMARY

The dried root of *Scutellaria baicalensis* has been used for centuries in Traditional Chinese Medicine, where it has been primarily used for its claimed antimicrobial effects. The flavonoid baicalein, derived from this root, and from some other related sources, has, in fact, demonstrated some notable antimicrobial effects. In one study, baicalein, in this case derived from the leaves of *Thymus vulgaris,* demonstrated a significant, strong synergetic effect with tetracycline against methicillin-resistant *Staphylococcus aureus* (MRSA) *in vitro.* Baicalein, by itself, exhibited weak anti-MRSA activity. In another *in vitro* study, baicalein inhibited, in a dose-dependent pattern, *Candida albicans* biofilms, suggesting that the substance might be useful in helping to prevent device-associated infections. This could be significant since microbial biofilm formation is often a problem with such devices as stents, pacemakers, shunts, various prostheses, implants, endotracheal tubes and dentures.

In both *in vitro* and animal studies, baicalein has shown anti-inflammatory and antioxidant effects sufficient to suggest that this substance might have broad-spectrum cytoprotective effects that could be useful in a broad spectrum of diseases, including cancer, heart disease, diabetes, stroke, neurodegenerative disorders, chronic inflammatory diseases and others. In one of these studies, baicalein was shown to be a potent scavenger of the powerful oxidant peroxynitrite, thought to be involved in the pathogenesis of various diseases. Protective effects were seen in renal cells, suggesting that baicalein might be useful in treating or preventing some forms of kidney disease. In a rat study, baicalein significantly protected against experimentally induced endotoxemia.

Cardioprotective effects were demonstrated in an *in vitro* model of ischemia-reperfusion injury. An antioxidative effect was said to partially explain baicalein's benefit in this context. Numerous other non-clinical tests have shown that baicalein has some neuroprotective capacity and may help protect the ischemic brain. In an *in vivo* experiment using a rabbit small clot embolic stroke model, baicalein significantly reduced behavioral deficits in these animals when it was administered by injection up to one hour following induced embolic stroke. A rat study suggested baicalein might protect against vascular dementia. More research is clearly indicated.

An anticancer effect was proposed in a recent study in which baicalein suppressed proliferation and induced apoptosis in human myeloma cells *in vitro.* Given the lack of effective treatments for multiple myeloma, this study warrants follow-up. Other experimental data exist showing that baicalein can help inhibit other cancers, as well, including prostate and bladder cancers.

Another study indicates that baicalein might have some antianxiety effects. This was suggested in an animal study. Previous studies had shown some sedative effects. It has been hypothesized that baicalein may exert an anxiolytic effect by acting as a benzodiazepine receptor agonist. More research is needed.

Among its various anti-inflammatory actions, baicalein has been shown, in one study, to inhibit experimentally induced inflammatory cytokine production in human mast cells. Whether it might thus have some usefulness in treating allergic rhinitis and some other allergic disorders remains to be elucidated by further study.

CONTRAINDICATIONS, PRECAUTIONS, ADVERSE REACTIONS

CONTRAINDICATIONS

Baicalein is contraindicated in those who are hypersensitive to any component of baicalein-containing dietary supplements.

PRECAUTIONS

Those who wish to try a baicalein supplement for the support of any health condition should first discuss its use with his or her physician.

Pregnant women and nursing mothers should avoid the use of baicalein-containing dietary supplements.

ADVERSE REACTIONS

None known.

INTERACTIONS

DRUGS

Baicalein and gentamicin have shown synergistic activity against vancomycin-resistant *Enterococcus in vitro.*

Baicalein and tetracycline, and baicalein and beta-lactams have shown synergistic activity against MRSA (methicillin-resistant *Staphylococcus aureus*) *in vitro.*

NUTRITIONAL SUPPLEMENTS

None known.

OVERDOSAGE

There are no reports of overdosage.

DOSAGE AND ADMINISTRATION

The optimal doses of baicalein or baicalin (baicalain-7-glucuronide) for health benefits are not known.

Several dietary supplements contain various amounts of baicalein and/or baicalin.

A number of teas are available containing various amounts of baicalin (baicalein-7-glucuronide).

A medical food is available containing baicalein and catechin.

Doses of baicalin of up to 750 mg daily, typically given in the form of an herbal extract, are used in TCM.

LITERATURE

Ahn HC, Lee SY, Kim JW, et al. Binding aspects of baicalein to HIV-1 integrase. *Mol Cells*. 2001;12(1):127-130.

Akao T, Hanada M, Sakashita Y, et al. Efflux of baicalin, a flavone glucuronide of Scutellariae Radix, on Caco-2 cells through multidrug resistance-associated protein 2. *J Pharm Pharmacol*. 2007;59(1):87-93.

Akao T, Kawabata K, Yanagisawa E, et al. Baicalin, the predominant flavone glucuronide of scutellariae radix, is absorbed from the rat gastrointestinal tract as the aglycone and restored to its original form. *J Pharm Pharmacol*. 2000;52(12):1563-1568.

Akao T, Sakashita Y, Hanada M, et al. Enteric excretion of baicalein, a flavone of Scutellariae Radix, via glucuronidation in rat: involvement of multidrug resistance-associated protein 2. *Pharm Res*. 2004;21(11):2120-2126.

Awad R, Arnason JT, Trudeau V, et al. Phytochemical and biological analysis of skullcap (Scutellaria lateriflora L.): a medicinal plant with anxiolytic properties. *Phytomedicine*. 2003;10(8):640-649.

Bonham M, Posakony J, Coleman I, et al. Characterization of chemical constituents in Scutellaria baicalensis with antiandrogenic and growth-inhibitory activities toward prostate carcinoma. *Clin Cancer Res*. 2005;11(10):3905-3914.

Cao Y, Dai B, Wang Y, et al. In vitro activity of baicalein against Candida albicans biofilms. *Int J Antimicrob Agents*. 2008;32(1):73-77.

Cha MH, Kim IC, Lee BH, et al. Baicalein inhibits adipocyte differentiation by enhancing COX-2 expression. *J Med Food*. 2006;9(2):145-153.

Chan FL, Choi HL, Chen ZY, et al. Induction of apoptosis in prostate cancer cell lines by a flavonoid, baicalin. *Cancer Lett*. 2000;160(2):219-228.

Chan HY, Chen ZY, Tsang DS, et al. Baicalein inhibits DMBA-DNA adduct formation by modulating CYP1A1 and CYP1B1 activities. *Biomed Pharmacother*. 2002;56(6):269-275.

Chang PC, Li HY, Tang HJ, et al. In vitro synergy of baicalein and gentamicin against vancomycin-resistant Enterococcus. *J Microbiol Immunol Infect*. 2007;40(1):56-61.

Chang WH, Chen CH, Gau RJ, et al. Effect of baicalein on apoptosis of the human Hep G2 cell line was induced by mitochondrial dysfunction. *Planta Med*. 2002;68(4):302-306.

Chao JI, Su WC, Liu HF. Baicalein induces cancer cell death and proliferation retardation by the inhibition of CDC2 kinase and survivin associated with opposite role of p38 mitogen-activated protein kinase and AKT. *Mol Cancer Ther*. 2007;6(11):3039-3048.

Chen CH, Huang LL, Huang CC, et al. Baicalein, a novel apoptotic agent for hepatoma cell lines: a potential medicine for hepatoma. *Nutr Cancer*. 2000;38(2):287-295.

Chen CJ, Raung SL, Liao SL, et al. Inhibition of inducible nitric oxide synthase expression by baicalein in endotoxin/cytokine-stimulated microglia. *Biochem Pharmacol*. 2004;67(5):957-965.

Chen HH, Hong HJ, Chou YH, et al. Inhibition of cyclic strain-induced endothelin-1 secretion by baicalein in human umbilical vein endothelial cells. *Planta Med*. 2006;72(14):1318-1321.

Chen S, Ruan Q, Bedner E, et al. Effects of the flavonoid baicalin and its metabolite baicalein on androgen receptor expression, cell cycle progression and apoptosis of prostate cancer cell lines. *Cell Prolif*. 2001;34(5):293-304.

Chen YC, Chow JM, Lin CW, et al. Baicalein inhibition of oxidative-stress-induced apoptosis via modulation of ERKs activation and induction of HO-1 gene expression in rat glioma cells C6. *Toxicol Appl Pharmacol*. 2006;216(2):263-273.

Cheng PY, Lee YM, Wu YS, et al. Protective effect of baicalein against endotoxic shock in rats in vivo and in vitro. *Biochem Pharmacol*. 2007;73(6):793-804.

Cho H, Lee HY, Ahn DR, et al. Baicalein induces functional hypoxia-inducible factor-1α (HIF-1α) and angiogenesis. *Mol Pharmacol*. 2008;74:70-81.

Chou DS, Lee JJ, Hsiao G, et al. Baicalein induction of hydroxyl radical formation via 12-lipoxygenase in human platelets: an ESR study. *J Agric Food Chem*. 2007;55(3):649-655.

Chow JM, Shen SC, Wu CY, et al. 12-o-Tetradecanoylphorbol 13-acetate prevents baicalein-induced apoptosis via activation of protein kinase C and JNKs in human leukemia cells. *Apoptosis*. 2006;11(11):1999-2011.

Deschamps JD, Kenyon VA, Holman TR. Baicalein is a potent in vitro inhibitor against both reticulocyte 15-human and platelet 12-human lipoxygenases. *Bioorg Med Chem*. 2006;14(12):4295-4301.

Dong QH, Zheng S, Xu RZ, et al. [Baicalein selectively induce apoptosis in human leukemia K562 cells] [Article in Chinese.] *Yao Xue Xue Bao*. 2003; 38(11):817-820.

Feng BY, Toyama BH, Wille H, et al. Small-molecule aggregates inhibit amyloid polymerization. *Nat Chem Biol*. 2008;4(3):197-199.

Fujita M, Shiota S, Kuroda T, et al. Remarkable synergies between baicalein and tetracycline, and baicalein and beta-lactams against methicillin-resistant Staphylococcus aureus. *Microbiol Immunol*. 2005;49(4):391-396.

Gao D, Tawa R, Masaki H, et al. Protective effects of baicalein against cell damage by reactive oxygen species. *Chem Pharm Bull* (Tokyo). 1998;46(9):1383-1387.

Gao H, Nishioka T, Kawabata J, et al. Structure-activity relationships for alpha-glucosidase inhibition of baicalein, 5,6,7-

trihydroxyflavone: the effect of A-ring substitution. *Biosci Biotechnol Biochem.* 2004;68(2):369-375.

Guo QL, Ding QL, Wu ZQ. Effect of baicalein on experimental prostatic hyperplasia in rats and mice. *Biol Pharm Bull.* 2004;27(3):333-337.

Hamada H, Hiramatsu M, Edamatsu R, et al. Free radical scavenging action of baicalein. *Arch Biochem Biophys.* 1993;306(1):261-266.

Heo HJ, Kim DO, Choi SJ, et al. Potent inhibitory effect of flavonoids in Scutellaria baicalensis on amyloid beta protein-induced neurotoxicity. *J Agric Food Chem.* 2004;52(13):4128-4132.

Hong T, Jin GB, Cho S, et al. Evaluation of the anti-inflammatory effect of baicalein on dextran sulfate sodium-induced colitis in mice. *Planta Med.* 2002;68(3):268-271.

Hsieh CJ, Hall K, Ha T, et al. Baicalein inhibits IL-1beta- and TNF-alpha-induced inflammatory cytokine production from human mast cells via regulation of the NF-kappaB pathway. *Clin Mol Allergy.* 2007;5:5.

Hsu SL, Hsieh YC, Hsieh WC, et al. Baicalein induces a dual growth arrest by modulating multiple cell cycle regulatory molecules. *Eur J Pharmacol.* 2001;425(3):165-171.

Huang Y, Tsang SY, Yao X, et al. Biological properties of baicalein in cardiovascular system. *Curr Drug Targets Cardiovasc Haematol Disord.* 2005;5(2):177-184.

Huang Y, Wong CM, Lau CW, et al. Inhibition of nitric oxide/ cyclic GMP-mediated relaxation by purified flavonoids, baicalin and baicalein, in rat aortic rings. *Biochem Pharmacol.* 2004;67(4):787-794.

Hwang JM, Tseng TH, Tsai YY, et al. Protective effects of baicalein on tert-butyl hydroperoxide-induced hepatic toxicity in rat hepatocytes. *J Biomed Sci.* 2005;12(2):389-397.

Ikemoto S, Sugimura K, Yoshida N, et al. Antitumor effects of Scutellariae radix and its components baicalein, baicalin, and wogonin on bladder cancer cell lines. *Urology.* 2000;55(6):951-955.

Im HI, Joo WS, Nam E, et al. Baicalein prevents 6-hydroxydopamine-induced dopaminergic dysfunction and lipid peroxidation in mice. *J Pharmacol Sci.* 2005;98(2):185-189.

Inoue T, Jackson EK. Strong antiproliferative effects of baicalein in cultured rat hepatic stellate cells. *Eur J Pharmacol.* 1999;378(1):129-135.

Kim JM, Lee SU, Kim YS, et al. Baicalein stimulates osteoblast differentiation via coordinating activation of MAP kinases and transcription factors. *J Cell Biochem.* 2008;104(5):1906-1917.

Kimura Y, Matsushita N, Okuda H. Effects of baicalein isolated from Scutellaria baicalensis on interleukin 1 beta-and tumor necrosis factor alpha-induced adhesion molecule expression in cultured human umbilical vein endothelial cells. *J Ethnopharmacol.* 1997;57(1):63-67.

Kimura Y, Okuda H, Arichi S. Effects of baicalein on leukotriene biosynthesis and degranulation in human polymorphonuclear leukocytes. *Biochim Biophys Acta.* 1987;922(3):278-286.

Ko WH, Law VW, Yip WC, et al. Stimulation of chloride secretion by baicalein in isolated rat distal colon. *Am J Physiol Gastrointest Liver Physiol.* 2002;282(3):G508-518.

Kotani A, Kojima S, Hakamata H, et al. HPLC with electrochemical detection to examine the pharmacokinetics of baicalin and baicalein in rat plasma after oral administration of a Kampo medicine. *Anal Biochem.* 2006;350(1):99-104.

Lai MY, Hsiu SL, Tsai SY, et al. Comparison of metabolic pharmacokinetics of baicalin and baicalein in rats. *J Pharm Pharmacol.* 2003;55(2):205-209.

Lapchak PA, Maher P, Schubert D, et al. Baicalein, an antioxidant 12/15-lipoxygenase inhibitor improves clinical rating scores following multiple infarct embolic strokes. *Neuroscience.* 2007;150(3):585-591.

Lebeau A, Esclaire F, Rostène W, et al. Baicalein protects cortical neurons from beta-amyloid (25-35) induced toxicity. *Neuroreport.* 2001;12(10):2199-2202.

Lee BH, Lee SJ, Kang TH, et al. Baicalein: an in vitro antigenotoxic compound from Scutellaria baicalensis. *Planta Med.* 2000;66(1):70-71.

Lee HJ, Noh YH, Lee DY, et al. Baicalein attenuates 6-hydroxydopamine-induced neurotoxicity in SH-SY5Y cells. *Eur J Cell Biol.* 2005;84(11):897-905.

Lee HZ, Leung HW, Lai MY, et al. Baicalein induced cell cycle arrest and apoptosis in human lung squamous carcinoma CH27 cells. *Anticancer Res.* 2005;25(2A):959-964.

Lee MJ, Wang CJ, Tsai YY, et al. Inhibitory effect of 12-O-tetradecanoylphorbol-13-acetate-caused tumor promotion in benzo[a]pyrene-initiated CD-1 mouse skin by baicalein. *Nutr Cancer.* 1999;34(2):185-191.

Lee SW, Song GS, Kwon CH, et al. Beneficial effect of flavonoid baicalein in cisplatin-induced cell death of human glioma cells. *Neurosci Lett.* 2005;382(1-2):71-75.

Leung HW, Yang WH, Lai MY, et al. Inhibition of 12-lipoxygenase during baicalein-induced human lung nonsmall carcinoma H460 cell apoptosis. *Food Chem Toxicol.* 2007;45(3):403-411.

Li QB, You Y, Chen ZC, et al. Role of Baicalein in the regulation of proliferation and apoptosis in human myeloma RPMI8226 cells. *Chin Med J* (Engl). 2006;119(11):948-952.

Li YC, Tyan YS, Kuo HM, et al. Baicalein induced in vitro apoptosis undergo caspases activity in human promyelocytic leukemia HL-60 cells. *Food Chem Toxicol.* 2004;42(1):37-43.

Li YC, Tyan YS, Lee YM, et al. N-acetyltransferase is involved in baicalein-induced N-acetylation of 2-aminofluorene and DNA-2-aminofluorene adduct formation in human leukemia HL-60 cells. *In Vivo.* 2005;19(2):399-405.

Liao JF, Hung WY, Chen CF. Anxiolytic-like effects of baicalein and baicalin in the Vogel conflict test in mice. *Eur J Pharmacol*. 2003;464(2-3):141-146.

Lin CC, Shieh DE. The anti-inflammatory activity of Scutellaria rivularis extracts and its active components, baicalin, baicalein and wogonin. *Am J Chin Med*. 1996;24(1):31-36.

Lin HY, Shen SC, Lin CW, et al. Baicalein inhibition of hydrogen peroxide-induced apoptosis via ROS-dependent heme oxygenase 1 gene expression. *Biochim Biophys Acta*. 2007;1773(7):1073-1086.

Liu JJ, Huang TS, Cheng WF, et al. Baicalein and baicalin are potent inhibitors of angiogenesis: Inhibition of endothelial cell proliferation, migration and differentiation. *Int J Cancer*. 2003;106(4):559-565.

Lu RH, Li Y, Zhang LJ, et al. [Effects of baicalein on the proliferation and differentiation of pig preadipocyte] [Article in Chinese.] *Sheng Wu Gong Cheng Xue Bao*. 2006;22(6):1002-1006.

Ma Z, Otsuyama K, Liu S, et al. Baicalein, a component of Scutellaria radix from Huang-Lian-Jie-Du-Tang (HLJDT), leads to suppression of proliferation and induction of apoptosis in human myeloma cells. *Blood*. 2005;105(8):3312-3318.

Machha A, Achike FI, Mohd MA, et al. Baicalein impairs vascular tone in normal rat aortas: role of superoxide anions. *Eur J Pharmacol*. 2007;565(1-3):144-150.

Matsuzaki Y, Kurokawa N, Terai S, et al. Cell death induced by baicalein in human hepatocellular carcinoma cell lines. *Jpn J Cancer Res*. 1996;87(2):170-177.

Mehendale S, Aung H, Wang CZ, et al. Scutellaria baicalensis and a constituent flavonoid, baicalein, attenuate ritonavir-induced gastrointestinal side-effects. *J Pharm Pharmacol*. 2007;59(11):1567-72.

Nakahata N, Kyo R, Kutsuwa M, et al. [Inhibition of mitogen-activated protein kinase cascade by baicalein, a flavonoid of natural origin] [Article in Japanese.] *Nippon Yakurigaku Zasshi*. 1999;114 Suppl 1:215P-219P.

Nakahata N, Tsuchiya C, Nakatani K, et al. Baicalein inhibits Raf-1-mediated phosphorylation of MEK-1 in C6 rat glioma cells. *Eur J Pharmacol*. 2003;461(1):1-7.

Nakajima T, Imanishi M, Yamamoto K, et al. Inhibitory effect of baicalein, a flavonoid in Scutellaria Root, on eotaxin production by human dermal fibroblasts. *Planta Med*. 2001;67(2):132-135.

Nakamura N, Hayasaka S, Zhang XY, et al. Effects of baicalin, baicalein, and wogonin on interleukin-6 and interleukin-8 expression, and nuclear factor-kappab binding activities induced by interleukin-1beta in human retinal pigment epithelial cell line. *Exp Eye Res*. 2003;77(2):195-202.

Nishioka T, Kawabata J, Aoyama Y. Baicalein, an alpha-glucosidase inhibitor from Scutellaria baicalensis. *J Nat Prod*. 1998;61(11):1413-1415.

Otsuyama KI, Ma Z, Abroun S, et al. PPARbeta-mediated growth suppression of baicalein and dexamethasone in human myeloma cells. *Leukemia*. 2007;21(1):187-190.

Piao XL, Cho EJ, Jang MH. Cytoprotective effect of baicalein against peroxynitrite-induced toxicity in LLC-PK(1) cells. *Food Chem Toxicol*. 2008;46(5):1576-1581.

Po LS, Chen ZY, Tsang DS, et al. Baicalein and genistein display differential actions on estrogen receptor (ER) transactivation and apoptosis in MCF-7 cells. *Cancer Lett*. 2002;187(1-2):33-40.

Roy MK, Nakahara K, Na TV, et al. Baicalein, a flavonoid extracted from a methanolic extract of Oroxylum indicum inhibits proliferation of a cancer cell line in vitro via induction of apoptosis. *Pharmazie*. 2007;62(2):149-153.

Sekiya K, Okuda H. Selective inhibition of platelet lipoxygenase by baicalein. *Biochem Biophys Res Commun*. 1982;105(3):1090-1095.

Shao ZH, Vanden Hoek TL, Qin Y, et al. Baicalein attenuates oxidant stress in cardiomyocytes. *Am J Physiol Heart Circ Physiol*. 2002;282(3):H999-H1006.

Shen YC, Chiou WF, Chou YC, et al. Mechanisms in mediating the anti-inflammatory effects of baicalin and baicalein in human leukocytes. *Eur J Pharmacol*. 2003;465(1-2):171-181.

Shieh DE, Liu LT, Lin CC. Antioxidant and free radical scavenging effects of baicalein, baicalin and wogonin. *Anticancer Res*. 2000;20(5A):2861-2865.

Suk K, Lee H, Kang SS, et al. Flavonoid baicalein attenuates activation-induced cell death of brain microglia. *J Pharmacol Exp Ther*. 2003;305(2):638-645.

Sun H, Zhang L, Chow EC, et al. A Catenary Model to Study Transport and Conjugation of Baicalein, a Bioactive Flavonoid, in the Caco-2 Cell Monolayer: Demonstration of Substrate Inhibition. *J Pharmacol Exp Ther*. 2008;326:117-126.

Taiming L, Xuehua J. Investigation of the absorption mechanisms of baicalin and baicalein in rats. *J Pharm Sci*. 2006;95(6):1326-1333.

Tsai TH, Liu SC, Tsai PL, et al. The effects of the cyclosporin A, a P-glycoprotein inhibitor, on the pharmacokinetics of baicalein in the rat: a microdialysis study. *Br J Pharmacol*. 2002;137(8):1314-1320.

Tu IH, Yen HT, Cheng HW, et al. Baicalein protects chicken embryonic cardiomyocyte against hypoxia-reoxygenation injury via mu- and delta- but not kappa-opioid receptor signaling. *Eur J Pharmacol*. 2008;588(2-3):251-258.

Uchiyama Y, Tagami J, Kamisuki S, et al. Selective inhibitors of terminal deoxyribonucleotidyltransferase (TdT): baicalin and genistin. *Biochim Biophys Acta*. 2005;1725(3):298-304.

van Leyen K, Kim HY, Lee SR, et al. Baicalein and 12/15-lipoxygenase in the ischemic brain. *Stroke*. 2006;37(12):3014-3018.

Wang J, Yu Y, Hashimoto F, et al. Baicalein induces apoptosis through ROS-mediated mitochondrial dysfunction pathway in HL-60 cells. *Int J Mol Med.* 2004;14(4):627-632.

Wang SY, Wang HH, Chi CW, et al. Effects of baicalein on beta-amyloid peptide-(25-35)-induced amnesia in mice. *Eur J Pharmacol.* 2004;506(1):55-61.

Woo AY, Cheng CH, Waye MM. Baicalein protects rat cardiomyocytes from hypoxia/reoxygenation damage via a prooxidant mechanism. *Cardiovasc Res.* 2005;65(1):244-253.

Woo KJ, Lim JH, Suh SI, et al. Differential inhibitory effects of baicalein and baicalin on LPS-induced cyclooxygenase-2 expression through inhibition of C/EBPbeta DNA-binding activity. *Immunobiology.* 2006;211(5):359-368.

Wu JY, Chung KT, Liu YW, et al. Synthesis and biological evaluation of novel C(6) modified baicalein derivatives as antioxidative agents. *J Agric Food Chem.* 2008;56(8):2838-2845.

Wu PH, Shen YC, Wang YH, et al. Baicalein attenuates methamphetamine-induced loss of dopamine transporter in mouse striatum. *Toxicology.* 2006;226(2-3):238-245.

Xing J, Chen X, Zhong D. Absorption and enterohepatic circulation of baicalin in rats. *Life Sci.* 2005;78(2):140-146.

Yang D, Hu H, Huang S, et al. [Study on the inhibitory activity, in vitro, of baicalein and baicalin against skin fungi and bacteria] [Article in Chinese.] *Zhong Yao Cai.* 2000;23(5):272-274.

Zhang L, Lin G, Chang Q, et al. Role of intestinal first-pass metabolism of baicalein in its absorption process. *Pharm Res.* 2005;22(7):1050-1058.

Zhang L, Lin G, Kovács B, et al. Mechanistic study on the intestinal absorption and disposition of baicalein. *Eur J Pharm Sci.* 2007;31(3-4):221-231.

Zhang L, Lin G, Zuo Z. Involvement of UDP-glucuronosyltransferases in the extensive liver and intestinal first-pass metabolism of flavonoid baicalein. *Pharm Res.* 2007;24(1):81-89.

Zhang L, Lin G, Zuo Z. High-performance liquid chromatographic method for simultaneous determination of baicalein and baicalein 7-glucuronide in rat plasma. *J Pharm Biomed Anal.* 2004;36(3):637-641.

Zhang XP, Li ZF, Liu XG, et al. Effects of emodin and baicalein on rats with severe acute pancreatitis. *World J Gastroenterol.* 2005;11(14):2095-2100.

Zhu M, Rajamani S, Kaylor J, et al. The flavonoid baicalein inhibits fibrillation of alpha-synuclein and disaggregates existing fibrils. *J Biol Chem.* 2004;279(26):26846-26857.

Bee Pollen

DESCRIPTION

Bee pollen consists of plant pollens collected by worker bees combined with plant nectar and bee saliva. The material is compacted into pellets, which are used as food for drone bees. Pollen consists of the male germ seeds of plants, flowers or blossoms on trees. As plants flower, pollen is transferred from the anther of a stamen to the stigma of a pistil; on reaching the ovary it brings about fertilization of the ovules and the growth of seeds. Flowers are mainly pollinated by insects, such as beetles, butterflies and bees. Palynology is the study of pollen.

Bee pollen is comprised of proteins (about 25-30%), carbohydrates (about 30-55%), lipids (about 1-20%), minerals, vitamins and trace amounts of other organic substances.

Bee pollen became popular as a nutritional supplement in the 1970s following testimonials by athletes claiming that its use increased stamina and improved athletic ability.

ACTIONS AND PHARMACOLOGY

ACTIONS

Putative anti-inflammatory, immunomodulatory, ergogenic and radioprotective actions.

PHARMACOKINETICS

Proteins, carbohydrates and lipids in bee pollen should be digested, absorbed and metabolized, as are similar substances found in foods. However, the shells of the individual grains of pollen are not readily digestible, and only a small percentage of the above substances may actually be processed by the body.

INDICATIONS AND USAGE

There is insufficient clinical research to suggest any indication for supplemental bee pollen. A few *in vitro* and animal studies suggest that it might protect against some forms of radiation damage, that it might have some immunomodulating effects and that it might have some benefit in pregnancy.

RESEARCH SUMMARY

In vitro studies indicate that bee pollen exerts protective effects against radiation in some animal tissues. A study of pregnant rats associated the addition of bee pollen to diet with improved body weight, hemoglobin levels and total protein, serum iron and albumin levels in the mother, as well as greater body weight and decreased fatality in the fetuses, compared with controls. Some favorable immunomodulating effects were seen in other very preliminary animal work.

CONTRAINDICATIONS, PRECAUTIONS, ADVERSE REACTIONS

CONTRAINDICATIONS

Bee pollen is contraindicated in those with pollen allergies. It is also contraindicated in those hypersensitive to bee pollen. (There are other proteins in bee pollen in addition to those from pollen.)

Children, pregnant women and nursing mothers should avoid bee pollen.

ADVERSE REACTIONS

Those who are allergic or hypersensitive to bee pollen can develop symptoms, including pruritis, rhinitis, conjunctivitis and bronchospasm and, in some cases, urticaria and anaphylaxis. Two cases of hepatitis have been reported following ingestion of bee pollen for several weeks. Hypereosinophilia, neurologic symptoms (decreased memory, headache) and gastrointestinal symptoms (nausea, abdominal pain, diarrhea) have also been reported following bee pollen ingestion.

OVERDOSAGE

No reported overdosage of bee pollen.

DOSAGE AND ADMINISTRATION

Typical doses used are 1 to 1.5 grams daily in divided doses.

LITERATURE

Anan'eva TV, Dvoretskii AI. [Effect of beta-carotene oil and bee pollen on ion transport in rat brain slices following radiation-chemical exposure.] [Article in Russian.] *Radiats Biol Radioecol.* 1999; 39:341-344.

Bevzo VV, Grygor'eva NP. [Effect of bee pollen extract on glutathione system activity in mice liver under X-ray irradiation.] [Article in Ukrainian.] *Ukr Biokhim Zh.* 1999; 69:115-117.

Cohen SH, Yunginger JW, Rosenberg N, Fink JN. Acute allergic reaction after composite pollen ingestion. *J Allergy Clin Immunol.* 1979; 64:270-274.

Dudov IA, Morenets AA, Artiukh VP, Starodub NF. [Immunotherapy effect of honeybee flower pollen load.] [Article in Russian.] *Ukr Biokhim Zh.* 1994; 66:91-93.

Geyman JP. Anaphylactic reaction after ingestion of bee pollen. *J Am Board Fam Pract.* 1994; 7:250-252.

Lin FL, Vaughan TR, Vandewalker ML, Weber RW. Hypereosinophilia, neurologic, and gastrointestinal symptoms after bee pollen ingestion. *J Allergy Clin Immunol.* 1989; 83:793-796.

Puente S, Iniquez A, Subirats M, et al. [Eosinophilic gastroenteritis caused by bee pollen sensitization.] [Article in Spanish.] *Med Clin (Barc).* 1997; 108:698-700.

Shad JA, Chinn CG, Brann OS. Acute hepatitis after ingestion of herbs. *South Med J.* 1999; 92:1095-1097.

Williams MH. Ergogenic and ergolytic substances. *Med Sci Sports Exerc.* 1992; 24 (9 Suppl):S344-S348.

Xie Y, Wan B, Li W. [Effect of bee pollen on maternal nutrition and fetal growth.] [Article in Chinese.] *Hua Hsi I Ko Hsueh Hsueh Pao.* 1994; 25:434-437.

Benfotiamine

DESCRIPTION

Benfotiamine, chemically, is an analogue of thiamin or vitamin B_1 (See Thiamin). Biochemically, benfotiamine is a precursor of thiamin. In that sense, benfotiamine is a prothiamine, or provitamin B_1. Benfotiamine was synthesized as part of a Japanese research project initiated over 60 years ago, originally led by the Japanese scientist M. Fujiwara and colleagues, whose mission was to discover and develop more bioavailable forms of thiamin for the treatment and prevention of beriberi, as well as for the treatment and prevention of alcoholic polyneuropathy.

The first compound discovered by these researchers was a disulfide derivative of thiamin, which was isolated from garlic and also found in other members of the allium or onion genus. The compound was named allithiamine and was given the chemical name thiamin tetrahydrofurfuryl disulfide (TTFD). TTFD was found to be more lipophilic than thiamin itself and appeared to have better bioavailability characteristics. Other disulfide derivatives of thiamin were synthesized, and, later, Japanese chemists went on to synthesize S-acyl-thiamin derivatives. One of the derivatives was given the chemical name S-benzoylthiamine monophosphate (BTMP). BTMP is better known by its common name, benfotiamine. Somewhere along the way benfotiamine was classified as a member of the allithiamine family. However, structurally speaking, benfotiamine is quite different from allithiamine. Also, there is no present evidence that benfotiamine is found in garlic or any other member of the allium or onion genus. In fact, to date, there is no evidence that benfotiamine is found naturally.

Along the way the idea was propagated that benfotiamine was significantly more lipophilic than thiamin and that it was perhaps the most bioavailable analogue of thiamin that had been synthesized by the Japanese chemists, much more so even than the disulfide analogues. It was also thought that it was the lipophilic character of a thiamin analogue that promoted greater bioavailability and favored its suitability, over thiamin itself, for therapeutic purposes. Part of this thinking was correct; part was not.

In a recent animal study, it was found that benfotiamine did strongly increase thiamin levels in the blood and liver, better than that found with thiamin itself, but also that very little passed into the brain. Further, physico-chemical data as well as studies with isolated cells strongly suggested that, in contrast to the disulfide derivatives of thiamin, benfotiamine had poor lipophilicity.

Benfotiamine is also known as S-benzoylthiamine monophosphate (BTMP); benzenecarbothioic acid S-[-2-[[(4-amino-2-methyl-5-pyrimidinyl)methyl]formylamino]-1-[2-(phosphonooxy)ethyl]-1-propenyl] ester; thiobenzoic acid S-ester with N-[(4-amino-2-methyl-5-pyrimidinyl)methyl]-N-(4-hydroxy-2-mercapto-1-methyl-1-butenyl)formamide O-phosphate. CAS registry number is 22457-89-2. Its molecular weight is 466.45, and its molecular formula is $C_{19}H_{23}N_4O_6$ PS. Benfotiamine is represented by the following chemical structure.

Benfotiamine

ACTIONS AND PHARMACOLOGY

ACTIONS

Benfotiamine is a precursor of thiamin, or vitamin B_1. Benfotiamine may have antioxidant activity. Benfotiamine may have antiglucotoxic activity, resulting in possible neuroprotective, retinoprotective, cardioprotective and renoprotective activities (see Thiamin for additional actions of thiamin).

MECHANISM OF ACTION

Benfotiamine is a provitamin of thiamin (prothiamin or provitamin B_1) and is converted to thiamin intracellularly. It is more bioavailable than is thiamin and it strongly increases thiamin levels in the blood and the liver when administered orally, but appears to have little effect on thiamin levels in the brain.

Benfotiamine was demonstrated to have direct antioxidative action and to prevent oxidative DNA damage *in vitro*. Benfotiamine prevented oxidative stress induced by the mutagen 4-nitroquinoline-1-oxide (NQO), known to form 8-hydroxydeoxyguanosine via reactive oxygen species (ROS), the uremic toxin indoxyl sulfate, and the peptide hormone angiotensin II. (Angiotensin II induces oxidative stress via its activation of NAD(P)H oxidase.) This was shown in a human embryonic kidney cell line, an epithelial rat kidney cell line and an epithelial porcine kidney cell line. Cell-free experiments also showed a direct antioxidant effect of benfotiamine. Oxidative damage induced by angiotensin II was completely prevented by benfotiamine. The exact mechanism of action of the antioxidant effect is unclear.

Although D-glucose is of utmost importance in cellular metabolism, glucose itself can be quite toxic to tissue when levels are higher than normal. The most serious complications of diabetes—diabetic peripheral neuropathy, diabetic retinopathy, diabetic nephropathy—peripheral vascular disease and cardiovascular disease are caused to a great degree by the toxicity (glucotoxicity) to tissue of high levels of D-glucose. Microvascular and macrovascular pathologies underlie all of these diabetic complications. Since thiamin plays a number of vital roles in the metabolism of glucose, it was thought that benfotiamine may have some therapeutic benefit in the prevention and treatment of these diabetic complications. Preliminary studies suggest that it may.

One of the major questions in pathophysiology is how all the diverse microvascular and macrovascular pathologies result from the toxic effects of elevated D-glucose levels. There are four hypotheses: by increased polyol pathway flux, by increased advanced glycation end products (AGEs) formation, by activation of protein kinase C (PKC) isoforms and by increased hexosamine pathway flux.

The first enzyme in the polyol pathway is aldose reductase. Aldose reductase catalyzes the reduced nicotanimide dinucleotide phosphate (NADPH)-dependent reduction of a wide variety of carbonyl compounds, including glucose. When D-glucose levels are high, aldose reductase reduces D-glucose to the sugar alcohol sorbitol. In the process, NADPH levels are lowered, sorbitol is oxidized to fructose via the enzyme sorbitol dehydrogenase and nicotinamide adenine dinucleotide (NAD+) is reduced to reduced nicotinamide dinucleotide (NADH). This leads to an increase in the cytosolic NADH:NAD ratio, which inhibits activity of the enzyme glyceraldehydes-3-phospate dehydrogenase (GAPDH) and increases the concentration of triose phosphate. Increased triose phosphate may increase concentrations of both methylglyoxal, one of the major precursors of advanced glycation end products (AGEs), and diacylglycerol (DAG). Elevated DAG may activate PCK isoforms (see below for further discussion).

AGEs are found in increased amounts in diabetic retinal blood vessels and renal glomeruli. In fact, the most important measure of long-term glucose control is the measurement of serum hemoglobin A1c. Hemoglobin A1c is glycated hemoglobin. The history of the discovery of AGEs goes back to the early 1900s and to the food chemist Louis-Camille Maillard. In 1912, Maillard described a chemical reaction that occurs with foods and which to a great extent imparts various flavors to foods. The reaction is now called the Maillard reaction or the browning reaction. The Maillard reaction is a nonenzymatic reaction that occurs when aldehydes, ketones and reducing sugars (eg, D-glucose) condense with the amino groups of proteins, peptides or amino acids. These reactions may impart flavor to foods but they do little worthwhile when they occur in the body. It is the Maillard or browning reaction that produces AGEs. Hemoglobin A1c was the first example that nonenzymatic reactions, specifically the Maillard reaction, can occur physiologically.

AGEs can arise from many sources: the auto-oxidation of glucose to glyoxal, the fragmentation of glyceraldehydes-3-

phosphate and dihydroxyacetone phosphate to methylglyox-al, among others. The dicarbonyls react with amino groups of intercellular and extracellular proteins to form AGEs via the Maillard reaction, which consists chemically of Schiff base formation leading to an Amadori derivative. Production of intracellular AGE precursors results in damage to cells and tissues, mainly by increasing oxidative stress. Recently, receptors for AGEs have been identified and called RAGEs, or receptors for advanced glycation end products. Association of AGEs with AGE receptors can either cause further havoc to tissue or neutralize the AGEs, depending on the type of receptor the AGEs bind to. The coupling of AGEs with certain receptors may cause the induction of severe oxidative stress. There is much ongoing research in AGEs and RAGEs

Shunting of excess D-glucose into the hexosamine pathway might also contribute to the severe manifestations of diabetic complications. In this pathway, fructose-6-phosphate is diverted from glycolysis to provide substrates to biochemical reactions that require UDP-N-acetylglucosamine, including proteoglycan synthesis and the formation of O-linked glycoproteins. Basically, activation of the hexosamine pathway by elevated D-glucose levels may result in many changes in both gene expression and protein function, which together contribute to the pathogenesis of diabetic complications.

The PKC family is comprised of at least 11 isoforms, nine of which are activated by the lipid second messenger diacylglycerol (DAG). Elevated levels of D-glucose in cells increase the amount of DAG in microvascular cells and in the retinal and renal glomeruli of diabetic animals. It does this by increasing *de novo* DAG synthesis from the glycolytic intermediate, dihydroxyacetone phosphate. Increases in DAG are thought to lead to activation of PKC, mainly the beta isoform of PKC. Activation of PKC-beta is thought to mediate retinal blood flow and renal blood flow abnormalities.

It is thought that each of the four different pathogenic mechanisms discussed above may reflect a single hyperglycemia-induced process—the overproduction of the reactive oxygen species superoxide by the mitochondrial electron transport chain. Much more research is necessary to establish this most interesting hypothesis.

Benfotiamine has been demonstrated to block three of the four pathways of hyperglycemic damage discussed above—the hexosamine pathway, the DAG-PKC pathway and the advanced glycation end products pathway. These studies were performed both *in vitro* in endothelial cells and *in vivo* in rats with experimental diabetic retinopathy. Benfotiamine was found to prevent diabetic retinopathy in the rats.

As a result of the reduced ability of glyceraldehyde-3-phosphate dehydrogenase to process upstream metabolites, the AGE pathway, the DAG-protein kinase C pathway and the hexosamine pathway are activated. Recently, it has been reported that benfotiamine blocks these pathways by activating the pentose phosphate pathway enzyme transketolase. Transketolase is a major enzyme in the pentose phosphate pathway, catalyzing the reaction of ribose-5-phosphate and xylulose-5-phosphate to glyceraldehyde-3-phosphate and sedoheptulose-7-phosphate. Transketolase requires cocarboxylase or thiamin diphosphate, the active form of thiamin, for its activity.

PHARMACOKINETICS

There is still much we don't know about the pharmacokinetics of benfotiamine. What follows is our present state of knowledge.

Benfotiamine is absorbed from the lumen of the small intestine, either intact as the monophosphate or dephosphorylated by intestinal alkaline phosphatase (found at the brush border of the small intestine) to S-benzoylthiamin. If benfotiamine is not dephosphorylated, then S-benzoylthiamin phosphate enters the circulation and is transported to various tissues, but especially to the liver. Once within the cells, benfotiamine is dephosphorylated to S-benzoylthiamin, the thiazole ring is formed and thiamin is produced. If the dephosphorylation step takes place in the intestine, then S-benzoylthiamin enters the cells, the thiazole ring is formed and thiamin is made. Recent evidence suggests that benfotiamine is dephosphorylated by brush border alkaline phosphatase before it enters the bloodstream. Intracellular thiamin is metabolized to thiamin monophosphate (TP, TMP), thiamin diphosphate (TDP, cocarboxylase) and thiamin triphosphate (TTP). Thiamin is phosphorylated directly to thiamin diphosphate by thiamin diphosphokinase, and thiamin diphosphate is dephosphorylated to thiamin monophosphate via thiamin diphosphatase. Approximately 80% of thiamin in blood is present in erythrocytes as TPP.

It is of interest to compare the pharmacokinetics of benfotiamine with that of thiamin itself. Thiamin is absorbed from the lumen of the small intestine—mainly the jejunum—by active transport and passive diffusion mechanisms. At lower amounts, absorption from the small intestine is by an active, carrier-mediated process that is energy-dependent as well as sodium-dependent. Passive diffusion occurs with higher amounts of thiamin. Absorption of thiamin appears to be limited by a saturable rate-limiting transport mechanism. Only a small percentage of a high dose of thiamin is absorbed. Benfotiamine does not appear to be subject to the rate-limiting transport mechanism. Thiamin is transported by the portal circulation to the liver and by the systemic circulation to various tissues in the body. The transport of thiamin into erythrocytes appears to occur by facilitated diffusion; it enters other cells by an active process. Total thiamin content in the adult body is about 30 milligrams. Thiamin and its metabolites are mainly excreted by the kidneys.

INDICATIONS AND USAGE

Benfotiamine, synthesized in the 1960s as an analogue and precursor of thiamin (vitamin B_1), has been reported to have greater bioavailability than thiamin itself and so has been postulated to have efficacy in various thiamin-related deficiencies and disorders. There is *in vitro* and *in vivo* experimental animal data, as well as some clinical data, suggesting that benfotiamine may be helpful in relieving inflammatory and neuropathic pain and especially diabetic neuropathy. There is also the suggestion in some research that benfotiamine might be beneficial in some hemodialysis patients, possibly reducing cancer risk in those patients. On the other hand, a recent study has called into question the mode of action through which benfotiamine was thought to achieve these benefits and, in so doing, has also questioned the extent to which some of the observed benefits are real.

RESEARCH SUMMARY

There have been many reports in the literature that benfotiamine is of benefit in diabetes. Among the more recent reports was one in which the researchers concluded that benfotiamine blocks three major pathways of hyperglycemic damage. They showed that through this blockage benfotiamine was able to prevent experimental diabetic retinopathy. They hypothesized that the substance might thus be useful in preventing the development and progression of diabetic complications generally. In an *in vitro* study of human endothelial progenitor cells (EPCs), another group of researchers demonstrated that benfotiamine can help correct hyperglycemic impairment of EPC differentiation into mature, healthy endothelial cells. Benfotiamine's ability to counteract glucose toxicity was again seen as an indication of the substance's ability to help curb diabetic damage generally. In a mouse study, benfotiamine was said to activate glucose metabolism and insulin synthesis in adult bone marrow-derived, insulin-producing cells and thus to prevent glucose toxicity resulting from high concentrations of blood glucose in diabetes mellitus. In a rat study, benfotiamine was reported to relieve inflammatory and neuropathic pain in both diabetic and nondiabetic animals.

A recent clinical test sought to determine whether benfotiamine could prevent some of the postprandial endothelial dysfunction that is a characteristic of diabetes. Thirteen people with type 2 diabetes were given a three-day trial of benfotiamine (1,050 mg per day) and challenged with a hyperglycemic diet. By several measures, the researchers concluded that benfotiamine had significantly prevented both macrovascular and microvascular endothelial dysfunction and oxidative stress in these subjects challenged with a meal rich in advanced glycation end products ages.

A still more recent study, this one related to hemodialysis, was inspired in part by the finding in prior studies that benfotiamine reduces AGEs, as noted above in the diabetes work. This is relevant to hemodialysis patients since they often suffer from thiamin (vitamin B_1) deficiency and accumulation of uremic toxins, including the glycation products. In this research, which comprised two related studies, the research concluded there were indications that benfotiamine helped prevent DNA damage in the peripheral blood lymphocytes of these patients. They speculated, based on some of their findings, that the benefits observed might have been due to a benfotiamine antioxidative effect. They further concluded that benfotiamine might, through this reduction of genomic damage, decrease the higher risk of cancer that dialysis patients experience.

Given the broad range of studies reporting positive effects from benfotiamine over a long period of research, it would seem unlikely that the substance is entirely without clinical merit, but one recent study has rejected one of the most important assumptions of the prior research and has thus called into question the validity of some of the positive conclusions of the earlier reports. This group reported that, contrary to all prior claims, there is little or no evidence that benfotiamine has bioavailability superior to the disulfide analogues. They reported that it is only slightly soluble in water under physiologic conditions and cannot be dissolved at all in some lipids. They claimed that it does not penetrate most cell membranes and that it could not be more effective than any of the other thiamin precursors in preventing or treating diabetic pathology. In their animal study, these researchers observed elevated levels of thiamin in peripheral tissues induced by benfotiamine but no elevation whatever in the brain. Thus they rejected the idea that benfotiamine could be helpful in central nervous system disorders. These researchers acknowledged the findings of others that benfotiamine exerts direct antioxidant effects but stated that it is not clear in what way, if any, this might have an impact on diabetic complications.

Clearly, more research is needed and warranted to try to resolve some of these conflicting findings and shed further light on the mode of action through which benfotiamine may confer some health benefits.

CONTRAINDICATIONS, PRECAUTIONS, ADVERSE REACTIONS
CONTRAINDICATIONS

Benfotiamine is contraindicated in those allergic to any component of a benfotiamine-containing product.

PRECAUTIONS

The use of benfotiamine for the support of any medical condition must be discussed with one's physician before starting supplementation.

ADVERSE REACTIONS

Oral benfotiamine is well tolerated at doses up to 600 milligrams daily or higher. There are rare reports of transient headaches.

INTERACTIONS

DRUGS

None known.

NUTRITIONAL SUPPLEMENTS

No known interactions.

FOODS

None known.

HERBS

No known interactions.

OVERDOSAGE

No reports.

DOSAGE AND ADMINISTRATION

Benfotiamine supplements have been recently introduced into the U.S. dietary supplement marketplace. Typical capsules contain 50 mg and 150 mg of benfotiamine, and those using this supplement take from one to four capsules daily (150 mg to 600 mg). However, doses that high need to be discussed with ones physician.

Benfotiamine has been available in Japan since 1961 and is marketed under the trade name Biotamin. Among other reasons, the Japanese take Biotamin (benfotiamine) for hearing disorders and alcohol-related neuropathy, sciatica and other painful nerve conditions. However, its most common use is the prevention and treatment of vitamin B_1 deficiencies.

Benfotiamine has been marketed in Germany since 1978 as 50 mg pills under the trade name Milgamma Mono. In Germany, it is considered a drug and is available in pharmacies without a prescription. Typical daily oral doses range from 50 mg to an authorized maximum of 900 mg. Milgamma Mono ((benfotiamine) is used to prevent and treat vitamin B_1 deficiencies. It is also used to treat painful nerve problems. In about 30 years of use in Germany, there have been only about ten reports of adverse events related to the use of Milgamma Mono, and those have mainly been transient headaches.

LITERATURE

Anisimova EI, Danilov AB. [Benfotiamine efficacy in alcoholic polyneuropathy therapy] [Article in Russian.] *Zh Nevrol Psikhiatr Im S S Korsakova.* 2001;101(12):32-36.

Babaei-Jadidi R, Karachalias N, et al. Prevention of incipient diabetic nephropathy by high-dose thiamin and benfotiamine. *Diabetes.* 2003;52(8):2110-2120.

Beltramo E, Berrone E, Buttiglieri S, et al. Thiamin and benfotiamine prevent increased apoptosis in endothelial cells and pericytes cultured in high glucose. *Diabetes Metab Res Rev.* 2004;20(4):330-336.

Brownlee M. The pathobiology of diabetic complications: a unifying mechanism. *Diabetes.* 2005;54(6):1615-1625.

Brownlee M. Biochemistry and molecular cell biology of diabetic complications. *Nature.* 2001;414(6865):813-820.

Ceylan-Isik AF, Wu S, Li Q, et al. High-dose benfotiamine rescues cardiomyocyte contractile dysfunction in streptozotocin-induced diabetes mellitus. *J Appl Physiol.* 2006;100(1):150-156.

Gadau S, Emanueli C, Van Linthout S, et al. Benfotiamine accelerates the healing of ischaemic diabetic limbs in mice through protein kinase B/Akt-mediated potentiation of angiogenesis and inhibition of apoptosis. *Diabetologia.* 2006;49(2):405-420.

Hammes HP, Du X, Edelstein D, et al. Benfotiamine blocks three major pathways of hyperglycemic damage and prevents experimental diabetic retinopathy. *Nat Med.* 2003;9(3):294-299.

Haupt E, Ledermann H, Köpcke W. Benfotiamine in the treatment of diabetic polyneuropathy—a three-week randomized, controlled pilot study (BEDIP study). *Int J Clin Pharmacol Ther.* 2005; 43(2):71-7. Erratum in: *Int J Clin Pharmacol Ther.* 2005;43(6):304.

Lin Y, Berg AH, Iyengar P, et al. The hyperglycemia-induced inflammatory response in adipocytes: the role of reactive oxygen species. *J Biol Chem.* 2005;280(6):4617-4626.

Loew D. Pharmacokinetics of thiamin derivatives especially of benfotiamine. *Int J Clin Pharmacol Ther.* 1996;34(2):47-50.

Marchetti V, Menghini R, Rizza S, et al. Benfotiamine counteracts glucose toxicity effects on endothelial progenitor cell differentiation via Akt/FoxO signaling. *Diabetes.* 2006;55(8):2231-2237.

Pomero F, Molinar Min A, La Selva M, et al. Benfotiamine is similar to thiamin in correcting endothelial cell defects induced by high glucose. *Acta Diabetol.* 2001;38(3):135-138.

Sánchez-Ramírez GM, Caram-Salas NL, Rocha-González HI, et al. Benfotiamine relieves inflammatory and neuropathic pain in rats. *Eur J Pharmacol.* 2006;530(1-2):48-53.

Schmid U, Stopper H, Heidland A, et al. Benfotiamine exhibits direct antioxidative capacity and prevents induction of DNA damage in vitro. *Diabetes Metab Res Rev.* 2008;24(5):371-377.

Schupp N, Dette EM, Schmid U, et al. Benfotiamine reduces genomic damage in peripheral lymphocytes of hemodialysis patients. *Naunyn Schmiedebergs Arch Pharmacol.* 2008;378(3):283-291.

Stracke H, Gaus W, Achenbach U, Federlin K, Bretzel RG. Benfotiamine in Diabetic Polyneuropathy (BENDIP): Results of a Randomised, Double Blind, Placebo-controlled Clinical Study. *Exp Clin Endocrinol Diabetes.* Epub: 2008 May 13.

Stirban A, Negrean M, Stratmann B, et al. Adiponectin decreases postprandially following a heat-processed meal in individuals with type 2 diabetes: an effect prevented by benfotiamine and cooking method. *Diabetes Care.* 2007;30(10):2514-2516.

Stirban A, Negrean M, Stratmann B, et al. Benfotiamine prevents macro- and microvascular endothelial dysfunction and oxidative stress following a meal rich in advanced glycation end products in individuals with type 2 diabetes. *Diabetes Care.* 2006;29(9):2064-2071.

Stracke H, Hammes HP, Werkmann D, et al. Efficacy of benfotiamine versus thiamin on function and glycation products of peripheral nerves in diabetic rats. *Exp Clin Endocrinol Diabetes.* 2001;109(6):330-336.

Uteshev BS, Lazareva GA, Prokopenko LG. The immunometabolic effects of benfotiamine and riboxine on hemolytic anemia] [Article in Russian.] *Eksp Klin Farmakol.* 2002;65(4):37-41.

Várkonyi T, Kempler P. Diabetic neuropathy: new strategies for treatment. *Diabetes Obes Metab.* 2008;10(2):99-108.

Volvert M-L, Seyen S, Piette M, et al. Benfotiamine, a synthetic S-acyl thiamin derivative, has different mechanisms of action and a different pharmacological profile than lipid-soluble thiamin disulfide derivatives. *BMC Pharmacology.* 2008; 8:10.

Woelk H, Lehrl S, Bitsch R, et al. Benfotiamine in treatment of alcoholic polyneuropathy: an 8-week randomized controlled study (BAP I Study). *Alcohol and Alcohol.* 1998;33(6):631-638.

Wu S, Ren J. Benfotiamine alleviates diabetes-induced cerebral oxidative damage independent of advanced glycation end-product, tissue factor and TNF-alpha. *Neurosci Lett.* 2006;394(2):158-162.

Bentonite

DESCRIPTION

Bentonite is occasionally used in nutritional supplements as a source of trace minerals. It is a type of clay, the major constituent of which is a hydrated aluminum silicate called montmorillonite. Minor constituents found in bentonite include calcium, magnesium and iron. Bentonite is found in certain areas of the United States and Canada. Wyoming bentonite, found in Wyoming and South Dakota, contains sodium and is composed of alternating layers of aluminum oxide and silicon dioxide. It is also known as sodium montmorillonite. Bentonite found in Mississippi is known as calcium montmorillonite.

Bentonite absorbs water readily to form highly viscous suspensions or gels. Bentonite itself is practically insoluble in water. Because of its water-absorbing property, bentonite has been used as a bulk laxative and is used in the pharmaceutical industry as a suspending and stabilizing agent, as well as an adsorbent or clarifying agent. A derivative of bentonite is used to block urushiols from the skins. Urushiols are the etiological factors causing contact dermatitis from poison ivy, poison oak and poison sumac. Bentonite itself may bind to some toxins, such as paraquat, by adsorbing them.

ACTIONS AND PHARMACOLOGY

ACTIONS

Bentonite may be a delivery form of small amounts of certain trace minerals and small amounts of magnesium and calcium. It may also bind to some toxins, such as pesticides.

MECHANISM OF ACTION

Certain toxins, such as paraquat, may be adsorbed by bentonite.

PHARMACOKINETICS

Little is reported on the pharmacokinetics of bentonite. Following ingestion, there is probably very little to no absorption of bentonite from the gastrointestinal tract, and it is excreted in the feces. Small amounts of trace minerals and small amounts of calcium and magnesium may be absorbed.

INDICATIONS AND USAGE

It is claimed that bentonite binds to a number of toxins and thus renders them harmless. There is some evidence of this effect in animal studies.

RESEARCH SUMMARY

Bentonite has been shown to protect against the effects of aflatoxins in broiler chickens and rats but did not alleviate locoweed toxicosis in rats. Bentonite has also been shown to prevent high radiocesium levels in animal products. Clinical trials are lacking.

CONTRAINDICATIONS, PRECAUTIONS, ADVERSE REACTIONS

CONTRAINDICATIONS

Bentonite is contraindicated in those who are hypersensitive to any component of a bentonite-containing product. It is also contraindicated in those whose gastrointestinal tract is not anatomically intact.

PRECAUTIONS

Pregnant women, nursing mothers and the elderly should avoid using bentonite.

Those who do use bentonite should ingest plenty of fluid (water, juice) concomitantly in order to avoid possible intestinal obstruction.

Bentonite should not be used concomitantly with drugs or nutritional supplements.

There is no documentation in humans that bentonite has any benefit as a trace mineral source or as an aid in removing toxins from the colon.

ADVERSE REACTIONS

At doses usually used in nutritional supplements—5 to 10 mg—there are no reports of adverse reactions. Higher doses, e.g., greater than 10 grams daily, may have a laxative effect—bentonite was used as a bulk laxative—and if not taken with plenty of fluids may cause intestinal obstruction.

INTERACTIONS

DRUGS

Bentonite may adsorb certain drugs. Bentonite should not be taken concomitantly with any drugs.

NUTRITIONAL SUPPLEMENTS

Bentonite may adsorb certain nutritional supplements and should not be used concomitantly with them.

FOODS

Bentonite may adsorb certain food components.

HERBS

Bentonite may adsorb certain herb components.

DOSAGE AND ADMINISTRATION

Bentonite is available in some nutritional supplements as a trace mineral source. Dosage is usually 5 to 10 mg daily. Those who use bentonite as a "colon cleanser" use one tablespoon once or twice a day, which must be taken with at least one glass of water or juice. This is not recommended. Drugs and nutritional supplements should not be used concomitantly with the higher doses.

LITERATURE

Abdel-Wahhab MA, Nada SA, Farag IM, et al. Potential protective effect of HSCAS and bentonite against dietary aflatoxicosis in rat: with special reference to chromosomal aberrations. *Nat Toxins*. 1998; 6:211-218.

Santurio JM, Mallmann CA, Rosa AP, et al. Effect of sodium bentonite on the performance and blood variables of broiler chickens intoxicated with aflatoxins. *Br Poult Sci*. 1999; 40:115-119.

Beta-Alanine

DESCRIPTION

Beta-alanine is a nonprotein amino acid that is a precursor of the peptides carnosine (beta-alanyl-L-histidine), anserine (beta-alanyl-N-methylhistidine) and balenine (beta-alanyl-N-tau-methylhistidine) or ophidine (beta-alanyl-3-methylhistidine). It is also a precursor in the synthesis of the vitamin pantothenic acid, itself the precursor of coenzyme A. All of the amino acids comprising proteins are alpha-amino acids, meaning that the amino group in the amino acid structure is attached to the carbon group adjacent to the carboxyl group. Beta-amino acids contain their amino group one carbon removed from that position. Beta-alanine is one of five beta-amino acids found in mammals. The other four are taurine (contains a sulfonic acid group in place of the carboxylic acid group), *R*-beta-aminoisobutyrate, *S*-beta-aminoisobutyrate and beta-leucine. Beta-alanine is a nonessential amino acid, meaning that it can be made in the body, which it is via the enzyme beta-ureidopropionase, also known as beta-alanine synthase. Beta-ureidopropionase is the third enzyme in the catabolic pathway of the pyrimidine bases uracil and thymine. Beta-alanine can also be produced from carnosine via the enzyme carnosinase, which exists in two isoforms. Beta-alanine is also an agonist for the strychnine-sensitive glycine receptor, suggesting a possible neurotransmitter role.

Recently, there has been interest in the athletic community in the use of beta-alanine as a precursor of carnosine (see Carnosine) to help delay skeletal muscle fatigue. This possible effect is attributed to some of the actions of the beta-alanine metabolite carnosine. Carnosine itself when used as a nutritional supplement is rapidly hydrolyzed in the plasma via carnosinase.

Beta-alanine is also known as beta-aminopropionic acid, 3-aminopropanoic acid and 3-aminopropionic acid. Its molecular formula is $C_3H_7NO_2$, its line formula is $NH_2CH_2CH_2CO_2H$ and its molecular weight is 89.09. The CAS registry number is 107-95-9. Beta-alanine is freely soluble in water and has a slightly sweet taste. Beta-alanine is represented by the following chemical structure.

Beta-Alanine

ACTIONS AND PHARMACOLOGY

ACTIONS

The following possible actions are attributed to beta-alanine: delays muscular fatigue, increases aerobic endurance, increases anaerobic endurance, increases muscle mass, increases muscular strength and power output.

MECHANISM OF ACTION

Oxidative stress is associated with heavy exercise, muscle fatigue and muscle injury. Specific sources of reactive oxygen species (ROS) during exercise include leakage of electrons from the mitochondrial electron transport chain and from activated neutrophils, among others. Exercise may also induce inflammatory reactions similar to the acute phase response occurring in injury, which in turn contributes to an increase in ROS production, particularly during fatiguing exercises. The beta-alanine metabolite carnosine demonstrates antioxidant activity. Studies show that carnosine scavenges reactive oxygen species and protects against lipid peroxidation. A few, but far from all, studies suggest that certain antioxidants may protect against muscle injury during exercise and improve overall performance. There is little evidence to date that either beta-alanine or carnosine supplementation can prevent muscle injury during exercise.

Carnosine is found in humans in type I or "slow twitch" muscle fibers and in type IIa and type IIx (formerly called type IIb) or "fast twitch" muscle fibers. Carnosine is highest in type IIx, followed by type IIa, and lowest in type I muscle fibers. Type I fibers are good for endurance and are slow to tire because they mainly obtain their energy via oxidative metabolism. That is, they get their ATP predominantly from the process of oxidative phosphorylation. Type II fibers are used for short bursts of speed and power. Type II fibers fatigue more quickly than type I fibers. Type IIa fibers obtain their energy by both aerobic (oxidative phosphorylation) and anaerobic (glycolysis) metabolism. Type IIx fibers obtain their energy mainly anaerobically (via glycolysis). Carnosine is present in higher concentration in glycolytic muscle fibers than it is in oxidative muscle fibers. The highest levels of carnosine in animals are found in those that perform prolonged hypoxic dives (whales), those that perform frequent sprints (greyhounds) and those that have explosive flight behavior (pheasants).

During high- to- moderate-intensity exercise, there is an accumulation of lactic acid in muscle tissue, causing an increase in hydronium cations and a lowering of muscle pH. Muscle pH can fall from 7.1 to 6.5 or even lower. The drop in pH can cause interference with calcium ion release from the sarcoplasmic reticulum and decreased ATP production, resulting in muscle fatigue. Carnosine with its pKa of 6.83 acts as an intramuscular hydronium cation buffer over the physiological range. It is known that carnosine is a major buffer for animals. Carnosine constitutes about 10% to 20% of the buffering capacity in muscle in humans. It appears to be important in its action as an intramuscular buffer in humans, but there are other factors that contribute to delaying muscular fatigue, as well, including other buffers. More research is needed and warranted to elucidate those factors.

PHARMACOKINETICS

Beta-alanine is absorbed from the small intestine and distributed to various tissues in the body, especially muscle and brain tissues. Beta-alanine is the rate limiting substrate in the carnosine synthase reaction that catalyzes the chemical reaction—Beta-alanine + L-histidine + ATP (adenosine triphosphate) > carnosine + AMP (adenosine monophosphate) + diphosphate.

The enzyme carnosinase converts carnosine to beta-alanine and L-histidine. There are two isoforms of carnosinase. Tissue carnosinase is found in the liver, kidney and spleen, and serum carnosinase is found in the plasma, brain and spinal fluid.

The first step in the catabolism of beta-alanine is the formation of malonic acid semialdehyde via the enzyme, beta-alanine:alpha-ketoglutarate aminotransferase. Malonic acid semialdehyde is subsequently metabolized by malonic semialdehyde dehydrogenase to acetyl-coenzyme A. Interestingly, the neurotransmitter GABA (gamma-aminobutyric acid) is transaminated by the same aminotransferase that transaminates beta-alanine.

INDICATIONS AND USAGE

A few recent studies have suggested that beta-alanine supplementation may enhance athletic performance in some circumstances.

RESEARCH SUMMARY

Beta-alanine is a nonproteogenic amino acid and precursor of carnosine, which is present in skeletal muscle and other excitable tissues, such as nervous tissue. Various studies have demonstrated that muscle-carnosine content is positively correlated with some high-intensity exercise performance parameters. Increased carnosine levels have been reported to help maintain optimal muscle pH, thought to be important since decreased pH has been associated with diminished muscular endurance. Carnosine supplementation itself, however, has not been effective in boosting carnosine concentrations in muscle owing to its hydrolyzation in plasma by the enzyme carnosinase. Thus researchers have concentrated on beta-alanine and have reported that supplementing with this amino acid for two to four weeks has increased carnosine concentration in human skeletal muscle by approximately 60%. Further study by the same group utilized beta-alanine supplements in 13 male subjects to determine, in part, whether the amino acid could positively affect performance on a high-intensity cycling endurance test. A significant increase in a measure called total work done (TWD) was observed in the experimental subjects. TWD in matched controls given placebo did not increase.

In a more recent study, 22 women were randomly assigned to either a beta-alanine regimen or placebo and then given a continuous, incremental cycle ergometry test to exhaustion in order to evaluate the possible effect of the amino acid on a number of performance parameters. The researchers reported that 28 days of beta-alanine supplementation (86 mg per kg of body weight per day) significantly delayed the onset of neuromuscular fatigue and ventilatory threshold and delayed the time to exhaustion in the experimental subjects. These researchers concluded that it would be premature to call for the use of this supplement until further clinical evidence accumulates.

Another group of researchers has also recently reported positive results, in this case using beta-alanine in trained sprinters. Fifteen male athletes participated in this double-blind, placebo-controlled study. Over a four-week period they received either placebo or 4.8 grams of beta-alanine daily. They were evaluated by their performance on knee extension tests, by endurance on muscular contractions and by 400 meter sprinting times. Magnetic resonance spectroscopy confirmed significant increases in carnosine concentration in calf muscles of beta-alanine-treated subjects, compared with controls. Fatigue was judged to be significantly attenuated during repeated isokinetic contraction bouts in the experimentals but not in the controls. Performance on the 400 meter race times, however, was not significantly enhanced, possibly, the researchers posited, because the challenge to these trained athletes in a 400 meter sprint was insufficient to reveal an experimental effect.

Though results to date are promising, the studies are small and few, and more research is needed and warranted to determine whether beta-alanine can be a significant aid in athletic performance.

Finally, a decline in carnosine of about 30% takes place between age 10 years and 70 years, which may be associated with the decline in muscle function and sarcopenia that generally occurs during aging. Research is also needed and warranted to determine if beta-alanine and carnosine have any effect in slowing this decline.

CONTRAINDICATIONS, PRECAUTIONS, ADVERSE REACTIONS

CONTRAINDICATIONS

Beta-alanine is contraindicated in those with known hypersensitivity to the supplement or its components, or with the very rare disease hyper-beta-alaninemia, thought to be due to a deficiency of beta-alanine pyruvate aminotransferase. There is a report of one infant death from inherited hyper-beta-alaninemia.

PRECAUTIONS

Pregnant women and nursing mothers should avoid beta-alanine supplements.

ADVERSE REACTIONS

Beta-alanine may cause paresthesia (a sensation of tingling and numbness in the skin) when ingested in amounts above 10 mg per kg body weight. Typically, paresthesia starts about 20 minutes after ingestion and may last for up to one hour. It is caused by the beta-alanine getting absorbed across the gut into the blood stream very rapidly and subsequently transported too quickly into muscle and CNS cells. Those who use beta-alanine supplements should thus take it in small doses up to eight times throughout the day. Controlled time-release pills are available which may avoid the paresthesia problem.

INTERACTIONS

DRUGS

None known.

NUTRITIONAL SUPPLEMENTS

Creatine and beta-alanine may increase skeletal creatine phosphate and carnosine and may work synergistically to delay fatigue and increase exercise performance, especially in trained athletes.

HERBS

None known.

FOOD

None known.

OVERDOSAGE

There are no reports of overdosage in those taking beta-alanine supplements.

DOSAGE AND ADMINISTRATION

Beta-alanine is available as a powder and in pill form. Controlled time-release pills are available. Athletes, based on a few studies, have been using around three grams to six grams daily. As mentioned above, ingestion of amounts above 10 mg per kg body weight may cause paresthesia. For those taking the powder form, it is recommended that beta-alanine be taken in doses up to eight times throughout the day.

The optimal dose of beta-alanine is unknown.

LITERATURE

Begum G, Cunliffe A, Leveritt M. Physiological role of carnosine in contracting muscle. *Int J Sport Nutr Exerc Metab*. 2005;15(5):493-514.

Derave W, Ozdemir MS, Harris RC, et al. Beta-alanine supplementation augments muscle carnosine content and attenuates fatigue during repeated isokinetic contraction bouts in trained sprinters. *J Appl Physiol*. 2007;103(5):1736-1743.

Hoffman J, Ratamess N, Kang J, et al. Effect of creatine and Beta-alanine supplementation on performance and endocrine responses in strength/power athletes. *Int J Sport Nutr Exerc Metab*. 2006;16(4):430-446.

Rozhkova EA, Ordzhonikidze ZG, Druzhinin AE, et al. [Using carnosine and natural antioxidants for the prophylaxis of acute post-loading oxidative stress.] [Article in Russian.] *Eksp Klin Farmakol*. 2007;70(5):44-46.

Stout JR, Cramer JT, Mielke M, et al. Effects of twenty-eight days of Beta-alanine and creatine monohydrate supplementation on the physical working capacity at neuromuscular fatigue threshold. *J Strength Cond Res*. 2006;20(4):928-931.

Stout JR, Cramer JT, Zoeller RF, et al. Effects of Beta-alanine supplementation on the onset of neuromuscular fatigue and ventilatory threshold in women. *Amino Acids*. 2007;32(3):381-386.

Zoeller RF, Stout JR, O'kroy JA, et al. Effects of 28 days of Beta-alanine and creatine monohydrate supplementation on aerobic power, ventilatory and lactate thresholds, and time to exhaustion. *Amino Acids*. 2007;33(3):505-510.

Beta-Carotene

DESCRIPTION

Beta-carotene is a member of a class of substances called carotenoids. Beta-carotene, similar to the other carotenoids, is a natural fat-soluble pigment found principally in plants, algae *(Dunaliella salina, Dunaliella bardawil)* and photosynthetic bacteria, where it serves as an accessory light-gathering pigment and to protect these organisms against the toxic effects of oxygen. Carotenoids are polyisoprenoids which typically contain 40 carbon atoms and an extensive system of conjugated double bonds. They usually show internal symmetry and frequently contain one or two ring structures at the ends of their conjugated chains. Beta-carotene contains a cyclic structure at each end of its conjugated chain. The structural formula for beta-carotene is:

Beta-Carotene

Carotenoids are the principal pigments responsible for the red, orange, yellow and green colors of vegetables and fruits. Beta-carotene is responsible for the color of carrots.

Beta-carotene along with alpha-carotene, lycopene, lutein, zeaxanthin and beta-cryptoxanthin are the principal dietary carotenoids. Three of these carotenoids, alpha-carotene, beta-carotene and beta-cryptoxanthin, can serve as dietary precursors of retinol (all-*trans* retinol, vitamin A). Collectively, these carotenoids are called provitamin A carotenoids or provitamin A. Dietary carotenoids that are not converted into retinol (lutein, zeaxanthin, lycopene) are referred to as nonprovitamin A carotenoids.

Beta-carotene occurs naturally as all-*trans* beta-carotene and 9-*cis* beta-carotene. Smaller amounts of 13-*cis* beta-carotene are also found naturally. Synthetic beta-carotene consists mainly of all-*trans* beta-carotene with smaller amounts of 13-*cis* beta-carotene and even smaller amounts of 9-*cis* beta-carotene. Carrots are the major contributors of beta-carotene in the diet. Beta-carotene is also found in cantaloupe, broccoli, spinach and collard greens. Palm oil, which is used as a food colorant, is rich in beta-carotene as well as alpha-carotene. Dietary intake of beta-carotene in the American diet ranges from 1.3 to 2.9 milligrams daily. The consumption of five or more servings of fruits and vegetables per day—which is recommended by a number of federal agencies and other organizations, including the National Cancer Institute—would provide 3 to 6 milligrams daily of beta-carotene.

Beta-carotene is considered a conditionally essential nutrient. Beta-carotene becomes an essential nutrient when the dietary intake of retinol (vitamin A) is inadequate. It is unclear whether beta-carotene has any biological function for humans other than as a precursor for vitamin A. There is some evidence that beta-carotene may play a beneficial role in human nutrition beyond its provitamin A function. Beta-carotene has antioxidant activity, at least *in vitro*, and it may enhance intercellular communication and may have immunomodulatory and anticarcinogenic activities in certain circumstances. However, the evidence for a unique role in human nutrition beyond its provitamin A function is, to date, not compelling.

The absorption efficiency of beta-carotene and the other carotenoids from food sources is highly variable. For this reason, it has been difficult to define a general numerical factor for converting provitamin A carotenoids to vitamin A. There are two systems of units which are currently used which do not agree with each other and which have caused confusion. In the first system, 1 IU (international unit) is equal to 0.6 micrograms of all-*trans* beta-carotene or 1.2 micrograms of mixed other provitamin A carotenoids. In this system, which is the one generally used for nutritional labeling, 3 milligrams of beta-carotene is equal to 5,000 IU. The U.S. RDA for vitamin A is 5,000 IU. The second system uses retinol equivalents in place of international units. In the second system, one retinol equivalent (RE) is defined as one microgram of all-*trans* retinol (vitamin A), six micrograms of all-*trans* beta-carotene or 12 micrograms of other provitamin A carotenoids. In the first system, two micrograms of all-*trans* beta-carotene are defined as being equal to one microgram of all-*trans* retinol. In the second system, six micrograms of dietary all-*trans* beta-carotene are assumed to be nutritionally equivalent to one microgram of all-*trans* retinol. It is clear that these two systems do not agree with each other. In any case, all-*trans* carotene, as found in nutritional supplements, should be converted according to the first system. That is, two micrograms of all-*trans* carotene are equal to one microgram of all-*trans* retinol (vitamin A) or 3.33 IU.

ACTIONS AND PHARMACOLOGY

ACTIONS

Beta-carotene may have antioxidant activity. It may also have immunomodulatory, anticarcinogenic and antiatherogenic activities in some cases.

MECHANISM OF ACTION

Beta-carotene has been found to have antioxidant activity *in vitro*. It has been demonstrated to quench singlet oxygen ($^1O_2$), scavenge peroxyl radicals and inhibit lipid peroxidation. The mechanism of beta-carotene's antioxidant activity is not clearly understood. Some, but not all, studies have shown a difference in the *in vitro* activities of the beta-carotene isomers. One study showed that 9-*cis* beta-carotene—a naturally occurring form of beta-carotene—protected methyl linoleate from oxidation more efficiently than all-*trans* beta-carotene. However, another study demonstrated that 9-*cis* beta-carotene and all-*trans* beta-carotene had equal antioxidant activities when assessed by enhanced human neutrophil chemiluminescence. Whether beta-carotene has significant antioxidant activity *in vivo* is unclear. Results from some human studies have shown improvement of measures of antioxidant activity (decreased copper-induced LDL oxidation, decreased DNA strand breaks and oxidized pyrimidine bases in lymphocytes, decreased serum lipid peroxide levels, decreased breath pentane, decreased serum malondialdehyde, increased red blood cell copper/zinc-superoxide dismutase activity) in those receiving relatively high intakes of beta-carotene. Studies of those receiving relatively low to modest levels of beta-carotene have shown no changes or inconsistent changes in the same antioxidant activities. Administration of beta-carotene to cystic fibrosis subjects was found to decrease serum malondialdehyde, in one study. Beta-carotene may have antioxidant activity in some with conditions of increased oxidative stress. Retinol itself appears to have low antioxidant activity. Therefore, possible *in vivo* antioxidant activity of beta-carotene is unlikely to be a consequence of its conversion to retinol.

Beta-carotene has demonstrated some immunomodulatory effects. In healthy male nonsmokers, beta-carotene supplementation (15 mg/day) was found to significantly increase the percentage of monocytes expressing the major histocompatibility complex class II molecule HLA-DR, to increase the expression of the adhesion molecules, intercellular adhesion molecule-1 and leukocyte function-associated antigen-3, and to increase *ex vivo* secretion of tumor necrosis factor (TNF)-alpha by blood monocytes. Beta-carotene supplementation has also been found to enhance natural killer cell activity in elderly men, to increase lymphocyte

response to mitogens in healthy male cigarette smokers and to increase the CD4 lymphocyte count in some subjects with AIDS. The mechanism of the possible immunomodulatory activity of beta-carotene is not known. It is thought that the possible immunomodulatory activity may be independent of beta-carotene's role as a precursor of retinol.

Beta-carotene has been found to inhibit the growth of some malignant cells, including human prostate cancer cells, *in vitro*. The mechanism of this activity is not well understood. It is speculated that beta-carotene may increase cellular differentiation, down-regulate epidermal growth factor receptors, reduce adenyl cyclase activity, enhance expression of gap junctional proteins and protect against oxidative damage. The ability of beta-carotene to modulate the carcinogenic process, at least *in vitro*, may be due, in part, to its conversion to retinoids. In this regard, there is evidence that beta-carotene may be converted to retinol and other related metabolites (e.g., retinoic acid) in human prostate cell lines.

Several observational epidemiological studies have shown an inverse association between dietary beta-carotene intake and a number of cancers, in particular lung cancer. Intervention trials, however, have not found beta-carotene to be protective against lung cancer. In fact, two intervention trials, the Alpha-Tocopherol, Beta-Carotene (ATBC) Cancer Prevention Study (the "Finnish study"), and the Carotene and Retinol Efficacy Trial (CARET), both reported an unexpected increase in the number of lung cancer cases in the groups that received supplemental beta-carotene. The subjects in the ATBC and CARET studies were smokers. In the case of these studies, the mechanism, not of the possible anticarcinogenic activity of beta-carotene, but of its possible procarcinogenic activity, at least for smokers, requires elucidation. Several possible explanations have been proposed to explain the unexpected increase in lung cancer in these studies. Beta-carotene may act as a prooxidant when present in high concentrations in an oxidative environment such as the lungs of smokers in the advanced promotional stage of the neoplastic process. (Beta-carotene may be effective in the prevention of lung cancer if chronically present before or during the phases of initiation and early promotion of the process). Supplemental beta-carotene is known to inhibit the absorption of the carotenoid lutein which itself may have chemopreventive activity. Beta-carotene may have a cocarcinogenic effect. Beta-carotene has been found in the rat lung to produce a booster effect on phase I carcinogen-bioactivating enzymes, including activators of polycyclic aromatic hydrocarbons (PAHs). Finally, oxidative metabolites of beta-carotene may diminish retinoid signaling and eventually enhance carcinogenesis. The mechanism of the possible effect of beta-carotene in enhancing lung cancer in smokers remains a mystery. The general opinion is that the effect is related to prooxidant activity of beta-carotene or oxidative metabolites of beta-carotene in the context of increased partial pressure of oxygen in smokers' lungs.

Beta-carotene may have anticarcinogenic activity in the case of prostate cancer. In the Physicians' Health Study, it was found that men with low baseline beta-carotene levels at the beginning of the study experienced a decreased risk of developing prostate cancer when supplemented with 50 milligrams of beta-carotene every other day. The mechanism of this possible anticarcinogenic effect is unclear. A review of the postulated mechanisms of possible anticarcinogenic activity in certain circumstances is as follows: beta-carotene may be metabolically converted to retinoids which modulate the gene expression of factors linked to differentiation and cell proliferation via retinoic acid. Beta-carotene may modulate the activity of enzymes that metabolize xenobiotics. The carotenoid has been found to increase the levels of phase II detoxifying enzymes such as glutathione S-transferase mu (GST-mu) and glutathione peroxidase. Beta-carotene's possible immunomodulatory activity may also play a role. Its possible antioxidant activity may result in prevention of oxidative damage to DNA and inhibition of lipid peroxidation as well as regulation of the expression of genes sensitive to the intracellular redox state that may be involved in carcinogenesis. Beta-carotene may modulate the gene expression of connexin 43 resulting in the induction of gap junctions with a consequent inhibition of neoplastic transformations. Finally, in animals, beta-carotene has been found to modulate the gene expression of the enzyme HMG-CoA reductase. This would inhibit the endogenous synthesis of cholesterol resulting in possible inhibition of cell proliferation and malignant transformation.

Epidemiological studies and some, but not all, intervention studies suggest an inverse association between coronary artery disease and beta-carotene intake. The possible antiatherogenic activity of beta-carotene may be accounted for, in part, by its possible antioxidant activity. Humans supplemented with beta-carotene, but not lycopene, were found to have low-density lipoproteins that were less oxidized than did controls using endothelial cell-initiated autoxidation.

PHARMACOKINETICS

The efficiency of absorption of beta-carotene is highly variable. The efficiency of absorption of beta-carotene from carrots and other beta-carotene containing raw foods is less than 5%. On the other hand, the efficiency of absorption of beta-carotene from beta-carotene-containing nutritional supplements can be as high as 70% or more. In foods, beta-carotene exists either as a solution in oil (e.g., red palm oil) or as part of a matrix within the vegetable or fruit. For example, in carrots, beta-carotene exists in a complex matrix,

comprised of indigestible polysaccharides, digestible polysaccharides and protein. Only a small percentage of beta-carotene is released from the matrix during the passage of foods such as carrots, through the gastrointestinal tract.

Beta-carotene from supplements, oils or foods is either solubilized in the lipid core of micelles (formed from bile salts and dietary fat) in the lumen of the small intestine or forms clathrate complexes with conjugated bile salts. Micelles and clathrate complexes deliver beta-carotene to the enterocytes. All of the beta-carotene isomers—all-*trans* beta-carotene, 9-*cis* beta-carotene and 13-*cis* beta-carotene—are absorbed from the lumen of the small intestine into the enterocytes. Within the enterocytes, a fraction of all-*trans* beta-carotene is oxidized to retinal and then reduced to retinol. Retinol is then esterified to form retinyl esters. It appears that 9-*cis* carotene is isomerized to the all-trans form before being released into the lymphatics. The principal enzyme involved in the oxidation of beta-carotene is called beta-carotene 15, 15' dioxygenase.

Beta-carotene and retinyl esters are released from the enterocytes into the lymphatics in the form of chylomicrons. (See Vitamin A for the pharmacokinetics of that substance.) Beta-carotene is transported by the lymphatics to the general circulation via the thoracic duct. In the circulation, lipoprotein lipase hydrolyzes much of the triglycerides in the chylomicrons, resulting in the formation of chylomicron remnants. Chylomicron remnants retain apolipoproteins E and B48 on their surfaces and are mainly taken up by hepatocytes and to smaller degrees by other tissues. Within hepatocytes, beta-carotene is incorporated into lipoproteins. Beta-carotene is released into the blood from the hepatocytes in the form of very low-density lipoproteins (VLDL) and low-density lipoproteins (LDL). In the plasma, VLDLs are converted by lipoprotein lipase to LDLs. Beta-carotene is transported in the plasma predominantly in the form of LDLs.

INDICATIONS AND USAGE

Beta-carotene may be protective against some forms of cancer in some populations. There is also evidence that it may act as a co-carcinogen in smokers and some others. It may also play a role in protecting against heart disease in some. Beta-carotene has demonstrated positive effects in the immune system. Diminished beta-carotene status has been observed in subjects with noninsulin-dependent diabetes, but supplementation with beta-carotene has so far produced no notable benefits in diabetic patients. Benefits sometimes attributed to beta-carotene in the prevention of cataracts and age-related macular degeneration may actually be due to other carotenoids, notably lutein and zeaxanthin.

RESEARCH SUMMARY

The epidemiologic evidence is overwhelming that those who consume three or more servings of fruits and vegetables daily have significantly lower risk of many forms of cancer and heart disease. The protective association is particularly strong for dietary carotenoids, especially with respect to protection against lung cancer in both men and women, smokers and non-smokers.

These epidemiologic findings have been fortified by other studies in which levels of carotenoids in blood and tissue have shown consistent inverse associations with cancer risks, especially lung-cancer risk. Plausible mechanisms of action in this context have further buttressed the case for a useful role of beta-carotene in cancer prevention.

Additionally, beta-carotene supplements have significantly inhibited oral leucoplakia and such other precancerous lesions as buccal cell micronuclei in subjects at risk of oral cancer. In the Linxian Interventive Trial, only a combination of beta-carotene, vitamin E and selenium, of four dietary regimens tested against placebo, had significant protective effects (principally against gastric and esophageal cancers). *In vitro* and animal studies have also shown significant beta-carotene anticancer effects. Recently it was shown *in vitro* that beta-carotene significantly inhibited growth of three different human prostate cancer cell lines.

While the large Linxian Intervention Trial found that a supplementary regimen that included beta-carotene, as noted above, significantly reduced mortality from gastric and total cancer in marginally malnourished subjects, three other large intervention studies in normally nourished subjects, long-term smokers, former smokers and those exposed to asbestos found no overall benefit from high-dose beta-carotene. Moreover, in one of these studies, there was a significant 18% excess incidence of lung cancer among those who received beta-carotene supplements.

These contrary and unexpected findings initially caused great consternation among researchers and physicians and provoked "panic" headlines in the lay press, leaving many with the impression that beta-carotene was categorically of no value and that it most likely was hazardous to health. As the dust from this uproar has begun to settle, some plausible explanations for the overall failure of beta-carotene in these particular studies have begun to emerge along with a rationale for the continued use of beta-carotene supplementation in some circumstances.

The study that most surprised the research and medical communities was the Alpha-Tocopherol, Beta-Carotene Prevention study (ATBC). This randomized, double-blind, placebo-controlled study tested beta-carotene (20 milligrams daily) or 50 milligrams of alpha-tocopherol, or both, against placebo in Finnish smokers aged 50-69 years of age over a period of five to eight years, primarily to see what impact, if any, supplementation might have on the incidence of lung cancer. Not only was no protective effect demonstrated but there was a significant increase in lung cancer incidence and mortality among the supplemented group. (Alpha-tocopherol also failed overall to protect smokers against lung cancer, except in the case of those who took it for five or more years. It was, however, associated with a significant reduction in risk of prostate cancer, a lesser reduction in colon cancer and increased risk of hemorrhagic stroke in smokers. See Vitamin E for more details.) It should be noted that there was evidence in this study that those with low beta-carotene status at baseline who received beta-carotene supplements had a 35% reduced incidence of pancreatic cancer, compared with controls who received placebo.

Another large intervention trial, the Beta-Carotene and Retinol Efficacy Trial (CARET), was halted prematurely in view of the ATBC findings and preliminary results demonstrating no benefit from supplemental beta-carotene and retinol in smokers, former smokers and those exposed to asbestos. Non-significant increases in cancer and cardiovascular incidence and mortality were noted. Doses used were 30 milligrams of beta-carotene and 25,000 IUs of retinyl palmitate.

In the Physicians' Health Study (PHS) which lasted 12 years, 22,071 healthy physicians, 11% of whom were current smokers and 39% of whom were former smokers, took high doses of beta-carotene, 50 milligrams every other day, or placebo. This was for a considerably longer period than supplements were taken in either the CARET or ATBC trials. Supplementation neither decreased nor increased overall risk of cancer. There was a non-significant decrease in the incidence of lung cancer among the smokers in this group receiving beta-carotene. In a subset of this population with low baseline blood levels of beta-carotene, there was, with supplements, a lower rate of total cancer and a 32% reduction in risk of prostate cancer. No toxic side effects were reported in this study.

How does one reconcile these confounding results? It appears, some researchers have concluded, that beta-carotene supplementation, even long-term and at doses as high as those used in these studies, while possibly not advisable or optimal, appears non-toxic in non-smoking and non-asbestos-exposed populations. Why even smokers in the PHS study suffered no harm, in contrast to some apparent harm in the CARET and ATBS studies, is unknown. It is possible that they smoked less, and that this well-educated, health-conscious population may have eaten more fruits and vegetables and may have more regularly consumed other vitamin-mineral preparations that favorably altered the activity of beta-carotene or that conferred some protection by themselves. Additionally, some others have pointed out that long-term, high-dose use of beta-carotene produced no toxic effects in the treatment of some with skin disorders.

As for why no overall benefit, as opposed to harm, was seen in the PHS group, some argue that this was due, in part, to the fact that this was a healthy, well-nourished population to begin with. In the Linxian Study, by contrast, the large number of subjects studied suffered from poor nutrition and showed significant benefit (in terms of cancer protection) from supplementation with beta-carotene, selenium and vitamin E. Even in the PHS study those with low baseline blood levels of beta-carotene apparently had some supplementation-associated reduction in prostate cancer risk.

Why might high-dose beta-carotene be helpful in some but harmful in smokers and others with significant lung impairment, such as that caused by asbestos exposure? Several researchers have now suggested that high concentrations of beta-carotene oxidize in the free-radical-rich milieu of the lungs of cigarette smokers and asbestos sufferers. More physiologic amounts of beta-carotene, such as that derived from diet, appear to have antioxidant effects, whereas, these researchers assert, the very high doses of beta-carotene used in these studies turned pro-oxidant in the lungs of smokers. Some experimental evidence *in vitro* and in animal models lends preliminary support to this hypothesis. Thus, the argument is made that doses of beta-carotene used were inappropriately high and that beta-carotene, without other nutrients to protect it against oxidation, could not be expected to have a beneficial effect in the lungs of long-term smokers.

It has been pointed out that other factors also may have conspired against beta-carotene in these studies. In the ATBC trial, for example, apparent adverse effects of beta-carotene were seen primarily in those who smoked and also consumed high quantities of alcohol, which also produces significant oxidative stress. In addition, others have noted that subjects studied in these largely negative interventive trials were mostly heavy smokers aged 50 or older who had been smoking for many years or were workers with long-term exposure to asbestos and were thus likely to be in the advanced promotional phase of carcinogenesis at the outset of the study. Many of these subjects had been smoking for decades, and the intervention, the argument goes, came too late and with doses so high they became pro-oxidant rather than antioxidant in these highly oxidative conditions.

Various researchers have proposed that beta-carotene be tested in more physiological doses and in combination with vitamins E and C and possibly some other antioxidant nutrients. In one recent study, the oxidative stress of environmental tobacco smoke was said to be reduced in humans supplemented with 3 milligrams of beta-carotene, 60 milligrams of vitamin C, 30 milligrams of alpha-tocopherol, 40 milligrams of zinc, 40 milligrams of selenium and 2 milligrams of copper. In another study, this one conducted double-blind, smokers and non-smokers received another mixture of antioxidants (35 milligrams of beta-carotene, 100 milligrams of vitamin C and 280 milligrams of vitamin E daily) for 20 weeks. Notable reductions were observed in endogenous oxidative base damage in the lymphocyte DNA of both smokers and non-smokers.

Others insist that more animal work should be done before more large interventive beta-carotene trials are launched.

One reviewer has stated that "the results of the major trials do not prove or disprove the value of antioxidant vitamins nor do they incriminate them as harmful." Another reviewer concurs, observing that "these results cannot be used as evidence to suggest that low-dose supplementation with beta-carotene would be harmful (or beneficial), but point out our lack of knowledge regarding the dose/response/toxicity of most prevention agents (certainly dietary supplements)." Both reviewers also note that the trials nonetheless signal caution. Other reviewers, while noting that beta-carotene has exhibited considerable, credible anti-cancer activity in a number of studies, conclude that "chronic pharmacological supplementation is not recommended for healthy populations, and the carotenoid may actually be deleterious to smokers."

Finally, another reviewer of the lung cancer research observes that recent data from follow-up in the same interventive trials that reported negative supplementation results show that "regardless of their intervention assignment, study participants with highest intake and serum concentrations of beta-carotene at baseline developed fewer subsequent lung cancers." In recent years, review articles continue to ask the same question: beta-carotene—cancer preventive or co-carcinogen? Little new data have emerged. CARET participants, however, continued to be followed after conclusion of the main thrust of that study. A report a few years ago stated that adverse effects seen in smokers and those exposed to asbestos continued to persist after supplementation was continued. Those effects, however, were found to be no longer statistically significant. The last of this controversy undoubtedly has yet to unfold. In the meantime, most clinicians remain reluctant to recommend beta-carotene, particularly for smokers or those exposed to environmental contaminants.

The situation with respect to beta-carotene and heart disease roughly parallels the beta-carotene-cancer story. A number of epidemiological studies, including several cohort and case-control studies, have reported significantly diminished risk of cardiovascular disease in those with high plasma/serum levels and/or high dietary intake of beta-carotene. Case-control studies showed significant protective effects in both smokers and non-smokers.

In the large interventive trials, however, no significant protective effects were seen with respect to heart disease. Some of the same arguments used in an attempt to explain inconsistent results in the beta-carotene cancer research have been put forward to try to explain inconsistencies in the heart-disease results. Obviously, more research is needed to resolve the issue.

Some animal, *in vitro* and human research persuasively suggests that beta-carotene has immune enhancing and anti-mutagenic effects independent of any vitamin A activity. Beta-carotene for example, had helped protect bone-marrow cells against mutagens in experiments in which vitamin A did not provide the same protection. Beta-carotene activity independent of any provitamin A activity has been credited in other experiments with enhancing both T- and B-lympho-cyte proliferative responses in mice fed nutritionally complete diets supplemented with beta-carotene.

T-helper cell counts were significantly increased in humans given very high dose (180 milligrams daily) beta-carotene for two weeks. Production of macrophage cytokines has been increased and tumor cell cytotoxicity enhanced in an animal model using beta-carotene supplementation. More tumor cells were killed by natural killer cells from human peripheral blood when incubated with beta-carotene, compared to killer cells not exposed to beta-carotene.

In another study, vegetarians were found to have twice the natural killer cell activity of non-vegetarians. Serum levels of vitamins A, E and C were equal in the two groups, but beta-carotene levels were about twice as high in the vegetarians as in the non-vegetarians.

Some effects have also been seen in autoimmune conditions. In one experiment, giving beta-carotene to autoimmune-prone mice resulted in reduced lymphadenopathy and prolonged lifespan.

Healthy non-smoking men receiving 15 milligrams of beta-carotene daily exhibited enhanced immune function of blood monocytes. Ultraviolet light suppression of one type of immune function was significantly inhibited in a randomized trial of healthy older men taking 30 milligrams of beta-carotene daily for 47 days while simultaneously consuming a low-carotenoid diet.

Though relationships have been reported between diminished beta-carotene status and increased risk of diabetes

mellitus, supplementation with beta-carotene has so far not been found to reduce the incidence of this disease.

Again, low beta-carotene status has been associated with higher risk of developing cataracts, but, once more, supplementation with beta-carotene has not been shown to reduce the incidence of cataracts. In the 12-year follow-up of the Nurses Health Study, involving 77,488 women aged 45-71 years, beta-carotene intake had no apparent impact on cataracts, but other carotenoids (lutein, zeaxanthin) were associated with a significant reduction in cataract risk.

With respect to age-related macular degeneration, higher dietary intake of carotenoids is associated with reduced risk. Again, lutein and zeaxanthin are the carotenoids that appear to provide the most protection. Beta-carotene is largely absent in the macula, whereas lutein and zeaxanthin are the dominant pigments of the macula.

CONTRAINDICATIONS, PRECAUTIONS, ADVERSE REACTIONS
CONTRAINDICATIONS
Beta-carotene is contraindicated in those hypersensitive to any component of a beta-carotene-containing preparation.

PRECAUTIONS
Pregnant women and nursing mothers should try to obtain an intake of beta-carotene from 3 to 6 milligrams daily from the consumption of five or more servings daily of fruits and vegetables. Pregnant women and nursing mothers should avoid intakes of beta-carotene greater than 6 milligrams/day from nutritional supplements.

Smokers should be made aware that supplemental intake of beta-carotene of 20 milligrams daily or greater were associated with a higher incidence of lung cancer in smokers. Smokers should avoid beta-carotene supplementation pending the establishment of a safe dose for smokers.

The use of beta-carotene for the treatment of vitamin A deficiency requires medical management.

ADVERSE REACTIONS
Beta-carotene is used for the treatment of erythropoietic protoporphyria. This is a photosensitivity disorder. Doses of up to 180 milligrams daily are used for the treatment of this disorder. No toxic effects are seen in those with this disorder taking this high dose. Doses of 30 milligrams/day or greater of beta-carotene taken for prolonged periods may cause carotenodermia. Carotenodermia is characterized by yellowish discoloration of the skin and is distinguished from jaundice by the absence of yellowed ocular sclerae, which are found in those with jaundice. Carotenodermia is considered harmless and reversible with the discontinuation of beta-carotene.

There is no evidence of hypervitaminosis A in those consuming high doses (up to 180 mg/d of beta-carotene).

There is an association of increased lung cancer in smokers taking 20 mg/d or greater of beta-carotene. In the Alpha-Tocopherol, Beta-Carotene (ATBC) Cancer Prevention Study, smokers supplemented with 20 mg/d of beta-carotene for five to eight years showed a higher incidence of lung cancer compared to the placebo group. In the Carotene and Retinol Efficacy Trial (CARET), smokers taking 30 milligrams of beta-carotene daily and 25,000 IUs/d of retinol were found to have a higher incidence of lung cancer when compared to the placebo group. It is at present unclear if there is a true link between increased lung cancer incidence in smokers taking beta-carotene supplements.

INTERACTIONS

DRUGS

Cholestyramine: Concomitant intake of cholestyramine and beta-carotene may decrease the absorption of beta-carotene.

Colestipol: Concomitant intake of colestipol and beta-carotene may decrease the absorption of beta-carotene.

Mineral Oil: Concomitant intake of mineral oil and beta-carotene may reduce the absorption of beta-carotene.

Orlistat: Orlistat may decrease the absorption of beta-carotene.

NUTRITIONAL SUPPLEMENTS

Lutein: Concomitant intake of the carotenoid lutein and beta-carotene may decrease the absorption of lutein.

Pectin: Concomitant intake of pectin and beta-carotene may decrease the absorption of beta-carotene.

FOODS

Olestra: Concomitant intake of olestra and beta-carotene may decrease the absorption of beta-carotene.

OVERDOSAGE

Beta-Carotene overdosage is not reported in the literature.

DOSAGE AND ADMINISTRATION

Beta-carotene supplements are available as synthetic beta-carotene and natural beta-carotene. Synthetic beta-carotene is comprised mainly of all-*trans* beta-carotene with smaller amounts of 13-*cis* beta-carotene and even smaller amounts of 9-*cis* beta-carotene. Natural beta-carotene is principally derived from the algae *Dunaliella salina* and is comprised of all-*trans* beta-carotene and 9-*cis* beta-carotene. Three milligrams of beta-carotene is equal to 5,000 IUs. Supplemental intake of beta-carotene ranges from 3-15 milligrams/day.

LITERATURE

Albanes D. Beta-carotene and lung cancer: a case study. *Am J Clin Nutr.* 1999;69:1345S-1350S.

Albanes D, Heinonen OP, Taylor PR, et al. Alpha-tocopherol and beta-carotene supplements and lung cancer incidence in the alpha-tocopherol, beta-carotene cancer prevention study: effects of base-line characteristics and study compliance. *J Natl Cancer Inst.* 1996;88:1560-1570.

Bendich A. Beta-carotene and the immune response. *Proc Nutr Soc.* 1991;50:263-274.

Bendich A. From 1989 to 2001: what have we learned about the "biological actions of beta-carotene"? *J Nutr.* 2004;134(1):225S-230S.

Blot WJ, Li JY, Taylor PR, et al. Nutrition intervention trials in Linxian, China: supplementation with specific vitamin/mineral combinations, cancer incidence, and disease-specific mortality in the general population. *J Natl Cancer Inst.* 1993;15:1483-1492.

Christen WG, Manson JE, Glynn RJ, et al. Beta carotene supplementation and age-related maculopathy in a randomized trial of US physicians. *Arch Ophthalmol.* 2007;125(3):333-339.

Dietary Reference Intakes for Vitamin C, Vitamin E, Selenium, and Carotenoids. Washington, DC: National Academy Press; 2000.

Duffield-Lillico AJ, Begg CB. Reflections on the landmark studies of beta-carotene supplementation. *J Natl Cancer Inst.* 2004;96(23):1729-1731.

Frieling UM, Schaumberg DA, Kupper TS, et al. A randomized, 12 year primary-prevention trial of beta carotene supplementation for nonmelanoma skin cancer in the Physicians' Health Study. *Arch Dermatol.* 2000;136:179-184.

Garewal HS, Katz RV, Meyskens F, et al. Beta-carotene produces sustained remissions in patients with oral leukoplakia. *Arch Otolaryngol Head Neck Surg.* 1999;125:1305-1310.

Gaziano JM. Antioxidants in cardiovascular disease: randomized trials. *Nutr Rev.* 1996;54:175-177.

Goodman GE. Prevention of lung cancer. *Crit Rev Oncol Hematol.* 2000;33:187-197.

Goodman GE, Thornquist MD, Balmes J, et al. The Beta-Carotene and Retinol Efficacy Trial: incidence of lung cancer and cardiovascular disease mortality during 6-year follow-up after stopping beta-carotene and retinol supplements. *J Natl Cancer Inst.* 2004;96(23):1743-1750.

Hennekens CH, Buring JE, Manson JE, et al. Lack of effect of long-term supplementation with beta carotene on the incidence of malignant neoplasms and cardiovascular disease. *N Engl J Med.* 1996;334:1145-1149.

Hughes DA, Wright AJ, Finglas PM, et al. The effect of beta-carotene supplementation on the immune function of blood monocytes from healthy male nonsmokers. *J Lab Clin Med.* 1997;129:309-317.

Kuntz E, Borlak J, Riss G, et al. Transcriptomics does not show adverse effects of beta-carotene in A/J mice exposed to smoke for 2 weeks. *Arch Biochem Biophys.* 2007;465(2):336-346.

Lee I-M, Cook NR, Manson JE, et al. Beta-carotene supplementation and incidence of cancer and cardiovascular disease: The Women's Health Study. *J Natl Cancer Inst.* 1999;91:2102-2106.

Liu S, Ajani U, Chae C, et al. Long-term beta-carotene supplementation and risk of type 2 diabetes mellitus. A randomized controlled trial. *JAMA.* 1999;282:1073-1075.

Liu Q, Suzuki K, Nakaji S, et al. Antioxidant activities of natural 9-*cis* and synthetic all-*trans* beta-carotene assessed by human neutrophil chemiluminescence. *Nutr Res.* 2000;20:5-14.

Mayne ST, Walter M, Cartmel B, et al. Supplemental beta-carotene, smoking, and urinary F2-isoprostane excretion in patients with prior early stage head and neck cancer. *Nutr Cancer.* 2004;49(1):1-6.

Naves MMV, Moreno FS. Beta-carotene and cancer chemoprevention: from epidemiological associations to cellular mechanisms of action. *Nutr Res.* 1998;18:1807-1824.

Omenn GS, Goodman GE, Thornquist MD, et al. Effects of the combination of beta carotene and vitamin A on lung cancer and cardiovascular disease. *N Engl J Med.* 1996;334:1150-1155.

Omenn GS, Goodman GE, Thornquist MD, et al. Risk factors for lung cancer and for intervention effects in CARET, the Beta-Carotene and Retinol Efficacy Trial. *J Natl Cancer Inst.* 1996;88:1550-1559.

Paolini M, Cantelli-Forti G, Perocco P, et al. Co-carcinogenic effect of beta-carotene. *Nature.* 1999;398:760-761.

Peto R, Doll R, Buckley JD, et al. Can dietary beta-carotene materially reduce human cancer rates? *Nature.* 1981;290:201-208.

Prabhala RH, Braune LM, Garewal HS, et al. Influence of beta-carotene on immune functions. *Ann NY Acad Sci.* 1993;691:262-263.

Pryor WA, Stahl W, Rock CL. Beta carotene: from biochemistry to clinical trials. *Nutr Rev.* 2000;58:39-53.

Rapola JM, Virtamo J, Ripatti S, et al. Effects of alpha tocopherol and beta carotene supplements on symptoms, progression, and prognosis of angina pectoris. *Heart.* 1998;79:454-458.

Rapola JM, Virtamo J, Ripatti S, et al. Randomized trial of alpha-tocopherol and beta-carotene supplements on incidence of major coronary events in men with previous myocardial infarction. *Lancet.* 1997;349:1715-1720.

Redlich CA, Chung JS, Cullen MR, et al. Effect of long-term beta-carotene and vitamin A on serum cholesterol and triglyceride levels among participants in the Carotene and Retinol Efficacy Trial (CARET). *Atherosclerosis.* 1999;145:425-432.

Santos MS, Gaziano JM, Leka LS, et al. Beta-carotene-induced enhancement of natural killer cell activity in elderly men: an investigation of the role of cytokines. *Am J Clin Nutr.* 1998;68:164-170.

Santos MS, Meydani SN, Leka L, et al. Natural killer cell activity in elderly men is enhanced by beta-carotene supplementation. *Am J Clin Nutr.* 1996;64:772-777.

Siems W, Wiswedel I, Salerno C, et al. Beta-carotene breakdown products may impair mitochondrial functions—potential side effects of high-dose beta-carotene supplementation. *J Nutr Biochem.* 2005;16(7):385-397.

Tavani A, La Vecchia C. Beta-carotene and risk of coronary heart disease. A review of observational and intervention studies. *Biomed Pharmacother.* 1999;53:409-416.

The Alpha-Tocopherol, Beta Carotene Cancer Prevention Study Group. The effect of vitamin E and beta-carotene on the incidence of lung cancer and other cancers in male smokers. *N Engl J Med.* 1994;330:1029-1035.

van Poppel G, Spanhaak S, Ockhiuizen T. Effect of beta-carotene on immunological indexes in healthy male smokers. *Am J Clin Nutr.* 1993;57:402-407.

Virtano J, Rapola JM, Ripatti S, et al. Effect of vitamin E and beta carotene on the incidence of primary nonfatal myocardial infarction and fatal coronary heart disease. *Arch Intern Med.* 1998;158:668-675.

Wang X-D, Liu C, Bronson RT, et al. Retinol signaling and activator protein-1 expression in ferrets given beta-carotene supplements and exposed to tobacco smoke. J *Natl Cancer Inst.* 1999;91:60-66.

Williams AW, Boileau T W-M, Zhou JR, et al. Beta-carotene modulates human prostate cancer cell growth and may undergo intracellular metabolism to retinol. *J Nutr.* 2000;130:728-732.

Beta-Hydroxy-Beta-Methylbutyrate (HMB)

DESCRIPTION

Beta-hydroxy-beta-methylbutyrate, abbreviated HMB, is found naturally in living matter as a metabolite of the essential amino acid L-leucine. There is preliminary evidence suggesting HMB may have anticatabolic, as well as immunomodulatory, properties. As a nutritional supplement, it is popular among athletes engaged in strenuous physical activity.

HMB is also known as hydroxymethylbutyrate, beta-hydroxyisovalerate and 3-hydroxyisovalerate.

ACTIONS AND PHARMACOLOGY

ACTIONS

HMB has putative anticatabolic and immunomodulatory activities.

MECHANISM OF ACTION

The mechanism of HMB's possible actions is unknown. There is, however, speculation. The branched-chain amino acids L-leucine, L-isoleucine and L-valine are known to be beneficial to catabolic patients (sepsis, trauma, burns, etc.) by improving hepatic protein synthesis and nitrogen economy. These amino acids make up about one-third of muscle protein. Of these amino acids, L-leucine has the highest oxidation rate. Further, L-leucine has been shown to stimulate protein synthesis in muscle, and decreases in leucine levels in skeletal muscle and in serum have been noted following exhaustive exercise. However, L-leucine supplementation has not been found to have a significant effect on athletic performance. It has been speculated that the L-leucine metabolite HMB may be responsible for the inhibitory effect of L-leucine on protein breakdown. How this may happen is unknown.

In pigs, HMB is produced from alpha-ketoisocaproate, a metabolite of L-leucine, via the enzyme alpha-ketoisocarproate dioxygenase, an enzyme that requires oxygen and iron for its activity. This pathway, located in the cytosol, may also exist in humans. L-leucine is also metabolized in mitochondria to produce HMB in the form of HMB-coenzyme A (HMB-CoA), rather than free HMB.

HMB has been found to induce chicken macrophage growth and enhance chicken macrophage function in culture. It has also been found to enhance both humoral and cellular immunity in young broilers. The mechanism of these immunomodulatory activities is unknown.

PHARMACOKINETICS

Little is reported on the pharmacokinetics of HMB in humans. Apparently, HMB is absorbed, and about 50% of an ingested dose is excreted unchanged in the urine. HMB may be metabolized to beta-hydroxy-beta-methylglutaryl-CoA, which is, in turn, metabolized to acetyl-CoA and acetoacetate.

INDICATIONS AND USAGE

It is claimed that HMB can increase lean muscle mass and exercise performance, but this is far from conclusively established. It appears to be useful in some muscle wasting conditions, such as occur in AIDS, cancer and bed-rest. It may also be of benefit in some critically ill trauma patients. There is the suggestion in some preliminary research that HMB may have some immunomodulating effects.

RESEARCH SUMMARY

One study has reported that HMB-supplemented subjects (receiving 1.5 or 3 grams daily) lifted more weight compared with unsupplemented subjects. The researchers concluded that either dose of HMB 'can partly prevent exercise-induced proteolysis and /or muscle damage and result in larger gains in muscle function associated with resistance training.'

Because the subjects in the above-described study were initiating training, another group of researchers sought to determine whether HMB might have effects similar to those reported in the first study — but this time in trained athletes. This was a double-blind study in which 40 experienced resistance-trained athletes were randomized to receive 0, 3 or 6 grams of HMB daily for 28 days. No significant differences were noted in whole body anabolic/catabolic status, muscle and liver enzyme efflux, fat/bone-free mass, fat mass, percent body fat, or leg press one repetition maximums(1RM) strength. More research is needed.

A recent review of the effects of HMB on exercise performance and body composition—across varying levels of age, sex and training experience—found conflicting results. On balance, the reviewers found "compelling evidence that HMB supplementation may be useful for clinical muscle wasting conditions, including AIDS, cancer, bed-rest, and during periods of caloric deficits." An enteral supplement that combines HMB with arginine and glutamine has recently been shown to restore muscle in cachetic AIDS and cancer patients. The reviewers found HMB supplementation to be generally safe and noted that some other benefits may accrue from it, such as lower blood pressure and LDL-cholesterol, although there is no definitive proof of these benefits. As an ergogenic aid in athletes, they suggested that the appropriate dose is 1 gram three times daily. They added, however, that more study is needed to see whether this dosage is indeed optimal and to determine whether HMB is truly efficacious in athletes. This review also examined the possible mechanisms through which HMB might achieve its putative effects. They found some evidence from cachetic cancer studies suggesting that HMB may inhibit the ubiquitin-proteasome proteolytic pathway responsible for the specific degradation of intracellular proteins and that it may directly stimulate protein synthesis via the mTOR pathway.

A recent study followed up on the findings related to use of HMB in AIDS and cancer patients with muscle wasting, to see if similar benefits could be achieved in critically ill trauma patients. Via tube feeds, trauma patients received HMB alone, HMB in combination with arginine and glutamine or placebo for 28 days. Favorable effects were seen on nitrogen balance in both the HMB and HMB/arginine/glutamine groups, but not in the placebo group. Further research is warranted.

Very preliminary research in some animal models suggests that HMB supplementation may improve several immunological functions that may result in decreased mortality in these animals.

CONTRAINDICATIONS, PRECAUTIONS, ADVERSE REACTIONS

CONTRAINDICATIONS

Known hypersensitivity to an HMB-containing product.

PRECAUTIONS

Pregnant women and nursing mothers should avoid supplemental HMB.

ADVERSE REACTIONS

None reported.

OVERDOSAGE

No reported overdosage.

DOSAGE AND ADMINISTRATION

Some athletes use 3 grams of HMB daily during periods of training.

LITERATURE

Eley HL, Russell ST, Baxter JH, et al. Signaling pathways initiated by beta-hydroxy-beta-methylbutyrate to attenuate the depression of protein synthesis in skeletal muscle in response to cachectic stimuli. *Am J Physiol Endocrinol Metab.* 2007;293(4):E923-931.

Kreider RB, Ferreira M, Wilson M, et al. Effects of calcium-beta hydroxy-beta-methylbutyrate (HMB) supplementation during resistance-training on markers of catabolism, body composition and strength. *Int J Sports Med.* 1999;20:503-509.

Kuhls DA, Rathmacher JA, Musngi MD, et al. Beta-hydroxy-beta-methylbutyrate supplementation in critically ill trauma patients. *J Trauma.* 2007 Jan;62(1):125-131;discussion 131-132.

Mero A. Leucine supplementation and intensive training. *Sports Med.* 1999;27:345-358.

Nissen S, Sharp R, Ray M, et al. Effect of leucine metabolite beta-hydroxy-beta-methylbutyrate on muscle metabolism during resistance exercise testing. *J Am Physiol.* 1996;81:2095-2104.

Peterson AL, Qureshi MA, Ferket PR, et al. Enhancement of cellular and humoral immunity in young broilers by the dietary supplementation of beta-hydroxy-beta-methylbutyrate. *Immunopharmacol Immunotoxicol.* 1999;21:307-330.

Peterson AL, Qureshi MA, Ferket PR, et al. In vitro exposure with beta-hydroxy-beta-methylbutyrate enhances chicken macrophage growth and function. *Vet Immunol Immunopathol.* 1999;67:67-78.

Wilson GJ, Wilson JM, Manninen AH. Effects of beta-hydroxy-beta-methylbutyrate (HMB) on exercise performance and body composition across varying levels of age, sex, and training experience: A review. *Nutr Metab (Lond).* 2008;5:1.

Beta-Sitosterol

DESCRIPTION

Beta-sitosterol is the most abundant phytosterol in the diet. (See Phytosterols.) It is also widely distributed in the plant kingdom and found in such botanicals as *Serenoa repens* (saw palmetto), *Curcurbita pepo* (pumpkin seed) and *Pygeum africanum.* These three botanicals are used in the herbal management of benign prostatic hypertrophy (BPH). There is some belief that beta-sitosterol plays some role in the possible benefits of these herbs in BPH. Beta-sitosterol itself is used as a medicine in Europe for BPH.

Chemically, beta-sitosterol is a very close relative of cholesterol. It differs from cholesterol by the presence of an ethyl group at the 24th carbon position of the side chain. It is also known as (3beta)-stigmast-5-en-3-ol; 22:23-dihydrostigmasterol; alpha-dihydrofucosterol; delta 5-stigmasten- 3beta-ol; 24beta-ethyl-delta 5-cholesten-3beta-ol; alpha-phytosterol; cinchol; cupreol; rhamnol; quebrachol; and sitosterin. Beta-sitosterol is extremely insoluble in aqueous media and poorly soluble in lipid media. It is found in nature in ester and glycoside forms, both of which forms are more soluble than beta-sitosterol itself. The chemical structure is:

Beta-Sitosterol

ACTIONS AND PHARMACOLOGY

ACTIONS

Beta-sitosterol has possible activity in promoting prostate health. It also has cholesterol-lowering activity.

MECHANISM OF ACTION

See Phytosterols for cholesterol discussion.

The mechanism of its possible action in promoting prostate health is unknown. In one report, beta-sitosterol was found to activate the sphingomyelin cycle and induce apoptosis in LNCaP human prostate cancer cells *in vitro.* There are also reports suggesting it has some anti-inflammatory activity in the prostate.

PHARMACOKINETICS

About 5% of an ingested dose of supplemental beta-sitosterol is absorbed from the gastrointestinal tract and is transported via the portal circulation to the liver. Some beta-sitosterol is glucuronidated in the liver. A portion is also metabolized to cholic acid and chenodesoxycholic acid. Beta-sitosterol is transported via the systemic circulation to other tissues in the body. Excretion is mainly via the biliary route.

INDICATIONS AND USAGE

Beta-sitosterol (the most abundant phytosterol—found in legumes and plentiful in such foods as peanut butter, pistachios and sunflower seeds) is reported to be of some benefit in some patients with benign prostatic hyperplasia (BPH). There are preliminary, non-clinical findings suggesting some possible benefit in some cancers, principally prostate cancer and breast cancer. There is one report indicating that in some circumstances beta-sitosterol might be neurotoxic. There is the suggestion that beta-sitosterol may have favorable immunomodulating effects.

RESEARCH SUMMARY

A review of four double-blind, placebo-controlled studies that tested the efficacy of beta-sitosterol in men with symptomatic benign prostatic hyperplasia concluded that the phytosterol significantly improved urological symptoms and flow measure in those subjects. These trials included 519 men and lasted four to 26 weeks.

Three studies reviewed used nonglucoside beta-sitosterols, and one used a preparation of pure beta-sitosterol-beta-D-glucoside. The latter did not improve flow volume. The reviewers cautioned that, despite positive results to date, "the existing studies are limited by short treatment and lack of standardized beta-sitosterol preparations. Their long-term effectiveness, safety and ability to prevent the complications of benign prostatic hyperplasia are unknown."

Generally, the findings have been that beta-sitosterol does not significantly reduce prostate size compared with placebo but does improve urinary flow measures in those with BPH. Recently there have been some indications that beta-sitosterol might have some direct anticancer potential; *in vitro* it has shown some ability to suppress the proliferation of prostate and breast cancer cells; *in vivo*, in some animal work, it inhibits metastases. There are reports that beta-sitosterol is an agonist for liver X receptors (LXR). LXR agonists have been shown to inhibit a number of cancers both *in vitro* and *in vivo*. One recent study found that beta-sitosterol is an effective apoptosis-promoting agent in a human breast cancer cell line. Another recent study similarly found that beta-sitosterol promotes cell death in both estrogen-receptor-positive and estrogen-receptor-negative human cancer cell lines. More research is needed and warranted.

One group of researchers has reported that when LXR-beta signaling is abnormal, ingestion of beta-sitosterol can lead to neuronal damage in both the spinal cord and substantia nigra, based upon findings in an animal study. They hypothesized that beta-sitosterol "could be a common etiological agent" in Parkinson's dementia and amyotrophic lateral sclerosis (ALS). They found some evidence that the LXR ligand beta-sitosterol depleted cholesterol in brain tissue. The issue needs further research and suggests caution in the use of beta-sitosterol.

A study conducted some years ago suggested that beta-sitosterol may have favorable immunomodulating effects. The researchers reported, among other things, an apparent beta-sitosterol induced enhancement of T-cell proliferative response *in vitro*. More recently, a group of researchers reported that dietary phytosterols, including beta-sitosterol, modulate T-helper immune response but do not induce anti-inflammatory effects in a mouse model of acute, aseptic inflammation. More research is needed.

CONTRAINDICATIONS, PRECAUTIONS, ADVERSE REACTIONS

CONTRAINDICATIONS

Beta-sitosterol is contraindicated in those with known hypersensitivity to the supplement or its components and in those with the genetic disorders sitosterolemia and cerebro-tendinotic xanthomatosis, both rare conditions.

PRECAUTIONS

Beta-sitosterol supplements should be avoided by pregnant women and nursing mothers.

ADVERSE REACTIONS

Reported adverse reactions include gastrointestinal problems, such as indigestion, gas, diarrhea and constipation.

INTERACTIONS

NUTRITIONAL SUPPLEMENTS AND FOODS

Some randomized trials have indicated that phytosterols—beta-sitosterol was the most abundant phytosterol in these studies—may lower serum levels of alpha- and beta-carotene, lycopene and vitamin E, probably by interfering with their absorption.

OVERDOSAGE

No reports of overdoses.

DOSAGE AND ADMINISTRATION

Beta-sitosterol typically comes in mixtures with other phytosterols and also with substances such as pumpkin seed oil and saw palmetto extract. In Europe, doses used for BPH are 20 to 130 milligrams of beta-sitosterol three times daily with meals. Maintenance doses are 10 to 65 milligrams of beta-sitosterol two to three times daily with meals.

LITERATURE

Awad AB, Barta SL, Fink CS, et al. beta-Sitosterol enhances tamoxifen effectiveness on breast cancer cells by affecting ceramide metabolism. *Mol Nutr Food Res.* 2008;52(4):419-426.

Awad AB, Burr AT, Fink CS. Effect of resveratrol and beta-sitosterol in combination on reactive oxygen species and prostaglandin release by PC-3 cells. *Prostaglandins Leukot Essent Fatty Acids.* 2005;72(3):219-226.

Awad AB, Chan KC, Downie AC, et al. Peanuts as a source of beta-sitosterol, a sterol with anticancer properties. *Nutr Cancer.* 2000;36(2):238-241.

Awad AB, Chinnam M, Fink CS, et al. beta-Sitosterol activates Fas signaling in human breast cancer cells. *Phytomedicine.* 2007;14(11):747-754.

Awad AB, Fink CS, Williams H, et al. In vitro and in vivo (SCID mice) effects of phytosterols on the growth and dissemination of human prostate cancer PC-3 cells. *Eur J Cancer Prev.* 2001;10(6):507-513.

Awad AB, Gan Y, Fink CS. Effect of beta-sitosterol, a plant sterol, on growth, protein phosphatase 2A, and phospholipase D in LNCaP cells. *Nutr Cancer.* 2000;36(1):74-78.

Berges RR, Windeler J, Trampisch HJ, et al. Randomized placebo-controlled, double-blind clinical trial of beta-sitosterol in patient with benign prostatic hyperplasia. Beta-sitosterol Study Group. *Lancet.* 1995;345;1529-1532.

Bradford PG, Awad AB. Phytosterols as anticancer compounds. *Mol Nutr Food Res.* 2007;51(2):161-170.

Cabeza M, Bratoeff E, Heuze I, et al. Effect of beta-sitosterol as inhibitor of 5 alpha-reductase in hamster prostate. *Proc West Pharmacol Soc.*2003;46:153-155.

Chuu CP, Kokontis JM, Hiipakka RA, et al. Modulation of liver X receptor signaling as novel therapy for prostate cancer. *J Biomed Sci.* 2007;14(5):543-553.

Kassen A, Berges R, Senge T. Effect of beta-sitosterol on transforming growth factor-beta-1 expression and translocation protein kinase C alpha in human prostate stromal cells in vitro. *Eur Urol.* 2000;37(6):735-741.

Kim HJ, Fan X, Gabbi C, et al. Liver X receptor beta (LXRbeta): a link between beta-sitosterol and amyotrophic lateral sclerosis-Parkinson's dementia. *Proc Natl Acad Sci U S A.* 2008 Feb;105(6):2094-2099.

Kobayashi Y, Sugaya Y, Tokue A. [Clinical effects of beta-sitosterol (phytosterol) on benign prostatic hyperplasia: preliminary study.] [Article in Japanese.] *Hinyokika Kiyo.* 1998;44:865-868.

Moon DO, Kim MO, Choi YH, et al. beta-Sitosterol induces G2/M arrest, endoreduplication, and apoptosis through the Bcl-2 and PI3K/Akt signaling pathways. *Cancer Lett.* 2008;264(2):181-191.

Moon DO, Lee KJ, Choi YH, et al. Beta-sitosterol-induced-apoptosis is mediated by the activation of ERK and the downregulation of Akt in MCA-102 murine fibrosarcoma cells. *Int Immunopharmacol.* 2007;7(8):1044-1053.

Normé n L, Dutta P, Lia A, et al. Soy sterol esters and beta-sitostanol ester as inhibitors of cholesterol absorption in human small bowel. *Am J Clin Nutr.* 2000;71:908-913.

Park C, Moon DO, Ryu CH, et al. Beta-sitosterol sensitizes MDA-MB-231 cells to TRAIL-induced apoptosis. *Acta Pharmacol Sin.* 2008;29(3):341-348.

von Holtz RL, Fink CS, Awad AB. Beta-sitosterol activates the sphingomyelin cycle and induces apoptosis in LNCaP human prostate cancer cells. *Nutr Cancer.* 1998;32:8-12.

Wilt T, Ishani A, MacDonald R, et al. Beta-sitosterols for benign prostatic hyperplasia. *Cochrane Database Syst Rev.* 2000;(2):CD001043.

Wilt TJ, MacDonald R, Ishani A. beta-sitosterol for the treatment of benign prostatic hyperplasia: a systematic review. *BJU Int.* 1999;83(9):976-983.

Betaine and Betaine Hydrochloride

DESCRIPTION

Betaine or trimethylglycine is a quarternary ammonium compound that was first discovered in the juice of sugar beets (*Beta vulgaris*). Betaine is a metabolite of choline (see Choline) and is a substrate in one of the two recycling pathways that convert homocysteine to L-methionine. The other and principal recycling reaction is catalyzed by the enzyme methionine synthase and uses methylcobalamin as a cofactor and 5-methyltetrahydrofolate as a cosubstrate (see Folate and Vitamin B_{12}).

Betaine, in the form of a white, granular, hygroscopic powder referred to as anhydrous betaine, is an orphan drug for the treatment of homocystinuria. Homocystinuria is a rare genetic disorder caused by any one of three inborn errors of metabolism. One type is known as cystathionine beta-synthase deficiency. Cystathionine beta-synthase is the enzyme that converts homocysteine to cystathionine, a precursor of cysteine. This is the most common genetic cause of homocystinuria. Cystathionine beta-synthase is a vitamin B_6-dependent enzyme, and deficiency of this enzyme may be responsive to treatment with vitamin B_6 (see Vitamin B_6).

A second type of inborn error of metabolism resulting in homocystinuria is due to deficiency of 5,10-methylenetetra-hydrofolate reductase. This enzyme catalyzes the conversion of 5-methylenetetrahydrofolate to 5-methyltetrahydrofolate, the cosubstrate in the methionine synthase reaction mentioned above. The third type of inborn error of metabolism that can result in homocystinuria is due to a defect in the synthesis of methylcobalamin, the cofactor in the methionine synthase reaction. Betaine therapy may be effective in the treatment of all three of these primary types of homocystinuria.

Betaine is also known as trimethylglycine, N-trimethylglycine, glycine betaine, glycocoll betaine, oxyneurine and lycine. Its chemical name is 1-carboxy-N,N,N-trimethylmethanaminium inner salt. The molecular formula of betaine is $C_5H_{11}NO_2$, its chemical formula is $(CH_3)_3N^+\text{-}CH_2COO^-$ and its molecular weight is 117.15 daltons. Betaine is very soluble in water and has a sweet taste. It is widely distributed in plants and animals. The hydrochloride of betaine is known as betaine hydrochloride, betaine HCL and pluchine. Its chemical name is 1-carboxy-N,N,N-trimethylmethanaminium chloride. The pH of a 5% aqueous solution of betaine hydrochloride is 1.

Betaine is represented by the following chemical structure:

Betaine

Both betaine and betaine hydrochloride are available as dietary supplements.

ACTIONS AND PHARMACOLOGY

ACTIONS

Betaine may lower elevated homocysteine levels in some. Betaine may also have lipotropic and hepatoprotective activity. Betaine hydrochloride is a delivery form of hydrochloric acid and may aid in digestion in some.

MECHANISM OF ACTION

Betaine-homocysteine methyltransferase (BHMT) is a zinc metalloenzyme which catalyzes the transfer of a methyl group from betaine to homocysteine in the formation of methionine. BHMT is found in the liver and kidneys and may also exist in brain tissue. Betaine acts to lower homocysteine levels in some with primary hyperhomocysteinemia/homocystinuria via this enzyme. Betaine has also been found to lower homocysteine levels in some animal studies, again, via BHMT. Mild to moderate elevation of homocysteine without homocystinuria is thought to be an independent risk factor for coronary heart disease. Betaine may lower elevated homocysteine levels in some with mild to moderate hyperhomocysteinemia, but this needs to be confirmed. A good group for such a study would be those with the C677T mutation for 5-methylenetetrahydrofolate reductase which occurs in approximately 10% of the population.

A lipotropic agent is defined as a substance that prevents the deposition of fat in the liver or accelerates its removal. The condition of fatty degeneration is called steatosis. Betaine, choline and L-methionine have been found to prevent or to reverse hepatic steatosis in experimental animals. It is thought that the lipotropic activity of betaine, choline and L-methionine is mediated via the body's principal transmethy-

lating agent, S-adenosylmethionine (SAMe). SAMe is involved in a number of biochemical functions that may promote liver health, including its role in the formation of phospholipids which are essential for normal cell membrane formation and function (see S-Adenosyl-L-Methionine). SAMe's methyl group is derived from betaine via the betaine-homocysteine methyltransferase reaction which provides the immediate precursor of SAMe, L-methionine. Choline is metabolized to betaine via the enzymes choline dehydrogenase and betaine aldehyde dehydrogenase. Thus, through a couple of transmethylations, the methyl group in choline winds up as the methyl group in SAMe.

Betaine has been found to protect the livers of experimental animals against the hepatotoxins ethanol and carbon tetrachloride. The hepatoprotective effect of betaine is thought to be mediated via SAMe, as discussed above. Betaine may have hepatoprotective activity as well as lipotropic activity in humans, but this has not been confirmed. Another possible hepatoprotective mechanism of betaine, at least in animals, may be due to its osmolyte activity. Betaine has been shown to be an intracellular osmolyte in rat liver macrophages (Kupffer cells) and sinusoidal endothelial cells, and may play an important role in the functions of these cells.

As an interesting aside, the osmoprotective effect of betaine has been found to be cytoprotective in the deep freezing of stallion sperm and also has been found to protect salmon from the physiological stress induced by transfer from fresh water to seawater. The osmoprotective effect of betaine may be due to an interaction between this substance and chloride ions. There is as yet no evidence that the osmoprotective effect of betaine has any consequence for humans.

Betaine hydrochloride is a delivery form of hydrochloric acid. Some with hypochlorhydria have used betaine hydrochloride alone, or in combination with pepsin, as a digestive aid.

PHARMACOKINETICS

Betaine is absorbed from the small intestines into the enterocytes. It is released by the enterocytes into the portal circulation which carries it to the liver where there is significant first-pass extraction and first-pass metabolism of betaine. The principal metabolic reaction is the transfer of a methyl group from betaine to homocysteine via the enzyme betaine-homocysteine methyltransferase. The products of the reaction are L-methionine and dimethylglycine. Betaine hydrochloride is converted to betaine in the alkaline environment of the small intestine.

INDICATIONS AND USAGE

Anhydrous betaine has been useful in the treatment of homocystinuria and betaine may be helpful in other conditions characterized by elevated plasma homocysteine levels.

Betaine hydrochloride is used as a digestive aid in some. There is some suggestion in animal research that betaine may be hepatoprotective in some circumstances.

RESEARCH SUMMARY

Betaine has been shown in numerous studies to be of significant benefit in all three primary types of homocystinuria. Clinical improvement has been reported in about 75% of the cases treated with betaine in these studies.

It has been suggested but not yet demonstrated that betaine might also be useful in other conditions characterized by elevated plasma homocysteine levels, such as those that have been noted in some with premature vascular disease and chronic renal failure.

Since hyperhomocysteinemia is thought to be an independent cardiovascular risk factor, betaine's role as a potential cardioprotector is suggested but, again, not yet demonstrated. Recently it was hypothesized that some of red wine's putative cardioprotective activity could be due to the fact that betaine is added to some wines via beet sugar used to increase alcohol content. More research is needed.

Several animal studies have indicated that betaine exerts some hepatoprotective effects. In one of these studies, betaine significantly speeded recovery of carbon tetrachloride-injured liver. It has also been credited with helping to protect against alcoholic steatosis resulting from dietary ethanol. Whether it might help similarly protect against or reverse fatty infiltration of the liver in humans has not yet been studied.

Betaine hydrochloride has been used for some time as a digestive aid. Those with excessive stomach acid should avoid this use.

CONTRAINDICATIONS, PRECAUTIONS, ADVERSE REACTIONS

CONTRAINDICATIONS

Betaine and betaine hydrochloride are contraindicated in those hypersensitive to any component of a betaine- or betaine hydrochloride-containing product.

PRECAUTIONS

Pregnant women and nursing mothers should avoid the use of betaine and betaine hydrochloride supplements.

Those with gastritis, gastroesophageal reflux disease (GERD) or peptic ulcer disease should avoid the use of betaine hydrochloride supplements.

ADVERSE REACTIONS

Occasional nausea, vomiting and diarrhea have been reported.

INTERACTIONS

NUTRITIONAL SUPPLEMENTS

Folic acid: Concomitant use of betaine and folic acid may be additive with regard to the possible lowering of serum homocysteine levels.

OVERDOSAGE

There are no reports of betaine overdosage in the literature.

DOSAGE AND ADMINISTRATION

Betaine and betaine hydrochloride are available as dietary supplements.

There are no typical doses for the management of mild to moderate hyperhomocysteinemia. Three grams taken twice daily were used in one small preliminary study showing a serum homocysteine-lowering effect.

Those who use betaine hydrochloride as a digestive aid, typically take a dose of 600 to 650 milligrams (usually in a combination product with pepsin) following a meal.

LITERATURE

Barak AJ, Tuma DJ. Betaine, metabolic by-product or vital methylating agent? *Life Sci.* 1983; 32:771-774.

Barak AJ, Beckenhauser HC, Tuma DJ. Betaine effects on hepatic methionine metabolism elicited by short-term ethanol feeding. *Alcohol.* 1996; 13:483-486.

Barak AJ, Beckenhauser HC, Tuma DJ. Betaine, ethanol and the liver: a review. *Alcohol.* 1996; 13:395-398.

Barak AJ, Beckenhauser HC, Badakhsh S, Tuma DJ. The effect of betaine in reversing alcoholic steatosis. *Alcohol Clin Exp Res.* 1997; 21:1100-1102.

Brower IA, Verhoef P, Urgert R. Betaine supplementation and plasma homocysteine in healthy volunteers. *Arch Inter Med.* 2000; 160:2546-2547.

Davies SEC, Chalmers RA, Randall EW, Iles RA. Betaine metabolism in human neonates and developing rats. *Clin Chim Acta.* 1988; 178:241-250.

Gahl WA, Bernardini I, Chen S, et al. The effect of oral betaine on vertebral body bone density in pyridoxine-non-responsive homocystinuria. *J Inher Metab Dis.* 1988; 11:291-298.

Holme E, Kjellman B, Ronge E. Betaine for treatment of homocystinuria caused by methylenetetrahydrofolate reductase deficiency. *Arch Dis Childhood.* 1989; 64:1064.

Junnila M, Barak AJ, Beckenhauer HC, Rahko T. Betaine reduces hepatic lipidosis induced by carbon tetrachloride in Sprague-Dawley rats. *Vet Hum Toxicol.* 1998; 40:263-266.

Junnila M, Rahko T, Sukura A, Lindberg L-A. Reduction of carbon tetrachloride-induced hepatotoxic effects by oral administration of betaine in male Han: Wistar rats. A morphometric histological study. *Vet Pathol.* 2000; 37:221-238.

Koskinen E, Junnila M, Katila T, Soini H. A preliminary study on the use of betaine as a cryoprotective agent in the deep freezing of stallion semen. *Zentralbl Veterinarmed A.* 1989; 36:110-114.

Millian NS, Garrow TA. Human betaine-homocysteine methyltransferase is a zinc metalloenzyme. *Arch Biochem Biophys.* 1998; 356:93-98.

Smolin LA, Benevenga NJ, Berlow S. The use of betaine for the treatment of homocystinuria. *J Pediatr.* 1981; 99:467-472.

Virtanen E, Junnila M, Soivio A. Effects of food containing betaine/amino acid additive on the osmotic adaptation of young Atlantic salmon, *Salmo Salar* L. *Aquaculture.* 1989; 83:109-122.

Wendel U, Bremer HJ. Betaine in the treatment of homocystinuria due to 5,10-methylenetetrahydrofolate reductase deficiency. *Eur J Pediatr.* 1984; 142:147-150.

Wettstein M, Haussinger D. Cytoprotection by the osmolytes betaine and taurine in ischemia-reoxygenation injury in the perfused rat liver. *Hepatology.* 1997; 26:1560-1566.

Wettstein M, Weik C, Holneicher C, Haussinger D. Betaine as an osmolyte in rat liver: metabolism and cell-to-cell interactions. *J Hepatol.* 1998; 27:787-793.

Wilcken DE, Dudman NP, Tyrrell PA. Homocystinuria due to cystathionine beta-synthase deficiency — the effects of betaine treatment in pyridoxine-responsive patients. *Metabolism.* 1985; 34:1115-1121.

Wilcken DE, Wilcken B, Dudman NP, Tyrrell PA. Homocystinuria — the effects of betaine in the treatment of patients not responsive to pyridoxine. *N Engl J Med.* 1983; 309:448-453.

Biochanin A

DESCRIPTION

Biochanin A (BCA) belongs to the isoflavone class of flavonoids. It is also classified as a phytoestrogen since it is a plant-derived nonsteroidal compound that possesses estrogen-like biological activity. Biochanin A has been found to have weak estrogenic activity.

Biochanin A is found in certain legumes, most notably red clover or *Trifolium pratense*. Red clover contains, in addition to biochanin A, the isoflavones genistein, daidzein and formononetin (methoxy daidzein). These isoflavones are present in red clover in the form of glycosides. However, when the leaves are crushed during the preparation of red clover isoflavone extracts, the glycosides undergo enzymatic hydrolysis, and the final preparation principally contains the aglycones.

Biochanin A is a solid substance that is virtually insoluble in water. Its molecular formula is $C_{16}H_{12}O_5$. It is the 4'-methyl ether of genistein. Biochanin A is also known as 5, 7-dihydroxy-4'-methoxyisoflavone and 5, 7-dihydroxy-4' -methoxy-3- (4-hydroxyphenyl)-4*H*-1-benzopyran-4-one.

ACTIONS AND PHARMACOLOGY

ACTIONS

Biochanin A has estrogenic activity. It may also have antioxidant, anticarcinogenic, anti-atherogenic and anti-osteoporotic activities.

MECHANISM OF ACTION

Biochanin A has weak estrogenic activity as measured in *in vivo* and *in vitro* assays.

Structurally, biochanin A would be expected to be able to scavenge reactive oxygen species and inhibit lipid peroxidation. However, there are few studies demonstrating this.

There are cell culture and animal studies indicating that biochanin A has anticarcinogenic activity.

Biochanin A has been found to have hypolipidemic activity in some animal models. Again the mechanism of this possible effect, as well as the mechanism of any anti-atherogenic activity, is unclear.

In comparison with other isoflavones, such as genistein and daidzein, biochanin A might be expected to have possible anti-osteoporotic activity. This might be due, in part, to its weak estrogenic activity.

PHARMACOKINETICS

Little is known about the pharmacokinetics of biochanin A in humans. Inferences can be drawn from some animal studies. Biochanin A appears to be absorbed from the small intestine from whence it is transported to the systemic circulation by the lymphatics. There is little information available on the tissue distribution of biochanin A. It appears that biochanin A delivered to the liver undergoes extensive conjugation with glucuronate and sulfate via hepatic UDP-glucuronosyl-transferases and sulfotransferases. The glucuronide and sulfate conjugates of biochanin A are excreted in the urine and the bile.

It is likely that there is considerable variation in the absorption and metabolism of ingested biochanin A.

INDICATIONS AND USAGE

There is very preliminary evidence that biochanin A may have some anti-atherosclerotic and anticarcinogenic effects. There are anecdotal reports that it may be helpful in ameliorating some of the problems associated with menopause, including osteoporosis.

RESEARCH SUMMARY

Biochanin A significantly reduced the incidence of chemically induced rat mammary cancer in a recent study. Multiplicity of tumors was also significantly decreased in biochanin A-supplemented animals, compared with unsupplemented controls. There is, additionally, some preliminary evidence that biochanin A may have some hypolipidemic effects. Clinical studies are lacking.

CONTRAINDICATIONS, PRECAUTIONS, ADVERSE REACTIONS

CONTRAINDICATIONS

Biochanin A is contraindicated in those who are hypersensitive to any component of a biochanin A-containing product.

PRECAUTIONS

Pregnant women and nursing mothers should avoid the use of biochanin A-containing supplements.

Women with estrogen receptor-positive tumors should exercise caution in the use of biochanin A-containing supplements and should use them only if they are recommended and monitored by a physician.

DOSAGE AND ADMINISTRATION

Biochanin A-containing supplements are derived from red clover and, in addition to biochanin A, usually contain the isoflavones genistein, daidzein and formononetin. A typical dose of such an isoflavone mixture—which also contains ingredients other than isoflavones—is 40 mg daily.

LITERATURE

Gotoh T, Yamada K, Yin H, et al. Chemoprevention of N-nitroso-N-methylurea-induced rat mammary carcinogenesis by soy foods or biochanin A. *Jpn J Cancer Res.* 1998; 89:137-142.

Lee YS, Kim TH, Cho KJ, Jang JJ. Inhibitory effects of biochanin A on benzo[a]pyrene induced carcinogenesis in mice. *In vivo.* 1992; 6:283-286.

Moon YJ, Shin BS, An G, Morris ME. Biochanin A inhibits breast cancer tumor growth in a murine xenograft model. *Pharm Res.* 2008;25(9):2158-2163.

Siddiqui MT, Siddiqui M. Hypolipidemic principles of *Cicer Arietnum*: biochanin A and formononetin. *Lipids.* 1976; 11:243-246.

Yanagihara K, Ito A, Toge T, Numoto M. Antiproliferative effects of isoflavones on human cancer cell lines established from the gastrointestinal tract. *Cancer Res.* 1993; 53:5815-5821.

Biotin

DESCRIPTION

Biotin, a member of the B-vitamin family, is an essential nutrient in human nutrition. It is involved in the biosynthesis of fatty acids, gluconeogenesis, energy production, the metabolism of the branched-chain amino acids (L-leucine, L-isoleucine, L-valine) and the *de novo* synthesis of purine nucleotides. Recent research indicates that biotin plays a role in gene expression, both at the transcriptional and translational levels, and that it may also play a role in DNA replication.

Biotin is widely distributed in natural foodstuffs. However, the absolute amounts of biotin in foodstuffs is relatively low when compared with the other B vitamins. Some of the better food sources of biotin, are egg yolk, liver, kidney, pancreas, milk, soya and barley. Brewer's yeast or *Saccharomyces cerevisiae* (see Brewer's Yeast), which is used as a nutritional supplement, is one of the richest sources of biotin, as well as the other B vitamins. Royal jelly, also used as a nutritional supplement (see Royal Jelly), is another rich source of biotin. Mammals and many plant species are unable to synthesize biotin. Biotin is synthesized by bacteria, yeast and other fungi, algae and certain plant species. In fact, the microflora of the human large intestine appear to contribute to the biotin requirements of the body.

The first demonstration of biotin deficiency in animals was observed in animals fed raw egg white. Rats fed egg white protein were found to develop dermatitis, hair loss and neuromuscular dysfunction. This syndrome was called egg white injury and was discovered to be caused by a glycoprotein found in egg white called avidin. It was subsequently found that egg white injury could be cured by a liver factor which was first called protective factor X and later determined to be biotin. Because biotin cured the skin disorder of egg white injury it was called vitamin H. H is for haut, the German word for skin. Avidin causes egg white injury because it binds very tightly to biotin, preventing its absorption. This is only true for native avidin, which is resistant to hydrolysis by proteolytic enzymes. When egg white is cooked, avidin is denatured and denatured avidin is digested by proteolytic enzymes.

Although clinical biotin deficiency in humans is rare, it does occur. Prolonged consumption of raw egg white, long-term total parenteral nutrition without biotin supplementation and malabsorption syndromes, such as short-gut syndrome, have resulted in biotin deficiency states. The symptoms and signs of biotin deficiency, include a generalized erythematous scaly skin eruption, alopecia, conjunctivitis and neurological abnormalities. The rash may be distributed around the eyes, nose, mouth, ears and perineal orifices. The facial appearance associated with the deficiency, with the rash around the eyes, nose and mouth along with an unusual distribution of facial fat, is called biotin deficiency facies. In biotin deficient infants, the neurological findings are hypotonia, lethargy and developmental delay. In adults, the neurological findings are lethargy, depression, hallucinations and paresthesias of the extremities. Marginal biotin status may occur under certain conditions, e.g., during the first trimester of pregnancy, and it is thought that this situation may be teratogenic. Functional biotin deficiency occurs in certain genetic disorders. These will be discussed below.

Biotin is the coenzyme for four carboxylases. Acetyl coenzyme A (CoA) carboxylase, found in both the mitochondria and cytosol, catalyzes the carboxylation of acetyl-CoA to malonyl-CoA. Malonyl-CoA is the immediate precursor of 14 of the 16 carbon atoms of the fatty acid palmitic acid. It is also the immediate precursor of all of the fatty acids up to palmitic acid. Further, the reaction catalyzed by acetyl-CoA carboxylase, a complex reaction, is the primary regulatory, or rate-limiting, step in the biosynthesis of fatty acids. Pyruvate carboxylase, which is located in the mitochondria, catalyzes the carboxylation of pyruvate to form oxaloacetate. Oxaloacetate can be metabolized in the tricarboxylic acid cycle or it can be converted to glucose in the liver and kidney and other tissues that are involved in gluconeogenesis. The formation of oxaloacetate from pyruvate is known as an anaplerotic reaction. Anaplerotic is from the Greek word anaplerosis, meaning filling up or restoration. The pyruvate carboxylate reaction is the principal reaction which replenishes tricarboxylic acid cycle intermediates. Methylcrotonyl-CoA carboxylase, also located in the mitochondria, is involved in the metabolism of L-leucine, while the mitochondrial enzyme propionyl-CoA carboxylase is involved in the metabolism of L-isoleucine and L-valine, as well as L-threonine and L-methionine.

All four of the carboxylase enzymes, which use bicarbonate as their one-carbon substrate, share a common biochemical mechanism. In all four carboxylases, biotin is covalently linked by an amide bond between the carboxyl group of the valeric side chain of biotin and an epsilon-amino group of a specific lysyl residue in the apocarboxylase. The enzyme that catalyzes the formation of the covalent bond is called holocarboxylase synthetase. Biotin is recycled by the enzyme biotinidase. Biotinidase, an hydrolase, functions to recycle biotin by cleaving biocytin (epsilon-N-biotinyl-L-lysine), or short-chain oligopeptides containing biotin-linked lysyl residues, products of the normal breakdown of the holocarboxylases, to free biotin. Biotinidase is also thought to play a critical role in the release of biotin from biotin-containing dietary proteins. Recently, biotinidase has been found to have biotinyl-transferase activity. All five classes of histones are selectively biotinylated via the biotinyl-transferase activity of biotinidase. It is thought that biotinylation of histones is involved in the regulation of gene transcription and may also play a role in the packaging of DNA. Interestingly, biotinylation is an important technique in molecular biology. Biotin can be covalently linked to both proteins and nucleic acids, and is used as a label in many molecular biology and biochemistry technologies.

Certain inborn errors of metabolism result in functional biotin deficiency. These disorders, include multiple carboxylase deficiency, holocarboxylase synthetase deficiency, biotinidase deficiency and propionic-CoA carboxylase deficiency. Those with these disorders require much greater cellular biotin levels than normal in order to activate these biotin-dependent enzymes. Biotinidase deficiency is the most common cause of late-onset multiple carboxylase deficiency. Features of late-onset multiple carboxylase deficiency, include skin rash, alopecia, seizures, hypotonia, ataxia, hearing loss, optic atrophy, developmental delay, immune deficiency and recurrent infections. Coma and death may occur if the disorder is not treated. The treatment is high-dose biotin, which results in pronounced, rapid clinical and biochemical improvement. Holocarboxylase deficiency is the most common form of multiple carboxylase deficiency in neonates. Features of neonatal multiple carboxylase deficiency, include lethargy, hypotonia, vomiting, alopecia, lactic acidosis, keratoconjunctivitis, perioral erosions and seizures. Again, the treatment is high-dose biotin, which may completely reverse the symptoms and signs of the disorder. There is a relatively high incidence or propionyl-CoA carboxylase deficiency among the Inuits of Greenland. Those with this deficiency may present early in life with a severe, often fatal metabolic acidosis, hyperglycinemia and hyperammonemia. The only known treatment for this disorder is high-dose biotin. All of the above inborn errors of metabolism are referred to as biotin-responsive disorders.

Biotin is a bicyclic compound. The tetrahydrothiophene ring contains sulfur and has a valeric acid side chain. The second ring contains a ureido group. Eight stereoisomers of biotin exist. However, only one is found naturally, and it is the only one that is enzymatically active. The natural stereoisomer of biotin is called d-(+)-biotin or just biotin. In addition to being known as vitamin H, biotin is also known as hexahydro-2-oxo-1*H*-thieno[3,4-*d*]imidazole-4-pentanoic acid; *cis*-5-(hexahydro-2-oxo-1*H*-thieno[3,4-*d*]imidazol-4-yl)valeric acid; *cis*-tetrahydro-2-oxothieno[3,4-*d*]imidazoline-4-valeric acid; *cis*-hexahydro-2-oxo-1*H*-thieno[3,4]imidazole-4-valeric acid; coenzyme R and bios IIb. Its molecular formula is $C_{10}H_{16}N_2O_3S$ and its molecular weight is 244.31 daltons. Biocytin or epsilon-N-biotinyl-L-lysine is a naturally occurring complex of biotin which has approximately the same biochemical activity as biotin.

ACTIONS AND PHARMACOLOGY

ACTIONS

Biotin is used for the treatment of biotin-responsive inborn errors of metabolism. It has putative glucose tolerance-modulating activity. It may also have activity in the management of brittle fingernails and the uncombable hair syndrome. There is some evidence that it may have antioxidant activity.

MECHANISM OF ACTION

Holocarboxylase synthetase catalyzes the biotinylation of the four biotin-dependent carboxylases in humans. Holocarboxylase synthetase deficiency is the most common cause of neonatal multiple carboxylase deficiency. Biotinidase catalyzes the recycling of biotin, among other reactions. Biotinidase deficiency is the most common cause of late-onset multiple carboxylase deficiency. Cellular biotin concentrations higher than are normally present, are required to activate the mutant holocarboxylase synthetase and biotinidase enzymes. Biotin does not bind to the mutant enzymes as strongly as it does to non-mutant enzymes and therefore, greater amounts of biotin are required for their activation. Biotin may also play a role in the regulation of the transcription of holocarboxylase synthetase.

Biotin supplementation has been found to improve glucose tolerance and decrease insulin resistance in a diabetic mouse model. It has also been found to influence hepatic glucokinase expression both at the transcriptional and translational levels in cell culture. More recently, biotin has been shown to affect pancreatic islet glucokinase activity and expression and insulin secretion in cultured rat islet cells. Glucokinase has a central regulatory role in glucose metabolism. The results of above studies suggest that the administration of supplementary biotin may improve the metabolism and/or utilization of glucose in those with type 2 diabetes mellitus. Clinical trials are needed.

Some studies have found that high doses of biotin are helpful in the management of brittle fingernails in women. The rationale to use biotin for this condition came from the finding that pathologic hoof changes in horses and swine can be treated with oral biotin. The mechanism of the possible effect of biotin in the management of brittle fingernails is not known. Biotin deficiency does cause skin changes. However, the subjects studied were not biotin deficient.

The uncombable hair syndrome, also known as spun-glass hair and cheveux incoiffables, is a rare congenital disorder. It is characterized by a longitudinal grooving of the hair shaft resulting in a triangular cross section (pili trianguli et canaliculi). There is a report of biotin reversing scaling, hair loss, hair fragility, and uncombability in a two-year old boy with the syndrome. The hair remained combable even after one year. The mechanism of action of biotin in this condition is not known. Perhaps some cases of uncombable hair syndrome are biotin-responsive. The uncombable hair syndrome should not be confused with cowlicks, localized patches of hair that will not comb down. The cowlick is not a forme fruste of the uncombable hair syndrome, nor is there any evidence that biotin has any effect on cowlicks.

Biotin has been found to inhibit the generation of reactive oxygen species, including superoxide anions, by neutrophils, *in vitro*. The mechanism of this antioxidant effect is unknown. Biotin does not appear to scavenge superoxide anions.

PHARMACOKINETICS

The intestine is exposed to biotin from a few sources: the diet, biotin supplements and biotin synthesized by bacteria in the large intestine. Dietary biotin exists in free and protein-bound forms. Protein-bound biotin is digested by proteases and peptidases to biotin-containing oligopeptides and biocytin (epsilon-N-biotinyl-L-lysine). Biocytin and the biotin-containing oligopeptides are converted to biotin via the enzyme biotinidase. Biotin—both dietary-derived biotin and supplementary biotin—is efficiently absorbed from the small intestine. At doses of biotin derived from food, biotin appears to be transported into enterocytes by a sodium-dependent carrier. At higher doses of biotin, absorption appears to occur by passive diffusion. Absorption of the biotin produced by the colonic microflora, appears to occur by a carrier mediated process in the proximal large intestine.

Biotin is transported to the liver via the portal circulation and by the systemic circulation, to the other tissues of the body. Biotin appears to be transported in the serum in both bound and unbound forms. Uptake of biotin by cells appears to occur by both a sodium-dependent carrier process and by passive diffusion. Transport of biotin across the blood-brain barrier appears to occur by a saturable transport mechanism. Placental transport of biotin appears to occur by a passive process. Within cells, the carboxylases (pyruvate carboxylase, acetyl-CoA carboxylase, 3-methylcrotonyl-CoA carboxylase, propionyl-CoA carboxylase) are biotinylated via holocarboxylase synthetase. Biotin and apocarboxylases are the substrates. ATP and magnesium also participate in the reaction. Biotin is recycled from the holocarboxylases via the action of proteolytic enzymes and biotinidase. Biotin is catabolized to a number of different metabolites, including bisnorbiotin, biotin sulfoxide, biotin sulfone, bisonorbiotin methylketone and tetranorbiotin-1-sulfoxide. Biotin is excreted in the urine as biotin, bisnorbiotin, biotin sulfoxide, biotin sulfone, bisnorbiotin methyl ketone and tetranobiotin-1-sulfoxide.

INDICATIONS AND USAGE

Biotin is used to treat the biotin-responsive inborn errors of metabolism holocarboxylase synthetase deficiency and biotinidase deficiency. Holocarboxylase deficiency is the most common cause of neonatal multiple carboxylase deficiency. Biotinidase deficiency is the most common cause of late-onset multiple carboxylase deficiency.

Recent studies have revealed that even marginal biotin deficiency is teratogenic in many mammals. This is of special concern since there is also now data showing that marginal biotin deficiency occurs in a significant proportion of pregnant women. It is too early to recommend widespread biotin supplementation during pregnancy, but the use of this vitamin might be indicated in some pregnant women whose physicians advise its use. There is very preliminary evidence that supplemental biotin might improve disordered glucose metabolism and thus might be helpful in some cases of diabetes. It may also be indicated in some cases of those on total parenteral nutrition and in some with brittle nails. There is some dated evidence that biotin can favorably affect lipids. There is no evidence that it can restore hair growth except in some cases of biotin deficiency. Nor will it reverse graying of hair. There is some evidence, however, that it may help manage the "uncombable hair syndrome," a rare condition seen in children. There is no evidence that biotin improves exercise performance.

RESEARCH SUMMARY

Biotin deficiency has been shown to cause birth defects in several animal, including mammalian, species. The level of deficiency required to be teratogenic is marginal, insufficient to produce any of the typical cutaneous and behavioral manifestations of more pronounced deficiency. These findings, coupled with recent disclosures that marginal biotin deficiency occurs in a significant proportion of pregnant women, raises serious concern.

A recent analysis of data from a multivitamin supplementation study has led one research group to conclude that there is at least indirect evidence of teratogenicity due to marginal biotin deficiency in humans. Adding to the concern are further findings that biotin deficiency can occur spontaneously in normal human gestation, that biotin transport by the human placenta is mainly passive and that proliferating cells have increased biotin requirements.

More research is required before biotin can be recommended for pregnant women as an antiteratogen, but physicians may find it appropriate to recommend its use in individual cases.

There are some recent preliminary animal studies suggesting that biotin may help improve glucose metabolism in ways that might be beneficial in some with diabetes. In one experiment, biotin supplemented diabetic mice had, compared with controls, lowered post-prandial glucose levels, improved glucose tolerance and decreased insulin resistance. Similar results were obtained in another animal study, leading the researchers to conclude that biotin may be helpful to patients with non-insulin-dependent diabetes mellitus (type 2 diabetes mellitus).

It has been claimed that supplemental biotin can reverse loss and graying of hair. In fact, biotin and pantothenic acid are widely used in cosmetic hair products. Except in cases of frank biotin deficiency, there appears to be no basis for this claim. There is a report, however, that severe hair loss secondary to biotin deficiency occurs in some patients receiving total parenteral nutrition (TPN). Supplementation with 200 micrograms of biotin daily has resulted in gradual regrowth of healthy hair in some of these patients.

There is also a report that supplemental biotin can help tame "uncombable hair syndrome" characterized by hair loss, hair fragility and uncombability, a rare disorder of children.

Biotin reportedly benefits some with brittle nails, as well. Supplementation with biotin resulted in a significant thickening of nail plates in 63% of subjects in a Swiss study.

There is a dated (1980) report that 0.9 milligrams of biotin daily for 71 days significantly and favorably affected lipids in 40 subjects aged 30-60. This isolated report needs follow-up.

CONTRAINDICATIONS, PRECAUTIONS, ADVERSE REACTIONS

CONTRAINDICATIONS

Biotin is contraindicated in those hypersensitive to any component of a biotin-containing product.

PRECAUTIONS

Pregnant women and nursing mothers should avoid supplemental doses of biotin greater than the adequate intakes (AI) recommended by the Food and Nutrition Board, unless higher doses are prescribed by their physicians. The AIs are 30 micrograms/day for pregnant women and 35 micrograms/day for nursing mothers.

The use of biotin for the treatment of a biotin-responsive medical conditions requires medical supervision.

ADVERSE REACTIONS

There are no reports of adverse reactions associated with biotin supplementation in the literature.

INTERACTIONS

DRUGS

Antibiotics: Antibiotic use may decrease the biotin contribution to the body made by the microflora of the large intestine.

Anticonvulsants (carbamazepine, phenytoin, phenobarbital, primidone): Carbamazepine, phenytoin and phenobarbital can accelerate biotin metabolism and may cause reduced biotin status. Long-term use of carbamazepine, phenytoin, phenobarbital and primidone has been associated with reduced plasma concentrations of biotin.

NUTRITIONAL SUPPLEMENTS

Pantothenic Acid: High-doses of pantothenic acid may inhibit the absorption of biotin produced by the microflora in the large intestine. Pantothenic acid and biotin appear to use the same uptake carrier in colonocytes.

DOSAGE AND ADMINISTRATION

Biotin is available in multivitamin and multivitamin/multimineral products as well as in single ingredient products. In single ingredient products, biotin is available as lozenges, tablets and capsules. Few prenatal vitamin/mineral formulas contain biotin. Those that do, typically contain biotin in doses of about 30 micrograms daily. Biotin is present in several combination products at doses of 30 to 60 micrograms daily. Intakes of biotin range from 30 to 1,000 micrograms/day.

The Food and Nutrition Board of the Institute of Medicine of the National Academy of Sciences has recommended the following Dietary Reference Intakes (DRI) for biotin:

Infants	Adequate Intake (AI)
0 through 6 months	5 micrograms/day ≈ 0.7 micrograms/Kg
7 through 12 months	6 micrograms/day ≈ 0.7 micrograms/Kg
Children	
1 through 3 years	8 micrograms/day
4 through 8 years	12 micrograms/day
Boys	
9 through 13 years	20 micrograms/day
14 through 18 years	25 micrograms/day
Girls	
9 through 13 years	20 micrograms/day
14 through 18 years	25 micrograms/day
Men	
19 years and older	30 micrograms/day
Women	
19 years and older	30 micrograms/day
Pregnancy	
14 through 50 years	30 micrograms/day
Lactation	
14 through 50 years	35 micrograms/day

The optimal intake values for biotin are not known. Those receiving hemodialysis, peritoneal dialysis or who have genetic abnormalities of biotin-dependent enzymes, such as biotinidase deficiency, have increased requirements for biotin. There are probably other such situations.

The DV (Daily Value) for biotin, which is used for determining percentage of nutrient daily values on nutritional supplement and food labels, is 300 micrograms. This is based on the U.S. RDA for biotin.

LITERATURE

Bonjour J-P. Biotin. In: Machlin, LJ, ed. *Handbook of Vitamins. Nutritional, Biochemical and Clinical Aspects.* New York, NY: Marcel Dekker, Inc; 1984:403-435.

Borboni P, Magnaterra R, Rabini RA, et al. Effect of biotin on glucokinase activity, mRNA expression and insulin release in cultured beta-cells. *Acta Diabetologica.* 1996; 33:154-158.

Casado de Frias E, Campos-Castello J, Careaga Maldonado J, Perez Cerda C. Biotinidase deficiency: result of treatment with biotin from age 12 years. *Europ J Paedriatr Neurol.* 1997; 1:173-176.

Colombo VE, Gerber F, Bronhofer M, Floersheim GL. Treatment of brittle fingernails and onychoschizia with biotin: scanning electron microscopy. *J Am Acad Dermatol.* 1990; 23(6 Pt 1):1127-1132.

Dabbaugh O, Brismar J, Gascon GC, Ozand PT. The clinical spectrum of biotin-treatable encephalopathies in Saudi Arabia. *Brain Dev.* 1994; 16Suppl:72-80.

Diamantopoulos N, Painter MJ, Wolf B, et al. Biotinidase deficiency: accumulation of lactate in the brain and response to physiologic doses of biotin. *Neurology.* 1986; 36:1107-1109.

Dietary Reference Intakes for Thiamin, Riboflavin, Niacin, Vitamin B_6, Folate, Vitamin B_{12}, Pantothenic Acid, Biotin, and Choline. Washington, DC: National Academy Press; 1998:374-389.

Dupuis L, Campeau E, Leclerc D, Gravel RA. Mechanism of biotin responsiveness in biotin-responsive multiple carboxylase deficiency. *Mol Genet Metab.* 1999; 66:80-90.

Floerscheim GL. [Treatment of brittle fingernails with biotin]. [Article in German]. *Z Hautkr.* 1989; 64:41-48.

Furukawa Y. [Enhancement of glucose-induced insulin secretion and modification of glucose metabolism by biotin]. [Article in Japanese]. *Nippon Rinsho.* 1999; 57:2261-2269.

Hochman LG, Scher RK, Meyerson MS. Brittle nails: response to daily biotin supplementation. *Cutis.* 1993; 51:303-305.

Hwu WL, Suzuki Y, Yang X, et al. Late-onset holocarboxylase synthetase deficiency with homologous R508W mutation. *J Formos Med Assoc.* 2000; 99:174-177.

Hymes J, Fleischauer K, Wolf B. Biotinylation of histones by human serum biotinidase: assessment of biotinyl-transferase activity in sera from normal individuals and children with biotinidase deficiency. *Biochem Mol Med.* 1995; 56:76-83.

Hymes J, Wolf B. Human biotinidase isn't just for recycling biotin. *J Nutr.* 1999; 129:485S-489S.

Innis SM, Allardyce DB. Possible biotin deficiency in adults receiving long-term total parenteral nutrition. *Am J Clin Nutr.* 1983; 37:185-187.

Jung U, Helbich-Endermann M, Bitsch R, et al. Are patients with chronic renal failure (CRF) deficient in biotin and is regular biotin supplementation required? *Z Ernä hrungswiss.* 1998; 37:363-367.

Keipert JA. Oral use of biotin in seborrhoeic dermatitis of infancy: a controlled trial. *Med J Aust.* 1976; 1:584-585.

Marshall MW, Kliman PG, Washington VA. Effects of biotin on lipids and other constituents of plasma of healthy men and women. *Artery.* 1980; 7:330-351.

Michalski AJ, Berry GT, Segal S. Holocarboxylase synthetase deficiency: 9-year follow-up of a patient on chronic biotin therapy and a review of the literature. *J Inher Metab Dis.* 1989; 12:312-316.

Mock DM. Biotin. In: Shils ME, Olson JA, Shike M, Ross AC, eds. *Modern Nutrition in Health and Disease.* Baltimore, MD: Williams and Wilkins; 1999:459-466.

Mock DM. Biotin status: which are valid indicators and how do we know? *J Nutr.* 1999; 129:498S-503S.

Mock DM, Mock NI, Nelson RP, Lombard KA. Disturbances in biotin metabolism in children undergoing long-term anticonvulsant therapy. *J Pediatr Gastroenterol Nutr.* 1998; 26:245-250.

Romero-Navarro G, Cabrera-Valladares G, German MS, et al. Biotin regulation of pancreatic glucokinase and insulin in primary cultured rat islets and in biotin-deficient rats. *Endocrinology.* 1999; 140:4595-4600.

Ravn K, Chloupkova M, Christensen E, et al. High incidence of propionic acidemia in Greenland is due to a prevalent mutation, 1540insCCC, in the gene for the beta-subunit of propionyl CoA carboxylase. *Am J Hum Genet.* 2000; 67:203-206.

Reddi A, DeAngelis B, Frank O, et al. Biotin supplementation improves glucose and insulin tolerances in genetically diabetic KK mice. *Life Sci.* 1988; 42:1323-1330.

Rodriguez Melendez R. [Importance of biotin metabolism]. [Article in Spanish]. *Rev Invest Clin.* 2000; 52:194-199.

Sekiguchi T, Nagamine T. Inhibition of free radical generation by biotin. *Biochem Pharmacol.* 1994; 47:594-596.

Shelley WB, Shelley ED. Uncombable hair syndrome: observations on response to biotin and occurrence in siblings with ectodermal dysplasia. *J Am Acad Dermatol.* 1985; 13:97-102.

Sugita Y, Shirakawa H, Sugimoto R, et al. Effect of biotin treatment on hepatic gene expression in streptozotocin-induced diabetic rats. *Biosci Biotechnol Biochem.* 2008;72(5):1290-1298.

Velazquez A, Baez TM, Gutierrez J, Rodriguez R. Biotin supplementation affects lymphocyte carboxylases and plasma biotin in severe protein-energy malnutrition. *Am J Clin Nutr.* 1995; 61:385-391.

Zempleni J, McCormick DB, Cook DM. Identification of biotin sulfone, bisnorbiotin methyl ketone, and tetranorbiotin-1-sulfoxide in human urine. *Am J Clin Nutr.* 1997; 65:508-511.

Zempleni J, Mock DM. Bioavailability of biotin given orally to humans in pharmacologic doses. *Am J Clin Nutr.* 1999; 69:504-508.

Zempleni J, Mock DM. Marginal biotin deficiency is teratogenic. *Proc Soc Exp Biol Med.* 2000; 223:14-21.

Zempleni J, Mock DM. Utilization of biotin in proliferating human lymphocytes. *J Nutr.* 2000; 130:335S-337S.

Blackcurrant Seed Oil

DESCRIPTION

Blackcurrant seed oil (BSO) is derived from the seeds of the plant *Ribes nigrum.* It is a rich source of the n-6 (omega-6) polyunsaturated fatty acid gamma-linolenic acid (GLA). Blackcurrant seed oil contains about 15 to 20% GLA. The n-3 (omega-3) polyunsaturated fatty acid alpha-linolenic acid (ALA) is also present in blackcurrant seed oil (12 to 14%) as is the fatty acid linoleic acid. Also present, in smaller amounts, is stearidonic acid or SDA (2 to 4%), an 18 carbon n-3 polyunsaturated fatty acid containing four double bonds. The various fatty acids are found in blackcurrant seed oil in the form of triacylglycerols (TAGs), also known as triglycerides. The stereospecific position of GLA varies among different oil sources. GLA is concentrated in the sn-3 position in blackcurrant seed oil as it is in evening primrose oil. In the case of borage oil, it is concentrated in the sn-2 position. The terms blackcurrant seed oil and blackcurrant oil are used interchangeably. (Also see monograph on gamma-linolenic acid [GLA].)

ACTIONS AND PHARMACOLOGY

ACTIONS

Blackcurrant oil, owing to its GLA, ALA and stearidonic acid content, may have antithrombotic and anti-inflammatory actions.

MECHANISM OF ACTION

Any anti-inflammatory or antithrombotic actions that blackcurrant oil possesses may be accounted for, principally, by the presence of GLA, ALA and SDA. GLA is a precursor in the synthesis of prostaglandin E_1 (PGE_1), and ALA is a precursor in the synthesis of eicosapentaenoic acid (EPA). EPA itself is a precursor of the series-3 prostaglandins, the series-5 leukotrienes and the series-3 thromboxanes. These eicosanoids possess antithrombotic and anti-inflammatory activity. Other mechanisms include inhibition of inflammatory cytokines.

PHARMACOKINETICS

GLA-, ALA- and linoleic acid-laden TAGs in blackcurrant oil, following ingestion, undergo hydroysis via lipases to form monoglycerides (MGs) and free fatty acids (FFAs). Once formed, the MGs and the FFAs are absorbed by the enterocytes. In the enterocytes, a reacylation takes place reforming TAGs, which are then assembled with phospholipids, cholesterol and apoproteins into chylomicrons (CM). The CM are released into the lymphatics and are transported to the systemic circulation. In the circulation the CM are degraded by lipoprotein lipase and the fatty acids are taken up in part by the endothelial tissues to be used for oxidation or for synthesis of phospholipids, components of cell membranes. GLA is metabolized to dihomo-gamma-linolenic acid, which is converted to prostaglandin E1. ALA is metabolized to EPA, which itself is a precursor in the synthesis of the series-3 prostaglandins, the series-5 leukotrienes and the series-3 thromboxanes. Linoleic acid, also contained in blackcurrant oil, is metabolized to ALA. Stearidonic acid is also metabolized to EPA. The metabolites of GLA and ALA are catabolized by oxidative processes, and the catabolic products are mostly excreted in the urine.

INDICATIONS AND USAGE

Blackcurrant seed oil may have cardioprotective effects as well as some efficacy in rheumatoid arthritis. It is not a useful cholesterol-lowering agent. (See gamma-linolenic acid [GLA] for other possible indications.)

RESEARCH SUMMARY

Claims made for blackcurrant seed oil are similar to those related to gamma-linolenic acid (GLA). But since blackcurrant seed oil is a source of both GLA and alpha-linolenic acid (ALA), it has carved out a separate niche for itself. Blackcurrant oil may be cardioprotective.

Many of the benefits noted with the use of GLA in rheumatoid arthritis may be observed with the use of blackcurrant oil.

CONTRAINDICATIONS, PRECAUTIONS, ADVERSE REACTIONS

CONTRAINDICATIONS

Known hypersensitivity to a blackcurrant oil-containing product.

PRECAUTIONS

Pregnant women, nursing mothers and children should avoid use of blackcurrant oil unless it is recommended by a physician. Because of possible antithrombotic activity, those with hemophilia and those taking warfarin (Coumadin) should use blackcurrant oil with caution.

ADVERSE REACTIONS

No significant adverse effects have been reported. Those taking blackcurrant oil may experience mild gastrointestinal symptoms such as diarrhea. Some cannot tolerate the number of capsules required to receive any benefit.

INTERACTIONS

No interaction between blackcurrant oil and aspirin, other NSAIDs, or herbs, such as *Allium sativum* (garlic) and *Ginkgo biloba* (ginkgo) have been reported. Such interactions, if they were to occur, might be manifested by nosebleeds and/or increased susceptibility to bruising. If this does occur, the blackcurrant oil dose should be lowered or stopped.

OVERDOSAGE

There are no reports of overdosage.

DOSAGE AND ADMINISTRATION

There are several blackcurrant seed oil supplements available, each differing slightly in the amount of GLA and ALA in a capsule. GLA ranges in these capsules from 60 to 90 milligrams and ALA 70 to 90 milligrams. The usual dose consumed is from three to six capsules, containing these amounts, daily, in divided doses.

LITERATURE

Deferne JL, Leeds AR. Resting blood pressure and cardiovascular reactivity to mental arithmetic in mild hypertensive males supplemented with blackcurrant seed oil. *J Hum Hyperten.* 1996; 10:531-537.

Diboune M, Ferard G, Ingenbleek V, et al. Composition of phospholipid fatty acids in red blood cell membranes of patients in intensive care units: effects of different intakes of soybean oil, medium chain triglycerides and blackcurrant oil. *J Parent Enteral Nutr.* 1992; 16:136-141.

Watson J, Byars ML, Mc Gill P, Kelman AW. Cytokine and prostaglandin production by monocytes of volunteers and rheumatoid arthritis patients treated with dietary supplements of blackcurrant seed oil. *Br J Rheumatol.* 1993; 32: 1055-1058.

Wu D, Meydani M, Leka LS, et al. Effect of dietary supplementation with blackcurrant seed oil on the immune response of healthy elderly subjects. *Am J Clin Nutr.* 1999; 70: 536-543.

Bone Meal

DESCRIPTION

Bone meal is used as a supplement for calcium and phosphorus. It is composed of finely crushed, processed bone, usually from cattle but sometimes also from horses. Bone marrow may also be added to the product. Calcium in bone meal occurs as a calcium phosphate compound known as hydroxyapatite or hydroxylapatite. Hydroxyapatite is an inorganic compound found in the matrix of bone and the teeth; it confers rigidity to these structures. The formula of hydroxyapatite is $(Ca_3 (PO_4)_2)_3 \bullet Ca (OH)_2$ or $Ca_{10} (PO_4)_6 (OH)_2$.

Bone meal was at one time a popular nutritional supplement for calcium. It is still marketed as a nutritional supplement, but it is no longer as popular. The reason for this is that in the 1980s analysis of bone meal supplements revealed them to contain substantial amounts of lead, as well as other toxic elements, such as arsenic, mercury and cadmium. A second-generation "bone meal" product called microcrystalline hydroxyapatite, or MCHA, is being marketed as a calcium supplement and is claimed to be free of contaminants.

Bone meal is also used as a high-phosphorus fertilizer and in some pet foods.

ACTIONS AND PHARMACOLOGY

MECHANISM OF ACTION

See Calcium and Phosphorus.

PHARMACOKINETICS

See Calcium and Phosphorus.

Hydroxyapatite is apparently well-absorbed from the gastrointestinal tract.

INDICATIONS AND USAGE

Bone meal is still sold as a "natural" source of calcium. Its use should be avoided owing to potential toxic-metal contamination.

RESEARCH SUMMARY

The use of bone meal as a calcium and phosphorus source is no longer recommended. Several researchers have reported that many bone meal preparations are contaminated with toxic metals. In one study, bone meal samples were contaminated with significant amounts of lead, arsenic, mercury and other metals. Dolomite and calcium carbonate supplements labeled "oyster shell" or "natural source" have also been found to be contaminated with these metals.

One researcher has advised that "physicians must consider the possibility of unrecognized self-poisoning from the consumption of such substances, especially in the context of unexplained neurologic, gastrointestinal, cutaneous and hematologic disorders."

The feeding of meat and bone meal to cattle, contaminated with bovine spongiform encephalopathy (BSE) tissue, led to an epidemic of BSE in the British cattle population in the 1990s.

CONTRAINDICATIONS, PRECAUTIONS, ADVERSE REACTIONS

CONTRAINDICATIONS

Bone meal is contraindicated in those with hypercalcemia. Conditions that cause hypercalcemia include hyperparathyroidism, hypervitaminosis D, some granulomatous diseases, sarcoidosis and cancer. Bone meal is also contraindicated in those with calcium pyrophosphate dihydrate (CPPD) deposition disease.

PRECAUTIONS

Bone meal is no longer recommended as a calcium and/or phosphorus supplement because of possible presence of toxic substances, such as lead. Children are especially sensitive to the effects of lead. Children, pregnant women and nursing mothers should absolutely avoid bone meal supplements.

ADVERSE REACTIONS

See Calcium. Prolonged use of bone meal contaminated with toxic elements, such as lead, may cause the typical toxic effects of these substances. Lead may produce abdominal pain, anemia and central nervous system damage.

OVERDOSAGE

There are no known reports of overdosage of bone meal.

DOSAGE AND ADMINISTRATION

No recommended dose. Second-generation "bone meal" supplements known as microcrystalline hydroxyapatite, or MCHA, are available as calcium supplements and are claimed to be free of contaminants.

LITERATURE

Boulos FM, von Smolinski A. Alert to users of calcium supplements as antihypertensive agents due to trace mineral contaminants. *Am J Hypterten.* 1988; 1(3 Pt 3):137S-142S.

Bourquin BP, Evans DR, Cornett JR, et al. Lead content of 70 brands of dietary calcium supplements. *Am J Public Health.* 1993; 83:1155-1160.

Groschup MH. [Bovine spongiform encephalopathy in ruminants and the new variant of Creutzfeldt-Jakob disease in humans.] [Article in German.] *DTW Dtsch Tierarzl Wochenschr.* 1999; 106:329-331.

Roberts HJ. Potential toxicity due to dolomite and bone meal. *South Med J.* 1983; 76:556-559.

Whiting SJ. Safety of some calcium supplements questioned. *Nutr Rev.* 1994; 52:95-97.

Borage Oil

DESCRIPTION

Borage oil is derived from the seeds of the borage plant (*Borago officinalis*), a member of the Boraginaceae family. Borage oil, also known as starflower oil and borage seed oil, is a rich source of the long-chain polyunsaturated fatty acid gamma-linolenic acid (GLA). The possible health benefits of borage oil are attributed to GLA. GLA is an unusual constituent of living matter and is found in very few plants. These include, in addition to borage, evening primrose, blackcurrant and hemp. The amount of GLA in borage oil, as the percentage of total fatty acid content, ranges from about 20% to 27%. Typical borage oil supplements contain approximately 24% GLA.

GLA is an all cis n-6 long-chain polyunsaturated fatty acid. It is comprised of 18 carbon atoms and three double bonds. GLA is also known as GLA; 18: 3n-6 and gamolenic acid. Chemically, it is known as 6, 9, 12-octadecatrienoic acid; (Z,

Z, Z)-6, 9, 12-octadecatrienoic acid, and cis-6, cis-9, cis-12-octadecatrienoic acid. GLA is present in borage oil in the form of triglycerides. GLA is concentrated in the sn-2 position in the triglycerides. GLA has the following chemical structure:

GLA (gamma-linolenic acid)

ACTIONS AND PHARMACOLOGY

ACTIONS

Borage oil may have anti-inflammatory and antithrombotic activities.

MECHANISM OF ACTION

The possible anti-inflammatory and anti-aggregatory actions of borage oil may be accounted for by examining the role of GLA in eicosanoid biochemistry. GLA is metabolized to the 20-carbon polyunsaturated fatty acid dihomo-gamma-linolenic acid (DGLA; 20: 3n-6), which is a precursor to the 1-series prostaglandins, such as prostaglandin E_1 (PGE$_1$). The action of PGE$_1$ on inflammatory cells (e.g. polymorphonuclear leukocytes or PMNs) is mostly inhibitory. PGE$_1$ increases intracellular cyclic AMP (cAMP). This increase reduces the release of lysosomal enzymes, PMN chemotaxis, and the margination and adherence of PMNs in the blood vessels. PGE$_1$ is also thought to inhibit lymphocyte function. PGE$_1$, in addition to its role in suppressing the inflammatory process, inhibits platelet aggregation and has vasodilatory activity.

GLA, via its metabolite DGLA, inhibits leukotriene (LT) synthesis. Leukotriene B$_4$ (LTB$_4$) is an inflammatory mediator. DGLA is metabolized to 15-hydroxyl DGLA, which blocks the conversion of arachidonic acid to LTs such as LTB$_4$.

In summary, GLA may suppress inflammation through its metabolism to DGLA, which in turn can competitively inhibit the pro-inflammatory 2-series prostaglandins and 4-series leukotrienes. The incorporation of GLA and its metabolites in cell membranes may also play a role in the possible anti-inflammatory, antithrombotic, anti-atherogenic and antiproliferative actions of borage oil.

PHARMACOKINETICS

GLA-laden triglycerides in borage oil are absorbed from the small intestine aided by bile salts. During this process, there is some deacylation of the fatty acid residues of the triglycerides. Reacylation takes place within the mucosal cells of the small intestine, and the GLA-laden triglycerides enter into the lymphatics in the form of chylomicrons. GLA-laden chylomicrons are transported from the lymphatics into the blood, where GLA is carried in lipid particles to the various tissues of the body.

GLA is metabolized to the 20-carbon polyunsaturated fatty acid dihomo-gamma-linolenic acid (DGLA), which is converted to prostaglandin E$_1$ (PGE$_1$). It may also be metabolized to eicosapentaenoic acid (EPA). GLA and DGLA are normally not found in cells as free fatty acids. They occur mainly in cell membranes as components of phopholipids, neutral lipids and cholesterol esters. PGE$_1$ is metabolized to smaller prostaglandin remnants, which are primarily polar dicarboxylic acids, most of which are excreted in the urine.

INDICATIONS AND USAGE

Borage oil appears to be effective in some cases of rheumatoid arthritis and may be indicated in some other inflammatory disorders, such as Sjogren's syndrome and ulcerative colitis. Possible other indications include osteoporosis, diabetic neuropathy, acute respiratory distress syndrome (ARDS), hypertension and elevated serum lipids. Borage oil has been used with some preliminary success in some cancers, principally cerebral gliomas. It has not proved useful for tardive dyskinesia, premenstrual syndrome or menopausal flushing. It may be indicated in some cases for atopic dermatitis, particularly to help with itching, as well as for uremic skin conditions in hemodialysis patients. It should probably not be used in efforts to enhance immunity, as it may be immunosuppressive.

RESEARCH SUMMARY

See Gamma-Linolenic Acid (GLA).

CONTRAINDICATIONS, PRECAUTIONS, ADVERSE REACTIONS

CONTRAINDICATIONS

Known hypersensitivity to a borage oil-containing product.

PRECAUTIONS

Pregnant women and nursing mothers should avoid using borage oil supplements. Those with a history of partial complex seizure disorders, such as temporal lobe epilepsy, should avoid using borage oil. Likewise, those with other types of seizure disorders and schizophrenics who are being treated with certain neuroleptic drugs, such as aliphatic phenothiazines (e.g. chlorpromazine), which may lower seizure threshold, should avoid using borage oil. Because of possible antithrombotic activity of borage oil, those with hemophilia or other hemorrhagic diatheses and those taking warfarin should exercise caution in the use of this supplement. Borage oil supplementation should be halted before any surgical procedure.

Because of its possible inhibition of lymphocyte function, those with immune deficiency disorders, such as AIDS, should exercise caution in the use of borage oil.

Pyrrolizidine alkaloids, such as amabiline, lycopsamine and thesinine, are found in various parts of the borage plant. The unsaturated pyrrolizidine alkaloids, such as amabiline, are potentially hepatotoxic and carcinogenic. Amabiline has not been detected in borage oil supplements down to five parts per million. However, chronic consumption of borage oil containing levels of amabiline of one part per million may prove harmful. Those who use borage oil chronically should only use products that are certified free of unsaturated pyrrolizidine alkaloids.

ADVERSE REACTIONS

Borage oil may cause such gastrointestinal symptoms as nausea, vomiting, flatulence, diarrhea and bloating. Similar to evening primrose oil, borage oil may precipitate symptoms of undiagnosed complex partial seizures and should be used, if at all, with extreme caution in those with a history of seizure disorders or those taking drugs that lower the seizure threshold, such as aliphatic phenothiazines (e.g., chlorpromazine).

INTERACTIONS

DRUGS

Use of borage oil in schizophrenics who are being treated with certain neuroleptic agents that lower seizure threshold — e.g. aliphatic phenothiazines, such as chlorpromazine — may cause partial complex seizures and possibly other types of seizures. Interactions may occur between borage oil and anticoagulants, such as warfarin, as well as antiplatelet drugs, such as aspirin and NSAIDs. Such interactions may enhance the effects of the anticoagulants and antiplatelet drugs. Manifestations of such interactions, if they were to occur, include nosebleeds, hematuria and increased susceptibility to bruising. Borage oil intake should be stopped if these symptoms occur.

NUTRITIONAL SUPPLEMENTS

Interactions may occur if borage oil is used with supplements that have antithrombotic activity, such as fish oils. This may be manifested by nosebleeds and increased susceptibility to bruising.

HERBS

Interactions may occur if borage oil is used with such herbs as garlic (*Allium sativum*) and ginkgo (*Ginkgo biloba*). Such interactions may be manifested by nosebleeds and easy bruising.

OVERDOSAGE

There are no reports of overdosage with borage oil.

DOSAGE AND ADMINISTRATION

Borage oil is available in capsules and bottles. Capsules of borage oil typically contain about 24% GLA. Doses used for the management of rheumatoid arthritis range from about 360 milligrams to 2.8 grams daily, in divided doses (expressed as GLA). For management of atopic dermatitis, doses of 320 to 480 milligrams (expressed as GLA) are used, taken daily in divided doses. Doses up to 2 grams daily (expressed as GLA) have been used by those with hypertriglyceridemia. For long-term use, borage oil should be certified free of unsaturated pyrrolizidine alkaloids. Borage oil supplements should contain an antioxidant, such as vitamin E, to protect the unsaturated fatty acids against oxidation.

LITERATURE

For additional literature, see Gamma-Linolenic Acid (GLA) and Evening Primrose Oil monographs.

Huang Y-S, Mills DE, eds. *Gamma-Linolenic Acid: Metabolism and its Roles in Nutrition.* Champaign, IL: American Oil Chemists Society Press; 1996.

Boron

DESCRIPTION

Boron, the fifth chemical element, is a dietary trace mineral found primarily in plant foods. It is essential for plant growth. Recently it has been shown to be essential in an animal species (zebra fish), and evidence is mounting that boron is probably essential for humans, as well. The first edition of *The Merck Manual* (1899) credits boric acid, the most common form of boron, with being a useful treatment for amenorrhea, dysmenorrhea, epilepsy and elevated uric acid. Boric acid has, in fact, proved to be ineffective for all of those disorders, but recent research lends some preliminary support for the use of boron for the promotion of bone and joint health. There is less evidence that it may be helpful in enhancing mental cognition.

ACTIONS AND PHARMACOLOGY

ACTIONS

Boron may have estrogen-mimetic and anti-osteoporotic activity. It may also participate in regulating the respiratory burst of neutrophils.

MECHANISM OF ACTION

The biochemical mechanism of boron is not yet known. Currently, two hypotheses have been advanced for the biochemical function of boron in animals, including humans. The first is that boron plays a role in cell-membrane functions that influence response to hormone action, trans-membrane signaling and trans-membrane movement of regulatory ions. Boron has been shown, in animal models, to influence the transport of extracellular calcium and the release of intracellular calcium in platelets activated by thrombin. It also influences redox actions involved in cellular membrane transport in plants.

A second hypothesis is that boron acts as a metabolic regulator in several enzymatic systems. Boron may play an important role in regulating the respiratory burst, which is the reactive-oxygen-species mechanism by which white blood cells kill micro-organisms. If boron does in fact regulate the respiratory burst, it assumes the role of a novel antioxidant, preventing some of the collateral damage that may occur when reactive oxygen species react with surrounding tissue.

The biochemistry of boron is essentially that of boric acid. Boric acid forms complexes with many of the chemical substances found in the body, such as carbohydrates (sugars and polysaccharides), nucleotides (such as adenosine monophosphate and niacinamide adenine dinucleotide) and vitamins (such as ascorbic acid, pyridoxine and riboflavin). Boric acid forms esters with hydroxyl groups found in many of these compounds. This occurs preferentially when the hydroxyl groups are next to each other and on the same side of the molecules. The most stable esters are those in which boric acid is the bridge between two carbohydrate molecules, e.g. fructose-boron-fructose. Such soluble boron complexes are found naturally in phloem saps and nectars in plants. Polysaccharides containing boron in similar linkages are found in plant cell walls in the form of pectins.

PHARMACOKINETICS

Nutritional forms of boron are readily and completely absorbed. They are either rapidly converted to boric acid and are absorbed as such or they are converted to boric acid following absorption. Absorbed boric acid is rapidly distributed throughout body water by passive diffusion. After being absorbed, boron's ratio of blood-to-soft-tissue concentration is approximately one. Concentrations of boron in bone, teeth and fingernails exceed those in blood by about a factor of four. Certain nutritional forms of boron (e.g., boron carbohydrate esters) are metabolized to boric acid. Boric acid itself does not undergo metabolism. It is eliminated unchanged in the urine. The half-life for elimination of boric acid, whether administered orally or intravenously, is about 21 hours.

INDICATIONS AND USAGE

Boron may be indicated for the promotion of bone and joint health, particularly in women. There is less evidence to support claims that boron enhances cognition and ameliorates the symptoms of arthritis. There is no evidence that it promotes the development of lean muscle mass. The evidence that boron may protect against prostate cancer is conflicting.

RESEARCH SUMMARY

Boron's potential therapeutic value in promoting bone and joint health is underscored by the widespread incidence of osteoporosis. There are more than 100 million afflicted by this disease worldwide, eight million of them in the United States. Postmenopausal women are mostly affected, but osteoporosis is also found in some men as they age. In the United States, osteoporosis is responsible for 300,000 hip fractures, 700,000 spine fractures and 250,000 wrist fractures each year. Associated health care costs are in the billions of dollars annually.

Adequate intake and metabolism of minerals can largely prevent osteoporosis. Dietary boron has been shown to affect several aspects of mineral metabolism in animal studies. And in a human study, 12 postmenopausal women were fed a diet deficient in boron (0.25 mg daily) for 119 days followed by a 48-day period in which they received supplements of 3 mg daily. On the boron-deficient diet, the women experienced increased loss of both calcium and magnesium. On the boron-supplemented diet, the opposite was true. Urinary excretion of calcium and magnesium was significantly diminished, and serum concentrations of 17 beta-estradiol, as well as testosterone, increased. The findings of the study suggest that maintaining adequate levels of boron, particularly in the presence of adequate levels of magnesium, can help prevent calcium loss and bone demineralization in postmenopausal women and, perhaps, others. The boron effect on testosterone levels, while possibly significant for women, would be too low to have any significance for men.

In a subsequent human study, boron supplementation increased serum levels of 25-hydroxycholecalciferol, a metabolite of vitamin D important in mineral metabolism, in postmenopausal women who were deficient in boron. There were also findings suggesting that estrogen replacement therapy used in conjunction with boron may have a synergistic effect. There is evidence to support the assertion that boron can both mimic and enhance some of the effects of estrogen in post-menopausal women.

Findings to date suggest that boron and calcium actions are inter-related or that the two elements affect similar systems, including the modification of hormone action, the alteration of cell membrane characteristics and/or trans-membrane signaling. Boron appears to be an important partner with calcium metabolism and as such might be expected to play an important role in the prevention of osteoporosis. Conclusive proof of this, however, remains to be demonstrated, though studies to date are suggestive of a positive effect.

Anecdotal reports, combined with some epidemiological findings, suggest that supplemental boron may alleviate the symptoms of osteoarthritis. There are reports that in those areas of the world where daily dietary intake of boron is 1 mg or less the estimated incidence of osteoarthritis ranges from 20 to 70%. In areas of the world where boron intakes are 3 to 10 mg daily, the estimated incidence of the disease ranges from 0 to 10%. This alone does not make a compelling argument for any role for boron in the prevention or treatment of osteoarthritis in the absence of clinical evidence. There is, however, one clinical study and one animal study that may justify further investigation.

The clinical trial involved 20 patients with radiographically confirmed osteoarthritis. This was a double-blind, placebo-controlled study in which half of the subjects were given 6 mg of boron daily while the other half received the placebo. The subjects were evaluated three times—prior to taking the tablets, after three weeks on the tablets and after eight weeks on the tablets. Patients were graded with respect to their symptoms as well as their use of a permitted analgesic. At the end of the eight-week period, 50% of those taking boron showed improvement, while only 10% of those on placebo showed similar improvement. The finding was declared statistically significant.

A recent study using rats indicated that dietary boron might be of benefit in adjuvant-induced arthritis. The benefits were evaluated by the amount of paw and joint swelling following adjuvant injection. A control group that did not receive boron was used for comparison. There was less swelling in the boron-supplemented animals. Measurements of natural killer cells, CD8 lymphocytes and neutrophils were also performed. The conclusion was that supplemental boron modulates the response to antigens of key immune cells and helps control the inflammatory process.

Further investigation is warranted and necessary before any conclusion can be made regarding the role of boron in the prevention and treatment of arthritis.

There is very preliminary evidence that supplemental boron may improve mental function. In one human study, subjects were first given a diet deficient in boron followed by a period in which they received supplemental boron in the amount of 3 mg daily. During the supplementation period, the subjects' electroencephalograms showed alterations suggesting improved behavioral activation (less drowsiness) and mental alertness. Improved psychomotor skills were also noted, along with improvement in attention and memory.

Studies have not supported the claim that boron can increase lean muscle mass. Studies show no effect on plasma testosterone levels or strength in male body builders. Claims to the contrary seem to have arisen from the studies on postmenopausal women, where boron may have induced a slight increase in plasma testosterone levels.

One observational study found an inverse relation between boron intake and prostate cancer. However, another observational study—the VITamins And Lifestyle (VITAL) cohort study—found no evidence among 35,244 males for a preventive role of boron intake on prostate cancer. Further research is needed to determine if boron has any role to play in the prevention of prostate cancer.

CONTRAINDICATIONS, PRECAUTIONS, ADVERSE REACTIONS

CONTRAINDICATIONS
Known hypersensitivity to a boron-containing product.

PRECAUTIONS
Because of the lack of long-term safety studies, supplemental boron should be avoided by pregnant women and nursing mothers except if recommended by their physicians.

ADVERSE REACTIONS
Doses up to 18 mg of boron daily appear to be safe for adults even if taken for prolonged periods of time. There is no evidence that boron is either carcinogenic or mutagenic. No adverse effects have been observed in either premenopausal or postmenopausal women using boron supplements.

OVERDOSAGE
The lowest levels at which boron supplementation may be toxic have not been established. In 1904, human volunteers consuming greater than 500 mg of boric acid daily (this is equivalent to about 180 mg of elemental boron) showed symptoms of poor appetite and digestive problems. Symptoms of acute toxicity typically include nausea, diarrhea and abdominal cramps. The symptoms of chronic toxicity include nausea, poor appetite and weight loss.

DOSAGE AND ADMINISTRATION
Except for tolerable upper intake levels (UL—see table), no DRI (dietary reference intake) has yet been established for boron. However, since there is some evidence for the essentiality of boron in humans, a DRI is likely to be established in the future. The DRI that is likely to be established for boron will probably be an AI (adequate intake) rather than an RDA (recommended dietary allowance).

Fruits and vegetables are the most important dietary sources of boron. A vegetarian diet is higher in boron than the typical American diet. The range of intake in the American diet is 0.5 to 3 mg daily. The average intake is about 1 mg daily. It is lower in the elderly. There is some evidence that this average intake may be too low; a more optimal intake of boron may be 2 to 3 mg daily.

Dietary supplements of boron now available include the following forms: sodium borate, boron citrate, boron aspartate, boron glycinate, calcium fructoborate. Once ingested, all of these forms are rapidly converted in the body to boric acid. Natural plant forms of boron or similar synthetic forms are not yet available, and whether they will have greater health benefits than the currently marketed forms remains to be seen.

Boron is often sold in supplements that combine a variety of nutrients. For example, it is found in products for bone and joint health that often combine such nutrients as vitamin D, calcium, magnesium, soy isoflavones, chondroitin sulfate, glucosamine, curcumin, boswellia, gelatin, ipriflavone, SAMe and others (see monographs on these substances). There's no evidence yet available that the therapeutic effects of boron are increased by such combinations.

The Food and Nutrition Board of the U.S. National Academy of Sciences has published the following Dietary Reference Intakes (DRI) for boron. A summary of DRIs for various age groups is as follows:

DRI values (milligrams/day)

Infants	Tolerable Upper Intake Level (UL)
0-6 months	ND
7-12 months	ND
Children	
1-3 years	3
4-8 years	6
Boys	
9-13 years	11
14-18 years	17
Girls	
9-13 years	11
14-18 years	17
Men	
19-30 years	20
31-50 years	20
51-70 years	20
70 years or older	20
Women	
19-30 years	20
31-50 years	20
51-70 years	20
70 years or older	20
Pregnancy	
14-18 years	17
19-30 years	20
31-50 years	20
Lactation	
14-18 years	17
19-30 years	20
31-50 years	20

ND = Not determinable. The value is not determinable because of the lack of data on adverse effects in this age group and concern regarding the lack of ability to handle excess amounts. To prevent high levels of intake, the only source of boron for infants should be from food and formula.

There are no Recommended Dietary Allowances (RDA), Estimated Average Requirements (EAR) or Adequate Intake Levels established for boron.

The UL is the Tolerable Upper Intake Level and usually represents the total intake from food, water and supplements.

LITERATURE

Chapin RE, Ku WW, Kenny MA, et al. The effects of dietary boron on bone strength in rats. *Fundam Appl Toxical.* 1997;35:205-215.

Gallardo-Williams MT, Chapin RE, King PE, et al. Boron supplementation inhibits the growth and local expression of IGF-1 in human prostate adenocarcinoma (LNCaP) tumors in nude mice. *Toxicol Pathol.* 2004;32(1):73-78.

Gonzalez A, Peters U, Lampe JW, et al. Boron intake and prostate cancer risk. *Cancer Causes Control.* 2007;18(10):1131-1140.

Green NR, Ferrando AA. Plasma boron and the effects of boron supplementation in males. *Environ Health Perspect.* 1994;102(Suppl 7):73-77.

Hu H, Penn SG, Lebrilla CB, et al. Isolation and characterization of soluble boron complexes in higher plants. The mechanism of phloem mobility of boron. *Plant Physiol.* 1997;113:649-655.

Hunt CD, Idso JP, Keehr KA. Dietary boron alleviates adjuvant-induced arthritis (AIA) and changes in the blood concentrations of neutrophil, CD8a, and natural killer cells in rats. *FASEBJ.* 1999;13:A545.

Hunt CD. Biochemical effects of physiological amounts of dietary boron. *J Trace Elem Exp Med.* 1999; 9:185-213.

Institute of Medicine, Food and Nutrition Board. Dietary Reference Intakes for vitamin A, vitamin K, arsenic, boron, chromium, copper, iodine, iron, manganese, molybdenum, nickel, silicon, vanadium, and zinc. Washington, DC: National Academy Press, 2001.

Linden CH, Hall AH, Kulig KW, et al. Acute ingestions of boric acid. *J Toxicol Clin Toxicol.* 1986;24:269-279.

Moore JA. An assessment of boric acid and borax using the IEHR evaluative process for assessing human developmental and reproductive toxicity of agents. *Reproduct Toxical.* 1997;11:123-160.

Murray FJ. A comparative review of the pharmacokinetics of boric acid in rodents and humans. *Biol Trace Elem Res.* 1998;66:331-341.

Murray FJ. A human health assessment of boron (boric acid and borax) in drinking water. *Regulat Toxical Pharmicol.* 1995;22:221-230.

Newnham RE. Essentiality of boron for healthy bones and joints. *Environ Health Perspect.* 102(Suppl 7):83-85.

Nielsen FH. Ultratrace minerals in Modern Nutrition in Health and Disease. In: Shils ME, Olson JA, Shike M., Ross AC, eds. *Modern Nutrition in Health and Disease.* 9th ed. Baltimore, MD: Williams & Wilkins; 1999:283-303.

Nielsen FH. Facts and Fallacies about Boron. *Nutrition Today.* 1992;27:6-12.

Nielsen FH. Biochemical and physiologic consequences of boron deprivation in humans. *Environ Health Perspect.* 1994;102(Suppl 7):59-63.

Nielsen FH, Gallagher SK, Johnson LK, et al. Boron enhances and mimics some effects of estrogen therapy in postmenopausal women. *J Trace Elem Exp Med.* 1992;5:237-246.

Nielsen FH, Hunt CD, Mullen LM, et al. Effect of dietary boron on mineral, estrogen, and testosterone metabolism in postmenopausal women. *FASEBJ.* 1987;1:394-397.

Penland JG. The importance of boron nutrition for brain and psychological function. *Biol Trace Elem Res.* 1998;66:299-317.

Rainey CJ, Nyquist LA, Christensen RE, et al. Daily boron intake from the American diet. *J Am Diet Assoc.* 1999;99:335-340.

Sheng MH, Taper LJ, Veit H, et al. Dietary boron supplementation enhanced the action of estrogen, but not that of parathyroid hormone, to improve trabecular bone quality in ovariectomized rats. *Biol Trace Elem Res.* 2001;82(1-3):109-123.

Sheng MH, Taper LJ, Veit H, et al. Dietary boron supplementation enhances the effects of estrogen on bone mineral balance in ovariectomized rats. *Biol Trace Elem Res.* 2001;81(1):29-45.

Further information in:

Proceedings of the 2nd International Symposium on the Health Effects of Boron and its Compounds. Irvine, California, U.S.A. October 22-24, 1997. *Biol Trace Elem Research.* 1998;66:1-473.

Health effects of boron. *Environmental Health Perspective Supplements.* 1994;102(Suppl 7):1-141.

Merck's 1899 Manual, Merck and Co., New York, 1899.

Bovine Cartilage

DESCRIPTION

Bovine cartilage is mainly comprised of the protein collagen and proteoglycans. Proteoglycans are composed of a core protein to which polysaccharides, known as glycosaminoglycans (GAGs) or mucopolysaccharides, are attached. The main glycosaminoglycan in bovine cartilage is chondroitin sulfate.

In 1976, Judah Folkman and his colleagues reported on the isolation of a factor from the scapular cartilage of calves that inhibited the growth of new blood vessels supporting implanted tumors in rabbits. It also stopped the growth of the tumors.

Subsequently, it was found that factors in shark cartilage had similar effects (see Shark Cartilage). Bovine cartilage, marketed as a nutritional supplement and for other indications, is primarily derived from bovine trachea.

ACTIONS AND PHARMACOLOGY

ACTIONS

Bovine cartilage has putative antitumor and anti-arthritic actions. Topical bovine cartilage may have wound-healing activity.

MECHANISM OF ACTION

The mechanism of the putative antitumor activity of bovine cartilage is unknown. Substances in bovine cartilage may have some anti-angiogenic activity. It has been suggested that chondroitin sulfate in bovine cartilage may have immunomodulatory activity and that such activity may play some role as well.

Bovine cartilage's putative anti-arthritic activity may be accounted for, in part, by the presence of chondroitin sulfate (see Chondroitin Sulfate).

Topical bovine cartilage appears to have wound-healing activity by stimulating granulation within the wound, thus establishing a matrix that induces wound repair.

PHARMACOKINETICS

The pharmacokinetics of collagen in bovine cartilage should be similar to those of dietary proteins. See Chondroitin Sulfate for pharmacokinetics of that substance.

INDICATIONS AND USAGE

As with shark cartilage, claims for bovine cartilage include anticancer, anti-inflammatory and anti-arthritic effects. Accelerated wound-healing effects are also claimed for oral bovine cartilage. There is little support for these claims. Topical bovine cartilage does appear to aid in wound healing.

RESEARCH SUMMARY

There are no well-controlled clinical studies showing efficacy of bovine cartilage in any cancer. There is one ongoing study on the effects of bovine cartilage in metastatic renal cell cancer. Similarly, there is no credible evidence that it is helpful in any form of arthritis. It contains chondroitin sulfate, which has been shown to be helpful in some with osteoarthritis, but studies showing similar activity with the use of bovine cartilage are lacking. Some anti-inflammatory and antitumor effects have been shown in animal and *in vitro* studies.

CONTRAINDICATIONS, PRECAUTIONS, ADVERSE REACTIONS

CONTRAINDICATIONS

Bovine cartilage supplements are contraindicated in those who are hypersensitive to any component of a bovine cartilage-containing product.

PRECAUTIONS

Pregnant women and nursing mothers should avoid using bovine cartilage supplements.

Those with renal failure or liver failure should exercise caution in the use of bovine cartilage.

Those with cancer who wish to try bovine cartilage must do so under medical supervision.

ADVERSE REACTIONS

These are occasional reports of gastrointestinal complaints, such as nausea, bloating and diarrhea. Also, fatigue has been associated with the use of this supplement.

DOSAGE AND ADMINISTRATION

Bovine cartilage is available in capsules and powders and in combination products. There are no typical doses. Bovine cartilage is also available as a wound dressing and as a dermatologic cream for skin care.

LITERATURE

Durie BG, Soehnlen B, Prudden JF. Antitumor activity of bovine cartilage extract (Catrix-S) in the human tumor stem cell assay. *J Biol Response Mod.* 1985; 4:590-595.

Langer R, Brem H, Falterman K, et al. Isolation of a cartilage factor that inhibits tumor neovascularization. *Science.* 1976; 193:70-72.

Prudden JF. The treatment of human cancer with agents prepared from bovine cartilage. *J Biol Response Mod.* 1985; 4:551-584.

Prudden JF, Balassa LL. The biological activity of bovine cartilage preparations. Clinical demonstration of their potent anti-inflammatory capacity with supplementary notes on certain relevant fundamental support studies. *Semin Arthritis Rheum.* 1974; 3: 287-321.

Puccio C, Mittelman A, Chun P, et al. Treatment of metastatic renal cell carcinoma with catrix. *Proc Amer Soc Clin Onc.* 1994; 13:A769.

Romano CF, Lipton A, Harvey HA, et al. A phase II study of Catrix-S in solid tumors. *J Biol Response Mod.* 1985; 4:585-589.

Rosen J, Sherman WT, Prudden JF, Thorbecke GJ. Immunoregulatory effects of catrix. *J Biol Resp Mod.* 1988; 7:498-512.

Sieper J, Kary S, Sorensen H, et al. Oral type II collagen treatment in early rheumatoid arthritis. A double-blind, placebo-controlled, randomized trial. *Arthritis Rheum.* 1996; 39:41-51.

Wolarsky ER, Finke SR, Prudden JF. Acceleration of wound healing with heterologous cartilage. Immunological considerations. *Proc Soc Exp Biol Med.* 1966; 123:556-561.

Bovine Colostrum

DESCRIPTION

Colostrum is the pre-milk fluid produced from the mother's mammary glands during the first few days after birth. Bovine colostrum is derived from cows. Colostrum is a rich source of antibodies, growth factors and nutrients for the suckling neonate and may provide passive immunity to the newborn against various infectious microorganisms, particularly those that affect the gastrointestinal tract. It may also have other health benefits.

The protein content of bovine colostrum is three to four times higher—up to 150 grams per liter compared to 30 to 40 grams per liter—than it is in regular cow's milk.

The greater part of this protein is comprised of whey proteins (see Whey Proteins). Immunoglobulins, mainly IgG, make up about 75% of the whey proteins. Other substances found in bovine colostrum include casein, lactoferrin, alpha-lactalbumin, beta-lactoglobulin, and the growth factors insulin-like growth factor-1 (IGF-1), insulin-like growth factor-2 (IGF-2), transforming growth factor beta (TGFbeta) and epidermal growth factor (EGF). In addition, bovine colostrum contains vitamins, minerals, lipids and lactose. Bovine colostrum may also contain colostrinin, also known as proline-rich polypeptide (PRP), a substance found in ovine (sheep) colostrum.

Bovine colostrum is marketed in several forms. Bovine colostrum prepared by microfiltration is mainly composed of whey proteins and their associated immunoglobulins and the growth factors IGF-1, IGF-2, TGFbeta and EGF.

Substances such as lactose, fats, casein and lactalbumin are significantly reduced in microfiltered bovine colostrum. Hyperimmune bovine colostrum is rich in immunoglobulins of the IgG type, which are protective against such infectious microorganisms as *Cryptosporidium parvum* (a major cause of AIDS-associated diarrhea), diarrheogenic *Escherichia coli* strains, *Shigella flexneri, Clostridium difficile,* and rotavirus, the most common cause of severe diarrhea in young children.

Hyperimmune bovine colostrum is prepared from cows previously immunized with specific antigens. Hyperimmune bovine colostrum IgG concentrate is an orphan drug for the treatment of diarrhea in AIDS patients caused by infection with *Cryptosporidium parvum.*

ACTIONS AND PHARMACOLOGY

ACTIONS

Bovine colostrum may have immunostimulatory and antimicrobial actions. It is reputed to have ergogenic activity as well.

MECHANISM OF ACTION

Hyperimmune bovine colostrum may have antimicrobial activity based on the ability of specific immunoglobulins of the IgG type to react with bacterial, viral and other microbiological antigens in the gut. Bovine colostrum contains a few immunostimulatory substances, including lactoferrin. It may also contain colostrinin or proline-rich polypeptide (PRP), another possible immunomodulatory substance. The combination of specific, as well as nonspecific, IgGs and such immunomodulatory factors as lactoferrin and PRP may afford general antimicrobial protection of the gastrointestinal tract.

Bovine colostrum's putative exercise-performance-enhancment is mainly attributed to such growth factors as IGF-1.

PHARMACOKINETICS

The pharmacokinetics of bovine colostrum, particularly with regard to the immunoglobulins, is unclear. It would be expected that immunoglobulins found in bovine colostrum would be rapidly inactivated by stomach acid and proteolytic action in the small intestine. Enteric coating would protect the proteins from acid in the stomach but not from proteolytic activity in the small intestine. However, following ingestion of bovine colostrum, some immunoglobulins are found to be excreted intact in the feces after a few days. This suggests that some immunoglobulins may be more resistant to degradation in the gut.

Growth factors and other peptides and proteins in bovine colostrum are most likely degraded by proteolytic enzymes and absorbed, distributed and metabolized in the same fashion as similar dietary substances. Colostrinin is resistant to intestinal proteolytic action.

INDICATIONS AND USAGE

Claims made for bovine colostrum are mostly unsubstantiated. Some preparations may have some antimicrobial effects. There is no credible evidence to support claims that bovine colostrum burns fat, builds muscle, speeds healing of injuries, regulates blood sugars, improves mood and fights depression or that it has anti-cancer effects.

RESEARCH SUMMARY

Well-designed, controlled clinical trials of bovine colostrum are largely lacking. A few small, usually uncontrolled or poorly controlled human studies have suggested that some components of some bovine colostrum preparations have significant antimicrobial activity. Immunoglobulins in colostrum derived from cows immunized against particular pathogens may help protect against those specific pathogens in some instances, but bovine colostrum supplements may vary widely in terms of specific constituents.

A bovine colostrum product derived from cows immunized against *Candida albicans* was reported to be effective in reducing levels of this fungal pathogen in severely immunocompromised patients. Similarly, AIDS patients with chronic *Cryptosporidium parvum* diarrhea were said to be helped by a formulation of concentrated bovine immunoglobulins given in dosages up to 40 grams daily.

Some bovine colostrum preparations pooled from many different cows may confer broad-spectrum antimicrobial activity, some animal research suggests. Better, designed, controlled clinical testing is needed to determine the safety and efficacy of bovine colostrum supplements.

CONTRAINDICATIONS, PRECAUTIONS, ADVERSE REACTIONS

CONTRAINDICATIONS

Bovine colostrum is contraindicated in those with hypersensitivity to any component of bovine colostrum-containing products.

PRECAUTIONS

Pregnant women and nursing mothers should avoid bovine colostrum supplements.

Bovine colostrum contains insulin-like growth factor-1 (IGF-1). IGF-1 levels are elevated in prostate, colorectal and lung cancer. Recent studies have found that IGF-1 levels correlate with risk of prostate cancer and colorectal cancer in men, premenopausal breast cancer in women and lung cancer in both men and women. Those with these types of cancer and those at risk for these cancers should exercise caution in the use of bovine colostrum supplements. It is unlikely that the amount of IGF-1 in bovine colostrum would be a problem, but caution should still be exercised.

ADVERSE REACTIONS

Adverse reactions to bovine colostrum supplements are mainly gastrointestinal and include nausea and vomiting, bloating and diarrhea. Bovine colostrum is generally well tolerated.

DOSAGE AND ADMINISTRATION

Bovine colostrum is available in several forms, including tablets, powders, bars and liquid solutions. Dosage is variable. Hyperimmune bovine colostrum used for AIDS-associated diarrhea usually caused by *Cryptosporidium parvum* is dosed at 10 grams four times daily for 21 days. This must only be taken under medical supervision.

LITERATURE

Bitzan MM, Gold BD, Philpott DJ, et al. Inhibition of Heliobacter pylori and Helicobacter mustelae binding to lipid receptors by bovine colostrum. *J Infect Dis.* 1998; 177:955-961.

Greenberg PD, Cello JP. Treatment of severe diarrhea caused by Crytosporidium parvum with oral bovine immunoglobulin concentrate in patients with AIDS. *J Acquir Immune Defic Syndr Hum Rretrovirol.* 1996; 13:348-354.

Huppertz HI, Rutkowski S, Busch DH, et al. Bovine colostrum ameliorates diarrhea in infection with diarrheagenic Escherichia coli, shiga toxin-producing E. coli, and E. coli expressing intimin and hemolysin. *J Pediatr Gastroenterol Nutr.* 1999; 29:452-456.

Lissner R, Thurmann PA, Merz G, Karch H. Antibody reactivity and fecal recovery of bovine immunoglobulins following oral administration of a colostrum concentrate from cows (Lactobin) to healthy volunteers. *Int J Clin Pharmacol Ther.* 1998; 36:239-245.

Merendino N, Prosperi S, Franci O, et al. Immunomodulatory activity of bovine colostrum on human peripheral blood mononuclear cells. *J Nutr Immunol.* 1996; 4:5-21.

Mero A, Miikkulainen H, Riski J, et al. Effects of bovine colostrum supplementation on serum IGF-1, IgG, hormone and saliva IgA during training. *J Appl Physiol.* 1997; 83: 1144-1151.

Playford RJ, Floyd DN, Macdonald CE, et al. Bovine colostrum is a health food supplement which prevents NSAID induced gut damage. *Gut.* 1999; 44:653-658.

Petschow BW, Talbott RD. Reduction in virus-neutralizing activity of a bovine colostrum immunoglobulin concentrate by gastric acid and digestive enzymes. *J Pediatr Gastroenterol Nutr.* 1994; 19:228-235.

Popik P, Bobula B, Janusz M, et al. Colostrinin, a polypeptide isolated from early milk, facilitates learning and memory in rats. *Pharmacol Biochem Behav.* 1999; 64:183-189.

Sarker SA, Caswall TH, Mahalanabis D, et al. Successful treatment of rotavirus diarrhea in children with immunoglobulin from immunized bovine colostrum. *Pediatr Infect Dis J.* 1998; 17:1149-1154.

Tacket CO, Binion SB, Bostwick E, et al. Efficacy of bovine milk immunoglobulin concentrate in preventing illness after Shigellla flexneri challenge. *Am J Trop Med Hyg.* 1992; 47:276-283.

Tacket CO, Losonsky G, Livio S, et al. Lack of prophylactic efficacy of an enteric-coated bovine hyperimmuune milk product against enterotoxigenic Escherichia coli challenge administered during a standard meal. *J Infect Dis.* 1999; 180:2056-2059.

Warny M, Fatimi A, Bostwick EF, et al. Bovine immunoglobulin concentrate-*Clostridium difficile* retains C. *difficile* toxin neutralizing activity after passage through the human stomach and small intestine. *Gut.* 1999; 44:212-217.

Branched-Chain Amino Acids (L-Leucine, L-Isoleucine, L-Valine)

DESCRIPTION

The branched-chain amino acids (BCAAs) comprise the three essential amino acids L-leucine, L-isoleucine and L-valine. These amino acids are found in proteins of all life forms. Dietary sources of the branched-chain amino acids are principally derived from animal and vegetable proteins. Vegetables and juices contain small amounts of the free amino acids, which are also found in fermented foods like yogurt and miso.

Several years ago the branched-chain amino acids created some interest in the neurological research community when a pilot study indicated that amyotrophic lateral sclerosis (ALS) patients showed symptomatic improvement when given large doses of BCAAs. It was theorized that BCAAs may protect against neuronal damage from the neuroexcitatory neurotransmitter glutamate. Based on this pilot study, branched-chain amino acids received orphan drug approval for the treatment of ALS. Unfortunately, most of the follow-up studies were negative, and one even suggested that BCAAs may increase mortality in those with ALS.

Branched-chain amino acids are sometimes used in enteral and parenteral feedings in the management of hepatic encephalopathy. They are also occasionally used enterally and parenterally in the management of extensive burns and other severe trauma conditions because of their possible anticatabolic action in these conditions.

L-leucine is also known as 2-amino-4-methylvaleric acid, alpha-aminoisocaproic acid and (*S*)-2-amino-4-methylpentanoic acid. It is abbreviated as Leu or by its one letter abbreviation L. Its molecular formula is $C_6H_{13}NO_2$, and its molecular weight is 131.17 daltons. The structural formula is:

L-leucine

L-isoleucine is also known as 2-amino-3-methylvaleric acid, alpha-amino-beta-methylvaleric acid and (2*S*, 3*S*)-2-amino-3-methylpentanoic acid. It is abbreviated as Ile or by its one letter abbreviation I. Its molecular formula is $C_6H_{13}NO_2$, and its molecular weight is 131.17 daltons. The structural formula is:

L-isoleucine

L-valine is also known as 2-aminoisovaleric acid, 2-amino-3-methylbutyric acid, alpha-aminoisovaleric acid and (S)-2-amino-3-methylbutanoic acid. It is abbreviated as Val, and its one letter abbreviation is V. Its molecular formula is $C_5H_{11}NO_2$, and its molecular weight is 117.15 daltons. The structural formula is:

L-valine

The branched-chain amino acids are sometimes classified as large neutral amino acids or LNAAs.

ACTIONS AND PHARMACOLOGY

ACTIONS

The branched-chain amino acids may have antihepatic encephalopathy activity in some. They may also have anticatabolic and antitardive dyskinesia activity in some.

MECHANISM OF ACTION

It has been theorized that some of the symptoms of hepatic encephalopathy are due to the accumulation of false neurotransmitters in the brain resulting, in part, from alterations in plasma levels of BCAAs. BCAAs may improve encephalopathy symptoms in some by decreasing the accumulation of these false neurotransmitters and perhaps other substances involved in the encephalopathy. The pathogenesis of hepatic encephalopathy is very complex and still poorly understood.

Although amino acids are not considered important energy sources, BCAAs serve as important fuel sources for skeletal muscle during periods of metabolic stress. Under such conditions, BCAAs may promote protein synthesis, suppress protein catabolism and serve as substrates for gluconeogenesis. BCAAs are mainly catabolized in skeletal muscle, stimulating the production of, among other substances, L-alanine and L-glutamine.

The BCAAs' possible antitardive dyskinesia activity may be accounted for, in part, by decreasing the availability of L-phenylalanine in the brain.

PHARMACOKINETICS

Following ingestion, the BCAAs are absorbed from the small intestine by a sodium-dependent active-transport process and transported to the liver via the portal circulation. In the liver, the BCAAs can serve as substrates for protein synthesis. Some catabolism of the BCAAs occurs in the liver. The catabolism of L-leucine, L-isoleucine and L-valine initially involves the same three reactions: the conversion of the amino acids to their corresponding alpha-keto acids; the conversion of the alpha-keto acids to their corresponding acyl-CoA thioesters and carbon dioxide; and the conversion of the acyl-CoA thioesters to their corresponding alpha, beta-unsaturated acyl-CoA thioesters. The enzyme deficiency in the inborn error of metabolism maple syrup urine disease is in the conversion of the acyl-CoA thioesters to the alpha, beta-unsaturated acyl-CoA thioesters, via the enzyme branched-chain alpha-keto acid decarboxylase.

L-leucine, L-isoleucine and L-valine are catabolized differently starting from their corresponding acyl-CoA thioesters. L-leucine, which is a ketogenic amino acid, is converted via a number of metabolic steps to beta-hydroxy-beta-methyl-glutaryl-CoA, which in turn is converted to acetoacetic acid and acetyl-CoA. The B vitamin biotin participates in this pathway. L-isoleucine, which is both glycogenic and ketogenic, is converted via a number of metabolic steps to alpha-methyl-acetoacetyl-CoA, which in turn is converted to acetyl-CoA (ketogenic) and propionyl-CoA (glycogenic). Finally, the glycogenic L-valine is converted via a number of steps to methylmalonyl-CoA and then, with the assistance of vitamin B_{12}, to succinyl-CoA.

The BCAAs are distributed to the various tissues of the body via the systemic circulation. The BCAAs appear to be preferentially taken up by skeletal muscle, where they undergo similar catabolic reactions to those described above. Skeletal muscle appears to be the major site of both BCAA transamination and oxidation in humans. BCAAs are also taken up by other organs, particularly the brain and kidney, where they also undergo oxidation.

INDICATIONS AND USAGE

BCAAs may be helpful in a minority of patients with hepatic encephalopathy. There is evidence that BCAA supplementation may decrease morbidity and duration of hospitalization in patients with chronic liver disease who undergo liver resection for hepatocellular carcinoma. There are some very preliminary indications BCAA might benefit some patients with chronic obstructive pulmonary disease (COPD) and that intravenous BCAA might benefit some with traumatic brain injury. There is preliminary evidence that BCAAs may prevent muscle catabolism and promote protein synthesis in some trauma subjects and, possibly, in some exercisers. There is no evidence that they are effective for enhancement of athletic performance. Neither have they proved useful in treating amyotrophic lateral sclerosis (ALS). In one trial, BCAAs reduced symptoms of tardive dyskinesia. They have also been used with some benefit in some with phenylketonuria.

RESEARCH SUMMARY

Meta-analyses have produced conflicting and largely ambiguous results with respect to the role, if any, that BCAAs may play in the prevention or treatment of hepatic encephalopathy. One group of researchers concluded several years ago that BCAAs might be helpful in treating some with advanced cirrhosis who are intolerant to alimentary proteins. More recently, a consensus review written under the auspices of the European society for parenteral and enteral nutrition, similarly concluded that BCAAs might be indicated in that small number of patients intolerant to the supplementary dietary proteins needed to achieve nitrogen balance in this condition.

A recent study found some benefit from BCAA supplementation in 30 liver cirrhosis patients. Improvement in energy metabolism and glucose tolerance was noted in this uncontrolled study. In another recent study, the effects of perioperative BCAA supplementation in patients undergoing liver resection for hepatocellular carcinoma, a disease usually accompanied by underlying liver cirrhosis, were tested. Compared with controls, the supplemented group enjoyed diminished postoperative complications, including diminished surgical site infection and bile leakage. Ascites appeared in significantly fewer of the supplemented subjects compared with controls. And hospitalization was considerably shorter in the supplemented patients. Further research is needed and warranted.

There is some preliminary evidence that BCAAs might help prevent muscle catabolism and promote protein synthesis in those with various forms of trauma. In one very small study, BCAAs were reported to inhibit protein breakdown in five men exercising the knee extensor muscles. Another very small study suggested that BCAAs might have inhibited muscle glycogen degradation during exercise.

On the other hand, there is no credible evidence that BCAAs have any significant effect on exercise performance. In a study of well-trained cyclists, BCAAs had no effect on performance in a 100-kilometer trial. No improvement in physical performance was seen in 12 sailors randomly assigned to a BCAA-supplemented standard diet or a standard diet alone during a 32-hour sailing race. Feeling of fatigue was said to be greater, however, in the non-supplemented group, which also performed less well on a short-term memory test.

There were some early reports suggesting that BCAAs might help ameliorate some of the symptoms of amyotrophic lateral sclerosis (ALS). In one of these studies, ALS patients receiving 12 grams of L-leucine, 8 grams of L-isoleucine and 6.4 grams of L-valine daily for one year showed significant benefit, as measured by maintenance of muscle strength in extremities and walking ability. Those receiving placebo in this small study showed a linear decline in these parameters consistent with the normal course of this disease.

More recently, however, most studies have produced negative results with respect to BCAA use in ALS. In one double-blind, placebo-controlled trial on the safety and efficacy of BCAAs in the treatment of ALS, there was a significant excess mortality in subjects randomized to BCAAs versus placebo. This finding, coupled with lack of apparent BCAA efficacy, resulted in early termination of the study.

In a two-center, double-blind, placebo-controlled trial of BCAAs in ALS patients, six months of treatment failed to produce results better than placebo. In fact, treatment with BCAAs in this study was associated with increased loss of pulmonary function. Decline in forced vital capacity (FVC) was said to be 2.5 times greater than in subjects receiving placebo.

In one recent study, BCAAs significantly decreased symptoms of tardive dyskinesia in nine men who had used neuroleptics for prolonged periods.

In a preliminary study, adolescents and young adults with phenylketonuria were said to benefit from BCAA treatment over a period of several months. Those receiving BCAAs performed better on neuropsychologic tests than did unsupplemented controls. More research is needed.

In a recent pilot study, researchers reported that 15 days of intravenous BCAA supplementation showed some signs of abetting recovery from a vegetative or minimally conscious state in patients with traumatic brain injury. Follow-up is needed. In another recent study, adding BCAA to soy protein was said to favorably alter protein metabolism in healthy elderly and to benefit even more those with chronic obstructive pulmonary disease. Again, more research is needed.

CONTRAINDICATIONS, PRECAUTIONS, ADVERSE REACTIONS

CONTRAINDICATIONS

Branched-chain amino acids are contraindicated in those with the rare inborn errors of metabolism maple syrup urine disease and isovaleric acidemia. BCAAs are also contraindicated in those with hypersensitivity to any component of a BCAA-containing supplement.

PRECAUTIONS

Pregnant women and nursing mothers should avoid BCAA supplementation except if prescribed by their physicians.

Treatment of hepatic encephalopathy, trauma and ALS or other diseases with BCAAs must only be done under qualified medical supervision.

Some recent research indicates that some ALS patients may get worse if treated with BCAAs.

ADVERSE REACTIONS

A recent study indicated increased mortality in ALS patients taking large doses of BCAAs.

OVERDOSAGE

No reports of overdosage.

DOSAGE AND ADMINISTRATION

Branched-chain amino acids are available for enteral and parenteral nutrition in the management of hepatic encephalopathy and metabolic stress conditions.

Nutritional supplements of BCAAs are available. Dosage is variable. Some combination BCAA products include other nutrients such as biotin and vitamin B_{12}, which are involved in the metabolism of the BCAAs.

LITERATURE

Abeta S, Inoue N, Matsui H, et al. Effect of branched-chain amino acids on glutamate neurotoxicity in primary cultured rat cerebral neurons. [Article in Japanese.] *Rinsho Shinkeigaku.* 1995;35:420-423.

Aquilani R, Boselli M, Boschi F, et al. Branched-chain amino acids may improve recovery from a vegetative or minimally conscious state in patients with traumatic brain injury: a pilot study. *Arch Phys Med Rehabil.* 2008;89(9):1642-1647.

Austic RE, Su C-L, Strupp BJ, et al. Effects of dietary mixtures of amino acids on fetal growth and maternal and fetal amino acid pools in experimental maternal phenylketonuria. *Am J Clin Nutr.* 1999;69:687-696.

Bastone A, Michel. A, Beghi E, et al. The imbalance of brain large-chain amino acid availability in amyotrophic lateral sclerosis patients treated with high doses of branched-chain amino acids. *Neurochem Int.* 1995;27:467-472.

Berry HK, Brunner RL, Hunt MM, et al. Valine, isoleucine and leucine. A new treatment for phenylketonuria. *Am J Dis Child.* 1990;144:539-543.

Engelen MP, Rutten EP, De Castro CL, et al. Supplementation of soy protein with branched-chain amino acids alters protein metabolism in healthy elderly and even more in patients with chronic obstructive pulmonary disease. *Am J Clin Nutr.* 2007;85(2):431-439.

Fabbri A, Magrini N, Bianchi G, et al. Overview of randomized clinical trials of oral branched-chain amino acid treatment in chronic hepatic encephalopathy. *J Parenter Enteral Nutr.* 1996;20:159-164.

Greer BK, Woodard JL, White JP, et al. Branched-chain amino acid supplementation and indicators of muscle damage after endurance exercise. *Int J Sport Nutr Exerc Metab.* 2007;17(6):595-607.

Kawaguchi T, Nagao Y, Matsuoka H, et al. Branched-chain amino acid-enriched supplementation improves insulin resistance in patients with chronic liver disease. *Int J Mol Med.* 2008;22(1):105-112.

MacLean DA, Graham TE, Saltin B. Stimulation of muscle ammonia production during exercise following branched-chain amino acid supplementation in humans. *J Physiol (Lond).* 1996;493(Pt 3):909-922.

Maddrey WC. Branched chain amino acid therapy in liver disease. *J Am Coll Nutr.* 1985;4:639-650.

Madsen K, Maclean DA, Kiens B, et al. Effects of glucose, glucose plus branched-chain amino acids, or placebo on bike performance over 100km. *J Appl Physiol.* 1996;81:2644-2650.

Marchesini G, Bianchi G, Rossi B, et al. Nutritional treatment with branched-chain amino acids in advanced liver cirrhosis. *J Gastroenterol.* 2000;35 Suppl 12:7-12.

Marchesini G, Zoli M, Dondi C, et al. Anticatabolic effect of branched-chain amino acid-enriched solutions with liver cirrhosis. *Hepatology.* 1982;2:420-425.

Okabayashi T, Nishimori I, Sugimoto T, et al. Effects of branched-chain amino acids-enriched nutrient support for patients undergoing liver resection for hepatocellular carcinoma. *J Gastroenterol Hepatol.* Epub: 2008 Aug 20.

Pelosi G, Proietti R, Magalini SI, et al. Anticatabolic properties of branched chain amino acids in trauma. *Resuscitation.* 1983;10:153-158.

Plaitakis A, Smith J, Mandeli J, et al. Pilot trial of branched-chain amino acids in amyotrophic lateral sclerosis. *Lancet.* 1988;1(8593):1015-1018.

Portier H, Chatard JC, Filaire E, et al. Effects of branched-chain amino acids supplementation on physiological and psychological performance during an offshore sailing race. *Eur J Appl Physiol.* 2008;104(5):787-794.

Richardson MA, Bevans ML, Weber JB, et al. Branched chain amino acids decrease tardive dyskinesia symptoms. *Psychopharmacol.* 1999;143:358-364.

Suryawan A, Hawes JW, Harris RA, et al. A molecular model of human branched-chain amino acid metabolism. *Am J Clin Nutr.* 1998;68:72-81.

Tandan R, Bromberg MB, Forshew D, et al. A controlled trial of amino acid therapy in amyotropic lateral sclerosis: I. Clinical, functional, and maximum isometric torque data. *Neurology.* 1996;47:1220-1226.

Testa D, Caraceni T, Fetoni V. Branched-chain amino acids in the treatment of amyotrophic lateral sclerosis. *J Neurol.* 1989;236:445-447.

The Italian ALS Study Group. Branched-chain amino acids and amyotrophic sclerosis: a treatment failure? *Neurology.* 1993;43:2466-2470.

Urata Y, Okita K, Korenaga K, et al. The effect of supplementation with branched-chain amino acids in patients with liver cirrhosis. *Hepatol Res.* 2007;37(7):510-516.

Brewer's Yeast

DESCRIPTION

Brewer's yeast is derived from the unicellular fungus *Saccharomyces cerevisiae*, which causes the fermentation process basic to the brewing of beer. Different strains of this yeast are used in the production of the various types of beer. Still other strains are used in the fermentation of dough to produce bread. The strains of *Saccharomyces cerevisiae* that are used for the production of bread are collectively called baker's yeast.

Dried brewer's yeast is a rich source of several nutrients, including the B vitamins thiamin, riboflavin, niacin, pyridoxine, pantothenic acid, folate, vitamin B_{12} and biotin, and such trace minerals as chromium and selenium. It also contains beta-glucans (see Yeast Beta-Glucan), ribonucleic acid or RNA (see Nucleic Acids/Nucleotides), para-aminobenzoic acid and myo-inositol. A substance isolated from brewer's yeast called skin respiratory factor or SRF has found application in some cosmetic and wound-healing products, as well as in some hemorrhoidal preparations. The chemical identity of SRF is unknown.

Brewer's yeast has been a popular nutritional supplement for many years. Much of the brewer's yeast marketed for nutritional supplement use is grown specifically for that marketplace. The supplements are prepared from dry, crushed cells of *Saccharomyces cerevisiae*. The cells are not alive. There are other yeast preparations, such as *Saccharomyces boulardii*, in which the cells are alive; they are used as probiotics. (See Probiotics.)

ACTIONS AND PHARMACOLOGY

ACTIONS

Brewer's yeast is a delivery form of the B vitamins and other nutrients, such as selenium and chromium. It is also a delivery form for beta-glucans and RNA. High-selenium brewer's yeast may have anticarcinogenic activity. High-chromium brewer's yeast has putative antidiabetic activity.

MECHANISM OF ACTION

High-selenium brewer's yeast given to deliver a daily dose of 200 micrograms of selenium was found to reduce the incidences of lung, prostate and colorectal cancer in one study. The mechanism of the possible anticarcinogenic activity is unclear. Selenium's antioxidant activity may account, in part, for its possible anticarcinogenic activity. (See Selenium.) The beta-glucans in yeast may also account, in part, for the possible anticarcinogenic activity via their possible immune-modulating activity. (See Yeast Beta-Glucan.)

High-chromium use has been found in a few, but not all, studies to improve glucose tolerance in those with hyperglycemia and in some with type 2 diabetes mellitus. Earlier, it was proposed that chromium acted via a so-called glucose tolerance factor, or GTF, in brewer's yeast. The chemical identity of this putative GTF has not been established. The mechanism of the putative antidiabetic effect of high-chromium yeast is unknown. (See Chromium.) RNA may also have immunomodulatory activity. (See Nucleic Acids/Nucleotides.)

PHARMACOKINETICS

See the various monographs on the B vitamins, as well as Selenium, Chromium, Yeast Beta-Glucan and Nucleic Acids and Derivatives, for pharmacokinetic information on these substances.

INDICATIONS AND USAGE

Claims that brewer's yeast is useful for diarrhea, acne, furunculosis, colds, coughs, dyspepsia, inflammatory conditions and various infections have little or no credible support.

Some have confused the brewer's yeast that is typically sold as a supplement with *Saccharomyces boulardii*, a probiotic (see Probiotics) that has demonstrated some of the benefits erroneously attributed to brewer's yeast, at least in very preliminary research. There is some suggestion that high-selenium brewer's yeast may have some anticarcinogenic effects and that high-chromium yeast might be helpful in some with type 2 diabetes.

RESEARCH SUMMARY

Supplementation with selenium-enriched brewer's yeast (delivering 200 micrograms of selenium a day) over a period of several years was associated, in one study, with significant reduction in the incidence of lung, colorectal, prostate and total cancer, as well as a reduction in total cancer mortality. It is not known with certainty which components in selenium-enriched brewer's yeast may exert anti-cancer effects. One recent animal study found that DL-selenomethionine lacked chemopreventive efficacy in colon carcinogenesis. (See Selenium.)

Some studies have shown that high-chromium brewer's yeast can improve glucose tolerance in some with type 2 diabetes. These results, however, are inconsistent. In one placebo-controlled study of elderly subjects with stable impaired glucose tolerance, chromium-rich yeast had no significant effects on glucose tolerance or serum lipids, compared with controls. In another study, brewer's yeast improved glucose tolerance and had beneficial effects on lipids in Chinese adults. More study is needed.

CONTRAINDICATIONS, PRECAUTIONS, ADVERSE REACTIONS

CONTRAINDICATIONS

Brewer's yeast is contraindicated in those hypersensitive to any component of a brewer's yeast containing-product. It is also contraindicated in those taking monoamine oxidase inhibitors.

PRECAUTIONS

Pregnant women and nursing mothers should avoid brewer's yeast supplements pending long-term safety studies.

ADVERSE REACTIONS

Brewer's yeast is generally well tolerated. Occasional allergic reactions have been reported. Some may develop flatulence when taking brewer's yeast. Some do not like the bitter taste.

INTERACTIONS

DRUGS

Monoamine oxidase (MAO) inhibitors: including phenelzine sulfate, tranylcypromine sulfate and pargyline HCl. Concomitant use of brewer's yeast and MAO inhibitors may cause hypertension.

OVERDOSAGE

No reports of overdosage.

DOSAGE AND ADMINISTRATION

Brewer's yeast is available as flakes, powder, tablets and capsules. These preparations are prepared from dried, crushed cells of *Saccharomyces cerevisiae*. Dosage is variable. Some marketed chromium and selenium preparations are derived from chromium-rich and selenium-rich baker's yeast, respectively. (See Chromium and Selenium.)

LITERATURE

See Chromium, Selenium, Yeast Beta-Glucan and Nucleic Acids/Nucleotides.

Also:

Clark LC, Combs GF Jr, Turnball BW, et al. Effects of selenium supplementation for cancer prevention in patients with carcinoma of the skin. A randomized controlled trial. Nutritional Prevention of Cancer Study Group. *JAMA.* 1996; 276:1957-1963.

Guan X, Matte JJ, Ku PK, et al. High chromium yeast supplementation improves glucose tolerance in pigs by decreasing hepatic extraction of insulin. *J Nutr.* 2000; 130:1274-1279.

Li YC. Effects of brewer's yeast on glucose tolerance and serum lipids in Chinese adults. *Biol Trace Elem Res.* 1994; 41:341-347.

Bromelain

DESCRIPTION

Bromelain is the collective term for enzymes (principally proteolytic enzymes) derived from the ripe and unripe fruit, as well as the stem and leaves, of the pineapple plant, *Ananas comosus*, a member of the Bromeliaceae family. Commercial bromelain is typically stem bromelain. Bromelain is mainly comprised of cysteine proteases, with smaller amounts of acid phosphatase, peroxidase, amylase and cellulase. Bromelain contains at least four distinct cysteine proteases. The principal stem protease is called stem bromelain or stem bromelain protease. Two additional proteases found in the stem are called ananain and comosain. Fruit bromelain is the name given to the principal protease found in the fruit. Stem protease is a basic glycoprotein with a molecular weight of 28,000 daltons.

Pineapple has been used as a folk medicine by the natives of the tropics for centuries. It has been used as a digestive aid, as a cleansing agent to improve the texture of the skin, and to promote the healing of wounds. It is used commercially in certain cosmetics and as a meat tenderizer and dietary supplement. Bromelain may have digestant activity and there is research suggesting that it may have wound healing, anti-inflammatory, antidiarrheal and anticarcinogenic effects, as well.

The activity of bromelain may be expressed in six different ways: Rorer units, FIP units, BTU (bromelain tyrosine units), CDU (casein digestion units), GDU (gelatin digestion units) or MCU (milk clotting units).

The most commonly used measures of activity are MCU or GDU. One GDU is equivalent to about 1.5 MCU.

An interesting aside, is that pineapple workers often have their fingerprints almost completely obliterated due to the proteolytic action of bromelain.

ACTIONS AND PHARMACOLOGY

ACTIONS

Bromelain may have digestant activity and has putative anti-inflammatory, immunomodulatory, antidiarrheal, anticarcinogenic and wound healing actions.

MECHANISM OF ACTION

Bromelain's digestant activity is based on its ability to hydrolyze proteins to oligopeptides and amino acids. Bromelain's proteolytic enzymes are cysteine proteases. Cysteine proteases cleave peptide bonds by nucleophilic attack via active-site cysteine residues. Other members of the cysteine protease family, include calpains and caspases.

The mechanism of the putative anti-inflammatory activity is not well understood. It may be accounted for, in part, by activation of plasmin production from plasminogen and reduction of kinin, via inhibition of the conversion of kininogen to kinin. Other possibilities, include proteolytic degradation of circulating immune complexes and inhibition of signaling by extracellular regulated kinase (ERK)-2 and p21^{ras}. It is speculated that the possible protective effect of bromelain in murine EAE (experimental allergic encephalomyelitis), the animal model of multiple sclerosis, is due to proteolytic cleavage of accessory molecules involved in the interaction of T lymphocytes and antigen presenting cells, thus increasing the activation threshold of the autoreactive T lymphocytes.

The mechanism of bromelain's putative immunomodulatory activity is likewise poorly understood. Bromelain has been shown to increase CD2-mediated T cell activation, to enhance antigen-independent binding to monocytes and to increase interferon (IFN)-gamma-dependent, tumor necrosis factor (TNF)-alpha, interleukin(IL)-1 beta, and interleukin(IL)-6 production in peripheral blood monocytes. These effects are thought to be due to bromelain's proteolytic activity at cell surfaces, whereby it either removes surface molecules or reveals ones that already exist on cell membranes, thereby altering receptor-ligand interactions. Recent studies have reported that bromelain proteolytically blocks activation of extracellular regulated kinase(ERK)-2 in T cells, resulting in inhibition of T cell signal transduction.

Bromelain has been found to reduce the incidence of enterotoxigenic *Escherichia coli* diarrhea in piglets. This effect is thought to be due to inactivation of enterotoxigenic *E. coli* receptors in the small intestine via proteolytic cleavage of the glycoprotein receptor.

The putative anticarcinogenic activity of bromelain is open to speculation. Possibilities include disruption of adhesion molecules on tumor and endothelial cells via its proteolytic activity and inhibition of signaling by ERK-2 and p21^{ras}. It has also been speculated that bromelain may play a role in the differentiation of malignant cells. Certain cysteine proteases (e.g., caspases) are involved in apoptosis. Were bromelain to enter cancer cells, one may speculate that it could induce apoptosis. On the other hand, bromelain entering normal cells does not appear to be desirable.

The putative wound healing activity of bromelain may be accounted for by its possible anti-inflammatory activity.

PHARMACOKINETICS

The pharmacokinetics of bromelain in humans are mostly unknown. Bromelain is active under a wide pH range (between pH3-10) and may not be inactivated by stomach acid. The putative anti-inflammatory, immunomodulatory and anticarcinogenic actions of bromelain most likely require that it gets absorbed from the intestine. It is conceivable that

unabsorbed bromelain may mediate some of these possible effects via a signal transduction mechanism. However, this is entirely speculative. There is some evidence from tissue culture studies that bromelain may be able to enter cells and some bromelain may be absorbed via the enteropancreatic circulation. Research is very much needed on the pharmacokinetics of bromelain.

INDICATIONS AND USAGE

There is some evidence that bromelain may be useful in speeding the healing time of some injuries and surgical wounds, that it is a digestive aid in some conditions, that it inhibits platelet aggregation and is helpful in some with thromboses and angina, that it has positive effects in some respiratory tract diseases, dysmenorrhea and some forms of diarrhea. It has also exhibited some immune-enhancing and anticancer effects.

RESEARCH SUMMARY

Bromelain has been shown to speed healing time and reduce pain following various surgical procedures, including oral surgical procedures and episiotomy. It has also been used with significant positive results in the treatment of various athletic injuries. In one open case observation study, high-dose bromelain was administered to 59 patients with blunt injuries to the musculoskeletal system. A clear reduction in swelling, pain at rest and during movement and in tenderness was reported. Positive bromelain studies related to oral surgery and episiotomy have been double-blind and placebo-controlled. Positive effects have been attributed by some to anti-inflammatory activity, rather than to an analgesic effect.

Bromelain has been used with some success as a substitute for trypsin and pepsin in cases of pancreatic insufficiency and post-pancreatectomy.

In vitro and *in vivo* studies show some bromelain-induced inhibition of platelet aggregation, and some positive bromelain-related effects have been reported in patients with thromboses and angina. In one double-blind study of 73 patients with acute thrombophlebitis, bromelain, used with analgesics, reduced pain, edema, redness, tenderness, elevated skin temperature and disability. The effective doses ranged between 60-160 milligrams daily of 1,200 MCU bromelain.

Bromelain's reported mucolytic activity has prompted some use of it in respiratory tract diseases. It has shown some benefit in chronic bronchitis and, in a double-blind study, in acute sinusitis.

Bromelain's reported efficacy (in combination with papain) in easing dysmenorrhea symptoms has been attributed to a smooth-muscle-relaxant effect since it has been observed to decrease spasms of contracted cervixes in these patients.

Some hypothesize that muscle-relaxing effects of bromelain on the uterus are due to modulation of various prostaglandins.

In animal models, bromelain has shown significant antidiarrheal activity. In these experiments, bromelain inhibited activity of enterotoxigenic *Escherichia coli* and *Vibrio cholerae*. It significantly reduced heat-stable and heat-labile enterotoxin-induced secretion, among other effects.

In the realm of immunity, bromelain is being tested for possible effects in T cell-mediated autoimmune diseases, including multiple sclerosis, type 1 diabetes and rheumatoid arthritis. In combination with trypsin and the flavonoid rutin, bromelain has been reported to protect against experimental allergic encephalomyelitis. This research is ongoing.

Bromelain has recently shown an ability to decrease lung metastases of Lewis lung cancer cells in mice. In another recent study, oral bromelain was administered to 16 breast cancer patients for ten days. The results of this study suggested that bromelain stimulated deficient monocyte cytotoxicity of mammary tumor patients. More research is needed.

CONTRAINDICATIONS, PRECAUTIONS, ADVERSE REACTIONS

CONTRAINDICATIONS

Bromelain is contraindicated in those hypersensitive to any component of a bromelain-containing product.

PRECAUTIONS

Bromelain supplements should be avoided by pregnant women and nursing mothers.

The use of bromelain for the treatment of any disorder must be medically supervised. The use of bromelain for the treatment of diarrhea caused by enteropathogenic *E. coli*, cancer or any inflammatory disorder is experimental.

Those on anticoagulants or antithrombotic agents should exercise caution in the use of bromelain. Bromelain may have blood-thinning activity in some.

ADVERSE REACTIONS

Gastrointestinal symptoms such as nausea and vomiting, diarrhea and cramping have been reported. There are occasional reports of metrorrhagia and menorrhagia.

INTERACTIONS

DRUGS

Antibiotics (amoxicillin, tetracycline): Concomitant use of bromelain and amoxicillin or tetracycline have been reported to increase the serum levels of these antibiotics.

Anticoagulants (e.g., warfarin): Bromelain may enhance the anticoagulant activity of such drugs as warfarin.

Antithrombotic agents (e.g., aspirin): Bromelain may enhance the antithrombotic activity of such drugs as aspirin.

OVERDOSAGE

There are no reports of bromelain overdosage in the literature.

DOSAGE AND ADMINISTRATION

Bromelain is available as a single ingredient product or in combination with other supplementary enzymes (see Supplementary Enzymes). Dosage ranges from 500-2,000 GDUs (gelatin digestion units) taken one to three times daily.

LITERATURE

Batkin S, Taussig SJ, Szekerezes J. Antimetastatic effect of bromelain with or without its proteolytic and anticoagulant activity. *J Cancer Res Clin Oncol.* 1988; 114:507-508.

Bock U, Kolac C, Borchard G, et al. Transport of proteolytic enzymes across Caco-2 cell monolayers. *Pharm Res.* 1998; 15:1393-1400.

Chandler DS, Mynott TL. Bromelain protects piglets from diarrhea caused by oral challenge with K88 positive enterotoxigenic Escherichia coli. *Gut.* 1998; 43:196-202.

Eckert K, Grabowska E, Strange R, et al. Effects of oral bromelain administration on the Impaired immunocytotoxicity of mononuclear cells from mammary tumor patients. *Oncol Rep.* 1999; 6:1191-1199.

Kumakura S, Yamashita M, Tsurufuji S. Effect of bromelain on kaolin-induced inflammation in rats. *Eur J Pharmacol.* 1988; 150:295-301.

Masson M. [Bromelain in blunt injuries of the locomotor system. A study of observed applications in general practice]. [Article in German]. *Fortschr Med.* 1995; 113:303-306.

Metzig C, Grabowska E, Eckert K, et al. Bromelain proteases reduce human platelet aggregation in vitro, adhesion to bovine endothelial cells and thrombus formation in rat vessels in vivo. *In Vivo.* 1999; 13:7-12.

Munzig E, Eckert K, Harrach T, et al. Bromelain protease F9 reduces the CD44 mediated adhesion of human peripheral blood lymphocytes to human umbilical vein endothelial cells. *FEBS Lett.* 1994; 351:215-218.

Mynott TL, Guandalini S, Raimondi F, Fasano A. Bromelain prevents secretion caused by Vibrio cholerae and Escherichia coli enterotoxins in rabbit ileum in vitro. *Gastroenterology.* 1997; 113:175-184.

Mynott TL, Ladhams A, Scarmato P, Engwerda CR. Bromelain from pineapple stems, proteolytically blocks activation of extracellular regulated kinase-2 in T cells. *J Immunol.* 1999; 163:2568-2575.

Rowan AD, Butte DJ, Barrett AJ. The cysteine proteinases of the pineapple plant. *Biochem J.* 1990; 266:869-875.

Targoni OS, Tary-Lehmann M, Lehmann PV. Prevention of murine EAE by oral hydrolytic enzyme treatment. *J Autoimmun.* 1999; 12:191-198.

Taussig SJ, Batkin S. Bromelain, the enzyme complex of pineapple (*Ananas comosus*) and its clinical application. *J Ethnopharmcol.* 1988; 22:191-203.

Bromine (Bromide)

DESCRIPTION

Bromine belongs to the halogen group of elements. Its atomic number is 35 and its symbol is Br. Bromine is a readily volatile, dark-reddish-brown liquid with a strong, disagreeable odor (*bromos* in Greek means stench) and an irritating effect on the eyes and throat. It is the only non-metallic element that is liquid under ordinary conditions. Many of the compounds of bromine are salts or bromides. Halogen comes from the Greek word meaning salt-producer. Bromine occurs in the form of salts in sea and ocean water, mineral springs and natural salt deposits.

Bromine is not considered an essential nutrient for humans. A bromine-deficiency state has been reported in goats. Goats fed diets low in bromide were found to have depressed growth, fertility and life expectancy. Also observed in these animals were decreased red-blood-cell count, increased milk fat and a greater number of spontaneous abortions. Dietary bromide has also been found to alleviate growth retardation caused by hyperthyroidism in mice and chicks and to substitute for part of the chloride requirement for chicks. Insomnia in some hemodialysis patients has been associated with bromide deficiency.

Bromide is the fifth most abundant inorganic anion in human plasma and tissues, following chloride, bicarbonate, phosphate and sulfate. In plasma, it is present at a concentration of 20-150 micromolar.

Bromine may play a role in the respiratory burst of eosinophils. Eosinophils play a central role in host defenses against helminthic parasites and other large invading metazoan pathogens, and possibly against some cancers. This is in contrast to neutrophils, which primarily ingest and kill relatively small microbes Eosinophil peroxidase catalyzes the oxidation of bromide to hypobromous acid and hypobromite, which may participate in the killing role of eosinophils. There is some evidence that this may occur by oxidative damage to proteins through bromination of tyrosine residues. Brominating oxidants may also participate in allergen-induced asthma.

Daily dietary intake of bromide is about 2 to 8 milligrams. Fish, grains and nuts are rich sources of bromide.

Potassium bromide had been used as a sedative drug in the United States and is still occasionally used as a sedative and anticonvulsant in Europe. Prolonged intake of potassium bromide can lead to bromide intoxication or bromism. Bromo-Seltzer does not contain bromine. Bromides are used in some homeopathic remedies such as kali bromatum.

The terms bromine and bromide are sometimes used interchangeably. Bromine is usually found as its bromide form.

ACTIONS AND PHARMACOLOGY

ACTIONS

None known for dietary bromine.

INDICATIONS AND USAGE

There are no indications for the supplemental use of bromine (bromide).

RESEARCH SUMMARY

An association has been made between insomnia experienced by some hemodialysis patients and bromide deficiency. This warrants followup.

CONTRAINDICATIONS, PRECAUTIONS, ADVERSE REACTIONS

CONTRAINDICATIONS

Supplemental bromide is not recommended for anyone.

PRECAUTIONS

Given our present state of knowledge regarding bromine, supplemental bromide is not recommended for anyone.

ADVERSE REACTIONS

Use of potassium bromide as a sedative drug may give rise to bromide intoxication or bromism. Symptoms include nausea, vomiting, slurred speech, memory impairment, drowsiness, irritability, ataxia, tremors, hallucinations, mania, delirium, psychoses, stupor and coma. Skin rashes of various types may occur, and toxic epidermal necrolysis has been reported.

OVERDOSAGE

Death after acute bromide poisoning is rare since vomiting follows the ingestion of large doses of potassium bromide. Ingestion of large doses of potassium bromide can lead to severe central nervous system depression, including coma.

DOSAGE AND ADMINISTRATION

No recommended dosage. Bromine as bromide may be found in colloidal or liquid mineral preparations and in some homeopathic remedies.

LITERATURE

Nielsen FH. Other trace elements. In: Ziegler EE, Filer LL Jr, eds. *Present Knowledge in Nutrition.* 7th ed. Washington, DC: ILSI Press; 1996:353-377.

Nielsen FH. Ultratrace minerals. In: Shils ME, Olson JA, Shike M, Ross AC, eds. *Modern Nutrition in Health and Disease.* 9th ed. Baltimore MD: Williams and Wilkins; 1999:283-303.

Thomas EL, Bozeman PM, Jefferson MM, King CC. Oxidation of bromide by the human leukocyte enzymes myeloperoxidase and eosinophil peroxidase. *J Biol Chem.* 1995; 270;2906-2913.

Wu W, Samoszuk MK, Comhair SAA, et al. Eosinophils generate brominating oxidants in allergen-induced asthma. *J Clin Invest*. 2000; 105:1455-1463.

Calcium

DESCRIPTION

Calcium is an essential mineral with a wide range of biological roles. Apart from being a major constituent of bones and teeth, calcium is crucial for muscle contraction, nerve conduction, the beating of the heart, blood coagulation, glandular secretion, the production of energy and the maintenance of immune function, among other things. Calcium is an alkaline-earth metal with atomic number 20 and an atomic mass of 40.08 daltons. Its atomic symbol is Ca.

Calcium is found in bone and teeth primarily in the form of the calcium phosphate compound hydroxyapatite. The molecular formula of hydroxyapatite is $Ca_{10}(PO_4)_6(OH)_2$. Over 99% of the total body calcium is found in bone and teeth, and calcium makes up from 1% to 2% of adult body weight.

Milk products are the most calcium-dense foods. Other foods rich in calcium include the vegetables collard greens, Chinese cabbage, mustard greens, broccoli and bok choy, as well as tofu and sardines with bones included. About 25% of women in the United States take calcium supplements. The average intake of calcium in the American diet is approximately 800 milligrams daily. Calcium intake is typically higher in males than it is in females.

ACTIONS AND PHARMACOLOGY

ACTIONS

Calcium has anti-osteoporotic activity. It may also have anticarcinogenic, antihypertensive and hypocholesterolemic activity.

MECHANISM OF ACTION

Inadequate calcium intake results in reduced bone mass and osteoporosis. Calcium exists in bone primarily in the form of hydroxyapatite ($Ca_{10}(PO_4)_6(OH)_2$). Hydroxyapatite comprises approximately 40% of the weight of bone. The skeleton has an obvious structural requirement for calcium. The skeleton also serves as a reservoir for calcium.

A number of studies suggest that calcium may reduce the risk of colorectal cancer. Calcium supplementation has been found to reduce colonic mucosal proliferation. Greater colonic mucosal proliferation is observed in those at high risk for colon cancer when compared with those at low risk. Calcium ions may precipitate bile acids and fatty acids that can stimulate the proliferation of colon cells.

Calcium supplementation has been found to have a modest effect on the reduction of systolic blood pressure in those with hypertension. Diastolic blood pressure does not appear to be affected by calcium, and calcium does not affect blood pressure in normotensives. The mechanism of the possible systolic blood pressure-lowering effect of supplemental calcium is unclear.

Some, but not all, studies have found supplemental calcium to lower serum cholesterol levels. A mechanism of this possible effect may be the binding of calcium ions with bile acids to form insoluble soaps, thus removing cholesterol entering the gut via the enterohepatic circulation.

PHARMACOKINETICS

Calcium is absorbed from the small intestine by both active and passive mechanisms. At low and moderate intakes of calcium, calcium is absorbed via active transfer. Active transfer depends on the action of the active form of vitamin D, 1,25-dihydroxycholecalciferol or $1,25(OH)_2 D_3$. Vitamin D-induced calcium transport involves the synthesis of the calcium-binding protein, calbindin. Calbindin serves as a calcium translocator. It also serves as a cytosolic calcium buffer. Calcium is typically freed from calcium complexes during digestion and is released in a soluble and probably ionized form for absorption. Low molecular weight complexes, such as calcium carbonate, may be absorbed intact.

As calcium intakes increase, the active transfer mechanism becomes saturated and an increasing proportion of calcium is absorbed via passive diffusion.

The absorption efficiency of calcium varies throughout the life span. It is highest during infancy when it is about 60%. In prepubertal children, it is about 28%. During early puberty, at the time of the growth spurt, it increases to about 34% and then drops to 25% two years later where it remains for several years. Absorption efficacy increases during the last two trimesters of pregnancy. It does decline with aging. In postmenopausal women, fractional absorption of calcium declines on the average of 0.21% yearly. Men lose absorption efficiency at about the same rate as women.

Absorption efficiency appears to vary with the different calcium complexes. In one study, absorption efficiency from a 250 milligram dose of calcium citrate malate was found to be 35%; from calcium carbonate, 27%; and from tricalcium phosphate, 25%. For comparison, calcium absorption efficiency from milk was found to be 29%. Some, but not all, studies suggest that calcium is more efficiently absorbed from calcium citrate and calcium citrate malate than it is from calcium carbonate. The efficiency of absorption of calcium from a calcium supplement is greatest when calcium is taken at doses of 500 milligrams or lower. Individuals with achlorhydria absorb calcium from calcium carbonate poorly unless the calcium carbonate supplement is taken with food.

Calcium that is unabsorbed from the intestine is excreted in the feces. Greater than 98% of calcium from the glomerular filtrate is reabsorbed. Renal reabsorption is primarily regulated by parathyroid hormone or PTH.

The colon plays an important role in calcium absorption after resection of the small intestine.

Approximately 40% of calcium in the plasma is bound to proteins, primarily albumin; about 50% of calcium in the plasma is diffusible ionic calcium and about 10% is diffusible, but is complexed with such anions as phosphate and citrate.

INDICATIONS AND USAGE

Calcium has long been assumed to be useful in preventing and treating osteoporosis and being beneficial for bone health in general. Recently, some highly publicized studies have cast some doubts on these claims, presenting conflicting and now controversial findings. The preponderance of evidence, however, continues to suggest an effective preventive role for calcium in osteoporosis in the aging population. Similarly, early findings that calcium significantly reduces risk of colorectal cancer were not supported by more-recent research. Again, however, there may be more evidence in support of a positive role than a neutral role; the issue is unresolved. Evidence continues to accumulate that calcium may help control blood pressure. There is also some evidence it may help reduce the risk of preeclampsia and maternal death during pregnancy. On the other hand, a recent study reported a higher incidence of myocardial infarction among healthy postmenopausal women who were taking calcium supplements (compared with placebo controls). There is weak and mixed evidence that calcium favorably affects lipids. An association has been made between higher intakes of calcium and lower incidence of stroke among women. A preliminary study some years ago suggested that calcium may help reduce the risk of obesity.

RESEARCH SUMMARY

In a review several years ago of 52 intervention trials investigating calcium's effects on osteoporosis, all but two were said to have shown beneficial effects, including better bone balance, greater bone gain during growth, reduced bone loss in the elderly and reduced risk of fracture. Observational studies have also, for the most part, associated higher calcium intake with enhanced bone health. Most of the intervention trials utilized calcium supplements; some used dairy products as the source of calcium. Most of these studies reported that high calcium intake augmented the osteoprotective effects of estrogen.

Some older studies have suggested that calcium citrate is better absorbed than calcium carbonate and that the citrate form might thus be more effective in helping to prevent or ameliorate osteoporosis. An analysis of 15 randomized trials concluded that calcium citrate was absorbed 22% to 27% better than calcium carbonate, whether taken on an empty stomach or with food. More research will be needed, however, to demonstrate conclusively that calcium citrate is more beneficial than calcium carbonate in osteoporosis.

Calcium has shown benefit in individuals who have lost bone mineral density due to long term corticosteroid therapy. In a double-blind, placebo-controlled study of subjects with rheumatoid arthritis, many of whom were being treated with corticosteroids, a combination of 1,000 milligrams of calcium carbonate and 500 IUs of vitamin D_3 daily was found to confer significant benefits. While subjects receiving placebo and prednisone lost bone mineral density in the lumbar spine and trochanter at a rate of 2% and 0.9%, respectively, per year, those getting prednisone and calcium gained bone mineral density in the lumbar spine and trochanter at a rate of 0.72% and 0.85% per year, respectively. No calcium-related improvements were seen, however, at any site in subjects who did not receive corticosteroids.

Recently, the results of some of these earlier studies have been partially contradicted by some, but not all, new research. In one major inquiry, 36,282 postmenopausal women, aged 50 to 79 years and enrolled in the Women's Health Initiative, were recruited for random assignment to either placebo or 1,000 milligrams of elemental calcium as calcium carbonate with 400 IU of vitamin D daily. The researchers sought to see what effect the calcium/D supplementation might have on risk of fractures in this aging population. Bone density was measured and fracture incidence followed up for seven years. A small but significant improvement in hip bone density was noted in the calcium/D group but not in the placebo group. The supplement group, however, had no fewer fractures than the placebo group. Incidence of kidney stones was higher in the supplement group. The result was unexpected, and the authors conceded that even a study involving this large a group of subjects with seven-year follow-up may not have been large enough or long enough in duration to detect at least a small but potentially significant benefit. Indeed, they reported that in a subgroup of women, over 60 years of age and judged by various measures to have a higher absolute risk of hip fracture, the calcium/D supplementation did significantly reduce the risk of hip fracture. Additionally, women who most closely complied with the supplement regimen had lower risk of fracture than those with lower levels of compliance.

An editorial accompanying publication of this important study in *The New England Journal of Medicine* noted that calcium supplements are the biggest seller in the multi-billion-dollar dietary-supplement marketplace, accounting for almost a billion dollars in sales per year in the United States alone. Thus, on financial as well as scientific grounds, the issue of what benefits, if any, accrue in terms of bone health warrants and demands close scrutiny. After taking into account the various weaknesses of the study, the editorialist nonetheless concluded that "calcium with vitamin D supplementation is not an effective means of preventing fractures in this population." Even if certain subgroups may benefit from this supplementation, the editorial cautioned women—and others at risk of fracture—about relying on this supplementation to significantly protect them: "Many women believe that they are completely protected against the development of osteoporosis if they are taking these supplements. This study should help correct this important misconception and allow more women to receive optimal therapy for bone health." Postmenopausal women, the editorial continued, might well be advised to continue taking the recommended daily levels of calcium and vitamin D (derived either through diet or supplementation or both), "but one message is clear: calcium with vitamin D supplementation by itself is not enough to ensure optimal bone health."

Some review authors concluded that there is evidence that calcium/vitamin D supplementation can be useful in preventing and ameliorating osteoporosis in the following groups: 1) patients with documented osteoporosis receiving antiresorptive or anabolic treatment, 2) individuals with or at high risk of calcium and/or vitamin D insufficiencies, especially elderly men and women, and 3) patients receiving glucocorticoids. They said benefits are most apparent when subjects are supplemented with 1,000-1,200 milligrams daily of elemental calcium combined with 800 IU daily of vitamin D. Level of compliance, they found, correlates with level of efficacy.

In a recent, double-blind, randomized trial, 930 generally healthy participants (mostly men, mean age: 61 years) received 1,200 milligrams of calcium daily for four years or placebo. Follow-up was for a mean of 10.8 years. The supplementation was found to significantly reduce the risk of all fractures and especially of minimal trauma fractures. The protective effect gradually dissipated after supplementation was discontinued. One of the purposes of this study was to see if calcium alone—not combined with vitamin D—could still exert bone-protective effects.

A recent meta-analysis published in *The Lancet* found support for the use of both calcium alone and calcium in combination with vitamin D in the preventive treatment of osteoporosis in people 50 years or older. This important meta-analysis was based upon data from 29 randomized trials involving 63,897 subjects. Main outcomes analyzed were fractures of all types and percentage change of bone-mineral density from baseline. A 12% reduction in risk of fractures of all types was reported. Bone-mineral density improvement was significantly associated with the supplementation, as measured at both the hip and the spine. Fracture-risk reduction was significantly correlated with compliance in these studies. And treatment effect was better with calcium doses of 1,200 milligrams or more daily than with doses lower than that; similarly, better results were consistently seen when vitamin D doses were 800 IU or greater. They found that, overall, calcium by itself was as effective as calcium with D. But in some subgroups of individuals (institutionalized elderly and those with clear vitamin D deficiency), the combination was more efficacious. Another meta-analysis, it should be noted, recently concluded that vitamin D is only effective in reducing risk of hip fracture when calcium is combined with it. The authors of *The Lancet* meta-analysis concluded that it is likely that calcium supplementation among postmenopausal women is cost-effective and that cost-effectiveness is likely to be better still in high-risk subjects who optimally comply with supplementation.

An editorial accompanying publication of this meta-analysis in *The Lancet* took note of some of the conflicting findings of other studies and the assertion by some authorities that calcium, with or without vitamin D, should not be systematically recommended for the primary or secondary prevention of fracture in the elderly. The editorial writer asserted that "most of these studies had poor long-term adherence to study drug." The editorial pointed out that the meta-analysis found that 50-60% of participants in the studies analyzed became non-compliant in taking their medication/supplementation properly. But in that subpopulation, where at least 80% remained compliant, the level of risk reduction was double that of those who were poorly compliant. The editorial found the cost-effectiveness conclusions of the meta-analysis encouraging but not definitive and concluded that these preliminary observations on cost-effectiveness emphasize "the need for extensive and sophisticated health-economic analyses to assess the incremental cost-effectiveness ratio of calcium or calcium with vitamin D supplementation in various doses, regimens, populations and settings."

An inverse relationship has been noted in epidemiological studies between colon cancer incidence and calcium intake. In the four-year, multicenter Calcium Polyp Prevention study, calcium supplementation was associated with a significant reduction in the risk of recurrent colorectal adenomas. This double-blind, randomized trial enrolled 930 subjects with a history of colorectal adenomas. Mean age was 61, and 72% of the subjects were men. Calcium was supplied in the carbonate form in a dose of 1,200 milligrams of elemental calcium daily. Follow-up continued for four years after initial examination.

Some other intervention trials, as well as several experimental studies, have provided further support for calcium benefit in modulating the rate of human colon cell proliferation and reducing the rate of colonic adematous polyps. It should be noted, however, that while many positive significant results have been reported, reduction in adenoma incidence has generally been modest in these studies.

More recently, some large studies and reviews have yielded far less promising results. One meta-analysis—while discerning some evidence in well-designed double-blind, placebo-controlled studies that calcium supplementation (1,200 milligrams daily for four years in one study, 2,000 milligrams daily for three years in another study) might confer a "moderate" preventive effect against colorectal adenomatous polyps—nonetheless concluded that "this does not constitute sufficient evidence to recommend the general use of calcium supplements to prevent colorectal cancer." In another recent study involving 36,282 postmenopausal women from 40 Women's Health Initiative centers, subjects were randomized to receive 500 mg of elemental calcium and 400 IU of vitamin D daily or placebo for an average of seven years. The supplementation was found to have no effect on the incidence of colorectal cancer in this group of postmenopausal women. The researchers conceded that, given the long latency associated with the development of colorectal cancer and the relatively short follow-up period, a significant effect could still not be entirely ruled out. Follow-up is ongoing to further assess this possibility. Some have criticized the study for using a dosage of both calcium and vitamin D that they believe is too low to deliver a significant effect; this shortcoming was acknowledged, as well, in an editorial accompanying publication of this paper in *The New England Journal of Medicine*.

There is some preliminary evidence that calcium supplementation may help some with PMS. A pilot study suggested that calcium might diminish some PMS symptoms. Subsequently, a placebo-controlled, multicenter study produced results showing that calcium-supplemented women had an overall reduction of 48% in severity of PMS symptoms, compared with a 30% reduction in those on placebo. Those in the calcium group reported a 54% reduction in aches and pains, compared with a 15% increase in pains reported by the placebo group. One of the researchers has speculated that women with PMS may have a functional hypocalcemia in which urine and blood levels of calcium are normal—but only because abnormally high levels of parathyroid hormone

constantly extract calcium from bone. More research is needed.

In a recent, randomized, double-blind, placebo-controlled study of the effects of calcium supplementation on serum cholesterol and blood pressure in 193 men and women aged 30 to 74 years, treatment with 1 and 2 grams daily of calcium for four months conferred no significant benefits, compared with placebo. No significant effects were seen with respect to blood pressure, total or HDL-cholesterol levels. In some earlier trials, however, some modest hypocholesterolemic effects were observed. And in an analysis of 14 studies, calcium supplementation in women (1.5 to 2 grams daily) was associated with a reduction of 5.40 mmHg in systolic blood pressure and a reduction of 3.44 mmHg in diastolic blood pressure, compared with controls. Some associated but inconclusive reduction in the incidence of preterm delivery, cesarean delivery, intrauterine growth retardation, perinatal death and preeclampsia has been reported.

In more recent work, one study found that intakes of low-fat dairy products, calcium and vitamin D were each inversely correlated with risk of hypertension in middle-aged and older women. A meta-analysis of 40 randomized, controlled studies found that a mean daily dose of 1,200 mg of calcium reduced systolic blood pressure by 1.86 mmHg and diastolic blood pressure by 0.99 mmHg. Greater improvement was seen in those with relatively low calcium intake at baseline. Those involved in the Dietary Approaches to Stop Hypertension Study (DASH), a large and well-designed inquiry, continue to stress the need for adequate dietary calcium intake via dairy products. Another recent study showed that calcium supplementation (1.5-2 grams daily) reduced the risk of high blood pressure, preeclampsia and maternal death or serious morbidity among women studied. The authors reported that calcium supplementation during pregnancy reduced the risk of preeclampsia by about half and was especially effective among those women with low calcium intake at baseline.

Yet another recent randomized, double-blind, placebo-controlled study reported an upward trend in cardiovascular event rates, including heart attack, in healthy postmenopausal women given calcium supplementation, compared with those receiving placebo. Mean age of subjects was 74. More research is clearly warranted to see if this negative finding can be confirmed.

In the ongoing Nurse's Health Study, supplementary intake of 400 or more milligrams daily of calcium has been associated with a significantly reduced risk of stroke among women. Supplementary intakes higher than 600 milligrams daily did not appear to confer further benefit. Authors of the study hypothesized that a possible hypocholesterolemic effect or some anti-clotting mechanism might account for the protective association observed in this population. Magnesium and potassium intakes were not associated with reduced risk of stroke in this study, although they have been thus associated in some other studies.

One group of researchers has recently reported that increasing the dietary calcium of obese subjects for one year produced a 4.9 kilogram loss of body fat. Experiments in mice showed that high calcium diets could reduce weight gain and foot pad mass by 26% to 39%. The same researchers examined epidemiological data in which they found a significant association between higher levels of body fat and lower intake of calcium. They concluded that "increasing dietary calcium suppresses adipocyte intracellular calcium and thereby modulates energy metabolism and attenuates obesity risk."

Prior laboratory research has shown that increased adipocyte intracellular calcium produces both stimulation of lipogenesis and inhibition of lipolysis. The high-calcium diets used in the studies of mice produced a 51% inhibition of adipocyte fatty acid synthase expression and activity and a 3.4- to 5.2-fold increase in lipolysis. More research is warranted.

CONTRAINDICATIONS, PRECAUTIONS, ADVERSE REACTIONS

CONTRAINDICATIONS

Calcium supplementation is contraindicated in those with hypercalcemia. Conditions causing hypercalcemia include sarcoidosis, hyperparathyroidism, hypervitaminosis D and cancer.

Calcium supplementation is contraindicated in those hypersensitive to any component of a calcium-containing supplement.

PRECAUTIONS

Supplemental calcium taken without food may increase the risk of kidney stones in women and possibly also in men. It is thought that taking supplemental calcium without food limits the opportunity for the beneficial effect that calcium may have in binding oxalate in the intestine. Therefore, it is advisable that supplemental calcium be taken with food.

Those who form calcium-containing kidney stones are generally advised not to take supplemental calcium.

Those with achlorhydria should take calcium carbonate with food.

ADVERSE REACTIONS

Calcium supplements are generally well tolerated. Use of calcium carbonate may cause such gastrointestinal side reactions as constipation, bloating, gas and flatulence. Prolonged use of large doses of calcium carbonate—greater than 12 grams daily (about 5 grams of elemental calcium)—

may lead to the milk-alkali syndrome, nephrocalcinosis and renal insufficiency.

INTERACTIONS

DRUGS

Biphosphonates (alendronate, etidronate, risedronate): Concomitant intake of a bisphosphonate and calcium may decrease the absorption of the bisphosphonate.

H_2 *blockers (cimetidine, famotidine, mizatidine, ranitidine):* Concomitant use of H_2 blockers and calcium carbonate or calcium phosphate can cause decreased absorption of these calcium salts.

Levothyroxine: Concomitant intake of levothyroxine and calcium carbonate was found to reduce levothyroxine absorption and to increase serum thyrotropin levels. Levothyroxine may adsorb to calcium carbonate in an acidic environment, which may block its absorption. There is no evidence that other forms of calcium block levothyroxine absorption if taken concomitantly.

Proton Pump Inhibitors (lansoprazole, omeprazole, rabeprazole sodium): Concomitant use of proton pump inhibitors and calcium carbonate or calcium phosphate can cause decreased absorption of these calcium salts.

Quinolones (ciprofloxacin, gatifloxacin, levofloxacin, lomefloxacin, moxifloxacin, norfloxacin, ofloxacin, sparfloxacin, trovafloxacin): Concomitant use of a quinolone and calcium may decrease the absorption of the quinolone.

Tetracyclines (doxycycline, minocycline, tetracycline): Concomitant intake of a tetracycline and calcium may decrease the absorption of the tetracycline. Tetracyclines may form nonabsorbable complexes with calcium.

Vitamin D Analogues (calcitriol, alfacalcidol): Concomitant use of these vitamin D analogues and calcium can cause increased absorption of calcium.

NUTRITIONAL SUPPLEMENTS

Inositol Hexaphosphate: Concomitant use of inositol hexaphosphate (phytic acid) and calcium may decrease the absorption of calcium.

Minerals (iron, fluoride, magnesium, phosphorous): Concomitant use of iron and calcium may inhibit the absorption of iron. Similarly, concomitant use of fluoride, magnesium, phosphorous or zinc and calcium may decrease the absorption of these minerals. However, these possible mineral interactions have not been shown to be of clinical significance.

Non-digestible oligosaccharides (fructo-oligosaccharides, inulin): Concomitant use of these oligosaccharides and calcium may increase the absorption of calcium in the colon.

Sodium Alginate: Concomitant intake of sodium alginate and calcium may decrease the absorption of calcium.

Vitamin D: Concomitant use of vitamin D and calcium may increase the absorption of calcium.

FOODS

Calcium may be poorly absorbed from foods rich in oxalic acid (spinach, sweet potatoes, rhubarb and beans) or phytic acid (unleavened bread, raw beans, seeds, nuts and grains and soy isolates). Concomitant intake of a calcium supplement with foods rich in oxalic acid or phytic acid may decrease the absorption of calcium. The phytate associated with dietary fiber appears to be the major factor involved in depressing absorption of calcium.

OVERDOSAGE

Overdosage has not been reported with calcium supplements.

DOSAGE AND ADMINISTRATION

There are several different calcium salts available as supplements. These include calcium carbonate, calcium citrate, calcium phosphate, calcium lactate and calcium gluconate. Calcium carbonate and calcium phosphate contain approximately 40% elemental calcium; calcium citrate, approximately 21% elemental calcium; calcium lactate, approximately 13% elemental calcium; calcium gluconate, approximately 9% elemental calcium. Some calcium preparations also contain vitamin D.

Adequate intake of calcium for women and men 19 through 50 years is 1,000 milligrams daily. Adequate intake of calcium for men and women 31 years through greater than 70 years is 1,200 milligrams daily. Adequate intake of vitamin D for women and men 19 to 50 years is 200 IU or 5.0 micrograms daily. Adequate intake of vitamin D for men and women 51 through 70 years is 400 IU or 10 micrograms daily. Adequate intake of vitamin D for men and women over 70 years is 600 IU or 15 picograms daily.

Absorption of calcium is greatest in doses of 500 milligrams or less and when taken with food.

There are several food products, including orange juice, that are now available which have added calcium. The salt calcium citrate malate is used to fortify some foods. Some physicians recommend 1,000 milligrams of supplement calcium daily for postmenopausal women taking estrogen replacement therapy (ERT) and 1,500 milligrams daily for postmenopausal women not taking ERT. An intake of 1,200 milligrams daily appears to be adequate for both groups. The Food and Nutrition Board of the Institute of Medicine of the U.S. National Academy of Sciences has recommended the following adequate intakes (AI) for calcium:

Infants	(AI)
0-6 months	210 mg/day
7-12 months	270 mg/day
Children	
1-3 years	500 mg/day
4-8 years	800 mg/day
Boys	
9-13 years	1,300 mg/day
14-18 years	1,300 mg/day
Girls	
9-13 years	1,300 mg/day
14-18 years	1,300 mg/day
Men	
19-30 years	1,000 mg/day
31-50 years	1,000 mg/day
51-70 years	1,200 mg/day
>70 years	1,200 mg/day
Women	
19-30 years	1,000 mg/day
31-50 years	1,000 mg/day
51-70 years	1,200 mg/day
>70 years	1,200 mg/day
Pregnancy	
14-18 years	1,300 mg/day
19-30 years	1,000 mg/day
31-50 years	1,000 mg/day
Lactation	
14-18 years	1,300 mg/day
19-30 years	1,000 mg/day
31-50 years	1,000 mg/day

A LOAEL (lowest-observed-adverse-effect level) in the range of 4 to 5 grams can be identified for adults. Based on this LOAEL and an uncertainty factor (UF) of 2 the Food and Nutrition Board of the Institute of Medicine has recommended the following tolerable upper intake levels (UL) for calcium:

Infants	(UL)
0-12 months	Not determinable
Children	
1-18 years	2,500 mg/day
Adults	
19-70 years	2,500 mg/day
>70 years	2,500 mg/day
Pregnancy	
14-50 years	2,500 mg/day
Lactation	
14-50 years	2,500 mg/day

The DV (Daily Value) for calcium, which is used for determining percentage of nutrient daily values on nutritional supplement and food labels, is 1,000 mg. The basis for the DV for calcium is the 1973 U.S. RDA.

LITERATURE

Allender PS, Cutler JA, Follman D, et al. Dietary calcium and blood pressure: meta-analysis of randomized clinical trials. *Ann Intern Med.* 1996;124:825-831.

Baron JA, Beach M, Mandel JS, et al. Calcium supplements for the prevention of colorectal adenomas. *N Engl J Med.* 1999;340:101-107.

Becker CB. Does supplementation with calcium alone or in combination with vitamin D reduce the risk of osteoporotic fracture? *Nat Clin Pract Endocrinol Metab.* 2008;4(4):190-191.

Bell L, Halstenson CE, Halstenson CJ, et al. Cholesterol-lowering effects of calcium carbonate in patients with mild to moderate hypercholesterolemia. *Arch Intern Med.* 1992;152:2441-2444.

Bolland MJ, Barber PA, Doughty RN, et al. Vascular events in healthy older women receiving calcium supplementation: randomised controlled trial. *BMJ.* 2008;336(7638):262-266.

Boonen S, Vanderschueren D, Haentjens P, et al. Calcium and vitamin D in the prevention and treatment of osteoporosis—a clinical update. *J Intern Med.* 2006;259(6):539-552.

Bostick RM, Fosdick L, Grandits GA, et al. Effect of calcium supplementation on serum cholesterol and blood pressure. A randomized, double-blind, placebo-controlled, clinical trial. *Arch Fam Med.* 2000;9:31-39.

Bronner F, Pansu D. Nutritional aspects of calcium absorption. *J Nutr.* 1999;129:9-12.

Buckley LM, Leib ES, Cartularo KS, et al. Calcium and vitamin D_3 supplementation prevents bone loss in the spine secondary to low-dose corticosteroids in patients with rheumatoid arthritis. *Ann Intern Med.* 1996;125:961-968.

Butner LE, et al. Calcium carbonate induced hypothyroidism. *Ann Intern Med.* 2000;132:595.

Curhan GC, Willett WC, Speizer FE, et al. Comparison of dietary calcium with supplemental calcium and other nutrients as factors affecting the risk of kidney stones in women. *Ann Intern Med.* 1997;126:497-504.

Dawson-Hughes B, Harris SS, Krall EA, et al. Effect of calcium and vitamin D supplementation on bone density on men and women 65 years of age and older. *N Engl J Med.* 1997;337:670-676.

Dickinson HO, Nicolson DJ, Cook JV, et al. Calcium supplementation for the management of primary hypertension in adults. *Cochrane Database Syst Rev.* 2006;(2):CD004639.

Finkelstein JS. Calcium plus vitamin D for postmenopausal women—bone appétit? *N Engl J Med.* 2006;354(7):750-752.

Forman MR, Levin B. Calcium plus vitamin D3 supplementation and colorectal cancer in women. *N Engl J Med.* 2006;354(7):752-754.

Garland CF, Garland FC, Gorham ED. Calcium and vitamin D. Their potential roles in colon and breast cancer prevention. *Ann NY Acad Sci.* 1999;889:107-119.

Heaney RP. Calcium, dairy products and osteoporosis. *J Am Coll Nutr.* 2000;19(2 Suppl):83S-99S.

Heaney RP, Dowell MS, Barger-Lux MJ. Absorption of calcium as the carbonate and citrate salts, with some observations on method. *Osteoporosis Int.* 1999;9:19-23.

Heller HJ, Stewart A, Haynes S, et al. Pharmacokinetics of calcium absorption from two commercial calcium supplements. *J Clin Pharmacol.* 1999;39:1151-1154.

Hofmeyr GJ, Atallah AN, Duley L. Calcium supplementation during pregnancy for preventing hypertensive disorders and related problems. *Cochrane Database Syst Rev.* 2006;3:CD001059.

Institute of Medicine, Food and Nutrition Board. Dietary Reference Intakes for calcium, phosphorous, magnesium, vitamin D, and fluoride. Washington, DC: National Academy Press, 1997.

Jackson RD, LaCroix AZ, Gass M, et al. Women's Health Initiative Investigators. Calcium plus vitamin D supplementation and the risk of fractures. *N Engl J Med.* 2006;354(7):669-683.

Jamal SA, Emanoilidis H. Review: calcium supplementation, with or without vitamin D, prevents osteoporotic fractures in older people. *Evid Based Med.* 2008;13(2):53.

Kruse H. Calcium supplementation and fracture risk—recent findings from the women's health initiative study. *S D Med.* 2006;59(5):207-208.

Levine RJ, Hauth JC, Curet LB, et al. Trial of calcium to prevent preeclampsia. *N Engl J Med.* 1997;337:69-76.

Lipkin M, Newmark H. Effect of added dietary calcium on colonic epithelial-cell proliferation in subjects at high risk for familial colonic cancer. *N Engl J Med.* 1985;313:1381-1384.

Oginni LM, Sharp CA, Worsfold M, et al. Healing of rickets after calcium supplementation. *Lancet.* 1999;353:296-297.

Passeri G, Vescovini R, Sansoni P, et al. Italian Multicentric Study on Centenarians (IMUSCE). Calcium metabolism and vitamin D in the extreme longevity. *Exp Gerontol.* 2008;43(2):79-87.

Recker RR. Calcium absorption and achlorhydria. *N Engl J Med.* 1985;313:70-73.

Reginster JY. Calcium and vitamin D for osteoporotic fracture risk. *Lancet.* 2007;370(9588):632-634.

Reid IR, Ames RW, Evans MC, et al. Effect of calcium supplementation on bone loss in postmenopausal women. *N Engl J Med.* 1993;328:460-464.

Singh N, Singh PN, Hershman JM. Effect of calcium carbonate on the absorption of levothyroxine. *JAMA.* 2000;283:2822-2825.

Talbot JR, Guardo P, Seccia S, et al. Calcium bioavailability and parathyroid hormone acute changes after oral intake of dairy and nondairy products in healthy volunteers. *Osteoporosis Int.* 1999;10:137-142.

Tan PC. Review: calcium supplementation during pregnancy reduces the risk of pre-eclampsia. *Evid Based Med.* 2008;13(3):83.

van Mierlo LA, Arends LR, Streppel MT, et al. Blood pressure response to calcium supplementation: a meta-analysis of randomized controlled trials. *J Hum Hypertens.* 2006;20(8):571-580.

Wactawski-Wende J, Kotchen JM, Anderson GL, et al. Women's Health Initiative Investigators. Calcium plus vitamin D supplementation and the risk of colorectal cancer. *N Engl J Med.* 2006;354(7):684-696.

Wang L, Manson JE, Buring JE, et al. Dietary intake of dairy products, calcium, and vitamin D and the risk of hypertension in middle-aged and older women. *Hypertension.* 2008;51(4):1073-1079.

Wargovich MJ, Eng VWS, Newmark HL. Calcium inhibits the damaging and compensatory proliferative effects of fatty acids on mouse colon epithelium. *Cancer Lett.* 1984;23:253-258.

Weaver CM, Heaney RP. Calcium. In: Shils ME, Olson JA, Shike M, Ross AC, eds. *Modern Nutrition in Health and Disease.* 9th ed. Baltimore, MD: Williams and Wilkins; 1999:141-155.

Weingarten MA, Zalmanovici A, Yaphe J. Dietary calcium supplementation for preventing colorectal cancer and adenomatous polyps. *Cochrane Database Syst Rev.* 2008;(1):CD003548.

Wolf RL, Cauley JA, Baker CE, et al. Factors associated with calcium absorption efficiency in pre- and perimenopausal women. *Am J Clin Nutr.* 2000;72:466-471.

Zemel MB, Shi H, Greer B, et al. Regulation of adiposity by dietary calcium. *FASEB J.* 2000;14:1132-1138.

Caprylic Acid

DESCRIPTION

Caprylic acid is a medium-chain 8-carbon saturated fatty acid. It is also known as octanoic acid. It occurs naturally in butterfat and palm and coconut oils in the form of triacylglcerols (TAG). It is represented by the following chemical structure:

$$CH_3(CH_2)_5CH_2-\overset{\overset{\displaystyle O}{\|}}{C}-OH$$

Caprylic acid

ACTIONS AND PHARMACOLOGY

ACTIONS

Caprylic acid was reported many years ago to have some antifungal activity *in vitro*. Other *in vitro* studies showed some activity against some viruses and bacteria. The monoglyceride of caprylic acid, monooctanin, given as an infusion into the bile duct, has been used for gallstone dissolution.

MECHANISM OF ACTION

The mechanism of caprylic acid's possible actions is unclear. Caprylic acid may affect the fluidity of viral and fungal cell membranes.

PHARMACOKINETICS

Caprylic acid is absorbed from the intestine and, in contrast with long-chain fatty acids, immediately enters into the portal circulation. It is carried by blood lipids. Most ingested caprylic acid undergoes beta-oxidation in the liver.

INDICATIONS AND USAGE

There is no significant clinical evidence to support an indication for the use of caprylic acid in the treatment or prevention of fungal infections such as *Candida albicans*.

RESEARCH SUMMARY

Some rather old studies reported antifungal activity of caprylic acid *in vitro*. However, clinical use of caprylic acid has not proved to be effective against *Candida albicans* or any other fungi. This is most likely due to the fact that caprylic acid is rapidly metabolized in the usual fatty acid pathways.

CONTRAINDICATIONS, PRECAUTIONS, ADVERSE REACTIONS

CONTRAINDICATIONS

Known hypersensitivity to a caprylic acid-containing product.

PRECAUTIONS

Infants, children, pregnant women, nursing mothers and those prone to stomach upsets should avoid caprylic acid supplementation.

ADVERSE REACTIONS

Caprylic acid has an unpleasant rancid taste and may cause mild gastrointestinal symptoms such as nausea and diarrhea.

DOSAGE AND ADMINISTRATION

The usual doses that are taken orally are 300 to 1200 milligrams daily.

LITERATURE

Abate MA, Moore TL. Monooctanin use for gallstone dissolution. *Drug Intell Clin Pharm.* 1985; 19:708-713.

Kabara JJ. Fatty acids and derivatives as antimicrobial agents. In: Kabara JJ, ed. *The Pharmacological Effect of Lipids I.* Champaign, IL: American Oil Chemists' Society; 1978; 1-14.

Wyss O, Ludwig BJ, Joiner RR. The fungistatic and fungicidal action of fatty acids and related compounds. *Arch Biochem.* 1943;7,415.

Capsiate and Capsaicin

DESCRIPTION

Capsiate, a nonpungent capsaicin analogue, and its dihydro and nordihydro derivatives, dihydrocapsiate and nordihydrocapsiate, respectively, are the major capsinoids of the nonpungent red pepper cultivar CH-19 Sweet. The capsinoids are fatty acid esters of vanillyl alcohol and are lipophilic.

Capsaicin, the main pungency compound of hot chili peppers, and its dihydro and nordihydro derivatives, dihydrocapsaicin and nordihydrocapsaicin, respectively, are the major capsaicinoids of hot chili peppers.

A number of health benefits have been ascribed to capsaicin and its derivatives, including anticancer activity, anti-inflammatory activity, anti-obesity activity and analgesia. Topical capsaicin is used in the treatment of postherpetic neuralgia, osteoarthritis and painful diabetic neuropathy. However, the strong pungency of these substances and potential for neurotoxicity limit their use in food, nutritional supplements and pharmaceuticals.

The pungency of chili peppers ranges from the coolness of bell and sweet pepper varieties to the mild to moderate heat of serranos to the earth-scorching habaneros, and has to do with the amount of capsaicin present in the chili pepper. In 1912, the chemist Wilbur Scoville developed a measure of the pungency of chili peppers which became known as the Scoville Organoleptic Test. The test, called a dilution-taste procedure, relies on the tongue of an experienced chili taster to determine the degree of heat (or Scoville unit) of the chili pepper. Recently, the experienced tongue has been replaced by HPLC (high pressure liquid chromatography) and ASTA (American Spice Trade Association) units. The ASTA units are then converted to Scoville units.

Scoville heat levels for a few chili peppers are: bell/sweet pepper varieties (*Capsicum annuum*), 0 Scoville Heat Units (SHU); ancho peppers (*Capsicum annuum*), 1,000-3,000 SHU; serrano peppers (*Capsicum annuum*), 4,000 SHU; New Mexican peppers (*Capsicum annuum*), 5,000 SHU; jalapeño peppers (*Capsicum annuum*), 5,000-25,000 SHU; cayenne peppers (*Capsicum annuum*), 23,000 SHU; Thai peppers (*Capsicum annuum*), 60,000 SHU; Tabasco peppers (*Capsicum frutescens*), 120,000 SHU; habanero peppers (*Capsicum chinense*), 200,000-300,000 SHU. The present Guinness Book of World Records holder is the Bhut Jolokia (*Capsicum frutescens*) chili from India, which weighed in at a blistering 1,001,304 SHU.

The SHU for pure capsaicin, the major pungent substance of the *Capsicum* family (hot chili peppers) is 16 million SHU, as is that of dihydrocapsaicin. The SHU of nordihydrocapsai-cin is 9.1 million. In contrast to the capsaicinoids, capsinoids are not pungent and have SHUs well below 100. Capsinoids are found in the various *Capsicum* species, but in very small amounts. A few years ago, a nonpungent cultivar of *Capsicum annuum* L was identified in Thailand. This cultivar was called CH-19 Sweet and was found to have much more capsiate in its fruit, as well as other capsinoids, than had ever before been found in chili peppers. CH-19 Sweet is virtually devoid of capsaicin and other pungent capsaicinoids. The SHU of CH-19 Sweet is well below 100.

The major capsinoids in CH-19 Sweet are capsiate (4-hydroxy-3-methoxybenzyl (*E*)-8-methyl-6-nonenoate; CAS No. 205687-01-0), dihydrocapsiate (4-hydroxy-3-methoxybenzyl 8-methylnonanoate; CAS No. 205687-03-2), and nordihydrocapsiate (4-hydroxy-3-methoxybenzyl 7-methyloctanoate; CAS No. 220012-5-3).

The capsinoids have an ester bond instead of the amide bond normally found in capsaicinoids between the vanillyl moiety and fatty acid chain. The difference between the sensory properties of capsaicin and capsiate is due to the way the vanillyl and acyl moiety of the basic structural motif is linked: by an amide bond in capsaicin-like compounds and by an ester bond in capsiate-type compounds.

The term capsiate is used either for the substance capsiate itself or for mixtures of capsiate with its analogues dihydrocapsiate and nordihydrocapsiate. The chemical structures below are described within this monograph.

Capsiate

Capsaicin

Dihydrocapsiate

Nordihydrocapsiate

ACTIONS AND PHARMACOLOGY

ACTIONS

Capsiate may have an anti-obesity effect. Capsiate has chemopreventive and anticancer potential.

MECHANISM OF ACTION

A two-week study with male mice administered capsiate (10 mg/kg body weight) reported increased metabolic rate and promotion of fat oxidation at rest. It was found that the two-week treatment of capsiate increased the levels of UCP-1 (uncoupling protein 1) and mRNA in brown adipose tissue (BAT), and UCP-2 (uncoupling protein 2) mRNA in white adipose tissue (WAT). Another study in mice by the same group found that continuous administration of capsiate suppressed body fat accumulation. Capsiate in the form of CH-19 Sweet extract has been reported to increase body temperature and oxygen consumption in humans.

A hypothetical model to explain the above results is as follows: Capsiate and other capsinoids activate TRPV1 (transient receptor potential vanilloid 1, the capsaicin receptor) found on the digestive tract surface, leading to activation of the sympathetic nervous system followed by activation of UCP-1 in BAT, UCP-3 in skeletal muscle and activation of lipolysis in WAT.

Capsinoids target a variety of pathways in cancer development. Nordihydrocapsiate was found to induce apoptosis in the Jurkat tumor cell line. Capsiate and dihydrocapsiate inhibited angiogenesis in human umbilical vascular endothelial cells. These capsinoids inhibited vascular endothelial growth factor (VEGF)-induced proliferation, chemotactic motility and capillary-like tube formation of primary cultured human endothelial cells. In addition, they inhibited sprouting of endothelial cells in the rat aorta and formation of new blood vessels in the mouse Matrigel plug assay in response to VEGF. VEGF, expressed by many cancer cell types and certain tumor stromal cells, is a potent proangiogenic factor that functions in tumor vascular development. The angiogenesis inhibitory activity of the capsinoids appears to be due to the suppression of VEGF-induced activation of Src kinase.

PHARMACOKINETICS

Pharmacokinetic studies with ^{14}C-labeled synthetic dihydrocapsiate have been performed in rats and with an oral ingestion of CH-19 Sweet extract in healthy male volunteers.

[14]C dihydrocapsiate is rapidly absorbed from the gastrointestinal tract, and radioactivity is found in several different tissues. Radioactivity reaches Cmax in plasma 0.67 hours after administration of a single dose of ^{14}C dihydrocapsiate. The apparent half-life is 2.4 hours. The dihydrocapsiate metabolites are excreted in the urine, bile and feces. Maximum concentrations of radioactivity were observed in most tissues two hours following single dose administration. Metabolism of dihydrocapsiate occurs very quickly after single dose administration, and it is thought that the metabolism takes place in the gastrointestinal tract, the intestinal mucosa and the liver. Metabolites include vanillyl alcohol, the glucuronide of vanillyl alcohol, the sulfate of vanillyl alcohol and the sulfate of vanillic acid.

Capsaicin is known to inhibit CYP3A4 (cytochrome P450 3A4). However, capsiate, dihydrocapsiate and nordihydrocapsiate were not found to inhibit CYP3A3 in human liver microsomes.

Further pharmacokinetic studies with single doses and repeated doses of dihydrocapsiate in both experimental animals and humans are necessary in order to completely elucidate the pharmacokinetics of the capsinoids.

INDICATIONS AND USAGE

Capsiate is said to have many of the same indications as its hotter cousin, capsaicin. Claims for it include: prevention and treatment of some cancers, anti-inflammatory, immunomodulator, useful in treating rheumatoid arthritis and other autoimmune diseases, analgesic, weight loss promoter, and athletic endurance enhancer.

RESEARCH SUMMARY

Recent research, principally in Japan, indicates that capsiate may be useful in inhibiting the pathologic angiogenesis (blood vessel formation) that characterizes and sustains some cancers. This evidence encompasses both *in vitro* and *in vivo* animal and human experiments which, while still very preliminary, show promising results. Like the pungent ("hot") capsaicin, cool capsiate demonstrates an ability to inhibit the vascular endothelial growth factor that promotes abnormal angiogenesis. Other dietary phytochemicals (eg, curcuminoids, resveratrol, etc.) have demonstrated similar abilities but, according to one group of Japanese researchers, capsiate is more potent in this regard.

It is hoped that this nonirritating capsaicinoid analogue will have broad-spectrum anti-inflammatory applications, for which capsaicin itself shows preliminary promise. The research that could establish it as efficacious in rheumatoid arthritis, psoriasis, diabetic retinopathy, atherosclerosis, hyperthyroidism and other conditions remains to be done. Already, however, there is evidence, based upon animal inflammation models, that capsiate may be effective in preventing and ameliorating such conditions as septic shock and inflammatory bowel disease. *In vitro* and animal experiments are yielding early evidence of positive immuno-modulatory effects that could have broad, positive implications.

Analgesic effects have not been established.

A few recent studies, again from Japan, suggest that capsiate, like capsaicin, may have thermogenic effects that could promote weight loss. There is a suggestion in this work that capsiate activates the sympathetic nervous system along pathways that increase energy expenditures at a level that inhibits the accumulation of fat. These findings have been observed in both animal and human experiments. One small human study compared male subjects matched to control subjects (and controlled for diet, smoking and several other relevant variables) over a period of just two weeks. In that time frame a significant reduction in body fat was reported among those receiving portions of CH-19 Sweet pepper prior to meals (0.4 grams per kilogram of body weight in the form of uncooked pepper three times per day) compared with the matched controls who did not receive the capsiate-containing sweet pepper. Unlike capsaicin, which has also been postulated to have weight-loss properties, capsiate did not, in these studies, accelerate heart rate or increase blood pressure. More rigorous follow-up, with larger cohorts, is warranted.

Another Japanese study demonstrated that mice that received orally administered capsiate were able to swim significantly longer than similar mice not fed capsiate. This suggests that the substance could promote athletic endurance. There was evidence in this study of enhanced fat oxidation and carbohydrate sparing. The experimentals showed increased residual muscle glycogen, higher serum free fatty acid concentration and significantly lower lactic acid concentration, as well as a lower respiratory exchange ratio during both rest and exercise, all consistent with the potential for greater physical endurance. This intriguing pilot study also needs follow-up.

In general, capsiate replicates many of the apparently beneficial effects of capsaicin but without the concomitant irritating properties than many researchers believe have impeded the use of these substances. It is hoped that capsiate will now provide a more attractive alternative and promote further research with capsaicinoids.

CONTRAINDICATIONS, PRECAUTIONS, ADVERSE REACTIONS

CONTRAINDICATIONS
Capsiate and all of the capsinoids are contraindicated in those hypersensitive to any component of a capsinoid preparation.

PRECAUTIONS
Those with chronic cough syndromes, including chronic cough due to the use of angiotensin-converting enzyme (ACE) inhibitors, may notice an increase in coughing when using capsinoids. To date, this has not been reported, but since capsinoids as well as capsaicin are agonists for the ligand-gated cation channel TRPV1, it is something to watch out for.

ADVERSE REACTIONS
There have been no reports of adverse events in those taking capsiate supplements.

INTERACTIONS
No interactions between capsiate and other dietary supplements, pharmaceuticals or foods have been reported.

OVERDOSAGE
There are no reports of overdosage in those taking capsiate supplements.

DOSAGE AND ADMINISTRATION
The presently marketed capsiate supplement contains one milligram per capsule, and the recommended dosage is three capsules every morning. The supplement contains the three capsinoids: capsiate, dihydrocapsiate and nordihydrocapsiate. Optimal dosage of capsiate is unknown. One human study using 30 milligrams of capsiate showed no adverse events.

LITERATURE
Faraut B, Giannesini B, Matarazzo V, et al. Downregulation of uncoupling protein-3 in vivo is linked to changes in muscle mitochondrial energy metabolism as a result of capsiate administration. *Am J Physiol Endocrinol Metab.* 2007;292(5):E1474-E1482.

Iida T, Moriyama T, Kobata K, et al. TRPV1 activation and induction of nociceptive response by a non-pungent capsaicin-like compound, capsiate. *Neuropharmacology.* 2003;44(7):958-967.

Ito, et al. Process of Producing a Capsinoid-Containing Food and Drink. US Patent Application. 20070264411, November 15, 2007.

Macho A, Lucena C, Sancho R, et al. Non-pungent capsaicinoids from sweet pepper synthesis and evaluation of the chemopreventive and anticancer potential. *Eur J Nutr.* 2003;42(1):2-9.

Macho A, Sancho R, Minassi A, et al. Involvement of reactive oxygen species in capsaicinoid-induced apoptosis in transformed cells. *Free Radic Res.* 2003;37(6):611-619.

Masuda Y, Haramizu S, Oki K, et al. Upregulation of uncoupling proteins by oral administration of capsiate, a nonpungent capsaicin analog. *J Appl Physiol.* 2003;95(6):2408-1415.

Ohnuki K, Haramizu S, Watanabe T, et al. CH-19 sweet, nonpungent cultivar of red pepper, increased body temperature in mice with vanilloid receptors stimulation by capsiate. *J Nutr Sci Vitaminol.* (Tokyo) 2001;47(4):295-298.

Ohnuki K, Haramizu S, Oki K, et al. Administration of capsiate, a non-pungent capsaicin analog, promotes energy metabolism and suppresses body fat accumulation in mice. *Biosci Biotechnol Biochem.* 2001;65(12):2735-2740.

Ohnuki K, Niwa S, Maeda S, et al. CH-19 sweet, a nonpungent cultivar of red pepper, increased body temperature and oxygen consumption in humans. *Biosci Biotechnol Biochem.* 2001; 65(9):2033-2036.

Pyun BJ, Choi S, Lee Y, et al. Capsiate, a nonpungent capsaicin-like compound, inhibits angiogenesis and vascular permeability via a direct inhibition of Src kinase activity. *Cancer Res.* 2008; 68(1):227-235.

Sancho R, Lucena C, Macho A, et al. Immunosuppressive activity of capsaicinoids: capsiate derived from sweet peppers inhibits NF-kappaB activation and is a potent anti-inflammatory compound in vivo. *Eur J Immunol.* 2002;32(6):1753-1763.

Tani Y, Fujioka T, Sumioka M, et al. Effects of capsinoid on serum and liver lipids in hyperlipidemic rats. *J Nutr Sci Vitaminol.* (Tokyo) 2004;50(5):351-355.

Yazawa, et al. Capsaicinoid-like substances having ester bond. US Patent 6 333 421. December 15, 2001.

The Ajinomoto Group. About Capsinoids. Available at: http://www.aboutcapsinoids.com/pages/home.htm. Accessed April, 2008.

The Ajinomoto Group. Capsinoids Mechanism. Available at: http://www.aboutcapsinoids.com/animation/index.html. Accessed April 2008.

The Ajinomoto Group. Capsinoids Research. http://www.capsinoidsresearch.com Accessed April 2008.

Carnosine

DESCRIPTION

Carnosine is a dipeptide comprised of the nonprotein amino acid beta-alanine (see Beta-Alanine) and the protein amino acid L-histidine. The dipeptide was first detected in 1900 by the chemists Gulewitsch and Amiradgibi in Liebig's meat extract. Liebig's meat extract was developed in 1840 by the German organic chemist Baron Justus von Liebig as a cheap and nutritious meat substitute for those who couldn't afford the real thing. It is a molasses-like black spread that contains only reduced meat stock and salt. It was widely used, including by European middle-class households, the Allied Forces of World War II and by the explorer Sir Henry Morton Stanley on his trip to Africa when he was searching for David Livingston. It is still marketed.

In addition to its presence in Liebig's meat extract, carnosine is also found in fairly high concentrations in vertebrate excitable tissues, including CNS tissue and skeletal muscle. Although the exact function of carnosine still remains unclear, it has been demonstrated to function as an antioxidant, an antiglycating agent and a skeletal muscle pH buffer, helping to delay muscle fatigue. It is a putative neurotransmitter and it is even speculated that carnosine might possess "antiaging" activity. It appears to be the first neuropeptide discovered.

Carnosine is chemically described as (2S)-2-(3-aminopropanoylamino)-3-(3H-imidazol-4-yl)propanoic acid. It is also known as beta-alanyl-L-histidine, beta-alanylhistidine and L-carnosine, and it is sometimes referred to as ignotine (in Australia) and karnozin (in Russia). Its CAS Registry Number is 305-84-0. Carnosine is a member of the histidine-containing dipeptide family. The other members include anserine (beta-alanyl-L-1-methylhistidine), also found in excitable tissues, balenine or ophidine (beta-alanyl-L-3-methylhistidine) and homocarnosine (gamma-amino-butyryl-histidine).

Carnosine is represented by the following chemical structure.

Carnosine

Carnosine's empirical formula is $C_9H_{14}N_4O_3$, its molecular weight is 226.23, its second pKa is 6.83, and it is soluble in water (one gram dissolves in 3.1 milliliters of water). Carnosine is found in skeletal muscles and CNS tissues at concentrations ranging from 2millimolar (2mM) to 25millimolar (25mM) or 0.45 mg per ml to 5.65 mg per ml. The dipeptide is synthesized in muscle and nervous tissues from beta alanine and L-histidine via the enzyme carnosine synthetase, which requires adenosine triphosphate (ATP). Vegetarian diets are lacking in carnosine, but carnosine is synthesized in the muscles and nervous tissues of vegetarians. N-acetylcarnosine eye drops are available, which are used by some for their putative anticataract action.

The predominance of carnosine and anserine in skeletal muscle is species-dependent. There is essentially no anserine in human muscle. In beef, turkey, pigs and goat, carnosine concentrations are higher than anserine concentrations. In chicken and rabbit skeletal muscle, anserine predominates. The human quadriceps contains about 362 mg of carnosine per 100 grams of tissue, a chicken breast, about 278 mg per

100 grams of tissue and a beef leg, about 150 mg per 100 grams of tissue. Salmon contains no carnosine.

ACTIONS AND PHARMACOLOGY

ACTIONS
Carnosine has possible antiglycating, antioxidant and pH-buffering activities.

MECHANISM OF ACTION
Antiglycating activity: Glycation of proteins comprises a series of nonenzymatic reactions between the carbonyl groups of reducing sugars with side-chain amino groups of proteins to yield a number of products, initially proceeding through the formation of Schiff bases—imines from the reaction of carbonyl groups with primary amino groups—and through Amadori rearrangements. Further gluco-oxidative degradation of the glycated proteins produces 1,2-dicarbonyl compounds (such as methylglyoxal), which react with other proteins, resulting in the formation of protein-protein cross-links, known as advanced glycation end products, or AGEs. The series of reactions responsible for the formation of AGEs is known as the Maillard reaction (also called the browning reaction), named for the food chemist Louis Camille Maillard, who reported on the reaction in 1912. AGEs have been implicated in the long-term complications of diabetes mellitus, such as atherosclerosis, retinopathy, nephropathy and cataracts. AGEs are also thought to be involved in neurodegenerative diseases, including Alzheimer's disease, and even in the process of aging itself. Hemoglobin A1c, which is used to test for long-term glucose control in diabetics, was the first example that non-enzymatic reactions, specifically the Maillard reaction, can occur physiologically.

The 1,2 dicarbonyl compound methylglyoxal is arguably the most important glycation agent. Methylglyoxal is the aldehyde form of pyruvic acid and is formed as a side-product of a number of metabolic reactions. The major source of methylglyoxal is from nonenzymatic phosphate elimination from the triose phosphates glyceraldehyde-3-phosphate and dihydroxyacetone phosphate.

Carnosine has been found to attenuate the formation of AGEs. The mechanism of carnosine's antiglycating activity is, however, unclear. One thought is that carnosine acts by sequestering the 1,2-dicarbonyl compounds.

Antioxidant activity: Carnosine has been demonstrated to have a number of antioxidant activities. The dipeptide has been shown to inhibit lipid oxidation catalyzed by iron, hydrogen peroxide-activated hemoglobin, singlet oxygen, lipoxygenase, peroxyl radicals, superoxide anion radicals and hydroxyl radicals. Antioxidant activity has been monitored by measuring a variety of lipid oxidation products, including thiobarbituric acid reactive-substances (TBARS), lipid peroxides and conjugated dienes. It also has been demonstrated to inhibit the oxidation of low-density lipoproteins (LDL) *in vitro.* Carnosine is able to form complexes with some redox metal ions, which are involved in the formation of reactive oxygen species (ROS) and reactive nitrogen species (RNS). While the mechanism of action of carnosine's antioxidant effects is still not completely understood, it can be partially explained by both its free radical scavenging activity and its ability to form chelates with certain metal ions. For example, its ability to form a chelate with copper ions would lead to inhibition of the formation of hydroxyl radicals via the Fenton reaction, which requires free copper ions. However, the ability of carnosine to inhibit iron-catalyzed lipid oxidation does not appear to be due to chelation of iron by carnosine, but to its ability to act as a free radical scavenger.

Trans-4-hydroxy-2-nonenal (HNE) is an aldehydic lipid peroxidation product. HNE is implicated in the pathogenesis of a number of degenerative diseases and is involved in the cross-linking of a variety of intracellular proteins and the induction of transversion mutations secondary to its attack on the nucleotide bases of DNA. HNE may induce neuronal death by altering the ATPases involved in calcium homeostasis. Interestingly, HNE has been found to be elevated in Alzheimer's disease patients. HNE can be detoxified by carnosine via Michael adduct formation.

Carnosine also protects against malondialdehyde (MDA) toxicity. Reactive oxygen species degrade polyunsaturated lipids, forming MDA. MDA is a very reactive aldehyde that can cause protein damage, nucleic acid damage and cellular toxicity. MDA reacts with deoxyguanosine and deoxyadenosine in DNA, forming DNA adducts, which are mutagenic and that can also be carcinogenic.

pH buffering activity: During high- to moderate-intensity exercise, there is accumulation of lactic acid in muscle tissue, causing an increase in hydronium cations and a lowering of muscle pH. Muscle pH can fall from 7.1 to 6.5 or even lower. The drop in pH can cause interference with calcium ion release from the sarcoplasmic reticulum and decreased ATP production, resulting in muscle fatigue. Carnosine with its pKa of 6.83 acts as an intramuscular hydronium cation buffer over the physiological range. Carnosine constitutes at least about 10% to 20% of the buffering capacity in muscle in humans. It appears to be important in its action as an intramuscular buffer in humans, but there are other factors that contribute to delaying muscular fatigue, including other buffers. More research is needed and warranted to elucidate those factors.

PHARMACOKINETICS

An intravenous dose of carnosine leads to a transient rise in the level of carnosine in muscle tissue. However, after 30 to 90 minutes, the renal excretion of carnosine and its metabolites beta-alanine and L-histidine is observed. The intracellular concentration of carnosine is regulated by the zinc metalloprotease carnosinase. There are two isoforms of carnosinase—the serum circulating form and tissue carnosinase. Tissue carnosinase is found in the liver, spleen and kidneys. Serum carnosinase is found in the plasma, brain and spinal fluid. Carnosinase catalyzes the conversion of carnosine to beta-alanine and L-histidine. The enzymatic hydrolysis of carnosine is the main limitation for its possible effective pharmacological applications.

There is some research on the development of delivery forms of carnosine that are resistant to hydrolysis. N-acetylcarnosine appears less susceptible to hydrolysis by carnosinase than is carnosine, and there are some carnosine cyclodextrin derivatives that appear very resistant to hydrolysis.

An oral dose of carnosine, following ingestion, is efficiently absorbed from the small intestine via an active transport mechanism. Carnosine enters the portal circulation which transports it to the liver. In the liver, as well as in the serum, a portion of the carnosine is hydrolyzed into beta-alanine and L-histidine. Carnosine that is not hydrolyzed enters the systemic circulation where it is transported to the muscles, kidneys and various other tissues. A transient rise in carnosine levels in muscle tissue is observed. Most of the carnosine that escaped hydrolysis in the plasma and the liver eventually undergoes hydrolysis to beta-alanine and L-histidine in the kidneys. The kidney seems to be the main organ responsible for the catabolism and excretion of carnosine.

Regarding the metabolism of beta-alanine and L-histidine, the first step in the metabolism of beta-alanine is the formation of malonic acid semialdehyde via the enzyme beta-alanine:alpha-ketoglutarate aminotransferase. Malonic acid semialdehyde is subsequently metabolized by malonic semialdehyde dehydrogenase to acetyl-coenzyme A. Interestingly, the neurotransmitter GABA (gamma-aminobutyric acid) is transaminated by the same aminotransferase that transaminates beta-alanine.

L-histidine is metabolized in a few ways. It can be converted to histamine. It can also be converted via the enzyme histidase to urocanic acid which in turn is converted via urocanase to imidazolonepropionic acid, then to alpha-formiminoglutamic acid. The formimino group of alpha-formiminoglutamic acid is transferred to the N5 position of tetrahydrofolic acid, and glutamic acid is formed.

INDICATIONS AND USAGE

Carnosine is said to be an antiaging agent and to have neuroprotective, antioxidant and anti-inflammatory properties. There is very preliminary information that it might: have antidepressive activity, be helpful in the treatment of cataracts, and be helpful in some ischemia/reperfusion-induced organ injuries. It has demonstrated some immunomodulating activity.

RESEARCH SUMMARY

Carnosine is a natural dipeptide (beta-alanyl-histidine) that is found only in animal tissue, principally in muscle. It was discovered more than 100 years ago. There is evidence that it is a potent hydrophilic antioxidant with a particular affinity for scavenging superoxide anion and hydroxyl radicals. Its antioxidative activity has been observed in many *in vitro* studies, as well as in several *in vivo* experiments conducted under hypoxic and ischemic conditions. In addition to protecting membrane lipids and proteins from oxidative assault, it also demonstrates antiglycating properties, which inhibit damage to cell structures from aldo- and keto-sugars. These properties, combined with other observed effects, have led several researchers to view carnosine as a potential antisenescence agent. Some have dubbed it "the antiaging peptide." Early *in vitro* work hinted at what some called a carnosine-influenced "rejuvenating" effect on cells. Cell lines exhibiting characteristic signs of senescence, when transferred to a carnosine-enriched medium, endured significantly longer than control cells and with greater non-senescent morphology. Additional studies more conclusively demonstrated that carnosine extends cellular life span in a dose-dependent manner.

The *in vitro* work has more recently been extended to animal inquiries. When used as a dietary supplement in the Accelerated Senescence Mice (SAM) line, administration of carnosine (100 mg/kg bodyweight daily in drinking water), though having no effect on maximum lifespan, nonetheless extended mean lifespan of the mice by 20%. Compared with controls, the carnosine-treated animals maintained a notably more youthful appearance and exhibited resistance to aging as measured by a number of physiological parameters. An antioxidative (reactive oxygen species-scavenging) mode of action alone was not believed to be wholly responsible for the observed effects. A favorable effect on the expression of certain genes was hypothesized, based, in part, upon prior research findings indicating that carnosine significantly reduced frequency of chromosomal aberrations in hamster cell cultures exposed to hyperoxia. Its antiglycating activity was also noted as a possible contributor. Interestingly, when other SAM mice were treated by these same researchers with a combination of beta-alanine and L-histidine taken in the same molar proportion as exists in carnosine, no antiaging effect was noted. Why this was the case is unknown. Far more animal, and, eventually, clinical work will be needed in order to determine whether carnosine can act as a genuine antiaging agent in humans.

There is growing evidence that carnosine has notable neuroprotective effects. There is hope, in some circles, that carnosine might help prevent/treat Alzheimer's disease and some other neurodegenerative processes. Carnosine has demonstrated neuroprotection in rat models of cerebral ischemia. Similarly, carnosine also proved to be of benefit in a mouse model of permanent focal cerebral ischemia. Infarct volume was reduced and neurological function improved in carnosine-treated mice, compared with controls. The authors asserted that carnosine is now an attractive candidate for testing as a potential therapy for stroke. In another study, dietary supplementation with carnosine significantly protected rats from ischemia/reperfusion-induced renal injury. These authors postulated a mode of action involving, among other things, a carnosine-induced suppression of renal sympathetic nerve activity that has been associated with renal injury. Another group of researchers has reported that carnosine can protect mast cells from degranulation and histamine release and may be a mast cell stabilizer in conditions of ischemia. Mast cells are involved in post-infarction inflammation and have been linked to processes related to Alzheimer's disease and other neurodegenerative disorders. In another study, carnosine was said to protect rat cells against amyloid beta peptide 42 (Ab42) neurotoxicity. Ab42 is believed by some to be the most important component of the amyloid plaques hypothesized to be the primary cause of Alzheimer's disease. (Carnosine was previously shown to protect rat brain vascular endothelial cells against some other amyloid plaques.) These researchers have presented some preliminary evidence that carnosine may be able to help regulate glutamatergic activity that they say could be disordered by Ab42. Glutamate is the most common brain neurotransmitter. It has been shown in still other research that carnosine is a copper and zinc chelator and that it can thus suppress zinc- and copper-induced neurotoxicity *in vitro*, specifically in cultured olfactory neurons. Intriguingly, olfactory dysfunction has been linked to some neurodegeneration. And elevated levels of zinc have been reported in individuals with Alzheimer's disease. Thus, one researcher has suggested that nasal administration of carnosine should be investigated "as a possible way of suppressing zinc/copper-mediated proteasome inhibition and consequent neurodegeneration." Research related to carnosine's neuroprotective effects deserves expansion into the clinical domain.

There is some evidence that carnosine might promote the health of the eye. N-acetylcarnosine (NAC) has been used as an ophthalmic prodrug of carnosine for clinical use. NAC is said to be more soluble than carnosine itself, and, in animal experiments, was able to deliver carnosine to the ocular lens tissues in significant amounts. In a canine model of cataract, NAC, delivered via eye drops, resulted in "striking" improvement in lens clarity. In a randomized, double-blind, placebo-controlled clinical trial, elderly patients with mild-to-severe cataracts received two NAC eyedrops twice daily or placebo eyedrops. Six months into the trial, the experimental subjects enjoyed marked improvement by several measures (including best corrected visual acuity). Controls, by contrast, mostly experienced continuing visual deterioration. A review author, however, noted that this study was small and, owing to that and other considerations, far from conclusive. Clearly more research is needed and warranted.

Recently researchers reported a carnosine-induced antidepressant-like activity in rats. Behavior that the authors of this study believe is related to depression was suppressed by carnosine administration. They hypothesized that a carnosine-induced stimulation of histaminergic neurons (an activity previously said to have been observed in mice) might be one possible mode of action. No conclusion can be drawn from this very preliminary investigation.

Finally, one researcher, noting that carnosine is found exclusively in animal tissue, has posed the question, "Are carnivorous diets beneficial?" and, by implication, the related question, 'Are vegetarian diets, devoid of carnosine, *not/less* beneficial?' One would assume that this is—or should be—presented as a null hypothesis, given the overwhelming experimental and epidemiological data in support of vegetarian diets versus diets high in animal tissue and low in fruits, vegetables and other plants. It is clearly disingenuous to suggest that a meat-based diet is superior to a vegetarian diet because the latter lacks carnosine, overlooking the broad spectrum of phytonutrients (for which the established health benefits far exceed any that can be claimed for carnosine) that are wholly lacking in meat and plentiful in a plant-based diet. Additionally, the author cites "anecdotal" evidence that carnivorous diabetic patients "appear to control their secondary complications better than vegetarian diabetics." These anecdotes are wholly unsupported by scientific evidence. Also, vegetarians do have the biochemical machinery to make a certain amount of carnosine.

There remains a very real question as to whether oral/dietary carnosine can be beneficial to human health. If it can be, it is most likely to be of benefit in supplement—not dietary—form.

CONTRAINDICATIONS, PRECAUTIONS, ADVERSE REACTIONS

CONTRAINDICATIONS

Carnosine dietary supplements are contraindicated in those who are hypersensitive to any component of a carnosine-containing supplement.

PRECAUTIONS

Those who wish to try a carnosine supplement for a health condition should first discuss its use with his or her physician.

Because of the lack of long-term safety studies on carnosine-containing dietary supplements, pregnant women and nursing mothers should avoid their use.

ADVERSE REACTIONS

None known.

INTERACTIONS

DRUGS

No known interactions.

NUTRITIONAL SUPPLEMENTS

No known interactions.

FOODS

No known interactions.

HERBS

No known interactions.

OVERDOSAGE

There are no reports of overdosage from use of carnosine supplements.

DOSAGE AND ADMINISTRATION

Carnosine supplements are available, typically in strengths of 100 to 500 milligrams. The optimal dosage of carnosine is not known. Doses higher than those recommended on the supplement label should not be exceeded.

The major dietary sources of carnosine are beef, chicken and pork. The concentration of carnosine in beef muscle meat ranges from 150 mg to 450 mg per 100 grams or 3.5 ounces. The concentration of carnosine in chicken muscle meat ranges from 50 mg to 279 mg per 100 grams.

LITERATURE

Antonini FM, Petruzzi E, Pinzani P, et al. The meat in the diet of aged subjects and the antioxidant effects of carnosine. *Arch Gerontol Geriatr Suppl.* 2002;8:7-14.

Aydogan S, Yapislar H, Artis S, et al. Impaired erythrocytes deformability in H(2)O(2)-induced oxidative stress: protective effect of L-carnosine. *Clin Hemorheol Microcirc.* 2008;39(1-4):93-98.

Bauchart C, Savary-Auzeloux I, Patureau Mirand P, et al. Carnosine concentration of ingested meat affects carnosine net release into the portal vein of minipigs. *J Nutr.* 2007;137(3):589-593.

Boldyrev AA, Gallant SC, Sukhich GT. Carnosine, the protective, anti-aging peptide. *Biosci Rep.* 1999;19(6):581-587.

Brownson C, Hipkiss AR. Carnosine reacts with a glycated protein. *Free Radic Biol Med.* 2000;28(10):1564-1570.

Chuang CH, Hu ML. L-Carnosine Inhibits Metastasis of SK-Hep-1 Cells by Inhibition of Matrix Metaoproteinase-9 Expression and Induction of an Antimetastatic Gene, nm23-H1. *Nutr Cancer.* 2008;60(4):526-533.

Cohen M, Hartlage PL, Krawiecki N, et al. Serum carnosinase deficiency: a non-disabling phenotype? *J Ment Defic Res.* 1985;29 (Pt 4):383-389.

Decker EA, Ivanov V, Zhu BZ, et al. Inhibition of low-density lipoprotein oxidation by carnosine histidine. *J Agric Food Chem.* 2001;49(1):511-516.

Dunnett M, Harris RC, Dunnett CE, et al. Plasma carnosine concentration: diurnal variation and effects of age, exercise and muscle damage. *Equine Vet J Suppl.* 2002;(34):283-287.

Fitzpatrick DW, Fisher H. Carnosine, histidine, and wound healing. *Surgery.* 1982;91(1):56-60.

Fleisher LD, Rassin DK, Wisniewski K, et al. Carnosinase deficiency: a new variant with high residual activity. *Pediatr Res.* 1980;14(4 Pt 1):269-271.

Fujii T, Takaoka M, Tsuruoka N, et al. Dietary supplementation of L-carnosine prevents ischemia/reperfusion-induced renal injury in rats. *Biol Pharm Bull.* 2005;28(2):361-363.

Gallant S, Semyonova M, Yuneva M. Carnosine as a potential anti-senescence drug. *Biochemistry* (Mosc). 2000;65(7):866-868.

Gjessing LR, Lunde HA, Mørkrid L, et al. Inborn errors of carnosine and homocarnosine metabolism. *J Neural Transm Suppl.* 1990;29:91-106.

Guo Y, Yan H. [Preventive effect of carnosine on cataract development][Article in Chinese.] *Yan Ke Xue Bao.* 2006;22(2):85-88.

Hipkiss AR. Could carnosine or related structures suppress Alzheimer's disease? *J Alzheimers Dis.* 2007;11(2):229-240.

Hipkiss AR. Would carnosine or a carnivorous diet help suppress aging and associated pathologies? *Ann N Y Acad Sci.* 2006;1067:369-374.

Hipkiss AR. Does chronic glycolysis accelerate aging? Could this explain how dietary restriction works? *Ann N Y Acad Sci.* 2006;1067:361-368.

Hipkiss AR. Glycation, ageing and carnosine: are carnivorous diets beneficial? *Mech Ageing Dev.* 2005;126(10):1034-1039.

Hipkiss AR. Could carnosine suppress zinc-mediated proteasome inhibition and neurodegeneration? Therapeutic potential of a non-toxic but non-patentable dipeptide. *Biogerontology.* 2005;6(2):147-149.

Hipkiss AR, Chana H. Carnosine protects proteins against methylglyoxal-mediated modifications. *Biochem Biophys Res Commun.* 1998;248(1):28-32.

Liu WH, Liu TC, Yin MC. Beneficial effects of histidine and carnosine on ethanol-induced chronic liver injury. *Food Chem Toxicol.* 2008;46(5):1503-1509.

Mahmood A, FitzGerald AJ, Marchbank T, et al. Zinc carnosine, a health food supplement that stabilises small bowel integrity and stimulates gut repair processes. *Gut.* 2007;56(2):168-175.

Min J, Senut MC, Rajanikant K, et al. Differential neuroprotective effects of carnosine, anserine, and N-acetyl carnosine against permanent focal ischemia. *J Neurosci Res.* 2008;86(13):2984-2991.

Muranov KO, Dizhevskaia AK, Boldyrev AA, et al. [Search for chaperon-like anticataract drugs, the antiaggregants of lens crystallins. Communication. 1. Chaperon-like activity of N-acetyl carnosine dipeptide: in vitro study on a model of ultraviolet-induced aggregation of betaL-crystallin] [Article in Russian.] *Vestn Oftalmol.* 2008;124(2):3-6.

Nagai K, Niijima A, Yamano T, et al. Possible role of L-carnosine in the regulation of blood glucose through controlling autonomic nerves. *Exp Biol Med* (Maywood). 2003;228(10):1138-1145.

Niijima A, Okui T, Matsumura Y, et al. Effects of L-carnosine on renal sympathetic nerve activity and DOCA-salt hypertension in rats. *Auton Neurosci.* 2002;97(2):99-102.

Quinn PJ, Boldyrev AA, Formazuyk VE. Carnosine: its properties, functions and potential therapeutic applications. *Mol Aspects Med.* 1992;13(5):379-444.

Reeve VE, Bosnic M, Rozinova E. Carnosine (beta-alanylhistidine) protects from the suppression of contact hypersensitivity by ultraviolet B (280-320 nm) radiation or by cis urocanic acid. *Immunology.* 1993;78(1):99-104.

Ririe DG, Roberts PR, Shouse MN, et al. Vasodilatory actions of the dietary peptide carnosine. *Nutrition.* 2000;16(3):168-172.

Sadikali F, Darwish R, Watson WC. Carnosinase activity of human gastrointestinal mucosa. *Gut.* 1975;16(8):585-589.

Seidler NW, Yeargans GS, Morgan TG. Carnosine disaggregates glycated alpha-crystallin: an in vitro study. *Arch Biochem Biophys.* 2004;427(1):110-115.

Shen J, Yao JF, Tanida M, et al. Regulation of sympathetic nerve activity by l-carnosine in mammalian white adipose tissue. *Neurosci Lett.* 2008;441(1):100-104.

Son DO, Satsu H, Kiso Y, et al. Characterization of carnosine uptake and its physiological function in human intestinal epithelial Caco-2 cells. *Biofactors.* 2004;21(1-4):395-398.

Tamaki N, Ikeda T, Fujimoto S, et al. Carnosine as a histidine source: transport and hydrolysis of exogenous carnosine by rat intestine. *J Nutr Sci Vitaminol* (Tokyo). 1985;31(6):607-618.

Tomonaga S, Hayakawa T, Yamane H, et al. Oral administration of chicken breast extract increases brain carnosine and anserine concentrations in rats. *Nutr Neurosci.* 2007;10(3-4):181-186.

Yan H, Harding JJ. Carnosine inhibits modifications and decreased molecular chaperone activity of lens alpha-crystallin induced by ribose and fructose 6-phosphate. *Mol Vis.* 2006;12:205-214.

CDP-Choline

DESCRIPTION

CDP-choline is a naturally occurring substance found in most life forms. It is an intermediate metabolite in the major pathway for the synthesis of phosphatidylcholine. Phosphatidylcholine is a phospholipid that is a major component of cell membranes. Phosphatidylcholine is necessary for the structure and function of all cells and is crucial for sustaining life.

CDP-choline is synthesized in cells by the reaction of the nucleotide cytidine triphosphate or CTP with phosphocholine. The enzyme catalyzing the reaction is called CTP: phosphocholine cytidyltransferase. This reaction is the rate-limiting step in the synthesis of phosphatidyl choline.

Phosphocholine is synthesized from choline, and, for the synthesis of phosphatidylcholine, CDP-choline reacts with diacylglyceride, catalyzed by the enzyme CDP-choline: 1,2-diacylglycerol cholinephosphotransferase.

CDP-choline is also known as cytidine-5′-diphosphate choline and citicoline, and has the following structural formula:

CDP-Choline

ACTIONS AND PHARMACOLOGY

ACTIONS

CDP-choline has putative activity as a cognition enhancer and in cell-membrane repair.

MECHANISM OF ACTION

Since the action of CDP-choline either as a pharmaceutical or nutraceutical agent has yet to be clarified, discussion of its mechanism of action is speculative. However, much is known about the biochemistry of endogenous CDP-choline. CDP-choline is an intermediate metabolite in the major pathway for the synthesis of the membrane phospholipid, phosphatidylcholine. Phosphatidylcholine is crucial for the maintenance of cell-membrane fluidity and cellular integrity. CDP-choline, hypothetically, may aid in cell-membrane repair, particularly neuronal cell membranes that have been damaged by trauma, ischemic events, toxins, infections or during the course of aging.

CDP-choline is also a delivery form of choline and cytidine. Choline is a precursor of acetylcholine and betaine. Acetylcholine is a neurotransmitter whose deficiency in certain regions of the brain is believed to be an etiological factor in certain dementia syndromes, including Alzheimer's disease. Betaine is involved in the conversion of the amino acid homocysteine to the essential amino acid L-methionine. L-methionine is a protein amino acid. Cytidine, following conversion to cytidine triphosphate, participates in a few reactions, including the formation of CDP-choline and nucleic acids.

PHARMACOKINETICS

Most pharmacokinetic studies have been performed in animals. Following oral intake, most CDP-choline is hydrolyzed in the small intestine to choline and cytidine. Choline and cytidine are absorbed and transported to the liver via the portal circulation. In the liver, choline may enter various metabolic pathways, resulting in the biosynthesis of various substances, including CDP-choline, betaine and phosphatidylcholine. Cytidine enters the cytidine nucleotide pool and may be incorporated into nucleic acids. Choline and cytidine not metabolized in the liver are distributed to various tissues in the body, where they undergo further metabolism. The uptake of CDP-choline by the brain is low. However, choline and cytidine may be taken up by the brain. Within the brain, cytidine and choline may be metabolized via a few steps to CDP-choline, which can serve as a substrate for phosphatidylcholine synthesis.

INDICATIONS AND USAGE

CDP-choline may be useful in the treatment of stroke and brain injury. There is some preliminary evidence that CDP-choline may be helpful in some with tardive dyskinesia, Parkinson's disease, Alzheimer's disease and other conditions characterized by impaired cognitive function, including memory loss. An indication may emerge for it to help improve visual acuity in those with amblyopia.

RESEARCH SUMMARY

In numerous studies of CDP-choline, favorable results have been obtained in cerebral ischemia and traumatic head injury. Its efficacy in these studies has been attributed to its apparent ability to increase phosphatidylcholine synthesis in the brain. In animal studies, it has been shown to enhance cell-membrane formation and repair, to restore intracellular enzyme function, to limit nerve damage and decrease edema.

The same mechanisms, generally, are said to account for favorable effects reported for it in the treatment of Parkinson's disease, Alzheimer's disease and a variety of cognitive disorders, including impaired memory associated with aging.

In a randomized, double-blind, placebo-controlled study, 259 patients with ischemic stroke received placebo or 500 to 2000 milligrams of CDP-choline daily for six weeks commencing within 24 hours of stroke. Among subjects who received 500 milligrams of CDP-choline daily, 53 percent achieved full or nearly-full recovery as measured by tests of neurolgic function. Among those receiving placebo, 33 percent achieved similar levels of recovery in the same time frame. The 500 milligram dose was as efficacious as higher doses and produced no significant side effects. Higher doses produced dizziness in some. Research continues.

One study showed that oral CDP-choline, administered within the first 24 hours after onset in patients with moderate to severe ischemic stroke, significantly increased the probability of complete recovery at three months. A recent rat study evidenced a synergistic effect on infarct size and neuronal death by CDP-choline and reperfusion induced by thrombolysis. (Thrombolysis is still the only generally accepted therapy in acute ischemic stroke.) This combined therapy was superior to either alone in reducing ischemic brain damage. A meta-analysis identified CDP-choline as the first clinically effective neuroprotective agent in ischemic stroke. The placebo-controlled, randomized, double-blind prospective trials evaluated in the meta-analysis used daily oral doses of CDP-choline in the 500-2,000 milligram range for six weeks and involved 1,500 patients in all. While functional recovery was significantly better than in placebo groups, there was less evidence of diminished neurological deficit. Larger trials are underway.

In one study, CDP-choline, given in a daily dose of 1000 milligrams for a month, slightly improved mental performance in subjects with Alzheimer's disease. Better results have been reported with similar doses of CDP-choline in patients with early-onset Alzheimer's disease. Both favorable immunogenic and neurotrophic effects are reported in many of these CDP-choline/Alzheimer's studies.

In a randomized, double-blind, placebo-controlled study, subjects, aged 50 to 85, received placebo or varying doses of CDP-choline, generally 1000 to 2000 milligrams a day, for several months. A subgroup of these subjects, shown to have relatively inefficient memories, benefited the most from CDP-choline, as measured by tests of logical memory. The researchers concluded: "Citicoline may prove effective in treating age-related cognitive decline that may be the precursor of dementia."

A review paper found evidence in current research that CDP-choline might improve cognitive function in elderly patients with memory deficits, mild cognitive impairment, and senile dementia of the Alzheimer's type. One recent study reported that dietary CDP-choline supplementation prevents memory impairment caused by impoverished environmental conditions in rats. And in a recent study using a rat model of birth asphyxia, CDP-choline attenuated brain damage.

There is preliminary evidence that CDP-choline might be useful in some disorders of vision. Statistically significant vision improvement was noted in a study of 50 patients with amblyopia treated with CDP-choline for 15 days. The improvement was sustained at a four-month follow-up. More research is warranted.

CONTRAINDICATIONS, PRECAUTIONS, ADVERSE REACTIONS

CONTRAINDICATIONS

Known hypersensitivity to a CDP-choline-containing product.

PRECAUTIONS

Because of lack of long-term safety studies, CDP-choline should be avoided by children, pregnant women and nursing mothers. Those who wish to try CDP-choline for a health condition should first discuss its use with his or her physician.

ADVERSE REACTIONS

Adverse reactions reported include epigastric distress, nausea, rash, headache and dizziness.

DOSAGE AND ADMINISTRATION

Citicoline (CDP-choline) is approved in some countries as a parenteral drug for the treatment of acute ischemic stroke. There are a number of ongoing clinical trials in the United States and other countries studying citicoline for acute stroke (ICTUS Study: International Citicoline Trial on acUte Stroke), for its effects on brain function and behavior in marijuana-dependent individuals, and as add-on therapy for patients with bipolar disorder and major depression. (See: ClinicalTrials.gov.)

CDP-choline is also being marketed by itself and along with other ingredients as a nutritional supplement, typically 250 milligrams, once or twice daily. Choline makes up approximately 21% of CDP-choline.

Stability is a concern with CDP-choline. Long-alkyl chain sulfonate salts of CDP-choline appear to show enhanced stability for oral use.

LITERATURE

Alonso de Leciñana M, Gutiérrez M, Roda JM, et al. Effect of combined therapy with thrombolysis and citicoline in a rat model of embolic stroke. *J Neurol Sci.* 2006;247(2):121-129.

Babb SM, Appelmans KE, Renshaw PF, et al. Differential effect of CDP-choline on brain cytosolic choline levels in younger and older subjects as measured by proton magnetic resonance spectroscopy. *Psychopharmacol.* 1996;127:88-94.

Conant R, Schauss AG. Therapeutic applications of citicoline for stroke and cognitive dysfunction in the elderly: a review of the literature. *Altern Med Rev.* 2004;9(1):17-31.

Dávalos A, Castillo J, Alvarez-Sabín J, et al. Oral citicoline in acute ischemic stroke: an individual patient data pooling analysis of clinical trials. *Stroke.* 2002;33(12):2850-2857.

Fiedorowicz M, Makarewicz D, Staczak-Mrozek KI, et al. CDP-choline (citicoline) attenuates brain damage in a rat model of birth asphyxia. *Acta Neurobiol Exp (Wars).* 2008;68(3):389-397.

Franco-Maside A, Coamano J, Gomez MJ, et al. Brain mapping activity and mental performance after treatment with CDP-choline in Alzheimer's disease. *Methods Find Exp Clin Pharmacol.* 1994;16:597-607.

Galletti P, DeRosa M, Cotticelli MG, et al (1991). Biochemical rationale for the use of CDPcholine in traumatic brain injury: pharmacokinetics of the orally administered drug. *J Neurol Sci.* 1991;103 Suppl:S19-S25.

Gimenez R, Soler S, Aquilar J. Cytidine diphosphate choline administration activates brain cytidine triphosphate: phosphocholine cytidyltransferase in aged rats. *Neurosci Lett.* 1999;273:163-166.

Overgaard K, Meden P. Citicoline—the first effective neuroprotectant to be combined with thrombolysis in acute ischemic stroke? *J Neurol Sci.* 2006;247(2):119-120.

Rema V, Bali KK, Ramachandra R, et al. Cytidine-5-diphosphocholine supplement in early life induces stable increase in dendritic complexity of neurons in the somatosensory cortex of adult rats. *Neuroscience.* 2008 Aug;155(2):556-564.

Spiers PA, Myers D, Hochanadel GS. Citicholine improves verbal memory in aging. *Arch Neurol.* 1996;53:441-448.

Teather LA, Wurtman RJ. Dietary CDP-choline supplementation prevents memory impairment caused by impoverished environmental conditions in rats. *Learn Mem.* 2005;12(1):39-43.

Weiss GB. Metabolism and actions of CDP-choline as an endogenous compound and administered exogenously as citicholine. *Life Sci.* 1995;56:637-660.

Cetyl Myristoleate

DESCRIPTION

Cetyl myristoleate is an ester comprised of the 16-carbon atom alcohol, 1-hexadecanol (cetyl alcohol), and the 14-

carbon monounsaturated fatty acid *cis*-9 tetradecenoic acid, or myristoleic acid. It was originally isolated from a NIH Swiss albino mouse strain that was resistant to adjuvant-induced arthritis. Cetyl myristoleate is known to exist naturally in sperm whale oil and in a small gland in the male beaver. It is marketed and used as an anti-osteoarthritis supplement. A waxy, lipid substance, it has the following chemical structure:

Cetyl myristoleate

ACTIONS AND PHARMACOLOGY

ACTIONS

Cetyl myristoleate has supposed anti-osteoarthritic activity.

PHARMACOKINETICS

No studies have been done on the pharmacokinetics of cetyl myristoleate. It is likely to be absorbed in the small intestine and transported from the lymph to the blood in lipid particles. Upon metabolism in the cells, it is likely that cetyl myristoleate undergoes enzymatic hydrolysis and that the component molecules, cetyl alcohol and myristoleic acid, are catabolized by normal cellular oxidative processes.

INDICATIONS AND USAGE

There is little credible support for claims that cetyl myristoleate is effective in arthritis, fibromyalgia, chronic fatigue syndrome and immune disorders.

RESEARCH SUMMARY

Claims for this substance have been sweeping, based upon an isolated finding that it provides protection against adjuvant-induced arthritis in a mouse strain (see above). In one animal study, high doses of cetyl myristoleate given parenterally were found to reduce the severity of arthritis in a rat adjuvant arthritis model. Another animal study found that cetyl myristoleate given in high doses orally had a modest antiarthritis effect in the mouse collagen-induced arthritis model. There are hardly any credible human clinical studies. A 68-day human placebo-controlled, single-blind, randomized controlled trial (RCT) of subjects having severe knee osteoarthritis reported an increase in knee flexibility in those receiving the study test article compared with those who received placebo. However, the study test article contained a number of substances, including olive oil, fish oil, lecithin and various cetylated fatty acids. Therefore, this was a low-quality RCT providing limited scientific evidence of efficacy for cetyl myristoleate. Until further positive research results are obtained from well-designed and well-executed clinical trials, the human use of cetyl myristoleate supplements has little scientific rationale. Claims that it is helpful in fibromyalgia, chronic fatigue syndrome and immune disorders have not been substantiated by credible research.

CONTRAINDICATIONS, PRECAUTIONS, ADVERSE REACTIONS

CONTRAINDICATIONS

Known hypersensitivity to a Cetyl myristoleate-containing product.

PRECAUTIONS

Children, pregnant women and nursing mothers should avoid cetyl myristoleate supplements.

ADVERSE REACTIONS

May cause mild gastrointestinal symptoms.

DOSAGE AND ADMINISTRATION

There are no typical doses.

LITERATURE

Diehl HW, May EL. Cetyl myristoleate isolated from Swiss albino mice: an apparent protective agent against adjuvant arthritis in rats. *J Pharm Sci.* 1994;83:296-299.

Hesslink R Jr, Armstrong D 3rd, Nagendran MV, et al. Cetylated fatty acids improve knee function in patients with osteoarthritis. *J Rheumatol.* 2002;29(8):1708-1712.

Hunter KW Jr, Gault RA, Stehouwer JS, et al. Synthesis of cetyl myristoleate and evaluation of its therapeutic efficacy in a murine model of collagen-induced arthritis. *Pharmacol Res.* 2003;47(1):43-47.

Kraemer WJ, Ratamess NA, Anderson JM, et al. Effect of a cetylated fatty acid topical cream on functional mobility and quality of life of patients with osteoarthritis. *J Rheumatol.* 2004;31(4):767-774.

Whitehouse MW, McGeary RP. Concerning the anti-arthritic action of cetyl myristoleate in rats: An interim report. *Inflammopharmacology.* 1999;7(3):303-310.

Chelated Minerals

DESCRIPTION

Chelated minerals are minerals complexed with various amino acids, oligopeptides or other organic molecules that can bind with minerals to form a molecular complex.

It is believed by some that chelated minerals are better absorbed than non-chelated minerals. There may be certain minerals, e.g., trivalent chromium and zinc, where this is possibly the case. However, in most cases chelated and non-chelated minerals are absorbed with equivalent efficiency.

ACTIONS AND PHARMACOLOGY

ACTIONS

Chelated minerals are delivery forms of minerals.

MECHANISM OF ACTION

See monographs on individual minerals. Chelated chromium forms appear to be better absorbed than non-chelated forms. The mechanism of this is not entirely clear.

PHARMACOKINETICS

See monographs on individual minerals.

INDICATIONS AND USAGE

See individual mineral monographs to determine whether chelated forms confer any advantage. The mere claim of "chelation" does not necessarily mean a superior product.

RESEARCH SUMMARY

The issue of mineral chelation is a complex one. See monographs on individual minerals.

CONTRAINDICATIONS, PRECAUTIONS, ADVERSE REACTIONS

See monographs on individual minerals.

OVERDOSAGE

The only mineral in which overdosage is a significant problem is iron. See monograph on Iron.

DOSAGE AND ADMINISTRATION

See monographs on individual minerals.

LITERATURE

See monographs on individual minerals.

Chicken Collagen II

DESCRIPTION

Chicken collagen II is type II collagen derived from the sternum of chickens. Type II collagen is the most abundant collagen found in hyaline cartilage (in synovial joints, sternum, respiratory tract), comprising 80 to 90% of the total collagen content. Chicken collagen II is also known as type II chicken collagen and is abbreviated as CCII.

Type II chicken collagen shares some similar antigenic regions with type II human collagen. Autoimmune response to type II collagen is thought to be a significant factor in the pathogenesis of rheumatoid arthritis. A few studies suggest that oral type II chicken collagen may be beneficial to some with rheumatoid arthritis, acting by a process known as oral tolerance.

ACTIONS AND PHARMACOLOGY

ACTIONS

Chicken collagen type II may have anti-rheumatoid arthritis activity in some.

MECHANISM OF ACTION

The mechanism of the possible anti-rheumatoid arthritis activity of chicken collagen type II may be through oral tolerance. Oral tolerance refers to the observation that if a protein is orally administered, subsequent immunization with the protein leads to a state of systemic hyporesponsiveness to it. Autoantibodies to type II collagen are thought to play a role in the pathogenesis of rheumatoid arthritis. Therefore, feeding antigenic type II collagen may be predicted to lead to the induction of immune tolerance to type II collagen, especially in the context of elevated autoantibodies to this substance.

The mechanism for oral tolerance appears to depend on the dose of the fed antigen. Low doses appear to induce active suppression, while high doses result in clonal anergy. Suppressive cytokines, such as interleukin-4 and transforming growth factor beta, appear to mediate active suppression. Studies in animals demonstrate the generation of regulatory lymphocytes in Peyer's patches, which subsequently migrate to mesenteric lymph nodes and spleen. Secretion of suppressive cytokines by these cells is believed to depend on antigen-specific stimulation with the fed antigen. Further, it is believed that active suppression of the inflammatory process by the regulatory lymphocytes requires their migration to the location where the fed antigen is present. Since the clinical studies to date indicate that low doses, but not high doses, have possible mild efficacy in rheumatoid arthritis, the mechanism responsible for oral tolerance would appear to be induction of active suppression, rather than clonal anergy.

PHARMACOKINETICS

There are no reports on the pharmacokinetics of chicken collagen type II. The pharmacokinetics of the substance should be similar to those of dietary proteins.

INDICATIONS AND USAGE

Chicken collagen II may offer some mild benefit for some with rheumatoid arthritis.

RESEARCH SUMMARY

A multicenter, randomized, controlled trial of oral type II collagen derived from chicken cartilage tested the substance in four different daily doses versus placebo in 273 rheumatoid arthritis patients. Various criteria were used to evaluate the results. The daily dose levels were 20 micrograms, 100 micrograms, 500 micrograms and 2,500 micrograms.

Results were negative at all dose levels except the lowest dose (20 micrograms daily). The difference in response between this dose level and placebo was significant only with respect to what was described as the weakest of the evaluative criteria. A *post hoc* analysis revealed that those who had antibodies reactive with type II collagen in their serum (at the baseline exam) were more likely to respond to collagen administration.

More research is needed, in part to investigate whether still lower doses might further improve efficacy of this antigenic substance.

CONTRAINDICATIONS, PRECAUTIONS, ADVERSE REACTIONS

CONTRAINDICATIONS

Chicken collagen II is contraindicated in those who are hypersensitive to any component of a chicken collagen II-containing product.

PRECAUTIONS

Because of lack of long-term safety studies, nutritional supplements containing chicken collagen II should be avoided by pregnant women and nursing mothers.

Those with rheumatoid arthritis who are interested in trying chicken collagen II should consult with their physicians before doing so.

ADVERSE REACTIONS

Chicken collagen type II supplements are generally well tolerated. There is one report of transient flushing in a patient with juvenile rheumatoid arthritis.

DOSAGE AND ADMINISTRATION

Chicken collagen II, derived from chicken sterum, is available as capsules and tablets. Some use 500 to 1000 mg daily. However, in the clinical trials showing possible mild effectiveness of chicken collagen type II, lower doses and different delivery forms were used. In these trials, the substance was first dissolved in 0.1 M acetic acid and added to orange juice prior to ingestion. The dose used in the trial of juvenile rheumatoid arthritics was 100 micrograms (0.1 mg) daily for one month followed by a dose of 500 micrograms (0.5 mg) daily. In a subsequent larger clinical trial involving rheumatoid arthritics, a dose of 20 micrograms (0.02 mg) daily appeared to have mild benefits in some. Higher doses did not.

LITERATURE

Barnett ML, Combitchi D, Trentham DE. A pilot trial of oral type II collagen in the treatment of juvenile rheumatoid arthritis. *Arthritis Rheum.* 1996; 39:623-628.

Barnett ML, Kremer JM, St Clair EW, et al. Treatment of rheumatoid arthritis with oral type II collagen. Results of a multicenter, double-blind, placebo-controlled trial. *Arthritis Rheum.* 1998; 41:290-297.

Trentham DE. Evidence that type II collagen feeding can induce a durable therapeutic response in some patients with rheumatoid arthritis. In: Weiner HL, Mayer LF, eds. *Oral Tolerance: Mechanisms and Applications. Ann NY Acad Sci.* 1996; 778:306-314.

Trentham DE. Oral tolerization as a treatment of rheumatoid arthritis. *Rheum Dis Clinc North Am.* 1998; 24: 525-536.

Trentham DE, Dynesius-Trentham RA, Orav EJ, et al. Effects of oral administration of type II collagen on rheumatoid arthritis. *Science.* 1993; 261:1727-1730.

Watson WC, Cremer MA, Wooley PH, Townes AS. Assessment of the potential pathogenicity of type II collagen autoantibodies in patients with rheumatoid arthritis. *Arthritis Rheum.* 1986; 29:1316-1321.

Chitosan

DESCRIPTION

Chitosan and chitin are polysaccharide polymers containing more than 5,000 glucosamine and acetylglucosamine units, respectively, and their molecular weights are over one million Daltons. Chitin is found in fungi, arthropods and marine invertebrates. Commercially, chitin is derived from the exoskeletons of crustaceans (shrimp, crab and other shellfish). Chitosan is obtained from chitin by a deacetylation process.

Chitin, the polysaccharide polymer from which chitosan is derived, is a cellulose-like polymer consisting mainly of unbranched chains of N-acetyl-D-glucosamine. Deacetylated chitin, or chitosan, is comprised of chains of D-glucosamine. When ingested, chitosan can be considered a dietary fiber. Chitosan has the following chemical structure:

Chitosan

Chitosan itself is the major source of the nutritional supplement glucosamine.

ACTIONS AND PHARMACOLOGY

ACTIONS

Chitosan may have hypocholesterolemic activity in some and may be beneficial in renal disease in some.

MECHANISM OF ACTION

Chitosan is, at the pH of the gastrointestinal tract, a positively charged polymer and can bind to negatively charged substances. It is believed that chitosan, similar to cholestryamine, has bile acid sequestration activity and that this may be the mechanism for its putative hypocholesterolemic effect. There is some evidence that chitosan binds to bile acids and some evidence that the polymer affects the metabolism of intestinal bile acids. However, in contrast to cholestyramine, chitosan does not have consistent hypocholesterolemic activity. There is also evidence that chitosan binds to fats in the intestine, blocking their absorption.

The mechanism of action of chitosan's possible beneficial effects on renal disease in some is unknown. Chitosan can absorb urea and ammonia, but it is unclear whether this mechanism has anything to do with its putative renal effects.

PHARMACOKINETICS

Ingested chitosan can be considered as a cellulose-like dietary fiber. After ingesting, there is minimal digestion and most of the ingested chitosan is excreted in the feces.

INDICATIONS AND USAGE

There is some evidence that supplemental chitosan may have favorable effects on lipids and may be of some use in renal failure. There is some suggestion from available research data that it might be helpful in preventing atherosclerosis and could play a role in wound healing, some types of diabetes and liver disease or injury. Claims that it can help reduce weight, fight cancer, heal ulcers, aid digestion and boost immunity are unsubstantiated.

RESEARCH SUMMARY

There are several studies, in both animals and humans, demonstrating chitosan's effect on lipids. These effects have generally been more dramatic in various animal models, possibly due to higher chitosan intake in many of those studies. Some of these animal studies show very dramatic reductions in cholesterol and in LDL-cholesterol. Some have observed increases in the HDL-cholesterol, as well.

In humans, results have been less clear-cut, though still suggestive of positive effects. In one recent placebo-controlled, double-blind study, there was a significant decrease in LDL-cholesterol among subjects receiving 2,400 milligrams of chitosan daily, compared with placebo subjects. Chitosan had no significant effect on serum total cholesterol or on HDL-cholesterol, but it slightly increased triglycerides. Others have reported similar effects: reduced LDL-cholesterol with little or no effect on HDL and total cholesterols. A few others, however, have reported no lipid effects. Differences may be due to dissimilar dosing.

In animal models of chronic renal failure, chitosan produced decreases in serum urea nitrogen, serum creatine and serum phosphate. It also ameliorated anemia and increased fecal weight, fecal water content, fecal nitrogen and fecal sodium. The apparent protein ratio was decreased in a dose-dependent pattern in some of these studies, and survival times were markedly and significantly extended.

In a human study of 80 patients with chronic renal failure, similarly encouraging results were obtained. Half of these patients received 30 chitosan tablets (each containing 45 milligrams of chitosan) three times a day for a total of 4,050 milligrams daily. After four weeks on this regiment, these subjects experienced significant reductions in urea and creatine levels in serum, compared with controls. Significant gains were also measured in physical strength, appetite and sleep patterns after 12 weeks of chitosan supplementation. It is interesting to note that chitosan at this dose also significantly reduced total serum cholesterol levels (and increased serum hemoglobin levels).

Favorable lipid results would suggest that supplemental chitosan might help prevent atherosclerosis. This idea has been tested in some animal models with promising results. Using the apolipoprotein E-deficient mouse model of atherosclerosis, for example, researchers recently showed that a 5% chitosan diet could produce "a highly significant inhibition of atherogenesis"—42% inhibition in the whole aorta and 50% inhibition in the aortic arch, compared with controls. These positive effects were attributed to a 65% reduction in blood cholesterol levels (after 20 weeks on the 5% chitosan diet).

Some research has demonstrated that topical preparations containing chitosan can help speed wound healing. Other preliminary studies suggest that chitosan might be useful in lean type non-insulin-dependent diabetes mellitus. In an animal model of this disease, chitosan significantly reduced blood glucose, cholesterol and triglycerides. (The same results, however, could not be obtained in obese type NIDDM.) Still other similarly preliminary studies suggest that chitosan might help protect the liver against some toxins. More research in these areas is needed.

Claims have been made that chitosan can help reduce weight. There is insufficient data to support this claim. Two recent studies failed to find any weight-loss effect from the use of chitosan in overweight subjects. In the larger and longer-term of these two studies, 51 healthy obese women were given either placebo or 2,400 milligrams of chitosan for eight weeks. No significant weight reduction was noted in the treatment group.

Similarly, there is insufficient data to support claims that chitosan fights cancer, heals ulcers, aids digestion, or boosts or otherwise modifies immunity.

CONTRAINDICATIONS, PRECAUTIONS, ADVERSE REACTIONS

CONTRAINDICATIONS

Known hypersensitivity to a chitosan-containing product.

PRECAUTIONS

Children, pregnant women and nursing mothers should avoid using chitosan.

Those with shellfish allergies should exercise caution in taking chitosan supplements.

ADVERSE REACTIONS

Occasionally, gastrointestinal side effects, such as nausea and diarrhea have been reported.

INTERACTIONS

DRUGS

No interactions are known. However, chitosan might bind to certain drugs, especially lipophilic drugs.

NUTRITIONAL SUPPLEMENTS

Vitamin C is believed to enhance the putative benefits of chitosan. Chitosan might bind to the fat soluble vitamins A, D, E and K, as well as carotenoids and flavonoids. It might also bind to some minerals such as zinc.

FOODS

Chitosan might bind some dietary lipids. It may also bind the fat-soluble vitamins A, D, E and K, as well as flavonoids, carotenoids and some minerals, such as zinc, found in foods.

OVERDOSAGE

There are no reports of overdosage.

DOSAGE AND ADMINISTRATION

There are several chitosan supplements available. Those who use chitosan for cholesterol-lowering effects typically use 1000 to 1200 milligrams twice a day, taken before or after meals and with a glass of water. Chitosan can be contaminated with such metals as lead, mercury, iron, copper and arsenic.

Chitosan supplements should not be consumed within two hours of taking the fat-soluble vitamins A, D, E and K, carotenoids (e.g., lycopene, lutein), flavonoids (e.g., genistein, quercetin, ipriflavone) or prescription medication.

LITERATURE

Ebihara K, Schneeman BO. Interaction of bile acids, phospholipids, cholesterol and triglyceride with dietary fibers in the small intestine of rats. *J Nutr.* 1989; 119 006700-1106.

Fukada Y, Kimura K, Ayaki Y. Effect of chitosan feeding on intestinal bile acid metabolism in rats. *Lipids.* 1991;26:395-399.

Han LK, Kimura Y Okuda H. Reduction in fat storage during chitin-chitosan treatment in mice fed a high-fat diet. *Int J Obes Relat Metab Disord.* 1999;23:174-179.

Jing SB, Li L, Ji D, et al. Effect of chitosan on renal function in patients with chronic renal failure. *J. Pharm Pharmacol* 1997; *49:* 721-723.

Lee JK, Kim SU, Kim JH. Modification of chitosan to improve its hypocholesterolemic capacity. *Biosci Biotechnol Biochem.* 1999;63:833-839.

LeHoux JG, Grondin F. Some effects of chitosan on liver function in the rat. *Endocrinology.* 1993; 132:1078-1084.

Miura T, Usami M, Tsuura Y, et al. Hypoglycemic and hypolipidemic effect of chitosan in normal and neonatal

streptozotacin-induced diabetic mice. *Biol Pharm Bull.* 1995; 18:1623-1625.

Nagano N, Yoshimoto H, Nishitoba T, et al. Pharmacological properties of chitosan-coated dialdehyde cellulose (chitosan DAC), a newly developed oral adsorbent (II). Effect of chitosan DAC on rats with chronic renal failure induced by adriamycin. [Article in Japanese]. *Nippon Yakurigaku Zasshi.* 1995; 106:123-133.

Omrod DJ, Holmes CC, Miller, TE. Dietary chitosan inhibits hypercholesterolcemia and atherosclerosis in the apolipoprotein E-deficient mouse model of atherosclerosis. *Atherosclerosis.* 1998; 138:329-334.

Pittler MH, Abbot NC, Harkness EF, Ernst E. Randomized, double-blind trial of chitosan for body weight reduction. *Eur J Clin Nutr.* 1999;53:379-381.

Sugano M, Watanabe S, Kishi A, et al. Hypocholesterolemic action of chitosans with different viscosity in rats. *Lipids.* 1988;23:187-191.

Wuolijoki E, Hirvela T, Ylitalo P. Decrease in LDL-cholesterol with microcrystalline chitosan. *Methods Find Exp Clin Pharmacol.* 1999;21:357-361.

Yoshimoto H, Nagano N, Nishitoba N, et al. Pharmacological properties of chitosan-coated dialdehyde cellulose (chitosan DAC), a newly developed oral adsorbent (I). Effect of chitosan DAC in normal rats. [Article in Japanese]. *Nippon Yakurigaku Zasshi.* 1995; 106 00673-122.

Chlorella

DESCRIPTION

Chlorella is a genus of unicellular green algae belonging to the Phylum *Chlorophyta.* Chlorophytes comprise a major component of the phytoplankton. Chlorella is a popular food supplement in Japan and is marketed as a nutritional supplement in the United States. Chlorella, along with wheat grass, barley grass and spirulina, are sometimes referred to as "green foods." There are several species of chlorella. Those most commonly used in nutritional supplements are *Chlorella vulgaris* and *Chlorella pyrenoidosa.*

Chlorella is rich in protein. In addition, it is rich in chlorophyll, carotenoids, such as astaxanthin, canthaxanthin, flavoxanthin, loraxanthin, neoxanthin and violaxanthin. Chlorella also contains the xanthophyll, echinenone.

ACTIONS AND PHARMACOLOGY

ACTIONS

Chlorella has putative anticarcinogenic, immunomodulatory, hypolipidemic, gastric mucosal-protective and detoxification activities.

MECHANISM OF ACTION

Glycoprotein-rich extracts of *Chlorella vulgaris* have been found to have antitumor activity against both spontaneous and experimentally induced metastasis in mice. The antitumor activity is thought to be mediated by an immunopotentiation mechanism. The glycoprotein-rich extracts may enhance the migration of T cells to the tumor sites.

The mechanism of the putative hypolipidemic and gastric mucosal-protective activities of chlorella, which again have only been found in animal studies, is unknown.

In rats, chlorella was found to promote the excretion of dioxin in the feces. The mechanism of this action is unknown.

PHARMACOKINETICS

The pharmacokinetics of chlorella in humans have not been studied. However, the proteins, lipids and carbohydrates in chlorella should be digested, absorbed and metabolized by normal physiological processes.

INDICATIONS AND USAGE

A chlorella extract has demonstrated antitumor and antimetastatic effects in animal experiments. Chlorella has shown some experimental antiatherogenic activity and some radio-protective and chemo-detoxifying effects. It has shown some preliminary benefit in immune function and in some with fibromyalgia.

RESEARCH SUMMARY

An extract of chlorella markedly increased survival time in mice injected with Meth-a tumor cells. A glycoprotein constituent of chlorella demonstrated antitumor properties *in vitro*. Recently, a glycoprotein extract exerted a pronounced antitumor effect against spontaneous and experimentally induced metastasis in mice. Immune-enhancement appeared to play a central role, particularly T cell activation in the peripheral lymph nodes of the tumor-bearing mice.

Chlorella has demonstrated an ability to protect against gamma-radiation, as well as against a number of drugs and various toxic chemicals. In one animal experiment, it alleviated some of the side effects of 5-fluorouracil. In another study, chlorella helped prevent gastrointestinal absorption and promoted the excretion of dioxin already present in tissues in rats.

Chlorella has exhibited hypolipidemic and antiatherogenic effects in some animal experiments. Aortic atheromatous lesions were significantly inhibited by chlorella in rabbits on a high-cholesterol diet.

In one animal model of peptic ulcer, oral administration of dry powder chlorella helped protect gastric mucosa.

In a recent clinical trial of chlorella, some patients with moderately severe symptoms of fibromyalgia syndrome were said to derive significant benefit from consumption, over a two-month period, of 10 grams daily of Sun chlorella tablets and 100 ml of liquid Wakasa Gold, two commercial chlorella products. Evaluation of improvement was largely subjective.

CONTRAINDICATIONS, PRECAUTIONS, ADVERSE REACTIONS

CONTRAINDICATIONS

Chlorella is contraindicated in those who are hypersensitive to any component of a chlorella-containing nutritional supplement.

PRECAUTIONS

Pregnant women and nursing mothers should avoid chlorella-containing supplements.

Some chlorella-containing supplements may be rich in vitamin K. Therefore those on warfarin should be cautious in the use of chlorella supplements.

Allergic reactions have been reported in some using chlorella supplements. Therefore, those with allergic diatheses should exercise caution in the use of chlorella supplements.

ADVERSE REACTIONS

Allergic reactions and photosensitivity reactions have been reported in some using chlorella supplements.

INTERACTIONS

Some chlorella supplements may be rich in vitamin K and may affect the INR of those on warfarin. Animal studies suggest that certain substances in chlorella may ameliorate some of the side effects of 5-fluorouracil. There is no human documentation of this.

OVERDOSAGE

No reports of overdosage.

DOSAGE AND ADMINISTRATION

There are various forms of chlorella, including capsules, tablets, softgels and granules. Most chlorella marketed in the U.S. is grown in Japan and Taiwan and is processed into the various supplemental forms. Chlorella is marketed as a stand-alone supplement or combined with other so-called "green foods," such as wheat grass, barley grass and spirulina. There is no typical dosage.

LITERATURE

Konishi F, Mitsuyama M, Okuda M, et al. Protective effect of an acidic glycoprotein obtained from culture of Chlorella vulgaris against myelosuppression by 5-fluorouracil. *Cancer Immunol Immunother.* 1996; 42:268-274.

Konishi F, Tanaka K, Kumamoto S, et al. Enhanced resistance against Escherichia coli infection by subcutaneous administration of the hot-water extract of Chlorella vulgaris in cyclophosphamide-treated mice. *Cancer Immunol Immunother.* 1990; 32:1-7.

Merchant RE, Carmack CA, Wise CM. Nutritional supplementation with Chlorella pyrenoidosa for patients with fibromyalgia syndrome: a pilot study. *Phytother Res.* 2000; 14:167-173.

Morita K, Matsueda T, Iida T, Hasegawa T. *Chlorella* accelerates dioxin excretion in rats. *J Nutr.* 1999; 129:1731-1736.

Noda K, Ohno N, Tanaka K, et al. A water-soluble antitumor glycoprotein from Chlorella vulgaris. *Planta Med.* 1996; 62:423-426.

Sano T, Kumanoto Y, Kamiya N, et al. Effect of lipophilic extract of Chlorella vulgaris on alimentary hyperlipidemia in cholesterol-fed rats. *Artery.* 1988; 15:217-224.

Sano T, Tanaka Y. Effect of dried, powdered Chlorella vulgaris on experimental atherosclerosis and alimentary hypercholesterolemia in cholesterol-fed rabbits. *Artery.* 1987; 76-84.

Tanaka K, Koga T, Konishi F, et al. Augmentation of host defense by unicellular green alga, Chlorella vulgaris, to Escherichia coli infection. *Infect Immun.* 1986; 53:267-271.

Tanaka K, Yamada A, Noda K, et al. Oral administration of a unicellular green algae, Chlorella vulgaris, prevents stress-induced ulcer. *Planta Med.* 1997; 63:465-466.

Tanaka K, Yamada A, Noda K, et al. A novel glycoprotein obtained from Chlorella vulgaris strain CK22 shows antimetastatic immunopotentiation. *Cancer Immunol Immunother.* 1998; 45:313-320.

Chlorophyll/Chlorophyllin

DESCRIPTION

Chlorophyll is the green pigment found in higher plants, as well as algae. Chlorophyll is the principal photoreceptor in photosynthesis, the light-driven process in which carbon dioxide is "fixed" to yield carbohydrates and oxygen. Chlorophyll is a cyclic tetrapyrolle, similar in structure to the heme group of globins (hemoglobin, myoglobin) and cytochromes. Chlorophyll differs from heme in a few major respects, most notably that the central metal ion in chlorophyll is magnesium while that in heme is iron.

There are a few types of chlorophyll. Higher plants and green algae, such as chlorella (see Chlorella) contain chlorophyll a and chlorophyll b in the approximate ratio of 3:1. The molecular formula of chlorophyll a is $C_{55}H_{72}MgN_4O_5$; the molecular formula of chlorophyll b is $C_{55}H_{70}MgN_4O_6$. The difference between the two chlorophylls is that a methyl side-chain in chlorophyll a is replaced by a formyl group in chlorophyll b. Chlorophyll a is found with chlorophyll c in many types of marine algae. Red algae contain principally chlorophyll a and also chlorophyll d.

Chlorophyllin is a semi-synthetic sodium/copper derivative of chlorophyll. In contrast to chlorophyll, chlorophyllin is water-soluble. Chlorophyllin, like chlorophyll, has deodorizing activity. It is used as an aid to reduce odor from a colostomy or ileostomy and also as an aid to reduce fecal odor due to incontinence. A topical ointment of chlorophyllin is used to reduce malodors in wounds and surface ulcers.

Chlorophyll and chlorophyllin are available as nutritional supplements. Preliminary evidence from *in vitro* and animal studies suggests that these substances may have anticarcinogenic activity.

ACTIONS AND PHARMACOLOGY

ACTIONS

Chlorophyll and chlorophyllin may have antimutagenic and anticarcinogenic activities.

MECHANISM OF ACTION

Chlorophyll and its metabolites pheophytin, pyropheophytin and pheophorbide, as well as chlorophyllin, have demonstrated antimutagenic effects *in vitro* against such mutagens as 3-methylcholanthrene, N-methyl-N'-nitro-N'-nitrosoguanidine (MNNG) and aflatoxin B1. Chlorophyll and chlorophyllin have also demonstrated anticarcinogenic effects in animal models against such carcinogens as aflatoxin B1, 1,2-dimethylhydrazine and dibenzo[a,1]pyrene.

The mechanism of the antimutagenic and anticarcinogenic activities of chlorophyll and chlorophyllin are unknown. It is speculated that antioxidant activity of chlorophyll/chlorophyllin may play a role in these activities. Another possible mechanism is the formation of complexes between the mutagen/carcinogen with chlorophyll/chlorophyllin through strong interactions between their planar unsaturated cyclic rings. The complexes would effectively inactivate the mutagens/carcinogens.

PHARMACOKINETICS

There is little on the pharmacokinetics of chlorophyll and its derivative chlorophyllin in humans. Some older studies showed that chlorophyll, following absorption, is converted into pheophytin, pyropheophytin and pheophorbide. These three derivatives of chlorophyll are tetrapyrolles.

INDICATIONS AND USAGE

Some experimental data suggests that chlorophyll and chlorophyllin may have some antimutagenic and anticarcinogenic potential, may help protect against some toxins, and may ameliorate some drug side effects. They are useful in reducing urinary and fecal odor in some circumstances. They may help ease constipation in some. There is some preliminary indication that they could be beneficial in the treatment of calcium oxalate stone disease and that they may have some anti-atherogenic activity.

RESEARCH SUMMARY

In one *in vitro* test, chlorophyllin demonstrated significant inhibition of several mutagens, including cigarette smoke, coal dust and diesel emission particles. Its antioxidant activity may have accounted for this effect. In another assay, chlorophyllin proved a more effective antimutagen than retinol, beta-carotene, vitamin C and vitamin E. In an animal study, chlorophyllin demonstrated both antimutagenic and anticarcinogenic activity, inhibiting 1,2-dimethylhydrazine-induced nuclear damage in rat colonic epithelium.

In another animal study, chlorophyllin significantly inhibited aflatoxin B1 hepatocacinogenesis. In a rainbow trout multi-organ tumor model, chlorophyllin markedly reduced liver, stomach and swimbladder cancer incidence.

Chlorophyllin has been used to reduce some of the side effects of cyclophosphamide. Chlorophyll consumption has been associated, in an animal study, with increased fecal excretion of polychlorinated dibenzo-p-dioxin (PCDD) congeners and polychlorinated dibenzofuran (PCDF). The researchers suggested that green vegetables rich in chlorophyll might be helpful in humans exposed to PCDD and PCDF congeners.

In a study of geriatric patients, chlorophyllin was said to be effective in helping control body and fecal odors and helped ease chronic constipation. It also reduced excessive flatus is some. In another study, this one involving incontinent geriatric patients, subjects received 100 mg of chlorophyllin daily or placebo for two weeks. A non-significant decrease in urinary odor was noted in those receiving chlorophyllin, compared with those on placebo.

One preliminary study indicated that chlorophyllin can inhibit the crystallisation and growth kinetics of calcium oxalate dihydrate in normal urine and that it might be helpful in the treatment of calcium oxalate stone disease.

Finally, chlorophyllin significantly decreased serum cholesterol and triglycerides in a study using rats with experimental atherogenesis. Followup is needed.

CONTRAINDICATIONS, PRECAUTIONS, ADVERSE REACTIONS

CONTRAINDICATIONS

Chlorophyll and chlorophyllin are contraindicated in those who are hypersensitive to any component in a chlorophyll-containing or chlorophyllin-containing preparation.

PRECAUTIONS

Supplemental chlorophyll and supplemental chlorophyllin should be avoided by pregnant women and nursing mothers.

ADVERSE REACTIONS

Use of chlorophyll and chlorophyllin supplements may cause discoloration of the urine (green urine), the feces (green stool) and the tongue (yellow to black tongue). There are occasional reports of diarrhea with use of these substances.

INTERACTIONS

In a mouse model, chlorophyllin ameliorated some of the side effects of cyclophosphamide.

OVERDOSAGE

No reports of overdosage.

DOSAGE AND ADMINISTRATION

There are a few chlorophyll and chlorophyllin nutritional supplements. Chlorophyllin is available as a liquid supplement. A typical dose is 100 mg daily. Those who use chlorophyllin to reduce fecal odor due to incontinence or to reduce odor from a colostomy or ileostomy typically take 100 mg daily.

LITERATURE

Breinholt V, Arbogast D, Loveland P, et al. Chlorophyllin chemoprevention: an evaluation of reduced bioavailability vs. target organ protective mechanisms. *Toxicol Appl Pharmacol*. 1999; 158:141-151.

Breinholt V, Hendricks J, Pereira C, et al. Dietary chlorophyllin is a potent inhibitor of aflatoxin B1 hepatocarcinogenesis in rainbow trout. *Cancer Res*. 1995; 55:57-62.

Chernomorsky S, Segelman A, Poretz RD. Effect of dietary chlorophyll derivatives on mutagenesis and tumor cell growth. *Teratogen Carcinogen Mutagen*. 1999; 19:313-322.

Dashwood RH, Breinholt V, Bailey GS. Chemopreventive properties of chlorophyllin: inhibition of aflatoxin B1 (AFB1)-DNA binding *in vivo* and antimutagenic activity against AFB1 and two heterocyclic amines in the Salmonella mutagenicity assay. *Carcinogenesis*. 1991; 12:939-942.

Nahata MC, Slencsak CA, Kamp J. Effect of chlorophyllin on urinary odor in incontinent geriartric patients. *Drug Intell Clin Pharm*. 1983; 17:732-734.

Ong TM, Whong WZ, Stewart J, Brockman HE. Chlorophyllin: a potent antimutagen against environmental and dietary complex mixtures. *Mutat Res*. 1986; 173:111-115.

Reddy AP, Harttig U, Barth MC, et al. Inhibition of dibenzo[*a,l*]pyrene-induced multi-organ carcinogenesis by dietary chlorophyllin in rainbow trout. *Carcinogenesis*. 1999; 20:1919-1926.

Robins EW, Nelson RL. Inhibition of 1,2-dimethylhydrazine-induced nuclear damage in rat colonic epithelium by chlorophyllin. *Anticancer Res*. 1989; 9:981-985.

Te C, Gentile JM, Baguley BC, et al. *In vivo* effects of chlorophyllin on the antitumot agent cyclophosphamide. *Int J Cancer*. 1997; 70:84-89.

Vlad M, Bordas E, Caseanu E, et al. Effect of cuprofilm on experimental atherosclerosis. *Biol Trace Elem Res*. 1995; 48:99-109.

Young RW, Beregi JS Jr. Use of chlorophyllin in the care of geriatric patients. *J Am Geriatr Soc*. 1980; 28:46-47.

Choline

DESCRIPTION

Choline is an essential nutrient that is widely distributed in foods, principally in the form of phosphatidylcholine but also as free choline. It is also found in foods in the form of the phospholipid sphingomyelin. Choline is necessary for the structure and function of all cells and is crucial for sustaining life.

Choline plays many roles in the body. The three major metabolic functions of choline are as a precursor for phosphatidylcholine biosynthesis, as a precursor for acetylcholine biosynthesis and as a methyl donor. In addition to serving as a precursor for phosphatidylcholine, choline is the precursor of the phospholipid sphingomyelin. Phosphatidylcholine and sphingomyelin are structural components of biological membranes. These phospholipids also serve as precursors for the intracellular messengers ceramide and diacylglycerol. Choline is also the precursor of the signaling lipids, platelet-activating factor (PAF) and sphingosylphosphoryl-choline.

An association between a low-choline diet and fatty infiltration of the liver in rats was first reported in 1935. Choline, as well as other substances, such as methionine, folic acid and vitamin B_{12}, that prevent deposition of fat in the liver are known as lipotropes. The primary criterion used to estimate the Adequate Intake (AI) for choline is the prevention of liver damage as assessed by measuring serum levels of the liver enzyme alanine aminotransferase or ALT. ALT was formerly called and is still referred to as SGPT (serum glutamate pyrutate transaminase).

The foods richest in phosphatidylcholine, the major delivery form of choline, are beef liver, egg yolks and soya. Beef liver, iceberg lettuce, peanut butter, peanuts and cauliflower are some foods that contain free choline.

Choline is also known as 2-Hydroxy-N,N,N-trimethylethanaminum; (beta-hydroxyethyl) trimethylammonium and bilineurine. The major commercial salts for supplementation are choline chloride and choline bitartrate. The chemical structure of Choline is:

$$CH_3 - N^+ - CH_2 - CH_2 - OH$$

with CH_3 groups above and below the N^+.

Choline

The major pathway for phosphatidylcholine synthesis in the body utilizes preformed or dietary choline. In an alternative pathway for phosphatidylcholine biosynthesis, phosphatidylcholine is sequentially methylated to form phosphatidylcholine, using S-adenosylmethionine as the methyl donor. This is probably the only pathway for *de novo* synthesis of choline in the body. However, *de novo* synthesis does not appear adequate to meet the demand for the nutrient.

ACTIONS AND PHARMACOLOGY

ACTIONS

Choline is a precursor for phosphatidylcholine, sphingomyelin, acetylcholine and the methyl donor betaine. Thus, choline is important for normal cellular membrane composition and repair, normal brain function and normal cardiovascular function.

MECHANISM OF ACTION

Choline is involved in several basic biological processes. Choline is a major part of the polar head group of phosphatidylcholine. Phosphatidylcholine's role in the maintenance of cell membrane integrity is vital to all of the basic biological processes: information flow, intracellular communication and bioenergetics. Inadequate choline intake would negatively affect all these processes. Choline is also a major part of another membrane phospholipid, sphingomyelin, also important for the maintenance of cell structure and function. It is noteworthy and not surprising that choline deficiency in cell culture causes apoptosis or programmed cell death. This appears to be due to abnormalities in cell membrane phosphatidylcholine content and an increase in ceramide, a precursor, as well as a metabolite, of sphingomyelin. Ceramide accumulation, which is caused by choline deficiency, appears to activate a caspase, a type of enzyme that mediates apoptosis.

Evidence is mounting that an elevated homocysteine level may be a significant risk factor for atherosclerosis, as well as other cardiovascular and neurological disorders. Betaine or trimethylglycine is derived from choline via an oxidation reaction. Betaine is one of the factors that maintains low levels of homocysteine by resynthesizing L-methionine from homocysteine.

Acetylcholine is one of the major neurotransmitters and requires choline for its synthesis. Adequate acetylcholine levels in the brain are believed to be protective against certain types of dementia, including Alzheimer's disease. Human studies are needed to determine whether dietary choline might be useful in the prevention of dementia.

The mechanism of the carcinogenic actions of choline deficiency are not known.

PHARMACOKINETICS

Choline is absorbed from the small intestine by means of transporter proteins in the intestinal cells. Some choline is metabolized in the gut to betaine (trimethylglycine) and trimethylamine, which are also absorbed by the gut. Choline, as well as betaine and trimethylamine, are transported to the liver via portal circulation. All tissues accumulate choline by diffusion and mediated transport.

In the liver, choline participates in various metabolic reactions, including the formation of CDP-choline, which combines with diacylglycerol to form phosphatidylcholine. Through oxidation, it forms the methyl donor betaine. Trimethylamine, a choline metabolite, is oxidized to trimethylamine oxide in the liver. Choline is transported across the blood-brain barrier by a specific carrier mechanism. Within the brain and other nervous tissue, choline is converted to acetylcholine by the enzyme choline acetyltransferase. Only a small fraction of dietary choline goes to form acetylcholine. The kidney also accumulates choline. Some appears in the urine unchanged but most is oxidized to form betaine.

INDICATIONS AND USAGE

Increased choline intake has recently been recommended by the Food and Nutrition Board of the National Academy of Sciences for pregnant and nursing women to help ensure normal fetal brain development. And, like phosphatidylcholine (see Phosphatidylcholine), choline may be helpful in some liver diseases, manic conditions, cognitive disorders, tardive dyskinesia and, possibly, some cancers.

RESEARCH SUMMARY

There is some evidence, derived from animal studies, that choline, if present in adequate amounts during pregnancy and breast feeding, can help ensure healthy fetal brain development. These studies further suggest that adequate prenatal choline can have long-lasting positive effects on cognitive function, including memory.

In a series of studies, the diets of pregnant rats have been supplemented with varying amounts of choline for variable periods of time during gestation. Supplementation, especially during the second half of pregnancy, has been strongly associated with positive cognitive effects (which are not seen in control animals receiving little or no choline).

Tested as adults, rats that had received approximately three times control amounts of choline during gestation were significantly superior in tasks that assess attention and spatial and temporal memory. Offspring of mothers that received no choline during pregnancy had attention and memory task impairment. And, even though both control and experimental animals were given the same standardized normal diet after birth, those whose mothers got higher levels of choline during pregnancy continued to exhibit significant cognitive superiority over controls throughout life. "Thus," one of the researchers concluded, "prenatal supplementation with choline prevented the normally observed memory decline of old age."

These significant studies are buttressed by neuroanatomical, neurophysiological and neurochemical studies that have similarly shown that choline has positive, long-lasting effects on prenatal brain development at the cellular level. Some of these studies have produced direct evidence that choline supplementation stimulates cell division in the embryonic brain, while choline deficiency increases apoptosis in areas of the brain, principally the hippocampus and septum, associated with memory processing. It has been hypothesized that choline supplementation during gestation may exert its apparent long-term effects through cellular and synaptic modifications that permanently increase memory-processing capacity.

Human studies have yet to be conducted on choline's effects on the fetus, but one researcher concludes that there is hope that "optimal dietary choline early in life may improve human cognitive development and slow cognitive declines associated with aging."

The Food and Nutrition Board of the National Academy of Sciences is impressed enough with research to date that it has recently recommended that pregnant and nursing women increase their intake of choline. The board recommends 425 milligrams of choline daily for women who are not pregnant, 450 milligrams daily for pregnant women and 550 milligrams daily for nursing women.

For information about other research related to choline, see Phosphatidylcholine.

CONTRAINDICATIONS, PRECAUTIONS, ADVERSE REACTIONS

CONTRAINDICATIONS

Known hypersensitivity to a choline-containing product.

PRECAUTIONS

Trimethylaminuria or fish-odor syndrome: Trimethylaminuria is a rare genetic metabolic disorder occurring in oil to 0.1 to 1% of the population. It is due to deficiency of the enzyme trimethylamine-N-oxide synthetase, which converts trimethylamine to trimethylamine-N-oxide. Trimethylamine, which is produced from choline, is excreted from the body via the urine, sweat, breath and other bodily secretions. It has a nauseating, rotten-fish-smelling odor. Trimethylamine-N-oxide, the metabolite of trimethylamine, is non-odorous. Those with primary genetic trimethyluria (the inherited enzyme deficiency) should restrict intake of supplemental choline. Also, those with certain types of liver disease caused by any of the hepatitis viruses or from other etiologies may develop fishy body odor when taking supplemental choline. Choline intake should be restricted in these cases.

ADVERSE REACTIONS

Choline doses of up to 3 grams daily are generally well tolerated with occasional reports of nausea, diarrhea and loose stools. Higher doses have been associated with fishy body odor—particularly in those with trimethylaminuria (fish-odor syndrome). Trimethylaminuria may also occur in those with liver damage who are using high doses of choline. High intakes of choline have been associated with excessive sweating and hypotension. There are some reports of depression or increased symptoms of depression in those using high doses of choline bitartrate.

There are no adequate data demonstrating a no-observed-adverse-effect level (NOAEL) for excess choline intake. Based on two clinical studies in humans, a lowest-observed-adverse-effect level (LOAEL) of 7.5 grams daily has been determined. At 7.5 grams of choline daily, nausea, diarrhea and a small decrease in blood pressure were reported in some patients. The upper limit (UL) for adults is 3.5 grams daily. Individuals that may be at increased risk of side effects with choline intakes at the UL include those with trimethylaminuria, liver disease, renal disease, depression and Parkinson's disease.

INTERACTIONS

DRUGS

Methotrexate: Methotrexate may diminish pools of all choline metabolites. Choline supplementation reverses fatty liver caused by methotrexate administration in rats.

NUTRITIONAL SUPPLEMENTS

Choline, via its metabolism to betaine, works in concert with vitamins B_6, B_{12} and folic acid in the metabolism of the potentially atherogenic substance homocysteine.

DOSAGE AND ADMINISTRATION

Typical doses of choline intake range from 300 to 1,200 milligrams daily. The major choline salt forms available are choline chloride and choline bitartrate.

Phosphatidylcholine is a delivery form of choline (see Phosphatidylcholine).

Choline is also added to some infant formulas and to some TPN formulations.

Adequate intakes (AI) of choline have been established by the Food and Nutrition Board of the Institute of Medicine of the National Academy of Sciences. The AI for adults is 550 milligrams daily for men and 425 milligrams daily for women. A summary of AIs for various age groups is as follows:

	(AI)
Infants	0-5 months, 125 mg/day or 8 mg/kg;
	6-11 months, 150 mg/day or 17 mg/kg.
Children	1-3 years, 200 mg/day;
	4-8 years, 250 mg/day;
	9-13 years, 375 mg/day.
Males	14-18 years, 550 mg/day;
Females	14-18 years, 450 mg/day.
Men	19 and older, 550 mg/day;
Women	19 and older, 425 mg/day.
Pregnant Women	450 mg/day.
Lactating Women All Ages	550 mg/day.

All of the above values are for the choline base. Values for choline salts are higher. For example, values for choline chloride would be 1.4 times as high and for choline bitartrate even higher. About 13 percent of phosphatidylcholine is choline.

LITERATURE

Albright CD, Liu R, Berthea TC, et al. Choline deficiency induces apoptosis in SV 40-immortalized CW SV-1 rat hepatocytes in culture. *FASEB J.* 1996; 10:510-516.

Blusztajn JK. Choline, a vital amine. *Science.* 1998; 281:794-795.

Canty DJ, Zeisel SH. Lecithin and choline in human health and disease. *Nutr Rev.* 1994; 52:327-339.

Cohen BM, Renshaw PF, Stoll, AL. Decreased brain choline uptake in older adults. An in vivo magnetic resonance spectroscopy study. *J Amer Med Ass.* 1995; 274:902-907.

Food and Nutrition Board. Institute of Medicine. *Dietary Reference Intakes for Thiamin, Riboflavin, Niacin, Vitamin B_6, Folate, Vitamin B_{12}, Pantothenic Acid, Biotin, and Choline* (National Academy Press, Washington, DC, 1998).

Pyapili GK, Turner DA, Williams, CL. Prenatal dietary choline supplementation decreases the threshold for induction of long-term potentiation in young adult rats. *J Neurophysiol.* 1998; 79:1790-1796.

Schocke Z, J, Kohlmueller D, Quak E, et al. Mild trimethylaminuria caused by common variants in FMO3 gene. *Lancet.* 1997; 354:834-835.

Shelly EP, Shelley WB. The fish odor syndrome. Trimethyluria. *J Amer Med Ass.* 1984; 251:253-255.

Wurtman RJ, Hefti F, Melamed E. Precursor control of neurotransmitter synthesis. *Pharmacol Rev.* 1981; 32:315-335.

Yen C-L, E Mar, M-H, Zeisel SH. Choline deficiency-induced apoptosis in PC 12 cells is associated with diminished membrane phosphatidylcholine and sphingomyelin, accumulation of ceramide and ciccylglycerol, and activation of a caspace. *FASEB J.* 1999; 13:135-142.

Chondroitin Sulfate

DESCRIPTION

Chondroitin sulfate belongs to a family of heteropolysaccharides called glycosaminoglycans or GAGs. Glycosaminoglycans were formerly known as mucopolysaccharides. GAGs in the form of proteoglycans comprise the ground substance in the extracellular matrix of connective tissue. Chondroitin sulfate is made up of linear repeating units containing D-galactosamine and D-glucuronic acid. Chondroitin sulfate is found in humans in cartilage, bone, cornea, skin and the arterial wall. This type of chondroitin sulfate is sometimes referred to as chondroitin sulfate A or galactosaminoglucuronoglycan sulfate. The amino group of galactosamines in the basic unit of chondroitin sulfate A is acetylated, yielding N-acetyl-galactosamine; there is a sulfate group esterified to the 4-position in N-acetyl-galactosamine. (Chondroitin sulfate A is also sometimes called chondroitin 4-sulfate.) The molecular weight of chondroitin sulfate ranges from 5,000 to 50,000 daltons and contains about 15 to 150 basic units of D-galactosamine and D-glucuronic acid. It is represented by the following structural formula:

Chondroitin sulfate A   R = SO_3H R^1 = H
Chondroitin sulfate C   R = H R^1 = SO_3H

Chondroitin sulfate C, primarily found in fish and shark cartilage, but also in humans, is also made up of linear repeating units of D-galactosamine and D-glucuronic acid. The amino group of D-galactosamine is acetylated to give N-acetyl-galactosamine, and, in the case of chondroitin sulfate C, the sulfate group is esterified to the 6-position in N-acetyl-galactosamine. Chondroitin sulfate C is sometimes called chondroitin 6-sulfate. Chondroitin sulfate B is also known as dermatan sulfate. It is abundant in skin and is also found in heart valves, tendons and arterial walls. Dermatan sulfate is made up of linear repeating units containing D-galactosamine and either L-iduronic acid or D-glucuronic acid. Its molecular weight ranges from 15,000 to 40,000 daltons.

The source of chondroitin sulfate used in nutritional supplements includes the cartilaginous rings of bovine trachea and pork byproducts (ears and snout). Shark cartilage and whale septum cartilage have also been used to obtain chondroitin sulfate. Chondroitin sulfate supplements are usually isomeric mixtures of chondroitin sulfate A(chondroitin 4-sulfate) and chondroitin sulfate C(chondroitin 6-sulfate).

ACTIONS AND PHARMACOLOGY

ACTIONS

The action of orally administered chondroitin sulfate has yet to be clarified. Possible actions include promotion and maintenance of the structure and function of cartilage (referred to as chondroprotection), pain relief of osteoarthritic joints and anti-inflammatory activity.

MECHANISM OF ACTION

Until the specific actions of supplemental chondroitin sulfate are determined, the mechanism of action is a matter of speculation. However, much is known about the biochemistry and physiology of chondroitin sulfate and similar molecules. Glycoproteins known as proteoglycans form the ground substance in the extracellular matrix of connective tissue. Proteoglycans are polyanionic substances of high molecular weight and contain heteropolysaccharide-side-chains covalently linked to a polypeptide-chain backbone. The polysaccharides, which include chondroitin sulfate and hyaluronic acid, make up as much as 95% of the proteoglycan structure.

The polysaccharides in proteoglycans are called glycosaminoglycans or GAGs. Chondroitin sulfate and hyaluronic acid are vital for the structure and function of articular cartilage. Chondroitin sulfate and hyaluronic acid are fundamental components of aggrecan found in articular cartilage. Aggrecan confers upon articular cartilage shock-absorbing properties. It does this by providing cartilage with a swelling pressure that is restrained by the tensile force of collagen fibers. This balance confers upon articular cartilage the deformable resilience vital to its function. Hyaluronic acid, which is also found in synovial fluid, has lubricating properties for the joint.

In the progression of degenerative joint disease or osteoarthritis, aggrecan synthesis is decreased, leading to the loss of cartilage resiliency and the pain and other symptoms that accompany osteoarthritis.

Intra-articular injections of hyaluronic acid, an FDA-approved drug, can relieve joint pain and improve mobility. This type of therapy is called viscotherapy and is believed to act by improving joint lubrication. If chondroitin sulfate were delivered into joints, some similar effects would be expected. Animal studies have shown that parenterally administered chondroitin sulfate does get into cartilage tissue as does orally administered chondroitin sulfate. There is some human data suggesting orally administered chondroitin sulfate, particularly low-molecular-weight chondroitin sulfate, is also delivered to articular tissue. There is some indication that orally administered chondroitin sulfate leads to increases in hyaluronic acid and viscosity of synovial fluid, as well as decreases in collagenase in synovial fluid. That is, glucosamine delivered into joints may inhibit enzymes involved in cartilage degradation and enhance the production of hyaluronic acid.

PHARMACOKINETICS
Earlier studies using high-molecular-weight chondroitin sulfate, concluded that there was no significant absorption of this high-molecular-weight version of chondroitin sulfate. More recent studies demonstrate that there is probably significant absorption of low-molecular-weight chondroitin sulfate. Absorption appears to occur from the stomach and small intestine. There is also an indication that some chondroitin sulfate, after absorption, does enter the joint space. Studies of the pharmacokinetics of orally administered chondroitin sulfate are ongoing.

It is of interest to note that a molecule similar in many resects to chondroitin sulfate, pertosan polysulfate, FDA-approved for the treatment of interstitial cystitis, is given orally and is absorbed to some extent.

INDICATIONS AND USAGE
Large, well-designed, recent studies have cast doubt on the claim that chondroitin sulfate may be generally beneficial in the treatment and prevention of osteoarthritis, either by itself or in combination with glucosamine (see Glucosamine). There is a suggestion that chondroitin sulfate may be helpful in atherosclerosis, but more research is needed to further support this.

RESEARCH SUMMARY
Chondroitin sulfate alone and in combination with glucosamine has become one of the biggest sellers in the supplement supermarket, used by millions for relief from arthritic symptoms and for joint/bone health generally. Some early studies indicated significant efficacy. These have now been confounded or contradicted by several well-designed new studies, some of which find no efficacy whatsoever. Older studies are analyzed first below, followed by summaries of the newer, mostly contradictory studies.

Two meta-analyses published several years ago indicated that chondroitin sulfate may be useful in the treatment of osteoarthritis. One of these meta-analyses included all double-blind, placebo-controlled trials that lasted four weeks or longer. This meta-analysis also included trials that studied the effects of glucosamine (see Glucosamine) on osteoarthritis. In all, there were 13 of these studies (six involving glucosamine and seven involving chondroitin sulfate).

All 13 studies found positive results in hip or knee osteoarthritis. The authors of the meta-analysis judged a trial positive if there was 25% or more improvement in the treatment group compared with placebo. The Levesque Index and global pain scores were used to assess improvement. Very significant improvement was associated with both glucosamine (39.5%) and chondroitin (40.2%), compared with placebo.

In another, now dated, meta-analysis of chondroitin sulfate, this one examining four randomized, double-blind, placebo- or NSAID-controlled studies of 227 patients, chondroitin sulfate supplemented subjects showed at least 50% improvement, compared with controls. Various studies have reported significant reduction in NSAID use among osteoarthritis subjects supplemented with chondroitin sulfate.

There is also radiological evidence of chondroitin's possible efficacy in osteoarthritis. Knee joint space decreased significantly in placebo subjects but remained unchanged in those receiving chondroitin sulfate for a year. And, in another study, those receiving chondroitin sulfate showed significantly fewer instances of erosive osteoarthritis (compared with placebo controls) on hand radiographs over a three-year period.

A significant synergistic effect was reported some years ago using combined glucosamine hydrochloride and chondroitin sulfate in an experimental study. The combination was more effective than either substance alone in inhibiting progression of degenerative cartilage lesions. Some postulated that chondroitin sulfate's possible efficacy in osteoarthritis derives from the fact that it is one of the two most abundant glycosaminoglycans (GAGs) in articular cartilage. Supplementation with this GAG seems, in part at least, to confer chondroprotection through its inhibitory action on some of the enzymes that damage cartilage. Further, by inhibiting other enzymes that can block transport of nutrients that nourish cartilage, this GAG may promote cartilage replacement.

It has been known for some time that injections of hyaluronic acid into arthritic joints can bring significant pain relief and enhanced mobility. Thus some said it is logical to assume that chondroitin sulfate, if it can reach the joints, may have similar effects since this substance has the ability to bind to receptor sites on synovial cell surfaces and thus induce production of hyaluronic acid, crucial to joint mobility.

The question for some time was whether a large molecule like chondroitin sulfate could achieve this penetration. Recent studies demonstrate that a low-molecular-weight version of oral chondroitin sulfate, of the sort used in all of the U.S. clinical trials, is absorbed.

In the last few years, several well-designed studies have largely contradicted the earlier positive data discussed above. The Glucosamine/chondroitin Arthritis Intervention Trial (GAIT) was a randomized, double-blind, placebo and active comparator (celecoxib) controlled trial of 1,583 individuals with symptomatic osteoarthritis of the knee. Those randomized to receive the drug celecoxib had significant reduction in knee pain, compared with placebo. The glucosamine/ chondroitin group, however, fared no better than those on placebo. This National Institutes of Health-funded study involved 16 participating clinics. Some subjects were randomized to receive only glucosamine hydrochloride (500 milligrams three times daily), only chondroitin sulfate (400 milligrams three times daily), combination chondroitin/glu- cosamine (in the same dosages) or 200 milligrams celecoxib daily. Study agents were mandated to be of pharmaceutical grade since previous inquiries have confirmed that both glucosamine and chondroitin products are not infrequently at variance with labeling (i.e. are inconsistent in content and potency from one product to another).

The study, though negative overall, was not wholly without some positive findings. In one subgroup of patients with moderate-to-severe knee pain at entry, some benefit was seen in those receiving the combination chondroitin/glucosamine supplement. An improvement in knee joint swelling that reached statistical significance was noted in those taking chondroitin sulfate alone. Notable, too, was the very high placebo-response level in this study, a finding that has plagued other studies of these substances in osteoarthritis patients. Some believe these findings make detection of positive responses more difficult. Nonetheless, the statistical robustness of the major negative finding was of high magnitude, imparting a high level of confidence in its accuracy. A *post hoc* analysis of the chondroitin sulfate subjects in whom knee swelling relief was statistically confirmed indicated that the best results were obtained in those with relatively milder symptoms and baseline radio- graphic changes.

An editorial accompanying the GAIT study in *The New England Journal of Medicine* said it was unfortunate that the inquiry did not use glucosamine sulfate instead of glucos- amine hydrochloride, since several other studies had previ- ously shown that the hydrochloride was not efficacious, whereas some other data seemed to indicate that the sulfate was. (See Glucosamine for more on this topic.) Nevertheless, the editorialist found the GAIT findings compelling and

concluded: "On the basis of the results from GAIT, it seems prudent to tell our patients with symptomatic osteoarthritis of the knee that neither glucosamine hydrochloride nor chon- droitin sulfate alone has been shown to be more efficacious than placebo for the treatment of knee pain." The editorialist further recommended that if individuals use glucosamine that they use glucosamine sulfate, rather than glucosamine hydrochloride and that they consider using a combination glucosamine sulfate and chondroitin sulfate for the possible additive effect. The editorial stated that there is no evidence that these substances can have any preventive effects in healthy persons or in persons with knee pain but normal radiographs. Three months of treatment was said to be adequate to test the substances for possible efficacy at the doses typically recommended.

A still more recent meta-analysis of chondroitin data related to osteoarthritis of the knee and hip concluded that "large- scale, methodically sound trials indicate that the symptomat- ic benefit of chondroitin is minimal or non-existent." The authors further concluded that "use of chondroitin in routine clinical practice should therefore be discouraged." The data, these researchers stated, left open some possibility that persons with low-grade osteoarthritis might obtain some benefit from chondroitin supplementation, although that is unproven. They found it very unlikely that those with more advanced osteoarthritis would benefit.

An accompanying editorial in *Annals of Internal Medicine* noted that $1 billion is spent each year on chondroitin in the United States alone. The editorial noted that one of the reasons chondroitin may fail is that it putatively targets cartilage; even assuming that it has some positive effect on cartilage, the editorial observed that osteoarthritis affects the whole joint, not just cartilage. And because cartilage is aneural, chondroitin would not be expected to alleviate the primary symptom of osteoarthritis: pain. The failure to alleviate pain also calls into question the claimed anti- inflammatory action of chondroitin, the editorial asserted. The editorial also noted that many previous, positive studies exhibited publication bias and numerous other shortcomings that have been commented on by many researchers in recent years. Sequence of random allocation was poorly concealed in many of the positive studies.

In a subset of large-scale trials that sought to avoid these shortcomings, findings were negative in all cases. The editorial also commented on individuals continuing to insist that chondroitin is of benefit to them, observing, as have others, that the very large placebo effect seen in so many studies must be considered.

Some years ago, chondroitin sulfate was investigated for its possible use in atherosclerosis. There was some evidence that it could favorably lower lipid levels and protect against blood clotting. Atheromatous aortic lesions were prevented in animals on high-cholesterol diets.

In a clinical trial, 60 patients suffering from coronary artery disease received 2 grams of oral chondroitin sulfate daily for 900 days. During that period, 16 of 60 unsupplemented control patients suffered acute coronary incidents. Only one of the chondroitin sulfate-treated subjects had an acute coronary incident. The same research group later followed up with similarly positive results.

More research is needed before any conclusions can be drawn with respect to a possible role for chondroitin sulfate in the treatment or prevention of atherosclerosis.

CONTRAINDICATIONS, PRECAUTIONS, ADVERSE REACTIONS

CONTRAINDICATIONS

Known hypersensitivity to a chondroitin sulfate-containing product.

PRECAUTIONS

Because of insufficient safety data, children, pregnant women and nursing mothers should avoid using chondroitin sulfate. Because of the theoretical possibility that chondroitin sulfate may have antithrombotic activity, those taking warfarin and those with hemophilia should exercise caution in its use. Those who need to restrict their salt intake should, if they use chondroitin sulfate, use salt-free preparations.

ADVERSE REACTIONS

Side effects that have been reported are mostly of the mild gastrointestinal variety, such as epigastric distress, nausea and diarrhea. No sulfa-allergic reactions or other allergic reactions have yet been reported.

INTERACTIONS

There are no known drug, nutrient, food or herb interactions. Chitosan (see Chitosan) may form complexes with chondroitin sulfate decreasing its absorption. Therefore, chondroitin sulfate should not be used concomitantly with chitosan.

OVERDOSAGE

Overdosage of chondroitin has not been reported in the literature.

DOSAGE AND ADMINISTRATION

Low-molecular-weight chondroitin sulfate is available as a stand-alone supplement or in combination with glucosamine (see Glucosamine). The usual dose used by those with osteoarthritis is 1,200 milligrams daily in divided doses.

It usually takes several weeks of supplementation before effects, if any, are experienced.

Chondroitin sulfate in combination with hyaluronic acid is available as an FDA-approved drug. It is used as a viscoelastic agent in cataract surgery. Hyaluronic acid itself is FDA approved for the treatment of osteoarthritis. The two forms presently available, Hylan G-F 20 (Synvisc, Wyeth-Ayerst) and sodium hyaluronate (Hyalgan, Sanofi/Orthologic), are given by intra-articular injection.

LITERATURE

Baici A, Horler D, Moser B, et al. Analysis of glycosaminoglycans in human serum after oral administration of chondroitin sulfate. *Rheum Int.* 1992;12:81-88.

Bartolucci C, Cellai L, Cordani D, et al. Chondroprotective action of chondroitin sulfate. Competitive action of chondroitin sulfate on the digestion of hyaluronan by bovine testicular hyaluronidase. *Int J Tiss Res.* 1991;13:311-317.

Bourgeois P, Chales G, Dehais J, et al. Efficacy and tolerability of chondroitin sulfate 1,200 mg/day vs. chondroitin 400 mg/day vs placebo. *Osteoarthritis Cartilage.* 1998;6 SupplA:25-30.

Busci L, Poor G. Efficacy and tolerability of oral chondroitin sulfate as a symptomatic slow-acting drug. for osteoarthritis (SYSADOA) in the treatment of knee osteoarthrosis. *Osteoarthritis Cartilage.* 1998;6 SupplA:31-36.

Conte A, Volpi N, Palmiera L, et al. Biochemical and pharmacokinetic aspects of oral treatment with chondroitin sulfate. *Drug Res.* 1995;45:918-925.

Deal CL, Moskowitz RW. Nutraceuticals as therapeutic agents in osteoarthritis. The role of glucosamine, chondroitin sulfate, and collagen hydrolysate. *Rheum Dis Clin North Am.* 1999;25:379-395.

Felson DT. Chondroitin for pain in osteoarthritis. *Ann Intern Med.* 2007;146(8):611-612.

Hochberg MC, Clegg DO. Potential effects of chondroitin sulfate on joint swelling: a GAIT report. *Osteoarthritis Cartilage.* 2008;16 Suppl 3:S22-24.

Iovu M, Dumais G, du Souich P. Anti-inflammatory activity of chondroitin sulfate. *Osteoarthritis Cartilage.* 2008 Jul 28.

Lamari FN. The potential of chondroitin sulfate as a therapeutic agent. *Connect Tissue Res.* 2008;49(3):289-292.

Leffler CT, Phillipi AF, Leffler SG, et al. Glucosamine, chondroitin, and manganese ascorbate for degenerative joint disease of the knee or low back: a randomized, double-blind, placebo-controlled pilot study. *Mil Med.* 1999;164:85-91.

McAlindon TE, LaValley MP, Gulin JP, et al. Glucosamine and chondroitin for treatment of osteoarthritis. A systematic quality assessment and meta-analysis. *JAMA.* 2000; 283:1469-1475.

Morrison LM, Enrick L. Coronary heart disease: reduction of death rate by chondroitin sulfate A. *Angiology.* 1973;24:269-287.

Morrison LM, Bajwa GS, Alfin-Slater RB, et al. Prevention of vascular lesions by chondroitin sulfate A in the coronary artery and aorta of rats induced by a hypervitaminosis D, cholesterol-containing diet. *Atherosclerosis.* 1972;16:105-118.

Pipitone VR. Chondroprotection with chondroitin sulfate. *Drugs Exp Clin Res.* 1991;17:3-7.

Reichenbach S, Sterchi R, Scherer M, et al. Meta-analysis: chondroitin for osteoarthritis of the knee or hip. *Ann Intern Med.* 2007;146(8):580-590.

Ronca F, Palmieri L, Panicucci P. et al. Anti-inflammatory activity of chondroitin sulfate. *Osteoarthritis Cartilage.* 1998;6 SupplA:14-21.

Tat SK, Pelletier JP, Vergés J, et al. Chondroitin and glucosamine sulfate in combination decrease the pro-resorptive properties of human osteoarthritis subchondral bone osteoblasts: a basic science study. *Arthritis Res Ther.* 2007;9(6):R117.

Towheed TE, Anastassiades TP. Glucosamine and chondroitin for treating symptoms of osteoarthritis. Evidence is widely touted but incomplete. *JAMA.* 2000;283:1483-1484.

Uebelhart D. Clinical review of chondroitin sulfate in osteoarthritis. *Osteoarthritis Cartilage.* 2008;16 Suppl 3:S19-21.

Uebelhart D, Thonar EJ, Delmas PD, et al. Effects of oral chondroitin sulfate on the progression of knee osteoarthritis: a pilot study. *Osteoarthritis Cartilage.* 1998;6 SupplA:39-46.

Yamanashi S, Toyoda H, Furuya N, et al. Metabolic study on chondroitin sulfate in rabbits. *Yakugaku Zasshi.* 1991;111:73-76.

Chromium

DESCRIPTION

Chromium is an essential trace mineral in human nutrition. Evidence suggests that it plays an important role in normal carbohydrate metabolism. In the 1950s it was found that chromium was necessary for the maintenance of normal glucose tolerance in rats; chromium-deficient rats had impaired glucose tolerance. Subsequently, it was found that patients receiving long-term total parenteral nutrition (TPN) without chromium developed glucose intolerance, weight loss and peripheral neuropathy. These symptoms were reversed when the patients were given intravenous chromium chloride.

Chromium is a metal with atomic number 24 and an atomic mass of 52 daltons. Its symbol is Cr. It occurs in nature chiefly as a chrome-iron ore. Chromium exists in several valence states, of which the trivalent and hexavalent states are the most common. Most chromium in the food supply is in the trivalent state. Hexavalent chromium compounds are recognized as toxic and are potential carcinogens. Chromium is found in many foods, typically in small amounts. Good food sources of chromium include whole grains, cereals, spices (black pepper, thyme), mushrooms, brown sugar, coffee, tea, beer, wine and meat products. Brewer's yeast is also a good source of chromium. Fruits and vegetables are generally poor sources of chromium, as are most refined foods.

ACTIONS AND PHARMACOLOGY

ACTIONS

Chromium may have glucose-regulatory activity. It may also have hypocholesterolemic and anti-atherogenic activities.

MECHANISM OF ACTION

The mechanism of chromium's possible glucose-regulatory activity is not well understood, but there are some theories. It is thought that the possible action of chromium on the control of blood glucose concentrations is the potentiation of insulin. Chromium is thought to be a cofactor necessary for optimal insulin action. One proposed mechanism involves increased insulin binding, increased insulin receptor number and increased insulin receptor phosphorylation. Chromium stimulates protein kinase activity of rat adipocytes in the presence of insulin. Chromium also inhibits phosphotyrosine phosphatase, a rat homolog of tyrosine phosphatase that inactivates the insulin receptor. The activation by chromium of insulin receptor kinase activity and the inhibition of insulin receptor tyrosine phosphatase would lead to increased phosphorylation of the insulin receptor, which is associated with increased insulin sensitivity.

It has also been suggested that chromium may decrease hepatic extraction of insulin and improve glucose tolerance by such a mechanism. Earlier, it was found that glucose tolerance could be restored in chromium-deficient rats by feeding them an extract of brewer's yeast. Brewer's yeast is rich in chromium, and it was proposed that it contained an organic factor which potentiated the action of insulin. This factor was called the glucose tolerance factor or GTF. GTF was hypothesized to contain trivalent chromium bound to nicotinic acid and the amino acids glycine, cysteine and glutamic acid. However, an organic glucose tolerance factor has, to date, not been isolated from brewer's yeast.

Recently, an oligopeptide low-molecular-weight chromium-binding substance (LMWCr) has been isolated from animal tissues. The oligopeptide is comprised of the amino acids glycine, cysteine, glutamic acid, and aspartic acid, with the two carboxylic acids (glutamic, aspartic) comprising more than half the amino acid residues. It is proposed that LMWCr is part of an insulin signal amplification system. Its possible participation in the glucose-regulatory activity may be as follows: chromium ions are transferred from transferrin to LMWCr. LMWCr normally exists in insulin-dependent cells in the apo or inactive form. Binding to chromic ions converts the inactive form to its holo or active form. Chromic-containing LMWCr then binds to insulin-activated insulin receptor, stimulating its tyrosine kinase activity and potentiating the activity of insulin. LMWCr is also called chromodulin because its proposed action is similar to that of calmodulin.

The mechanism of the possible hypocholesterolemic activity of chromium is unknown. The possible anti-atherogenic activity of chromium may be accounted for by its possible glucose-regulatory activity.

PHARMACOKINETICS

Very little chromium in the form of inorganic compounds, such as chromic chloride, is absorbed. The efficiency of absorption of chromium from chromic chloride is less than 2%. The efficiency of absorption of chromium from organic compounds is higher. For example, approximately 2.8% of an ingested dose of chromium picolinate is absorbed. Following absorption, chromium is bound to transferrin and albumin. Chromium is transported primarily by transferrin.

Chromium is distributed to various tissues of the body but appears to have a preference for bone, spleen, liver and kidney. Pharmacokinetic studies indicate that chromium is distributed into four different compartments that have rapid, medium, slow and very slow turnover, respectively. Bone, spleen, liver and kidney appear to contain all four compartments. The half-life of the rapid compartment is less than one day, that of the medium compartment approximately one week and that of the slow compartment from 7 to 12 weeks. The half-life of chromium in the compartment which appears to turn over most slowly is approximately one year. This compartment is probably related to long-term tissue deposition.

Most of an ingested dose of chromium is excreted in the feces. Chromium that has been absorbed is excreted mainly in the urine. Little excretion occurs via the biliary route.

There is much that remains unknown regarding the pharmacokinetics of chromium and its various trivalent forms in humans. More research in this area is needed.

INDICATIONS AND USAGE

There is some evidence that chromium may improve glucose tolerance and may be helpful in some with diabetes. There is preliminary evidence it may have some favorable effects on lipids. Claims that it boosts athletic performance, builds muscle and promotes weight loss have little, if any, credible support. The Federal Trade Commission has, in fact, declared such claims to be unsubstantiated and deceptive. Evidence is mixed with respect to claims that chromium picolinate may be mutagenic. The suggestion that chromium is nephrotoxic is based on isolated case studies and requires further investigation.

RESEARCH SUMMARY

The American Diabetes Association asserted in 1996 that "chromium supplementation has no known benefit in patients who are not chromium deficient." Some patients on long-term parenteral nutrition have developed chromium deficiency and diabetic symptoms that were reversed with chromium supplementation. In general, plasma chromium levels are about 40% lower in diabetic subjects, compared with healthy individuals.

A double-blind, placebo-controlled study of 180 subjects with type 2 diabetes demonstrated that supplemental chromium significantly improved fasting glucose, postprandial glucose, insulin, hemoglobin A_{1c} and cholesterol levels. Subjects in this study, conducted in China, received placebo, 200 micrograms of chromium picolinate or 1,000 micrograms of chromium picolinate daily. Subjects had suffered from diabetes for five to eight years. Better results were achieved with the higher dose of chromium.

This trial, while encouraging, was flawed in that baseline chromium status was not assessed; neither was postsupplemental status evaluated. Extrapolation of these results to Western populations is not possible. Additionally, the best designed prior studies have failed to show consistent results. Two of the best studies were largely negative. Variations may be due to divergence in chromium status at baseline and to the type and dose of chromium used. No beneficial effect was seen in diabetic patients taking 200 micrograms of chromium chloride, for example, but some positive effects were noted in those getting 400 micrograms or more of chromium chloride daily. With respect to the study in China, some hypothesized that the more dramatic effects achieved in that trial may be due to possible greater chromium deficiency in that country. More research is needed.

Chromium picolinate supplementation (200 micrograms daily) significantly decreased levels of total cholesterol, LDL-cholesterol and apolipoprotein B, compared with controls, in one small study. There was no significant effect on HDL-cholesterol. In a subsequent trial, 600 micrograms of chromium daily reportedly increased serum levels of HDL-cholesterol in patients taking beta-blockers. Again, however, studies have produced mixed results so that no persuasive conclusion can yet be reached with respect to chromium's effects on lipids.

One study reported that six weeks of chromium supplementation resulted in a significant increase in lean body mass and a decrease in body fat among athletes. Numerous, better designed follow-up studies, however, failed to confirm this finding. The original study used skinfold measurements (anthropometry) to assess changes in body composition. The subsequent studies used more sensitive measures, e.g., dual x-ray absorptiometry (DXA) and underwater weighing (hydrodensitometry). Even a study using the same anthropometry measurements that were employed in the original study also produced negative results.

Claims that chromium can be useful in treating obesity have similarly met with largely negative results. In some of these studies subjects have actually gained weight. Claims related to obesity were fueled by a study in which 200 micrograms of chromium daily reportedly led to weight loss even without alterations in food intake and exercise. In fact, however, weight loss in this small study was very modest, with a consequent high dropout rate. The same researchers conducted another study in which greater weight loss was achieved, but in this study chromium supplementation was used in conjunction with caloric restriction, dietary fiber and other nutritional support, making it impossible to assess the role of chromium, if any, in the final results.

There are two *in vitro* reports that, in high concentrations, chromium picolinate, but not chromium chloride or chromium nicotinate, is clastogenic. Thus some have concluded that picolinate, rather than chromium itself, might be mutagenic and should thus be avoided. Some have suggested that long-term use of chromium picolinate, particularly at doses higher than 200 micrograms daily, could be hazardous. More research is needed to clarify this issue.

Additional warnings have been issued based upon scattered case reports. In one of these cases, a 33-year-old woman taking 1,200-2,400 micrograms of chromium picolinate daily for four to five months in an effort to lose weight developed renal failure. In another case, a 49-year-old woman who took 600 micrograms of chromium picolinate daily for six weeks was also diagnosed with chronic renal failure.

It has not been demonstrated conclusively that chromium picolinate caused the renal failure, but some have speculated that the greater absorbability of the picolinate form of chromium may, when used at higher doses long term, increase the incidence of any possible side effects. One researcher has speculated that supplementation with 600 micrograms of chromium picolinate daily for five years could result in tissue accumulation of chromium picolinate possibly sufficient to cause chromosomal damage similar to that seen in *in vitro* studies.

Though these precautions need to be further investigated, the observation of one reviewer should also be noted. In reviewing the safety data, he concluded, "in contrast, better evidence exists that chromium is safe rather than toxic at very high doses." In contrast with the *in vitro* studies showing clastogenic effects, experimental *in vivo* results have differed. In one of these experiments, rats were fed either chromium chloride or chromium picolinate at high doses for 20 weeks. These doses were calculated to be several thousand times greater than the ESSADI (Estimated Safe and Adequate Daily Dietary Intake) for humans. After being killed, the animals were examined for toxic effects.

Whether the animals received 0, 5, 25, 50 or 100 mg/kg of chromium, there were no significant differences in body weight, organ weight or blood variables. Histologic evaluations of liver and kidneys of controls and those fed the highest chromium doses, whether chloride or picolinate, also failed to find significant differences. Again, more research is needed.

The FDA recently gave chromium picolinate the food-related qualified health claim that "it may reduce the risk of insulin resistance, and therefore may reduce the risk of type 2 diabetes . . . however, the existence of such a relationship between chromium picolinate and either insulin resistance or type 2 diabetes is highly uncertain."

Finally, a recent systematic review of randomized controlled trials on the effect of chromium supplementation on glucose metabolism and lipids came to the following conclusions: supplementation in patients with type 2 diabetes may have a modest beneficial effect on glycemia and dyslipidemia; there was no beneficial effect of chromium supplementation on serum glucose or lipid levels on those without diabetes; 41 studies met the criteria for the review, almost half of which were of poor quality; larger effects were more commonly observed in poor-quality studies; and future studies that address the limitations in the current evidence are needed before definitive claims can be made about the effect of chromium supplementation. And, it should be added, future research should focus on how to determine which patients are chromium deficient. It is very important and certainly warranted to develop a good method to define an individual's chromium status.

CONTRAINDICATIONS, PRECAUTIONS, ADVERSE REACTIONS

CONTRAINDICATIONS

Chromium is contraindicated in those hypersensitive to any component of a chromium-containing supplement.

PRECAUTIONS

Pregnant women and nursing mothers should avoid doses of chromium above the upper limit of the estimated safe and adequate daily dietary intake (ESADDI). The ESADDI for chromium is 50 to 200 micrograms daily.

Those with a history of hypoglycemia should exercise caution in the use of chromium supplements.

Those with a history of hyperglycemia or type 2 diabetes mellitus should only use chromium supplements for the possible management of abnormal glucose tolerance under medical supervision.

ADVERSE REACTIONS

Chromium supplements are generally well tolerated. There are a few reports of adverse reactions particularly with use of chromium picolinate. There is one report of a 24-year-old body builder who developed rhabdomyolysis after ingesting 1,200 micrograms of chromium in the form of chromium picolinate. Acute generalized exanthematous pustulosis was reported to be associated with the use of chromium picolinate. A case of interstitial nephritis was reported to occur five months after a subject received a six-week course of 600 micrograms of chromium in the form of chromium picolinate daily. Another report described anemia, thrombocytopenia, hemolysis, liver dysfunction, renal failure and weight loss after the use of 1,200-2,400 micrograms of chromium picolinate daily for four to five months.

INTERACTIONS

DRUGS

Beta-Blockers: One study reported that those on beta-blockers who took 600 micrograms daily of chromium in the form of high-chromium yeast were found to have modestly elevated HDL-cholesterol levels after two months of chromium use.

NUTRITIONAL SUPPLEMENTS

Ascorbate: Concomitant intake of ascorbate and chromium may increase the absorption of chromium.

FOODS

Concomitant intake of chromium with foods rich in phytic acid (unleavened bread, raw beans, seeds, nuts and grains and soy isolates) may decrease the absorption of chromium.

DOSAGE AND ADMINISTRATION

There are a few forms of chromium available for nutritional supplementation. They include chromium picolinate, chromium polynicotinate, chromium chloride and high-chromium yeast. These forms are available as stand-alone supplements or in combination products. Typical doses of chromium range from 50 to 200 micrograms daily, expressed as elemental chromium.

Dietary intake of chromium is approximately 25 micrograms daily.

The Food and Nutrition Board of the U.S. National Academy of Sciences has recommended the following Dietary Reference Intakes (DRI) for chromium. A summary of DRIs for various age groups is as follows:

DRI values (micrograms/day)

Infants	Adequate Intake (AI)
0-6 months	0.2
7-12 months	5.5

Children	
1-3 years	11
4-8 years	15

Boys	
9-13 years	25
14-18 years	35

Girls	
9-13 years	21
14-18 years	24

Men	
19-30 years	35
31-50 years	35
51-70 years	30
Older than 70 years	30

Women	
19-30 years	25
31-50 years	25
51-70 years	20
Older than 70 years	20

Pregnancy	
14-18 years	29
19-30 years	30
31-50 years	30

Lactation	
14-18 years	44
19-30 years	45
31-50 years	45

The DV (Daily Value) for chromium, which is used for determining percentage of nutrient daily values on nutritional supplement and food labels, is 120 micrograms. The basis for the DV for chromium is the 1989 Estimated Safe and Adequate Daily Dietary Intake (ESADDI).

LITERATURE

Anderson RA. Chromium, glucose intolerance and diabetes. *J Amer Coll Nutr.* 1998;17:548-555.

Anderson RA. Effects of chromium on body composition and weight loss. *Nutr Rev.* 1998;56:266-270.

Anderson RA, Bryden NA, Polansky MM. Lack of toxicity of chromium chloride and chromium picolinate in rats. *J Amer Coll Nutr.* 1997;16:273-279.

Anderson RA, Cheng N, Bryden NA, et al. Elevated intakes of supplemental chromium improve glucose and insulin variables in individuals with type II diabetes. *Diabetes.* 1997;46:1786-1791.

Balk EM, Tatsioni A, Lichtenstein AH, et al. Effect of chromium supplementation on glucose metabolism and lipids: a systematic review of randomized controlled trials. *Diabetes Care.* 2007;30(8):2154-2163.

Cerulli J, Grabe DW, Gauthier I, et al. Chromium picolinate toxicity. *Ann Pharmacother.* 1998;32:428-431.

Donaldson RM Jr, Barreras RF. Intestinal absorption of trace quantities of chromium. *J Lab Clin Med.* 1966;68:484-493.

Guan X, Matte JJ, Ku PK, et al. High chromium yeast supplementation improves glucose tolerance in pigs by decreasing hepatic extraction of insulin. *J Nutr.* 2000;130:1274-1279.

Institute of Medicine, Food and Nutrition Board. Dietary Reference Intakes for vitamin A, vitamin K, arsenic, boron, chromium, copper, iodine, iron, manganese, molybdenum, nickel, silicon, vanadium, and zinc. Washington, DC: National Academy Press, 2001.

International Symposium on the Health Effects of Dietary Chromium. J Trace Elem Exp Med. 1999;12:53-169.

Jeejeebhoy KN. The role of chromium in nutrition and therapeutics and as a potential toxin. *Nutr Rev.* 1999;57:329-335.

Kaats GR, Blum K, Fisher JA, et al. Effects of chromium picolinate supplementation on body composition: a randomized, double-masked, placebo-controlled study. *Curr Therap Res.* 1996;57:747-756.

Lukaski HC. Chromium as a supplement. *Annu Rev Nutr.* 1999;19:279-302.

Martin WR, Fuller RE. Suspected chromium picolinate-induced rhabdomyolysis. *Pharmacotherapy.* 1998;18:860-862.

Merz W. Chromium in human nutrition: a review. *J Nutr.* 1993;123:626-633.

Nielsen FH. Controversial chromium. *Nutr Today.* 1996;31:226-233.

Press RI, Geller J, Evans GW. The effect of chromium picolinate on serum cholesterol and apolipoprotein fractions in human subjects. *West J Med.* 1990;152:41-45.

Porter DJ, Raymond LW, Anastasio GD. Chromium: Friend or foe? *Arch Fam Med.* 1999;8:386-390.

Roeback JR Jr, Hla KM, Chambless LE, et al. Effects of chromium supplementation on serum high-density lipoprotein cholesterol levels in men taking beta-blockers. *Ann Intern Med.* 1991;115:917-924.

Speetjens JK, Collins RA, Vincent JB, et al. The nutritional supplement chromium (III) tris (picolinate) cleaves DNA. *Chem Res Toxicol.* 1999;12:483-487.

Stallings DM, Hepburn DD, Hannah M, et al. Nutritional supplement chromium picolinate generates chromosomal aberrations and impedes progeny development in Drosophila melanogaster. *Mutat Res.* 2006;610(1-2):101-113.

Stearns DM, Belbruno JJ, Wetterhahn KE. A prediction of chromium (III) accumulation in humans from chromium dietary supplements. *FASEB J.* 1995;9:1650-1657.

Stearns DM, Wise JP Sr, Patierno SR, et al. Chromium (III) picolinate produces chromosome damage in Chinese hamster ovary cells. *FASEB J.* 1995;9:1643-1649.

Stoecker BJ. Chromium. In: Shils ME, Olson JA, Shike M, Ross AC, eds. *Modern Nutrition in Health and Disease.* 9th ed. Baltimore, MD: Williams and Wilkins; 1999:277-282.

Verhage AH, Cheong WK, Jeejeebhoy KN. Neurologic symptoms due to possible chromium deficiency in long-term parenteral nutrition that closely mimic metronidazole-induced syndromes. *J Parenter Enter Nutr.* 1996;20:123-127.

Vincent J. The biochemistry of chromium. *J Nutr.* 2000;130:715-718.

Vincent JB. Quest for the molecular mechanism of chromium action and its relationship to diabetes. *Nutr Rev.* 2000;58:67-72.

Wasser WG, Feldman NS, D'Agati VD. Chronic renal failure after ingestion of over-the-counter chromium picolinate [letter]. *Ann Intern Med.* 1997;126:410.

Young PC, Turiansky GW, Bonner MW, et al. Acute generalized exanthematous pustulosis induced by chromium picolinate. *J Am Acad Dermatol.* 1999;41(5 pt 2):820-823.

Chrysin

DESCRIPTION

Chrysin belongs to the flavone class of flavonoids. Chrysin is found naturally in various plants including the *Pelargonium* species, which are germanium-like plants; the *Passiflora* or passion flower species, which include tropical passion fruit; and the *Pinaceae* species, including pine trees.

Chrysin, principally obtained from the plant *Passiflora coerulea*, is marketed as a nutritional supplement and is especially popular among male body builders and other athletes because of its possible action in inhibiting the conversions of androgens to estrogens.

Chrysin is a solid substance with the molecular formula $C_{15}H_{10}O_4$. Its molecular weight is 254.24 daltons. It is practically insoluble in water. Chrysin is also known as 5,7-dihydroxyflavone and 5,7-dihydroxy-2-phenyl-4*H*-1-benzopyran-4-one. Chrysin is found in plants as such but is mainly found naturally in the form of a glucoside. Chrysin has the following chemical structure:

Chrysin

ACTIONS AND PHARMACOLOGY

ACTIONS

Chrysin may have aromatase-inhibitory action. It may also have phytoestrogenic, antioxidant and anxiolytic activities.

MECHANISM OF ACTION

Aromatase is a cytochrome P-450 enzyme that catalyzes the rate-limiting step in estrogen synthesis, the conversion of androgens to estrogens. Androstenedione and testosterone serve as substrates for aromatase. Aromatase, also known as estrogen synthase or synthetase, is inhibited by chrysin *in vitro*.

Chrysin has been demonstrated to bind weakly to estrogen receptors alpha and beta, again *in vitro*.

Chrysin's antioxidant potential has been shown by its ability to inhibit xanthine oxidase and consequently suppress the formation of uric acid and certain reactive oxygen species. It may also, under some conditions, inhibit lipid peroxidation.

Other *in vitro* studies have shown that chrysin binds to an area of the $GABA_A$ receptor known as the benzodiazepine receptor.

PHARMACOKINETICS

Little is known of the pharmacokinetics of chrysin in humans. Intestinal and hepatic cell cultures indicate that chrysin can get into cells but that it undergoes extensive glucuronidation and sulfation within the cells. If oral chrysin were to be extensively metabolized following absorption, one would expect that it would be essentially inactivated. Human pharmacokinetic studies are needed to clarify this. Chrysin does appear to be absorbed and to have activity in certain animal models.

INDICATIONS AND USAGE

Chrysin's aromatase-inhibiting effects have made it popular among some body builders and athletes who use androgens. Very preliminary research suggests that chrysin may emerge as a useful anxiolytic agent, that it might aid in the control of morphine withdrawal and that it might have some chemopreventive properties in cardiovascular disease and cancer.

RESEARCH SUMMARY

Chrysin's ability to inhibit the aromatization of androstenedione and testosterone to estrogens has been demonstrated in the laboratory. Chrysin has been shown to be among the most potent of the natural and synthetic flavone inhibitors of human estrogen aromatase. There are no studies directly demonstrating that chrysin makes the use of testosterone and related steroids less likely to produce estrogenic side effects.

A study using rats has shown that various flavonoids, including chrysin, can selectively bind to the central benzodiazepine receptor and thus exert potent anxiolytic and other benzodiazepine effects. More research is warranted.

Another study, this one *in vitro*, has suggested that chrysin might be helpful in controlling morphine withdrawal. Still other *in vitro* studies have found some chrysin-related chemopreventive effects in cardiovascular disease and cancer. No conclusions can yet be drawn from these very early studies.

CONTRAINDICATIONS, PRECAUTIONS, ADVERSE REACTIONS

CONTRAINDICATIONS

Chrysin is contraindicated in those with prostate cancer. It is also contraindicated in those hypersensitive to any component of a chrysin-containing product.

PRECAUTIONS

Pregnant women, nursing mothers, children and adolescents should avoid using chrysin. Women generally should avoid its use.

Hormonal manipulation may have unforeseen consequences. Those interested in chrysin supplementation should exercise caution in its use.

Women with hormone dependent malignancies (breast, uterine, ovarian) should only use chrysin if they are in a clinical study or if chrysin is prescribed and monitored by their physicians.

ADVERSE REACTIONS

No reported adverse reactions.

INTERACTIONS

Aromatase inhibitors: Chrysin may be addictive to the effects of such aromatase inhibitors as aminoglutethimide, anastrozole, exemestane and letrozole.

OVERDOSAGE

There are no reports of overdosage.

DOSAGE AND ADMINISTRATION

Body builders and athletes—typically male—who use chrysin take about one gram daily during training.

LITERATURE

Capasso A, Piacente S, Pizza C, Sorrentino L. Flavonoids reduce morphine withdrawal *in vitro*. *J Pharm Pharmacol.* 1998; 50:561-564.

Galijatovic A, Otake Y, Walle UK, Walle T. Extensive metabolism of the flavonoid chrysin by human Caco-2 and Hep G2 cells. *Xenobiotica.* 1999; 29:1241-1256.

Jeong HJ, Shin YG, Kim IH, Pezzuto JM. Inhibition of aromatase activity by flavonoids. *Arch Pharm Res.* 1999; 22:309-312.

Kellis JT Jr, Vickery LE. Inhibition of human estrogen synthetase (aromatase) by flavones. *Science.* 1984; 225:1032-1034.

Kuiper GG, Lemmen JG, Carlsson B, et al. Interaction of estrogenic chemicals and phytoestrogens with estrogen receptor beta. *Endocrinology.* 1998; 139:4256-4263.

Nagao A, Seki M, Kobayashi H. Inhibition of xanthine oxidase by flavonoids. *Biosci Biotechnol Biochem.* 1999; 63:1787-1790.

Paladini AC, Marder M, Viola H, et al. Flavonoids and the central nervous system: from forgotten factors to potent anxiolytic compounds. *J Pharm Pharmacol*. 1999; 51:519-526.

Salgueiro JB, Ardenghi P, Dias M, et al. Anxiolytic natural and synthetic flavonoid ligands of the central benzodiazepine receptor have no effect on memory tasks in rats. *Pharmacol Biochem Behav*. 1997; 58:887-891.

Walle UK, Galijatovic A, Walle T. Transport of the flavonoid chrysin and its conjugated metabolites by the human intestinal cell line Caco-2. *Biochem Pharmacol*. 1999; 58:431-438.

Cocoa Flavonoids

DESCRIPTION

Cocoa and chocolate are products derived from cacao beans, the seeds of the *Theobroma cacao* tree. Polyphenols comprise about 12 to 18% of the dry weight of cacao beans. About 60% of the polyphenols are in the form of procyanidins (also known as leucocyanidins).

Procyanidins in cocoa and chocolate are mainly homodimers and homotrimers of (-)-epicatechin or heterodimers of (-)-epicatechin and (+)-catechin. (-)-Epicatechin and (+)-catechin belong to the flavan-3-ol class of flavonoids. Procyanidins containing up to 10 subunits (decamers) are found in fresh cacao beans and in dark chocolate. These are also called oligomeric procyanidins.

In addition to containing (-)-epicatechin, (+)-catechin and procyanidins, cocoa and chocolate contain other flavonoids, including other catechins and the flavanol quercetin and its glycosides. Collectively, these flavonoids are known as cocoa flavonoids or cocoa polyphenols.

Interestingly, the Mayans and Aztecs used cacao beans for the preparation of various remedies. The cocoa flavonoids appear to have potent antioxidant activity and may eventually turn out to have health-promoting benefits.

ACTIONS AND PHARMACOLOGY

ACTIONS

Cocoa flavonoids have antioxidant activity. They also may have anti-inflammatory and immunomodulatory activities.

MECHANISM OF ACTION

Cocoa flavonoids have been demonstrated to scavenge reactive oxygen and reactive nitrogen species. They may also chelate metals, such as ferrous cations, which participate in reactive oxygen species-generating reactions. Further, there is some evidence that the larger procyanidin oligomers have greater antioxidant potential.

Cocoa flavonoids have been shown to inhibit the oxidation of LDL. The oxidation of LDL is thought to be a crucial event in the pathogenesis of atherosclerosis.

Some of the cocoa flavonoids appear to reduce the expression of phytohemagglutinin-induced interleukin 2 (IL-2) mRNA, as well as the expression of interleukin 1beta (IL-1B), in peripheral blood mononuclear cells (PBMC).

Reduction of IL-2 and IL-1beta in PBMC could account, in part, for possible anti-inflammatory and immunomodulatory activities of cocoa flavonoids. The mechanism of these actions could again be due to the antioxidant action of cocoa flavonoids. Reactive oxygen species can activate nuclear transcription factor-Kappa B (NF-Kappa B). NF-Kappa B, in turn, may stimulate the production of such pro-inflammatory factors as IL-2 and IL-1 beta.

PHARMACOKINETICS

Little is known about the pharmacokinetics of cocoa polyphenols in humans. It appears that they do, at least partially, get absorbed. However, the extent of absorption appears to vary widely, not only among the different cocoa flavonoids, but also among subjects.

It also appears that the cocoa flavonoids undergo extensive glucuronidation, sulfation and methylation following and/or during absorption.

INDICATIONS AND USAGE

Cocoa flavonoids have been shown, in some mostly small, preliminary studies, to have possible benefit in blood pressure and in heart health generally.

RESEARCH SUMMARY

The cocoa bean is a rich source of polyphenols that exhibit significant antioxidant activity *in vitro*. These polyphenols are found in cocoa, baking chocolate and milk chocolate, among other foods. In one *in vitro* study, all three of these showed some ability to inhibit oxidation of LDL-cholesterol. Cocoa was the most potent of the three in this respect. In the decade since cocoa polyphenols have been investigated, some further small studies have demonstrated some benefits in humans, including lower platelet aggregation in one study and increased HDL-cholesterol in another.

In a few studies, improved insulin sensitivity was noted and blood pressure was improved. In a recent review of studies conducted over the past decade, the authors questioned the value of many of these studies since so many of them were small, poorly controlled and utilized healthy, well-nourished subjects. They also questioned whether observed effects were from cocoa polyphenols or from some other components in the agents used, such as caffeine or magnesium, or from synergistic effects of several components with cocoa. They noted that the majority of the studies were industryfunded and designed, but also observed that since they were published in peer-reviewed journals the industry factor should not invalidate them. They called for more and better-designed studies in the future and suggested that endpoints other than just vascular endpoints be investigated. And, they concluded, "The *bona fide* health effects of cocoa polyphenols will not be answered short of a large-scale epidemiological study or long-term intervention." At present, they stated, there is insufficient data to know whether cocoa has any real public health benefit.

The review authors provided this checklist, which they propose for future planning of cocoa and chocolate trials:

1. Where possible, conduct randomized, controlled, cross-over, multi-dose trials.

2. Use well-defined cocoa or chocolate (if possible, for industry to allow similar cocoa/chocolate to be available for independent researchers for future studies/repeating work).

3. Ensure bioavailability of the active component from its matrix.

4. Use an appropriate control of no-polyphenol chocolate.

5. Recruit volunteers with at least one non-optimal biomarker or disease risk factor.

6. Use a dose of cocoa or chocolate that can readily be incorporated into the daily diet, giving appropriate dietary advice to volunteers on balancing energy.

7. Measure composition, including the polyphenol profile of the cocoa or chocolate before and after the trial (check for stability on storage or batch variations).

8. Ensure the final publication contains the analytical results along with the appropriate description of analytical methodology.

9. Carefully assess the biological relevance of the chosen biomarker, with special attention to antioxidant biomarkers.

10. Strive for transparency by registering human trials, before they start, with a recognized database, eg, www.clinicaltrials.gov.

11. Attempt to publish null or negative results, to enable balancing of the literature and preventing needless duplication of work. Challenge journals if papers are rejected on this basis.

In one recent study involving a cohort of elderly men, cocoa intake was inversely associated with blood pressure and 15-year cardiovascular and all-cause mortality. The data used were derived from 470 elderly men participating in the Zutphen Elderly Study who were free of chronic diseases at baseline. Blood pressure was measured at baseline and at five-year intervals.

Another recent study found that supplementing diet in 34 elderly males with flavonol-rich cocoa increased cerebral blood flow velocity in the middle cerebral artery in these subjects, compared with controls. This, the researchers said, suggested some possible role for cocoa products in cerebrovascular ischemic syndromes, including dementia and stroke. Far more research will be needed, however, to establish clinical significance.

CONTRAINDICATIONS, PRECAUTIONS, ADVERSE REACTIONS

Cocoa polyphenols are contraindicated in those who are hypersensitive to any component of a cocoa polyphenol-containing product.

OVERDOSAGE

There are no reports of overdosage.

DOSAGE AND ADMINISTRATION

Chocolate bars and beverage mixtures that are rich in cocoa flavanols are available. Dark chocolate is generally higher in cocoa flavanols than milk chocolate. This is because the flavanols come from the cocoa liquor and milk chocolate generally contains less cocoa liquor than dark chocolate. White chocolate contains no cocoa liquor and hence no flavanols at all.

No dosage recommendations at this time.

LITERATURE

Aron PM, Kennedy JA. Flavan-3-ols: nature, occurrence and biological activity. *Mol Nutr Food Res.* 2008;52(1):79-104.

Arteel GE, Sies H. Protection against peroxynitrite by cocoa polyphenol oligomers. *FEBS Left.* 1999;462:167-170.

Arts ICW, Hollman PCH, Kromhout D. Chocolate as a source of tea flavonoids. *Lancet.* 1999;354:488.

Balzer J, Rassaf T, Heiss C, et al. Sustained benefits in vascular function through flavanol-containing cocoa in medicated diabetic patients a double-masked, randomized, controlled trial. *J Am Coll Cardiol.* 2008;51(22):2141-2149.

Buijsse B, Feskens EJ, Kok FJ, et al. Cocoa intake, blood pressure, and cardiovascular mortality: the Zutphen Elderly Study. *Arch Intern Med.* 2006;166(4):411-417.

Cooper KA, Donovan JL, Waterhouse AL, et al. Cocoa and health: a decade of research. *Br J Nutr.* 2008;99(1):1-11.

Ding EL, Hutfless SM, Ding X, et al. Chocolate and prevention of cardiovascular disease: a systematic review. *Nutr Metab* (Lond). 2006;3:2.

Engler MB, Engler MM. The emerging role of flavonoid-rich cocoa and chocolate in cardiovascular health and disease. *Nutr Rev.* 2006;64(3):109-118.

Erdman JW Jr, Carson L, Kwik-Uribe C, et al. Effects of cocoa flavanols on risk factors for cardiovascular disease. *Asia Pac J Clin Nutr.* 2008;17 Suppl 1:284-287.

Fisher ND, Hughes M, Gerhard-Herman M, et al. Flavanol-rich cocoa induces nitric-oxide-dependent vasodilation in healthy humans. *J Hypertens.* 2003;21(12):2281-2286.

Hammerstone JF, Lazarus SA, Mitchell AE, et al. Identification of procyanidins in cocoa (*Theobroma Cacao*) and chocolate using high-performance liquid chromatography/mass spectrometry. *J Agric Food Chem.* 1999;47:490-496.

Heiss C, Schroeter H, Balzer J, et al. Endothelial function, nitric oxide, and cocoa flavanols. *J Cardiovasc Pharmacol.* 2006;47 Suppl 2:S128-135; discussion S172-176.

Holt RR, Actis-Goretta L, Momma TY, et al. Dietary flavanols and platelet reactivity. *J Cardiovasc Pharmacol.* 2006;47 Suppl 2:S187-196; discussion S206-209.

Keen CL, Holt RR, Oteiza PI, et al. Cocoa antioxidants and cardiovascular health. *Am J Clin Nutr.* 2005;81(1 Suppl):298S-303S.

Kwik-Uribe C, Bektash RM. Cocoa flavanols—measurement, bioavailability and bioactivity. *Asia Pac J Clin Nutr.* 2008;17 Suppl 1:280-283.

Lazarus SA, Hammerstone JF, Schmitz HA. Chocolate contains additional flavonoids not found in tea. *Lancet.* 1999;354:1825.

Mao TK, Powell J, Van de Water J, et al. The effect of cocoa procyanidins on the transcription and secretion of interleukin 1beta in peripheral blood mononuclear cells. *Life Sci.* 2000;66:1377-1386.

Mao TK, Powell JJ, Van de Water J, et al. The influence of cocoa procyanidins on the transcription of interleukin-2 in peripheral blood mononuclear cells. *Int J Immunotherapy.* 1999;15:23-29.

Mehrinfar R, Frishman WH. Flavanol-rich cocoa: a cardioprotective nutraceutical. *Cardiol Rev.* 2008;16(3):109-115.

Sanbongi C, Suzuki N, Sakane T. Polyphenols in chocolate, which have antioxidant activity, modulate immune function in humans *in vitro. Cell Immunol.* 1997;177:129-136.

Schroeter H, Heiss C, Balzer J, et al. (-)-Epicatechin mediates beneficial effects of flavanol-rich cocoa on vascular function in humans. *Proc Natl Acad Sci USA.* 2006;103(4):1024-1029.

Selmi C, Mao TK, Keen CL, et al. The anti-inflammatory properties of cocoa flavanols. *J Cardiovasc Pharmacol.* 2006;47 Suppl 2:S163-171; discussion S172-176.

Sorond FA, Lipsitz LA, Hollenberg NK, et al. Cerebral blood flow response to flavanol-rich cocoa in healthy elderly humans. *Neuropsychiatr Dis Treat.* 2008;4(2):433-440.

Taubert D, Roesen R, Lehmann C, et al. Effects of low habitual cocoa intake on blood pressure and bioactive nitric oxide: a randomized controlled trial. *JAMA.* 2007;298(1):49-60.

Vinson JA, Proch J, Zubik L. Phenol antioxidant quantity and quality in foods: cocoa, dark chocolate and milk chocolate. *J Agric Food Chem.* 1999;47:4821-4824.

Coenzyme Q10 (CoQ10)

DESCRIPTION

Coenzyme Q_{10} or CoQ_{10} belongs to a family of substances called ubiquinones. Ubiquinones, also known as coenzymes Q and mitoquinones, are lipophilic, water-insoluble substances involved in electron transport and energy production in mitochondria. The basic structure of ubiquinones consists of a benzoquinone "head" and a terpinoid "tail." The "head" structure participates in the redox activity of the electron transport chain. The major difference among the various coenzymes Q is in the number of isoprenoid units (5-carbon structures) in the "tail." Coenzymes Q contain one to 12 isoprenoid units in the "tail"; 10 isoprenoid units are common in animals.

Coenzymes Q occur in the majority of aerobic organisms, from bacteria to plants and animals. Two numbering systems exist for designation of the number of isoprenoid units in the terpinoid "tail": coenzyme Qn and coenzyme Q(x). N refers to the number of isoprenoid side chains, and x refers to the number of carbons in the terpinoid "tail" and can be any multiple of five. Thus, coenzyme Q_{10} refers to a coenzyme Q having 10 isoprenoid units in the "tail." Since each isoprenoid unit has five carbons, coenzyme Q_{10} can also be designated coenzyme Q(50). The structures of coenzymes Q are analogous to those of vitamin K2.

Coenzyme Q_{10} is also known as Coenzyme Q(5O), CoQ_{10}, CoQ(50), ubiquinone (50), ubiquinol—10 and ubidecarerone. Chemically, CoQ_{10} is known as 2, 3-dimethyoxy-5-methyl-6-decaprenyl-1,4-benzoquinone, and its structural formula is:

CoEnzyme Q_{10}

It is a solid wax-like substance. CoQ_{10} is the predominant form in humans, and CoQ_9 is the predominant form in rats.

Supplemental CoQ_{10} is typically derived from tobacco leaf extracts and fermented sugar cane and beets.

ACTIONS AND PHARMACOLOGY

ACTIONS

Supplemental CoQ_{10} may have cardioprotective, cytoprotective and neuroprotective activities.

MECHANISM OF ACTION

Since the actions of supplemental CoQ_{10} have yet to be clarified, the mechanism of these actions is a matter of speculation. However, much is known about the biochemistry of CoQ_{10}. CoQ_{10} is an essential cofactor in the mitochondrial electron transport chain, where it accepts electrons from complex I and II, an activity that is vital for the production of ATP.

CoQ_{10} has antioxidant activity in mitochondria and cellular membranes, protecting against peroxidation of lipid membranes. It also inhibits the oxidation of LDL-cholesterol. LDL-cholesterol oxidation is believed to play a significant role in the pathogenesis of atherosclerosis.

CoQ_{10} is biosynthesized in the body and shares a common synthetic pathway with cholesterol. CoQ_{10} levels decrease with aging in humans. Why this occurs is not known but may be due to decreased synthesis and/or increased lipid peroxidation which occurs with aging.

PHARMACOKINETICS

CoQ_{10} is absorbed from the small intestine into the lymphatics; from there it enters the blood. Absorption of CoQ_{10} is poor. Well over 60% of an oral dose is excreted in the feces. Furthermore, absorption of CoQ_{10} is highly variable and depends not only on food intake but also on the amount of lipids present in the food. Absorption is lower on an empty stomach and greater when taken with food of high lipid content. In the blood, CoQ_{10} is partitioned into the various lipoprotein particles, including VLDL, LDL and HDL.

It takes about three weeks of daily dosing with CoQ_{10} to reach maximal serum concentrations, which then plateau with continuous daily dosing. CoQ_{10} is distributed to the various tissues of the body and is able to enter the brain. The main elimination of CoQ_{10} occurs via bile.

INDICATIONS AND USAGE

Coenzyme Q_{10} is of benefit, either alone or in combination with other therapies, in hypertension and heart failure. Its efficacy in ischemic heart disease may be less pronounced. Its usefulness as concomitant therapy with statins is unclear. It may be of benefit in some neurodegenerative diseases. It may also be helpful in the management of periodontal disease in some. There is very preliminary evidence it might reduce muscular injury in some athletes. There is no evidence it can inhibit obesity and only scant evidence of usefulness in cancer, muscular dystrophy and immune dysfunction.

RESEARCH SUMMARY

There are many studies, spanning more than two decades, reporting positive results from the use of CoQ_{10} as adjunctive therapy in the treatment of congestive heart failure. CoQ_{10} has been an approved drug in Japan for use in congestive heart failure since 1974. It has also been approved for this use in some other countries. Several studies have demonstrated a strong correlation between severity of heart disease and severity of CoQ_{10} deficiency. Some have suggested that this deficiency is the primary cause of some variations of heart muscle dysfunction, while others believe it plays a secondary role in the etiology of heart failure.

Early studies of congestive heart failure focused on idiopathic dilated cardiomyopathy, testing CoQ_{10} against placebo using echocardiography to assess heart function. Echocardiographic improvement seen in these studies was generally slow but sustained and was accompanied by diminished fatigue, chest pain, dyspnea and palpitations. Normal heart size and function were restored in some patients using only CoQ_{10}; this occurred primarily in patients with recent onset of congestive heart failure.

Subsequently, nearly all of the several placebo-controlled studies investigating CoQ_{10}'s effects on heart muscle function have reported significant positive results. One multicenter Italian study included 2,664 patients with congestive heart failure. No notable adverse effects on drug interactions have been reported in these studies except for one report that noted a slight diminution in coumadin activity.

Many studies to date have examined CoQ_{10} as an addition to standard medical treatments. In several studies involving hypertension and other manifestations of cardiovascular disease, there was a significant reduction in the use of concomitant drug therapies when CoQ_{10} was added to the treatment regimen.

The most recent reviews and meta-analyses continue to find support for the use of coenzyme Q_{10} in heart failure and hypertension. These results led one group of reviewers to recommend recently that patients who have symptomatic heart failure despite conventional therapy, or those who experience side effects of conventional therapy, take 150-300 mg of CoQ_{10} daily and to monitor CoQ_{10} blood levels and clinical response.

A recent meta-analysis of CoQ_{10} in the treatment of hypertension found that subjects in 12 clinical trials who received the supplement had significant reductions in blood pressure, compared with controls. Those who were enrolled in randomized controlled trials had systolic blood pressure of 167.7 mmHg at the outset of supplementation and 151.1 mmHg at the end of the trials. Diastolic pressure went from 103 mmHg to 94.8 mmHg. There was no significant change in the placebo groups.

The routine use of CoQ_{10} in combination with HMG-CoA reductase inhibitors (statins) to reduce cholesterol levels is not recommended by some researchers. Statins have been shown to reduce CoQ_{10} levels. It has been hypothesized that statin-induced CoQ_{10} deficiency may be involved in the pathogenesis of statin myopathy. A recent review found insufficient consistent data to demonstrate this involvement. Nonetheless, given the lack of CoQ_{10} side effects, these reviewers suggested that CoQ_{10} could be tested in persons who develop statin myalgia and who cannot be satisfactorily treated with other agents. Another group agreed recently that studies indicating a protective CoQ_{10} effect in this context are too small and dissimilar to allow for any definitive conclusion. But, given the lack of side effects and the other data suggesting usefulness in heart failure, they stated that some subpopulations might benefit from taking the supplement, including those with familial hypercholesterolemia, heart failure and those 65 years and older.

There is emerging evidence that CoQ_{10} may be helpful in some neurodegenerative diseases. Coenzyme Q_{10} is believed to ameliorate some of the oxidative stress and impaired mitochondrial function that characterizes some of these diseases. A randomized, placebo-controlled, double-blind, multi-center trial of CoQ_{10} is underway to see if the agent can be of help in subjects with amyotrophic lateral sclerosis (ALS). Prior studies in an animal model of ALS suggested benefit. Animals treated with CoQ_{10} had increased survival. Coenzyme Q_{10} was identified in a recent systematic review of candidate agents for ALS treatments as one of 20 priority agents for clinical investigation. Similarly, CoQ_{10} delayed onset of motor deficits and prolonged survival in an animal model of Huntington's disease. One randomized, placebo-controlled study has demonstrated some CoQ_{10} benefit in patients with Huntington's, though this did not rise to a level of statistical significance. Larger trials have been called for and are underway. Some early animal data have suggested possible benefit from CoQ_{10} in those with Parkinson's disease. Efficacy trials are underway. There are also plans to investigate the use of CoQ_{10} in Alzheimer's patients.

Significant CoQ_{10} deficiencies have been noted in diseased gingiva. CoQ_{10}'s efficacy in reducing gingival inflammation and periodontal pocket-depth has been demonstrated in placebo-controlled trials. Claims that CoQ_{10} might be an effective anti-cancer agent are based upon a few suggestive case histories that will require far more rigorous clinical investigation before these claims can be properly evaluated. Similarly, claims that CoQ_{10} might be useful in AIDS and some other immune dysfunctions are premature.

It is not unreasonable to hypothesize that CoQ_{10} might be helpful in muscular dystrophy—and there is some very preliminary animal and clinical data suggesting that it might be. Muscular dystrophy is usually associated with cardiac disease. Research is ongoing but, to date, is inconclusive.

There is some preliminary evidence that CoQ_{10} might boost energy and speed recovery of exercise-related muscle exhaustion and damage. A recent report found that oral administration of CoQ_{10} improved subjective fatigue and physical performance during fatigue-producing workload trials among 17 healthy volunteers who were randomized to receive either CoQ_{10} (100 or 300 mg daily) or placebo for eight days. Results significantly better than placebo were obtained with the 300-mg daily dose. A recent Japanese trial reported that supplementation with CoQ_{10} reduced exercise-induced muscular injury among kendo athletes. (Kendo is a traditional Japanese sport that involves dueling with a sword-like stave made of bamboo.)

Recently, beneficial effects were seen in a rat model of metabolic syndrome supplemented with CoQ_{10}. These benefits, however, did not extend to weight loss, and there is no indication that CoQ_{10} is an effective antiobesity agent.

CONTRAINDICATIONS, PRECAUTIONS, ADVERSE REACTIONS

CONTRAINDICATIONS

Known hypersensitivity to a CoQ_{10}-containing product.

PRECAUTIONS

There is one report of CoQ_{10} decreasing the effectiveness of warfarin. Those taking warfarin should be aware of this possibility.

Because of lack of long-term safety studies, pregnant women and nursing mothers should avoid CoQ_{10} supplements.

Clinical reports from Japan suggest that supplemental CoQ_{10} may improve beta-cell function and glycemic control in type II diabetics. CoQ_{10} does not appear to improve glycemic control in type I diabetics. Diabetics should be made aware of this possibility, and those diabetics who do use supplemental CoQ_{10} should determine by appropriate monitoring if they need to make any adjustments in their diabetic medications.

ADVERSE REACTIONS

Mild gastrointestinal symptoms such as nausea, diarrhea and epigastric distress have been reported, particularly with higher doses (200 milligrams or more daily).

INTERACTIONS

DRUGS

Antidiabetic medications: CoQ_{10} may improve glycemic control in some type II diabetics. If this were to occur, antidiabetic medications might need appropriate adjusting.

Beta Blockers: Some beta blockers, in particular propanolol, have been reported to inhibit some CoQ_{10}-dependent enzymes

Corticosteroids: One study found that CoQ_{10} reduced corticosteroid dosage in patients with bronchial asthma.

Doxorubicin: CoQ_{10} may help ameliorate the cardiotoxicity of doxorubicin.

Statins: CoQ_{10} and cholesterol share the same metabolic pathways. Inhibition of the enzyme 3-hydroxyl-3-methylglutonyl coenzyme A (HMG-CoA) reductase would be expected to decrease CoQ_{10} levels. The statin drugs lovastatin, simvastatin and pravastatin are known to decrease CoQ_{10} levels in humans. It is likely that all statins have this effect.

Warfarin: There is one report of CoQ_{10} decreasing the effectiveness of warfarin.

DIETARY SUPPLEMENTS

Alpha-Tocopherol: Elevation in CoQ_{10} levels in mitochondria by dietary supplementation is linked to a corresponding rise in α-tocopherol content.

FOOD

Piperine: Piperine, found in black pepper, may increase plasma levels of CoQ_{10}. Piperine is also available as a dietary supplement.

DOSAGE AND ADMINISTRATION

CoQ_{10} is available in different formulations: oil-based capsules, powder-filled capsules, and tablets and solubilized softgels (microemulsions and others). The solubilized softgels are claimed to give higher absorption.

Daily doses of CoQ_{10} range from 5 to 300 milligrams. Those who use CoQ_{10} for periodontal health take 100 to 150 milligrams daily. Effectiveness, if any, is thought to be obtained with doses of 50 to 200 milligrams daily. The same dose range applies to those who take statin drugs for treatment of hypercholesterolemia.

CoQ_{10} is best taken with food. About three weeks of daily dosing are necessary to reach maximal serum concentrations of CoQ_{10}.

CoQ_{10} is also available topically in some toothpastes and skin creams.

LITERATURE

Ankola DD, Viswanad B, Bhardwaj V, et al. Development of potent oral nanoparticulate formulation of coenzyme Q10 for treatment of hypertension: can the simple nutritional supplements be used as first line therapeutic agents for prophylaxis/therapy? *Eur J Pharm Biopharm.* 2007;67(2):361-369.

Atar D, Mortensen SA, Flachs H, et al. Coenzyme Q_{10} protects ischemic myocardium in an open-chart swine model. *Clin Investig.* 1993;71(Suppl):S103-S111.

Baggio E, Gandini R, Plancher AC, et al. Italian multicenter study on the safety and efficacy of coenzyme Q_{10} as adjunctive therapy in heart failure. *Mol Aspects Med.* 1994;15(Suppl):287-294.

Belardinelli R, Muçaj A, Lacalaprice F, et al. Coenzyme Q10 and exercise training in chronic heart failure. *Eur Heart J.* 2006;27(22):2675-2681.

Bergossi AM, Grossi G, Fioletta PL, et al. Exogenous CoQ_{10} supplementation prevents plasma ubiquone reduction induced by HMG-CoA reductase inhibitors. *Mol Aspects Med.* 1994;15(Suppl):187-193.

Bliznakov EM, Wilkins DJ. Biochemical and clinical consequences of inhibiting coenzyme Q_{10} biosynthesis by lipid-lowering HMG-CoA reductase inhibitors (statins). *Advanc Therap.* 1998;15:218-228.

Chopra RK, Goldman R, Sinatra ST, et al. Relative bioavailability of coenzyme Q_{10} formulations in human subjects. *Int J Vitam Nutr Res.* 1998;68:109-113.

Crane FL, Sun IL, Sun EE. The essential functions of coenzyme Q. *Clin Investig.* 1993;71(Suppl):S55-S59.

Folkers K. Critique of 30 years of research on hematopoietic and immunological activities of coenzyme Q_{10} and potentiality for therapy of AIDS and cancer. *Med Chem Res.* 1992;2:48-60.

Folkers K, Hanioka T, Xia L-J, et al. Coenzyme Q_{10} increase T4/T8 ratios of lymphocytes in ordinary subjects and relevance to patients having the AIDS related complex. *Biochem Biophys Res Comm.* 1991;176:786-791.

Folkers K, Langsjoen P, Willis R, et al. Lovastatin decreases coenzyme Q levels in humans. *Proc Natl Acad Sci USA.* 1990;87:8931-8934.

Folkers K, Mortensen SA, Littarru GP, et al. The biochemical and clinical aspects of coenzyme Q. *Clin Investig.* 1993;71(Suppl):S51-S178.

Folkers K, Vadhanavikit S, Mortensen SA. Biochemical rationale and myocardial tissue data on the protective therapy of cardiomyopathy with coenzyme Q_{10}. *Proc Natl Acad Sci USA.* 1985;82:901-904.

Galpern WR, Cudkowicz ME. Coenzyme Q treatment of neurodegenerative diseases of aging. *Mitochondrion.* 2007;7(Suppl):S146-153.

Ghirlanda G, Oradei A, Manto A, et al. Evidence of plasma CoQ_{10} -lowering effect by HMG-CoA reductase inhibitors: a double-blind, placebo-controlled study. *J Clin Pharmacol.* 1993;33:226-229.

Gvozdjáková A, Kucharská J, Bartkovjaková M, et al. Coenzyme Q10 supplementation reduces corticosteroids dosage in patients with bronchial asthma. *Biofactors.* 2005;25(1-4):235-240.

Hanaki Y, Sugiyama S, Ozawa T, et al. Coenzyme Q_{10} and coronary artery disease. *Clin Investig.* 1993;71(Suppl):S112-S115.

Hanioka T, Tanaka M, Oijima M, et al. Effect of topical application of coenzyme Q_{10} on adult periodontitis. *Molec Aspects Med.* 1994;15(Suppl):S241-S248.

Henriksen JE, Andersen CB, Hother-Nielsen O, et al. Impact of ubiquinone (coenzyme Q10) treatment on glycaemic control, insulin requirement and well-being in patients with type 1 diabetes mellitus. *Diabet Med.* 1999;16:312-318.

Hofman-Bang C, Rehnqvist N, Swedberg K, et al. Coenzyme Q_{10} as an adjunctive in the treatment of chronic congestive heart failure. The Q_{10} study group. *J Card Fail.* 1995;1:101-107.

Kishi H, Kishi T, Folkers K. Bioenergetics in clinical medicine. III. Inhibition of coenzyme Q10-enzymes by clinically used anti-hypertensive drugs. *Res Commun Chem Pathol Pharmacol.* 1975;12:533-540.

Kishi T, Watanabe T, Folkers K. Bioenergetics in clinical medicine XV. Inhibition of coenzyme Q10-enzymes by clinically used adrenergic blockers of beta-receptors. *Rev Commun Chem Pathol Pharmacol.* 1977;17:157-164.

Kon M, Tanabe K, Akimoto T, et al. Reducing exercise-induced muscular injury in kendo athletes with supplementation of coenzyme Q10. *Br J Nutr.* 2008;100(4):903-909.

Kucharská J, Gvozdjáková A, Simko F. Simvastatin decreased coenzyme Q in the left ventricle and skeletal muscle but not in the brain and liver in L-NAME-induced hypertension. *Physiol Res.* 2007;56(Suppl 2):S49-54.

Kunitomo M, Yamaguchi Y, Kagota S, et al. Beneficial effect of coenzyme Q10 on increased oxidative and nitrative stress and inflammation and individual metabolic components developing in a rat model of metabolic syndrome. *J Pharmacol Sci.* 2008;107(2):128-137.

Lampertico M, Comis S. Italian multicenter study on the efficacy and safety of coenzyme Q_{10} as adjuvant therapy in heart failure. *Clin Investig.* 1993;71(Suppl):S129-S133.

Lass A, Sohal RS. Effect of coenzyme Q_{10} and alpha-tocopherol content of mitochondria on the production of superoxide anion radicals. *FASEB J.* 2000;14:87-94.

Levy HB, Kohlhaas HK. Considerations for supplementing with coenzyme Q10 during statin therapy. *Ann Pharmacother.* 2006;40(2):290-294.

Littarru GP, Langsjoen P. Coenzyme Q10 and statins: biochemical and clinical implications. Mitochondrion. 2007;7(Suppl):S168-174.

Lucker PW, Werzelberger N, Hennings G, et al. Pharmacokinetics of coenzyme ubidecarenone in healthy volunteers. In: Folkers K, Yamamura Y, eds. *Biomedical and clinical aspects of coenzyme Q.* Vol 4. Amsterdam: Elsevier Sci. Publ. BV. 1984;143-148.

Marcoff L, Thompson PD. The role of coenzyme Q10 in statin-associated myopathy: a systematic review. *J Am Coll Cardiol.* 2007;49(23):2231-2237.

Matthews RT, Yang L, Browne S, et al. Coenzyme Q_{10} administration increases mitochondrial concentrations and exerts neuroprotective effects. *Proc Natl Acad Sci USA.* 1998;95:8892-8897.

Mizuno K, Tanaka M, Nozaki S, et al. Antifatigue effects of coenzyme Q10 during physical fatigue. *Nutrition.* 2008;24(4):293-299.

Morisco C, Trimarco B, Condorelli M. Effect of coenzyme Q_{10} therapy in patients with congestive heart failure: a long-term multi-center randomized study. *Clinic Investig.* 1993;71(Suppl):S134-S136.

Pepe S, Marasco SF, Haas SJ, et al. Coenzyme Q10 in cardiovascular disease. *Mitochondrion.* 2007;7(Suppl):S154-167.

Pozzi F, Longo A, Lazzarini C, et al. Formulations of ubidecarenone with improved bioavailabiltity. *Eur J Pharm Biopharm.* 1991;37:243-246.

Rosenfeldt FL, Haas SJ, Krum H, et al. Coenzyme Q10 in the treatment of hypertension: a meta-analysis of the clinical trials. *J Hum Hypertens.* 2007;21(4):297-306.

Sander S, Coleman CI, Patel AA, et al. The impact of coenzyme Q10 on systolic function in patients with chronic heart failure. *J Card Fail.* 2006;12(6):464-472.

Shults CW, Haas R. Clinical trials of coenzyme Q10 in neurological disorders. *Biofactors.* 2005;25(1-4):117-126.

Singh U, Devaraj S, Jialal I. Coenzyme Q10 supplementation and heart failure. *Nutr Rev.* 2007;65(6 Pt 1):286-293.

Sohal RS. Coenzyme Q and vitamin E interactions. *Methods Enzymol.* 2004;378:146-151.

Sohal RS, Forster MJ. Coenzyme Q, oxidative stress and aging. *Mitochondrion.* 2007;7(Suppl):S103-111.

Spigset O. Reduced effect of warfarin caused by ubidecarenone. *Lancet.* 1994;344:1372-1373.

Stocker R, Bowry VW, Frei B. Ubiquinol-$_{10}$ protects human low-density lipoprotein more efficiently against lipid peroxidation than does alpha-tocopherol. *Proc Natl Acad Sci USA.* 1991;88:1646-1650.

Tomasetti M, Littaru GP, Stocker R, et al. Coenzyme Q_{10} enrichment decreases oxidative DNA damage in human lymphocytes. *Free Rad Biol Med.* 1999;27:1027-1032.

Tomono Y, Hasegawa J, Seki T, et al. Pharmacokinetic study of deuterium-labeled coenzyme Q_{10} in man. *Int J Clin Pharmacol Ther Toxicol.* 1986;24:536-541.

Watts GF, Castellucio CLA, Riceevans CLA, et al. Plasma coenzyme Q (ubiquinone) concentration in patients treated with simvastatin. *J Clin Pathol.* 1995;46:1055-1057.

Watts TLP. Coenzyme Q_{10} and periodontal treatment: is there any beneficial effect? *Br Dent J.* 1995;178:209-213.

Colloidal Minerals

DESCRIPTION

Colloidal mineral supplements refer to liquid extracts of minerals mainly derived from humic shale deposits or from aluminosilicate-containing clays. Humic shale extracts predominantly contain sulfates of iron and aluminum and traces of colloidal metal hydroxides. The term colloidal mineral is derived from the presence in these preparations of colloidal metal hydroxides. However, many of the minerals are present in ionic forms.

In addition to the sulfates of iron and aluminum, colloidal minerals from humic shale deposits contain zinc, nickel, manganese, magnesium, calcium, chromium, boron, copper, lithium and silicon. They also contain traces of several other elements including arsenic, vanadium, strontium, selenium, iodine and praseodymium. Similar minerals may be found in colloidal minerals derived from clay and from plant sources. Humic and fulvic acids are found in some preparations. Interestingly, humic acids convert minerals into more useable forms for plants. It is believed by some that minerals in colloidal form are more easily absorbable than minerals in solid form (tablets and capsules).

Colloidal minerals are sometimes referred to as liquid minerals. However, some supplements marketed as liquid minerals are generally different from the so-called colloidal mineral supplements. They are liquid mixtures comprised of chelated minerals, ocean minerals and mineral citrates, as well as some colloidal minerals.

Note: Products called "colloidal silver" should not be confused with the colloidal mineral supplements. Colloidal silver may pose health threat and should be avoided (see Colloidal Silver).

ACTIONS AND PHARMACOLOGY

ACTIONS
Colloidal minerals are delivery forms of trace minerals. They have putative enhanced-absorption capability.

MECHANISM OF ACTION
It is speculated that because colloidal minerals do not have to undergo disintegration and dissolution, in contrast with minerals taken in the form of tablets and capsules, they are better absorbed.

PHARMACOKINETICS
There is little on the pharmacokinetics of colloidal minerals, and there are no adequate studies comparing mineral absorption in this form with minerals in tablet or capsule form.

INDICATIONS AND USAGE
There is no credible evidence to support claims that colloidal minerals are effective in the prevention and treatment of arthritis, diabetes, cancer, cardiovascular disease, immune disorders or any other disease condition. Safety data are lacking on most or all of them. Some have been found to contain varying levels of mercury, lead, aluminum, cadmium and arsenic, among other substances.

RESEARCH SUMMARY
There is no credible research showing benefits from colloidal minerals. Claims that they are more absorbable are also unsubstantiated.

CONTRAINDICATIONS, PRECAUTIONS, ADVERSE REACTIONS

CONTRAINDICATIONS
Colloidal minerals are contraindicated in those who are hypersensitive to any component of a colloidal mineral supplement.

PRECAUTIONS
Pregnant women and nursing mothers should avoid supplementing with colloidal minerals.

Those with hemochromatosis or those with any condition of iron overload should avoid colloidal mineral supplementation. Iron is one of the richest minerals in these supplements.

Those with hepatolenticular degeneration (Wilson's disease) should avoid colloidal mineral supplementation because of the presence of copper in these supplements.

Those who do use colloidal minerals should refrigerate the bottle after opening.

Those who require mineral supplementation should be aware of the great variability of minerals in these supplements from batch to batch.

ADVERSE REACTIONS
There are no reports of adverse reactions in those ingesting colloidal minerals. Earlier reports of colloidal minerals containing radioactivity and unusually high levels of strontium have not been confirmed. Some earlier preparations contained high levels of aluminum. Some preparations contain potentially toxic minerals (e.g., arsenic, lead), but in very small amounts.

INTERACTIONS
No known interactions with drugs, nutritional supplements, food or herbs.

OVERDOSAGE
There are no reports of overdosage.

DOSAGE AND ADMINISTRATION
No recommended dosage.

LITERATURE
Schauss A. Colloidal minerals: clinical implications of clay suspension products sold as dietary supplements. *Am J Nat Med.* 1997; 4:3-10.

Schrauzer GN. An evaluation of liquid vitamin-mineral supplement technology. *J Med Food.* 1998; 1:207-216.

Colloidal Silver

DESCRIPTION

Silver is a metallic element with atomic number 47 and atomic symbol Ag. It occurs in nature in ores and as a free metal and is also found in living matter. Ultratrace amounts of silver occur in the diet. The daily dietary intake of silver from food and water is approximately 300 micrograms. However, silver is not an essential nutrient for humans. Nor does it appear to be essential for any living organism.

Silver is highly toxic to most microbial cells and can be used as an antimicrobial agent. Silver-containing compounds, such as silver sulfadiazine, which has broad antimicrobial as well as antifungal activity, and silver nitrate, are used in medicine as topical agents. Colloidal silver is a suspension of extremely small silver particles and was used in medicine until the 1940s as both a topical and an internal antiseptic. Colloidal silver was also known as argentum colloidale, argentum credé and collargolum. Argentum is Latin for silver.

Colloidal silver no longer has a role in medicine but reappeared in the 1990s as a nutritional supplement. Neither colloidal silver nor any form of silver has any valid role in nutrition as a nutritional or dietary supplement.

ACTIONS AND PHARMACOLOGY

ACTIONS

There are no known actions of supplemental colloidal silver.

PHARMACOKINETICS

There are no reported studies on the pharmacokinetics of colloidal silver.

INDICATIONS AND USAGE

There are no indications for use of supplemental silver. In 1999, the Food and Drug Administration issued a final rule establishing that all over-the-counter products containing colloidal silver ingredients or silver salts for external or internal use are not generally recognized as safe and effective and are misbranded. These products are being marketed for numerous disease conditions, and the FDA states that it is "not aware of any substantial scientific evidence that supports the use of OTC colloidal silver ingredients or silver salts for these disease conditions."

RESEARCH SUMMARY

Silver has long been used as a topical antiseptic. Doses that could have internal antiseptic effects are not considered safe. There are many documented cases of argyria, a condition in which the skin of the entire body assumes a grayish-blue pigmentation that is irreversible and permanent. It is often attended by permanent discoloration of hair, nails and oral and gingival mucosae. Not only quantity of silver intake but also individual sensitivity to silver and other factors, such as exposure to sunlight, contribute to the appearance of argyriasis.

A number of case studies shed light on the etiology of this disfiguring condition. A 34-year old woman, for example, developed it when she took colloidal silver for 25 months in an effort to treat intestinal dyspepsia with diarrheic episodes. Some others have developed it after treating themselves with silver nitrate eye drops or to treat oral ulcers. Cases have resulted from the use of silver acetate chewing gum used as a putative, unproved smoking deterrent. One schizophrenic patient developed argyria and convulsive seizures, which some researchers also associated with prolonged silver use.

Current research makes it clear that there are no safe uses for over-the-counter silver products.

CONTRAINDICATIONS, PRECAUTIONS, ADVERSE REACTIONS

CONTRAINDICATIONS

Supplemental colloidal silver is not advised for anyone.

ADVERSE REACTIONS

Prolonged intake of colloidal silver can cause argyria, a condition in which the skin of the entire body assumes a blue-gray discoloration, particularly in areas exposed to light. Argyria is permanent and irreversible. Argyria also affects the lips, cheeks and gums.

OVERDOSAGE

There are no reports of overdosage of colloidal silver.

DOSAGE AND ADMINISTRATION

Supplemental colloidal silver is not recommended. Colloidal or liquid minerals often contain silver.

LITERATURE

Anon. Over the-counter drug products containing colloidal silver ingredients or silver salts. Department of Health and Human Services (HHS), Public Health Service (PHS), Food and Drug Administration (FDA). Final rule. *Fed Regist.* 1999; 64:44653-44658.

Fung MC, Bowen DL. Silver products for medical indications: risk-benefit assessment. *J Toxicol Clin Toxicol.* 1996; 34:119-126.

Hollinger MA. Toxicological aspects of topical silver pharmaceuticals. *Crit Rev Toxicol* 1996; 26:255-260.

Ohbo Y, Fukuzako H, Takeuchi K, Takigawa M. Argyria and convulsive seizures caused by ingestion of silver in a patient with schizophrenia. *Psychiatry Clin Neurosci.* 1996; 50:89-90.

Pardo-Peret P, Sans-Sebrafen J, Boleda Relats M. [Argyriasis. Report of a case.] [Article in Spanish.] *Med Clin (Barc).* 1979; 73:386-389.

Russell AD, Hugo WB. Antimicrobial activity and action of silver. *Prog Med Chem.* 1994; 31:351-370.

Slawson RM, Lee H, Trevors JT. Bacterial interactions with silver. *Biol Met.* 1990; 3:151-154.

Colosolic Acid

DESCRIPTION

Colosolic acid, sometimes called corosolic acid, is a triterpene compound extracted from the leaves of the plant *Lagerstroemia speciosa*. The leaves of *Lagerstroemia speciosa* are used in Southeast Asia as an herbal remedy for a number of disorders, including diabetes and obesity. In the Philippines, the plant is known by the Tagalog name of banaba.

Colosolic acid has been reported to activate glucose transport in cell cultures and to lower glucose in diabetic mice. There are a few reports that colosolic acid lowers blood glucose levels in type 2 diabetic subjects. However, none of these reports has appeared in peer-reviewed scientific literature.

Colosolic acid is also known as 2alpha-hydroxyursolic acid, corosolic acid and botanical insulin. A similar triterpene called corosolic acid has been isolated from the fruit of *Crataegus pinnatifida* var. pilosa, a member of the hawthorn family.

ACTIONS AND PHARMACOLOGY

ACTIONS

Supplemental colosolic acid is reputed to activate glucose transport, resulting in hypoglycemic activity.

MECHANISM OF ACTION

The mechanism of action of colosolic's putative hypoglycemic action is not known.

PHARMACOKINETICS

There are no reported pharmacokinetics on colosolic acid.

INDICATIONS AND USAGE

It is claimed that colosolic acid lowers blood glucose in type 2 diabetics, burns fat, lowers elevated blood pressure and boosts energy, among other things. Currently, there is no credible evidence to support any claim for the use of this substance in humans.

RESEARCH SUMMARY

Colosolic acid is reported to activate glucose transport in Ehrlich ascites tumor cells. Extracts from *Lagerstroemia speciosa*. Leaves have been reported to have hypoglycemic activity in genetically diabetic KK-AY mice. There are no credible reports that colosolic acid can lower blood glucose in type 2 diabetics, boost energy, burn fat or lower blood pressure in hypertensives.

CONTRAINDICATIONS, PRECAUTIONS, ADVERSE REACTIONS

CONTRAINDICATIONS

Known hypersensitivity to a colosolic acid-containing product.

PRECAUTIONS

Children, pregnant women and nursing mothers should avoid using products called colosolic acid or corosolic acid. Those with diabetes should be extremely cautious about using colosolic/corosolic acid. Those with hypoglycemia should avoid using colosolic/corosolic acid.

ADVERSE REACTIONS

None reported.

INTERACTIONS

If colosolic acid were to lower blood glucose, it could have additive effects with drugs used in the management of diabetes, and therefore blood glucose must be closely monitored.

OVERDOSAGE

None reported.

DOSAGE AND ADMINISTRATION

No recommended dose. Colosolic acid is marketed in stand-alone supplements and in combination products. Colosolic acid in these products is usually from extracts of *Lagerstroemia speciosa* leaves.

LITERATURE

Ahn KS, Hahm MS, Park EJ, et al. Corosolic acid isolated from the fruit of *Crataegus pinnatifida* var. pilosa is a protein kinase inhibitor a well as a cytotoxic agent. *Planta Med.* 1998; 64:468-470.

Kakuda T, Sakane I, Takhara T, et al. Hypoglycemic effect of extracts from *Lagerstroemia speciosa* L. leaves in genetically diabetic KK-AY mice. *Biosci Biotechnol Biochem.* 1996; 60:204-208.

Murakami C, Myoga K, Kasai R, et al. Screening of plant constituents for effect on glucose transport activity in Ehrlich ascites tumour cells. *Chem Pharm Bull.* 1993; 41:2129-2131.

Conjugated Linoleic Acid (CLA)

DESCRIPTION

Conjugated linoleic acid or CLA refers to a group of positional and geometric octadecadienoic acid isomers of linoleic acid. CLA is not a single substance. In contrast to linoleic acid, all the CLA isomers have conjugated bonds. In an unsaturated organic compound, two double bonds separated by a single bond are said to be conjugated. CLA is represented by the following structural formulas:

Conjugated linoleic acid (CLA)

A. $CH_3(CH_2)_5$ ————————————COOH

trans,9-cis,11-octadecadienoic acid

B. $CH_3(CH_2)_4$ ————————————COOH

trans,10-cis,12-octadecadienoic acid

CLA is found naturally in animal tissues and food sources, including ruminant meats, poultry, eggs and dairy products, such as cheeses, milk and yogurt that have undergone heat processing treatments. Vegetable fats are generally poorer sources of CLA. However, CLA is produced from linoleic acid in safflower oil and sunflower oil by special treatment of these oils. CLA was originally found in milk fat where it exists in the form of phospholipids and triglycerides. Also, there is evidence that human milk contains CLA.

The principal dietary isomer of CLA is cis-9, trans-11 CLA, also known as rumenic acid and RA. This isomer is produced in the rumen of ruminant animals by microbial metabolism of linoleic and linolenic acids. Cis-9, trans-11 CLA may be absorbed directly or undergo further metabolism. Another CLA isomer, also found in ruminant tissue, is trans-10, cis-12 CLA. Most of the animal studies to date with CLA have used mixtures of CLA isomers that are mostly cis-9, trans-11 CLA and trans-10, cis-12 CLA in approximately equal amounts. Most commercial preparations of CLA contain cis-9, trans-11 CLA and trans-10, cis-12 CLA along with smaller amounts of other CLA isomers, including trans-9, cis-11 CLA, cis-10, cis-12 CLA, trans-9, trans-11 CLA, trans-10, trans-12 CLA and other isomers with conjugated double bonds at the 8, 10 and 11, 13 positions. The various isomers may produce different biologic effects.

Cis-9, trans-11 CLA is also known as c9, t11-octadecadienoic acid; trans-10, cis-12 CLA is also known as t10, c12-octadecadienoic acid. The term octadecadienoates is sometimes used synonymously with CLA.

ACTIONS AND PHARMACOLOGY

ACTIONS

CLA may have anti-carcinogenic, anti-atherogenic, anti-diabetagenic and body composition-modifying activities in humans. These activities have been reported in experimental animals.

MECHANISM OF ACTION

The mechanism(s) of actions of CLA are not clearly understood. To reach a better understanding, it is necessary to determine the specific, possibly varying, effects of the different isomers. For example, the CLA-associated body composition changes observed in animals appear to be associated mainly with the trans-10, cis-12 CLA isomer. In mouse tissue culture, the trans-10, cis-12 CLA isomer was found to reduce lipoprotein lipase activity and concentrations of intracellular triglyceride. The trans-10, cis-12 isomer also decreased the expression of hepatic steroyl-CoA desaturase mRNA in one mouse study and the expression of stearoyl-CoA desaturase activity in mouse adipocytes in tissue culture in another study. Inhibition of stearoyl-CoA desaturase activity may depress fat synthesis.

Both cis-9, trans-11 and trans-10, cis-12 CLA isomers show anti-cancer activity. It is speculated that CLA may modulate eicosanoid activity as well as the activity of such cytokines as tumor necrosis factor-alpha. It is also speculated that activation of peroxisome proliferator-activated receptor-gamma (PPAR-gamma) may play some role in the putative anti-diabetic activity of CLA. Activation of PPAR-gamma and/or PPAR-alpha may account, in part, for the anti-carcinogenic, lipid-lowering and anti-atherogenic effects of CLA reported in animal studies. The enzymes to produce the major isomers are being cloned in bacteria, and it is expected that with the availability of larger amounts of these materials, the effects and mechanisms of actions of these isomers, alone or in combination, will become clearer.

PHARMACOKINETICS

Little is currently known about the pharmacokinetics of CLA in humans. In experimental animals, the CLA isomers do get absorbed following digestion, but not much is known about CLA's metabolism subsequent to absorption. Some CLA appears to get incorporated into the phospholipids of cell membranes.

INDICATIONS AND USAGE

A hoped-for and early indicated CLA antiobesity effect is not supported by recent research. Similarly, inconsistent results make it impossible to conclude at present that CLA is an effective antiatherogenic agent. Some data suggest harmful effects from some CLA isomers. There is some evidence of anticancer activity and some suggestion of possible benefit in diabetes in a preliminary animal study. There is also, however, some equally preliminary evidence that CLA might be prodiabetic.

RESEARCH SUMMARY

Much of the early media "buzz" about CLA was related to claims that it could "burn fat" and fight obesity. In some early trials using animal obesity models, it was reported that CLA-enriched diets reduced body weight independent of food intake. Some CLA isomers were said to be more effective than others in fighting fat. Now, many years later, it appears that CLA does, in fact, reduce weight in some animal models but shows very little efficacy in humans. One recent review concluded: "Experiments in humans have not been able to show a significant effect on body weight, body composition or weight regain related to either of the CLA isomers" commonly promoted for this purpose. The trans-10, cis-12 and cis-9, trans-11 isomers have been combined in some weight-loss products. And, these reviewers cautioned, there is some data suggesting possible harm from the trans-10, cis-12 isomer in terms of negative effects on lipid profile, glucose metabolism and insulin sensitivity. Another recent review of CLA weight studies concluded that body weight loss is "rarely observed" with CLA supplementation in humans. These reviewers further make reference to "the absence of confirmed or even plausible mechanisms" by which CLA might promote weight loss in humans. They stated that CLA should not be recommended for this purpose.

CLA has shown some anticancer effects in a number of animal and *in vitro* studies. Proliferation of human malignant breast, colorectal, prostate, melanoma and lung cell lines has been inhibited by CLA. CLA has inhibited mammary tumorogenesis in a number of studies that demonstrate its efficacy in animal models independent of the amount and type of fat in the diet. In other experimental animal studies, it has significantly inhibited mouse forestomach neoplasia, epidermal tumors in mice and aberrant crypt foci in rat colon.

The mechanisms by which CLA exerts its anti-cancer effects are not yet understood, but it is evident that, in some cases, it appears to interact directly with carcinogens to reduce their potency and that, in other instances, it protects specific tissues through its interaction with those tissues, independent of the carcinogen. It appears to modulate carcinogenesis in all of its separate stages: initiation, promotion, progression.

At one time it was believed that CLA's anti-cancer and other therapeutic effects were largely due to an anti-oxidant property. More recent research demonstrated no significant CLA anti-oxidant effect. Instead, it is now believed by some that CLA exerts beneficial complex regulatory effects at the molecular level through its influence, among other things, on peroxisome proliferator-activated receptors (PPAR). The PPARs are nuclear receptors that modulate gene expression in response to fatty acids, some drugs and other substances. It is also believed to modulate eicosanoid and cytokine activity as well.

One group of researchers recently reported that high-CLA diets reduce the quantity of terminal end buds out of which mammary tumors develop. They further observe that CLA seems to inhibit cancer by selectively inhibiting rapidly dividing cells and by promoting programmed cell death or apoptosis.

More animal data have continued to accumulate, but, so far, meaningful clinical data related to a possible role of CLA in human cancers is lacking. Safety studies in human cancer conditions are needed before clinical trials can be launched. Some have expressed fear that some isomers or combination of CLA isomers might pose peril.

CLA's widely reported hypolipidemic effects (in animal studies) are also believed to be linked to the substance's influence on PPAR subtypes involved with lipid metabolizing enzymes and the modulation of plasma triglyceride clearance, among other things. Beneficial effects on lipids have been reported in rats, mice, rabbits, chickens, hamsters and in other animal models. Atheromatous lesions have regressed significantly in CLA-supplemented animals. And CLA has significantly reduced free fatty acids and triglycerides in Zucker diabetic fatty rats compared with fatty rats on control diets.

Despite some preliminary positive results, as discussed above, a recent review of the CLA atherosclerosis data concluded that after a decade of research no consensus has yet been reached on the potential for CLA to meaningfully modify atherosclerosis in animals, let alone in humans, where data is almost wholly lacking. There is no convincing evidence at this time, these reviewers concluded, that CLA reduces the incidence or severity of atherosclerotic lesions or that CLA can improve plasma lipid and lipoprotein levels. Moreover, as noted above, some researchers have observed that, in some circumstances, at least one CLA isomer exerted negative effects on lipid profile, glucose metabolism and insulin sensitivity.

In view of the latter, some preliminary indications that CLA might have benefit in a pre-diabetic animal model will need particularly careful follow-up.

CONTRAINDICATIONS, PRECAUTIONS, ADVERSE REACTIONS

CONTRAINDICATIONS

CLA is contraindicated in those hypersensitive to any component of the preparation.

PRECAUTIONS

Because of lack of long-term safety data, CLA supplements should be avoided by children, pregnant women and nursing mothers.

ADVERSE REACTIONS

At doses of up to 2 grams daily, occasional gastrointestinal complaints, such as nausea, have been noted.

DOSAGE AND ADMINISTRATION

There are a few products with CLA available. The amounts of the two most studied isomers of CLA, cis-9, trans-11 and trans-10, cis-12 CLA, vary. Also, there are different amounts of other isomers of CLA in the various preparations. Typical doses are 1 to 2 grams daily. Some use doses up to 6 grams daily.

CLA is also being developed for use in functional foods.

LITERATURE

Banni S, Angioni E, Stefania M, et al. Conjugated linoleic acid and oxidative stress. *J Am Oil Chem Soc.* 1998;75:261-267.

Belury MA. Conjugated linoleate: a polyunsaturated fatty acid with unique chemopreventive properties. *Nutr Rev.* 1995;53:83-89.

Cesano A, Visonneau S, Scimeca JA, et al. Opposite effects of linoleic acid and conjugated linoleic acid on human prostate cancer in SCID mice. *Anticanc Res.* 1998;18:833-838.

de Deckere EA, van Amelsvoort JM, Mc Neill GP, Jones P. Effects of conjugated linoleic acid (CLA) isomers on lipid levels and peroxisome proliferation in the hamster. *Br J Nutr.* 1999;82:309-317.

Gavino VC, Gavino G, Leblanc MJ, Tuchweber B. An isomeric mixture of conjugated linoleic acids but not pure cis-9, trans-11-octadecadienoic acid affects body weight gain and plasma lipids in hamsters. *J Nutr.* 2000;130:27-29.

Houseknecht KL, Vanden Heuvel JP, Moya-Camarena SY, et al. Dietary conjugated linoleic acid normalizes impaired glucose tolerance in the Zucker diabetic fatty fa/fa rat. *Biochem Biophys Res Commun.* 1998;244:678-682.

Kelley NS, Hubbard NE, Erickson KL. Conjugated linoleic acid isomers and cancer. *J Nutr.* 2007;137(12):2599-2607.

Lee KN, Kritchevsky D, Pariza MW. Conjugated linoleic acid and atherosclerosis in rabbits. *Atherosclero.* 1994;108:19-25.

Lee KN, Pariza MW, Ntambi JM. Conjugated linoleic acid decreases hepatic stearoyl-CoA desaturase mRNA expression. *Biochem Biophys Res Commun.* 1998;248:817-821.

McCarty MF. Downregulaton of macrophage activation by PPAR gamma suggests a role for conjugated linoleic acid in prevention of Alzheimer's disease. *J Med Food.* 1998;1:217-226.

Mitchell PL, McLeod RS. Conjugated linoleic acid and atherosclerosis: studies in animal models. *Biochem Cell Biol.* 2008;86(4):293-301.

Moya-Camarena SY, Belury MA. Species differences in the metabolism and regulation of gene expression by conjugated linoleic acid. *Nutr Rev.* 1999;57:336-340.

Ostrowski E, Muralitharan M, Cross RF. Dietary conjugated linoleic acids increase lean tissue and decrease fat deposition in growing pigs. *J Nutr.* 1999;129:2037-2042.

Pariza MW, Park Y, Cook ME. Conjugated linoleic acid and the control of cancer and obesity. *Toxicol Sci.* 1999;51(2 Suppl):107-110.

Pariza MW, Park Y, Cook ME. Mechanisms of action of conjugated linoleic acid: evidence and speculation. *Proc Soc Exp Biol Med.* 2000;223:8-13.

Pariza MW, Park Y, Kim S, et al. Mechanism of body fat reduction by conjugated linoleic acid. *FASEB J.* 1997;11:A139.

Park Y, Albright KJ, Liu W, et al. Effect of conjugated linoleic acid on body composition in mice. *Lipids.* 1997;32:853-858.

Plourde M, Jew S, Cunnane SC, Jones PJ. Conjugated linoleic acids: why the discrepancy between animal and human studies? *Nutr Rev.* 2008;66(7):415-421.

Silveira MB, Carraro R, Monereo S, et al. Conjugated linoleic acid (CLA) and obesity. *Public Health Nutr.* 2007;10(10A):1181-1186.

van den Berg JJ, Cook NE, Tribble DL. Reinvestigation of the antioxidant properties of conjugated linoleic acid. *Lipids.* 1995;30:599-605.

West DB, Delany JP, Camet PM, et al. Effects of conjugated linoleic acid on body fat and energy metabolism in the mouse. *Am J Physiol.* 1998;275(3 Pt 2):R667-R672.

Yurawecz MP, Mossoba MM, Kramer JKG, Pariza MW, Nelson GJ, eds. *Advances in Conjugated Linoleic Acid Research.* Volume 1. Champaign, IL:AOCS Press;1999.

Further information:

To keep track of CLA progress, an updated listing can be found on the Internet at http://www.wisc.edu/fri/clarefs.htm.

Copper

DESCRIPTION

Copper is an essential trace mineral in animal and human nutrition. Anemia, neutropenia and osteoporosis are found with frank copper deficiency. Copper deficiency in humans is rare but it does occur under certain circumstances, such as in patients receiving long-term total parenteral nutrition (TPN). Mild copper deficiency due to marginal copper intake over a long period may also occur. In addition to possible anemia, neutropenia and osteoporosis, manifestations of mild copper deficiency may include abnormal glucose tolerance, hypercholesterolemia, arthritis, myocardial disease, arterial disease, cardiac arrhythmias, loss of pigmentation and neurological problems.

Copper is a transition metal with atomic number 29 and an atomic weight of 63.55 daltons. Its symbol is Cu. Copper participates in metabolism as a component of many metalloenzymes, including ceruloplasmin or ferroxidase I, cytochromecoxidase, copper/zinc superoxide dismutase, dopamine beta-hydroxylase, tyrosinase, monoamine oxidase, diamine oxidase, lysyl oxidase (protein-lysine 6-oxidase), peptidylglycine-alpha-amidating monoxygenase and ferroxidase II.

Copper essentiality for humans was first demonstrated in malnourished children in Peru. The children had an anemia that was not responsive to iron therapy, as well as neutropenia and bone abnormalities. The anemia, neutropenia and bone abnormalities were responsive to copper supplementation. Copper is required for normal infant development, red and white blood cell maturation, iron transport, bone strength, cholesterol metabolism, myocardial contractility, glucose metabolism, brain development and immune function, among other things.

Although copper is clearly essential for a wide range of biochemical processes that are necessary for the maintenance of good health, copper is also a potentially toxic substance. Copper exists in the oxidation states Cu(I) or Cu+ (cuprous), and Cu(II) or Cu2+ (cupric) under physiological conditions. The shift back and forth between these two oxidation states via single-electron-transfer reactions is the property that makes copper such an essential component of the enzymes mentioned above. However, this redox property also contributes to its potential toxicity. Redox cycling between Cu+ and Cu2+ can generate the highly reactive oxygen species hydroxyl radicals, which can damage lipids, DNA and proteins. Recently, intracellular proteins have been discovered that protect against the potential toxicity of copper ions. These proteins escort copper ions directly to enzymes that require them in order to function. Free copper ions are involved in the formation of hydroxyl radicals. The proteins that protect cells from copper toxicity are called copper chaperones and essentially keep the cells free of free copper ions. Wilson's disease, or hepatolenticular degeneration, is an autosomal recessive disorder that results from pathological accumulation of copper, principally in liver and brain tissues.

The richest dietary sources of copper include nuts, seeds, legumes, the bran and germ portions of grains, liver, kidneys, shellfish, oysters and crustaceans. Cow's milk has little copper.

ACTIONS AND PHARMACOLOGY
ACTIONS
Copper may have antioxidant activity.

MECHANISM OF ACTION
Copper deficiency has been found to increase the susceptibility of lipoproteins to peroxidation in rats and to increase oxidative DNA damage in lymphocytes in culture. Supplemental copper was found to prevent oxidative DNA damage in lymphocytes in culture. Copper supplementation in middle-aged volunteers was found to protect red blood cells against oxidation. Copper is a cofactor for copper/zinc superoxide dismutase and ceruloplasmin, two important antioxidant enzymes, and the possible antioxidant activity of copper may be accounted for, at least in part, by its role in these enzymes. However, the study with human volunteers

mentioned above did not show increased copper/zinc superoxide activity with copper supplementation. The mechanism of the possible antioxidant activity of supplemental copper is unclear.

PHARMACOKINETICS
Copper is principally absorbed in the small intestine. A small amount of copper is absorbed in the stomach. Copper appears to be absorbed by both active and passive processes. At low and moderate intakes of copper, it appears to be absorbed by a saturable active transport mechanism. At high copper intakes the active transport mechanism becomes saturated, and copper is absorbed by passive diffusion. The absorption efficiency of copper ranges from 15% to 97% and appears to depend on the level of dietary copper intake. As dietary copper increases, the fractional absorption of copper decreases.

Following absorption from the small intestine, copper is transported in the blood primarily bound to albumin. Copper is mainly taken up by the liver where it is principally incorporated into ceruloplasmin. Copper-containing ceruloplasmin is released from the liver into the blood and delivered to cells containing ceruloplasmin receptors.

Copper containing ceruloplasmin binds to these receptors and releases copper into the cell. The major route of copper excretion is via bile into the gastrointestinal tract.

INDICATIONS AND USAGE
There is some experimental indication that supplemental copper may have some anticancer effects and may be of benefit in some with arthritis. Claims that it is protective against cardiovascular disease apply primarily to those with copper deficiency. There is preliminary evidence that copper may have beneficial effects on immunity in those with copper deficiency and perhaps in those with marginal copper deficiency.

RESEARCH SUMMARY
There are some dated reports that supplementary copper significantly protected rats against chemically-induced cancers. Another study reported that a copper-salicylate derivative inhibited tumor promotion in mice. In an *in vitro* study, several copper-containing compounds prevented the malignant transformation of chick-embryo cells by the Rous sarcoma virus. Further research may be warranted.

Copper bracelets have been worn by many in an effort to ameliorate symptoms of arthritis. A study of this folk remedy found that some of those who had worn the bracelets for prolonged periods and then discontinued wearing them became significantly worse, compared with controls who wore placebo bracelets that also appeared to be made of copper. The subjects in this study suffered primarily from osteoarthritis. There was evidence that copper from the bracelets, dissolved in sweat, was absorbed through the skin.

There is also evidence from animal studies that copper complexes of aspirin, tryptophan and penicillamine have anti-inflammatory effects. Injections of copper/zinc superoxide dismutase directly into the joints of some patients with osteoarthritis and rheumatoid arthritis have reportedly produced some relief. More research is needed.

There is no doubt that copper deficiency can contribute to cardiovascular disease. It seems likely that supplemental copper might be helpful in preventing and treating cardiovascular disease even in those with marginal copper deficiency. This hypothesis needs further investigation. Animal studies have shown that copper deficiency increases the susceptibility of lipoproteins and tissues to peroxidation. There are also indications that copper deficiency may play a role in hypertension, in weakening of the structural integrity of the heart and blood vessels and in reduced ability of the heart to contract, among other negative effects.

Similarly, copper appears to play some important roles in immunity, and supplemental copper might thus be beneficial in even those with slight or marginal copper deficiency. Copper deficiency has been shown to increase vulnerability to and mortality from infection in some animal studies. Recently, it has been shown that neutrophils in human peripheral blood are significantly diminished both in number and in their ability to create superoxide anions and kill ingested micro-organisms in conditions of marginal, as well as overt, copper deficiency. Animal and *in vitro* studies have also demonstrated that even marginal copper deficiency reduces levels of interleukin 2 and diminishes T cell proliferation.

CONTRAINDICATIONS, PRECAUTIONS, ADVERSE REACTIONS
CONTRAINDICATIONS
Supplemental copper is contraindicated in those with Wilson's disease (hepatolenticular degeneration), a disease of abnormal copper accumulation.

Supplemental copper is also contraindicated in those hypersensitive to any component of a copper-containing nutritional supplement.

PRECAUTIONS
Pregnant women and nursing mothers should avoid doses of copper above the U.S. RDA for copper unless advised to do so by their physicians. The U.S. RDA for copper is 2 mg daily.

Accidental copper poisoning has occurred among children. Others have ingested several grams in suicide attempts.

ADVERSE REACTIONS
Excessive copper intake produces nausea and vomiting, epigastric pain and diarrhea.

INTERACTIONS
DRUGS
Penicillamine: Concomitant use of penicillamine and copper can cause decreased absorption of both substances. Those who use penicillamine for the treatment of Wilson's disease should avoid the use of supplemental copper (see Contraindications).

NUTRITIONAL SUPPLEMENTS
Iron: Excessive intake of nonheme iron may decrease copper status.

Molybdenum: Excessive intake of molybdenum may decrease copper status.

Zinc: Excessive use of zinc may cause decreased absorption of copper. One explanation for this interaction is that high dietary zinc induces intestinal metallothionein. Copper has a stronger affinity for intestinal metallothionein than does zinc and displaces zinc in intestinal metallothionein and is trapped. Copper depletion was observed when supplements of 50 milligrams or more of zinc were given for extended periods. Copper absorption was not affected by zinc doses of 16.5 milligrams daily for extended periods.

Vitamin C: Vitamin C supplementation of 1,500 milligrams daily caused the activity of the copper transporting protein ceruloplasmin to decline. Vitamin C supplementation of 600 milligrams daily also caused a decline in ceruloplasmin, but copper absorption was not impaired.

FOODS
Concomitant intake of copper with foods rich in phytic acid (unleavened bread, raw beans, seeds, nuts and grains and soy isolates) may decrease the absorption of copper.

Diets high in fructose may decrease copper status.

OVERDOSAGE
Gram amounts of copper can cause coma, oliguria, hepatic necrosis, vascular collapse and death.

DOSAGE AND ADMINISTRATION
Copper supplements are available in several forms, including cupric oxide, copper gluconate, copper sulfate and copper amino acid chelates. Copper supplements are typically found in combination products. Typical doses range from 1.5 to 3.0 milligrams daily. There is no reason to use higher amounts of copper.

The Food and Nutrition Board of the U.S. National Academy of Sciences has recommended the following Dietary Reference Intakes (DRI) for copper. A summary of DRIs for various age groups is as follows:

DRI values (micrograms/day)

Infants	Adequate Intake (AI)
0-6 months	200
7-12 months	220

Children	Recommended Daily Allowance (RDA)
1-3 years	340
4-8 years	440

Boys	
9-13 years	700
14-18 years	890

Girls	
9-13 years	700
14-18 years	890

Men	
19-30 years	900
31-50 years	900
51-70 years	900
Older than 70 years	900

Women	
19-30 years	900
31-50 years	900
51-70 years	900
Older than 70 years	900

Pregnancy	
14-18 years	1,000
19-30 years	1,000
31-50 years	1,000

Lactation	
14-18 years	1,300
19-30 years	1,300
31-50 years	1,300

The following summarizes the Tolerable Upper Intake Level (UL) for various age groups and conditions:

Children	
1-3 years	1,000
4-8 years	3,000
9-13 years	5,000

Adolescents	
14-18 years	8,000

Adults	
19 years and older	10,000

Pregnancy	
14-18 years	8,000
19 years and older	10,000

Lactation	
14-18 years	8,000
19 years and older	10,000

The DV (Daily Value) for copper, which is used for determining percentage of nutrient daily values on nutritional supplement and food labels, is 2 mg. The basis for the DV for copper is the 1973 U.S. RDA.

LITERATURE

Fields M, Lewis CG. Starch diets high in iron can duplicate the severity of copper deficiency in rats fed fructose. *J Med Food.* 1998;1:193-199.

Harris ED. Cellular copper transport and metabolism. *Annu Rev Nutr.* 2000;20:291-310.

Harrison MD, Jones CE, Solioz M, et al. Intracellular copper routing: the role of copper chaperones. *Trends Biochem Sci.* 2000;25:29-32.

Institute of Medicine, Food and Nutrition Board. Dietary Reference Intakes for vitamin A, vitamin K, arsenic, boron, chromium, copper, iodine, iron, manganese, molybdenum, nickel, silicon, vanadium, and zinc. Washington, DC: National Academy Press, 2001.

Johnson WT, Thomas AC. Copper deprivation potentiates oxidative stress in HL-60 cell mitochondria. *Proc Soc Exp Biol Med.* 1999;221:147-152.

Klevay LM. Cardiovascular disease from copper deficiency—a history. *J Nutr.* 2000;130:489S-492S.

Klevay LM. Coronary heart disease: the zinc/copper hypothesis. *Am J Clin Nutr.* 1975;28:764-774.

Rayssiguier Y, Gueux E, Bussiere L, et al. Copper deficiency increases the susceptibility of lipoproteins and tissues to peroxidation in rats. *J Nutr.* 1993;123:1343-1348.

Rock E, Mazur A, O'Connor JM, et al. The effect of copper supplementation on red blood cell oxidizability and plasma antioxidants in middle-aged healthy volunteers. *Free Rad Biol Med.* 2000;28:324-329.

Saari JT, Sahuschke DA. Cardiovascular effects of dietary copper deficiency. *Biofactors.* 1999;10:359-375.

Toyama T, Kubuki Y, Suzuki M, et al. Copper deficiency anemia and neutropenia secondary to total gastrectomy. [Article in Japanese]. *Rinsho Ketsueki.* 2000;41:441-443.

Turnlund Jr. Copper. In: Shils ME, Olson JA, Shike M, Ross AC, eds. *Modern Nutrition in Health and Disease,* 9th ed. Baltimore, MD: Williams and Wilkins; 1999:241-252.

Waggoner DJ, Bartnikas TB, Gitlin JD. The role of copper in neurodegenerative disease. *Neurobiology of Disease.* 1999;6:221-230.

Creatine

DESCRIPTION

Creatine is a non-protein amino acid found in animals and, in much lesser amounts, plants. Creatine is synthesized in the kidney, liver and pancreas from the amino acids L-arginine, glycine and L-methionine. Following its biosynthesis, creatine is transported to the skeletal muscle, heart, brain and other tissues. Most of the creatine is metabolized in these tissues to phosphocreatine (creatine phosphate). Phosphocreatine is a major energy storage form in the body.

Creatine is known chemically as N-(aminoiminomethyl)-N-methyl glycine and its structural formula is:

$$HOOC-CH_2-N(CH_3)-C(=NH)-NH_2$$

Creatine

Supplemental creatine is typically a synthetic substance. It is a solid and is water-soluble.

ACTIONS AND PHARMACOLOGY

ACTIONS

Supplemental creatine may have an energy-generating action during anaerobic exercise and may also have neuroprotective and cardioprotective actions.

MECHANISM OF ACTION

Since the action of supplemental creatine has yet to be clarified, the mechanism of action is a matter of speculation. Much is known, however, about the biochemistry of endogenous creatine. Creatine is mainly synthesized in the kidney, liver and pancreas. In its synthesis, the guanidino group of L-arginine is transferred to glycine to form guanidinoacetate and ornithine by a transamidinase reaction, a reaction that takes place in the pancreas, liver and kidney. Guanidinoacetate is methylated by S-adenosylmethione (SAMe) to form creatine. About 1 to 2 grams of creatine are biosynthesized daily and another 1 to 2 grams are obtained from diet.

In muscle and nerve, most of the creatine is phosphorylated to phosphocreatine (PCr) in a reaction that is catalyzed by the enzyme creatine kinase (CK). There are three isoforms (isoenzymes) of CK. CK-MM is the skeletal muscle isoform; CK-BB, the brain isoform, and CK-MB, the isoform found in cardiac muscle. Most of the PCr in the body is in skeletal muscle.

Creatine, creatine kinase and phosphocreatine make up an intricate cellular energy buffering and transport system connecting sites of energy production in the mitochondria with sites of energy consumption. CK is a key enzyme involved in cellular energy homeostasis. It reversibly catalyzes the transfer of the high-energy phosphate bond in PCr to adenosine diphosphate (ADP) to form adenosine triphosphate (ATP), and it catalyzes the transfer of the high-energy phosphate bond in ATP to creatine to form PCr. During periods of intense exercise and skeletal muscle contraction, bioenergetic metabolism switches from one in which oxidative phosphorylation is the major pathway of ATP production to one in which so-called anaerobic glycolysis becomes dominant. Much less ATP would be generated during this period if it were not for phosphocreatine (PCr) being the only fuel available to regenerate ATP during this period. Thus the availability of PCr is the limiting factor of skeletal-muscle performance during high intensity and brief bursts (about 10 seconds) of activity. Supplemental creatine may increase PCr levels in skeletal muscle and hypothetically enhance ATP turnover during maximal exercise.

Creatine supplementation of transgenic amyotrophic lateral sclerosis (ALS) mice carrying the superoxide dismutase (SOD)1 mutation has reportedly produced improvement in motor performance and extension of survival, as well as protection against loss of both motor neurons and substantia nigra neurons. Mitochondrial dysfunction is among the earliest features found in these mice models of familial ALS. Creatine administration to these mice appears to stabilize mitochondrial CK and inhibits opening of the mitochondrial transition pores.

Creatine, as well as a creatine analogue called cyclocreatine, inhibit growth of a broad range of solid tumors in rat models of cancer; these tumors express high levels of CK. Although the mechanism of tumor inhibition is unknown, there is speculation about what it may be. Creatine feedback inhibits the transamidination step in its biosynthesis. This results in sparing L-arginine, the limiting precursor in creatine synthesis. More available L-arginine can lead to increased levels of nitric oxide (NO), which is a factor in macrophage activation. Another possibility is that glycolysis is inhibited in these tumors. Phosphocreatine inhibits enzymes in the glycolitic pathway, including glyceraldehyde-3-phosphate dehydrogenase, phosphofructokinase and pyruvate kinase.

PHARMACOKINETICS

Creatine is absorbed from the small intestine and enters the portal circulation and is transported to the liver. The ingested creatine, along with creatine made in the liver, is then transported into the systemic circulation and distributed to various tissues of the body, including muscle and nerves, by crossing the cell membrane via a specific creatine-transporter system against a 200:1 gradient. Chronic creatine supplementation in rats down-regulates creatine transporter protein expression. If this is also the case in humans, then chronic creatine supplementation would lead to lower amounts entering cells at any given time.

Within muscle and nerve cells, about 60 to 67% of the creatine entering the cells gets converted to phosphocreatine via the enzyme creatine kinase. About 2% of creatine is converted to creatinine, and both creatine and creatinine are excreted by the kidneys.

INDICATIONS AND USAGE

There is some evidence that supplemental creatine may enhance performance in a limited number of high-intensity, short-term physical activities, but the data are mixed, and no ergogenic effect has been convincingly demonstrated outside of laboratory settings. Adequate safety data are still lacking. There is some very preliminary data that creatine may be helpful in treating muscular dystrophy and amyotrophic lateral scleroses and may improve skeletal muscle function in some with congestive heart failure and gyrate atrophy of the retina. Creatine has inhibited the growth of some solid tumors in rats, but no human cancer data exist.

RESEARCH SUMMARY

Limited muscle function benefit has been noted in some early studies of creatine. All of these studies have been of short duration (mostly lasting one or two weeks and, in no case, more than eight weeks). Many other studies have found no benefit.

A recent review article summarized the results of 71 trials published between 1993 and 1997. Of those that studied effects of supplemental creatine (usually 20 grams daily for 4 to 21 days) on short term, high-intensity performance, 23 reported positive effects and 20 reported no effect. Studies examining the effects of creatine on oxidative energy systems, muscle isokinetic torque and isometric force produced similarly mixed results. Among the few field tests that have been conducted (all related to swim sprints) none detected any effect on athletic performance. Only among studies of cycle ergometer performance was there any superiority of creatine over placebo (11 trials reported improvement, while six others reported no improvement).

Since this review was published there have been a few more positive than negative reports, but, again, the positive effects are almost entirely seen in laboratory settings and are confined to short-term, high-intensity performance.

One author recently reviewed the creatine data and has concluded that supplemental creatine achieves an ergogenic effect, at least in the laboratory, in repeated stationary cycling sprints. But he found no convincing evidence that it does so in single sprints. He also discerned a possible ergogenic effect in weightlifting, but none in running or swimming sprints of any kind. He and others have speculated that the weight gain that typically accompanies creatine supplementation offsets any ergogenic effect that might otherwise benefit runners and swimmers.

Some have claimed that this weight gain, typically 0.5 to 1.6 kilograms occurring in the first few days to first two weeks of creatine supplementation, is evidence of increased muscle mass. Most researchers, however, believe that this weight gain is accounted for by creatine-induced water retention. The longer-term studies needed to confirm or refute claims that chronic creatine supplementation can result in greater muscle mass have not been conducted.

Another caveat offered by several researchers is that almost all of the positive creatine effects so far noted have been achieved in laboratory tests of elite athletes and were observed only in the sort of maximal intermittent exercise that non-athletes can rarely achieve. No benefit for any aerobic activity has been demonstrated.

In addition, safety data are lacking and are urgently needed, especially for long-term use of creatine and for use among the pediatric population (including adolescents) and among those in poor health. There are some reports that long-term use of creatine may be nephrotoxic. This needs further investigation before long-term creatine supplementation can be recommended under any circumstance.

Possible additional uses for creatine have been suggested by preliminary work. There is some evidence of creatine synthesis in the retina, and supplementation with 1.5 grams of creatine daily for a year has been reported to bring improvement in genetic gyrate atrophy—not in the blindness that results from this condition but in the skeletal muscle abnormalities that also characterize it. Giving 5 grams of creatine four times a day for a period of five days has similarly been reported to improve skeletal muscle function in some with congestive heart failure. The effect was small.

In a mouse model of amyotrophic lateral sclerosis (ALS), supplemental creatine significantly prolonged survival. Improvement was seen on motor-performance tests, and there was histologic evidence of neuron protection associated with creatine supplementation. Because creatine protected neurons in the substantia nigra, there is speculation that the supplement could also have positive effects in Parkinson's disease.

These researchers have suggested that creatine may exert the favorable results seen in the mouse model through an intracellular energy-buffering effect that may help prevent the sort of mitochondrial dysfunction that they postulate plays a role in neuronal cell death. More research is needed.

Another recent, preliminary report asserts a positive role for supplemental creatine in the treatment of muscular dystrophy and some other neuromuscular disorders. This study tested 10 grams of creatine daily for five days, followed by 5 grams daily for an additional 5 to7 days, against placebo. Increases were noted in handgrip, ankle and knee strength among those taking creatine. Again, more research is needed.

CONTRAINDICATIONS, PRECAUTIONS, ADVERSE REACTIONS

CONTRAINDICATIONS

Creatine is contraindicated in those with renal failure and renal disorders such as nephrotic syndrome and to those with known hypersensitivity to a creatine-containing product.

PRECAUTIONS

Creatine supplements should be avoided by children, adolescents, pregnant women, nursing mothers and anyone at risk for renal disorders such as diabetics. Those taking creatine should have serum creatinine levels monitored.

ADVERSE REACTIONS

The deaths of three American college wrestlers had been linked to the use of creatine supplements. However, results of post mortem tests led to the conclusion that the deaths were caused by severe dehydration and renal failure, and were not due to creatine. Apparently, the wrestlers were trying to lose enough weight through perspiration to allow them to compete in lower-weight classes. Typical adverse effects are gastrointestinal and include nausea, diarrhea and indigestion. Also common are muscle cramping and strains. Weight gain may occur from water retention. During a five day loading period, weight gains of 1.1 to 3.5 pounds have been reported. There are reports of elevated serum creatinine, a metabolite of creatine and a marker of kidney function, in some who take creatine and have normal renal function. This is reversible upon discontinuation of creatine.

Anecdotal reports of adverse events to FDA have included rash, dyspnea, vomiting, diarrhea, nervousness, anxiety, migraine, fatigue, polymyositis, myopathy, seizures and atrial fibrillation.

INTERACTIONS

There are as yet no known drug, nutritional supplement or herb interactions. Caffeine (in coffee, tea and caffeinated beverages) appears to interfere with any beneficial effects of creatine supplementation.

DOSAGE AND ADMINISTRATION

The typical form of creatine available is a creatine monohydrate powder.

The dosing for those who use creatine to attempt to improve performance in brief, high-intensity activities, is a loading dose of 20 grams or 0.3 grams per kilogram in divided doses four times a day for two to five days, followed by a maintenance dose of no more than 2 grams daily or 0.03 grams per kilogram. Those who use creatine supplements should take them with adequate water, six to eight glasses per day.

LITERATURE

Feldman EB. Creatine: a dietary supplement and ergogenic aid. *Nutr Rev.*1999; 57:45-50.

Greenhoff PL. Creatine and its application as an ergogenic aid. *Int J Sport Nutr.* 1995; 5:S100-S110.

Juhn MS. Oral creatine supplementation. *Phys Sports Med.* 1999; 27;47-45.

Klivenyi P, Ferrante RJ, Matthews RT, et al. Neuroprotective effects of creatine in a transgenic animal model of amyotrophic lateral sclerosis, *Nat Med.* 1999; 5:47-350.

Koshy KM, Griswald E, Sneeberger EE. Interstitial nephritis in a patient taking creatine. *N Engl J Med.* 1999; 340:814-815.

Miller EE, Evans AE, Cohn M. Inhibitions of rate of tumor growth by creatine and cyclocreatine. *Proc Natl Accd Sci USA.* 1993; 90:3304-3308.

Poortman JR, Augier H, Renaut V, et al. Effect of short-term creatine supplementation on renal responses in men. *Eur J Appl Physiol.* 1997; 76:566-567.

Sipila I, Rapola J, Simell O, et al. Supplemental creatine as a treatment for gyrate atrophy of the choroid and retina. *N Engl J Med.* 1981; 304:867-870.

Tarnopolsky M, Martin J. Creatine monohydrate increases strength in patients with neuromuscular disease. *Neurology.* 1999; 52:854-857.

Toler SM. Creatine is an ergogenic for anaerobic exercise. *Nutr Rev.* 1997; 55:21-23.

Vandenberghe K, Gillis N. Van Leemputte M, et al. Caffeine counteracts the ergogenic action of muscle creatine loading. *J Appl Physiol.* 1996; 80:452-457.

Williams MH, Branch JD. Creatine supplementation and exercise performance: an update. *J Am Coll Nutr.* 1998; 17:216-234.

Curcuminoids

DESCRIPTION

Curcuminoids are polyphenolic pigments found in the spice turmeric. The term turmeric is used both for the plant *Curcuma longa* L. and the spice derived from the rhizomes of the plant. The major curcuminoids are curcumin, demethoxycurcumin and bisdemethoxycurcumin. These substances comprise 3 to 6% of *Curcuma longa*. Curcumin makes up 70 to 75% of the curcuminoids, demethoxycurcumin 15 to 20% and bisdemethoxycurcumin about 3%.

Curcuma longa is a tropical plant native to south and southeast tropical Asia. It is a member of the ginger or *Zingiberaceae* family. Turmeric is widely consumed in the countries of origin for a variety of uses, including use as a dietary spice, as a dietary pigment and as an Indian folk medicine for the treatment of various illnesses. It is also used in Hindu religious ceremonies in one form or another as part of the religious rites.

Curcuminoids are responsible for the yellow color of turmeric, as well as the yellow color of curry.

Curcuminoids are derived from turmeric by extraction with ethanol. Curcumin is the most studied of the curcuminoids. In pure form, it is an orange-yellow, crystalline powder that is insoluble in water. It is also known as diferuloylmethane and turmeric yellow. Its chemical name is (*E, E*) —1, 7-bis(4-hydroxy-3- methoxyphenyl)-1,6-heptadiene-3, 5 dione. The molecular formula of curcumin is $C_{21}H_{20}O_6$, its molecular weight is 368.39 daltons, and its structural formula is:

Curcumin

Curcumin and the other curcuminoids have been found to have antioxidant and anti-inflammatory activities and have been entered into Phase I clinical trials for cancer chemoprevention by the National Cancer Institute.

ACTIONS AND PHARMACOLOGY

ACTIONS
Curcumin, demethoxycurcumin and bisdemethoxycurcumin have antioxidant activity. They may also have anticarcinogenic, anti-inflammatory, antiviral and hypocholesterolemic activities.

MECHANISM OF ACTION
The curcuminoids have been found to have a number of antioxidant activities, including scavenging of such reactive oxygen species as superoxide anions and hydrogen peroxide, inhibition of lipid peroxidation and inhibition of the oxidation of low-density lipoprotein (LDL). The reduced derivative of curcumin, tetrahydrocurcumin, has been found to have even stronger antioxidant activity. Tetrahydrocurcumin may be formed from curcumin following ingestion; however, this is unclear.

The possible anticarcinogenic activity of curcumin and the other curcuminoids may be accounted for by a few mechanisms. These include inhibition of angiogenesis, upregulation of apoptosis, interference with certain signal transduction pathways that are critical for cell growth and proliferation, inhibition of colonic mucosa cyclooxygenase (COX) and lipoxygenase (LOX) activities and inhibition of farnesyl protein transferase. In addition to its possible activity in preventing malignant transformation and inhibiting tumor growth, curcumin may have antimetastatic potential, as well. In this regard, curcumin has been found to inhibit matrix metalloproteinase-9 in a human hepatocellular carcinoma cell line. The possible anticarcinogenic activity of the curcuminoids may be attributed, at least in part, to their ability to inhibit activation of the transcription factors NF-KappaB and AP-1. Curcuminoids have also been found to target the fibroblast growth factor-2 (FGF-2) angiogenic signaling pathway and inhibit expression of gelatinase B in the angiogenic process.

In the final analysis, the curcuminoids' antioxidant activity may underlie many of the above mechanisms. Reactive oxygen species (ROS) can activate AP-1 and NF-KappaB. Further, FGF-2 induces AP-1 activation via ROS produced through NADPH oxidase. The curcuminoids, acting as antioxidants, may interfere with the ability of FGF-2 to stimulate AP-1, and they may generally inhibit the activation of NF-KappaB and AP-1.

The possible anti-inflammatory activity of the curcuminoids may also be accounted for by several mechanisms, including inhibition of COX and LOX, reduction of the release of ROS by stimulated neutrophils, inhibition of AP-1 and NF-KappaB, and inhibition of the activation of the pro-inflammatory cytokines TNF (tumor necrosis factor) -alpha and IL (interleukin)-1 beta.

Curcumin has modest anti HIV-1 activity. It has been found to inhibit HIV-1 and HIV-2 proteases, HIV-1 LTR (long terminal repeat)-directed gene expression, Tat-mediated transactivation of HIV-1-LTR and HIV-1 integrase. All of these actions have been demonstrated *in vitro*. There is no evidence that curcumin or the other curcuminoids significantly inhibit the replication of HIV-1 *in vivo*. The mechanism of the possible hypocholesterolemic effect of the curcuminoids is unclear.

PHARMACOKINETICS
The pharmacokinetics of the curcuminoids remains incompletely understood. Of the curcuminoids, curcumin has been most studied, mainly in animals. Curcumin is poorly absorbed following ingestion in mice and rats. In these animals, 38 to 75% of an ingested dose is excreted directly in the feces. Absorption appears to be better with food. In mice, the major metabolites of curcumin are curcumin glucuronoside, dihydrocurcumin glucuronoside, tetrahydrocurcumin glucuronoside and tetrahydrocurcumin. These metabolites

are formed in the liver. Animal studies and the pharmacokinetics of curcumin are continuing. Human pharmacokinetic studies are needed.

INDICATIONS AND USAGE

The curcuminoids may have anticarcinogenic, anti-atherosclerotic, anti-inflammatory (including anti-arthritic), antiviral, antifungal and immune-modulating effects. They appear to help detoxify some drugs and other chemicals. There is some evidence the curcuminoids may help prevent cataracts and ameliorate chronic anterior uveitis. They may also help speed wound healing. Claims that the curcuminoids may be helpful in gall bladder disease are poorly supported. There is emerging evidence that curcuminoids may be beneficial in the treatment of gastric inflammation, including ulcer and reflux esophagitis, in cystic fibrosis. It may also be neuroprotective and possibly of benefit in Alzheimer's disease and in some forms of depression. Indications for curcuminoids are likely to expand considerably in coming years as these substances are enjoying an explosion of research interest.

RESEARCH SUMMARY

The curcuminoids have exhibited significant anticarcinogenic effects in numerous *in vitro* and animal studies. They have inhibited progression of chemically induced colon and skin cancers through, it has been suggested, their ability to inhibit angiogenesis, among other possible mechanisms. In some of these studies, curcumin has reduced the size and number of tumors as well as the incidence of tumorigenesis. Curcumin appears to have significant inhibitory effects in both the promotional and progression stages of colon cancer.

In *in vitro* studies, curcumin has induced apoptosis in human leukemia cells, a variety of B lymphoma cells and others. It has been used topically *in vitro* and in some animal work to inhibit some skin cancers.

Turmeric, the activity of which may be due to constituents in addition to, or other than, the curcuminoids, has been used in various parts of the world to treat everything from abdominal bloating and flatulence to gonorrhea and hepatitis. Evidence in support of these uses is largely anecdotal. The German commission E, however, has approved turmeric for the treatment of liver and gall bladder disorders and for appetite loss.

Turmeric, administered in 1-gram doses daily for nine months, reportedly conferred significant protection against palatal cancer in a study of subjects at risk of this malignancy owing to reverse smoking. Significant regression of precancerous lesions was noted. Curcumin has also been reported to diminish the toxic effects of a number of cancer drugs and other chemicals, including cisplatin, doxorubicin, carbon tetrachloride, paraquat and ethanol. This work has

been conducted using animals. Marked neuroprotective, hepatoprotective and pulmonary-protective effects have been seen.

In one study, curcumin significantly reduced the total amount of chromosomal damage in nontumor cells of rats given cisplatin. This effect was attributed to curcumin's free radical-scavenging activity. Similarly, curcumin was shown to significantly prevent the nephrotoxicity of doxorubicin in rats.

Research in recent years has continued to support a role for curcuminoids in the treatment/prevention of some cancers. One of the many recent reviews of the rapidly expanding curcuminoid research around the world found evidence in recent trials of curcuminoid activity against several cancers and cancer precursor conditions. In a small clinical trial, supplementation with 480 mg of curcumin and 20 mg of quercetin three times daily for six months significantly decreased the number and size of familial adematous polyps in patients suffering from this autosomal-dominant polyposis disorder. These polyps, which often lead to colorectal cancer, were diminished in number by 60% and in size by about 50%. In a recent Phase II trial in subjects with advanced pancreatic cancer, 8 grams of oral curcumin daily resulted in some favorable biological activity. This dose was well tolerated. Prior work by this and other groups had shown both *in vitro* and *in vivo* animal activity by curcumin against pancreatic cell lines and animal models of this highly treatment-resistant cancer. Antitumor activity was noted in two of the 21 subjects evaluated. One subject had a 73% tumor reduction. The researchers suggested that a liposomal encapsulated form of curcumin, with greater bioavailability, might yield still better results.

Chemoprevention trials of curcumin in hepatocellular carcinoma, gastric cancer and colon cancer are ongoing in Japan. In the U.S., a variety of trials are underway or planned to investigate possible curcuminoid activity against a number of other cancers. Other research is further elucidating the modes of action through which the curcuminoids exert their anticancer effects. Another recent review discusses data showing curcuminoid activity against leukemia and lymphoma, gastrointestinal cancers, genitourinary cancers, breast cancer, ovarian cancer, head and neck squamous cell carcinoma, lung cancer, melanoma, neurological cancers and sarcoma—mostly in non-clinical or clinical pilot studies.

The anti-inflammatory properties of the curcuminoids have been demonstrated in a number of *in vitro* and in some animal studies. These substances are widely used in India and Indonesia for various inflammatory conditions. *In vitro*, curcumin inhibits the production of such pro-inflammatory cytokines as tumor necrosis factor-alpha (TNF-alpha), interleukin-1 beta (IL-1 beta) and interleukin-8, among other anti-inflammatory actions.

Some preliminary evidence that one or more constituents of turmeric may be helpful in some forms of arthritis has emerged from a few animal studies and some human work. Curcumin itself was administered to rheumatoid arthritis patients (400 milligrams of curcumin three times a day for a total daily dose of 1,200 milligrams) for two weeks in a randomized, double-blind, crossover study. Significant subjective improvement was reported in terms of morning stiffness, walking time and joint swelling. No significant improvement was observed, however, in any objective measurement. Some have suggested that curcuminoids might be helpful in osteoarthritis, but there is no supporting evidence.

The anti-inflammatory properties of the curcuminoids continue to become more evident. These substances have been found to be effective in two rare inflammatory diseases—chronic anterior uveitis (CAU) and idiopathic inflammatory orbital pseudotumors (IIOT). Oral doses of 375 mg of curcumin three times a day for 12 weeks in CAU subjects resulted in improvement and reduced recurrence rates. In a small study with five IIOT patients, four recovered completely on a dose of curcumin (again, 375 mg three times daily), this time for 6-22 months. There were no recurrences. There is also the suggestion from one study that the curcuminoids might benefit some patients with psoriasis. In a partially blinded, randomized pilot study, one or two tablets of a standardized turmeric extract daily for eight weeks resulted in significantly diminished symptoms of irritable bowel syndrome. Clinical pilot studies have demonstrated positive effects from curcuminoids in the treatment of Crohn's disease and ulcerative colitis. Animal studies show positive effects in ameliorating gastric esophageal reflux disease (GERD). In a rat model of reflux esophagitis, curcumin was more effective than the proton pump inhibitor lansoprazole in inhibiting mixed reflux of gastroduodenal contents. Mixed reflux is said to inflict more free radical damage in esophageal mucosa than pure acid reflux does. Curcumin has also exerted antiulcerogenic effects in animal models.

In a mouse model of cystic fibrosis, curcumin administered by oral gavage enjoyed dramatically increased survival. This has caused some excitement in the research world due to the progressive and ultimately fatal course of this inherited disorder characterized by, among other things, breathing difficulties and respiratory infections. The exact mechanism by which curcumin appears to help correct defects in the mutant gene encoding for cystic fibrosis is unknown. Clinical trials have been called for, are needed and are warranted.

Another area of growing interest relates to the possible neuroprotective effects of the curcuminoids. It has been shown that curcumin can bind beta-amyloids and thus reduce plaque burdens associated with cognitive dysfunction, including Alzheimer's disease. In a recent large population-based study, 1,010 elderly Asian individuals without diagnosed dementia were placed in several categories, depending upon how much curry, rich in curcumin, they consumed. Those with higher consumption levels scored better than those with lower levels on the Mini-Mental State Examination (MMSE). The MMSE is an often used, established test of cognitive function. Studies are ongoing to try to determine whether curcumin can be clinically effective.

One recent study found very preliminary evidence of an antidepressive effect in an animal depression model.

Claims that the curcuminoids may have anti-atherosclerotic effects are supported by some preliminary animal studies. Curcumin has shown some antithrombotic, anti-platelet aggregating activity in some *in vitro* and animal studies. It has also inhibited vascular smooth muscle cell proliferation *in vitro*. A turmeric extract was recently shown to significantly inhibit LDL-cholesterol oxidation in rabbits with experimental atherosclerosis.

The curcuminoids have demonstrated antiviral, anti-fungal and immunomodulating effects, mostly *in vitro*. Curcumin has been described as having HIV-1-inhibiting effects *in vitro*. In a clinical trial of curcumin in 40 subjects with HIV-1 infection, however, the substance was ineffective in reducing viral load or increasing CD4 counts. The low bioavailability of curcumin may account, in part, for its lack of *in vivo* antiviral activity. There is no credible clinical data to support claims that curcumin is helpful in those with hepatitis C. Some of the curcuminoids and turmeric extracts have exhibited some *in vitro* anti-fungal activity, specifically against *Candida albicans, Candida kruseii* and *Candida parapsilosis*. Recently, curcumin was shown to have various immunomodulating effects *in vitro*, which the researchers concluded might indicate some therapeutic potential for curcumin in T helper 1(Th1)-mediated immune diseases. Research is ongoing.

It was demonstrated in an animal study that naphthalene-initiated cataracts can be significantly prevented by curcumin. Naphthalene-initiated cataract is used as a model for studying senile human cataract. The study showed for the first time that these experimental cataracts are associated with apoptosis of lens epithelial cells and that curcumin prevents some of the apoptotic activity.

Finally, curcumin has enhanced cutaneous wound-healing in diabetic mice. Previous studies showed that curcumin could enhance cutaneous wound-healing in rats and guinea pigs. Both oral and topical curcumin were effective in the diabetic mice. Earlier re-epithelialization and improved neovascularization were among the healing processes observed in curcumin-treated animals. The researchers concluded that curcumin might be of benefit in helping to overcome diabetic-impaired healing processes.

CONTRAINDICATIONS, PRECAUTIONS, ADVERSE REACTIONS

CONTRAINDICATIONS

Curcuminoids should be avoided by those hypersensitive to any component of a curcuminoid-containing supplement.

Curcuminoids may stimulate bile production in some. The volatile oil of turmeric is thought to be responsible for the bile-stimulating activity of turmeric, but this has not been conclusively established. Therefore, curcuminoids are contraindicated in those with bile duct obstructions and those with gallstones.

PRECAUTIONS

Pregnant women and nursing mothers should avoid curcuminoid supplementation.

Those with gastroesophageal reflux disease (GERD) and those with a history of peptic ulcer disease should exercise caution in the use of curcuminoid supplements.

Curcuminoids may have antithrombotic activity in some. Therefore, those on warfarin or anti-platelet drugs should exercise caution in their use. Cancer patients should only use curcuminoid supplements under medical supervision.

Curcuminoid supplements must be taken with food. Curcuminoids may cause gastric irritation and ulceration if taken on an empty stomach.

ADVERSE REACTIONS

Adverse reactions of supplements principally comprised of curcuminoids are mainly gastrointestinal and include epigastric distress and nausea. There is one report of transient giddiness following curcuminoid ingestion. Abnormal liver tests have been reported in rats but not humans, and transient hypotension has been reported in dogs but, again, not in humans.

Curcuminoids may cause gastritis and peptic ulcer disease if taken without food.

INTERACTIONS

DRUGS

Chemotherapeutic agents: In animal studies, curcumin was found to enhance the antitumor effect of cisplatin against fibrosarcoma. It was also found to decrease the clastogenic effect of cisplatin. Also in animal studies, curcumin was found to decrease the nephrotoxicity due to doxorubicin and to decrease chromosomal aberrations due to bleomycin.

Anti-platelet drugs: Curcuminoids may enhance the action of anti-platelet drugs.

Warfarin: Curcuminoids may enhance the anticoagulant effect of warfarin.

NUTRITIONAL SUPPLEMENTS

Bromelain: Bromelain (see Bromelain) is reputed to enhance the absorption of curcuminoids. However, there is no credible documentation of this.

Piperine: Piperine (see Piperine) may enhance the absorption of curcuminoids.

DOSAGE AND ADMINISTRATION

Curcuminoid supplements are available that contain curcumin at 70 to 75%, demethoxycurcumin at 15 to 20% and bisdemethoxycumin at about 3%. Doses used range from 500 to 4000 milligrams daily, and they are taken with meals.

Curcuminoids taken on an empty stomach may cause gastric distress.

LITERATURE

Anand P, Sundaram C, Jhurani S, et al. Curcumin and cancer: an "old-age" disease with an "age-old" solution. *Cancer Lett.* 2008;267(1):133-164.

Antunes LMG, Araújo MCP, Darin JD, et al. Effects of the antioxidants curcumin and vitamin C on cisplatin-induced clastogenesis in Wistar rat bone marrow cells. *Mutat Res.* 2000;465:131-137.

Arbiser JL, Klauber N, Rohan R, et al. Curcumin is an in vivo inhibitor of angiogenesis. *Mol Med.* 1998;4:376-383.

Barthelmy S, Vergnes L, Moynier M, et al. Curcumin and curcumin derivatives inhibit Tat-mediated transactivation of type 1 human immunodeficiency virus long terminal repeat. *Res Virol.* 1998;149:43-52.

Bharti AC, Donato N, Singh S, et al. Curcumin (diferuloylmethane) down-regulates the constitutive activation of nuclear factor-kappa B and IkappaBalpha kinase in human multiple myeloma cells, leading to suppression of proliferation and induction of apoptosis. *Blood.* 2003;101(3):1053-1062.

Chan MM-Y. Inhibition of tumor necrosis factor by curcumin, a phytochemical. *Biochem Pharmacol.* 1995;49:1551-1556.

Dhillon N, Aggarwal BB, Newman RA, et al. Phase II trial of curcumin in patients with advanced pancreatic cancer. *Clin Cancer Res.* 2008;14(14):4491-4499.

Egan ME, Pearson M, Weiner SA, et al. Curcumin, a major constituent of turmeric, corrects cystic fibrosis defects. *Science.* 2004;304(5670):600-602.

Goel A, Kunnumakkara AB, Aggarwal BB. Curcumin as "Curecumin": from kitchen to clinic. *Biochem Pharmacol.* 2008;75(4):787-809.

Hellinger JA, Cohen CJ, Dugan ME, et al. Phase I/II randomized, open-label study of oral curcumin safety, and antiviral effects on HIV-RT PCR in HIV+ individuals. *Third Conference on Retroviruses and Opportunistic Infections.* Washington, DC; 1996:Abstract #140.

Huang MT, Newmark HL, Fenkel K. Inhibitory effects of curcumin on tumorigenesis in mice. *J Cell Biochem Suppl.* 1997;27:26-34.

Kang BY, Song YJ, Kim KM, et al. Curcumin inhibits Th1 cytokine profile in CD4+ T cells by suppressing interleukin-12 production in macrophages. *BR J Pharmacol.* 1999;128:380-384.

Kawamori T, Lubet R, Steele VE, et al. Chemopreventive effect of curcumin, a naturally occurring anti-inflammatory agent, during the promotion/progression stages of colon cancer. *Cancer Res.* 1999;59:597-601.

Khopde SM, Priyadarsini KI, Guha SN, et al. Inhibition of radiation-induced lipid peroxidation by tetrahydrocurcumin: possible mechanisms by pulse radiolysis. *Biosci Biotechnol Biochem.* 2000;64:503-509.

Kulkarni SK, Bhutani MK, Bishnoi M. Antidepressant activity of curcumin: involvement of serotonin and dopamine system. *Psychopharmacology* (Berl). Epub: 2008 Sep 3.

Kulkarni AP, Ghebremariam YT, Kotwal GJ. Curcumin inhibits the classical and the alternate pathways of complement activation. *Ann N Y Acad Sci.* 2005;1056:100-112.

Kuo ML, Huang TS, Lin JK. Curcumin, an antioxidant and anti-tumor promoter, induces apoptosis in human leukemia cells. *Biochim Biophys Acta.* 1996;1317:95-100.

Li M, Zhang Z, Hill DL, et al. Curcumin, a dietary component, has anticancer, chemosensitization, and radiosensitization effects by down-regulating the MDM2 oncogene through the PI3K/mTOR/ETS2 pathway. *Cancer Res.* 2007;67(5):1988-1996.

Liu Y, Dargusch R, Maher P, et al. A broadly neuroprotective derivative of curcumin. *J Neurochem.* 2008;105(4):1336-1145.

Mazumder A, Raghavan K, Weinstein J, et al. Inhibition of human immunodeficiency virus type-1 integrase by curcumin. *Biochem Pharmacol.* 1995;49:1165-1170.

Mohan R, Sivak J, Ashton P, et al. Curcuminoids inhibit the angiogenic response stimulated by fibroblast growth factor-2, including expression of matrix metalloproteinase gelatinase B. *J Biol Chem.* 2000;275:10405-10412.

Pan M-H, Huang T-M, Lin J-K. Biotransformation of curcumin through reduction and glucuronidation in mice. *Drug Metab Disp.* 1999;27:486-494.

Pandya U, Saini MK, Jin GF, et al. Dietary curcumin prevents ocular toxicity of naphthalene in rats. *Toxicol Lett.* 2000;115:195-204.

Pari L, Tewas D, Eckel J. Role of curcumin in health and disease. *Arch Physiol Biochem.* 2008;114(2):127-149.

Park EJ, Jeon CH, Ko G, et al. Protective effect of curcumin in rat liver injury induced by carbon tetrachloride. *J Pharm Pharmacol.* 2000;52:437-440.

Ramiré z-Tortosa MC, Mesa MD, Aguilera MC, et al. Oral administration of a turmeric extract inhibits LDL oxidation and has hypocholesterolemic effects in rabbits with experimental atherosclerosis. *Atherosclerosis.* 1999;147:371-378.

Ringman JM, Frautschy SA, Cole GM, et al. A potential role of the curry spice curcumin in Alzheimer's disease. *Curr Alzheimer Res.* 2005;2(2):131-136.

Sidhu GS, Mani H, Gaddipati JP, et al. Curcumin enhances wound healing in streptozotocin induced diabetic rats and genetically diabetic mice. *Wound Rep Reg.* 1999;7:362-374.

Strimpakos AS, Sharma RA. Curcumin: preventive and therapeutic properties in laboratory studies and clinical trials. *Antioxid Redox Signal.* 2008;10(3):511-545.

Tsvetkov P, Asher G, Reiss V, et al. Inhibition of NAD(P)H:quinone oxidoreductase 1 activity and induction of p53 degradation by the natural phenolic compound curcumin. *Proc Natl Acad Sci U S A.* 2005;102(15):5535-5540.

Venkatesan N. Pulmonary protective effects of curcumin against paraquat toxicity. *Life Sci.* 2000;66:PL21-PL28.

Venkatesan N, Punithavathi D, Arumugam V. Curcumin prevents adriamycin nephrotoxicity in rats. *Br J Pharmacol.* 2000;129:231-234.

Zeitlin P. Can curcumin cure cystic fibrosis? *N Engl J Med.* 2004;351(6):606-608.

Zhang F, Altorki NK, Mestre JR, et al. Curcumin inhibits cyclooxygenase-2 transcription in bile acid-and phorbol ester-treated human gastrointestinal epithelial cells. *Carcinogenesis.* 1999;20:445-451.

D-Glucarate

DESCRIPTION

D-glucarate is the anionic form of D-glucaric acid, a dicarboxylic sugar acid derived from the oxidation of D-gluconic acid. It is naturally found in some vegetables and fruits, including cruciferous vegetables, bean sprouts and apples. D-glucarate may have cancer-chemopreventive activity.

D-glucarate is also known as D-saccharate. D-glucarate, in the form of its calcium salt, calcium D-glucarate, is marketed as a nutritional supplement. The molecular formula of calcium D-glucarate is $C_6H_8C_9O_8$, and its molecular weight is 248.20 daltons.

ACTIONS AND PHARMACOLOGY

MECHANISM OF ACTION

The mechanism of D-glucarate's possible anticarcinogenic activity is not entirely clear. One possibility is the inhibition of beta-glucuronidase via the D-glucarate derivative D-glucaro-1, 4-lactone (1, 4-GL). A major mechanism for the detoxification of certain carcinogens is via glucuronidation, which is catalyzed by glucuronyl transferase. The glucuronide conjugates are excreted in the urine and bile. However, deconjugation can occur via the enzyme beta-glucuronidase. Inhibition of beta-glucuronidase prevents deconjugation. D-glucarate may have anticarcinogenic activity independent of 1, 4-GL. D-glucarate has been demonstrated to inhibit protein kinase, and this is a possible mechanism for a direct anticarcinogenic effect of the substance.

D-glucarate has been shown to lower cholesterol in rats. The mechanism of this effect is unknown.

PHARMACOKINETICS

There is little on the pharmacokinetics of D-glucarate in humans. Rat studies indicate that D-glucarate is converted to 1, 4-GL in the stomach. 1, 4-GL, again in rats, appears to be absorbed, transported by the blood to various tissues and excreted in the urine and, to a lesser extent, in the bile. Calcium-D-glucarate is claimed to be a sustained or slow release precursor of 1, 4-GL, but there are few human data to substantiate this.

INDICATIONS AND USAGE

Animal and *in vitro* work suggest that D-glucarate may have some anticancer and lipid-lowering effects. Clinical data, however, are lacking.

RESEARCH SUMMARY

D-glucarate has exhibited significant anticarcinogenic effects in numerous *in vitro* and animal experiments. It has shown some efficacy when used alone or in combination with some other putative anticancer substances, notably some of the retinoids. It has shown preventive and therapeutic activity against a number of cancers, including mammary, liver, prostate and colon cancer. There is evidence it may protect against a number of chemical carcinogens.

In one experiment, D-glucarate was found to be particularly effective in inhibiting chemically induced cancer in animals when fed during the promotional phase of carcinogenesis, but it was also effective when fed during the initiation phase. A more recent study also found that D-glucarate seems to be most effective in the post-initiation phases of cancer, as assessed, in this study by its inhibiting effects on carcinogen-induced aberrant crypt foci in the colons of rats. Research is ongoing.

Data related to claims that D-glucarate is an effective lipid-lowering agent are not as plentiful as the cancer data. Some animal data, however, suggest that D-glucarate may reduce total cholesterol and LDL-cholesterol. It does not appear to affect HDL-cholesterol. More research is needed.

CONTRAINDICATIONS, PRECAUTIONS, ADVERSE REACTIONS

CONTRAINDICATIONS

D-glucarate is contraindicated in those hypersensitive to any component of a D-glucarate-containing product.

PRECAUTIONS

Pregnant women and nursing mothers should avoid D-glucarate supplementation pending long-term safety studies.

INTERACTIONS

DRUGS

Retinoids: D-glucarate has shown synergistic chemopreventive effects with retinoids in some tumor models.

5-Fluorouracil: D-glucarate and 5-fluorouracil exhibited synergistic antitumor activity in a rat-tumor model.

DOSAGE AND ADMINISTRATION

D-glucarate is available in supplemental form as calcium-D-glucarate. A usual dose is 200 mg once or twice daily.

LITERATURE

Abou-Issa H, Moeschberger M, el-Masry W, et al. Relative efficacy of glucarate on the initiation and promotion phases of rat mammary carcinogenesis. *Anticancer Res.* 1995; 15:805-810.

Curley RW Jr, Humphries KA, Koolemans-Beyman A, et al. Activity of D-glucarate analogues: synergistic antiproliferative effects with retinoid in cultured human mammary tumor cells appear to specifically require the D-glucarate structure. *Life Sci.* 1994; 54:1299-1303.

Dwivedi C, Heck WJ, Downie AA, et al. Effect of calcium glucarate on beta-glucuronidase activity and glucarate content of certain vegetables and fruits. *Biochem Med Metab Biol.* 1990; 43:83-92.

Heerdt AS, Young CW, Borgen PI. Calcium glucarate as a chemopreventive agent in breast cancer. *Isr J Med Sci.* 1995; 31:101-105.

Oredipe OA, Barth RF, Dwivedi C, Webb TE. Dietary glucarate-mediated inhibition of initiation of diethylnitrosamine-induced hepatocarcinogenesis. *Toxicology.* 1992; 74:209-222.

Schmittgen TD, Koolesmans-Beynen A, Webb TE, et al. Effects of 5-fluorouracil, leucovorin, and glucarate in rat colon-tumor explants. *Cancer Chemother Pharmacol.* 1992; 30:25-30.

Walaszek A, Szemraj J, Hanausek M, et al. D-glucaric acid content of various fruits and vegetables and cholesterol-lowering effects of dietary D-glucarate in the rat. *Nutr Res.* 1996; 16:673-682.

Walaszek Z. Potential use of D-glucaric acid derivatives in cancer prevention. *Cancer Lett.* 1990; 54:1-8.

Walaszek Z, Szemraj J, Narog M, et al. Metabolism, uptake, and excretion of D-glucaric acid salt and its potential use in cancer prevention. *Cancer Detect Prev.* 1997; 21:178-190.

D-Ribose

DESCRIPTION

D-ribose is a naturally occurring five-carbon sugar found in all living cells, as well as in RNA-containing viruses. It is not an essential nutrient, since it can be made in the body from other substances, such as glucose. D-ribose, however, is very essential for life. Some of the most important biological molecules contain D-ribose, including ATP (adenosine triphosphate), all the nucleotides and nucleotide coenzymes and all forms of RNA (ribonucleic acid). D-ribose, in the form of ribonucleoside diphosphates, is converted to deoxyribonucleoside diphosphates, precursor molecules for DNA. D-ribose in RNA and D-deoxyribose in DNA may be considered genetic sugars.

Since D-ribose is ubiquitous in living matter, it is ingested in our diets. Such nutritional substances as brewers yeast are rich in RNA and are thus rich sources of D-ribose. Some recent research suggests that supraphysiological amounts of this sugar may have cardioprotective effects, particularly for the ischemic heart.

D-ribose is a sweet, solid, water-soluble substance that is also known as alpha-D-ribofuranoside. L-ribose does not have biological activity. D-ribose is sometimes referred to as just ribose. Supplemental D-ribose is produced from the fermentation of corn syrup. D-ribose has the following structural formula:

D-ribose

ACTIONS AND PHARMACOLOGY

ACTIONS

Supplemental D-ribose may have metabolic cardioprotective activity. It may also enhance *de novo* purine biosynthesis.

MECHANISM OF ACTION

Following a cardiac ischemic event, ATP levels in the heart decline rapidly and are slow to rebound. 5-Phosphoribosyl 1-pyrophosphate (PRPP) is a key intermediate in the *de novo* and salvage pathways of purine nucleotide formation, as well as a key intermediate in synthesis of pyrimidine nucleotides. PRPP is the biochemically activated form of D-ribose and is synthesized from D-ribose-5-phosphate, which is produced in the oxidative pentose phosphate pathway (PPP). The limiting step in the PPP is the glucose-6-phosphate dehydrogenase (G-6-PD) reaction. The G-6-PD reaction can be bypassed with D-ribose. In supraphysiological amounts, D-ribose may serve as a precursor to PRPP, which then allows for *de novo* synthesis of purine nucleotides, including ATP. D-ribose infusion has been shown to significantly enhance the recovery of energy levels in the post-ischemic myocardium in animal models.

PHARMACOKINETICS

About 88% to 100% of an oral dose of D-ribose, up to 200 milligrams per kilogram per hour, is absorbed from the small intestine, from whence it is distributed to various tissues of the body, including cardiac muscle and skeletal muscle. Very little first-pass metabolism occurs in the liver. Following transport into cells, D-ribose is phosphorylated to D-ribose-5-phosphate. D-ribose-5-phosphate is metabolized via a number of pathways, including the pentose phosphate pathway and glycolytic pathway. Its metabolism is complex. It is also metabolized to PRPP, which is the precursor to purine nucleotides, as well as L-histidine and pyrimidine nucleotides. Those receiving very high doses of D-ribose excrete a small fraction of the administered dose unchanged in the urine.

INDICATIONS AND USAGE

D-ribose may have some protective effects in cardiac ischemia. Claims that it is an effective "energizer" and exercise-performance enhancer are not substantiated by credible evidence. D-ribose may also be beneficial in some rare genetic diseases, such as adenylosuccinase deficiency and myoadenylade deaminase deficiency.

RESEARCH SUMMARY

In a study of 20 men (aged 45 to 69 years) with documented severe coronary artery disease and a history of angina induced by normal daily activities, 60 grams of ribose (in four doses of 15 grams each) were tested against placebo. Treated subjects exhibited improvement as measured electrocardiographically, and time to onset of moderate angina (during exercise testing) increased significantly in those ribose-treated subjects. There was no significant electrocardiograph improvement in the placebo group, and there was no significant difference between the groups in time to onset of moderate angina. The authors concluded: "In patients with CAD, administration of ribose by mouth for three days improved the heart's tolerance to ischemia. The presumed effects on cardiac energy metabolism offer new possibilities for adjunctive medical treatment of myocardial ischemia."

Claims that supplemental ribose is an energy booster and exercise/athletic-performance enhancer are unfounded. Studies sometimes cited in support of these claims fall far short of being substantiating. It has been shown that administration of ribose in patients with myoadenylate deaminase deficiency disease can reduce cramping and stiffness caused by exercise. On the other hand, in a double-blind, placebo-controlled crossover trial of ribose in McArdle's disease, 60 grams of ribose daily for seven days failed to improve exercise tolerance in these subjects. Finally, there is one case report of a patient with adenylosuccinate deficiency whose neurological symptoms (behavior and seizure frequency) improved with supplemental D-ribose.

CONTRAINDICATIONS, PRECAUTIONS, ADVERSE REACTIONS

CONTRAINDICATIONS

Known hypersensitivity to a D-ribose-containing product.

PRECAUTIONS

Pregnant women and nursing mothers should avoid supplemental D-ribose.

Supplemental D-ribose may cause hypoglycemia and elevation in uric acid levels. Those with gout should avoid supplemental D-ribose, and those with elevated uric acid levels and hypoglycemics should exercise extreme caution in its use. Those with diabetes should also exercise extreme caution in its use. And those diabetics who decide to try D-ribose must be under a physician's supervision and have their blood glucose levels closely monitored and their antidiabetic medications appropriately adjusted, if necessary.

ADVERSE REACTIONS

Reported adverse reactions include hypoglycemia, hyperuricemia, hyperuricosuria, diarrhea, nausea and headache.

INTERACTIONS

Antidiabetic drugs: D-ribose may cause hypoglycemia. Diabetics who use D-ribose must have their blood glucose levels closely monitored and their antidiabetic medicines appropriately adjusted, if necessary.

OVERDOSAGE

No reports of overdosage.

DOSAGE AND ADMINISTRATION

No typical dosage. Most experimental studies with ribose used very high doses, usually about 60 grams daily.

LITERATURE

Gross M, Dormann B, Zollner N. Ribose administration during exercise: effects on substrates and products of energy metabolism in healthy subjects and a patient with myoadenylate deaminase deficiency. *Klin Wochenschr.* 1991; 69:151-155.

Priml W, von Arnim T, Stablein A, et al. Effects of ribose on exercise-induced ischaemia in stable coronary artery disease. *Lancet.* 1992; 340:507-510.

Salerno C, D'Eufermia P, Finocchiaro R, et al. Effect of D-ribose on purine synthesis and neurological symptoms in a patient with adenylsuccinase deficiency. *Biochim Biophys Acta.* 1999; 1453:135-140.

Steele IC, Patterson VH, Nicholls DP. A double-blind, placebo-controlled, crossover trial of D-ribose in McArdle's disease. *J Neurol Sci.* 1996; 136:174-177.

Tullson PC, Terjung RL. Adenine nucleotide synthesis in exercising and endurance-trained skeletal muscle. *Am J Physiol.* 1991; 261:C342-C347.

Zimmer HG. The oxidative pentose phosphate pathway in the heart: regulation, physiological significance and clinical implications. *Basic Res Cardiol.* 1992; 87:3003-316.

Zimmer HG. Regulation of and intervention into the oxidative pentose phosphate pathway and adenine nucleotide metabolism in the heart. *Mol Cell Biochem.* 1996; 160/161:101-109.

Zimmer HG. Significance of the 5-phosphoribosyl-1-pyrophosphate pool for cardiac purine and pyrimidine nucleotide synthesis: studies with ribose, adenine, inosine, and orotic acid in rats. *Cardiovasc Drugs Ther.* 1998; 12 Suppl 2:179-187.

Zollner N, Reiter S, Gross M, et al. Myoadenylate deaminase deficiency: successful symptomatic therapy by high dose oral administration of ribose. *Klin Wochenschr.* 1986; 64:1281-1290.

Daidzein

DESCRIPTION

Daidzein belongs to the isoflavone class of flavonoids. It is also classified as a phytoestrogen since it is a plant-derived nonsteroidal compound that possesses estrogen-like biological activity. Daidzein has been found to have both weak estrogenic and weak anti-estrogenic effects.

Daidzein is the aglycone (aglucon) of daidzin. The isoflavone is found naturally as the glycoside daidzin and as the glycosides 6″-O-malonylgenistin and 6″-O-acetyldaidzin. Daidzein and its glycosides are mainly found in legumes, such as soybeans and chickpeas. Soybeans and soy foods are the major dietary sources of these substances. Daidzein glycosides are the second most abundant isoflavones in soybeans and soy foods; genistein glycosides are the most abundant. Nonfermented soy foods, such as tofu, contain daidzein, principally in its glycoside forms. Fermented soy foods, such as tempeh and miso, contain significant levels of the aglycone.

Daidzein and daidzin are also found in *Radix puerariae* (RP). RP is an herbal medicine prepared from the root of the legume *Pueraria lobata,* commonly known as kudzu. RP has been used for centuries in traditional Chinese medicine for the treatment of a wide range of disorders. It has also been used in traditional Chinese medicine since 600 AD for its "anti-drunkenness" effect and is still used by traditional Chinese physicians for the treatment of those who abuse alcohol. It is thought that the antidipsotropic (anti-drinking) effect of RP is due to daidzein and daidzin.

Daidzein is a solid substance that is virtually insoluble in water. Its molecular formula is $C_{15}H_{10}O_4$, and its molecular weight is 254.24 daltons. Daidzein is also known as 7-

hydroxy-3- (4-hydroxyphenyl)-4*H*-1-benzopyran-4-one and 4′, 7-dihydroxyisoflavone. Daidzin, which has greater water solubility than daidzein, is the 7-beta glucoside of daidzein. The structural formula of daidzein is:

Daidzein

When marketed as a nutritional supplement, daidzein is mainly present in the form of its beta-glucoside, daidzin.

See also Soy Isoflavones and Equol.

ACTIONS AND PHARMACOLOGY

ACTIONS
Daidzein may have estrogenic, antiestrogenic and antioxidant activities. It may also have antidipsotropic, anticarcinogenic, anti-atherogenic and anti-osteoporotic activity.

MECHANISM OF ACTION
Daidzein has weak estrogenic activity as measured *in vivo* and *in vitro* assays. *In vivo,* its estrogenic activity is the lowest of the soy isoflavones.

Daidzein is a scavenger of reactive oxygen species. Genistein is the most studied of the soy isoflavones with regard to antioxidant activity. It is thought that genistein may be a more potent antioxidant than daidzein. There are few studies comparing the antioxidant activity of the two isoflavones.

The proposed mechanism of daidzein's possible antidipsotropic activity is as follows. Daidzein inhibits the class I isoenzymes of human alcohol dehydrogenase (ADH), especially the gamma-type ADH. Inhibition of human class I ADH may suppress ethanol consumption by increasing the bioavailability of ingested ethanol. Daidzin is an inhibitor of human mitochondrial aldehyde dehydrogenase (ALDH)-2. Inhibition of ALDH-2 could also suppress ethanol consumption by increasing the bioavailability of ingested ethanol. Finally, daidzin has been found to inhibit the metabolism of serotonin via its inhibition of ALDH-2. This inhibition is accompanied by a concomitant accumulation of 5-hydroxy-indole-3-acetaldehyde (S-HIAL) and 3, 4-dihydroxyphenyla-cetaldehyde (DOPAL). 5-HIAL and DOPAL may be involved in mediating the possible antidipsotropic action of daidzein. In contrast to the broad-acting ALDH inhibitor disulfiram, daidzein/daidzin does not appear to block acetaldehyde metabolism.

The mechanism of daidzein's possible anticarcinogenic activity, as well as its possible anti-atherogenic activity, is

unclear. Daidzein's weak estrogenic effect may play some role in the possible activity of soy isoflavones against prostate cancer. Likewise, daidzein's weak estrogenic effect, as well as its possible antioxidant activity, may contribute to its possible anti-atherogenic activity.

Daidzein's weak estrogenic effect may also be involved in its possible anti-osteoporotic activity. Daidzein has been found to have an anabolic effect in an osteoblastic cell line in culture, suggesting that it may be able to stimulate osteoblastic bone formation. Also, the major metabolite of the synthetic isoflavone ipriflavone is daidzein. Ipriflavone has demonstrated a significant ability to prevent osteoporosis in both animal models and humans.

PHARMACOKINETICS
The pharmacokinetics of daidzein in humans is complex and not well understood. Pharmacokinetics of daidzein and daidzin are available from animal models, and some inferences can be made. The aglycone daidzein may be absorbed from the small intestine from whence it is transported to the systemic circulation by the lymphatics. There is little information available on the tissue distribution of daidzein. That which is delivered to the liver mainly undergoes conjugation with glucuronate and sulfate via hepatic phase II enzymes (UDP-glucuronosyltransferases and sulfotransferases). The glucoronide and sulfate conjugates of daidzein are excreted in the urine and in the bile. The daidzein conjugates may be deconjugated to release daidzein, which may be reabsorbed via the enterohepatic circulation.

Most of ingested daidzin, the major dietary and supplemental form of daidzein, is delivered to the large intestine intact. In the large intestine, bacterial beta-glucosidases hydrolyze daidzin to daidzein. Daidzein is either absorbed and processed as described above or further metabolized in the large intestine to dihydrodaidzein, which is then metabolized to equol or O-desmethylangolensin.

There is considerable individual variation in the absorption and metabolism of ingested daidzein and daidzin. The extent of absorption of the daidzein beta-glucoside daidzin is also unclear.

In addition to the above, and to make the pharmacokinetics even more complex, about 20 to 35% of the adult population forms equol from daidzin, the so-called equol producers. See Equol.

INDICATIONS AND USAGE
Daidzein, like the other soy isoflavones, may have some anticancer and anti-atherogenic effects. It may also help to suppress "hot flashes" in some menopausal women and may help prevent osteoporosis. Preliminary animal work suggests

that it might help curb ethanol intake in those who are alcohol-dependent.

RESEARCH SUMMARY

It has been demonstrated that daidzein can promote bone formation and mineralization *in vitro*. A recent study found that daidzein, but not other phytoestrogens, including genistein, preserved bone architecture in ovariectomized female rats *in vivo*. Human trials are needed and warranted. It also appears to share the anti-atherogenic and anticancer properties of the other soy isoflavones. Some of these effects may be due to the conversion, by equol producers, of daidzein to equol in the large intestine. (See Soy Isoflavones, Equol, Glycitein and Genistein.)

Daidzein has been shown to suppress free-choice ethanol intake in Syrian Golden hamsters. *Radix puerariae,* a herb rich in daidzein and daidzin, the 7-glucoside of daidzein, has long been used in traditional Chinese medicine to treat those who are alcohol-dependent. Both daidzein and daidzin themselves were effective in significantly reducing ethanol intake by more than 50% in hamsters dependent on alcohol. The treatment did not significantly affect body weight, water or food intake.

More recent work has confirmed that daidzin, which is the major delivery form of daidzein, successfully and significantly suppresses ethanol intake in all rodent models tested. A recent study showed that daidzin inhibits serotonin and dopamine metabolism in isolated mitochondria. The researchers involved in this study believe this inhibition may be one of the mechanisms by which this soy isoflavone suppresses ethanol intake. Clinical testing is needed to evaluate the possible benefits of daidzein/daidzin in human dipsomaniacs.

CONTRAINDICATIONS, PRECAUTIONS, ADVERSE REACTIONS

CONTRAINDICATIONS

Daidzein is contraindicated in those who are hypersensitive to any component of a daidzin- or daidzein-containing product.

PRECAUTIONS

Pregnant women and nursing mothers should avoid the use of daidzein/daidzin-containing supplements pending long-term safety studies.

Men with prostate cancer should discuss the advisability of the use of daidzein/daidzin-containing supplements with their physicians before deciding to use them.

Women with estrogen receptor-positive tumors should exercise caution in the use of daidzein/dadzin-containing supplements and should only use them if they are recommended and monitored by a physician.

INTERACTIONS

Ethanol: Daidzein/daidzin may increase the bioavailability of ingested ethanol.

OVERDOSAGE

There are no reports of overdosage.

DOSAGE AND ADMINISTRATION

Daidzein is available in a few different isoflavone formulas. A standard soy isoflavone formula contains daidzein principally in the form of daidzin, as well as genistin and glycitin, with much smaller amounts of the aglycones daidzein, genistein and glycitein. The percentages of the soy isoflavones present in such a supplement reflect the percentages of these substances as found in soybeans and are: daidzin, about 38%; genistin, about 50%; and glycitin, about 12%. A 50-mg dose of soy isoflavone supplement—a typical daily dose—delivers 19 mg of daidzin, 25 mg of genistin and about 6 mg of glycitin. Usually, 40% of the formula is comprised of soy isoflavones. Therefore, to get a dose of 50 mg of soy isoflavones, 125 mg of the soy preparation are required.

Smaller amounts of daidzein in the aglycone form are available in some red clover preparations (see Biochanin A).

LITERATURE

Keung WM, Lazo O, Kunze L, et al. Daidzin suppresses ethanol consumption by Syrian golden hamsters without blocking acetaldehyde metabolism. *Proc Natl Acad Sci USA.* 1995;92:8990-8993.

Keung WM, Lazo O, Kunze L, et al. Potentiation of the bioavailability of daidzin by an extract of *Radix puerariae. Proc Natl Acad Sci USA.* 1996;93:4284-4288.

Keung WM, Vallee BL. Daidzin and daidzein suppress free-choice ethanol intake by Syrian Golden hamsters. *Proc Natl Acad Sci USA.* 1993;90:10008-10012.

Keung WM, Vallee BL. Daidzin and its antidipsotropic analogs inhibit serotonin and dopamine metabolism in isolated mitochondria. *Proc Natl Acad Sci USA.* 1998;95:2198-2203.

Lo FH, Mak NK, Leung KN. Studies on the anti-tumor activities of the soy isoflavone daidzein on murine neuroblastoma cells. *Biomed Pharmacother.* 2007;61(9):591-595.

Mao Z, Zheng YL, Zhang YQ, et al. The anti-apoptosis effects of daidzein in the brain of D-galactose treated mice. *Molecules.* 2007;12(7):1455-1470.

Raimondi S, Roncaglia L, De Lucia M, et al. Bioconversion of soy isoflavones daidzin and daidzein by Bifidobacterium strains. *Appl Microbiol Biotechnol.* Epub: 2008 Sep 27.

Somjen D, Katzburg S, Kohen F, et al. Daidzein but not other phytoestrogens preserves bone architecture in ovariectomized female rats in vivo. *J Cell Biochem.* 2008;103(6):1826-1832.

Sugimoto E, Yamaguchi M. Stimulatory effect of daidzein in osteoblastic MC3T3-E1 cells. *Biochem Pharmacol.* 2000;59:471-475.

For additional references, see Soy Isoflavones.

Deanol

DESCRIPTION

Deanol or dimethylaminoethanol is presently marketed as a dietary supplement, but at one time it was used as a drug for the treatment of hyperactivity in children and was also used for such conditions as neuroleptic-induced tardive dyskinesia. Deanol was thought to affect tardive dyskinesia because it was believed to be a cholinergic precursor and to enhance acetylcholine synthesis in the brain. It is now known that, although deanol is a precursor to choline, very little of the choline formed from it is converted to acetylcholine in the brain.

Deanol or dimethylaminoethanol is also known as 2-(dimethylamino)ethanol, beta-dimethylaminoethyl alcohol and N, N-dimethyl-2-hydroxy ethylamine. It is abbreviated DMAE. When deanol was on the market as a drug, it was called Deaner and was in the form of deanol acetamidobenzoate. Deanol is itself a liquid. The most common form of deanol supplement is deanol bitartrate.

Another deanol-containing substance, deanol 4-chlorphenoxyacetate hydrochloride or centrophenoxine hydrochloride, is used in Europe, Japan, Australia and Mexico as a cognition enhancer in the elderly.

ACTIONS AND PHARMACOLOGY

ACTIONS

Deanol may increase choline levels.

MECHANISM OF ACTION

Deanol is a precursor to choline.

PHARMACOKINETICS

There is limited information on the pharmacokinetics of deanol in humans. Deanol is absorbed from the small intestine from whence it is transported to the liver where much of it is metabolized to choline. Very little of this choline appears to be converted to acetylcholine in the brain. In fact, it is reported that deanol inhibits the uptake of choline into the brain. Deanol also appears to inhibit the oxidation of choline to betaine and may inhibit other reactions of choline metabolism.

INDICATIONS AND USAGE

Results with deanol in the treatment of tardive dyskinesia are mostly negative. Claims that deanol is helpful in Alzheimer's disease, age-related cognitive deficits and in aging itself are without foundation.

RESEARCH SUMMARY

Given the assumption that deanol is an acetylcholine precursor and that it might thus enhance the cholinergic neurotransmitter system, deanol has been used in numerous trials investigating it as a possible treatment for tardive dyskinesia. The results have been mixed but mostly negative. A recent meta-analysis showed that it is no more effective than placebo in this disorder.

Deanol has similarly been shown to have no significant effect in the treatment of Alzheimer's disease, amnesic disorders, age-related cognitive impairment and Tourette's syndrome. Effects on aging in animal models have been contradictory; one study showed decreased life span.

CONTRAINDICATIONS, PRECAUTIONS, ADVERSE REACTIONS

CONTRAINDICATIONS

Known hypersensitivity to a deanol-containing product.

PRECAUTIONS

Deanol should be avoided by pregnant women and nursing mothers. Those with elevated homocysteine should avoid deanol.

ADVERSE REACTIONS

Reported adverse reactions include headache, cramps, constipation, insomnia and the induction of lucid dreams. There is one report of a subject who was treated for 10 years with deanol for essential tremor who developed a marked dyskinesia syndrome affecting predominantly orofacial and respiratrory musculature. This was partially reversed upon discontinuation of deanol.

DOSAGE AND ADMINISTRATION

Deanol is available as a liquid or as deanol bitartrate. Typical doses are 100 milligrams daily.

LITERATURE

Andriamampandry C, Freysz L, Kanfer JN, et al. Conversion of ethanolamine, monomethylethanolamine and dimethylethanolamine to choline-containing compounds by neurons in culture and by the rat brain. *Biochem J.* 1989; 264:555-562.

Cherkin A, Exhardt MJ. Effects of dimethylaminoethanol upon life-span and behavior of aged Japanese quail. *J Geront.* 1977; 32:38-45.

de Montigny C, Chouinard G, Annable L. Ineffectiveness of deanol in tardive dyskinesia: a placebo-controlled study. *Psychopharmacology.* 1979; 65:219-223.

Fisman M, Mersky H, Holmes H. Double-blind trial of 2-dimethylaminoethanol in Alzheimer's disease. *Am J Psychiatry.* 1981; 138:970-972.

Haubrich DR, Gerber NH, Pflueger AB. Deanol affects choline metabolism in peripheral tissues of mice. *J Neurochem.* 1981; 37:476-482.

Jope RS, Jenden DJ. Dimethylaminoethanol (deanol) metabolism in rat brain and its effect on acetylcholine synthesis. *J Pharamacol Exp Ther.* 1979; 211:472-479.

Millington WR, Mc Call AL, Wurtman RJ. Deanol acetamidobenzoate inhibits the blood-brain barrier transport of choline. *Ann Neurol.* 1978; 4:302-306.

Penovich P, Morgan JP, Kerzner B, et al. Double-blind evaluation of deanol in tardive dyskinesia. *JAMA.* 1978; 239:1997-1998.

Sergio W. Use of DMAE (dimethylaminoethanol) in the induction of lucid dreams. *Med Hypotheses.* 1988; 26:255-257.

Soares KV, McGrath JJ. The treatment of tardive dyskinesia—a systematic review and meta-analysis. *Schizophr Res.* 1999; 39:1-16.

Zahniser NR, Chou D, Hanin I. Is 2-dimethylaminoethanol (deanol) indeed a precursor of brain acetylcholine? A gas chromotographic evaluation. *J Pharmacol Exp Ther.* 1977; 200:545-549.

Deglycyrrhizinated Licorice (DGL)

DESCRIPTION

Deglycyrrhizinated licorice, commonly abbreviated DGL, is an extract of the root of true licorice, *Glycyrrhiza glabra*, which has significantly reduced mineralocorticoid activity. Licorice has a number of medicinal properties, including peptic ulcer healing, anti-inflammatory, antimicrobial and antioxidant activities. Glycyrrhizinic acid and its metabolite, glycyrrhetinic acid, have mineralocorticoid-like, as well as testosterone-reducing, activities. The use of licorice for the management of peptic ulcer disease is associated with hypertension, water retension and hypokalemia. The removal of most of the glycyrrhizinic and glycyrrhetinic acids yields a product without these undesirable effects.

ACTIONS AND PHARMACOLOGY

ACTIONS
DGL may have peptic ulcer-healing activity.

MECHANISM OF ACTION
The mechanism of action of the peptic ulcer-healing activity of DGL is not entirely understood. DGL was found to stimulate and/or accelerate the differentiation of glandular cells in the forestomach of the rat, as well as stimulate mucus formation and secretion. The stimulation of mucus secretion in the stomach is believed to account, at least in part, for the activity of DGL. DGL contains some flavonoids that have antimicrobial activity, including activity against the ulcer-causing bacterium *Helicobacter pylori*. This too could account, at least in part, for DGL's activity. New substances are continually being discovered in licorice, and it is possible that some of these may also play a role in DGL's activity.

PHARMACOKINETICS
There is very little known about the pharmacokinetics of DGL.

INDICATIONS AND USAGE
DGL has been shown to be useful in the management of gastric and duodenal ulcers.

RESEARCH SUMMARY
Several studies in animals and humans have demonstrated positive effects from the use of DGL in gastric and duodenal ulcer conditions. DGL, administered in chewable doses of 760 milligrams a day for one month, was significantly superior to placebo in reducing peptic ulcer size and in hastening healing in human subjects, compared with the placebo control subjects. DGL produced complete healing in 44% of those receiving it, compared with complete healing in 6% of controls.

Subsequent studies have shown that DGL is about as effective as cimetidine and ranitidine for both treatment and maintenance therapy of gastric ulcers. Comparison studies have not been made with DGL and famotidine, lansoprazole, omeprazole and other more recent anti-ulcer drugs.

DGL appears to confer significant protection against the gastric mucosal damage caused by aspirin and other nonsteroidal anti-inflammatory drugs. Gastric bleeding induced by aspirin intake can also be reduced with DGL supplementation.

DGL has also demonstrated significant efficacy in the treatment of duodenal ulcers. In one study, 40 patients who had suffered from severe duodenal ulcers for four to 12 years (and who had experienced more than six relapses in the previous year) were treated with either 3 grams of DGL daily for eight weeks or with 4.5 grams daily for 16 weeks. All showed significant improvement, but more improvement was seen with the higher-dose regimen. None of the patients required surgery during a one-year follow-up period. In other research, DGL had a therapeutic effect in duodenal ulcers equal to that of cimetidine.

DGL's protective activity is attributed by some to its ability to stimulate the formation and secretion of mucus. It has been shown, in rats, to stimulate epithelial proliferation in the forestomach. More recently, it has been demonstrated that several flavonoids that are present in DGL can inhibit *Helicobacter pylori* growth.

CONTRAINDICATIONS, PRECAUTIONS, ADVERSE REACTIONS

CONTRAINDICATIONS
Known hypersensitivity to a DGL-containing product.

PRECAUTIONS

Because of lack of long-term safety studies, DGL should be avoided by children, pregnant women and nursing mothers.

Those with hypertension, congestive heart failure, arrhythmias, water retention and low potassium and/or magnesium levels should discuss the use of DGL with their physicians and should be certain that any DGL they use is free of glycyrrhizinic acid.

ADVERSE REACTIONS

There are significant adverse effects with licorice extracts containing glycyrrhizinic and glycyrrhetinic acid when used for the management of peptic ulcer disease, including hypokalemia, hypomagnesemia, hypertension, headache, cardiac arrhythmias, water retention and congestive heart failure. DGL, however, should be free of these side effects. There are occasional reports of gastrointestinal side effects, such as diarrhea and nausea.

INTERACTIONS

The excretion rate of nitrofurantoin was found to be significantly higher in patients receiving the drug along with DGL. No interactions with drugs used in the treatment of peptic ulcer disease are known.

OVERDOSAGE

There are no reports of overdosage with DGL.

DOSAGE AND ADMINISTRATION

In Europe, Canada and South Africa, DGL is available as a medicinal preparation called Caved-S. In the U.S., DGL is available as a nutritional supplement in the form of chewable tablets. Typically, those who use DGL for management of peptic ulcer disorders chew from one to four 380-milligram tablets or the equivalent before each meal.

LITERATURE

Armanini D, Bonanni G, Palermo M. Reduction of serum testosterone in men by licorice. *N Engl J Med.* 1999; 341:1158.

Balackrishnan V, Pillai MV, Raveendran PM, Nair CS. Deglycyrrhizinated liquorice in the treatment of chronic duodenal ulcer. *J Assoc Physicians India.* 1978; 26:811-814.

Bardham KD, Cumberland DC, Dixon RA, Holdsworth CD. Proceedings: deglycyrrhizinated liquorice in gastric ulcer: a double-blind controlled study. *Gut.* 1976; 17:397

Beil W, Birkholz C, Sewing KF. Effects of flavonoids on parietal cell acid secretion, gastric mucosal prostaglandin production and *Helicobactee pylori* growth. *Arzneimittelforschung.* 1995; 45:697-700.

Bennett A, Clark-Wibberley T, Stamford IF, Wright JE. Aspirin-induced gastric mucosal damage in rats: cimetidine and deglycyrrhizinated liquorice together give greater protection than low doses of either drug alone. *J Pharm Pharmacol.* 1980; 32:151.

Dalta R, Rao SR, Murthy KJ. Excretion studies of nitrofurantoin and nitrofurantoin with deglycyrrhizinated liquorice. *Indian J Physiol Pharmacol.* 1981; 25:59-63.

Farese Jr RV, Biglieri EJ, Shackleton CHL, et al. Licorice-induced hypermineralocorticoidism. *N Engl J Med.* 1991; 325:1223-1227.

Glick L. Deglycyrrhizinated liquorice for peptic ulcer. *Lancet* 1982; 2:817.

Li W, Asada Y, Yoshikawa T. Antimicrobial compounds from *Glycyrrhiza glabra* hairy root cultures. *Planta Med.* 1998; 64:746-747.

Morgan AG, McAdam WA, Pascoo C, Darnborough A. Comparison between cimetidine and Caved-S in the treatment of gastric ulceration and subsequent maintenance therapy. *Gut.* 1982; 23:545-551.

Morgan AG, Pacsoo C, McAdam WA. Comparison between ranitidine and ranitidine plus Caved-S in the treatment of gastric ulceration. *Gut.* 1985; 26:1377-1379.

Morgan AG, Pacsoo C, McAdam WA. Maintenance therapy: a two year comparison between Caved-S and cimetidine treatment in the prevention of symptomatic gastric ulcer recurrence. *Gut.* 1985; 26:599-602.

Rees WD, Rhodes J, Wright JE, et al. Effect of deglycyrrhizinated liquorice on gastric mucosal damage by aspirin. *Scand J Gastroenterol.* 1979; 14:605-607.

Stewart PM, Wallace AM, Vallentino R, et al. Mineralocorticoid activity of liquorice: 11-beta-hydroxysteroid dehyrdogenase deficiency comes of age. *Lancet.* 1987; 2:821-824.

van Marle J, Aarsen PN, Lind A, van Weeren-Kramer, J. Deglycyrrhizinated liquorice (DGL) and the renewal of rat stomach epithelium. *Eur J Pharmacol.* 1981; 72:219-225.

DHEA (Dehydroepiandrosterone)

DESCRIPTION

Dehydroepiandrosterone, commonly abbreviated as DHEA, is a natural substance produced in the adrenal glands, gonads and in the brain. DHEA is a steroid prohormone and a precursor for both androgens and estrogens. DHEA and its metabolite dehydroepiandrosterone-3-sulfate, or DHEAS, are the major secretory steroidal products of the adrenal gland and the most abundant circulating steroids in the human adult. The ratio of DHEAS to DHEA in serum is approximately 300:1 to 500:1, and the concentration of DHEAS in the serum is approximately 20 times higher than that of any other steroid hormone. It is noteworthy that the mean concentration of DHEAS in serum decreases progressively from a peak at age 25 to less than 20% of that peak before the age of 70. Further, DHEAS serum levels are typically low in those with chronic diseases, such as cancer and AIDS. While DHEA levels follow a circadian rhythm with a peak in the morning, DHEAS levels are relatively stable throughout the day and therefore are used as a marker for DHEA levels and adrenal androgen secretion.

To date, the unique physiological roles of DHEA and DHEAS remain largely unknown.

DHEA is synthesized in the adrenal cortex in the region known as the zona reticularis. It is produced from cholesterol. Pregnenolone and 17-hydroxy pregnenolone are intermediates, and oxygen and cytochrome P450a17 are involved in the pathway. DHEA itself has weak androgenic activity. It is metabolized in the adrenal gland to other androgenic substances, including androstenediol, androstenedione and testosterone. It is also metabolized to the estrogens, estrone and estradiol. DHEA is converted to DHEAS via a reversible biochemical reaction. DHEA and DHEAS have also been found in the brain, and there appears to be synthetic pathways to their production present in the nervous system. Neurosteroids are steroids that accumulate in the nervous system independently, at least in part, of supply produced by the steroidogenic endocrine glands. These can be synthesized *de novo* in the nervous system from sterol precursors. DHEA and DHEAS in the nervous system are classified as neurosteroids. Neurosteroids include 3-alpha-hydroxy compounds (e.g. pregnenolone, DHEA and DHEAS) and metabolites of progesterone. The expression of the enzyme P450c17 and the biosynthesis of DHEA have been found to interact by way of a tripartite contribution of astrocytes, oligodendrocytes, and neurons. DHEA and DHEAS act as modulators of the gamma-aminobutyric acid type A receptor and of the N-methyl-D-aspartate receptor and may have memory-enhancing, anxiolytic and sleep-inducing (rapid eye movement or REM sleep) properties.

DHEA and DHEAS are being developed by some biotechnology companies as possible pharmaceuticals. Prestara, a synthetic form of DHEA, is an orphan drug for the prevention of loss of bone mineral density in systemic lupus erythematosus (SLE) patients on glucocorticoids. DHEA is also being developed as a possible treatment for systemic lupus erythematosus. Injectable DHEAS is being developed for the possible treatment of acute asthmatic attacks and severe burns. Injectable DHEA is being developed to help preserve neuronal and myocardial tissue from the harmful effects of ischemia/reperfusion injury associated with heart attacks, stroke and cardiovascular surgery. Whether these drugs will prove to be safe and effective and be marketed remains to be seen.

DHEA is known as dehydroepiandrosterone and prasterone. DHEAS is known as dehydroepiandrosterone sulfate, dehydroepiandrosterone-3-sulfate and prasterone sulfate. DHEA has the following structural formula:

DHEA
(Dehydroepiandrosterone)

DHEA can be synthesized in the laboratory from the steroid sapogenin diosgenin, which is extracted from the tubers of the *Dioscorea* wild yam plants, such as cabeza de negro and barbasco. Much of supplemental DHEA is produced in this manner. In fact, these Mexican wild yam extracts served as the starting points for the synthesis of the components of the oral contraceptive pill (OCP).

Extracts of the wild yam plants *Dioscorea mexicana*, *Dioscorea villosa* or other *Dioscorea* species are not converted to DHEA following their ingestion. Information that markets wild yam as "natural DHEA" is inaccurate.

ACTIONS AND PHARMACOLOGY

ACTIONS

Oral DHEA has weak androgenic activity. DHEA and DHEAS have several putative actions, including anti-inflammatory, anticancer, antiobesity, antidiabetogenic, immunomodulating, memory-enhancing and antiaging.

MECHANISM OF ACTION

Some of the reported effects of oral DHEA may be due to its weak androgenic activity and to the fact that it is metabolized to androstenedione which, in turn, is metabolized to androgens and estrogens. The observed benefits of DHEA in post-menopausal women, for example, may be accounted for by this weak androgenic activity. Administration of DHEA in physiologic doses increases androgens in women, but not in men. Circulating estrogens are increased in both men and women.

DHEA is an inhibitory modulator of the gamma-aminobutyric acid-benzodiazepine receptor complex in rats, and DHEA enhances the effect of excitatory amino acids on the NMDA receptors, also in rats. How this relates to any effect of oral DHEA in humans is entirely speculative.

The decline in the human immune system that occurs with aging is known as immunosenescence. Although not the only factor, an increased cortisol/DHEA ratio appears to be a contributing factor to immunosenescence. The two adrenal steroid hormones appear to have opposing effects on immune function. In general, cortisol is an immunosuppressant, while DHEA enhances immune function. Supplementation with DHEA in the elderly may be beneficial to immune function, although human clinical studies are needed to confirm this. Again, this is speculative.

With aging, several changes occur in inflammatory signaling pathways and in the various inflammatory mediators. These changes have been associated with a number of different degenerative diseases, including cardiovascular disease and neurodegenerative diseases. It has been speculated that DHEA and DHEAS may be able to modulate some of these changes. It has been reported that treatment of human aortic endothelial cells with DHEAS dramatically inhibited the tumor necrosis factor-alpha (TNF-alpha)-induced activation of the major inflammatory transcription factor NF-kappaB and also increased levels of the NF-kappaB inhibitor IkappaB-alpha. It was thought that the peroxisome proliferator-activated receptor alpha (PPAR-alpha) was involved with the inhibition.

In another study, DHEAS, but not DHEA, has been reported to induce peroxisome gene expression via the activation of the PPAR-alpha. Therefore, DHEAS may serve as an important endogenous regulator of hepatic PPAR-alpha-mediated pathways, which maintain lipid homeostasis and prevent the decline in cellular PPAR-alpha expression during aging. There is some evidence that in aging men and women, DHEAS levels are negatively correlated with serum concentrations of the inflammatory cytokine interleukin-6 (IL-6). The increase in IL-6 production during aging might be related to decreased DHEAS secretion. Administration of DHEAS to aging animals has been found to activate PPAR-alpha and reverse the proinflammatory effects of IL-6. Human clinical trials are needed to determine if DHEAS and DHEA have anti-inflammatory activity, and, if they do, by what mechanism. There are some ongoing human studies on the effect of DHEA in systemic lupus erythematosus (SLE), but all of the results are not yet in.

PHARMACOKINETICS

DHEA is absorbed from the small intestine and is transported to the liver, where it is metabolized mainly to DHEAS by the enzyme sulfotransferase. DHEA and DHEAS are distributed to the various tissues in the body where metabolites, including androstenedione, testosterone, estrogens (estrone and estradiol), androstenediol and 7-oxo-DHEA, are synthesized. There is great individual variability in the metabolism

of oral DHEA. Excretion of DHEA and its metabolites is primarily via the urinary route.

INDICATIONS AND USAGE

Regarded as a drug by many researchers, a controlled drug in the United Kingdom and a prescription drug in Canada, the use of DHEA as a supplement is not indicated for the treatment or prevention of any condition without qualified medical recommendation and monitoring. The best available research suggests that DHEA, particularly at the high doses many have reported are being used, poses potentially serious health risks.

There is some evidence that DHEA, in monitored doses in selected subjects, may be of some help in easing some of the symptoms of systemic lupus erythematosus (SLE), may enhance immune response in some others and may be indicated in some women with adrenal insufficiency. There is very preliminary evidence that DHEA can have a positive impact on mood and memory. DHEA replacement after menopause has been proposed.

There is no credible evidence that DHEA can burn fat and build lean muscle mass, that it can boost sexual performance or that it can fight cancer, heart disease, fatigue, diabetes, osteoporosis and aging itself.

RESEARCH SUMMARY

Recent research has raised hopes that DHEA may provide some benefit to those with systemic lupus erythematosus (SLE). Studies, both completed and underway, indicate that DHEA, at dose levels that most researchers regard as risky for the general population, enabled some lupus patients to reduce their reliance on prednisone while still achieving equivalent relief from pain, fatigue and inflammation.

In vitro and animal studies have shown that DHEA can inhibit the cytokine molecular signaling that directs release of some of the inflammatory substances implicated in lupus. A synthesized DHEA product called Prestara is currently being tested as a drug for treatment of lupus.

DHEA may have other useful immune-modulating properties. In some studies of immune function in older humans, DHEA has boosted natural killer (NK)-cell activity and has dampened immune-damaging interleukin-6 activity. It has also increased levels of circulating insulin-like growth factor-1 and, when given concomitantly with influenza vaccine, it has boosted antibody titers in an elderly subgroup with particularly low levels of DHEA to begin with. It did not have similar effects when combined with tetanus vaccine. More study is needed to see whether DHEA might be an effective vaccine adjuvant.

DHEA's use in adrenal insufficiency was tested recently in a double-blind study of 24 women with this disorder who were randomized to receive either placebo or 50 milligrams of oral DHEA daily for four months. These subjects were all DHEA-deficient at baseline. Treatment with DHEA normalized serum concentrations of DHEA, androstenedione and testosterone. Researchers noted a significant correlation between DHEA supplementation and overall "well-being." DHEA-treated women were said to be significantly less depressed and anxious, compared with controls. Sexual thoughts and interest were also found to significantly increase.

Some androgenic effects were observed in this study, but only one subject had to be given a reduced dose of DHEA for this reason. The researchers noted, however, that lower doses in general might be required in the longer-term studies that will be needed to confirm the findings of this preliminary study. They cautioned that DHEA should be used only with medical supervision and carefully monitored to see whether it initiates or promotes breast or prostatic cancer.

In a few aged and severely depressed subjects with diminished baseline DHEA, supplemental DHEA (30 milligrams to 90 milligrams orally each day for four weeks) produced significant improvement. This open-label study involved only six subjects, but some other equally preliminary research, largely confined to animal models, similarly suggests that supplemental DHEA, in some subgroups, might elevate mood and improve age-related declines in memory. One study, however, in which subjects took 100 milligrams of DHEA daily for six months, found no mood-elevating effects. There is no evidence at this time that DHEA is useful in Alzheimer's disease. Recently the DHEA and Well-Ness (DAWN) trial involving 110 men and 115 women aged 55 to 85 concluded that DHEA supplementation has no benefit on cognitive performance or well-being in healthy older adults and stated that "it should not be recommended for that purpose in the general population." This placebo-controlled study used six cognitive function tests. Previous cognitive DHEA tests showed mixed, mostly neutral results; a few showed negative DHEA effects on cognition. In one test, DHEA supplementation was associated with significant impairment on a visual memory recall test. In another test, no DHEA effect was noted on cognition in 46 men aged 62 to 76 during three months of DHEA supplementation.

It has been proposed that DHEA be used (much as estrogen replacement therapy is used) in post-menopausal women to compensate for endogenous age-related and menopause-accelerated declines in DHEA. A dose of 50 milligrams daily has been suggested for this purpose, but there are no clinical trials demonstrating that this regimen would either be effective or safe long-term. It has been noted that DHEA can bring estrogen levels in postmenopausal women to levels equal to that observed in standard hormone-replacement therapy. This may prove risky inasmuch as it has been shown that taking estrogen without concomitant use of progesterone is an established risk factor for uterine cancer.

A number of positive effects have been seen in some DHEA-treated animal models but usually at doses that are considered dangerous in humans. Additionally, these studies have been short-term for the most part, and animal models are considered by many researchers to be poor predictors of human effects since these animals, unlike humans, have little endogenous DHEA and do not exhibit the kind of age-related DHEA declines that are found in humans.

There is no convincing evidence that DHEA boosts sexual performance, retards aging in general or fights cancer and osteoporosis, or that it builds muscle. After 12 weeks of supplementation with DHEA, no improvement was noted in muscle strength in ambulatory myotonic dystrophy type 1 patients. There is one recent study involving old female rats in which DHEA supplementation may have favorably affected insulin sensitivity and may have induced some weight loss. There is also some recent evidence in animal work indicating that DHEA might inhibit chronic hypoxic pulmonary artery hypertension via its effects on smooth muscle cells. Another recent study found an association between lower DHEA plasma levels and risk of impaired endothelial function in postmenopausal women with coronary artery risk factors. There is no evidence, however, that supplementation with DHEA can safely or effectively diminish this risk.

Several studies have failed to find any benefit from DHEA in breast cancer. On the contrary, two studies have found an association between higher levels of DHEA and higher incidence of breast cancer.

Another study has found no correlation between bone density and DHEA levels.

A 19-year follow-up study of nearly 2,000 people reported only a modest decrease in cardiac risk for men and a slight, nonsignificant increase in risk for women associated with DHEA levels. Some small studies have shown that DHEA can inhibit platelet aggregation. But other studies have also shown that supplemental DHEA can lower levels of HDL-cholesterol in some women.

A report in 1988 that high-dose DHEA could favorably affect lipids and induce weight loss in young males was not confirmed in two subsequent trials. In another trial, using the same 1,600-milligram daily dosage of DHEA used in the 1988 study but this time in women, there was, again, no weight loss. The women subjects suffered androgenic effects and developed insulin resistance and adverse changes in lipoprotein.

Other serious adverse effects noted in DHEA studies include transient jaundice and adverse hepatic effects, increased risk of uterine, breast, ovarian and prostate cancers.

CONTRAINDICATIONS, PRECAUTIONS, ADVERSE REACTIONS

CONTRAINDICATIONS

DHEA supplementation is contraindicated in those with prostate, breast, uterine and ovarian cancer. Known hypersensitivity to a DHEA-containing product.

PRECAUTIONS

DHEA supplementation should be avoided by children, adolescents, pregnant women and nursing mothers. The use of DHEA for any health condition should be discussed with one's physician.

ADVERSE REACTIONS

Various androgenic effects, including acne, deepening of the voice, hirsutism and hair loss have been reported in women using supplemental DHEA. Hirsutism and voice changes may be irreversible. There is a report of transient hepatitis associated with DHEA use by a woman. Decreased HDL-cholesterol levels have been reported in women using oral DHEA. This could increase risk of cardiovascular disease. Elevated IGF (insulin-like growth factor)-1 levels have been noted in both men and women taking oral DHEA. Elevated IGF-1 levels have been associated with increased risk of certain types of cancer, e.g. prostate cancer. Oral DHEA has also been observed to increase insulin resistance when taken by women. Manic symptoms and palpitations have been reported with continued use.

INTERACTIONS

DHEA inhibits CYP3A4 *in vitro*, and could increase serum concentrations of the many drugs metabolized by this isozyme.

In some individuals taking alprazolam, or diltiazem, serum DHEA and DHEAS levels may increase. These individuals could be at higher risk of any adverse effects from supplemental DHEA. Danazol, dexamethasone, insulin and morphine may lower endogenous DHEA and DHEAS levels.

DHEA may have additive adverse effects if used along with 4-androstenedione, 4-androstenediol, 5-androstenedione, 19-4-norandrostenedione and 19-5-norandrostenediol

DHEA could have additive adverse effects if used along with testosterone replacement therapy.

OVERDOSAGE

There are no reports of overdosage.

DOSAGE AND ADMINISTRATION

The physiological replacement dose of DHEA is usually considered to be about 25-50 mg/day. Use of DHEA should be discussed with one's physician. Moreover, a physician should closely monitor doses above 50 milligrams daily for any of the possible adverse effects mentioned above.

In March 2007, Senator Charles Grassley introduced a bill in the U.S. Senate (S.762) that that would classify DHEA, if passed, as a controlled substance under the Anabolic Steroid Control Act of 2004. (DHEA had been specifically exempted from the list of controlled anabolic substances.) On December 13, 2007, Senator Grassley introduced the Dehydroepiandrosterone Abuse Reduction Act of 2007 (S.2470). This bill would amend the Controlled Substances Act to impose civil penalties for knowingly selling, causing another to sell, or conspiring to sell a product containing dehydroepiandrosterone to an individual under the age of 18, including any such sale using the Internet. As of September 2008, neither bill has yet been passed.

DHEA is banned by the International Olympic Committee, the National Collegiate Athletic Association, the National Football League and other sports organizations.

LITERATURE

Akishita M, Hashimoto M, Ohike Y, et al. Association of plasma dehydroepiandrosterone-sulfate levels with endothelial function in postmenopausal women with coronary risk factors. *Hypertens Res*. 2008;31(1):69-74.

Allolio B, Arlt W, Hahner S. DHEA: why, when, and how much—DHEA replacement in adrenal insufficiency. *Ann Endocrinol* (Paris). 2007;68(4):268-273.

Altman R, Motton DD, Kota RS, et al. Inhibition of vascular inflammation by dehydroepiandrosterone sulfate in human aortic endothelial cells: roles of PPARalpha and NF-kappaB. *Vascul Pharmacol*. 2008;48(2-3):76-84.

Araghiniknan M, Chung S, Nelson-White T, et al. Antioxidant activity of Dioscorea and dehydroepiandrosterone (DHEA) in older humans. *Life Sciences*. 1996;59:147-157.

Arlt W, Callies F, van Vlijmen JC, et al. Dehydroepiandrosterone replacement in women with adrenal insufficiency. *N Engl J Med*. 1999;341:1013-1020.

Barrett-Connor E, Khaw K-T, Yen SSC. A prospective study of dehydroepiandrosterone sulfate, mortality, and cardiovascular disease. *N Engl J Med*. 1986;315:1519-1524.

Baulieu EE. Dehydroepiandrosterone (DHEA): a fountain of youth? *J Clin Endocrinol Metab*. 1996;81(9):3147-3151.

Baulieu EE, Robel P. Dehydroepiandrosterone (DHEA) and dehydroepiandrosterone sulfate (DHEAS) as neuroactive neurosteroids (Commentary). *Proc Natl Acad Sci*. 1998;95:4089-4091.

Berr C, Lafont S, Debuire B, et al. Relationships of dehydroepiandrosterone sulfate in the elderly with functional, psychological, and mental status, and short-term mortality: a French community-based study. *Proc Natl Acad Sci*. 1996;93:13410-13415.

Bhagra S, Nippoldt TB, Nair KS. Dehydroepiandrosterone in adrenal insufficiency and ageing. *Curr Opin Endocrinol Diabetes Obes.* 2008;15(3):239-243.

Buford TW, Willoughby DS. Impact of DHEA(S) and cortisol on immune function in aging: a brief review. *Appl Physiol Nutr Metab.* 2008;33(3):429-433.

Cardounel A, Regelson W, Kalimi M. Deyhydroepiandrosterone protects hippocampal neurons against neurotixin-induced cell death: mechanism of action. *Proc Soc Exp Biol Med.* 1999;222:145-149.

Chang AY, Ghayee HK, Auchus RJ. Dehydroepiandrosterone replacement therapy—panacea, snake oil, or a bit of both? *Nat Clin Pract Endocrinol Metab.* 2008;4(8):442-443.

Chen H, Lin AS, Li Y, et al. DHEA stimulates phosphorylation of FoxO1 in vascular endothelial cells via PI3-kinase- and PKA-dependent signaling pathways to regulate ET-1 synthesis and secretion. *J Biol Chem.* Epub: 2008 Aug 21.

Cleary, MP. The antiobesity effect of dehydroepiandrosterone in rats. *Proc Soc Exp Biol Med.* 1991;196:8-16.

Compagnone NA, Mellon SH. Dehydroepiandrosterone: a potential signalling molecule for neocortical organization during development. *Proc Natl Acad Sci.* 1998;95:4678-4683.

Davis SR, Shah SM, McKenzie DP, et al. Dehydroepiandrosterone sulfate levels are associated with more favorable cognitive function in women. *J Clin Endocrinol Metab.* 2008;93(3):801-808.

Debonneuil EH, Quillard J, Baulieu EE. Hypoxia and dehydroepiandrosterone in old age: a mouse survival study. *Respir Res.* 2006;7:144.

Dessouroux A, Akwa Y, Baulieu EE. DHEA decreases HIF-1alpha accumulation under hypoxia in human pulmonary artery cells: potential role in the treatment of pulmonary arterial hypertension. *J Steroid Biochem Mol Biol.* 2008;109(1-2):81-89.

Dwell T, Norton SD, Araneo BA. Method for reducing mast cell medicted allergic reactions. 1999. U.S. Patent Number 585900. Issued Jan 12, 1999.

Ebeling P, Koivisto VA. Physiological importance of dehydroepiandrosterone. *Lancet.* 1994;343:1479-1481.

Enomoto M, Adachi H, Fukami A, et al. Serum dehydroepiandrosterone sulfate levels predict longevity in men: 27-year follow-up study in a community-based cohort (Tanushimaru study). *J Am Geriatr Soc.* 2008;56(6):994-998.

Friedrich N, Völzke H, Rosskopf D, et al. Reference Ranges for Serum Dehydroepiandrosterone Sulfate and Testosterone in Adult Men. *J Androl.* Epub: 2008 Jul 3.

Genud R, Merenlender A, Gispan-Herman I, et al. DHEA Lessens Depressive-Like Behavior via GABA-ergic Modulation of the Mesolimbic System. *Neuropsychopharmacology.* Epub: 2008 May 21.

Grimley Evans J, Malouf R, Huppert F, et al. Dehydroepiandrosterone (DHEA) supplementation for cognitive function in healthy elderly people. *Cochrane Database Syst Rev.* 2006;(4):CD006221.

Kasperska-Zajac A, Brzoza Z, Rogala B. Dehydroepiandrosterone and dehydroepiandrosterone sulphate in atopic allergy and chronic urticaria. *Inflammation.* 2008;31(3):141-145.

Kimonides VG, Khatibi NH, Svendsen CN, et al. Dehydrocepiandrosterone (DHEA) and DHEA-sulfate (DHEAS) protect hippocampal neurons against excitatory amino acid-induced neurotoxicity. *Proc Natl Acad Sci.* 1998;95:1852-1857.

Kritz-Silverstein D, von Mühlen D, Laughlin GA, et al. Effects of Dehydroepiandrosterone Supplementation on Cognitive Function and Quality of Life: The DHEA and Well-Ness (DAWN) Trial. *J Am Geriatr Soc.* 2008 Jul;56(7):1292-1298.

Kroboth PD, Salek FS, Pittenger AL, et al. DHEA and DHEA-S: A review. *J Clin Pharmacol.* 1999;39:327-348.

McIntosh M, Bao, H Lee, C. Opposing actions of dehydroepiandrosterone and cortocosterone in rats. *Proc Soc Exp Biol Med.* 1999;221:198-206.

Morales AJ, Nolan JJ, Nelson JC, et al. Effects of replacement dose of dehydroepiandrosterone in men and women of advancing age. *J Clin Endocrinol Metab.* 1994;78:1360-1367.

Mori I, Ishizuka T, Morita H, et al. Comparison of Biochemical Data, Blood Pressure and Physical Activity Between Longevity and Non-Longevity Districts in Japan. *Circ J.* 2008;72(10):1680-1684.

Mortola JF, Yen SSC. The effects of oral dehydroepiandcosterone on endocrine-metabolic parameters in postmenopausal women. *J Clin Endocrinol Metab.* 1990;71:696-704.

Naylor JC, Hulette CM, Steffens DC, et al. Cerebrospinal fluid dehydroepiandrosterone levels are correlated with brain dehydroepiandrosterone levels, elevated in Alzheimer's disease, and related to neuropathological disease stage. *J Clin Endocrinol Metab.* 2008;93(8):3173-3178.

Oelkers W. Dehydroepiandrosterone for adrenal insufficiency (editorial). *N Engl J Med.* 1999;341:1073-1074.

Pénisson-Besnier I, Devillers M, Porcher R, et al. Dehydroepiandrosterone for myotonic dystrophy type 1. *Neurology.* 2008;71(6):407-412.

Sánchez J, Pérez-Heredia F, Priego T, et al. Dehydroepiandrosterone prevents age-associated alterations, increasing insulin sensitivity. *J Nutr Biochem.* Epub: 2008 May 13.

Sawalha AH, Kovats S. Dehydroepiandrosterone in systemic lupus erythematosus. *Curr Rheumatol Rep.* 2008;10(4):286-291.

Skolnick AA. Scientific verdict still out on DHEA. *J Am Med Assoc.* 1996;276:1365-1367.

Solano ME, Sander V, Wald MR, et al. Dehydroepiandrosterone and metformin regulate proliferation of murine T lymphocytes. *Clin Exp Immunol.* 2008;153(2):289-296.

Strous RD, Gibel A, Maayan R, et al. Hormonal response to dehydroepiandrosterone administration in schizophrenia: findings from a randomized, double-blind, placebo-controlled, crossover study. *J Clin Psychopharmacol.* 2008;28(4):456-459.

Van Vollenhaven RF, Morabito LM, Engleman EG, et al. Treatment of systemic lupus erythematosus with dehydroepiandrosterone: 50 patients treated up to 12 months. *J Rheumatol.* 1998;25:285-289.

Yen SS. Dehydroepiandrosterone sulfate and longevity: new clues for an old friend. *Proc Natl Acad Sci USA.* 200;98(15):8167-8169.

Dimethylglycine (DMG)

DESCRIPTION

Dimethylglycine or DMG is a non-protein amino acid found naturally in animal and plant cells. DMG is produced in cells as an intermediate in the metabolism of choline to glycine.

There has been much confusion surrounding the history of DMG as a nutritional supplement. DMG appeared as a supplement in the 1960s under the names vitamin B15, pangamic acid and calcium pangamate. Calcium pangamate was originally a mixture of calcium gluconate and DMG. Calcium pangamate was intended as a delivery form of DMG. However, several products entered the supplement marketplace called pangamic acid or calcium pangamate, and these did not contain DMG. Some of these products contained, instead of DMG, a substance called diisopropylammonium dichloroacetate. At present, DMG supplements are available that do contain dimethylglycine.

DMG-containing calcium pangamate was popular with Russian athletes and cosmonauts because it was reputed to enhance oxygenation at the cellular level, reduce fatigue and enhance physical stamina. None of those claims, however, was ever substantiated. DMG is neither a vitamin nor an essential nutrient. DMG is also known as N, N-dimethylglycine, (dimethylamino)acetic acid and N-methylsarcosine. Its chemical structure is:

Dimethylglycine (N,N-Dimethylglycine)

DMG is a solid, water-soluble substance. DMG should not be confused with TMG (trimethylglycine or betaine). TMG is involved in the methylation of homocysteine to form methionine (see Trimethylglycine).

ACTIONS AND PHARMACOLOGY

ACTIONS

There are no known actions of supplemental DMG.

PHARMACOKINETICS

DMG is absorbed from the small intestine and from there transported by the portal circulation to the liver. DMG is metabolized in the liver to monomethylglycine or sarcosine which, in turn, is converted to glycine. Dimethylglycine dehydrogenase, a flavoprotein, is the enzyme that catalyzes the oxidative demethylation of DMG to sarcosine. The methyl group produced in this reaction returns to the one carbon pool at the level of N^{10}-hydroxymethyl-tetrahydrofolic acid. DMG itself is formed from trimethylglycine or betaine. DMG that is not metabolized in the liver is transported by the circulatory system to various tissues in the body.

INDICATIONS AND USAGE

It is too early to say whether DMG might eventually be indicated as an immune enhancer or in the management of autism. It is not indicated as an anticonvulsant, in epilepsy or for any condition characterized by seizures. Nor is it indicated as an energy booster or athletic-performance enhancer.

RESEARCH SUMMARY

Based on claims that DMG is a highly potent "oxygenator" of body/brain tissues, this supplement has been touted as a panacea for years.

Several studies show that DMG has no anticonvulsant value and is thus of no help in epilepsy or other conditions characterized by seizures. Persistent claims that DMG is useful in autism are thus far anecdotal.

Claims that DMG can boost energy and athletic performance have been refuted by human and animal studies. Tests on exercising thoroughbred horses found "no beneficial effects on cardiorespiratory function or lactate production." And male track athletes supplemented with DMG exhibited no significant changes in short-term maximal treadmill performance.

On the other hand, an early finding that DMG can enhance both humoral and cell-mediated immune responses has been fortified by some subsequent research. This animal research needs to be extended to humans.

Early fears that DMG might be mutagenic now appear to be unfounded.

CONTRAINDICATIONS, PRECAUTIONS, ADVERSE REACTIONS

CONTRAINDICATIONS

Those with hypersensitivity to any component of the preparation should not use DMG.

PRECAUTIONS

DMG is not advised for pregnant women or nursing mothers and should only be used in children under medical supervision.

ADVERSE REACTIONS

Those with the rare disorder of dimethylglycine dehydrogenase deficiency may complain of a fish odor when taking DMG supplements. No other significant adverse reactions have been reported with DMG.

INTERACTIONS

There are no known drug, nutritional supplement, food or herb interactions. There is no known interaction with alcohol.

OVERDOSAGE

There are no known reports of overdose with DMG.

DOSAGE AND ADMINISTRATION

Use of DMG should be restricted to items specifically labeled DMG or dimethylglycine. Items labeled pangamic acid, calcium pangamate and vitamin B15 should be avoided. DMG comes in tablets, capsules and sublingual preparations, typically at a dose of 125 milligrams. The usual dose is 125 milligrams daily with meals.

LITERATURE

Bolman WM, Richmond JA. A double-blind, placebo-controlled crossover pilot trial of low dose dimethylglycine in patients with autistic disorder. *J Autism Dev Disord.* 1999; 29:191-194.

Gascon G, Patterson B, Yearwood K, Slotnick H. N, N-dimethylglycine and epilepsy. *Epilepsia.* 1989; 30:90-93.

Graber CD, Goust JM, Glassman AD, et al. Immunomodulating properties of dimethylglycine in humans. *J Infect Dis.* 1981; 143:101-105.

Gray ME, Titlow LW. The effect of pangamic acid on maximal treadmill performance. *Med Sci Sports Exerc.* 1982; 14:424-427.

Hoorn AJ. Dimethylglycine and chemically related amines tested for mutagenicity under potential nitrosation conditions. *Mutat Res.* 1989; 222:343-350.

Moolenaar SH, Paggi-Bach J, Engelke UF, et al. Defect in dimethylglycine dehydrogenase, a new inborn error of metabolism: NMR spectroscopy study. *Clin Chem.* 1999; 45:459-464.

Reap EA, Lawson JW. Stimulation of the immune response by dimethylglycine, a nontoxic metabolite. *J Lab Clin Med.* 1990; 115:481-486.

Rose RJ, Schlierf HA. Knight PK, et al. Effects of N, N-dimethylglycine on cardiorespiratory function and lactate performance in thoroughbred horses performing incremental treadmill exercise. *Vet Rec.* 1989; 125; 268-271.

Dimethyl Sulfoxide (DMSO)

DESCRIPTION

Dimethyl sulfoxide or DMSO is a very hygroscopic, sulfur-containing organic compound. It is a colorless liquid with a faint scent of sulfur and mixes readily with a wide range of water-insoluble and water-soluble substances, including water itself. DMSO is rapidly absorbed into the body if ingested or even if touched by the hands, very quickly producing a garlic-like taste. It occurs naturally in small amounts in vegetables, grains, fruits and animal products. DMSO is formed as a byproduct of wood pulp processing and is used as an industrial solvent.

Up until the 1970s DMSO was sold in vitamin stores and used both externally and internally, primarily for various aches and pains. DMSO is approved by the FDA for the palliative treatment of interstitial cystitis and for limited veterinary use. It is not allowed for use as a dietary supplement. A second-generation DMSO, methylsulfonylmethane or MSM (see Methylsulfonylmethane), which is a metabolite of DMSO, is marketed as a dietary supplement.

DMSO is also known as sulfinylbismethane and methyl sulfoxide. The inclusion of DMSO, which is not a nutritional supplement in this PDR, is for historical and informational purposes, and because one of its metabolites, methylsulfonylmethane or MSM, is marketed as a nutritional supplement. The claims for MSM are related to claims made for DMSO.

ACTIONS AND PHARMACOLOGY

ACTIONS

DMSO may have anti-inflammatory, antioxidant and analgesic activities. DMSO also readily penetrates cellular membranes.

MECHANISM OF ACTION

The mechanism of DMSO's actions is not well understood. DMSO has demonstrated antioxidant activity in certain biological settings. For example, the cardiovascular protective effect of DMSO in copper-deficient rats is thought to occur by an antioxidant mechanism. It is also thought that DMSO's possible anti-inflammatory activity is due to antioxidant action. The membrane-penetrating ability of DMSO may enhance diffusion of other substances through the skin. For this reason, mixtures of idoxuridine and DMSO have been used for topical treatment of herpes zoster in the United Kingdom.

PHARMACOKINETICS

DMSO is readily and rapidly absorbed following administration by all routes and distributed throughout the body. It is metabolized in part by oxidation to methylsulfonylmethane and by reduction to dimethyl sulfide. These metabolites are excreted in the urine and feces. Most of administered DMSO is excreted in the urine as such. Dimethyl sulfide is excreted through the lungs and skin, producing a characteristic sulfuric odor.

Following ingestion by Rhesus monkeys, DMSO was rapidly absorbed, reached a steady state blood level after one day and was cleared from the blood within 72 hours after ending treatment. Urinary excretion of unmetabolized DMSO and methylsulfonylmethane accounted for about 60% and 16%, respectively, of the ingested dose.

INDICATIONS AND USAGE

The medical use of DMSO is currently restricted by the FDA to the palliative treatment of interstitial cystitis and to certain experimental applications. It may have shown some usefulness in some forms of arthritis and connective tissue injuries, in amyloidosis, in scleroderma, in the prevention of skin ulceration induced by some antineoplastic agents, in reversing cerebral edema and intracranial hypertension and in the topical treatment of herpes zoster. It may have some anti-cancer, neuroprotective and cardioprotective effects. It has not been established that it can halt progression of degenerative joint disease.

RESEARCH SUMMARY

DMSO has been used for years to treat the symptoms of interstitial cystitis. Dermal applications often bring quick relief from pain caused by arthritis and connective tissue injury. It has not been established, however, that DMSO has any effect on the degenerative processes of arthritis. There is some preliminary evidence that DMSO diminishes destructive changes in the joints in a spontaneous arthritis animal model. This warrants followup. In another animal model, DMSO did not suppress the clinical manifestations of arthritis.

DMSO has exerted favorable effects in the treatment of amyloidosis, possibly, it has been hypothesized, by helping to move amyloid deposits out of tissue and into urine. In one case study, a girl with secondary amyloidosis, which was a complication of juvenile rheumatoid arthritis, was treated with topical DMSO. Gastrointestinal symptoms and massive proteinuria improved. There was marked improvement of decreased left ventricular function and creatinine clearance.

Topical preparations containing high concentrations of DMSO have helped resolve cutaneous manifestations of scleroderma in some.

In a multi-center, placebo-controlled study, 157 patients with acute tenopathies were randomized to treatment with 10% DMSO gel applied three times daily or gel excipient for 14 days. Treatment in all cases started within 72 hours after onset of acute symptoms. Pain and mobility were significantly improved in the DMSO group, beginning as early as three days after onset of treatment. After 14 days, 44% of DMSO subjects were pain free, compared with 9% of placebo subjects.

Skin ulcers have been prevented by a topical application of DMSO and alpha-tocopherol in patients under treatment with anti-neoplastic agents that typically induce these ulcers. In other studies, topical DMSO has alleviated some of the symptoms of herpes zoster. It has demonstrated neuroprotective effects in experimental cerebral ischemia, significantly reducing infarction volume compared with controls. It has also demonstrated some efficacy in reversing cerebral edema and intracranial hypertension. Chronic treatment with DMSO has experimentally protected against cardiovascular—but not renal—effects of copper deficiency.

Some animal studies have further suggested that DMSO might have some anti-cancer effects. A 3% concentration of DMSO added to the drinking water of a strain of mice that spontaneously develop a series of diseases, including some cancers, had significant beneficial effects. Commencing at 10 weeks of age, mice were given the DMSO, and 90% of them were still alive at 40 weeks compared with 50% of controls. Incidence of tumors was far lower in 40-week-old treated mice than in 20-week-old untreated mice. Significant tumor regression has been seen in other DMSO-treated mice. Followup research is needed.

CONTRAINDICATIONS, PRECAUTIONS, ADVERSE REACTIONS

CONTRAINDICATIONS

DMSO should not be used as a dietary supplement by anyone.

PRECAUTIONS

DMSO is neither a nutritional supplement nor an over-the-counter medicinal product; its use for the treatment of interstitial cystitis—performed by interstitial instillation—requires a physician with expertise in this procedure. Bladder instillation may be harmful in patients with urinary-tract malignancy. Those who receive long-term treatment with intravesical DMSO should have liver and renal function tests as well as ophthalmologic evaluation performed every six months during treatment. DMSO has been associated with lens changes in animals.

Pregnant women and nursing mothers should avoid using DMSO.

DMSO used as an industrial solvent is not medical grade.

ADVERSE REACTIONS

Adverse reactions reported in those using DMSO for treatment of interstitial cystitis include garlic-like taste, transient chemical cystitis, bladder spasm, discomfort, allergic reactions and anaphylactoid reactions. Adverse reactions for topical use include garlic-like taste, local dermatitis, nausea, vomiting, headache, burning eyes and sedation. Concomitant use of DMSO and sulindac may cause peripheral neuropathy.

INTERACTIONS
Sulindac may decrease the pharmacologic effects of DMSO. DMSO may impair sulindac's conversion to its sulfide metabolite by competitive inhibition of sulfide reductase. Peripheral neuropathy has been reported with the simultaneous use of DMSO and sulindac.

DOSAGE AND ADMINISTRATION
No recommended dose. DMSO is not a nutritional supplement. It is used as a treatment for interstitial cystitis, and treatment must be performed by a qualified physician. DMSO is metabolized to methylsulfonylmethane, which is available as a nutritional supplement. See Methylsulfonylmethane.

DMSO sold as an industrial solvent is not medical grade.

LITERATURE
Eberhardt R, Zwingers T, Hoffman R. [DMSO in patients with active gonarthrosis. A double-blind, placebo-controlled phase III study.] [Article in German.] *Fortschr Med.* 1995; 113:446-450.

Jacob SW, Herschler R. Pharmacology of DMSO. *Cryobiology.* 1986; 23:14-27.

Jacob SW, Wood DC. Dimethyl sulfoxide (DMSO) toxicology, pharmacology and clinical experience. *Am J Surg.* 1967; 114:414-426.

Kolb KH, Jaenicke G, Kramer M, Schulze PE. Absorption, distribution and elimination of labeled dimethyl sulfoxide in man and animals. *Ann NY Acad Sci.* 1967; 141:85-95.

Layman DL, Jacob SW. The absorption, metabolism and excretion of dimethyl sulfoxide by Rhesus monkeys. *Life Sci.* 1985; 37:2431-2437.

Ludwig CU, Stoll HR, Obrist R, Obrecht JP. Prevention of cytotoxic drug induced skin ulcers with dimethyl sulfoxide (DMSO) and alpha-tocopherol. *Eur J Cancer Clin Oncol.* 1987; 23:327-329.

Milner LS, de Chadaré vian J-P, Goodyer PR, et al. Amelioration of murine lupus nephritis by dimethylsulfoxide. *Clin Immun Immunopathol.* 1987; 45:259-267.

Perez-Marrero R, Emerson LE, Feltis JT. A controlled study of dimethyl sulfoxide in interstitial cystitis. *J Urol.* 1988; 140:36-39.

Shimizu S, Simon RP, Graham SH. Dimethyl sulfoxide (DMSO) treatment reduces infarction volume after permanent focal cerebral ischemia in rats. *Neurosci Lett.* 1997; 239:125-127.

Swanson BN. Medical use of dimethyl sulfoxide (DMSO). *Rev Clin Basic Pharm.* 1985; 5:1-33.

Trentham DE, Rowland D. Dimethyl sulfoxide does not suppress the clinical manifestations of collagen arthritis. *J Rheumatol.* 1983; 10:114-116.

Yokoi K, Kimura M, Itokawa Y. Cardiovascular but not renal effects of copper deficiency are inhibited by dimethyl sulfoxide. *Nutr Res.* 1990; 10:467-477.

DL-Phenylalanine

DESCRIPTION
DL-phenylalanine refers to a racemic mixture consisting of 50% D-phenylalanine and 50% L-phenylalanine. L-phenylalanine is an essential protein amino acid. (See L-Phenylalanine.) D-phenylalanine is the enantiomer of L-phenylalanine. D-phenylalanine is a nonprotein amino acid, meaning that it does not participate in protein biosynthesis. D-phenylalanine and other D-amino acids are, however, found in proteins, in small amounts, particularly aged proteins and food proteins that have been processed. The biological functions of D-amino acids remain unclear. Some D-amino acids, such as D-phenylalanine, may have pharmacologic activity.

DL-phenylalanine is marketed as a nutritional supplement for its putative analgesic and antidepressant activities. D-phenylalanine is not available as a nutritional supplement.

ACTIONS AND PHARMACOLOGY
DL-phenylalanine has putative analgesic and antidepressant activities.

MECHANISM OF ACTION
The putative analgesic activity of DL-phenylalanine may be explained by the possible blockage by D-phenylalanine of enkephalin degradation by the enzyme carboxypeptidase A.

The mechanism of DL-phenylalanine's putative antidepressant activity may be accounted for by the precursor role of L-phenylalanine in the synthesis of the neurotransmitters norepinephrine and dopamine. Elevated brain norepinephrine and dopamine levels are thought to be associated with antidepressant effects.

PHARMACOKINETICS
See L-Phenylalanine for the pharmacokinetics of this amino acid. D-phenylalanine is absorbed from the small intestine, following ingestion, and transported to the liver via the portal circulation. A fraction of D-phenylalanine appears to be converted to L-phenylalanine. D-phenylalanine is distributed to the various tissues of the body via the systemic circulation. D-phenylalanine appears to cross the blood-brain barrier with less efficiency than L-phenylalanine. A fraction of an ingested dose of D-phenylalanine is excreted in the

urine. There is much about the pharmacokinetics in humans that is unknown.

INDICATIONS AND USAGE

There is very preliminary evidence that DL-phenylalanine might be helpful in some with depression. It may also have some analgesic properties. It has not shown benefit in the treatment of attention deficit disorder.

RESEARCH SUMMARY

In a small open trial, depressed subjects were treated with 75 to 200 mg of DL-phenylalanine daily for 20 days. Significant benefit was reported. The same researchers subsequently conducted a double-blind study in which depressed patients were given either 150 to 200 mg of DL-phenylalanine or 150 to 200 mg of imipramine daily for 30 days. There was no significant difference in the antidepressant activity of the two substances. Both of these studies are dated. There are a few studies showing that D-phenylalanine, not available as a supplement, has some analgesic effects. Thus, DL-phenylalanine, an equal mixture of D-phenylalanine and L-phenylalanine, may have some of the same activity, although this has not been persuasively demonstrated to date.

CONTRAINDICATIONS, PRECAUTIONS, ADVERSE REACTIONS

CONTRAINDICATIONS

DL-phenylalanine is contraindicated in those with phenylketonuria. It is also contraindicated in those taking non-selective monoamine oxidase (MAO) inhibitors. DL-phenylalanine is contraindicated in those hypersensitive to any component of a DL-phenylalanine-containing supplement.

PRECAUTIONS

Pregnant women and nursing mothers should avoid supplementation with DL-phenylalanine.

Tardive dyskinesia has been reported to be exacerbated after ingestion of L-phenylalanine by schizophrenics. Therefore, those with schizophrenia should exercise extreme caution in the use of DL-phenylalanine.

Those with hypertension should exercise caution in the use of DL-phenylalanine.

ADVERSE REACTIONS

L-phenylalanine will exacerbate symptoms of phenylketonuria if used by phenylketonurics. L-phenylalanine was reported to exacerbate tardive dyskinesia when used by some with schizophrenia.

INTERACTIONS

DRUGS

Non-selective monoamine oxidase (MAO) inhibitors: including phenelzine sulfate, tranylcypromine sulfate and pargyline HCl — Concomitant use of L-phenylalanine and non-selective MAO inhibitors may cause hypertension.

Selegiline: L-phenylalanine and the selective MAO inhibitor selegiline may have synergistic antidepressant activity if used concomitantly.

Neuroleptic drugs: L-phenylalanine may potentiate the tardive dyskinesia side effects of neuroleptic drugs if used concomitantly.

OVERDOSAGE

No reports of overdosage.

DOSAGE AND ADMINISTRATION

Those who use DL-phenylalanine supplements typically use 375 mg to 2.25 grams daily.

LITERATURE

Beckman H, Athen D, Olteanu M, Zimmer R. DL-phenylalanine versus imipramine: a double-blind controlled study. *Arch Psychiatr Nervenkr.* 1979; 227:49-58.

Beckman H, Ludolph E. [DL-phenylalanine as an antidepressant. Open study.] [Article in German.] *Arzneimittelforschung.* 1978; 28:1283-1284.

Beckman H, Strauss MA, Ludolph E. DL-phenylalanine in depressed patients: an open study. *J Neural Transm.* 1977; 41:123-134.

Dove B, Morgenstern E, Gores E. [Analgesic effect, tolerance development and dependence potential of D-phenylalanine.] [Article in German.] *Pharmazie.* 1985; 40:648-650.

Ehrenpreis S. Pharmacology of enkephalinase inhibitors: animal and human studies. *Acupunct Electrother Res.* 1985; 10:203-208.

Halpern LM, Dong WK. D-phenylalanine: a putative enkephalinase inhibitor studied in a primate acute pain model. *Pain.* 1986; 24:223-237.

Lehmann WD, Theobald N, Fischer R, Heinrich HC. Stereospecificity of phenylalanine plasma kinetics and hydroxylation in man following oral application of a stable isotope-labeled pseudo-racemic mixture of L- and D-phenylalanine. *Clin Chim Acta.* 1983; 128:181-198.

Walsh NE, Ramamurthy S, Schoenfeld L, Hoffman J. Analgesic effectiveness of D-phenylalanine in chronic pain patients. *Arch Phys Med Rehabil.* 1986; 67:436-439.

Wood DR, Reimherr FW, Wender PH. Treatment of attention deficit disorder with DL-phenylalanine. *Psychiatry Res.* 1985; 16:21-26.

Docosahexaenoic Acid (DHA)

DESCRIPTION

Docosahexaenoic acid, or DHA, is a major component of fish oil. It is a long-chain polyunsaturated fatty acid (LCPUFA) of the n-3 or omega-3 type. DHA is an all cis polyunsaturated fatty acid containing 22 carbon atoms and 6 double bonds. It has the following structural formula:

DHA (cis-4,7,10,13,16,19-Docosahexaenoic Acid)

DHA is also known as DHA; C22: 6n-3 and cis-4, 7, 10, 13, 16, 19-docosahexaenoic acid. DHA is a vital component of the phospholipids of human cellular membranes, especially those in the brain and retina. It is necessary for optimal neural development and visual acuity. DHA is the most abundant omega-3 fatty acid in human breast milk. DHA occurs naturally in the form of triacylglycerols (TAGs).

ACTIONS AND PHARMACOLOGY

ACTIONS
Supplemental DHA may lower triglyceride levels and in some, may elevate HDL-cholesterol levels. DHA is vital for normal brain development for the fetus and infant and for the maintenance of normal brain function throughout life. Supplemental DHA may have anti-inflammatory and immune-modulating activities.

MECHANISM OF ACTION
DHA's triglyceride-lowering property results from the combined effects of inhibition of lipogenesis and stimulation of fatty acid oxidation. Fatty acid oxidation of eicosapentaenoic (EPA) acid occurs mainly in the mitochondria, while DHA undergoes fatty acid oxidation in the peroxisomes.

DHA is taken up by the brain in preference to other fatty acids and is incorporated into the phospholipids of the cell membranes of brain cells and the retina. DHA-containing phospholipids in the cell membranes of the neurons appear to be necessary for neurite elongation and formation of synapses. DHA-containing phospholipids in these cells are believed to be vital for cell signaling. DHA is the prominent structural fatty acid in the gray matter of the brain and retinal tissues of humans, as well as other animals.

PHARMACOKINETICS
DHA-laden TAGs, following ingestion, undergo hydrolysis via lipases to form monoglycerides (MG) and free fatty acids (FFA). Once formed, the MG and the FFA are absorbed by the enterocytes. In the enterocytes, reacylation takes place reforming TAGs, which are then assembled with phospholipids, cholesterol and apoproteins into chylomicrons. The chylomicrons are released into the lymphatics and from there transported to the systemic circulation. In the circulation, the chylomicrons are degraded by lipoprotein lipase, and the fatty acids, including DHA, are taken up in part by the

endothelial tissues. DHA is transported via the circulation to various tissues in the body, where it is used for the synthesis of phospholipids. These phospholipids are incorporated into the cell membranes of red blood cells, platelet cells and cells of the brain and retina. DHA is taken up by the brain in preference to other fatty acids. During fetal development, DHA is preferentially transported across the placenta into the fetal circulation. About 10% of DHA is retroconverted to eicosapentaenoic acid (EPA).

INDICATIONS AND USAGE
DHA is indicated to lower triglycerides in some hypertriglyceridemic individuals. It may also be indicated for pregnant women and nursing mothers, for those with peroxisomal disorders (such as Zellweger's syndrome), for cystic fibrosis sufferers, for those with attention deficit disorder, dyslexia and, possibly, those with cognitive impairment and dementia (including Alzheimer's disease). There is a preliminary indication that DHA might be helpful in atopic eczema. It may benefit eye health, helping to prevent retinopathy and age-related macular degeneration.

RESEARCH SUMMARY
A double-blind placebo-controlled study was performed to determine the triglyceride-lowering effect of DHA compared with EPA. In this seven-week study, 234 healthy men were randomly given: DHA in the ethyl ester form at a dose of 3.6 grams daily, the ethyl ester of EPA at 3.18 grams daily or corn oil at 4 grams daily. Triglycerides decreased by 26% in the DHA group and 21% in the EPA group compared with placebo. Some retroconversion of DHA to EPA was noted, but no significant conversion of EPA to DHA was observed. A slight, but significant, increase in HDL-cholesterol was seen in the DHA group.

In another study on the effect of DHA on serum triglycerides, 27 hypertriglyceridemic subjects were randomized to receive either 1.25 grams of DHA daily, 2.5 grams of DHA daily or a vegetable oil placebo. The DHA was in the natural form derived from microalgae, and the study lasted six weeks. Serum triglycerides decreased 17 to 21% and were of similar magnitude in both DHA groups. HDL-cholesterol increased by 6% and again was of similar magnitude in both DHA groups. LDL-cholesterol increased by 9.3% in the 1.25 gram DHA group. This was not significant. An increase of LDL-cholesterol of 13.6% was noted in the 2.5-gram DHA group, which was statistically significant.

A recent review of the fish oil supplementation data has indicated that there is no convincing evidence that one of the two long-chain omega-3 fatty acids is more cardioprotective than the other. Some studies seemed to indicate that DHA might have more blood-pressure benefits than eicosapentaenoic acid (EPA) and that EPA might have more triglyceride-lowering ability, but this review found little evidence of this. The best cardioprotective data have emerged from studies utilizing the two fatty acids in combination. Some other recent studies have further elucidated DHA's modes of action in cardioprotection related to its anti-inflammatory and possible plaque-stabilizing effects.

DHA is essential for the growth and functional development of the fetal and infant brain and visual system. Human breast milk contains DHA but, unless supplemented with DHA, infant formulas in the U.S. do not contain any significant amounts. (The DHA level in the breast milk of the average American woman is among the lowest in he world.) In Europe and Japan, by contrast, infant formulas are routinely supplemented with DHA.

Whether to supplement these formulas in the U.S. continues to be a matter of considerable controversy. A recent double-blind, randomized, controlled efficacy and safety trial of infant formulas with and without DHA failed to resolve the controversy. No beneficial effects were noted, but more long-term studies are needed to settle the issue. No adverse safety outcomes, measured by growth, infection, atopy and gastrointestinal tolerance, were noted.

The data for supplementation of DHA in infant-formula milk for pre-term infants are more compelling. One study compared pre-term infants on formula without supplemental DHA with infants getting breast milk. The breast-fed infants had an IQ 8.3 points higher at $7^1/_2$ to 8 years of age.

Another study comparing pre-term infants receiving formula supplemented with DHA with those receiving formula unsupplemented with DHA demonstrated a significantly higher Bayley Mental Development Index at 12 months in the infants receiving the DHA-supplemented formula. Large scale retrospective studies have shown that pre-term breast-fed infants have an average 5- to 12-point higher IQ later in life than babies fed formula milk without supplemental DHA. The difference in term infants is 2 to 5 IQ points.

The authors of a recent review noted that experiments most relevant to this issue have yielded mixed findings. But they stated that results from human breastfeeding studies, though seriously confounded in some respects, "are not inconsistent with a need for supplementation." A recent Canadian study associated increased DHA intake during pregnancy with improved motor function in offspring later in life.

Recent studies have suggested that DHA might be able to play some role in preventing Alzheimer's disease. In an aged Alzheimer mouse model, a diet enriched with DHA reduced beta-amyloid burden by greater than 40%. DHA levels have been found to be low in serum in brains of Alzheimer's patients. In a randomized, double-blind, placebo-controlled study, 174 Alzheimer's patients received daily either 1.7 grams DHA and 0.6 grams EPA or placebo for six months. Though it is difficult to draw clinically useful conclusions from this study, there were indications in the results that the DHA modified cytokine activity in ways that may be helpful in those with Alzheimer's disease. Some of the cytokines and growth factors impacted in this study are reportedly strong predictors of Alzheimer's development. It is far from established that DHA (or EPA) can be of real benefit in Alzheimer's, although ongoing clinical trials have yielded some early results suggesting a benefit that manifests in some stabilization of disease progression at the earliest stages of cognitive decline. Another trial showed no benefit in those with more advanced disease and greater cognitive dysfunction. One reviewer recently observed that the clinical trials using DHA have relied upon doses that may have been insufficient to obtain a potentially more favorable result.

DHA is known to benefit eye health and may help protect nerve cells in the retina. Increased dietary intake of omega-3 fatty acids was said to reduce pathological retinal angiogenesis in one study. Some studies suggest DHA may protect against age-related macular degeneration (AMD). Increased consumption of both DHA and EPA was associated in one recent study with an approximate 70% reduction in risk of AMD.

Preliminary research suggests that some other therapeutic roles might emerge for DHA. There is some indication that, in both humans suffering from cystic fibrosis and in the cystic fibrosis mouse model, in cell membranes of the lung, pancreas and intestine (the organs most affected by this disease) there are abnormally elevated levels of arachidonic acid and abnormally diminished levels of DHA. In a pilot animal study, daily supplementation of the mouse diet with DHA corrected the lipid imbalance and reversed the progression of the disease after one week. These results have prompted a human clinical trial, the results of which are not yet available.

DHA is similarly deficient, this time in the brain, as well as in the blood and all body tissues, in those suffering from congenital peroxisomal disorders. This includes those with Zellweger cerebro-hepato-renal syndrome, neonatal adreno-leukodystrophy (made famous by the film Lorenzo's Oil) and infantile Refsum disease, characterized by severe psychomotor retardation, retinopathy, liver disease and early death.

In one very encouraging early study of Zellweger Syndrome patients, the ethyl ester of DHA in daily doses of 100 to 500 milligrams was given to 13 patients. Blood DHA levels became normal within a few weeks, liver enzymes returned nearly to normal, and most of the patients showed improvement in vision, liver function, muscle tone and social skill. Normalization of brain myelin was confirmed by MRI in three patients.

DHA deficiencies have been established in the plasma phospholipids of those with attention deficit disorder.

A small study suggests that DHA might prove beneficial in the treatment of dyslexia. Dark adaptation was found to be impaired in 10 dyslexic subjects—compared with a non-dyslexic control group. A fish oil high in DHA improved dark adaptation in five subjects after one month of supplementation.

A recent randomized, double-blind, controlled study suggested that DHA supplementation might benefit some patients with atopic eczema. DHA dosage in this study was 5.4 grams daily for eight weeks. Subjects receiving DHA, compared with controls, enjoyed significant clinical improvement by several measures. Follow-up is warranted.

CONTRAINDICATIONS, PRECAUTIONS, ADVERSE REACTIONS

CONTRAINDICATIONS
Known hypersensitivity to a DHA-containing product.

PRECAUTIONS
Infants, pregnant women or nursing mothers should use DHA only if recommended and monitored by a physician.

Because DHA may have antithrombotic activity, those taking warfarin (Coumadin) and those with hemophilia should exercise caution in its use. Similarly, DHA supplementation should be stopped before any surgery.

ADVERSE REACTIONS
There have been no reports of serious adverse events in those taking DHA supplements. Those side effects that have been reported include mild gastrointestinal upsets such as nausea and diarrhea, eructation and "fishy" smelling breath. To date, there have been no significant reports of nosebleeds and easy bruising. One study performed in healthy adult male volunteers found no observable physiological changes in blood coagulation, platelet function or thrombotic tendencies in those consuming 6 grams daily of supplemental DHA for 90 days. Studies have not yet been done on those with hemophilia or those taking warfarin (Coumadin).

INTERACTIONS
No interactions between DHA and aspirin, other NSAIDs or herbs, such as *Allium sativum* (garlic) and *Ginkgo biloba* (ginkgo), have been reported. Such interactions, if they were to occur, might be manifested by nosebleeds and increased susceptibility to bruising.

OVERDOSAGE
None reported.

DOSAGE AND ADMINISTRATION
There are several forms of DHA supplements. These include DHA as the triacylglycerol ester derived from fish or from phytoplankton and DHA as the ethyl ester. Infant formulas containing DHA are available in Europe and Japan, but not yet approved in the U.S. Functional foods high in DHA, such as eggs, are now available.

Recommended DHA products should contain antioxidants, such as tocopherol, to protect against their oxidation.

Usual doses consumed by pregnant and nursing women are 100 to 200 milligrams daily. Doses of DHA for hypertrigly-ceridemics range from 1 to 4 grams. The dose needs to be determined by optimization of triglyceride levels. In those with elevated triglycerides and elevated cholesterol, doses of 1 to 2 grams daily may lower triglyceride levels and increase HDL-cholesterol levels in some. DHA is best tolerated with meals.

LITERATURE
Akbar M, Calderon F, Wen Z, et al. Docosahexaenoic acid: a positive modulator of Akt signaling in neuronal survival. *Proc Natl Acad Sci U S A*. 2005;102(31):10858-10863. in: *Proc Natl Acad Sci U S A*. 2005;102(36):12997.

Chapkin RS, Seo J, McMurray DN, et al. Mechanisms by which docosahexaenoic acid and related fatty acids reduce colon cancer risk and inflammatory disorders of the intestine. *Chem Phys Lipids*. 2008;153(1):14-23.

Davidson MH, Maki KC, Kalkowski J, et al. Effects of docosahexaenoic acid on the serum lipoproteins with combined hyperlipidemia: a randomized, double-blind, placebo-controlled trial. *J Am Coll Nutr*. 1997;16:236-243.

Eriksson PS, Perfilieva E, Bjork-Eriksson T, et al. Neurogenesis in the adult human hippocampus. *Nat Med*. 1998;4:1313-1317.

Freedman SD, Katz MH, Parker EM, et al. A membrane lipid imbalance plays a role in the phenotypic expression of cystic fibrosis in aftr -/-mice. *Proc Natl Acad Sci USA*. 1999;96:13995-14000.

Grimsgaard S, Bonaa KH, Hansen J-B, et al. Highly purified eicosapentaenoic acid and docosahexaenoic acid in humans have similar triacylglycerol- lowering effects but divergent effects on serum fatty acids. *Am J Clin Nutr*. 1997;66:649-959.

Horrocks LA, Yeo YK. Health benefits of docosahexaenoic acid. *Pharma Res*. 1999;40:211-225.

Koch C, Dölle S, Metzger M, et al. Docosahexaenoic acid (DHA) supplementation in atopic eczema: a randomized, double-blind, controlled trial. *Br J Dermatol*. 2008;158(4):786-792.

Lim GP, Calon F, Morihara T, et al. A diet enriched with the omega-3 fatty acid docosahexaenoic acid reduces amyloid burden in an aged Alzheimer mouse model. *J Neurosci*. 2005;25(12):3032-3040.

Lucas A, Stafford M, Morley R, et al. Efficacy and safety of long-chain polyunsaturated fatty acid supplementation of infant-formula milk: a randomized trial. *Lancet.* 1999;354:1948-1954.

Ma QL, Teter B, Ubeda OJ, et al. Omega-3 fatty acid docosahexaenoic acid increases SorLA/LR11, a sorting protein with reduced expression in sporadic Alzheimer's disease (AD): relevance to AD prevention. *J Neurosci.* 2007;27(52):14299-14307.

Madsen L, Rustan AC, Vaagenes H, et al. Eicosapentaenoic and docosahexaenoic acid affect mitochondrial and peroxisomal fatty acid oxidation in relation to substrate preference. *Lipids.* 1999;34:951-963.

Malcolm CA, McCulloch DL, Montgomery C, et al. Maternal docosahexaenoic acid supplementation during pregnancy and visual evoked potential development in term infants: a double blind, prospective, randomized trial. *Arch Dis Child Fetal Neonatal Ed.* 2003;88(5):F383-390.

Martinez M, Vazquez E, Garcia-Silva MT, et al. Therapeutic effects of docosahexaenoic acid ethyl ester in patients with generalized peroxisomal disorders. *Am J Clin Nutr.* 2000;71:376S-385S.

Massaro M, Habib A, Lubrano L, et al. The omega-3 fatty acid docosahexaenoate attenuates endothelial cyclooxygenase-2 induction through both NADP(H) oxidase and PKC epsilon inhibition. *Proc Natl Acad Sci U S A.* 2006;103(41):15184-15189.

McCann JC, Ames BN. Is docosahexaenoic acid, an n-3 long-chain polyunsaturated fatty acid, required for development of normal brain function? An overview of evidence from cognitive and behavioral tests in humans and animals. *Am J Clin Nutr.* 2005;82(2):281-295.

Nelson GJ, Schmidt PS, Bartolini GL, et al. The effect of dietary docosahexaenoic acid on platelet function, platelet fatty acid composition, and blood coagulation in humans. *Lipids.* 1997;32:1129-1136.

Orr SK, Bazinet RP. The emerging role of docosahexaenoic acid in neuroinflammation. *Curr Opin Investig Drugs.* 2008;9(7):735-743.

Plourde M, Fortier M, Vandal M, et al. Unresolved issues in the link between docosahexaenoic acid and Alzheimer's disease. *Prostaglandins Leukot Essent Fatty Acids.* 2007;77(5-6):301-308.

Soderberg M, Edlund C, Kristennson K, et al. Fatty acid composition of brain phospholipids in aging and Alzheimer's disease. *Lipids.* 1991;26:421-425.

Stordy BJ. Dark adaptation, motor skills, docosahexaenoic acid, and dyslexia. *Am J Clin Nutr.* 2000;71:323S-326S.

Vedin I, Cederholm T, Freund Levi Y, et al. Effects of docosahexaenoic acid-rich n-3 fatty acid supplementation on cytokine release from blood mononuclear leukocytes: the OmegAD study. *Am J Clin Nutr.* 2008;87(6):1616-1622.

Dolomite

DESCRIPTION

Dolomite, named for the French geologist D.G. Dolomieu, is a mineral containing calcium and magnesium carbonate, as well as trace heavy metals. It is a double salt made up of approximately 60% calcium carbonate (equivalent to 24% calcium) and 40% magnesium carbonate (equivalent to 12% magnesium). Dolomite is also known as magnesium lime-stone and earlier was called compound-spar, bitter-spar, rhomb-spar and pearl-spar. The Dolomites, a mountain region in the South Tyrolese Alps, are named for the presence of dolomite in the mountains.

Dolomite was at one time a popular nutritional supplement for calcium and magnesium. It is still marketed as a nutritional supplement, but is no longer popular. The reason for this is that in the early 1980s analysis of dolomite nutritional supplements revealed them to contain substantial amounts of lead, as well as other toxic elements, such as mercury, arsenic and cadmium. In addition, much better supplementary forms of calcium and magnesium are available. Dolomite is still used in several parts of the world as a liming agent, to raise the pH of the soil, and as a fertilizer to maintain soil magnesium levels. It is also used to make magnesia, which has medical applications.

ACTIONS AND PHARMACOLOGY

ACTIONS

Dolomite is a delivery form of calcium and magnesium.

MECHANISM OF ACTION

See Calcium and Magnesium.

PHARMACOKINETICS

See Calcium and Magnesium. Noteworthy is that magnesium from magnesium carbonate is more poorly absorbed than it is from most other magnesium supplements.

INDICATIONS AND USAGE

Dolomite is no longer recommended as a calcium or magnesium source because it may be contaminated with toxic metals such as lead.

RESEARCH SUMMARY

Several studies have revealed significant toxic metal contamination of many randomly selected and analyzed dolomite supplements (the same is true of some other "natural" calcium sources, e.g., bonemeal and "oyster shell" or "natural source" calcium carbonate). In one study of randomly selected dolomite tablets, aluminum, arsenic, zinc, cadmium and lead were among the metals found. The researchers cautioned that "these trace metals could pose health risks to the public such as lead poisoning, dementia and hypertension due to cadmium. Also, zinc can potentiate cadmium-hypertensive effects."

Another researcher has pointed out that "physicians must consider the possibility of unrecognized self-poisoning from the consumption of such substances, especially in the context of unexplained neurologic, gastrointestinal, cutaneous and hematologic disorders."

CONTRAINDICATIONS, PRECAUTIONS, ADVERSE REACTIONS

CONTRAINDICATIONS

Those with hypercalcemia should not take calcium supplements. Conditions that cause hypercalcemia include hyperparathyroidism, hypervitaminosis D, some granulomatous diseases, sarcoidosis and cancer.

Those with renal failure and high-grade atrioventricular blocks should not take magnesium supplements.

PRECAUTIONS

Dolomite is no longer recommended as a calcium and magnesium supplement because of possible presence of toxic metals, such as lead, Children are especially sensitive to the effects of lead. Children, pregnant women and nursing mothers should absolutely avoid dolomite.

INTERACTIONS

See Calcium and Magnesium for adverse reactions of supplements containing these minerals. Prolonged use of dolomite containing toxic elements, such as lead, may cause the typical toxic effects of those substances.

OVERDOSAGE

There are no known reports of overdosage of dolomite.

DOSAGE AND ADMINISTRATION

No recommended dose.

LITERATURE

Boulos FM, von Smolinski A. Alert to users of calcium supplements as antihypertensive agents due to trace mineral contaminants. *Am J Hypterten*. 1988; 1(3 Pt 3):137S-142S.

Bourquin BP, Evans DR, Cornett JR, et al. Lead content of 70 brands of dietary calcium supplements. *Am J Public Health*. 1993; 83:1155-1160.

Roberts HJ. Potential toxicity due to dolomite and bone meal. *South Med J*. 1983; 76:556-559.

Whiting SJ. Safety of some calcium supplements questioned. *Nutr Rev*. 1884; 52:95-97.

Eicosapentaenoic Acid (EPA)

DESCRIPTION

Eicosapentaenoic acid, or EPA, is a major component of fish oil. It is a long-chain polyunsaturated fatty acid of the n-3 or omega-3 type. EPA is an all cis polyunsaturated fatty acid containing 20 carbons and 5 double bonds. EPA is also known as EPA; C20: 5n-3 and cis-5, 8, 11, 14,17-eicosapentaenoic acid. The structural formula is as follows:

EPA (5,8,11,14,17-Eicosapentaenoic Acid)

EPA is a precursor of the series-3 prostaglandins, the series-5 leukotrienes and the series-3 thromboxanes, which are anti-atherogenic and anti-thrombogenic. EPA is found naturally in the form of triacylglycerols (TAGs).

ACTIONS AND PHARMACOLOGY

ACTIONS

Supplemental EPA may have anti-inflammatory, antithrombotic and immunomodulatory activities. It may also have triglyceride-lowering activity.

MECHANISM OF ACTION

The possible anti-inflammatory, antithrombotic and immunomodulatory actions of supplemental EPA are probably due mostly to EPA's role in eicosanoid physiology and biochemistry.

Eicosanoids are produced by the metabolism of the n-3 or omega-3 polyunsaturated fatty acids, and in particular the 20 carbon n-3 polyunsaturated fatty acid, arachidonic acid. These eicosanoids are of the leukotriene 4 series and thromboxane 2 series. Leukotriene B_4 (LTB_4) and thromboxane A_2 (TXA_2) stimulate leukocyte chemotaxis, platelet aggregation and vasoconstriction. These eicosanoids are thrombogenic and atherogenic.

On the other hand, EPA is metabolized to leukotriene B_5 (LTB_5) and thromboxane A_3 (TXA_3), eicosanoids that promote vasodilation, inhibit platelet aggregation and leukocyte chemotaxis and are anti-atherogenic and anti-thrombotic.

The triglyceride-lowering effect of EPA results from inhibition of lipogenesis and stimulation of fatty acid oxidation. Fatty acid oxidation of EPA occurs mainly in the mitochondria.

(For further discussion on the action of EPA, see the Fish Oil monograph.)

PHARMACOKINETICS

See the Fish Oils monograph.

INDICATIONS AND USAGE

EPA may be indicated for lowering elevated triglycerides in those who are hyperglyceridemic. EPA may play some therapeutic role in those with cystic fibrosis to reduce disease severity and may similarly play a role in type 2 diabetics in retarding the progression of diabetic nephropathy. However, the latter two indications require clinical trials and documentation to establish this.

There is conflicting evidence about a possible EPA benefit in depression. There is evidence in recent studies that EPA may have some neuroprotective properties. In that regard it has been investigated with some positive results for possible use in Huntington's disease, multiple sclerosis and some other disorders with neurodegenerative aspects. It might be of help in very mild, early Alzheimer's disease.

See the monograph on Fish Oils for further information.

RESEARCH SUMMARY

A double-blind, placebo-controlled study was performed to determine the triglyceride-lowering effect of EPA and DHA by themselves. In the seven-week study, 234 healthy men were randomly given the following: EPA in the ethyl ester at a dose of 3.8 grams daily, the ethyl ester of DHA at 3.6 grams daily or corn oil at 4 grams daily as a placebo. Triglycerides decreased by 21% in the EPA group and by 26% in the DHA group when compared with placebo. Some retroconversion of DHA to EPA was found, but no significant conversion of EPA to DHA was observed. A small, but significant increase in HDL-cholesterol was seen in the DHA group, and a small, but significant, decrease of total cholesterol and apolipoprotein A1 (Apo A1) was noted in the EPA group.

A randomized, double-blind, placebo-controlled crossover trial comparing fish oil supplementation against placebo was performed to determine fish oil effects on markers of clinical state, neutrophil function and lung inflammation in 16 patients with cystic fibrosis who were colonized with *Pseudomonas aeruginosa*. The fish oil used in this trial contained 2.7 grams of EPA (the amount of DHA in the capsules was not mentioned), which the subjects received daily for a six-week period. The placebo group received olive oil. The fish oil-supplemented group showed a significant reduction in disease severity and sputum volume and in the pathogenesis of lung damage.

The study also showed that EPA-rich fish oil dampens the damaging effects of the circulating neutrophils in the chronic inflammatory process. There is a reduction of leukotriene B4, which is believed to play an important role in the pathogenesis of lung damage in cystic fibrosis.

The effect of EPA on the progression of diabetic nephropathy has been studied in rats and humans. Measurement of urinary albumin is a key marker in determining renal function in diabetics. In a six-month study with Wister rats made diabetic by administration of streptozotocin, the ethyl ester of EPA was given to 16 rats, while an equal number served as the control. The mean microalbuminuria of the EPA group was significantly lower than that of the control group after four months, and this significant difference persisted for the remaining two months of the trial.

In a human study with type 2 diabetics, administration of 900 milligrams daily of the ethyl ester of EPA resulted in a significant decrease in urinary albumin excretion at three months after start of treatment; this reduction was sustained for a year after the start of treatment. These studies suggest that EPA supplementation of diabetics with albuminuria might retard the progression of diabetic nephropathy.

Like DHA, EPA has shown some very preliminary signs of possible benefit in some disorders of mental decline, including very mild Alzheimer's disease (with no impact on more established disease). There have been mixed results reported concerning the use of EPA to favorably modify behavior/learning in children. A recent French study reported that plasma EPA was inversely related to severity of depression in elderly subjects taking antidepressants; no other fatty acid was thus associated. Another research group, however, found that the data, at least so far, generally do not provide a convincing role for omega-3 fatty acids in the treatment of depression. More research is needed to further elucidate this issue.

Another recent review of relevant studies cited an open label trial in which EPA was used in subjects with Huntington's disease, a fatal autosomal dominant neurodegenerative disease characterized by progressive motor, cognitive and psychiatric abnormalities. Motor function improved in this study, compared with placebo controls. In another study, patients with advanced Huntington's disease also improved on a six-month EPA regimen, compared with controls who continued to deteriorate. Notable were 3D magnetic resonance imaging scans showing continuing progressive cerebral atrophy in the controls, while the EPA group showed some reversal of atrophy in these scans. In contrast with these findings, however, a larger, more recent trial, in which subjects received 2 grams daily of EPA, revealed no significant benefit in the experimentals versus the placebo group. There were statistically non-significant indications, however, of some stabilization or improvement in motor function in the EPA group. The review authors believe that more study is warranted and that EPA might yet demonstrate some significant benefit in subgroups of patients—or as an adjuvant treatment.

EPA has also been tested in multiple sclerosis (MS) patients. Multiple sclerosis is a chronic neurodegenerative demyelinating disease with autoimmune/inflammatory components. Many years ago, an association was made between high dietary fish intake and a lower incidence of multiple sclerosis (in coastal communities). And there is evidence that the omega-3 fatty acids may enhance *in vivo* myelinogenesis. Injected EPA, more potently than injected DHA, stimulated the expression of specific myelin proteins in rats. In a small open-label study, some omega-3 benefit was seen in MS patients followed for two years. They were supplemented with 0.9 grams daily of omega-3 and various vitamins. Annual exacerbation of symptoms rate was said to be significantly reduced in the EPA supplemented group. Two double-blind, placebo-controlled, randomized studies using EPA and DHA have been conducted in MS patients. In one of these, there was a non-statistically significant risk of disease progression among subjects receiving 10 grams of fish oil daily over two years, compared with subjects receiving olive oil placebo. A second smaller trial again resulted in statistically non-significant benefit in the EPA/DHA group, compared with placebo. The review authors concluded that the omega-3 fatty acids may be of moderate benefit in MS patients, although only further investigation can determine this with certainty.

A number of animal experiments have shown that omega-3 fatty acids may also be of benefit in neurologic injury. Some of these benefits have been demonstrated in animal models of ischemia/reperfusion injury and kainic acid-induced epileptic seizures. Again, more research is needed to see whether these substances can be helpful in a clinical context.

See the monograph on Fish Oils for further discussion.

CONTRAINDICATIONS, PRECAUTIONS, ADVERSE REACTIONS

CONTRAINDICATIONS
Known hypersensitivity to an EPA-containing product.

PRECAUTIONS
Because of possible antithrombotic activity of EPA, it should be used with caution in those who take warfarin (Coumadin) and by those with hemophilia. Similarly, EPA should be stopped before surgical procedures.

EPA supplements should be used by children, pregnant women and nursing mothers only if recommended and monitored by a physician.

ADVERSE REACTIONS
There have been no reports of serious adverse events in those taking EPA supplements, even up to 15 grams daily, for prolonged periods of time. Those side effects that have been reported include mild gastrointestinal upsets such as nausea and diarrhea, halitosis, eructation, "fishy" smelling breath, skin and even urine. The blood-thinning effects can cause occasional nosebleeds and easy bruising.

INTERACTIONS
Interactions may occur between EPA supplements and aspirin and other non-steroidal anti-inflammatory drugs and herbs such as garlic (*Allium sativum*) and ginkgo (*Ginkgo biloba*). Such interactions might be manifested by increased susceptibility to bruising, nosebleeds, hemoptysis, hematemesis, hematuria and blood in the stool. Most who take EPA supplements and the above drugs or herbs do not suffer from these problems and if they occur, they are rare. If they do occur, the EPA dose should be lowered or discontinued.

Conflicting results have been reported regarding the effects of EPA supplements on glycemic control in non-diabetics with glucose intolerance, and those with type 2 diabetes. Some early studies indicated that EPA supplements might have detrimental effects in those groups. Recent, better designed studies have not reported these adverse effects. There is no evidence that EPA supplements have detrimental effects on glucose tolerance, insulin secretion or insulin resistance in non-diabetic subjects. Diabetics should discuss the use of these supplements with their physicians and note if the supplements affect their glycemic control. Diabetics who take EPA supplements should be monitored by their physicians.

OVERDOSAGE
None known.

DOSAGE AND ADMINISTRATION
EPA is typically available in fish oil in combination with DHA. The usual ratio of EPA to DHA in these preparations is about 1.5. Fish oil preparations are available with higher ratios up to about 3. There is an ethyl ester form of EPA.

See Fish Oil monograph for further discussion.

LITERATURE
Féart C, Peuchant E, Letenneur L, et al. Plasma eicosapentaenoic acid is inversely associated with severity of depressive symptomatology in the elderly: data from the Bordeaux sample of the Three-City Study. *Am J Clin Nutr*. 2008;87(5):1156-1162.

Fujikawa M, Yamazaki K, Hamazaki T, et al. Effect of eicosapentaenoic acid ethyl ester on albuminuria in streptozotocin-induced diabetic rats. *J Nutr Sci Vitaminol*. 1994;40:49-61.

Grimsgaard S, Bønaa KH, Hansen JB, et al. Highly purified eicosapentaenoic acid and docosahexaenoic acid in humans have similar triacylglycerol-lowering effects but divergent effects on serum fatty acids. *Am J Clin Nutr*. 1997;66:649-659.

Jazayeri S, Tehrani-Doost M, Keshavarz SA, et al. Comparison of therapeutic effects of omega-3 fatty acid eicosapentaenoic acid and fluoxetine, separately and in combination, in major depressive disorder. *Aust N Z J Psychiatry*. 2008;42(3):192-198.

Kohno M, Ohmori K, Wada Y, et al. Inhibition by eicosapentaenoic acid of oxidized-LDL- and lysophosphatidylcholine-induced human coronary artery smooth muscle cell production of endothelin. *J Vasc Res*. 2001;38(4):379-388.

Lawrence R, Sorrell T. Eicosapentaenoic acid in cystic fibrosis: evidence of a pathogenic role for leukotriene B$_4$. *Lancet*. 1993;342:465-469.

Madsen L, Rustan QC, Vaagenes H, et al. Eicosapentaenoic and docosahexaenoic acid affect mitochondrial and peroxisomal fatty acid oxidation in relation to substrate preference. *Lipids*. 1999;34:951-963.

Otsuji S, Shibata N, Hirota H, et al. Highly purified eicosapentaenoic acid attenuates tissue damage in experimental myocardial infarction. *Jpn Circ J*. 1993;57(4):335-343.

Shimizu H, Ohtani K, Tanaka Y, et al. Long-term effect of eicosapentaenoic acid ethyl (EPA-E) on albuminuria of non-insulin dependent diabetic patients. *Diabetes Res Clin Pract*. 1995;28:35-40.

Terano T, Hira A, Hamazaki T, et al. Effect of oral administration of highly purified eicosapentaenoic acid on platelet function, blood viscosity and red blood cell deformability in healthy human subjects. *Atheroscler*. 1983;46:321-331.

Wada M, DeLong CJ, Hong YH, et al. Enzymes and receptors of prostaglandin pathways with arachidonic acid-derived versus eicosapentaenoic acid-derived substrates and products. *J Biol Chem*. 2007;282(31):22254-22266.

See Fish Oils monograph for further literature.

Equol

DESCRIPTION

Equol, an isoflavan, was first isolated in 1932 by Marrian and Haslewood from pregnant mare's urine and was named equol because of its equine source and the fact that it is a phenolic compound. In the early 1980s, equol was discovered in the urine of adults consuming soy foods and was found to be a metabolite of daidzein, the aglycone of daidzin, an isoflavone found in soy foods. (See Daidzein.)

Equol is formed from daidzein via colonic bacterial transformation. It is important to note that only about 20% to 35% of the adult population produces equol following soy consumption, the so-called equol producers. The frequency of equol producers in vegetarians is about 59% compared to the frequency of equol producers in nonvegetarian adults, which is about 25%. The frequency of equol producers among Japanese adults consuming soy is also about 59%. The nature of the colonic bacteria responsible for equol production remains unclear.

It is speculated that equol may be largely responsible for the putative health benefits of soy consumption, including a lower risk of breast cancer, lower risk of prostate cancer, lower risk of cardiovascular disease, better bone health, and decreased menopausal symptoms. The variance in the reported data on the putative health benefits of soy may have to do with whether one is an equol producer or an equol non-producer. This is known as the equol hypothesis. Interestingly, certain groups with a higher percentage of equol producers—for example, the Japanese and vegetarians—do have lower incidences of prostate and breast cancer, and cardiovascular disease.

Equol has a chiral center—equol has a chiral carbon atom at position C-3 of the furan ring—and consequently exists as two distinct, optically-active isomers (diastereoisomers), R-equol and S-equol. The enantiomer produced by metabolic reduction from daidzein is S-(-)equol. S-equol is also known as 7-hydroxy-3-(4'-hydroxyphenyl)-chroman; 3,4-dihydro-3-(4-hydroxyphenyl)-2*H*-1-benzopyran-7-ol; 4'.7-isoflavandiol, and 4',7-dihydroxyisoflavan. Its molecular formula is $C_{15}H_{14}O_3$. Equol is a non-steroidal estrogen, but, in contrast to the isoflavones genistein, daidzein and glycetein, equol is not a phytoestrogen, since it is not derived directly from soy, but is a metabolite of the phytoestrogen daidzein. Equol is represented by the following chemical structure.

S-(-)equol

To date, most of the studies on equol have been done on experimental animals or are *in vitro* studies. Human studies have been done comparing equol producers with equol non-producers. Equol itself is expected to enter the dietary supplement marketplace by 2009.

ACTIONS AND PHARMACOLOGY

ACTIONS

Equol has estrogenic activity, anti-androgen activity and antioxidant activity. Equol may have antiatherogenic, antiosteoporotic and anticarcinogenic activities.

MECHANISM OF ACTION

S-equol has a high affinity for estrogen receptor-beta. The affinity of S-equol for estrogen receptor-alpha is relatively poor. R-equol is relatively inactive with both estrogen receptor-beta and estrogen receptor-alpha.

S-equol is an antagonist of 5-alpha-dihydrotestosterone (DHT). S-equol is unique in being both a selective estrogen receptor agonist and an androgen antagonist. Equol binds DHT with high affinity, preventing DHT from binding to the androgen receptor. This could be beneficial for preventing growth of prostate tissue. Equol itself is not an androgen receptor blocker, nor does it inhibit the conversion of testosterone to DHT via the enzyme 5-alpha-DHT reductase. The nature of the putative binding of equol to DHT is unclear.

Equol has more potent antioxidant activity than the soy isoflavones daidzein and genistein. Equol's antioxidant capacity is basically due to its ability to donate hydrogen atoms/electrons from its phenolic hydroxyl group to free radicals.

Nitric oxide (NO) is produced in the body via the action of the constitutive nitric oxide synthases (NOS), endothelial NOS (eNOS) and neuronal NOS (nNOS), or by the inducible NOS (iNOS). NO produced by eNOS is crucial for the maintenance of healthy vascular tone and structure. However, NO produced via iNOS increases vascular oxidative stress, leading to decreased vascular bioavailability of NO. Equol has been shown to increase the vascular endothelial bioavailability of NO by affecting both eNOS and iNOS.

Vascular endothelial bioavailability of nitric oxide (NO) is key to vascular tone. Vascular tone is regulated by endothelial NO, which causes vascular relaxation by increasing intracellular cGMP (cyclic guanosine monophosphate) and activating cGMP-dependent protein kinase 1 (PKG1). Equol has been shown to enhance the bioavailability of endothelial NO through the downregulation of superoxide formation, mainly originating from NADPH oxidase activity. Among other things, this could result in lower levels of oxidatively modified low-density lipoprotein (LDL) and a decrease in inflammatory processes that could lead to atherosclerosis. The reactive oxygen species superoxide itself can react with NO to produce the highly reactive nitrogen species peroxynitrite. Production of peroxynitrite decreases vascular endothelial bioavailability of NO.

Equol was administered to male Sprague-Dawley rats and found to reduce prostate and epididymal weight and to increase luteinizing hormone (LH) levels. Equol was found to specifically bind to 5-alpha-dihydrotestosterone (DHT). It did not bind to the prostatic androgen receptor, nor did it bind to testosterone. Equol also has affinity for the estrogen receptor-beta, but has no affinity for the estrogen receptor-alpha. The decrease of prostate and epididymal weight and change in LH levels were attributed to the anti-androgen effect of equol via its binding to DHT and sequestering of DHT from the androgen receptor. Equol was also found to

have antiproliferative effects on benign and malignant prostatic epithelial cells, *in vitro*.

In another study looking at the effect of equol on mouse cell transformation, it was found that equol inhibited malignant transformation of the mouse cells by targeting an MEK (a type of mitogen activated kinase) signaling pathway. The putative antiandrogen activity of equol appeared not to be involved with the inhibition of malignant transformation of the cells in this case.

Ovariectomized mice were given doses of equol, and bone mineral density was measured by dual-energy X-ray absorptiometry. It was found that equol inhibited bone loss in the ovariectomized mice. A possible estrogenic effect of the equol was ruled out and the reason for the inhibition of bone loss was not clear.

PHARMACOKINETICS

The pharmacokinetics of equol in humans is complex and not well understood. The oral administration of both S-equol and R-equol to three healthy humans yielded similar pharmacokinetic profiles, confirming that the two diastereoisomers are similarly bioavailable. There were no statistical differences in maximum plasma concentration, time to reach maximum plasma concentration, terminal elimination half life, AUC (area under the curve), apparent volume of distribution, and systemic clearance between R-equol and S-equol, and no difference in the absorption rates between the two enantiomers. The data indicated that both enantiomeric forms of equol were absorbed without change and that no racemization occurred during or after intestinal uptake.

There are few detailed studies on the metabolism of equol. It has been thought that equol was the end product of the biotransformation of daidzein. Intact equol is found in the urine. However, recent research of the phase I metabolism of equol using human microsomes found that equol was converted to six metabolites with 3'-hydroxy-equol and 6-hydroxy-equol as the main products.

See Daidzein for the pharmacokinetics of daidzin and daidzein.

INDICATIONS AND USAGE

Claims for equol are similar to those for daidzein (see Daidzein), other soy isoflavones and soy products, in general. The principal claims for equol are that it may alleviate some menopausal symptoms, such as "hot flushes," and that it may help protect against osteoporosis and some cancers, as well as cardiovascular disease. It has also been postulated that it might even help prevent hair loss or promote hair regrowth by binding to 5-alpha dihydrotestosterone. Credible clinical evidence for these claims is lacking at this time. In fact, there are hardly any human clinical studies that have been performed with equol itself.

RESEARCH SUMMARY

After many years of researching the soy isoflavones with mixed and largely disappointing results, investigators recently concluded that they may have discovered why these products have yielded such inconsistent results. The discovery was made that equol, the major metabolite of daidzein, a phytoestrogen claimed by some to be a safer alternative to hormone replacement therapy (HRT) in menopausal women, is produced in the colon of only *some*, not all, humans. Indeed, only about one third of all humans have the ability to produce equol from the consumption of soy products. Much research has recently focused on investigating the effects of these products in both equol producers and equol non-producers.

Even taking this into account, however, effects being reported in equol producers remain inconclusive. One recent double-blind, placebo-controlled clinical trial in Taiwan divided a group of healthy menopausal women into equol producers and equol non-producers and tested the effects of soy isoflavones over a six-month period. There was a significant alleviation of hot flushes, excessive sweating and some other menopausal symptoms among the equol producers but not the equol non-producers. The researchers acknowledged that the effects were modest since the estrogenic activity of these isoflavones is significantly less than that of estrogen itself.

The preponderance of evidence to date suggests that even among equol producers, soy isoflavones, owing to their weaker estrogenic effects, are unlikely to provide a satisfactory alternative to standard HRT for most women suffering menopausal symptoms. Nor is the premise that soy isoflavones can provide a *safe* alternative to the standard therapy established. Some recent animal and *in vitro* studies show, on the contrary, that equol may promote changes in uterine and mammary tissues that could contribute to pre-cancerous and possibly even cancerous conditions. In one such study, using an animal menopause model, dietary supplementation over a three-month period with equol resulted in cellular mammary features of estrogenic stimulation similar to that found with estrogenic drugs.

Another recent animal study in which female rats were dosed with equol resulted in observations of uterine changes, again consistent with the sort of estrogenic stimulation seen with the estrogenic drugs. It is unclear as to the significance of these mammary and uterine changes for women, since the main estrogen receptors in uterine and mammary tissue are the alpha receptors and equol has low affinity for these receptors.

There is epidemiological evidence that dietary intake of soy products is positively correlated with a lower incidence of some cancers, cardiovascular disease and osteoporosis. There is no convincing human clinical evidence, however, that supplementation with equol is of benefit in these diseases. Some research suggests, but does not prove, that soy isoflavones may be of benefit in prostate cancer and its prevention. Trials are ongoing and may eventually yield some positive evidence of efficacy, but this remains to be seen. The possibility of using these isoflavones in the treatment and prevention of cervical and ovarian cancers is also under investigation.

Similarly, there is some evidence of bone-protective and cardiovascular-protective effects but none to date that rises to the level of convincing clinical results. Again, results have been highly inconsistent and the effects observed, at best, modest. Finally, there is no credible evidence that equol affects hair growth. Clinical research with equol will be more meaningful when equol itself becomes available, which should be in the near future.

CONTRAINDICATIONS, PRECAUTIONS, ADVERSE REACTIONS

CONTRAINDICATIONS

Equol is contraindicated in those who are hypersensitive to any component of an equol-containing product.

PRECAUTIONS

Pregnant women and nursing mothers should avoid the use of equol-containing supplements. All women should discuss the use of equol-containing supplements with their physicians before initiating their use.

Men with prostate cancer should discuss the advisability of the use of equol-containing supplements with their physicians before deciding to use them.

Women with estrogen receptor-positive tumors should exercise caution in the use of equol-containing supplements and should only use them if they are recommended and monitored by a physician.

ADVERSE REACTIONS

None known.

INTERACTIONS

DRUGS

Antibiotics may decrease equol formation.

DIETARY SUPPLEMENTS, FOODS

Green tea, fructooligosaccharides and potato starch may promote the formation of equol.

OVERDOSAGE

There are no reports of overdosage.

DOSAGE AND ADMINISTRATION

Equol dietary supplements are newly entering the dietary supplement marketplace. Doses higher than those recommended should be avoided.

LITERATURE

Akaza H, Miyanaga N, Takashima N, et al. Comparisons of percent equol producers between prostate cancer patients and controls: case-controlled studies of isoflavones in Japanese, Korean and American residents. *Jpn J Clin Oncol.* 2004;34(2):86-89.

Appt S, Clarkson TB, Groop PH, et al. Equol production capability is associated with favorable vascular function in postmenopausal women using tibolone; no effect with soy supplementation. *Atherosclerosis.* 2008;198(1):174-178.

Bolca S, Possemiers S, Herregat A, et al. Microbial and dietary factors are associated with the equol producer phenotype in healthy postmenopausal women. *J Nutr.* 2007;137(10):2242-2246.

Decroos K, Eeckhaut E, Possemiers S, et al. Administration of equol-producing bacteria alters the equol production status in the Simulator of the Gastrointestinal Microbial Ecosystem (SHIME). *J Nutr.* 2006;136(4):946-952.

Fuhrman BJ, Teter BE, Barba M, et al. Equol status modifies the association of soy intake and mammographic density in a sample of postmenopausal women. *Cancer Epidemiol Biomarkers Prev.* 2008;17(1):33-42.

Fujioka M, Uehara M, Wu J, et al. Equol, a metabolite of daidzein, inhibits bone loss in ovariectomized mice. *J Nutr.* 2004;134(10):2623-2627.

Fujimoto K, Tanaka M, Hirao Y, et al. Age-stratified serum levels of isoflavones and proportion of equol producers in Japanese and Korean healthy men. *Prostate Cancer Prostatic Dis.* 2008;11(3):252-257.

Hedlund TE, Johannes WU, Miller GJ. Soy isoflavonoid equol modulates the growth of benign and malignant prostatic epithelial cells in vitro. *Prostate.* 2003;54(1):68-78.

Hwang J, Wang J, Morazzoni P, et al. The phytoestrogen equol increases nitric oxide availability by inhibiting superoxide production: an antioxidant mechanism for cell-mediated LDL modification. *Free Radic Biol Med.* 2003;34(10):1271-1282.

Jackman KA, Woodman OL, Sobey CG. Isoflavones, equol and cardiovascular disease: pharmacological and therapeutic insights. *Curr Med Chem.* 2007;14(26):2824-2830.

Jackman KA, Woodman OL, Chrissobolis S, et al. Vasorelaxant and antioxidant activity of the isoflavone metabolite equol in carotid and cerebral arteries. *Brain Res.* 2007;1141:99-107.

Jou HJ, Wu SC, Chang FW, et al. Effect of intestinal production of equol on menopausal symptoms in women treated with soy isoflavones. *Int J Gynaecol Obstet.* 2008;102(1):44-49.

Joy S, Siow RC, Rowlands DJ, et al. The isoflavone Equol mediates rapid vascular relaxation: Ca2+-independent activation of endothelial nitric-oxide synthase/Hsp90 involving ERK1/2 and Akt phosphorylation in human endothelial cells. *J Biol Chem.* 2006;281(37):27335-27345.

Kang NJ, Lee KW, Rogozin EA, et al. Equol, a metabolite of the soybean isoflavone daidzein, inhibits neoplastic cell transformation by targeting the MEK/ERK/p90RSK/activator protein-1 pathway. *J Biol Chem.* 2007;282(45):32856-32866.

Kang JS, Yoon YD, Han MH, et al. Equol inhibits nitric oxide production and inducible nitric oxide synthase gene expression through down-regulating the activation of Akt. *Int Immunopharmacol.* 2007;7(4):491-499.

Lund TD, Munson DJ, Haldy ME, et al. Equol is a novel anti-androgen that inhibits prostate growth and hormone feedback. *Biol Reprod.* 2004;70(4):1188-1195.

Maruo T, Sakamoto M, Ito C, et al. Adlercreutzia equolifaciens gen. nov., sp. nov., an equol-producing bacterium isolated from human faeces, and emended description of the genus Eggerthella. *Int J Syst Evol Microbiol.* 2008;58(Pt 5):1221-1227.

Miyanaga N, Akaza H, Takashima N, et al. Higher consumption of green tea may enhance equol production. *Asian Pac J Cancer Prev.* 2003;4(4):297-301.

Rachoń D, Menche A, Vortherms T, et al. Effects of dietary equol administration on the mammary gland in ovariectomized Sprague-Dawley rats. *Menopause.* 2008;15(2):340-345.

Rachoń D, Vortherms T, Seidlová-Wuttke D, et al. Uterotropic effects of dietary equol administration in ovariectomized Sprague-Dawley rats. *Climacteric.* 2007;10(5):416-426.

Rachoń D, Vortherms T, Seidlová-Wuttke D, et al. Effects of dietary equol on the pituitary of the ovariectomized rats. *Horm Metab Res.* 2007;39(4):256-261.

Setchell KD, Brown NM, Lydeking-Olsen E. The clinical importance of the metabolite equol-a clue to the effectiveness of soy and its isoflavones. *J Nutr.* 2002;132(12):3577-3584.

Setchell KD, Clerici C, Lephart ED, et al. S-equol, a potent ligand for estrogen receptor beta, is the exclusive enantiomeric form of the soy isoflavone metabolite produced by human intestinal bacterial flora. *Am J Clin Nutr.* 2005;81(5):1072-1079.

Setchell KD, Cole SJ. Method of defining equol-producer status and its frequency among vegetarians. *J Nutr.* 2006;136(8):2188-2193.

Törmälä RM, Appt S, Clarkson TB, et al. Individual differences in equol production capability modulate blood pressure in tibolone-treated postmenopausal women: lack of effect of soy supplementation. *Climacteric.* 2007;10(6):471-479.

Vatanparast H, Chilibeck PD. Does the effect of soy phytoestrogens on bone in postmenopausal women depend on the equol-producing phenotype? *Nutr Rev.* 2007;65(6 Pt 1):294-299.

Wu J, Oka J, Ezaki J, et al. Possible role of equol status in the effects of isoflavone on bone and fat mass in postmenopausal Japanese women: a double-blind, randomized, controlled trial. *Menopause.* 2007;14(5):866-874.

Yuan JP, Wang JH, Liu X. Metabolism of dietary soy isoflavones to equol by human intestinal microflora—implications for health. *Mol Nutr Food Res.* 2007;51(7):765-781.

Evening Primrose Oil

DESCRIPTION

Evening primrose oil (EPO) is derived from the seeds of the evening primrose plant also known as *Oenthera biennis*. The evening primrose is native to North America, where it is regarded as a weed. This biennial plant is thought to be a complex of several closely related species belonging to the *Onagraceae* family.

EPO is a rich source of the long-chain fatty acid gamma-linolenic acid (GLA). The health benefits of EPO are attributed to GLA. GLA is an unusual constituent of living matter and is found in very few plants. These include, in addition to evening primrose, black currant, borage and hemp. GLA content in EPO ranges from approximately 7 to 14%. Typical EPO supplements contain about 9% GLA.

GLA is an all cis n-6 long-chain polyunsaturated fatty acid. It is comprised of 18 carbon atoms and three double bonds. GLA is also known as GLA; 18: 3n-6 and gamolenic acid, and chemically it is known as 6, 9, 12-octadecatrienoic acid; (Z, Z, Z)-6, 9, 12-octadecatrienoic acid, and cis-6, cis-9, cis-12-octadecatrienoic acid. GLA is present in EPO in the form of triglycerides. One such triglyceride in EPO contains two linoleic acid residues and one of GLA. This triglyceride, called di-linoleoyl-mono-gamma-linenyl-glycerol (DLMG), makes up about 18 to 19% of the triglycerides in EPO. GLA is concentrated in the sn-3 position in the triglycerides. GLA is represented by the following chemical structure:

GLA (gamma-linolenic acid)

EPO is approved in the United Kingdom as a pharmaceutical treatment for atopic dermatitis and mastalgia.

ACTIONS AND PHARMACOLOGY

ACTIONS

EPO may have anti-inflammatory and antithrombotic activities.

MECHANISM OF ACTION

The possible anti-inflammatory and anti-aggregatory actions of EPO may be accounted for by examining the role of GLA in eicosanoid biochemistry. GLA is metabolized to the 20-carbon polyunsaturated fatty acid dihomo-gamma-linolenic acid (DGLA; 20: 3n-6), which is a precursor to the 1-series prostaglandins, such as prostaglandin E_1 (PGE_1). The action of PGE_1 on inflammatory cells (e.g., polymorphonuclear leukocytes or PMNs) is mostly inhibitory. PGE_1 increases intracellular cyclic AMP (cAMP). This increase reduces the release of lysosomal enzymes, PMN chemotaxis and the margination and adherence of PMNs in the blood vessels. PGE_1 is also thought to inhibit lymphocyte function.

PGE_1, in addition to its role in suppressing the inflammatory process, inhibits platelet aggregation and has vasodilatory activity.

GLA, via its metabolite DGLA, has an inhibitory effect on leukotriene (LT) synthesis. Leukotriene B_4 (LTB_4) is an inflammatory mediator. DGLA is metabolized to 15-hydroxyl DGLA, which blocks the conversion of arachidonic acid to LTs, such as LTB_4.

In summary, GLA may suppress inflammation through its metabolism to DGLA, which, in turn, can competitively inhibit the pro-inflammatory 2-series prostaglandins and 4-series leukotrienes. The incorporation of GLA and its metabolites in cell membranes may also play a role in the possible anti-inflammatory, antithrombotic, anti-atherogenic and antiproliferative actions of EPO.

PHARMACOKINETICS

GLA-laden triglycerides in EPO are absorbed from the small intestine aided by bile salts. During this process, there is some deacylation of the fatty acids of the triglycerides. Reacylation takes place within the mucosal cells of the small intestine, and the GLA-laden triglycerides enter into the lymphatics in the form of chylomicrons. GLA-laden chylomicrons are transported from the lymphatics into the blood where GLA is carried in lipid particles to the various tissues of the body.

GLA is metabolized to the 20-carbon polyunsaturated fatty acid dihomo-gamma-linoleic acid (DGLA), which is converted to prostaglandin E_1 (PGE_1). It may also be metabolized to eicosapentaenoic acid (EPA). GLA and DGLA are normally not found as free fatty acids in cells. They occur mainly in cell membranes as components of phospholipids, neutral lipids and cholesterol esters. PGE_1 is metabolized to smaller prostaglandin remnants, which are primarily polar dicarboxylic acids, most of which are excreted in the urine.

INDICATIONS AND USAGE

EPO appears to be effective in some cases of rheumatoid arthritis and may be indicated in some other inflammatory disorders, such as Sjogren's syndrome and ulcerative colitis. Possible other indications include diabetic neuropathy, osteoporosis, acute respiratory distress syndrome (ARDS), hypertension and elevated serum lipids. EPO has been used with some preliminary success in some cancers, principally cerebral gliomas. It has not proved useful for tardive dyskinesia, premenstrual syndrome or menopausal flushing. It may be indicated in some cases for atopic dermatitis, particularly to help with itching, as well as for uremic skin conditions in hemodialysis patients. It should probably not be used in efforts to enhance immunity as it may be immunosuppressive.

RESEARCH SUMMARY

See GLA.

CONTRAINDICATIONS, PRECAUTIONS, ADVERSE REACTIONS

CONTRAINDICATIONS

Known hypersensitivity to an EPO-containing product.

PRECAUTIONS

Pregnant women and nursing mothers should avoid EPO supplements. Those with a history of partial complex seizure disorders, such as temporal lobe epilepsy, should avoid using EPO. Likewise, those with other types of seizure disorders and schizophrenics who are being treated with certain neuroleptic drugs, such as aliphatic phenothiazines (e.g., chlorpromazine), which may lower seizure threshold, should avoid using EPO. Because of possible antithrombotic activity of EPO, those with hemophilia or other hemorrhagic diatheses and those taking warfarin should exercise caution in the use of this supplement.

EPO supplementation should be halted before any surgical procedure. Because of its possible inhibition of lymphocyte function, those with immune deficiency disorders, such as AIDS, should exercise caution in the use of EPO.

ADVERSE REACTIONS

EPO may cause gastrointestinal symptoms like nausea, vomiting, flatulence, diarrhea and bloating. Headaches have also been reported in those taking EPO. It may precipitate symptoms of undiagnosed complex partial seizures and should be used, if at all, with extreme caution in those with a history of seizure disorder or those taking drugs that lower the seizure threshold, such as aliphatic phenothiazines.

INTERACTIONS

DRUGS

Use of EPO in schizophrenics who are being treated with certain neuroleptic agents which lower seizure threshold e.g., aliphatic phenothiazines, such as chlorpromazine, may cause partial complex seizures (e.g., temporal lobe epilepsy), as well as other types of seizures. Interactions may occur between EPO and warfarin, aspirin and NSAIDs. Such interactions, if they were to occur, might be manifested by nosebleeds, increased susceptibility to bruising and hematuria. If these symptoms occur, EPO intake should be stopped.

NUTRITIONAL SUPPLEMENTS

Interactions may occur if EPO is used with supplements that have antithrombotic activity, such as fish oils. This may be manifested by nosebleeds and increased susceptibility to bruising.

HERBS

Interactions may occur if EPO is used with such herbs as garlic (*Allium sativa*) and ginkgo (*Ginkgo biloba*). Such interactions may be manifested by nosebleeds and easy bruising.

OVERDOSAGE

There are no reports of overdosage with EPO.

DOSAGE AND ADMINISTRATION

EPO is available in capsules and also in topical preparations for cosmetic use. A capsule of EPO typically contains about 9% GLA. Doses used for the management of rheumatoid arthritis range from about 360 milligrams to 2.8 grams daily in divided doses (expressed as GLA). For management of atopic dermatitis, doses of 320 to 480 milligrams daily are used in divided doses (expressed as GLA). Doses of up to 2 grams daily (expressed as GLA) have been used by those with hypertriglyceridemia. EPO supplements should contain an antioxidant, such as vitamin E, to protect the unsaturated fatty acids against oxidation.

LITERATURE

See GLA monograph for additional literature.

Belch JJF, Hill A. Evening primrose oil and borage oil in rheumatologic conditions. *Am J Clin Nutr.* 2000; 71(suppl):352S-355S.

Holman CP, Bell AFJ. A trial of evening primrose oil in the treatment of chronic schizophrenia. *J Orthomol Psychiatry.* 1983; 12; 302-304.

Huang Y-S, Mills DE, eds. *Gamma-linolenic Acid: Metabolism and its Roles in Nutrition.* Champaign IL: American Oil Chemists Society Press; 1996.

Newall CA, Anderson LA, Phillipson, JD. Herbal Medicines: *A Guide for Health-Care Professionals.* London: The Pharmaceutical Press; 1996, pp110-113.

Vaddahi KS. The use of gamma-linolenic acid and linoleic acid to differentiate between temporal lobe epilepsy and schizophrenia. *Prostaglandins Med.* 1981; 6:375-379.

Fisetin

DESCRIPTION

Fisetin is a member of the flavonol subclass of flavonoids. Related members of the subclass include kaempferol, myricetin and quercetin. Fisetin is found in fruits, including strawberries, persimmons, kiwi fruit, peaches, grapes, apples and tomatoes, and in vegetables, including onions and cucumbers. Fisetin was a little known flavonoid until October 2006, when scientists from the Salk Institute reported that fisetin was found to boost memory in mice by stimulating the signaling pathways that enhance long-term memory and also play an important role in memory formation. Since cognitive deficits are common in those 60 years and older, this finding was looked upon as being a very significant one. Interestingly, older rats fed a diet enriched in strawberry extract for two months did much better in a test that measured cognitive performance than rats fed a control diet. Strawberries appear to be the highest natural source of fisetin.

Research is ongoing on the neuroprotective and cognitive-enhancing activities of fisetin. In addition, fisetin has also been found to have possible anticancer activity, including against prostate cancer.

Fisetin is chemically described as 2-(3,4-dihydroxyphenyl)-3,7-dihydroxy-4*H*-1-benzopyran-one and 3,3′,4,7-tetrahydroxy-2-phenylchromen-4-one. It is also called 3,3′,4′,7-tetrahydroxyflavone, 6-desoxyquercetin and fisidenolon. Its CAS registry number is 528-48-3, its empirical formula is $C_{15}H_{10}O_6$ and its molecular weight is 286.24

Fisetin usually is found in plants as the glycoside fisetin-8-glucoside.

All flavonoids possess a basic 15-carbon skeleton that can be represented as C_6-C_3-C_6 (see figure). The common structure is that of a diphenylpropane molecule, consisting of two aromatic rings linked through the three carbons. Flavonoids differ in the saturation of the heteroatomic ring C, in the placement of the aromatic ring B at positions C-2 or C-3 of ring C and in the overall hydroxylation or methoxylation patterns.

Flavonols possess a hydroxyl group on position 3 of the C ring (see figure), and fisetin possesses an additional three hydroxyl groups, one on position 7 of the A ring and the other two on the B ring (see figure). The chemical structures below are described within this monograph.

Fisetin

Flavonoid Skeleton

Flavonol Skeleton

ACTIONS AND PHARMACOLOGY
ACTIONS
Fisetin has antioxidant activity and possible antiallergy, anticancer, anti-inflammatory, cognition-enhancing and neurotropic activities.

MECHANISM OF ACTION
Antiallergy effects: Fisetin was found to inhibit T helper (Th) 2-type cytokine production by activated human basophils. The flavonoid was also demonstrated to have anti-inflammatory activity in activated human mast cells.

Activation of basophils via allergen stimulation releases cytokines, including interleukin (IL)-4, interleukin (IL)-13 and interleukin (IL)-5. These T helper 2-type cytokines are major participants in the allergic response and are key substances related to Ig (immunoglobulin) E production.

Mast cells also play a major role in the pathogenesis of allergic disorders. Activation of mast cells releases a number of inflammatory mediators, including histamine, cysteinyl leukotrienes, cytokines and chemokines. Fisetin was shown to modulate the inflammatory reaction in activated human mast cells.

The mechanism of fisetin's possible antiallergy action is unclear.

Anticancer activity: Fisetin has been shown to decrease the viability of three human prostate cancer cell lines: LNCaP, PC-3 and CWR22Rv1, and to have minimal effect on normal prostate epithelial cells. Fisetin demonstrated both cell-cycle arrest and apoptosis in human prostate cancer LNCaP cells.

The cell cycle is regulated by the cyclins in partnership with the cyclin-dependent kinases (CDKs). Fisetin was shown to induce arrest in the G1 phase of the cell cycle, accompanied by decreased levels of cyclins and CDKs and concomitant induction of the CDK inhibitors p21 and p27. Fisetin also was found to induce apoptosis in the LNCaP cells, associated with the release of mitochondrial cytochrome c into the cytosol of the cells. The caspases, also known as "executioner" proteins, play essential roles in programmed cell death, or apoptosis. Eleven human caspases have so far been described. Fisetin treatment of LNCaP cells activated caspases-3,-8 and -9. Pretreatment of the cells with a caspase inhibitor blocked the fisetin activation of these caspases.

Fisetin has also been demonstrated to inhibit the proliferation of the human cancer cell line HT-29. The inhibition of proliferation of these cells was accompanied by decreases in the activities of the cyclin-dependent kinases (CDKs) CDK2 and CDK4, as well as decreases in the levels of cyclin E and D1, and an increase in the CDK inhibitor p21.

Antioxidant activity: Fisetin is a polyphenol and, like other polyphenols, it can scavenge reactive oxygen and nitrogen species such as hydroxyl radicals, superoxide anions and peroxynitrite radicals. It can also inhibit the peroxidation of lipids. However, it has more specific antioxidant activities that it does not share with other polyphenolics, such as the ability to maintain reduced glutathione (GSH) levels in nerve cells and the ability to activate the transcription factor Nrf2, which in turn activates the antioxidant response element (ARE). GSH is the major intracellular antioxidant.

Peroxynitrite is one of the most potent of the reactive oxygen and reactive nitrogen species that cells encounter. Treatment of rat neurons with the peroxynitrite donor, SIN-1 (3-morpholino-sychonimine), was demonstrated to decrease intracellular GSH levels and cell viability. Extracellular signal-related kinases 1/2 (ERK 1/2) are kinases downstream from Ras, Raf and MEK that are ultimately responsible for the phosphorylation of key activator proteins within the cell. The peroxynitrite treatment of the neurons led to hyperphosphorylation of ERK 1/2 and decreases in the phosphorylation of c-Myc, decreased expression of glutamate cysteine ligase (GCL) levels, the rate-limiting enzyme for GSH biosynthesis, decreases in the levels of intracellular GSH and a reduction in the nuclear expression of the transcription factor Nrf-2, which activates the antioxidant response element (ARE). Fisetin was found to abolish all of these peroxynitrite-mediated changes. More study is required to completely understand this unique antioxidant mechanism of fisetin.

Anti-inflammatory activity: Fisetin has been reported to suppress the inflammatory effects of lipopolysaccharide (LPS)-induced microglial activation and neurotoxicity in microglial cells in *vitro*.

Microglial cells are innate immune cells in the central nervous system (CNS) and are the CNS's first and main form of active immune defense. However, activation of glial cells can also have negative effects, such as causing CNS neuroinflammation, which plays an important role in neurodegenerative diseases, including Alzheimer's disease and Parkinson's disease. Activation of microglial cells can produce various proinflammatory cytokines and nitric oxide (NO). Fisetin was found to suppress the production of tumor necrosis factor (TNF)-alpha, NO and prostaglandin (PGE$_2$), and to inhibit the gene expression of TNF-alpha, interleukin (IL)-1beta, cyclooxygenase (COX)-2 and inducible nitric oxide synthase (iNOS) at both mRNA (transcription) and protein (translation) levels in LPS-stimulated microglial cells.

Cognition-enhancing activity: Fisetin has been demonstrated to have significant effects on memory in a mouse object-recognition task assay study.

As discussed above, fisetin has been found to have neurotrophic activity, promoting the differentiation of nerve cells. The induction of nerve differentiation by fisetin depends to a large degree on the activation of the Ras-ERK (extracellular signal-regulated kinase) cascade. ERK activation ultimately leads to the phosphorylation and activation of the transcription factor CREB (cyclic AMP response element-binding) protein, and CREB activation appears to be a critical step in the signaling cascade that leads to the structural changes underlying the development of long-term potentiation.

Long-term potentiation (LTP) is the long-lasting enhancement in communication between two neurons that results from stimulating them simultaneously. LTP results in the strengthening of synaptic connections. LTP is considered to be an important model as to how memory is formed at the cellular level. Thus, the activation of the Ras-ERK cascade in neuronal cells by fisetin could result in changes in the brain that form the cellular basis of memory. Since neurons communicate by chemical synapses, LTP and its opposite process, long-term depression, are arguably the major cellular mechanisms that underlie learning and memory. Clearly, many more studies in this important area are necessary and warranted.

Neurotrophic activity: Neurotrophic factors comprise a family of proteins that play critical roles in the development, growth, maintenance and survival of nerve cells. Changes in the levels of these factors and/or their receptors are involved in the pathophysiology of neurodegenerative diseases, including Alzheimer's disease, Parkinson's disease, multiple sclerosis, amyotrophic lateral sclerosis and Huntington's disease. However, the use of these factors in the treatment of neurodegenerative disease has been less than successful. Proteins are not easy to deliver to the brain and their bioavailability in the brain is poor. In a study looking at various small molecules that had possible neurotrophic properties, fisetin emerged as a strong candidate. Using an assay for neurotrophic factor withdrawal with primary cortical neurons derived from rat embryos, it was demonstrated that these cells, which typically die within 24 hours in the absence of neurotrophic factors, survived when treated with fisetin and produced long neurites (immature or developing neurons).

PC12 is a rat pheochromocytoma cell line used as a model system for neuronal differentiation. In a study with PC12 cells, it was shown that fisetin promoted neuronal differentiation and was found to promote neuronal survival when exposed to oxidative stress.

In both of the above studies, the neurotrophic activity of fisetin (3,7,3',4' tetrahydroxyflavone [THF]) was compared with seven derivatives of fisetin: 3,3' dihydroxyflavone, 3,4' dihydroxyflavone, 3'4' dihydroxyflavone, 3,3',4' trihydroxyflavone, 3,7,3' trihydroxyflavone, 3,7,4' trihydroxyflavone and 7,3'4' trihydroxyflavone. In both protection from oxidative stress-induced death and in induction of PC12 cell differentiation, it turned out that although fisetin had good neuronal differentiation activity and good neuronal survival activity when faced with an oxidative stress challenge, both of these activities were somewhat better in the hands of 3,3',4' trihydroxyflavone. However, in the neurotrophic factor withdrawal assay, fisetin was found to be more effective than 3,3',4 trihydroxyflavone. Analysis of the chemical structural requirements for the neurotrophic activity lead to the following conclusions: The best activity is obtained when there is a phenolic hydroxyl group in the C3 position, when there is 3',4' dihydroxy or catechol structure in the B ring and when there is unsaturation in the C ring. Also, the more hydrophilic the structure, the better the penetration into the nerve cells. Further, the 3-hydroxyl structure appears to antagonize the survival-promoting effects of fisetin, while the 7-hydroxyl structure enhances the survival-promoting effects, and a minimum of three hydroxyl groups seems optimal for both the differentiation effect and the promotion of survival effect in the neurotrophic factor withdrawal assay.

Although the mechanism of the neurotrophic effect of fisetin is not completely understood, there are a few things that can be said. The effect may be a result of antioxidant activity; there may be activation of signaling pathways, for example, the Ras-ERK cascade; glutathione levels may increase; and there may be increased proteasome activity in the neurons.

One can look at biological antioxidation in a number of ways. Fisetin and the fisetin derivatives are polyphenols, and polyphenols are known to be scavengers of superoxide anions and hydroxyl radicals and to protect against lipid peroxidation. Fisetin and the fisetin derivatives do all of that, but does that have anything to do with its neurotrophic activity? There are a number of assays for antioxidant activity, including TEAC, or the Trolox equivalent activity concentration. There was no correlation with antioxidant activity of fisetin and the various derivatives, as determined by the TEAC value, and protection from oxidative stress-induced death. The tripeptide, reduced glutathione (GSH), is the major cellular antioxidant. Fisetin can increase intracellular levels of GSH, while stress secondary to neurotrophic withdrawal can decrease levels. However, enhancement of GSH levels did not appear to play a significant role in the survival-promoting activity of fisetin or any of the fisetin derivatives.

Cells possess a number of different endogenous antioxidant mechanisms. Induction of phase II detoxification enzymes, including heme oxygenase (HO-1), can provide significant antioxidant protection of cells. The activation of the transcription of the genes for the phase II detoxification enzymes is via the *cis* acting enhancer, the antioxidant response element (ARE). Activation of the ARE is via the leucine zipper transcription factor Nfr2. A good way to determine if induction of heme oxygenase-1 by fisetin and its derivatives plays a role in their neurotrophic activity is to assay the activity of heme oxygenase-1. Activation of ARE and subsequently of heme oxygenase-1 does not appear to play a significant role in the neurotrophic activity of these flavonoids.

Fisetin and its derivatives activate several signaling pathways, some of which may be involved in protection of cortical neurons from trophic factor withdrawal. Fisetin, as well as some of its derivatives, can activate the Ras-ERK signaling pathway, and it appears that this mechanism may play a role in the neurotrophic activity of fisetin.

The proteasome is a large protein complex whose main role is to degrade unneeded or damaged proteins by proteolysis. Proteins are tagged for degradation by a small protein called ubiquitin, catalyzed by the enzyme ubiquitin ligase. This is a major biological housekeeping function. Recently, it has been learned that proteasomes have other functions, as well. Proteasome activity appears to be required for axon initiation, elongation and maintenance in primary, postmitotic neurons. Also, recently, it has been observed that proteasome activity is decreased in a number of degenerative neurological disorders, including Alzheimer's disease and Parkinson's disease. Therefore, increasing proteasome activity might play a critical role in the elimination of abnormal and oxidized proteins. Fisetin and several of its derivatives appear to enhance proteasome activity in a nerve cell line and this may account, in part, for the neurotrophic activity of fisetin. It is clear that much work needs to be done, and is certainly warranted, in order to better understand the mechanism of action of the neurotrophic activity of fisetin.

PHARMACOKINETICS

Very little is known about the pharmacokinetics of fisetin. The major food form of fisetin appears to be the glycan, fisetin-8-glucoside. After oral intake of fisetin-8-glucoside, it is likely that some is absorbed at the level of the small intestine and some may travel to the large intestine and undergo metabolism by bacterial enzymes and then get absorbed. The fisetin produced from the metabolism of fisetin-8-glucone and the fisetin-8-glucoside absorbed from the small intestine are likely to be very rapidly metabolized to form glucuronides and sulfates. The various metabolites are likely to be transported to various tissues of the body. Based on murine studies on the cognition-enhancing effects of fisetin, it is very likely that fisetin can cross the blood-brain barrier and be transported into nerve cells. Much work is needed and warranted on the pharmacokinetics of fisetin.

INDICATIONS AND USAGE

There are preliminary indications in the research that the flavonoid fisetin may have neuroprotective, anti-inflammatory and anticancer effects.

RESEARCH SUMMARY

In a number of *in vitro* investigations, fisetin demonstrated potent neuroprotective effects. In one of these studies, fisetin suppressed activation of microglia, immune cells found in the central nervous system. Activation of these cells has been associated with production of proinflammatory cytokines and nitric oxide which can exert neurotoxic effects leading to various neurodegenerative diseases, including, it is claimed, Alzheimer's disease. Based upon the exhibited strong anti-inflammatory activity of fisetin in these microglia, the researchers concluded that fisetin might ultimately prove a useful therapeutic agent in the treatment of many neuro-inflammatory diseases. In another study, fisetin helped protect retinal ganglion cells from oxidative-induced death. The researchers suggested that fisetin might thus become a candidate for preventing/treating such ocular diseases as glaucoma, diabetic retinopathy and age-related macular degeneration. And in a test of fisetin in the small clot embolism model of cerebral ischemia in rabbits, the flavonoid significantly reduced behavioral deficits following stroke, further reinforcing the idea that this substance may have broad-spectrum neuroprotective effects. There is also experimental animal data indicating that fisetin might have the ability to enhance long-term memory through its neuroprotective actions. Clinical data in support of these findings are entirely lacking at this time. Studies in the clinical domain are needed and warranted.

There is also very preliminary *in vitro* evidence that fisetin might be helpful in disorders characterized by allergic inflammation. In one study related to this, fisetin was reported to strongly downregulate human mast cell activation. Mast cell activation is associated with release of such inflammatory mediators as histamine, cytokines, chemokines and leukotrienes. Here, too, more research is needed.

Though again very preliminary, there is some evidence emerging that fisetin might have useful anticancer effects. In an *in vitro* study of human colon-cancer cells, fisetin, in a dose-dependent manner, inhibited cancer cell growth. In another *in vitro* trial, fisetin induced apoptosis and cell-cycle arrest in human prostate cancer cells. Follow-up in animal and clinical trials is clearly warranted.

CONTRAINDICATIONS, PRECAUTIONS, ADVERSE REACTIONS

CONTRAINDICATIONS

Fisetin is contraindicated in those who are hypersensitive to any component of a fisetin-containing product.

PRECAUTIONS

Those who wish to try fisetin supplements for the support of any health condition should first discuss its use with his or her physician.

The use of fisetin-containing supplements by pregnant and nursing women should be avoided.

ADVERSE REACTIONS

None known.

INTERACTIONS

DRUGS

None known.

DIETARY SUPPLEMENTS

None known.

OVERDOSAGE

There are no reports of overdosage.

DOSAGE AND ADMINISTRATION

The optimal dose of fisetin for health benefits is not known.

Several dietary supplements contain low and probably insignificant amounts of fisetin as part of a blend.

Dietary supplements containing only fisetin are expected to enter the nutritional supplement marketplace in the near future.

Strawberries are probably the richest natural source of fisetin. However, it would probably require consuming pounds of strawberries daily to achieve the various health benefits claimed for fisetin. Obviously, this is not recommended.

LITERATURE

Burdo J, Schubert D, Maher P. Glutathione production is regulated via distinct pathways in stressed and non-stressed cortical neurons. *Brain Res*. 2008;1189:12-22.

Chen YC, Shen SC, Lee WR, et al. Wogonin and fisetin induction of apoptosis through activation of caspase 3 cascade and alternative expression of p21 protein in hepatocellular carcinoma cells SK-HEP-1. *Arch Toxicol.* 2002;76(5-6):351-359.

Hanneken A, Lin FF, Johnson J, et al. Flavonoids protect human retinal pigment epithelial cells from oxidative-stress-induced death. *Invest Ophthalmol Vis Sci.* 2006; 47(7):3164-3177.

Higa S, Hirano T, Kotani M, et al. Fisetin, a flavonol, inhibits TH2-type cytokine production by activated human basophils. *J Allergy Clin Immunol.* 2003;111(6):1299-1306.

Hou DX, Fukuda M, Johnson JA, et al. Fisetin induces transcription of NADPH:quinone oxidoreductase gene through an antioxidant responsive element-involved activation. *Int J Oncol.* 2001;18(6):1175-1179.

Khan N, Afaq F, Syed DN, et al. Fisetin, a novel dietary flavonoid causes apoptosis and cell-cycle arrest in human prostate cancer LNCaP cells. *Carcinogenesis.* 2008;29(5):1049-1056.

Lee WR, Shen SC, Lin HY, et al. Wogonin and fisetin induce apoptosis in human promyeloleukemic cells, accompanied by a decrease of reactive oxygen species, and activation of caspase 3 and Ca(2+)-dependent endonuclease. *Biochem Pharmacol.* 2002;63(2):225-236.

Lu X, Jung J, Cho HJ, et al. Fisetin inhibits the activities of cyclin-dependent kinases leading to cell cycle arrest in HT-29 human colon cancer cells. *J Nutr.* 2005;135(12):2884-2890.

Maher P. The flavonoid fisetin promotes nerve cell survival from trophic factor withdrawal by enhancement of proteasome activity. *Arch Biochem Biophys.* 2008;476(2):139-144.

Maher P. A comparison of the neurotrophic activities of the flavonoid fisetin and some of its derivatives. *Free Radic Res.* 2006;40(10):1105-1111.

Maher P, Akaishi T, Abe K. Flavonoid fisetin promotes ERK-dependent long-term potentiation and enhances memory. *Proc Natl Acad Sci U S A.* 2006;103(44):16568-16573.

Maher P, Salgado KF, Zivin JA, et al. A novel approach to screening for new neuroprotective compounds for the treatment of stroke. *Brain Res.* 2007;1173:117-125.

Park HH, Lee S, Oh JM, et al. Anti-inflammatory activity of fisetin in human mast cells (HMC-1). *Pharmacol Res.* 2007; 55(1):31-37.

Sengupta B, Banerjee A, Sengupta PK. Interactions of the plant flavonoid fisetin with macromolecular targets: insights from fluorescence spectroscopic studies. *J Photochem Photobiol B.* 2005;80(2):79-86.

Sengupta B, Banerjee A, Sengupta PK. Investigations on the binding and antioxidant properties of the plant flavonoid fisetin in model biomembranes. *FEBS Lett.* 2004;570(1-3):77-81.

Zbarsky V, Datla KP, Parkar S, et al. Neuroprotective properties of the natural phenolic antioxidants curcumin and naringenin but not quercetin and fisetin in a 6-OHDA model of Parkinson's disease. *Free Radic Res.* 2005;39(10):1119-1125.

Zheng LT, Ock J, Kwon BM, et al. Suppressive effects of flavonoid fisetin on lipopolysaccharide-induced microglial activation and neurotoxicity. *Int Immunopharmacol.* 2008;8(3):484-494.

Fish Oils

DESCRIPTION

Fish oils, also known as marine oils, are lipids found in fish, particularly cold water fish, and other marine life such as phytoplankton. These oils are rich sources of long-chain polyunsaturated fatty acids (LCPUFA) of the n-3 (omega-3) type. The two most studied fish oils are the 20 carbon eicosapentaenoic acid (EPA; C20:5n-3) and the 22-carbon docosahexaenoic acid (DHA; C22:6n-3). EPA contains five double bonds and DHA, six double bonds. These double bonds are all in the cis configuration. DHA is a vital component of the phospholipids of human cellular membranes, especially those in the brain and retina.

Both EPA and DHA are found naturally in the form of triacylglycerols or TAGs. The docosahexaenate in the triacylglycerols of fish oil appears to be primarily in the sn-2 position (the middle carbon) of glycerol whereas there is more random distribution of eicosapantaenoate over all three positions of glycerol.

In September 2004, the Food and Drug Administration (FDA) announced the following qualified health claim for EPA and DHA omega-3 fatty acids: "Supportive but not conclusive research shows that consumption of EPA and DHA omega-3 fatty acids may reduce the risk of coronary heart disease. One serving of (name of food, typically an oily fish, such as salmon, tuna and herring) provides (x) grams of EPA and DHA fatty acids." In 2000, the FDA announced a similar qualified health claim for dietary supplements containing EPA and DHA omega-3 fatty acids and the reduced risk of coronary heart disease (CHD). The FDA recommended that consumers not exceed more than a total of 3 grams per day of EPA and DHA omega-3 fatty acids, with no more than 2 grams from a nutritional supplement.

ACTIONS AND PHARMACOLOGY

ACTIONS

Supplemental fish oils have triglyceride-lowering activity. They may also have anti-inflammatory, anti-thrombotic and immunomodulatory actions.

MECHANISM OF ACTION

EPA and DHA have several actions in a number of body systems. EPA and DHA lower elevated triglyceride levels. In the cardiovascular system, EPA and DHA have anti-arrhythmic properties. EPA and DHA have anti-inflammatory and immune-modulating properties and are beneficial for the musculoskeletal, gastrointestinal and immune systems. EPA and DHA are also important for maintenance of normal blood flow as they lower fibrinogen levels and prevent platelets from sticking to each other. DHA is vital for normal brain development for the fetus and infant and for the maintenance of normal brain function throughout life. DHA appears to be a major determinant of membrane fluidity in brain cells, and this could play a major role in the maintenance of normal cognition and mood.

The triglyceride-lowering effect of EPA and DHA appears to result from the combined effects of inhibition of lipogenesis and stimulation of fatty acid oxidation in liver. EPA and DHA inhibit the transcription of genes coding for lipogenesis enzymes and increase the transcription of the regulatory enzymes of fatty acid oxidation. Stimulation of fatty acid oxidation is through activation of PPAR (peroxisome proliferator-activated receptor)- alpha. Inhibition of lipogenesis is through down-regulation of SREBP (sterol regulatory element binding protein) -1c messenger RNA.

Several mechanisms are believed to account for the anti-inflammatory activity of EPA and DHA. The two competitively inhibit the conversion of arachidonic acid to the pro-inflammatory eicosanoids PG (prostaglandin)E_2 and LT(leukotiene)B_4, thus reducing their synthesis. EPA and DHA also inhibit the synthesis of the inflammatory cytokines TNF (tumor necrosis factor)-alpha and IL(interleukin)-1 beta in both healthy volunteers and rheumatoid arthritis patients. EPA and DHA inhibit the 5-LOX (lipoxygenase) pathway responsible for the conversion of arachidonic acid to inflammatory leukotrienes in neutrophils and monocytes and can suppress phospholipase C-mediated signal transduction, also involved in inflammatory events. EPA and DHA may possess disease-modifying activity. Incorporation of EPA and DHA into articular cartilage chondrocyte membranes results in a dose-dependent reduction in the expression and activity of the proteoglycan-degrading enzymes known as aggrecanases. This similarly results in decreased expression of interleukin IL-1 alpha and TNF-alpha as well as COX (cyclooxygenase) -2, but not COX-1.

EPA and DHA have both similar and dissimilar physiologic roles. EPA appears to be more important in those roles where the eicosanoids are involved, whereas DHA seems to play its most important roles in the membranes of CNS cells and in the PPAR system. EPA is the precursor to series-3 prostaglandins (PG), the series-5 leukotrienes (LT) and the series-3 thromboxanes (TX). Specifically, EPA is the precursor of TXA_3 and LTB_5, eicosanoids, which reduce platelet aggregation and increase vasodilation. This could account in part for those fish oil effects that may lead to reduced clotting activity and decreased blood pressure.

Fish oils appear to have mood-stabilizing properties when used in the treatment of bipolar disorder. Overactive cell-signaling pathways may be involved in the pathophysiology of bipolar disorder. EPA and DHA may dampen signal transduction associated with phosphatidylinositol and arachidonic acid. These LCPUFAs, especially DHA, are incorporated into the phospholipids of the membranes of cells involved in cell-signaling pathways.

The mechanism by which fish oils appear to prevent cardiac arrhythmia is unclear but also may have something to do with the incorporation of these LCPUFAs into the cell membranes of the heart.

Fish oils may have cancer chemopreventive effects, but clinical chemoprevention studies are needed to determine if this is the case. *In vitro* and animal studies have shown EPA and DHA to suppress neoplastic transformation, inhibit cancer growth, enhance apoptosis or programmed cell death and to have anti-angiogenic activity. A common mechanism underlying all of the above activity could be the role of the LCPUFAs in modulating eicosanoid production and activity. Fats other than from fish sources are known risk factors for cancer as well as cardiovascular disease. Those fats may direct the eicosanoid pathways toward situations in which cancer cells can flourish, whereas the opposite may be the case for the fish oils.

PHARMACOKINETICS

Different forms of fish oil are commercially available. The natural forms of EPA and DHA, as found in fish and phytoplankton, exist in the form of triacylglycerols (TAGs). These are the forms most commonly available at present. More concentrated forms of EPA and DHA are the EPA and DHA ethyl esters and free (i.e. unesterified) EPA and DHA. The pharmacokinetics of these forms is similar.

EPA- and DHA-laden triacylglycerols, following ingestion, undergo hydrolysis via lipases to form monoglycerides and free fatty acids. In the enterocytes, reacylation takes place reforming TAGs, which are then assembled with phospholipids, cholesterol and apoproteins into chylomicrons. The chylomicrons are released into the lymphatics from whence they are transported to the systemic circulation. In the circulation, the chylomicrons are degraded by lipoprotein lipase, and EPA and DHA are transported by the circulation to various tissues of the body where they are used mainly for the synthesis of phospholipids. These phospholipids are incorporated into the cell membranes of red blood cells, platelets and CNS cells, among others. EPA and DHA are mainly found in the phospholipid components of the cell membranes. DHA is taken up by the brain in preference to other fatty acids. DHA can partially retroconvert to EPA, and EPA may partially convert to DHA.

Enteral absorption of EPA and DHA is at least as good from semi-synthetic ethyl esters as it is from the natural forms.

INDICATIONS AND USAGE

Fish oils may primarily be indicated to lower triglyceride levels in those with hypertriglyceridemia. Another important indication may be to prevent death in those who have suffered myocardial infarctions. Fish oils are used to decrease clotting tendencies of the blood. They may also be indicated for lowering blood pressure, for preventing restenosis following coronary angioplasty, for alleviating some of the symptoms of rheumatoid arthritis and for ulcerative colitis. The claim that they can help prevent relapse in Crohn's disease is questioned by recent research. They may help stabilize mood in bipolar disorder and may have beneficial effects in IgA nephropathy. There is evidence they may help prevent rejection in renal transplant patients, and they are used in enteral feeding of various patient categories.

There is some evidence that fish oils have neuroprotective properties and may be useful in very mild, early stages of Alzheimer's disease. They may also be beneficial for eye health.

There is very little evidence in support of an indication for use in angina and no convincing evidence to support claimed indications for asthma, hay fever and psoriasis. There is insufficient data to make any judgment about possible use of fish oil in cancer.

RESEARCH SUMMARY

A meta-analysis of several studies to determine the effect of fish oil supplementation on serum triglyceride levels consistently shows a significant triglyceride-lowering effect. Doses of fish oil in the studies ranged from 0.5 grams to 25 grams daily with an average intake of about 6 grams daily. These numbers refer to the amount of EPA and DHA received. The average ratio of EPA to DHA in these studies was about 1.5, and the studies lasted from two weeks to two years. The triglyceride-lowering effect was dose-related. Overall, cholesterol levels did not change. Some of the studies reported an increase in LDL cholesterol and some showed an increase in HDL cholesterol.

A double-blind, placebo-controlled study was performed to determine the triglyceride-lowering effect of EPA and DHA by themselves. In this seven-week study, 234 healthy men were randomly given the following: EPA, in the ethyl ester at a dose of 3.8 grams daily, the ethyl ester of DHA at 3.6 grams daily or corn oil at 4 grams daily. Triglycerides decreased by 21% in the EPA group and by 26% in the DHA group when compared to placebo. Some retroconversion from DHA to EPA was noted, but no significant conversion of EPA to DHA was observed. A slight, but significant, increase in HDL-cholesterol was seen in the DHA group, and a slight, but significant, decrease of total cholesterol and apolipoprotein A1 was noted in the EPA group.

Another study looked at the effect on serum lipids of fish oil supplements by themselves and in combination with fish oils and garlic powder. Fifty men with moderately elevated cholesterol were assigned to one of four treatment groups and followed for 12 weeks. The fish oil used in this study was a natural triacylglycerol, and those receiving fish oil took 12 grams containing 30% of a mixture of EPA and DHA in a 1.5 ratio for a total of 2.16 grams of EPA and 1.44 grams of DHA daily. One group received fish oil and garlic powder, another group received fish oil and a placebo powder, a third group received powder and a placebo oil, and the remaining group was given a placebo oil and a placebo powder.

The fish oil group registered a 3.73% lowering of serum triglycerides, no significant change in total cholesterol and an 8.5% increase in LDL-cholesterol. No significant changes were noted in this group in the ratios of total cholesterol over HDL-cholesterol and LDL-cholesterol over HDL-cholesterol. The fish oil and garlic powder group were found to have a 34.3% lowering of triglycerides, a 12% lowering of total cholesterol, a 9.5% decrease in LDL cholesterol, a 16% decrease in the total cholesterol over HDL-cholesterol ratio and a 19% decrease in the LDL-cholesterol over HDL-cholesterol ratio. The garlic group showed no change in the serum triglyceride value, and 11.5% decrease in total cholesterol, a 14% decrease in LDL cholesterol, a 12.5% decrease in the total cholesterol to HDL-cholesterol ratio and a 15% decrease in the LDL-cholesterol ratio. No change in HDL-cholesterol was observed in the fish oil group. A slight non-significant increase in HDL-cholesterol was noted in the garlic group.

The GISSI-Prevenzione study examined the effect of dietary fish oil and vitamin E supplementation on mortality and morbidity in over 11,000 subjects who had suffered a myocardial infarction within three months of entering the trial. The subjects (85% men, 51% younger than 60) were randomly assigned to one of four groups. One group, consisting of 2,836 subjects, received 1 gram of fish oil daily containing 850 to 882 milligrams of EPA and DHA in the form of the ethyl esters and in a ratio of EPA to DHA of 1 to 2. A second group, consisting of 2,830 subjects, received 300 milligrams of vitamin E in the form of synthetic D alpha-tocopherol. A third group of 2,830 subjects received both the fish oils and vitamin E, while the fourth group of 2,828 acted as the control. The trial lasted for 42 months.

The primary combined endpoint was death, non-fatal myocardial infarction and stroke. Treatment with fish oil, but not vitamin E, significantly lowered the risk of the primary endpoint. The effect of the combined treatment was similar to that of fish oil alone. Although vitamin E did show a trend toward a reduction in mortality, the trend did not show significance. No adverse effects were reported except for some mild gastrointestinal symptoms. The dose of fish oil used in the trial lowered serum triglycerides by 3.4%.

The most significant result of this trial was the reduction in risk for overall and sudden cardiac death. It is believed that the reduction of sudden cardiac death was due to the anti-arrhythmic effect of the LCPUFAs. The study suggests that up to 20 lives per 1,000 post-MI patients could be saved by consuming daily doses of less than 1 gram of EPA and DHA.

Meta-analysis of 17 controlled studies with fish oil indicates that supplementation with 3 or more grams of fish oil daily can lead to clinically relevant systolic and diastolic blood pressure reductions in individuals with untreated hypertension but not in normotensives. The EPA plus DHA doses used in these trials ranged from 1 to 15 grams with an EPA to DHA ratio of about 1.5.

A meta-analysis of the effect of fish oils following coronary angioplasty indicated that subjects who had undergone successful angioplasty had a significantly lower rate (13.9%) of restenosis when given 4 to 5 grams daily of mixtures of EPA and DHA for three months to one year following the angioplasty.

In contrast to these positive findings, one meta-analysis conducted a few years ago failed to find a clear effect of long-chain and shorter-chain omega-3 fats on total mortality, combined cardiovascular events or cancer. These researchers went so far as to say that "clinically important harm could not be excluded" based on their analysis of the data reviewed. More recently, however, the GISSI group, using new data, found that the omega-3 fatty acids "can provide a small beneficial advantage in terms of mortality and admission to hospital for cardiovascular reasons in patients with heart failure in a context of usual care." An editorial accompanying this study's publication concluded that "supplementation with n-3 polyunsaturated fatty acids should join the short list of evidence-based life-prolonging therapies for heart failure."

Another recent review cited three large controlled, randomized trials involving 32,000 participants in which supplementation with DHA and EPA resulted in significant reductions in cardiovascular events. These findings, they concluded, show that intake of fish oils should be increased, especially among those at risk of cardiovascular disease. They recommended consuming both DHA and EPA in a combined dose of about 500 mg for those without disease and 1,000 mg in those with known coronary artery disease. They further recommended that those with hypertriglyceridemia take 3 to

4 grams of DHA/EPA daily, a dosage that they say can reduce triglyceride levels by 25 to 50%. They further suggested that blood levels of DHA and EPA could one day be used to identify patients with insufficient levels and to individualize treatment protocols.

And yet another recent review of the data related to omega-3 fatty acids and their use in coronary heart disease concluded that the relevant studies demonstrate a definite benefit. The American Heart Association currently recommends about 1 gram of fish oils per day for those with known coronary artery disease. And people with no known heart disease, it suggests, should eat oily fish at least twice a week. Because of possible mercury and other contaminants in some fish and fish oils, the FDA has cautioned pregnant women to avoid any probable contaminated source. Daily ingestion of at least 3 grams of EPA and DHA mixtures for a period of 12 weeks or longer has been found to reduce the number of tender joints and amount of morning stiffness in subjects with rheumatoid arthritis. Those with rheumatoid arthritis consuming these supplements have been reported to lower or discontinue use of nonsteroidal anti-inflammatory drugs or disease-modifying anti-rheumatic drugs. The supplements appeared to be well tolerated in these individuals, and no serious toxicity was reported.

A one-year double-blind trial of subjects with Crohn's disease randomized these subjects into two groups. One group received a mixture of 2.7 grams of EPA and DHA daily. The fish oil was in the form of enterically coated free fatty acids and provided 1.8 grams of EPA and 0.9 grams of DHA daily. It was noted that the subjects taking the fish oil supplement had a significantly reduced relapse rate. No significant adverse effects were reported. More recently, however, two randomized, placebo-controlled studies conducted at 98 centers in Canada, Europe, the U.S. and Israel found that the omega-3 fatty acids are not effective for the prevention of relapse in Crohn's disease. Rate of relapse was similar in both fatty acid and placebo groups at one year.

Supplementation of fish oils in subjects with ulcerative colitis has shown some encouraging trends. In one study, six patients with active ulcerative colitis were given 3 to 4 grams of a mixture of EPA and DHA daily in the form of natural triacylglycerols for a period of 12 weeks. Significant results were reported regarding the subjects' symptoms and histological appearance of the rectal mucosa by the end of the 12 weeks.

A few open studies with few subjects have suggested that fish oil supplements positively affect the clinical course of psoriasis. The best study to date, a double-blind, placebo-controlled, multi-center trial of 155 subjects with moderate-to-severe psoriasis showed no clinically important difference between subjects receiving 5 grams daily of EPA and DHA in ethyl ester form and the placebo group over a four-month period.

A four-month, double-blind, placebo-controlled study of 30 subjects with bipolar disorder compared the effects of fish oil supplements with placebo. Fourteen subjects received 9.6 grams daily of fish oil consisting of 6.2 grams of EPA and 3.4 grams of DHA, and 16 subjects received olive oil as a placebo. This study showed improvement in the short-term course of the disorder with fish oil supplementation. Among those taking fish oils, longer periods of remission were observed in nearly every outcome category, and the results were statistically significant. Mild gastrointestinal side effects were reported in the fish oil group.

The author of a recent review article concluded that omega-3 shows positive results as an adjunctive treatment for depressive—but not manic—symptoms in bipolar disorder. The author cautioned that the data are few and called for larger, well-designed studies to further investigate. With respect to other depressive disorders, there is some evidence that fish oils may be of some benefit, although a recent review concluded that no meaningful determinations can be made at this time based on available research results. More study is clearly warranted.

There is evidence that fish oils have some neuroprotective properties that could be significant. EPA has shown some efficacy in ameliorating such neurodegenerative disorders as Huntington's disease, multiple sclerosis and others. (See EPA.) The fish oils also show some evidence of being able to impede very mild, early manifestations of Alzheimer's disease. Again, more research is needed and warranted.

Increased consumption of EPA and DHA may reduce the risk of age-related macular degeneration by about 70% according to some recent research.

Immunoglobulin (Ig) A nephropathy is the most common glomerular disease worldwide. Beneficial effects with fish oil supplements have been reported in two studies, while two other studies showed no beneficial effects. In the largest and longest study to date, daily supplementation with fish oil showed protection against progressive renal disease. This blinded, placebo-controlled trial included 51 subjects who received a daily mixture of EPA and DHA at 1.87 grams and 1.36 grams, respectively. The study lasted two years, and the placebo group used olive oil as the control. It was concluded that fish oil retarded the rate of renal function loss.

There is some epidemiological and animal data suggesting that fish oils may have some anticancer effects. There are no data, however, to directly establish any efficacy for fish oil supplements in any cancer.

CONTRAINDICATIONS, PRECAUTIONS, ADVERSE REACTIONS

CONTRAINDICATIONS
Known hypersensitivity to a fish oil-containing product.

PRECAUTIONS
Fish oil supplements should be used by children, pregnant women and nursing mothers only if recommended and monitored by a physician. Because of the possible anti-thrombotic effect of fish oil supplements, hemophiliacs and those taking warfarin (Coumadin) should exercise caution in their use. Fish oil supplements should be stopped before any surgical procedure. Conflicting results have been reported regarding the effects of fish oil supplements on glycemic control in those with glucose intolerance including type 2 diabetics. Some early studies indicated that fish oil supplements might have detrimental effects in those groups. Recently, better designed studies have not reported these adverse effects. There is no evidence that fish oil supplements have detrimental effects on glucose tolerance, insulin secretion or insulin resistance in non-diabetic subjects. Diabetics should discuss the use of these supplements with their physicians and note if the supplements affect their glycemic control. Diabetics who take fish oil supplements should be monitored by their physicians.

ADVERSE REACTIONS
There have been no reports of serious adverse events in those taking fish oil supplements, even up to 15 grams daily for prolonged periods of time. Those side effects that have been reported include mild gastrointestinal upsets such as dyspepsia, nausea and diarrhea, halitosis, eructation and "fishy" smelling breath, skin and even urine. The blood-thinning effects can cause occasional nosebleeds and easy bruising. Diabetics may experience worsening of glycemic control.

INTERACTIONS
Interactions may occur between fish oil supplements and aspirin and other non-steroidal anti-inflammatory drugs and herbs such as garlic (Allium sativum) and ginkgo (Ginkgo biloba). Such interactions might be manifested by increased susceptibility to bruising, nosebleeds, hemoptysis, hematemesis, hematuria and blood in the stool. Most who take fish oil supplements and the above drugs or herbs do not suffer from these problems, and, if they occur, they are rare. If they do occur, the dose should be lowered or discontinued.

OVERDOSAGE
Not reported.

DOSAGE AND ADMINISTRATION
There are several forms of fish oil supplements. The most common form is natural fish oil, usually produced from the body of cold-water fish. These fish oils are, typically, 30% EPA and DHA with a ratio of EPA to DHA of 1.5. A typical 1 gram softgel capsule of fish oil contains 180 milligrams of

EPA and 120 milligrams of DHA. Natural EPA and DHA are chemically triacylglycerols. Natural fish oil capsules containing 50% EPA and DHA in a 1.5 ratio are now available. Some natural fish oil supplements contain EPA and DHA in a higher ratio, i.e. higher EPA. There are also fish oil supplements with a lower ratio, i.e. higher DHA.

A more concentrated form of fish oil is the semi-synthetic ethyl ester product containing 85% EPA/DHA. One such product contains 490 milligrams of EPA ethyl ester and 350 milligrams of DHA ethyl ester per 1 gram capsule.

Enteric coated EPA and DHA as the free fatty acids are also available. These capsules are more concentrated in EPA and DHA. Emulsions of fish oils are now available that can be used as constituents for salad dressings and other foods. Functional foods, including bars containing fish oil, are becoming available. Infant formulas containing DHA are available in Europe and Japan. Certain enteral supplements contain EPA and DHA as well as other immune-modulating nutrients such as L-arginine, L-glutamine and RNA.

Recommended fish oil products must contain antioxidants such as tocopherol to protect against their oxidation. Further, fish oil products that contain high quantities of vitamin A and D, which could be toxic, should not be used.

The usual oral dose of fish oil for use in hypertriglyceridemia is about 5 grams of combined EPA/DHA daily. The values expressed in this section refer to the amounts of EPA plus DHA. The actual weight of the capsule is typically much higher. Labels should be checked in order to determine the actual EPA/DHA content. The daily intake should be taken in divided doses; the supplements are best tolerated with meals. The usual dose for hypertensives who have not previously been treated is about 3 grams of EPA/DHA daily. About 3 grams daily is also the usual dose for those with rheumatoid arthritis, Crohn's disease and ulcerative colitis. Those who have had successful angioplasty and are trying to prevent restenosis might use 4 to 5 grams daily. Based on the GISSI-Prevenzione trial, a dose of 1 gram daily of EPA and DHA might have protective value for those who have had an MI.

In 2005, the FDA approved a highly concentrated omega-3 polyunsaturated fatty acid preparation (*Lovaza*) as an adjunct to diet for treatment of very high plasma triglyceride concentrations. The product is a combination of the ethyl esters of EPA and DHA. The recommended daily dosage for *Lovaza* is 4 grams once daily or 2 grams twice a day, taken with meals.

LITERATURE

Adler AJ, Holub BJ. Effect of garlic and fish-oil supplementation on serum lipid and lipoprotein concentrations in hypercholesterolemic men. *Am J Clin Nutr.* 1997;65:445-450.

Appel LJ, Miller ER III, Seidler AJ, et al. Does supplementation of diet with "fish oil' reduce blood pressure? A meta-analysis of controlled clinical trials. *Arch Intern Med.* 1993;153:1429-1438.

Ariel A, Serhan CN. Resolvins and protectins in the termination program of acute inflammation. *Trends Immunol.* 2007;28(4):176-183.

Ariza-Ariza R, Mestanza-Peralta M, Cardiel MH. Omega-3 fatty acid in rheumatoid arthritis: an overview. *Semin Arthritis Rheum.* 1998;27:366-370.

Bays HE, Tighe AP, Sadovsky R, et al. Prescription omega-3 fatty acids and their lipid effects: physiologic mechanisms of action and clinical implications. *Expert Rev Cardiovasc Ther.* 2008;6(3):391-409.

Belluzi A, Brignola C, Campieri M, et al. Effect of an enteric-coated fish-oil preparation on relapses in Crohn's disease. *N Engl J Med.* 1996;334:1557-1560.

Connor KM, SanGiovanni JP, Lofqvist C, et al. Increased dietary intake of omega-3-polyunsaturated fatty acids reduces pathological retinal angiogenesis. *Nat Med.* 2007;13(7):868-873.

Connor WE, Prince MJ, Ullman D, et al. The hypotriglyceridemic effect of fish oil in adult-onset diabetes without adverse glucose control. *Ann N Y Acad Sci.* 1993;683:337-340.

Curtis CL, Hughes CE, Flannery CR, et al. n-3 Fatty acids specifically modulate catabolic factors involved in articular cartilage degradation. *J Biol Chem.* 2000;275:721-724.

da Cunha DN, Hamlin RL, Billman GE, et al. n-3 (omega-3) polyunsaturated fatty acids prevent acute atrial electrophysiological remodeling. *Br J Pharmacol.* 2007;150(3):281-285.

Den Ruijter HM, Berecki G, Verkerk AO, et al. Acute administration of fish oil inhibits triggered activity in isolated myocytes from rabbits and patients with heart failure. *Circulation.* 2008;117(4):536-544.

Donadia Jr, JV, Bergstralh MS, Offard MS, et al. A controlled trial of fish oil in Iga nephropathy. *N Engl J Med.* 1994;331:1194-1199.

Dyall SC, Michael-Titus AT. Neurological Benefits of Omega-3 Fatty Acids. *Neuromolecular Med.* Epub: 2008 Jun 10.

Feagan BG, Sandborn WJ, Mittmann U, et al. Omega-3 free fatty acids for the maintenance of remission in Crohn disease: the EPIC Randomized Controlled Trials. *JAMA.* 2008;299(14):1690-1697.

Flower RJ, Perretti M. Controlling inflammation: a fat chance? *J Exp Med.* 2005;201(5):671-674.

Gapinski JP, VanRuiswyk JV, Heudebert GR, et al. Preventing restenosis with fish oils following coronary angioplasty: a meta-analysis. *Arch Intern Med.* 1993;153:1595-1601.

GISSI-HF Investigators. Effect of n-3 polyunsaturated fatty acids in patients with chronic heart failure (the GISSI-HF trial):

a randomised, double-blind, placebo-controlled trial. *Lancet.* Epub: 2008 Aug 29.

GISSI-Prevenzione Investigators. Dietary supplementation with n-3 polyunsaturated fatty acids and vitamin E after myocardial infarction: results of the GISSI-Prevenzione trial. *Lancet.* 1999;354:447-455.

Grimsgaard S, Bonaa KH, Hansen J-B, et al. Highly purified eicosapentaenoic acid and docosahexaenoic acids in humans have similar triacylglycerol-lowering effects but divergent effects on serum fatty acids. *Am J Clin Nutr.* 1997;66:649-659.

Harris WS. Fish oils and plasma lipid and lipoprotein metabolism in humans: a critical review. *J Lipid Res.* 1989;30:785-807.

Homan van der Heide JJ, Bilo HGJ, Donker JM, et al. Effect of dietary fish oil on renal function and rejection in cyclosporine-treated recipients of renal transplants. *N Engl J Med.* 1993;329:769-773.

Hooper L, Thompson RL, Harrison RA, et al. Risks and benefits of omega 3 fats for mortality, cardiovascular disease, and cancer: systematic review. *BMJ.* 2006;332(7544):752-760.

Hudert CA, Weylandt KH, Lu Y, et al. Transgenic mice rich in endogenous omega-3 fatty acids are protected from colitis. *Proc Natl Acad Sci U S A.* 2006;103(30):11276-11281.

Jacobson TA. Role of n-3 fatty acids in the treatment of hypertriglyceridemia and cardiovascular disease. *Am J Clin Nutr.* 2008;87(6):1981S-1990S.

Jung UJ, Torrejon C, Tighe AP, et al. n-3 Fatty acids and cardiovascular disease: mechanisms underlying beneficial effects. *Am J Clin Nutr.* 2008;87(6):2003S-2009S.

Kim H-J, Takahashi M, Ezaki O. Fish oil feeding decreases mature sterol regulatory element-binding protein 1 (SREBP-1) by down-regulation of SREBP-1c mRNA in mouse liver. *J Biol Chem.* 1999;274:25892-25898.

Kremer JM. n-3 Fatty acid supplements in rheumatoid arthritis. *Am J Clin Nutr.* 2000;71:349s-351s.

Leaf A. Historical overview of n-3 fatty acids and coronary heart disease. *Am J Clin Nutr.* 2008;87(6):1978S-1980S.

Lee JH, O'Keefe JH, Lavie CJ, et al. Omega-3 fatty acids for cardioprotection. *Mayo Clin Proc.* 2008;83(3):324-332.

McKenney JM, Sica D.Role of prescription omega-3 fatty acids in the treatment of hypertriglyceridemia. *Pharmacotherapy.* 2007;27(5):715-728.

McManus RM, Jumpson J, Finegood DT, et al. A comparison of the effects of n-3 fatty acids from linseed oil and fish oil in well-controlled type II diabetes. *Diabetes Care.* 1996;9:463-467.

Montgomery P, Richardson AJ. Omega-3 fatty acids for bipolar disorder. *Cochrane Database Syst Rev.* 2008;(2):CD005169.

O'Keefe JH Jr, Abuissa H, Sastre A, et al. Effects of omega-3 fatty acids on resting heart rate, heart rate recovery after exercise, and heart rate variability in men with healed myocardial infarctions and depressed ejection fractions. *Am J Cardiol.* 2006;97(8):1127-1130.

Opthof T, Den Ruijter HM. Omega-3 polyunsaturated fatty acids (PUFAs or fish oils) and atrial fibrillation. *Br J Pharmacol.* 2007;150(3):258-260.

Stoll AL, Severus WE, Freeman MP, et al. Omega 3 fatty acids in bipolar disorder. *Arch Gen Psychiatry.* 1999;56:407-412.

Toft I, Bonaa KH, Ingebresten OC, et al. Effects of n-3 polyunsaturated fatty acids on glucose homeostasis and blood pressure in essential hypertension. *Ann Intern Med.* 1995;123:911-918.

Torrejon C, Jung UJ, Deckelbaum RJ. n-3 Fatty acids and cardiovascular disease: actions and molecular mechanisms. *Prostaglandins Leukot Essent Fatty Acids.* 2007;77(5-6):319-326.

van de Rest O, Geleijnse JM, Kok FJ, et al. Effect of fish oil on cognitive performance in older subjects: a randomized, controlled trial. *Neurology.* 2008;71(6):430-438.

Von Schacky C, Angerer P, Kothny W, et al. The effect of dietary omega-3 fatty acids on coronary atherosclerosis. A randomized, double-blind, placebo-controlled trial. *Ann Intern Med.* 1999;130:554-562.

Flaxseed Lignans

DESCRIPTION

Lignans are phenylpropanoid dimers widely distributed in the plant kingdom. Flaxseed (*Linum usitatissimum* L.) is one of the richest sources of dietary lignans. Plant lignans comprise one of the two main groups of phytoestrogens, the other group being the isoflavonoids.

The major flax lignan is secoisolariciresinol diglucoside (SDG). Flaxseed is the richest food source of SDG. Flaxseed also contains much smaller amounts of matairesinol, lariciresinol and pinoresinol. The plant lignans are converted by the intestinal microflora in the proximal or upper part of the large intestine to enterodiol (END) and enterolactone (ENL). END and ENL are not themselves plant lignans and are called mammalian lignans or enterolignans. Plant lignans are precursors of mammalian lignans. It is thought that many of the possible biological actions of SDG are due to its conversion to END and ENL.

SDG is a dibenzylbutyrolactone. This is one of the two major structural types of plant lignans. The spruce lignan 7-hydroxymatairesinol also possesses this type of chemical structure. (See Spruce Lignans.) The other major chemical type is the tetrahydrofuran type that can be found in the sesame seed lignans sesamin and sesaminol. (See Sesame Seed Lignans.) The biphenolic nature of SDG resembles many of the substances known to exert estrogenic action or to block estrogen receptor sites. Lignans have been observed in some epidemiological studies to be correlated with reductions in prostate cancer and breast cancer incidence. Experimental evidence in animals has shown anticarcinogenic effects of SDG as well as cardiovascular and renal protective effects. Plant lignans began receiving much attention in the field of natural product chemistry ever since the discovery of the plant lignan podophyllotoxin, which is used as the starting compound for a few cancer drugs, including etoposide.

The chemical name for SDG is beta-D-Glucopyranoside, 2,3-bis[(4-hydroxy-3-methoxyphenyl methyl]-1,4-butanediyl bis-,[R-(R*,R*)]. Its molecular formula is $C_{32}H_{46}O_{16}$ and its molecular weight is 686.7. Its CAS number is 158932-33-3. END is also known as 2,3-bis[(3-hydroxyphenyl)methyl]-1,4-Butanediol and has a molecular weight of 302. ENL is also known as *trans*-dihydro-3,4-bis[(3-hydroxyphenyl)methyl]-2(3H)-Furanone and has a molecular weight of 298. The aglycone of SDG is secoisolariciresinol (SECO). SECO is also known as [R-(R*¹,R*)-2,3-bis[(4-hydroxy-3-methoxy phenyl)methyl]-1,4-Butadiol and has a molecular weight of 362. The chemical structures below are described within this monograph.

Enterodiol

Enterolactone

Secoisoariciresinol

Seicoisolariciresinol-diglucoside

Lignans should not be confused with lignins. A lignin is a cross-linked phenolic polymer which combines with cellulose to give woody plant tissue its rigidity.

ACTIONS AND PHARMACOLOGY

ACTIONS
SDG has antioxidant activity. It also may have hypoglycemic, hypocholesterolemic, estrogenic, anti-estrogenic, anticancer, antiproliferative and renoprotective properties.

MECHANISM OF ACTION
SDG, SECO and the enterolignans END and ENL have been shown to be effective antioxidants against lipid peroxidation and oxidative DNA damage, potentially due to their free radical scavenging activity.

SDG was found to be protective against streptozotocin-induced diabetes in rats, an animal model of type 1diabetes. It delayed the onset of diabetes in the rats and was thought to act by an antioxidant mechanism. Streptozotocin is known to induce oxidative stress. SDG was also found to delay the development of type 2 diabetes in Zucker rats, an animal model of type 2 diabetes. Again, it was thought this effect was due to SDG acting as an antioxidant.

SDG was found in a human study which took place in China to lower total cholesterol and LDL-cholesterol. The mechanism of this effect is unclear.

SDG, END and ENL may block some of the cancer-inducing effects of estrogen and may have selective estrogen receptor modulating (SERM) activity.

END and ENL may also have anti-platelet-activating factor activity, which would produce anti-thrombotic activity.

END and ENL have been shown to have anti-proliferative activity against the human breast carcinoma cell line, ZR-75-1. These enterolignans also inhibit the growth of estrogen-independent human colon tumor cells.

SDG has been found to reduce chemically-induced mammary and colon tumorigenesis in rats. SDG inhibits the initiation, promotion and progression of mammary carcinogenesis in rats and inhibits tumor growth and metastasis in nude mice. SDG has also been shown to reduce experimental metastasis of melanoma cells in mice.

The mechanism of the anticancer activity of SDG is unclear. Biological properties of SDG may be responsible for its anticancer properties. These include antioxidant, estrogenic, antiestrogenic, antiproliferative and anti-aromatase activities. Further research on this is warranted and needed.

The MRL/lpr mouse model is an animal model of systemic lupus erythematosus (SLE). Lupus nephritis is one of the most serious manifestations of SLE. SDG was found to significantly delay the onset of proteinuria and preserve the glomerular filtration rate (GFR) and renal size in this mouse model. Platelet activating factor (PAF) has been implicated in the immunopathogenesis of SLE and in renal injury. The renoprotective effect of SDG may be explained by the dibenzylbutyl skeleton in the chemical structure of SDG. This type of structure has been shown to reversibly inhibit PAF.

In a human study that took place in China, SDG was found to significantly alleviate the lower urinary tract symptoms associated with benign prostatic hyperplasia (BPH). The mechanism of this effect remains unclear. Possibilities include inhibition of 5-alpha reductase, the enzyme that converts testosterone to dihydrotestosterone (DHT) or by androgen receptor blockade. However, it is not clear if these possible mechanisms have anything to do with the observed effect.

PHARMACOKINETICS

The pharmacokinetics for SDG in humans is incomplete. After ingestion, SDG is converted to SECO. Deglycosylation of SDG can occur from the small intestine onward either via enzymatic activity at the brush border of the small intestine or via bacterial enzymatic activity.

SECO is then converted by the intestinal microflora in the proximal or upper part of the large intestine to END via demethylation and dehydroxylation, and END is converted into ENL via dehydrogenation. Following conjugation by colon epithelial cells or within the liver, SECO, END and ENL, but not SDG, are found in the portal circulation, plasma and urine as glucuronides and sulfates.

HT29 human colon cells show that measurable amounts of intracellular free END can be detected within up to four hours of incubation whereas ENL appears to be rapidly conjugated by the HT29 cells.

The pharmacokinetics of SDG in flaxseed is even more complex. In flaxseed, SDG occurs as a macromolecular structure bound by the linker molecule hydroxymethyl glutaric acid. Ferulic acid glucoside, herbacetin diglucoside, and coumaric acid glucoside are also found in the macromolecule. It is not known in which part of the gastrointestinal tract SDG is released from the macromolecule. Once it is released, the pharmacokinetics should be similar to that described above.

INDICATIONS AND USAGE

There are claims that the flaxseed lignan SDG may be useful in preventing heart disease, some cancers, insulin-dependent diabetes mellitus and obesity; that is has kidney-protective effects; that it may favorably alter estrogen metabolism in postmenopausal women to an equal or greater extent than supplementation with soy products; and that it may relieve the symptoms of benign prostatic hyperplasia (BPH). The best-supported claims relate to heart disease, BPH and cancer.

RESEARCH SUMMARY

A variety of research efforts, spanning more than 20 years, indicates that flaxseed and flaxseed oil have the ability to favorably modify lipid metabolism and to exert cardioprotective effects. One recent, eight-week, randomized, double-blind, placebo-controlled study sought to determine whether the SDG component of flaxseed can duplicate favorable lipid-modifying results seen with flaxseed and flax oil. The study enrolled 55 hypercholesterolemic subjects who were given various doses of an SDG-rich flaxseed extract. Effects related to LDL-cholesterol levels and glucose concentrations were measured. Compared with controls, who received no SDG, the experimental subjects exhibited significant reductions in LDL-cholesterol and fasting plasma glucose concentrations in a dose-dependent manner. Doses administered were 300 mg and 600 mg daily.

In another recent study, this one utilizing several *in vitro* and *in vivo* animal models of ischemia-reperfusion injury, SDG was reported to have potent favorable angiogenic and antiapoptotic effects that the investigators believe help explain its cardioprotective properties. They further stated that this was the first time favorable myocardial neovascularization was achieved in this manner. They concluded that SDG may have the potential to improve the management of ischemic heart failure in patients with coronary artery disease. Follow-up is needed and warranted

Yet another recent study tested SDG for possible effects on diet-induced obesity in mice. Groups of animals were variously administered a low-fat diet, a high-fat diet or a high-fat diet that included SDG over a four-week period. Effects were noted that were said to significantly and favorably regulate gene expressions involved in the genesis of fat. The researchers concluded that SDG might thus have the potential to help control obesity and reduce the risk of dietary-induced diseases, including hypertension, atherosclerosis and diabetes. Further investigation of these possible gene expression effects is needed.

Flaxseed lignans, like flaxseed and flaxseed oil, have been postulated as possible agents for the prevention and treatment of some cancers, principally breast and prostate cancers. Previously, animal and human studies indicated that supplementation with flaxseed products could slow prostate tumor growths, but the substances were used in these studies with a low-fat diet. More recently one group of researchers presented results of a clinical study that they believe demonstrates that flaxseed alone can significantly slow prostate tumor growth. Yet another recent clinical study of 87 men with benign prostatic hyperplasia has also yielded positive results. In this study the men were given placebo or 300 mg- or 600 mg-doses of SDG daily over a four-month period. Appreciable improvement in lower urinary tract symptoms was seen in the SDG-dosed subjects. The efficacy of SDG in this context was hypothesized to be due to its estrogenic effects, although this was not clear.

Another group demonstrated that dietary flaxseed could inhibit experimental metastases of melanoma cells in mice. More recently, the same group has extended this research to see if SDG can similarly inhibit these metastases. Pulmonary metastases of melanoma cells were significantly inhibited by varying doses of SDG in a dose-dependent manner in this study. In addition, some animal studies have suggested that SDG may have positive effects in mammary and colon cancers. *In vitro* studies revealed that SDG has anti-proliferative, antiestrogenic, estrogenic, anti-aromatase and antioxidant effects, all or any of which may help inhibit some cancers. Research is ongoing.

Flaxseed has shown some renoprotective effects in both animals and humans. In one study, SDG exhibited renoprotection in a dose-dependent fashion in an animal model of lupus nephritis. Further research is needed.

One recent study concluded that supplementation with flaxseed alters estrogen metabolism to a possible less mitogenic form of estrogen to a greater extent in menopausal women than does soy. Experimentation with SDG itself in this context has apparently not been performed.

CONTRAINDICATIONS, PRECAUTIONS, ADVERSE REACTIONS

CONTRAINDICATIONS
Flax lignans are contraindicated in those who are hypersensitive to any component of a flax lignan-containing product.

PRECAUTIONS
Pregnant women and nursing mothers should avoid the use of flax lignan supplements pending long-term safety studies.

Men with prostate cancer or BPH should discuss the advisability of the use of flax lignan supplements with their physicians before deciding to use them.

Women with estrogen receptor-positive tumors should exercise caution in the use of flax lignan supplements and should only use them if they are recommended and monitored by a physician.

ADVERSE REACTIONS
None known.

INTERACTIONS

DRUGS
Antibiotics may decrease the production of END and ENL from SDG.

NUTRITIONAL SUPPLEMENTS
No known interactions.

FOODS
No known interactions.

HERBS
No known interactions.

OVERDOSAGE
There are no reports of flaxseed lignan overdosage.

DOSAGE AND ADMINISTRATION
SDG has been studied at doses of 300 mg to 600 mg daily for prolonged periods of time without any significant adverse events noted.

Doses of SDG of 300 mg to 600 mg daily have been used in clinical trials for hypercholesterolemia and BPH.

Doses of 25 mg to 50 mg of SDG daily are frequently used.

Pills typically contain at least 35% SDG by weight.

The amount of SDG in flaxseed varies from about 6 to 13 mg per gram of flaxseed.

LITERATURE
Adlercreutz H. Lignans and human health. *Crit Rev Clin Lab Sci.* 2007;44(5-6):483-525.

Bergman Jungeström M, Thompson LU, Dabrosin C. Flaxseed and its lignans inhibit estradiol-induced growth, angiogenesis, and secretion of vascular endothelial growth factor in human breast cancer xenografts in vivo. *Clin Cancer Res.* 2007;13(3):1061-1067.

Brooks JD, Ward WE, Lewis JE, et al. Supplementation with flaxseed alters estrogen metabolism in postmenopausal women to a greater extent than does supplementation with an equal amount of soy. *Am J Clin Nutr.* 2004;79(2):318-325.

Clark WF, Muir AD, Westcott ND, et al. A novel treatment for lupus nephritis: lignan precursor derived from flax. *Lupus*. 2000;9(6):429-436.

Danbara N, Yuri T, Tsujita-Kyutoku M, et al. Enterolactone induces apoptosis and inhibits growth of Colo 201 human colon cancer cells both in vitro and in vivo. *Anticancer Res*. 2005;25(3B):2269-2276.

Fukumitsu S, Aida K, Ueno N, et al. Flaxseed lignan attenuates high-fat diet-induced fat accumulation and induces adiponectin expression in mice. *Br J Nutr*. 2008:1-8.

Hosseinian FS, Muir AD, Westcott ND, et al. AAPH-mediated antioxidant reactions of secoisolariciresinol and SDG. *Org Biomol Chem*. 2007;5(4):644-654.

Hu C, Yuan YV, Kitts DD. Antioxidant activities of the flaxseed lignan secoisolariciresinol diglucoside,its aglycone secoisolariciresinol and the mammalian lignans enterodiol and enterolactone in vitro. *Food Chem Toxicol*. 2007;45(11):2219-2227.

Jenab M, Thompson LU. The influence of flaxseed and lignans on colon carcinogenesis and beta-glucuronidase activity. *Carcinogenesis*. 1996;17(6):1343-1348.

Kitts DD, Yuan YV, Wijewickreme AN, et al. Antioxidant activity of the flaxseed lignan secoisolariciresinol diglycoside and its mammalian lignan metabolites enterodiol and enterolactone. *Mol Cell Biochem*. 1999;202(1-2):91-100.

Li X, Yuan JP, Xu SP, et al. Separation and determination of secoisolariciresinol diglucoside oligomers and their hydrolysates in the flaxseed extract by high-performance liquid chromatography. *J Chromatogr A*. 2008;1185(2):223-232.

Li D, Yee JA, Thompson LU, et al. Dietary supplementation with secoisolariciresinol diglycoside (SDG) reduces experimental metastasis of melanoma cells in mice. *Cancer Lett*. 1999;142(1):91-96.

Muir AD. Flax lignans—analytical methods and how they influence our understanding of biological activity. *J AOAC Int*. 2006;89(4):1147-1157.

Pan A, Sun J, Chen Y, et al. Effects of a flaxseed-derived lignan supplement in type 2 diabetic patients: a randomized, double-blind, cross-over trial. *PLoS ONE*. 2007;2(11):e1148.

Penumathsa SV, Koneru S, Thirunavukkarasu M, et al. Secoisolariciresinol diglucoside: relevance to angiogenesis and cardioprotection against ischemia-reperfusion injury. *J Pharmacol Exp Ther*. 2007;320(2):951-959.

Prasad K. A study on regression of hypercholesterolemic atherosclerosis in rabbits by flax lignan complex. *J Cardiovasc Pharmacol Ther*. 2007;12(4):304-313.

Prasad K. Secoisolariciresinol diglucoside from flaxseed delays the development of type 2 diabetes in Zucker rat. *J Lab Clin Med*. 2001;138(1):32-39.

Prasad K, Mantha SV, Muir AD, et al. Protective effect of secoisolariciresinol diglucoside against streptozotocin-induced diabetes and its mechanism. *Mol Cell Biochem*. 2000;206(1-2):141-149.

Rickard SE, Yuan YV, Chen J, et al. Dose effects of flaxseed and its lignan on N-methyl-N-nitrosourea-induced mammary tumorigenesis in rats. *Nutr Cancer*. 1999;35(1):50-57.

Serraino M, Thompson LU. Flaxseed supplementation and early markers of colon carcinogenesis. *Cancer Lett*. 1992;63(2):159-165.

Serraino M, Thompson LU. The effect of flaxseed supplementation on early risk markers for mammary carcinogenesis. *Cancer Lett*. 1991;60(2):135-142.

Sung MK, Lautens M, Thompson LU. Mammalian lignans inhibit the growth of estrogen-independent human colon tumor cells. *Anticancer Res*. 1998;18(3A):1405-1408.

Thompson LU. Experimental studies on lignans and cancer. *Baillieres Clin Endocrinol Metab*. 1998;12(4):691-705.

Thompson LU, Rickard SE, Orcheson LJ, et al. Flaxseed and its lignan and oil components reduce mammary tumor growth at a late stage of carcinogenesis. *Carcinogenesis*. 1996;17(6):1373-1376.

Thompson LU, Seidl MM, Rickard SE, et al. Antitumorigenic effect of a mammalian lignan precursor from flaxseed. *Nutr Cancer*. 1996;26(2):159-165.

Zhang LY, Wang XL, Sun DX, et al. Regulation of zinc transporters by dietary flaxseed lignan in human breast cancer xenografts. *Mol Biol Rep*. Epub: 2007 Sep 5.

Zhang W, Wang X, Liu Y, et al. Effects of Dietary Flaxseed Lignan Extract on Symptoms of Benign Prostatic Hyperplasia. *J Med Food*. 2008;11(2):207-214.

Zhang W, Wang X, Liu Y, et al. Dietary flaxseed lignan extract lowers plasma cholesterol and glucose concentrations in hypercholesterolaemic subjects. *Br J Nutr*. 2008;99(6):1301-1309.

Flaxseed Oil

DESCRIPTION

Flaxseed, also known as flax oil and linseed oil, is derived from the seeds of the plant *Linium usitatissimum*. Flaxseed oil is a very rich source of alpha-linolenic acid. Alpha-linolenic acid concentration in flaxseed oil ranges from approximately 40 to 60%. Lower amounts of linoleic acid and oleic acid (each about 15%) are also present in flaxseed oil. In addition, flaxseed oil contains varying amounts of the lignan, secoisolariciresinol diglycoside (SDG).

Alpha-linolenic acid (ALA) is an n-3(omega-3), all-cis polyunsaturated fatty acid containing 18 carbon atoms and three double bonds. It is also known as ALA; ALA, 18:3n-3; 9,12,15-octadecatrienoic acid and (Z, Z, Z)-9, 12, 15 octadecatrienoic acid. ALA has the following structural formula:

$$H_3C \diagup\diagdown\diagup\diagdown\diagup\diagdown (CH_2)_6 COOH$$

Alpha-linolenic acid

ALA is present in flaxseed oil in the form of a triglyceride. The Mediterranean diet, high in ALA, appears to lower the risk of coronary artery disease and certain types of cancer.

The lignan SDG belongs to a group of plant substances known as phytoestrogens.

See also Flaxseed Lignans and Secoisolariciresinol Diglycoside (SDG).

ACTIONS AND PHARMACOLOGY

ACTIONS

Flaxseed oil may have anti-inflammatory, anti-atherogenic, anti-thrombotic and anti-proliferative activities.

MECHANISM OF ACTION

ALA is metabolized to eicosopentaenoic acid (EPA). EPA is a precursor of the series-3 prostaglandins, the series-5 leukotrienes and the series-3 thromboxanes. These eicosanoids have anti-inflammatory and anti-atherogenic properties. ALA metabolites may also inhibit the production of the pro-inflammatory eicosanoids, prostaglandin E_2 (PGE2) and leukotriene B4 (LTB4), as well as the pro-inflammatory cytokines, tumor necrosis factor-alpha (TNF-alpha) and interleukin-1 beta (IL-1 beta). Incorporation of ALA and its metabolites in cell membranes can affect membrane fluidity and may play a role in anti-inflammatory activity, inhibition of platelet aggregation and possibly in anti-proliferative actions of ALA.

Secoisolaricoresinol diglycoside (SDG) is metabolized to enterolactone and enterodiol. These substances may have anti-platelet-activating factor activity, which would produce anti-thrombotic activity. SDG metabolites may also block some of the cancer-inducing effects of estrogen and may have selective estrogen receptor modulating (SERM) activity.

PHARMACOKINETICS

ALA-laden triglycerides in flaxseed oil are absorbed from the small intestine aided by bile salts. During this process, there is some deacylation of the fatty acids of the triglycerides. Reacylation takes place within the mucosal cells of the small intestine, and the ALA-laden triglycerides enter the lymph system in the form of chylomicrons. ALA-laden chylomicrons are transported from the lymph into the blood, where ALA is then carried in various lipid particles to the various cells of the body, where it gets metabolized to EPA and series-3 prostaglandins, series-5 leukotrienes and series-3 thromboxanes.

The flaxseed oil lignan SDG is metabolized by bacteria in the colon to enterolactone and enterodiol. These substances are absorbed from the colon and metabolized to several hydroxylated metabolites in the body.

INDICATIONS AND USAGE

Flaxseed and flaxseed oil may be indicated in hyperlipidemia, to decrease platelet aggregation, to lower blood pressure, to help prevent heart attacks and stroke, and to ameliorate some of the symptoms of arthritis. There is a suggestion that it may be helpful in some cancers. Claims that it can be useful in the treatment of anxiety, constipation, vaginitis and weight loss are unsubstantiated.

RESEARCH SUMMARY

Though high in alpha-linolenic acid (ALA), flaxseed and flaxseed oil may have beneficial effects that may sometimes be independent of their ALA content. In animal models, flaxseed-enriched diets have significantly reduced hypercholestemic atherosclerosis; this has been true even when CDC-flaxseed (Type II flaxseed), which contains quantities of oil and lignan similar to that of standard flaxseed but with very little ALA content, has been used. Lignan content could be responsible for some of the positive effects. Lignans have been shown, in various studies, to contain anti-platelet-activating factor activity and possess antioxidant properties. Development of atherosclerosis has been reduced by up to 69% in some of these studies using flaxseed-enriched diets.

To what extent research findings using flaxseed itself can be extended to the use of flaxseed oil remains to be determined. There is preliminary clinical evidence suggesting that the oil can decrease platelet aggregation, that it may lower cholesterol (but probably not triglycerides) and that it might have some ability to lower blood pressure and have some anti-inflammatory effects in some with arthritis.

Some animal studies have suggested a possible role for flaxseed in the treatment of some cancers, particularly mammary cancers. Lignans have been shown to block some of the cancer-inducing effects of endogenous estrogens. Human trials are underway.

Recently, some poultry farmers have begun feeding chickens diets rich in flaxseed, boosting the omega-3 fatty acid content of the eggs of these chickens to levels eight to 10 times that of regular eggs. These functional foods have already captured four percent of the Canadian egg market. It has been reported that two of these eggs supply half of Health Canada's recommended daily intake of omega-3 fatty acids for adults.

A researcher at the Center for Genetics, Nutrition and Health, Washington, D.C., has concluded: "The availability of omega-3 fatty acid-enriched products should lead to improvements in the food supply...studies with omega-3-enriched eggs lower cholesterol levels, platelet aggregation and blood pressure."

Claims that flaxseed and flaxseed oil are useful in treating anxiety, vaginitis and weight loss are not substantiated by the available research data. Veterinarians reportedly use these products to treat some animals for constipation, but human data are lacking. And, regarding animals, flaxseed oil fed to broiler chickens has been found to reduce pulmonary hypertension and right ventricular hypertrophy in birds raised under hypoxic conditions. No human data are available.

CONTRAINDICATIONS, PRECAUTIONS, ADVERSE REACTIONS

CONTRAINDICATIONS
Flaxseed oil is contraindicated in those who are hypersensitive to any component of a flaxseed oil-containing product.

PRECAUTIONS
Infants, young children, pregnant women and nursing mothers should avoid supplemental flaxseed oil pending long-term safety studies. Because of possible antithrombotic activity, those with hemophilia and those taking warfarin should be cautious about the use of supplemental flaxseed or flaxseed oil. Flaxseed oil intake should be halted in those having surgical procedures.

ADVERSE REACTIONS
Flaxseed oil may cause mild gastrointestinal symptoms, such as diarrhea.

INTERACTIONS

DRUGS
Interactions may occur between flaxseed oil-ALA and its metabolites and warfarin, aspirin and NSAIDs. Such interactions, if they were to occur, might be manifested by nosebleeds and increased susceptibility to bruising. If this does occur, consideration should be given to lowering or stopping intake.

NUTRITIONAL SUPPLEMENTS
Interactions may occur if flaxseed oil is used with other nutritional supplements, such as fish oils, which have antithrombotic activity.

HERBS
Interactions may occur between ALA and its metabolites with such herbs as garlic (*Allium sativa*) and ginkgo (*Ginkgo biloba*). Such interactions might be manifested by nosebleeds and easy bruising.

OVERDOSAGE
There are no reports of flaxseed oil overdosage.

DOSAGE AND ADMINISTRATION
Flaxseed oil comes in a few forms: capsules containing from 40-60 percent ALA, oils and in functional foods. Regarding the latter, ALA-laden eggs are available from laying hens fed flaxseed diets.

Three to four grams of ALA is approximately equivalent to the 0.3 grams of EPA, which one would derive from a fish-rich diet. Six 1-gram capsules of flaxseed oil that are 50% ALA contains 3 grams of ALA. A tablespoon of 50% ALA-containing flaxseed oil provides about 7.5 grams of ALA.

Many use flaxseed oil as a component in salad dressings. Since flaxseed oil is easily oxidized, it is important that it contains an antioxidant, such as vitamin E.

The amounts of flaxseed lignan in flaxseed oil are highly variable.

LITERATURE
Allman MA, Penna MM, Pang D. Supplementation with flaxseed oil versus sunflower seed oil in healthy young men consuming a low fat diet: effects on platelet composition and function. *Eur J Clin Nutr.* 1995;49:169-178.

Fisher S, Honigmann G, Hora C, et al. Results of linseed oil and olive oil therapy in hyperlipoproteinemia patients. [Article in German]. *Dtsch Z Verdau Stoffwechselkr.* 1984;44:245-251.

Indu M, Ghafoorunissa. n-3 fatty acids in Indian diets: comparison of the effects of precursor (alpha-linolenic acid) vs. product (long-chain n-3 polyunsaturated fatty acids). *Nutr Res.* 1992;12:569-582.

James MJ, Gibson RA, Cleland LG. Dietary polyunsaturated fatty acids and inflammatory mediator production. *Am J Clin Nutr.* 2000;71(Suppl):343S-348S.

Jenkins DJ, Kendall CW, Vidgen E, et al. Health aspects of partially defatted flaxseed, including effects on serum lipids, oxidative measures, and ex vivo androgen and progestin activity: a controlled crossover trial. *Am J Clin Nutr.* 1999;69:395-402.

Prasad K, Mantha SV, Muir AD, Westcott ND. Reduction of hypercholesterolemic atherosclerosis by CDC-flaxseed with very low alpha-linolenic acid. *Atherosclerosis.* 1998;136:367-375.

Prasad K. Dietary flaxseed in prevention of hypercholesterolemic atherosclerosis. *Atherosclerosis.* 1997;132:69-76.

Rozanova IA, Pogozheva AV, Kupakova SN, et al. Effect of anti-atherosclerotic diet, containing polyunsaturated fatty acids of the omega-3 family from flax oil, on fatty acid composition of cell membranes of patients with ischemic heart disease, hypertensive disease and hyperlipoproteinemia. [Article in Russian]. *Vopr Pitan.* 1997;(5):15-17.

Simopoulos AP. New products from the agri-food industry: the return of n-3 fatty acids into the food supply. *Lipids.* 1999;34 Suppl:S297-S301.

Singer P, Wirth M, Berg, I. A possible contribution of decrease in free fatty acids to low serum triglyceride after diets supplemented with n-6 and n-3 polyunsaturated fatty acids. *Atherosclerosis.* 1990;83:167-175.

Tou JC, Thompson LU. Exposure to flaxseed or its lignan component during different developmental stages influences rat mammory gland structures. *Carcinogenesis.* 1999;20:1831-1835.

Walton JP, Bond JM, Julian RJ, et al. Effect of dietary flax oil and hypobaric hypoxia on pulmonary hypertension and haematological variables in broiler chickens. *Br Poult Sci.* 1999;40:385-391.

Flower Pollen

DESCRIPTION

The supplement flower pollen is an extract of pollen. Pollen consists of the male germ seeds of plants, flowers or blossoms on trees. As plants flower, pollen is transferred from the anther of a stamen to the stigma of a pistil; on reaching the ovary it brings about fertilization of seeds. Entomophilus pollen refers to pollen that is spread by insects such as bees; anemophilous pollen refers to pollen spread by wind.

In contrast to bee pollen, which is collected from bees (see Bee Pollen), flower pollen is harvested directly from plants. The major flower pollen supplement in the marketplace is harvested from a number of organically grown specially selected flowers. The harvested pollen then undergoes extraction and fermentation processes in order to produce a better-absorbable product. Substances found in this product include vitamins, carotenoids, minerals, amino acids, lipids, enzymes, flavonoids, long-chain alcohols and phytosterols, among others.

ACTIONS AND PHARMACOLOGY

ACTIONS

Supplemental flower pollen may promote prostate health and may have anti-inflammatory activity.

MECHANISM OF ACTION

The mechanism of these possible activities is not known.

PHARMACOKINETICS

There is little information on the pharmacokinetics of flower pollen in humans. The various components present in flower pollen should be digested, absorbed and metabolized as are similar substances found in food.

INDICATIONS AND USAGE

Flower pollen may have some effectiveness in benign prostatic hyperplasia and in prostatitis. It has reported hepato and gastroprotective effects and may have some ability to inhibit some cancers, ameliorate symptoms of rheumatoid arthritis and protect against cardiovascular disease.

RESEARCH SUMMARY

Several studies have demonstrated positive effects for flower pollen extracts in the management of benign prostatic hyperplasia. In one double-blind, placebo-controlled study, a flower pollen extract taken for six months achieved significant subjective improvement in 69% of patients receiving it, compared with 30% improvement in placebo subjects. Treated subjects had significantly decreased residual urine and significantly decreased antero-posterior diameter of the prostate on ultrasound. In some other studies, average and maximum urine flow rates have also significantly improved with flower pollen supplementation.

In an open British study, 13 of 15 patients with chronic abacterial prostatitis and prostatodynia that had resisted other treatments enjoyed marked-to-complete relief of symptoms with flower pollen extract treatment. Experimental studies suggesting that flower pollen has anti-inflammatory and anti-androgenic properties may explain some of its apparent efficacy in these prostatic disorders.

There have also been numerous studies indicating that flower pollen and its extracts have hepatoprotective effects and have increased survival rates in animals exposed to such potential toxins as acetaminophen, organic solvents, ammonium fluoride, methionine, carbon tetrachloride, galactosamine and allyl alcohol. Protective effects in the lungs have been seen with exposure to ammonium fluoride. Gastroprotective effects of flower pollen have been seen in some with gastroduodenal disorders.

Some improvement in clinical manifestations of rheumatoid arthritis has been reported in one study using flower pollen. There are a few *in vitro* studies indicating that flower pollen extracts may inhibit prostate cancer cells. And in animals with experimental atherosclerosis, pollen extracts have been reported to significantly lower serum lipid levels and to decrease arterial lipid deposits.

CONTRAINDICATIONS, PRECAUTIONS, ADVERSE REACTIONS

CONTRAINDICATIONS

Flower pollen is contraindicated in those allergic or hypersensitive to flower pollen.

PRECAUTIONS

Flower pollen supplements should be avoided by pregnant women and nursing mothers.

ADVERSE REACTIONS

No adverse reactions have been reported. However, those who are allergic or hypersensitive to flower pollen may develop symptoms, including rhinitis, conjunctivitis, pruritis and bronchospasm and, in some cases, urticaria and anaphylaxis.

OVERDOSAGE

No reports of overdosage.

DOSAGE AND ADMINISTRATION

Those who take flower pollen for prostate health typically use about 360 milligrams daily taken in divided doses.

LITERATURE

Buck AC, Cox R, Rees RW, et al. Treatment of outflow tract obstruction due to benign-prostatic hyperplasia with the pollen extract, cernilton. A double-blind, placebo-controlled study. *Br J Urol.* 1990; 66:398-404.

Buck AC, Rees RW, Ebeling L. Treatment of chronic prostatitis and prostadynia with pollen extract. *Br J Urol.* 1989; 64:496-499.

Czarnecki R, Librowski T, Polanski M. [Hepatoprotective effect of flower pollen lipid extract in paracetamol-induced hepatotoxicity in mice.] [Article in Polish.] *Folia Med Cracov.* 1997; 38:53-61.

Dutkiewicz S. Usefulness of Cernilton in the treatment of benign prostatic hyperplasia. *Int Urol Nephrol.* 1996; 28:49-53.

Habib FK, Ross M, Buck AC, et al. *In vitro* evaluation of the pollen extract, cernitin T-60, in the regulation of prostate cell growth. *Br J Urol.* 1990; 66:393-397.

Habib FK, Ross M, Lewenstein A, et al. Identification of a prostate inhibitory substance in a pollen extract. *Prostate.* 1995; 26:133-139.

Polanski M, Czarnecki R, Woron J. [The hepatoprotective and hypolipidemic effect of flower pollen lipid extract in androgenized rats.] [Article in Polish.] *Folia Med Cracov.* 1996; 37:89-95.

Roberts KP, Iyer RA, Prasad G, et al. Cyclic hydroxamic inhibitors of prostate cell growth: selectivity and structure activity relationships. *Prostate.* 1998; 34; 92-99.

Voloshym OI, Pishak OV, Seniuk BP, Cherniavs'ka NB. [The efficacy of flower pollen in patients with rheumatoid arthritis and concomitant diseases of the gastrointestinal and hepatobiliary systems.] [Article in Ukrainian.] *Lik Sprava.* 1998; 4:151-154.

Yasumoto R, Kawanishi H, Tsujino T, et al. Clinical evaluation of long-term treatment using cernitin pollen extract in patients with benign prostatic hyperplasia. *Clin Ther.* 1995; 17:82-87.

Fluoride

DESCRIPTION

In the 1930s, it was discovered that high fluoride intake was responsible for a dental condition which is characterized by mottled enamel and which is known as dental fluorosis. Observational studies at the time led to the conclusion that those who lived in areas with a high incidence of dental fluorosis also had a lower incidence of caries than those who lived in areas where the fluoride intake was low.

In 1945, water fluoridation began in Grand Rapids, Michigan as a public health measure to reduce the incidence of caries. Presently, approximately 60% of community water supplies in the United States contain fluoride from 0.7 to 1.2 parts per million or 0.7 to 1.2 milligrams per liter.

Fluoride is the anionic form of fluorine. Fluorine is a halogen gas with atomic number 9 and an atomic weight of 19 daltons. Its symbol is F. Fluorine is the most electronegative element in the periodic table and, in size, it is very similar to the first element, hydrogen.

Even though fluoride has a beneficial role in the protection against caries, there is no evidence that fluoride is an essential nutrient for humans. The only evidence that it may be essential for higher animals is a recent report that fluoride deficiency in goats decreased life expectancy and caused pathological findings in the kidneys and endocrine organs. Fluoride, in addition to being found in municipal drinking water, is found in many foods. Particularly rich sources of fluoride are teas and marine fish.

ACTIONS AND PHARMACOLOGY

ACTIONS

Fluoride may have cariostatic and anti-osteoporotic activities.

MECHANISM OF ACTION

The mechanism of the cariostatic activity of fluoride is not completely understood. It is thought that fluoride interacts with hydroxyapatite to form the less acid soluble fluorhydroxyapatite. Fluorhydroxyapatite is believed to be more resistant to dissolution by the acids produced by bacteria found in plaque. Fluoride may also promote the remineralization of enamel in early caries. Finally, fluoride may reduce oral concentrations of cariogenic bacteria or reduce the metabolism of bacteria in plaque.

The mechanism of the possible anti-osteoporotic activity of fluoride is also incompletely understood. Fluoride is thought to have osteoblastic activity and, in partnership with calcium, stimulates the production of new bone. Insufficient intake of calcium at the time that fluoride is administered could lead to osteoid formation and osteomalacia. Fluoride is incorporated in the crystalline structure of bone as fluoroapatite. Fluoride may also slow the resorptive phase of the remodeling process and promote calcification.

PHARMACOKINETICS

Approximately 75% to 90% of ingested fluoride is absorbed from the gastrointestinal tract. About 50% of ingested fluoride is absorbed after 30 minutes. Absorption appears to occur by passive diffusion. A large fraction of ingested fluoride is absorbed from the stomach. Fluoride absorbed from the stomach appears to be absorbed as hydrofluoric acid. Fluoride absorbed from the small intestine is absorbed as fluoride. Slow-release sodium fluoride preparations are principally absorbed from the small intestine as fluoride. Concomitant intake of fluoride with antacids of the aluminum hydroxide type or high doses of calcium can cause decreased absorption of fluoride. Fluoride may form insoluble compounds with aluminum hydroxide and calcium.

For healthy, young, or middle aged adults, approximately 50% of absorbed fluoride is deposited in calcified tissues and 50% is excreted in the urine. For young children, up to 80% is deposited in bone and developing teeth. From 5% to 10% of ingested fluoride is excreted in the feces.

INDICATIONS AND USAGE

Fluoride, in appropriate doses, protects against dental caries. Its use in the treatment of osteoporosis remains controversial and experimental. A trend toward increased fluoride exposure has heightened concerns related to enamel and skeletal fluorosis, the incidences of which, however, still remain low.

RESEARCH SUMMARY

Sodium fluoride is approved by the Food and Drug Administration (FDA) for the prevention of dental caries. Fluoride is often added to public water supplies to achieve concentrations of 0.7 to 1.2 ppm. Higher concentrations (in the maximum 1.2 ppm range) are used in colder climates and lower concentrations in warmer climates where more water is typically consumed.

Epidemiological data show that low fluoride consumption is significantly associated with a higher incidence of dental caries. Experimental and clinical studies provide further substantial support for these epidemiologic findings. Numerous studies have shown that benefits are greatest when teeth get adequate pre-eruptive, as well as posteruptive, fluoride exposure.

Concerns have grown in recent years, however, that some children may be over-exposed to fluoride. Despite some reduction in exposure levels recommended by the American Academy of Pediatrics, incidence of dental fluorosis, while small, has continued to increase, a finding that some attribute to increased opportunities for fluoride exposure, not only from water but also from oral supplements, toothpastes, rinses, gels and some processed foods and beverages. Further modifications in recommended exposure levels are under consideration.

Because it is an effective osteoblast stimulator, fluoride has been investigated as a treatment for osteoporosis. It has shown some usefulness in this regard, particularly when given in the earliest stages of osteoporosis and particularly in patients with intact trabecular bone. Its effectiveness appears to be enhanced when combined in low doses with vitamin D and calcium.

Fluoride's efficacy in osteoporosis, however, is far from established. Where benefit has been demonstrated it has often been modest. Some studies have shown that it has no benefit. In one study, fluoride plus calcium decreased vertebral fracture rates, compared with calcium alone, in postmenopausal women with moderate osteoporosis. The dose of fluoride was 20 milligrams per day. In another recent study, a fluoride/calcium/vitamin D regimen was no more effective than a calcium/vitamin D regimen in preventing new vertebral fractures in women with postmenopausal osteoporosis.

Some have reported that fluoride-stimulated bone has abnormal texture and is less mineralized and durable than healthy bone. In some studies, despite increased bone mineral density, an increased incidence of fracture has been reported. Additionally, some have reported upper gastrointestinal discomfort and, of greater concern, lower extremity pain syndrome said to be caused by stress fractures. Thus, the benefits of fluoride in the treatment of osteoporosis remain in doubt. And its use in this context remains experimental.

There have been some cases of skeletal fluorosis associated with fluoride supplementation, particularly in those with various forms of renal failure. Two cases of bilateral hip fracture were reported involving women (aged 69 and 78) receiving 40 to 60 milligrams of fluoride daily for 11 to 21 months, in combination with calcium and vitamin D. Both women had moderate renal failure. Histological examination of a bone specimen from the 69-year-old patient revealed severe fluorosis. A specimen from the 78-year-old patient revealed osteomalacia and skeletal fluorosis. Researchers concluded that the fractures were caused by excessive fluoride retention due to renal insufficiency.

CONTRAINDICATIONS, PRECAUTIONS, ADVERSE REACTIONS

CONTRAINDICATIONS

Use of fluoride supplements is contraindicated in areas where fluoride water content is greater than 0.6 parts per million (ppm) or 0.6 milligrams per liter.

Fluoride supplements are contraindicated in those who are hypersensitive to any component of a fluoride-containing supplement.

PRECAUTIONS

Fluoride supplementation is not recommended in children under six months of age.

Excess fluoride intake may result in dental fluorosis in children and skeletal fluorosis in children and adults. Fluoride is not presently approved for the prevention or treatment of osteoporosis.

Pregnant women and nursing mothers should avoid intake of fluoride greater than adequate intake (AI) amounts.

ADVERSE REACTIONS

At the amounts recommended for fluoridation of drinking water and at the recommended doses used for caries prophylaxis, fluoride (sodium fluoride) is generally well tolerated and has not been found to have significant adverse reactions.

Recommended adequate intake for adult males is 4 milligrams daily and for adult females, 3 milligrams daily.

Adverse reactions are occasionally reported at doses of 5 to 10 milligrams daily and are more frequently reported at doses of 10 to 20 milligrams daily and higher. Adverse reactions include nausea, vomiting, mouth sores, rashes, and upper gastrointestinal complaints, such as abdominal distress. Gastrointestinal side effects (nausea, vomiting, abdominal distress) are generally less frequent with slow-acting fluoride preparations than with immediate-release preparations.

A single dose of sodium fluoride of 5 to 10 grams may be lethal. Less than one gram of sodium fluoride has caused serious poisoning.

Chronic fluoride poisoning may result in dental fluorosis and skeletal fluorosis. Symptoms of skeletal fluorosis include bone pain, stiffness and limited movement. A so-called lower extremity pain syndrome has been reported which was caused by stress fractures. Dental fluorosis is characterized by mottled enamel.

INTERACTIONS

DRUGS

Aluminum hydroxide: Concomitant intake of aluminum hydroxide antacids and fluoride can cause decreased absorption of fluoride.

NUTRITIONAL SUPPLEMENTS

Calcium: Concomitant intake of a calcium supplement and fluoride can cause decreased absorption of fluoride.

FOODS

Concomitant intake of foods rich in calcium, such as milk or dairy products, can cause decreased absorption of fluoride.

OVERDOSAGE

Symptoms of acute overdosage include nausea, bloody vomiting, increased salivation, watery eyes, weakness, tremors, tarry stools, drowsiness, faintness, shallow breathing, hypocalcemia, hyperkalemia, convulsions, cardiac arrhythmias, shock, respiratory arrest and cardiac arrest. Death may occur within two to four hours. A single oral dose of 5 to 10 grams of sodium fluoride may be lethal.

DOSAGE AND ADMINISTRATION

Sodium fluoride is available as a prescription supplement, either as a stand-alone product or in combination with vitamins and other minerals. High-fluoride waters are also available containing up to 3 parts per million (3 milligrams per liter) of fluoride. Intakes of fluoride of higher than 4 milligrams daily for adult males and 3 milligrams daily for adult females are not recommended.

The recommendations for fluoride supplementation by the Council on Dental Therapeutics of the American Dental Association are as follows:

Fluoride supplements are not recommended for infants under six months of age. If the fluoride content of the drinking water contains less than 0.3 parts per million (ppm) or 0.3 mg per liter, children aged six months to three years may be given 0.25 mg of fluoride daily; those aged three to six years, 0.5 mg of fluoride daily, and those aged six years and older, 1 mg daily. When the drinking water contains 0.3 to 0.6 ppm or 0.3 to 0.6 mg per liter of fluoride, lower doses should be considered. Specifically, it is recommended that no additional fluoride should be given to children less than three years of age. For children aged three to six years, 0.25 mg of fluoride daily is recommended, and for those aged six years and older, 0.5 mg daily is recommended. Again, if the fluoride content of the drinking water is greater than 0.6 ppm, fluoride supplementation is not recommended.

For calculation purposes, 1.1 milligrams of sodium fluoride are equivalent to 0.5 milligram of fluoride. Fluoride comprises approximately 45% of sodium fluoride.

The Food and Nutrition Board of the Institute of Medicine of the U.S. National Academy of Sciences has recommended the following adequate intakes (AI) for fluoride:

Infants	(AI)
0 through 6 months	0.01 mg/day
7 through 12 months	0.5 mg/day
Children	
1 through 3 years	0.7 mg/day
4 through 8 years	1 mg/day
Boys	
9 through 13 years	2 mg/day
14 through 18 years	3 mg/day

Girls

9 through 13 years	2 mg/day
14 through 18 years	3 mg/day

Males

19 and over	4 mg/day

Females

19 and over	3 mg/day

Pregnancy

14 through 18 years	3 mg/day
19 through 50 years	3 mg/day

Lactation

14 through 18 years	3 mg/day
19 through 50 years	3 mg/day

The Food and Nutrition Board of the Institute of Medicine has recommended the following tolerable upper limits (UL) for fluoride.

Infants

	(UL)
0 through 6 months	0.7 mg/day
7 through 12 months	0.9 mg/day

Children

1 through 3 years	1.3 mg/day
4 through 8 years	2.2 mg/day

Children and Adults

More than 8 years	10 mg/day

Pregnancy and Lactation

14 through 50 years	10 mg/day

LITERATURE

Adair SM. Overview of the history and current status of fluoride supplementation schedules. *J Public Health Dent.* 1999; 59:252-258.

Angelillo IF, Torre I, Nobile CG, Villari P. Caries and fluorosis prevalence in communities with different concentrations of fluoride in the water. *Caries Res.* 1999; 33:114-122.

Dietary Reference Intakes for Calcium Phosphorus, Magnesium, Vitamin D, and Fluoride. Washington, DC: National Academy Press; 1997.

Guañabens N, Farrerons J, Perez-Edo L, et al. Cyclical etidronate versus sodium fluoride in established postmenopausal osteoporosis: a randomized 3 year trial. *Bone.* 2000; 27:123-128.

Hillier S, Cooper C, Kelligray S, et al. Fluoride in drinking water and risk of hip fracture in the UK: a case-control study. *Lancet.* 2000; 355:265-269.

Horowitz HS. The role of dietary fluoride supplements in caries prevention. *J Public Health Dent.* 1999; 59:205-210.

Leverett DH, Adair SM, Vaughan BW, et al. Randomized clinical trial of the effect of prenatal fluoride supplements in preventing dental caries. *Caries Res.* 1997; 31:174-179.

Lips P. [Fluoride in osteoporosis: still an experimental and controversial treatment]. [Article in Dutch]. *Ned Tijdschr Geneeskd.* 1998; 142:1913-1915.

Meunier PJ, Sebert JL, Reginster JY, et al. Fluoride salts are no better at preventing new vertebral fracture than calcium-vitamin D in postmenopausal osteoporosis: the FAVO Study. *Osteoporosis Int.* 1998; 8:4-12.

Nielsen FH. Ultratrace minerals. In: Shils ME, Olson JA, Shike M, Ross AC, eds. *Modern Nutrition in Health and Disease,* 9th ed. Baltimore, MD: Williams and Wilkins; 1999:283-303.

Pak CYC, Sakhaee K, Adams-Huet B, et al. Treatment of postmenopausal osteoporosis with slow-release sodium fluoride. *Ann Int Med.* 1995; 123:401-408.

Pak CYC, Sakhaee K, Piziak V, et al. Slow-release sodium fluoride in the management of postmenopausal osteoporosis. *Ann Int Med.* 1994; 120:625-632.

Reginster JY, Meurmans L, Zegels B, et al. The effect of sodium monofluorophosphate plus calcium on vertebral fracture rate in postmenopausal women with moderate osteoporosis. A randomized, controlled trial. *Ann Intern Med.* 1998; 129:1-8.

Schulz W. [Fluoride treatment of osteoporosis]. [Article in German]. *Wien Med Wochenschr.* 2000; 150:42-52.

Folate

DESCRIPTION

The term folate is used in two different ways. Folate, a member of the B-vitamin family, is a collective term for a number of chemical forms which are structurally related and which have similar biological activity to folic acid. Folate is also the term which is used for the anionic form of folic acid. Folic acid or pteroylglutamic acid (PGA) is comprised of *para*-aminobenzoic acid linked at one end to a pteridine ring and at the other end to glutamic acid. The pteridine-*para*-aminobenzoic acid portion of the molecule is called the pteroyl group. Folic acid is a synthetic folate form which is used for food fortification and nutritional supplements. It is not one of the principal naturally occurring forms of folate, used in the collective sense.

The naturally occurring forms of folate differ in the extent of the reduction state of the pteroyl group, the nature of the substituents on the pteridine ring and the number of glutamyl residues attached to the pteroyl group. The naturally occurring folates, include 5-methyltetrahydrofolate (5-MTHF), 5-formyltetrahydrofolate (5-formyl-THF), 10-formyltetrahydrofolate (10-formyl-THF), 5,10-methylenetetrahydrofolate (5,10-methylene-THF), 5,10-methenyltetrahydrofolate (5,10-methenyl-THF), 5-formiminotetrahydrofolate (5-formimino-THF), 5,6,7,8-tetrahydrofolate (THF) and dihydrofolate (DHF). Most naturally occurring folates are pteroylpolyglutamates, containing two to seven glutamates joined in amide (peptide) linkages to the gamma-carboxyl of glutamate. The principal intracellular folates are pteroylpentaglutamates, while the principal extracellular folates are pteroylmonoglutamates. Pteroylpolyglutamates with up to 11 glutamic acid residues exist naturally. Folate is represented by the following chemical structure.

Folic Acid

Folate participates in several key biological processes, including the synthesis of DNA, RNA and proteins. It is necessary for DNA replication and repair, the maintenance of the integrity of the genome, and is involved in the regulation of gene expression, among other things. Folate deficiency leads to an anemia, called megaloblastic anemia, which is very similar to that caused by vitamin B_{12}. However, folate deficiency does not result in the neurological symptoms and signs that occur with vitamin B_{12} deficiency. Other symptoms and signs of folate deficiency, include weakness, fatigue, irritability, headache, difficulty concentrating, cramps, palpitations, shortness of breath and atrophic glossitis. Laboratory findings of folate deficiency, include decreased serum folate and erythrocyte folate concentrations, elevated serum homocysteine concentration, hypersegmentation of the neutrophils, decreased hemoglobin and erythrocyte concentrations, decreased hematocrit and macrocytic, hyperchromic erythrocytes. Marginal folate deficiency appears to increase the risk of cardiovascular disease, certain types of cancer, Alzheimer's disease and depression. Marginal folate deficiency in pregnant women results in an increased incidence of neural tube defects, including meningomyelocele (e.g., spina bifida), anencephaly, meningocele and craniorachischisis, in their neonates.

A number of conditions can lead to folate deficiency. Chronic alcohol users can become deficient in the vitamin secondary to inadequate intake as well as to ethanol's impairment of folate absorption and hepatobiliary metabolism, as well as to increased renal folate excretion caused by ethanol. Malabsorption syndromes, including Crohn's disease, lymphoma or amyloidosis of the small intestine, diabetic enteropathy, tropical sprue and non-tropical sprue (gluten-sensitive enteropathy), can result in folate deficiency

secondary to inadequate absorption of the vitamin, as can small intestinal resections or diversions for the same reason. Some conditions or situations, such as chronic hemolytic anemias (e.g., sickle cell disease), chronic hemodialysis or peritoneal dialysis, chronic exfoliative skin disorders and pregnancy, cause increased demand for folate and folate deficiency will result if the increased demand is not met. Certain drugs, e.g., methotrexate, trimethoprim, pyrimethamine, sulfasalazine and phenytoin, interfere with folate metabolism and may cause functional folate deficiencies. In fact, the mechanism of action of certain antimetabolites, including methotrexate, 5-fluoruracil and the newer multitargeted antifolates, depends on their creating a functional folate deficiency. Some genetic disorders result in folate deficiency and are responsive to folate treatment. Folate-induced remission has been reported in aplastic anemia with familial defect of cellular folate uptake.

Recognizing the increased demand of folate during pregnancy and the increased risk of neural tube defects in neonates born to pregnant women with marginal folate status, the United States Food and Drug Administration (FDA) mandated that folic acid be added to all enriched cereal grains in order to prevent neural tube defects. The mandate became effective on January 1, 1998. The level of folic acid adopted for enriched cereal grain fortification was 140 micrograms per 100 grams. The U.S. Public Health Service recommends that all women of childbearing age in the U.S. consume 400 micrograms of folic acid daily to reduce their risk of having a baby affected with spina bifida or other neural tube defects. This is one of the few health claims allowed by the FDA for nutritional supplementation. The FDA determined 400 micrograms of folic acid daily to be an optimal dose for the prevention of neural tube defects. Those women who already have had a child with a neural tube defect require higher doses.

Natural folates are found in dark green leafy vegetables (spinach, kale, mustard greens, turnip greens, escarole, chard, arugula, beet greens, bok choy, dandelion green, mache, radicchio, rapini or broccoli de rabe, Swiss chard), oranges, lentils, pinto beans, garbanzo beans, asparagus, orange juice, broccoli, cauliflower, liver and brewer's yeast. The absorption efficiency of natural folates is approximately 50% that of folic acid (see Pharmacokinetics). Interestingly, folate was named because of its presence in green leafy vegetables (folium is Latin for leaf) and was originally isolated from four tons of spinach, such was the crudity of isolation techniques more than seven decades ago.

The principal biochemical function of folates is the mediation of one-carbon transfer reactions. 5-Methyltetrahydrofolate donates a methyl group to homocysteine, in the conversion of homocysteine to L-methionine. The enzyme that catalyzes the reaction is methionine synthase. Vitamin B_{12} is a cofactor in the reaction. This reaction is of great importance in the regulation of serum homocysteine levels and is the only reaction in the body in which folate and vitamin B_{12} are coparticipants. (See Vitamin B_{12}). The L-methione produced in the reaction can participate in protein synthesis and is also a major source for the synthesis of S-adenosyl-L-methionine (SAMe). The methyl group that was donated by 5-methyltetrahydrofolate to homocysteine in the formation of L-methionine is used by SAMe in a number of transmethylation reactions involving nucleic acids, phospholipids and proteins, as well as for the synthesis of epinephrine, melatonin, creatine and other molecules (see S-Adenosyl-L-Methionine). Tetrahydrofolate is the folate product of the methionine synthase reaction. 5-Methyltetrahydrofolate can be generated in only one way: conversion of 5,10-methylenetetrahydrofolate into 5-methyltetrahydrofolate via the enzyme methyleneterahydrofolate reductase (MTHFR). 5,10-Methylenetetrahydrofolate is regenerated from tetrahydrofolate via the enzyme serine hydroxymethyltransferase, a reaction, which in addition to producing 5,10-methylenetetrahydrofolate, yields glycine.

5,10-Methylenetetrahydrofolate, in addition to its role in the metabolism of homocysteine, supplies the one-carbon group for the methylation of deoxyuridylic acid to form the DNA precursor thymidylic acid. This reaction is catalyzed by thymidylate synthase and the folate product of the reaction is dihydrofolate. Dihydrofolate is converted to tetrahydrofolate via the enzyme dihydrofolate reductase.

Folates are also involved in reactions leading to *de novo* purine nucleotide synthesis, interconversion of serine and glycine, generation and utilization of formate, the metabolism of L-histidine to L-glutamic acid, the metabolism of dimethylglycine to sarcosine and the metabolism of sarcosine to glycine.

One of the natural folates, folinic acid, is used as a pharmaceutical agent. Folinic acid, also known as leucovorin, citrovorum factor and 5-formyltetrahydrofolate, is used as rescue therapy following high-dose methotrexate in the treatment of osteosarcoma. It is also used to diminish the toxicity of methotrexate. It is used in the treatment of megaloblastic anemia due to folate deficiency and in the prevention or treatment of the toxic side effects of trimetrexate and pyrimethamine. The combination of folinic acid and 5-fluorouracil has until recently been standard therapy for metastatic colorectal cancer. Folinic acid increases the affinity of flurouracil for thymidylate synthase. Folinic acid is available as a calcium salt for parenteral or oral administration. See *Physicians' Desk Reference* for further discussion of folinic acid.

In addition to being known as pteroylglutamic acid or PGA, folic acid is known chemically as *N*-[4-[[(2-amino-1,4-dihydro-4-oxo-6-pteridinyl)methyl]amino]benzoyl]-L-glutamic acid. Older names for folic acid are vitamin B_9, folicin, vitamin Bc and vitamin M. Its molecular formula is $C_{19}H_{19}N_7O_6$ and its molecular weight is 441.40 daltons. Folic acid forms yellowish-orange crystals. The color is imparted by the pteridine ring of folic acid. Pteridine also imparts color to butterfly wings.

ACTIONS AND PHARMACOLOGY

ACTIONS

Folic acid lowers the risk of neural tube defects and possibly other types of birth defects. It may also have antiatherogenic, anticarcinogenic, neuroprotective and antidepressant actions.

MECHANISM OF ACTION

Animal and epidemiologic studies have shown that folate deficiency is associated with defects of neural tube closure. Human studies have shown that folic acid, when taken by women planning to become pregnant, can greatly reduce the risk of bearing a child with spina bifida or other neural tube defects. The exact mechanism by which folic acid reduces the risk of neural tube defects and possibly other types of birth defects is not known. It is likely that this effect of folic acid is due to its role in nucleic acid synthesis and/or its role in the metabolism of homocysteine to methionine. Along a different line, it is hypothesized by some that folic acid may not prevent the occurrence of neural tube defects, but may instead selectively increase the abortion rate of affected fetuses.

A central feature of fetal development is widespread and sustained cell division. Folate plays a central role in the formation of nucleic acid precursors, such as thymidylic acid and purine nucleotides, which are essential for nucleic acid synthesis and cell division. The requirement for folate increases during times of rapid tissue growth. The teratogenic effect of folate deficiency may be a result of an insufficient supply of nucleic acid precursors in the rapidly dividing embryonic cells. Increasing folate tissue concentrations might overcome a metabolic deficiency of the vitamin in the production of nucleic acids, and possibly also proteins, at the time of neural tube closure, which typically occurs 24 to 28 days after conception. An insufficient supply of nucleic acid precursors, however, might be expected to cause more general birth defects than the highly specific and predictable nature of the congenital defects caused by folate deficiency. Although derivatives of the neural ectoderm are affected more than other tissues by folate deficiency, all of the embryonic tissues are dividing rapidly during the susceptible developmental period. An insufficient supply of nucleic acid precursors may play some role in the mechanism of folate deficiency-induced neural tube defects, but it is not a sufficient explanation for these congenital disorders.

Some studies have found that homocysteine levels in pregnant women who subsequently gave birth to children with neural tube defects, were significantly higher than those of pregnant women who gave birth to normal children. This would be expected to occur in pregnant women with low folate status. The enzyme that metabolizes homocysteine to methionine, methionine synthase, uses 5-methyltetrahydrofolate, as well as vitamin B_{12}, as a cofactor. There is some evidence that pregnant women with elevated homocysteine levels have a defect in the methionine synthase enzyme. A defect in the enzyme would lead to decreased production of methionine and S-adenosylmethione (SAMe). SAMe is involved in a number of transmethylation reactions, including reactions involved in the formation of myelin. Further, increased homocysteine levels could result in increased oxidative stress which might be contributory to a teratogenic effect. Homocysteine has been found to be teratogenic in avian embryos. Avian embryos treated directly with D,L-homocysteine or with L-homocysteine thiolactone showed neural tube defects which were prevented with folic acid, indicating that homocysteine *per se* can cause dysmorphogenesis of the neural tube.

Hyperhomocysteinemia is associated with cardiovascular disease, cerebrovascular disease and carotid artery stenosis in adults. Folic acid can lower homocysteine blood levels by converting homocysteine to methionine. A high intake of folate has been associated with a lower risk of coronary events. There is evidence that hyperhomocysteinemia is a risk factor for coronary heart disease independent of other known risk factors (hypercholesterolemia, hypertension, diabetes, smoking). Folic acid, as mentioned above, can lower homocysteine blood levels, but the mechanism by which hyperhomocysteinemia might increase the risk of vascular disease is unclear. A number of hypotheses have been proposed. Homocysteine may promote atherogenesis through endothelial dysfunction and oxidative stress. Elevated homocysteine levels may result in increased oxidation of low-density lipoprotein cholesterol (LDL-C). Oxidized LDL-C is thought to be a major etiological factor in atherogenesis. Homocysteine can promote the growth of smooth muscle cells and increase platelet adhesiveness and affect several factors in the coagulation cascade. Thus, homocysteine can be thrombogenic.

Approximately 10% of the population have a defective folate metabolizing enzyme called methylenetetrahydrofolate reductase (MTHFR). MTHFR catalyzes the reduction of 5,10-methylenetetrahydrofolate to 5-methyltetrahydrofolate. 5-Methyltetrahydrofolate transfers its methyl group to homocysteine in the formation of methionine, in a reaction catalyzed by methionine synthase. Flavin adenine dinucleotide (FAD), derived from riboflavin (vitamin B_2) and reduced nicotinamide adenine dinucleotide phosphate (NADPH), derived from niacin, are cofactors in the reaction. Deficiency of MTHFR is the most common inborn error of folate metabolism and is a major genetic cause of hyperhomocysteinemia. The polymorphism A222V (alanine to valine substitution at residue 222 of the enzyme), in which there is a base change at position 677 of its gene, of cytosine to thymine, is homozygous in about 10% of the population. Those homozygous for the T677 allele are found to have elevated homocysteine levels which appear to be associated with an increased risk of vascular disease. The mutant enzyme is thermolabile and does not bind as tightly to its cofactor FAD as does the normal enzyme. Addition of folate to the mutant enzyme stabilizes its binding to FAD and also stabilizes the enzyme against heat inactivation.

Folic acid may have antiatherogenic mechanisms other than that of lowering homocysteine levels. Impaired availability of endothelium-derived nitric oxide (NO), produced by the enzyme endothelial nitric oxide synthase (eNOS), has been identified as a mediator of atherosclerosis. Folic acid and 5-methyltetrahydrofolate have been demonstrated to restore impaired NO status in hypercholesterolemic subjects. In cultured endothelial cells, 5-methyltetrahydrofolate was found to enhance the enzymatic activity of partially tetrahydrobiopterin (BH_4)-repleted eNOS, enhancing NO formation. BH_4 is the cofactor for eNOS. The enhancement of eNOS activity may be another mechanism for the possible antiatherogenic activity of folic acid.

5-Methyltetrahydrofolate has been found to directly scavenge superoxide radicals *in vitro*. Activated eNOS also decreases the production of superoxide. Uncoupling of eNOS, which occurs under conditions of hypercholesterolemia, results in decreased production of NO and increased production of superoxide. Folate appears to restore impaired NO availability by an ameliorative effect on eNOS uncoupling.

Epidemiologic studies have shown that diminished folate status is associated with colorectal, lung, esophageal, brain, cervical and breast cancers. Data supporting the effect of folate status on carcinogenesis are most compelling for colorectal cancer. The mechanism of the possible anticarcinogenic activity of folate is not well understood. Folate deficiency may induce DNA hypomethylation and gene "unsilencing." Folate is critical for the synthesis of the transmethylating agent S-adenosylmethione (SAMe). SAMe methylates certain bases in DNA leading to gene silencing. Gene "unsilencing" alters gene expression and can disrupt the integrity of the genome. DNA hypomethylation appears to be an early, and consistent event in carcinogenesis, including that of colorectal cancer. Folate deficiency may lead to increased uracil incorporation in DNA. Folate is critical for the formation of thymidylic acid from deoxyuridylic acid. Increased uracil incorporation in DNA can lead to disruption of the integrity of DNA. Folate deficiency may also result in diminished DNA repair, impaired natural killer cell surveillance, secondary choline deficiency, decreased stimulation of T lymphocytes by phytohemagglutinin and activation of tumorigenic viruses. A recent report demonstrated that folate deficiency produced progressive DNA strand breaks in the highly conserved region of the p53 tumor-suppressor gene in rat colon.

Low concentrations of folate in the blood have been associated with poor cognitive function, dementia and Alzheimer's disease-related neurodegeneration of the brain. A recent report from the "Nun Study" showed that low serum folate was strongly associated with atrophy of the cerebral cortex. The mechanism of the neuroprotective effect of folate is not well understood. It has been suggested that elevated homocysteine levels secondary to folate deficiency may account, in large part, for neurodegeneration via increased oxidative stress and endothelial dysfunction, among other things. Elevated serum homocysteine levels were associated with progressive atrophy of the medial temporal lobe in subjects with Alzheimer's disease, in one study.

Folate deficiency has been associated with depression and other psychiatric symptoms. Consistent findings in major depression have been low plasma and low erythrocyte folate levels which have been linked to poor response to antidepressants. Subjects with low plasma folate levels responded less well to the antidepressant fluoxetine than did those with normal folate levels. A recent study reported that folic acid enhanced the antidepressant action of fluoxetine in subjects who did not appear to be folate deficient. The mechanism by which folate affects brain functions is unclear. It is thought that the most likely explanation is folate's role in the synthesis of S-adenosylmethione (SAMe). 5-Methyltetrahydrofolate is the methyl donor in the formation of methionine from homocysteine. It is thought that this reaction is important for the maintenance of the SAMe pool (SAMe is formed from methionine). SAMe is the methylating agent in the formation of the catecholamine neurotransmitters in the brain. These neurotransmitters are important in maintaining the affective state. SAMe itself has been found to have mood-modulating activity (see SAMe).

PHARMACOKINETICS

Folic acid or pteroylglutamic acid (PGA) is the form of folate used in food fortification and the principal form of folate found in nutritional supplements. Natural food folates are pteroylpolyglutamate derivatives. Pteroylpolyglutamate derivatives are hydrolyzed to pteroylmonoglutamate forms prior to absorption from the small intestine. The enzyme that catalyzes the cleavage is called folate conjugase or gamma-glutamylhydrolase. The monoglutamate forms of folate, including folic acid, are transported across the proximal small intestine via a saturable pH-dependent process. Higher doses of the pteroylmonoglutamates, including folic acid, are absorbed via a nonsaturable passive diffusion process. The efficiency of absorption of the pteroylmonoglutamates is greater than that of the pteroylpolyglutamates.

Because of the difference in absorption efficiency between natural food folate and folic acid, the concept of dietary folate equivalents (DFEs) has been introduced. Folic acid taken on an empty stomach is twice as available as food folate. Folic acid taken with food is 1.7 times as available as food folate. For example, 400 micrograms of folic acid taken on an empty stomach is equivalent to 470 micrograms of folic acid taken with food and is equivalent to 800 micrograms of food folate. DFEs can be calculated as follows:

1 microgram of DFEs = 1 microgram of food folate = 0.5 micrograms of folic acid taken on an empty stomach = 0.6 micrograms of folic acid taken with meals.

Following absorption of physiological amounts of folic acid into the enterocytes, a certain percentage undergoes reduction. Reduced folate is transported to the liver via the portal circulation. Much of a pharmacological dose of folic acid is transported to the liver as such, without first undergoing metabolism in the enterocytes. The various natural pteroylmonoglutamate forms undergo some metabolism in the enterocytes to pteroylpolyglutamate forms, but for the most part are also transported as their unmetabolized forms via the portal circulation to the liver. The folates are taken up by the liver and metabolized to polyglutamate derivatives (principally pteroylpentaglutamates), via the action of folylpolyglutamate synthase. Folates are stored in tissue in their polyglutamate forms. Folate is metabolized to its various metabolic forms in the liver. The various pteroylpolyglutamate forms are the active cellular cofactor forms of folate. Folate polyglutamates are released from the liver to the systemic circulation and to the bile. When released from the liver into the circulation, the polyglutamate forms are hydrolyzed by gamma-glutamylhydrolase and reconverted to the monoglutamate forms.

The principal folate in the plasma is 5-methyltetrahydrofolate in its monoglutate form. 5-Methyltetrahydrofolate circulates in erythrocytes in its polyglutamate form. Approximately two-thirds of folate in plasma is protein bound. All tissue forms of folate are polyglutamates, while circulating forms of folate are monoglutamates. When pharmacological doses of folic acid are administered, a significant amount of unchanged folic acid is found in the plasma. The liver contains approximately 50% of the body stores of folate, or about 6 to 14 milligrams. The total body store of folate is about 12 to 28 milligrams.

Folate is excreted in the urine as folate cleavage products. Intact folate enters the glomerulus and is reabsorbed into the proximal renal tubule. Very little intact folate is excreted in the urine. Folate is excreted in the bile and much of it is reabsorbed via the enterohepatic circulation.

INDICATIONS AND USAGE

Folic acid is indicated for the prevention of some birth defects. Its widely heralded usefulness in cardiovascular disease has recently been called into question by results from some large, long-term studies. Its use in cancer has now also become controversial, with some data suggesting that it may actually be tumorigenic in some circumstances. While available evidence suggests significant preventive/protective effects against various cancers, the use of folic acid as an interventive treatment for cancer is too premature to recommend due to some preliminary findings that it might promote growth of some established cancers. There is very preliminary evidence that folic acid might be helpful in reducing the symptoms of some psychiatric disorders. It has been hypothesized that folic acid supplementation might help prevent Alzheimer's disease and recurrent spontaneous early pregnancy loss, but the research that might confirm or refute these suggestions has not been performed. There is some recent data suggesting that supplemental folate might help preserve hearing function in the aged.

RESEARCH SUMMARY

So strong are the data indicating that folic acid can protect against neural tube birth defects that the Food and Drug Administration issued a regulation that became effective in 1998 requiring fortification of all uncooked cereal grain products and all flour with folic acid.

Several studies have shown that women with low plasma folate and vitamin B_{12} concentrations are at significantly increased risk of giving birth to babies with neural tube defects, as well as some other birth defects. Moreover, several double-blind, placebo-controlled studies have demonstrated that neural tube defects can be significantly prevented when women take folic acid supplements during the periconceptional period. A dose of 400 micrograms of folic acid daily is now widely recommended for women of reproductive age.

Additional studies have shown that multivitamin supplements containing folic acid also significantly reduce the incidence of neural tube defects. There is some preliminary indication that periconceptional supplementation with these preparations may reduce the incidence of orofacial clefts, limb defects and cardiovascular anomalies. For some time, folic acid and various B vitamins have been credited with having significant impact in the prevention of cardiovascular disease. The American Heart Association went so far as to declare that these vitamins were playing a significant role in preventing 17,000 deaths from coronary causes each year in this country. Recently, however, a succession of large, long-term studies have failed to find benefit from B vitamins in heart disease. The older positive data are discussed first and then are followed by a discussion of the more recent and more negative findings.

In a meta-analysis of studies conducted some years ago of the relationship between folic acid intakes and plasma homocysteine levels and between the incidence of coronary heart disease, cerebrovascular and peripheral vascular disease and homocysteine levels, these conclusions were reached: The association between elevated homocysteine and these diseases is "consistent and very strong." Folic acid intakes up to 600 micrograms daily significantly reduce homocysteine levels in a dose-dependent fashion.

Based upon findings from this updated meta-analysis, it has been estimated that, for every 50 microgram daily increase in average food folate intake, 4,000 to 18,000 deaths due to cardiovascular disease could be prevented annually. It was further estimated that with population-wide consumption of 400 micrograms daily of supplemental folic acid, 3,000 to 23,000 deaths from cardiovascular disease could be prevented each year. Another group of researchers has estimated that ten percent of all U.S. heart disease is attributable to elevated homocysteine levels.

It was demonstrated in a prospective, randomized, placebo-controlled trial that folic acid can help prevent some of the deleterious effects of triglyceride-rich lipoproteins on endothelium-dependent vasodilation in healthy volunteers challenged with an acute oral fat load. These protective effects were achieved with oral doses of folic acid (10 milligrams daily for two weeks). These same researchers had previously demonstrated that parenteral administration of folic acid could restore endothelial function *in vivo* in subjects with elevated LDL-cholesterol levels.

In a study of 45 subjects with established cardiovascular disease, folic acid intake was significantly inversely correlated with multiple indices of oxidized LDL-cholesterol. This correlation remained significant even when adjusted for potential confounding variables, including consumption of other vitamins and nutrients.

Evidence for a causal link between homocysteine and cardiovascular disease was further fortified in recent years via mendelian randomization studies showing that about

10% of the population has a genotype that leads to 25% higher homocysteine concentrations and also to higher cardiovascular disease risk. This and other evidence discussed above resulted in a statement a few years ago from the American Heart Association asserting that "the lowering of the population mean level of total homocysteine is estimated to have prevented 17,000 deaths from coronary causes each year." Some other authorities called for adding folic acid to a polypill designed to prevent heart disease and stroke.

Despite all of this, folic acid, and the B vitamins in general, are not winning universal praise from the medical establishment for their use in heart disease. Several large, randomized long-term studies are now failing to find benefit from B vitamin therapies in this context. These negative studies include the Vitamins Intervention for Stroke Prevention (VISP) trial and the Heart Outcomes Prevention Evaluation (HOPE-2) trial. Neither found any vitamin B benefit overall—with the exception of some significant protection against stroke seen in the HOPE-2 trial, but not in the VISP trial. The VISP trial, it should be noted, was designed specifically to look for a homocysteine effect on stroke, whereas the HOPE-2 trial was not. Overseas, several large trials have similarly failed to find benefit. These include the Cambridge Heart Antioxidant Study (CHAOS-2), Norwegian Vitamin Trial (NORVIT) and the Western Norway B-Vitamin Intervention Trial (WENBIT). More recently still, no benefit from vitamin B supplements was seen with respect to either coronary heart disease or stroke in the Women's Antioxidant and Folic Acid Cardiovascular Study (WAFACS). It had longer follow-up than other studies: 7.3 years.

In view of all these negative results, an editorial in *JAMA* asked: "Is there a role for additional trials or should researchers close yet another chapter, which seemed promising but has failed to deliver?" Possible reasons for the failure, the editorial continued, include, among other things, doses used in the various studies and even "potential unexpected proatherosclerotic effects of folic acid supplementation, which may have counteracted benefits associated with homocysteine lowering." A number of large trials are still ongoing, and many consider the jury still to be out. But as the *JAMA* editorial observed: "until further data become available it is important to remain fully grounded on the available evidence and to admit that once again experimental and observational data do not always translate into therapeutic benefits . . . In conclusion, vitamin B supplements cannot currently be recommended for the prevention of CVD events (with the exception of rare genetic disorders) and there is no role for routine screening for elevated homocysteine levels."

A recent editorial in *Circulation*, on the other hand, has urged researchers and the medical world, generally, not to "close the book" on folic acid and its use in cardiovascular disease. The editorialist noted that there are several reports in which folic acid improves endothelial function independent of homocysteine-lowering effects. In the same issue of *Circulation,* a report found a "dramatic" cardioprotective effect of folic acid that the editorial said "could potentially bring folic acid to the center stage in the management of ischemic heart disease." This was a rat study in which very high-dose folic acid was administered for one week. The rats were subjected to myocardial ischemia for 30 minutes. The hearts of the treated rats maintained cardiac function during ischemia and developed almost no infarct after reperfusion, while untreated rats suffered severe injury, including infarct in 60% of the area at risk. This high-dose treatment was said to be comparable to or exceeding ischemic preconditioning, "the most powerful protection against ischemic injury demonstrated so far." The study suggested that this result could also be achieved via acute intravenous delivery of folic acid 10 minutes after the onset of ischemia. The dose used was 400 times greater than the high recommended clinical dose. Evidence of antioxidant activity was noted, but the researchers said that this activity alone was unlikely to be responsible for the marked benefits observed. The researchers hypothesized that high concentrations of folate might increase purine synthesis and thus sustain ATP levels in the heart during ischemia. Loss of purines from ischemic myocardium has been noted for some time and is a major hallmark of ischemia. The editorialist observed that "identifying ways to prevent the loss of purines or to increase *de novo* purine synthesis is the holy grail of cardiac biochemistry."

There is precedent in other recent animal research for preservation of the total adenine nucleotide pool with a long-term supply of high doses of folate (in this case in combination with ribose in a rat model of right heart hypertrophy). The *Circulation* editorial, while stressing "the remarkable, almost magical, effect of folate on the ischemic myocardium" in the report contained in that journal, admitted that the new study raises as many questions as it answers and concluded: "As the effects demonstrated here are so powerful and as folic acid is highly affordable, further investigations are certainly warranted for both scientific and social causes."

Folic acid appears to protect against a number of cancers, particularly colorectal cancers. Some 20 epidemiologic studies suggest that those with the highest folate intake have an approximately 40% reduction in risk of this cancer. In the Nurses Health Study, involving 88,756 women, there was a 75% reduction in risk of colorectal cancer among those using multivitamin supplements containing 400 or more micrograms of folic acid for 15 or more years, compared with those not using these supplements. This benefit was calculated after controlling for all relevant potential confounding factors.

Long-term folate supplementation was found, in another study, to reduce the incidence of colorectal neoplasia by 62% in subjects with extensive chronic ulcerative colitis. Such subjects, without this supplementation, typically have a 10-fold to 40-fold increased risk of developing colorectal neoplasia.

In a double-blind, placebo-controlled studies, administration of 5 to 10 milligrams of folic acid daily for six months to a year had several positive effects, as measured, for example, by a reduced biomarker of colorectal cancer development in patients with either colorectal cancer or adenomas. Another placebo-controlled study involved subjects who were given 1 milligram of folic acid daily following polypectomy. At two years post-surgery, the supplemented group had a recurrence rate half that of the placebo group. Larger multi-center, prospective studies are now in progress to test the effects of 1-5 milligrams of folic acid daily on recurrence of colorectal adenoma.

Effects of folic acid on uterine cervical cancer are in doubt. Earlier reports that folic acid supplementation can bring about reversal or regression of cervical dysplasia have not been confirmed in recent, well-controlled human trials using 5-10 milligrams of folic acid daily for three to six months.

Epidemiological studies hint at the possibility that folic acid might be helpful in preventing cancers of the brain, stomach and esophagus. Other such studies have recently shown considerably stronger evidence that, in both premenopausal and postmenopausal women who consume 15 grams of alcohol daily (the equivalent of one drink), total folate intake of at least 600 micrograms daily is significantly protective against breast cancer. The same protection is not evident in women who consume less than 15 grams of alcohol daily. Two of three case-control studies have also found evidence that folate might be protective against breast cancer in some women.

Another case-control study suggests that folate may be protective against pancreatic cancer in male smokers. Higher baseline serum folate concentrations were associated with a 55% reduction in pancreatic cancer risk, compared with those with lower baseline serum levels of folate.

There have been two studies showing that folic acid, in combination with vitamin B_{12}, can reverse a precursor of bronchial squamous cell cancer of the lung. In one of these randomized, placebo-controlled studies, both of which in-volved heavy smokers, 10 milligrams of folic acid daily, combined with 500 micrograms of vitamin B_{12} daily, resulted, after four months, in a significant reduction in the number of subjects exhibiting abnormal bronchial cells said to be cancer precursors.

One folate researcher, while observing that "folate appears to be an ideal candidate for chemoprevention given its proven safety and cost," nonetheless cautions that "the optimal dose, duration, and timing, as well as the appropriate target population, of folate chemoprevention need to be clearly defined." This researcher adds that "some animal studies have suggested that supraphysiologic levels of folate supplementation do not confer protection and, in some cases, may enhance carcinogenesis."

In a genetic murine model of colon cancer, for example, folate supplementation prevented development of tumors when administered prior to the presence of any microscopic neoplastic foci. But when supplementation began after the appearance of such foci, it promoted tumor development in this experiment. "Therefore," this researcher concluded, "it appears that folate supplementation should be implemented before the development of precursor lesions in the target organ or in individuals free of any evidence of neoplastic foci."

The controversy over folate use in cancer has continued in recent years. A recent editorial in *JAMA* emphasized that when it comes to this issue "timing is everything." It noted that "recent experiments have suggested that the time of folate administration during cancer progression can modify outcomes. Folate administered prior to the existence of preneoplastic lesions can prevent tumor development, whereas provision of folate once early lesions are established appears to increase tumorigenesis." The explanation for this may be that rapidly proliferating tissues, such as those that arise in tumors, have increased the need for nucleotides, which folate helps synthesize. Thus some antifolate drugs are efficacious in some cancer treatments. Some recent studies have provided further evidence that folate can increase colorectal neoplasia and cancer, when the agent is administered after lesions are present.

Recently a report was published in the *American Journal of Clinical Nutrition* demonstrating a strong inverse relationship between dietary intakes of folate and invasive breast cancer, with reductions of 40% and more in the highest quintile of intake compared with the lowest. An accompanying editorial, however, again cautioned that timing is of the essence in the use of folate in cancer treatment and that, at present, too little is known for the medically unsupervised use of this vitamin in cancer patients or in those at risk of cancer. Much more study is clearly needed and warranted.

Since there is a reported high incidence of folate deficiency in some psychiatric patients, including those with depression, dementia and schizophrenia, some have suggested that supplemental folic acid might be beneficial in some of these individuals. Some open studies have shown some benefit from folic acid supplementation. Placebo-controlled studies have generally shown no therapeutic effect. These have often used very high doses (15-20 milligrams a day) with what one reviewer has called effects toxic enough to cause, rather than ameliorate, mental symptoms. Two placebo-controlled studies using smaller doses produced benefits in patients with psychopathology associated with folate deficiency and in another group of patients on long-term lithium therapy. The latter were treated with 200 micrograms of folic acid daily.

It has been hypothesized that, since folic acid deficiency is associated with reduced brain levels of S-adenosylmethionine and 5-hydroxytryptamine, supplemental folic acid might be helpful in some with depression. Studies have, in fact, confirmed that serum folate levels are often deficient in those suffering from depression. Whether supplemental folic acid would be of benefit remains unknown.

Similarly, an association has been made recently between low serum folate levels and the severity of atrophy of the neocortex in Alzheimer's disease subjects. But whether supplemental folic acid can be of any help in this disease has not been determined.

In a recent randomized, double-blind, placebo-controlled study, supplementation with 800 micrograms of folic acid daily for three years resulted in significantly improved cognitive function in men and women aged 50-70 years. Assessment measures used in this study included change in memory, information processing speed and sensorimotor speed. By all of these measures the supplemented group did significantly better than the placebo group.

Observational studies have suggested a relationship between age-related hearing loss and low folate levels. In one study, administration of 800 micrograms of folate daily helped reduce hearing loss over a three-year period in subjects thus supplemented, compared with those receiving placebo. Further research is needed to determine whether this observed effect can be replicated.

Finally, there has been a report that elevated homocysteine and reduced serum folate concentrations are significantly associated with recurrent spontaneous early pregnancy losses in humans. The suggestion has thus been made that folic acid supplementation might help prevent these recurrent early pregnancy losses. Again, this hypothesis has not yet been tested.

CONTRAINDICATIONS, PRECAUTIONS, ADVERSE REACTIONS

CONTRAINDICATIONS

Folic acid is contraindicated in those who are hypersensitive to any component of a folic acid-containing product.

PRECAUTIONS

Women of childbearing age, pregnant women and nursing mothers should ensure that their intake of folic acid from nutritional supplements and/or fortified food is 400 micrograms/day. A number of pre- and postnatal supplements deliver 1 milligram (1,000 micrograms) daily of folic acid. Doses higher than 1 milligam/day should only be used by the above groups if prescribed by their physicians.

The use of folic acid for the treatment of folate deficiency or for the treatment of any medical condition requires medical supervision.

The use of folic acid doses above 1 milligram/day may precipitate or exacerbate the neurological damage of vitamin B_{12} deficiency. Those who use folic acid doses above 1 milligram/day should only do so under medical supervision.

Those with undiagnosed anemia, should exercise caution in the use of supplementary folic acid. Doses of folic acid greater than 100 micrograms daily may result in hematologic improvement in those with vitamin B_{12} deficiency.

ADVERSE REACTIONS

Folic acid doses of up to 1 milligram daily are well tolerated. There are more than 100 reported cases in which vitamin B_{12}-deficient subjects who were receiving oral doses of folic acid of 5 milligrams daily or more experienced progression of neurological symptoms and signs. There are very few such reports in those receiving doses of folic acid less than 5 milligrams daily. There are rare reports of hypersensitivity reactions to oral folic acid. There is one report of a trial using oral doses of folic acid of 15 milligrams daily for one month in which some subjects experienced sleep disturbances, mental changes and gastrointestinal effects. Studies using comparable or higher doses, longer duration, or both, failed to confirm these findings.

INTERACTIONS

DRUGS

Anticonvulsants (carbamazepine, fosphenytoin, phenytoin, phenobarbital, primidone valproic acid): These first-generation anticonvulsants may cause decreased serum folate levels and increased serum homocysteine levels. High doses of folic acid may result in decreased serum levels of these drugs.

Cholestyramine: Concomitant use of cholestyramine and folic acid may cause decreased absorption of folic acid.

Colestipol: Concomitant use of colestipol and folic acid may cause decreased absorption of folic acid.

Colchicine: Colchicine is reported to depress blood folate levels.

Fluoxetine: The use of folic acid at a dose of 500 micrograms/day was found to enhance the antidepressant action of fluoxetine given at a dose of 20 milligrams daily in one study.

Lithium: The use of folic acid at a dose of 200 micrograms daily was found to improve the efficacy of maintenance lithium in one study.

Lometrexol: ("T64") Folic acid supplementation in mice was found to augment the therapeutic activity and ameliorate the adverse reactions of the experimental antifolate cancer chemotherapeutic agent lometrexol.

Metformin: Long-term use of metformin has been associated with elevated homocysteine levels which are reduced with folic acid administration.

Methotrexate: The use of folic acid at a dose of 1 milligram daily may significantly reduce the toxic side effects with no reduction in drug efficacy in those undergoing chronic methotrexate therapy for rheumatoid arthritis.

Nonsteroidal anti-inflammatory drugs (NSAIDS), including ibuprofen, indomethacin, naproxen, mefenamic acid, piroxicam, sulindac: When taken in large therapeutic doses, these NSAIDS may exert antifolate activity.

Phenytoin: Phenytoin may decrease serum folate levels and negatively affect folate status. High doses of folic acid may cause a decrease in serum phenytoin levels.

Pyrimethamine: The use of high doses of folic acid concomitantly with pyrimethamine to prevent bone marrow depression may cause a pharmacodynamic antagonism of the antiparasitic effect of pyrimethamine.

Sulfasalazine: Sulfasalazine may reduce the absorption of folic acid when used concomitantly.

NUTRITIONAL SUPPLEMENTS

Vitamin B_6: Vitamin B_6 may work synergistically with folic acid in lowering serum homocysteine levels.

Vitamin B_12: Vitamin B_{12} may work synergistically with folic acid in lowering homocysteine levels.

Zinc: Supplemental folic acid has been said to adversely affect the absorption of zinc. However, a review of the literature reveals no effect of folic acid supplementation on zinc nutriture.

FOODS

Administration of folic acid with food marginally decreases its availability.

OVERDOSAGE

There are no reports of folic acid overdosage in the literature.

DOSAGE AND ADMINISTRATION

The principal form of supplementary folate is folic acid. Folate triglutamate (pteroyltriglutamate) is also available. Folic acid is available in single ingredient and in combination products. A typical daily dose is 400 micrograms. Unit doses of one milligram or greater require a prescription.

The Food and Nutrition Board of the Institute of Medicine of the National Academy of Sciences has recommended the following Dietary Reference Intakes (RDI) for folate, expressed as dietary folate equivalents (1 microgram of dietary folate equivalents [DFEs]=1 microgram of food folate = 0.5 micrograms of folic acid taken on an empty stomach = 0.6 micrograms of folic acid with meals):

Infants	Adequate Intakes (AI)
0 through 6 months	65 micrograms/day ~ 9.4 micrograms/Kg
7 through 12 months	80 micrograms/day ~ 8.8 micrograms/Kg
Children	Recommended Dietary Allowances (RDA)
1 through 3 years	150 micrograms/day
4 through 8 years	200 micrograms/day
Boys	
9 through 13 years	300 micrograms/day
14 through 18 years	400 micrograms/day
Girls	
9 through 13 years	300 micrograms/day
14 through 18 years	400 micrograms/day
Men	
19 years and older	400 micrograms/day
Women	
19 years and older	400 micrograms/day
RDA for Pregnancy	
14 through 50 years	600 micrograms/day
Lactation	
14 through 50 years	500 micrograms/day

The DV (Daily Value) for folate, which is used for determining percentage of nutrient daily values on nutritional supplement and food labeling purposes, is 400 micrograms. This is based on the U.S. RDA for folate.

A Lowest-Observed-Adverse-Effect Level (LOAEL) for folate is set by the Food and Nutrition Board at 5 milligrams/day. Based on this LOAEL and assuming an uncertainty factor (UF) of 5, the Food and Nutrition Board has recommended the following Tolerable Upper Intake Levels (UL) for folate from fortified foods or supplements (folic acid):

Adults	(UL)
19 years and older	1,000 micrograms/day

Infants	
0 through 12 months	Not possible to establish for supplemental folic acid

Children	
1 through 3 years	300 micrograms/day
4 through 8 years	400 micrograms/day
9 through 13 years	600 micrograms/day
14 through 18 years	800 micrograms/day

Pregnancy	
14 through 18 years	800 micrograms/day
19 years and older	1,000 micrograms/day

Lactation	
14 through 18 years	800 micrograms/day
19 years and older	1,000 micrograms/day

LITERATURE

Aarsand AK, Carlsen SM. Folate administration reduces circulating homocysteine levels in NIDDM patients on long-term metformin treatment. *J Intern Med*. 1998;244:169-174.

Alati T, Worzalla JF, Shih C, et al. Augmentation of the therapeutic activity of lometrexol [(6-*R*)5,10-dideazetetra-hydrofolate] by oral folic acid. *Cancer Res*. 1996;56:2331-2335.

Alpert JE, Fava M. Nutrition and depression: the role of folate. *Nutr Rev*. 1997;55:145-149.

Anon. How folate fights disease. *Nature Struct biol*. 1999;6:293-294.

Anon. Recommendations for the use of folic acid to reduce the number of cases of spina bifida and other neural tube defects. *MMWR Morb Mortal Wkly Rep*. 1992;42(RR-14):1-7.

Berry RJ, Li Z, Erickson JD, et al. Prevention of neural-tube defects with folic acid in China. *N Engl J Med*. 1999;341:1485-1490.

Boushey CJ, Beresford SA, Omenn GS, et al. A quantitative assessment of plasma homocysteine as a risk factor for vascular disease. Probable benefits of increasing folic acid intakes. *JAMA*. 1995;274:1049-1057.

Branda RF, Moldow CF, MacArthur JR, et al. Folate-induced remission in aplastic anemia with familial defect of cellular folate uptake. *N Engl J Med*. 1978;298:469-475.

Butterworth CE Jr, Bendich A. Folic acid and the prevention of birth defects. *Annu Rev Nutr*. 1996;16:73-97.

Butterworth CE Jr, Hatch KD, Macaluso M, et al. Folate deficiency and cervical dysplasia. *JAMA*. 1992;267:528-533.

Butterworth CE Jr, Hatch KD, Soong SJ, et al. Oral folic acid supplementation for cervical dysplasia: a clinical intervention trial. *Am J Obstet Gynecol*. 1992;166:803-809.

Campbell NRC. How safe are folic acid supplements? *Arch Intern Med*. 1996;156:1638-1644.

Charles D, Ness AR, Campbell D, et al. Taking folate in pregnancy and risk of maternal breast cancer. *BMJ*. 2004;329(7479):1375-1376.

Choi S-W, Mason JB. Folate and carcinogenesis: An integrated scheme. *J Nutr*. 2000;130:129-132.

Cole BF, Baron JA, Sandler RS, et al. Folic acid for the prevention of colorectal adenomas: a randomized clinical trial. *JAMA*. 2007;297(21):2351-2359.

Coppen A, Bailey J. Enhancement of the antidepressant action of fluoxetine by folic acid: a randomized, placebo controlled trial. *J Affect Disord*. 2000;60:121-130.

Coppen A, Chaudhry S, Swade C. Folic acid enhances lithium prophylaxis. *J Affect Disord*. 1986;10:9-13.

Czeizel AE, Dudás I. Prevention of the first occurrence of neural-tube defects by periconceptional vitamin supplementation. *N Engl J Med*. 1992;327:1832-1835.

Dietary Reference Intakes for Thiamin, Riboflavin, Niacin, Vitamin B_6, Folate, Vitamin B_{12}, Pantothenic Acid, Biotin, and Choline. Washington, DC: National Academy Press;1998.

Dobie RA. Folate supplementation and age-related hearing loss. *Ann Intern Med*. 2007;146(1):63-64.

Durga J, van Boxtel MP, Schouten EG, et al. Effect of 3-year folic acid supplementation on cognitive function in older adults in the FACIT trial: a randomised, double blind, controlled trial. *Lancet*. 2007;369(9557):208-216.

Durga J, Verhoef P, Anteunis LJ, et al. Effects of folic acid supplementation on hearing in older adults: a randomized, controlled trial. *Ann Intern Med*. 2007;146(1):1-9.

Ericson U, Sonestedt E, Gullberg B, et al. High folate intake is associated with lower breast cancer incidence in postmenopausal women in the Malmö Diet and Cancer cohort. *Am J Clin Nutr*. 2007;86(2):434-443.

Forman JP, Rimm EB, Stampfer MJ, et al. Folate intake and the risk of incident hypertension among US women. *JAMA*. 2005;293(3):320-329.

Giovannucci E, Stampfer MJ, Colditz GA, et al. Multivitamin use, folate, and colon cancer in women in the Nurses' Health Study. *Ann Intern Med*. 1998;129:517-524.

Gisondi P, Fantuzzi F, Malerba M, et al. Folic acid in general medicine and dermatology. *J Dermatolog Treat*. 2007;18(3):138-146.

Glade MJ. Workshop on folate, B_{12}, and choline. Sponsored by the Panel on Folate and other B Vitamins of the Standing

Committee on the Scientific Evaluation of Dietary Reference Intakes, Food and Nutrition Board, Institute of Medicine, Washington, D.C., March 3-4, 1997. *Nutrition*. 1999;15:92-96.

Guenther BD, Sheppard CA, Tran P, et al. The structure and properties of methylenetetrahydrofolate reductase from *Escherichia coli* suggest how folate ameliorates human hyperhomocysteinemia. *Nature Struct Biol*. 1999;6:359-365.

Heimburger DC, Alexander CB, Birch R, et al. Improvement in bronchial squamous metaplasia in smokers treated with folate and vitamin B_{12}. Report of a preliminary randomized, double-blind intervention trial. *JAMA*. 1988;259:1525-1530.

Herbert V. Folic acid. In: Shils ME, Olson JA, Shike M, Ross AC, eds. *Modern Nutrition in Health and Disease*. 9th ed. Baltimore, MD: Williams and Wilkins;1999:433-446.

Homocysteine Lowering Trialists' Collaboration. Lowering blood homocysteine with folic acid based supplements: meta-analysis of randomized trials. *Brit Med J*. 1998;316:894-898.

Hopkins PN, Wu LL, Wu J, et al. Higher plasma homocysteine and increased susceptibility to adverse effects of low folate in early familial coronary artery disease. *Arterioscler Thromb Vasc Biol*. 1995;15:1314-1320.

Jacob RA. Folate, DNA methylation, and gene expression: factors of nature and nurture. *Am J Clin Nutr*. 2000;72:903-904.

Jacques PF, Selhub J, Bostom AG, et al. The effect of folic acid fortification on plasma folate and total homocysteine concentrations. *N Engl J Med*. 1999;340:1449-1454.

Kim Y-I. Folate and Cancer Prevention: A new medical application of folate beyond hyperhomocysteinemia and neural tube defects. *Nutr Rev*. 1999;57:314-321.

Kim Y-I. Folate and carcinogenesis: Evidence, mechanisms, and implications. *J Nut Biochem*. 1999;10:66-88.

Kim Y-I. Methyletetrahydrofolate reductase polymorphisms, folate and cancer risk: a paradigm of gene-nutrient interactions in carcinogenesis. *Nutr Rev*. 2000;58:205-209.

Kim Y-I, Shirwadkar S, Choi S-W, et al. Effects of dietary folate on DNA strand breaks within mutation-prone exons of the p53 gene in the rat colon. *Gastroenterol*. 2000;119:151-161.

Lucock M. Folic acid: nutritional biochemistry, molecular biology, and role in disease processes. *Mol Genet Metab*. 2000;71:121-138.

Lucock M. Is folic acid the ultimate functional food component for disease prevention? *BMJ*. 2004;328(7433):211-214.

Malinow MR, Duell PB, Hess DL, et al. Reduction of plasma homocyst(e)ine levels by breakfast cereal fortified with folic acid in patients with heart disease. *N Engl J Med*. 1998;338:1009-1015.

Marini NJ, Gin J, Ziegle J, et al. The prevalence of folate-remedial MTHFR enzyme variants in humans. *Proc Natl Acad Sci U S A*. 2008;105(23):8055-8060.

Mills JL. Fortification of foods with folic acid-how much is enough? *N Engl J Med*. 2000;342:1442-1445.

Moens AL, Champion HC, Claeys MJ, et al. High-dose folic acid pretreatment blunts cardiac dysfunction during ischemia coupled to maintenance of high-energy phosphates and reduces postreperfusion injury. *Circulation*. 2008;117(14):1810-1819.

Moens AL, Claeys MJ, Wuyts FL, et al. Effect of folic acid on endothelial function following acute myocardial infarction. *Am J Cardiol*. 2007;99(4):476-481.

Morgan SL, Baggott JE, Vaughn WH, et al. Supplementation with folic acid during methotrexate therapy for rheumatoid arthritis. A double-blind, placebo-controlled trial. *Ann Intern Med*. 1994;121:833-841.

MRC Vitamin Study Research Group Prevention of neural tube defects: results of the Medical Council Vitamin Study. *Lancet*. 1991;388:131-137.

Nakata Y, Katsuya T, Takami S, et al. Methylenetetrahydrofolate reductase gene polymorphism: relation to blood pressure and cerebrovascular disease. *Am J Hypertens*. 1998;11(8 Pt 1):1019-1023.

Nelen WL, Blom HJ, Steegers EA, et al. Homocysteine and folate levels as risk factors for recurrent early pregnancy loss. *Obstet Gynecol*. 2000;95:519-524.

Oakley GP Jr. Eat right *and* take a multivitamin. *N Engl J Med*. 1998;338:1060-1061.

Rampersaud GC, Kauwell GPA, Hutson AD, et al. Genomic DNA methylation decreases in response to moderate folate depletion in elderly women. *Am J Clin Nutr*. 2000;72:998-1003.

Rimm EB, Willett WC, Hu FB, et al. Higher intake of folate and vitamin B_6 is associated with low rates of coronary artery disease in women. *JAMA*. 1998;279:359-364.

Rosenquist TH, Ratashak SA, Selhub J. Homocysteine induces congenital defects of the heart and neural tube: Effect of folic acid. *Proc Natl Acad Sci USA*. 1996; 93:15227-15232.

Sato Y, Honda Y, Iwamoto J, et al. Effect of folate and mecobalamin on hip fractures in patients with stroke: a randomized controlled trial. *JAMA*. 2005;293(9):1082-1088.

Scholl TO, Johnson WG. Folic acid: influence on the outcome of pregnancy. *Am J Clin Nutr*. 2000;71:1295S-1303S.

Snowdon DA, Tully CL, Smith CD, et al. Serum folate and the severity of atrophy of the neocortex in Alzheimer disease: findings from the Nun Study. *Am J Clin Nutr*. 2000;71:993-998.

Song J, Sohn KJ, Medline A, et al. Chemopreventive effects of dietary folate on intestinal polyps in Apc+/-Msh2-/-mice. *Cancer Res*. 2000;60:3191-3199.

Stroes ESG, van Faassen EE, Yo M, et al. Folic acid reverts dysfunctional nitric oxide synthase. *Circ Res*. 2000;86:1129-1134.

Tian R, Ingwall JS. How does folic acid cure heart attacks? *Circulation*. 2008;117(14):1772-1774.

Title LM, Cummings PM, Giddens K, et al. Effect of folic acid and antioxidant vitamins on endothelial dysfunction in patients with coronary artery disease. *J Amer Coll Cardiol.* 2000;36:758-765.

Ulrich CM. Folate and cancer prevention: a closer look at a complex picture. *Am J Clin Nutr.* 2007;86(2):271-273.

Ulrich CM, Potter JD. Folate and cancer—timing is everything. *JAMA.* 2007;297(21):2408-2409.

Voutilainen S, Lakka TA, Porkkala-Sarataho E, et al. Low serum folate concentrations are associated with an excess incidence of acute coronary events: the Kuopio Ischaemic Heart Disease Risk Factor Study. *Eur J Clin Nutr.* 2000;54:424-428.

Wilmink HW, Stroes ESG, Erkelens WD, et al. Influence of folic acid on postprandial endothelial dysfunction. *Arterioscler Thromb Vasc Biol.* 2000;20:185-188.

Woo KS, Chook P, Lolin YI, et al. Folic acid improves arterial endothelial function in adults with hyperhomocysteinemia. *J Am Coll Cardiol.* 1999;34:2002-2006.

Zhang S, Hunter DJ, Hankinson SE, et al. A prospective study of folate intake and the risk of breast cancer. *JAMA.* 1999;281:1632-1637.

Fructo-oligosaccharides

DESCRIPTION

Fructo-oligosaccharides (FOS) typically refer to short-chain oligosaccharides comprised of D-fructose and D-glucose, containing from 3 to 5 monosaccharide units. Similar molecules are obtained by partial enzymatic hydrolysis of inulins (see Inulins). Those are called oligofructose. FOS, also called neosugar and short-chain FOS (scFOS), are produced on a commercial scale from sucrose using a fungal fructosyltransferase enzyme.

FOS are comprised of one molecule of D-glucose in the terminal position and from 2 to 4 D-fructose units. FOS containing 2 fructose residues are abbreviated GF_2 (G is for glucose, F, for fructose). Those with 3 fructoses are abbreviated GF_3, and those with 4 fructoses, GF_4. GF_2 is also called 1-kestose and GF_3 is called nystose. The linkage between fructose units in FOS is a beta-(2-1) glycosidic link. The structural formula is represented below.

Fructo-oligosaccharides
(The top sugar is glucose. n = 2-4 fructose residues)

FOS are resistant to digestion in the stomach and small intestine. The reason for this is the presence of the beta configuration of the anomeric C_2 in the D-fructose residues. The human digestive enzymes sucrase, maltase-isomaltase and alpha-glucosidase are specific for alpha-glycosidic linkages. FOS are considered nondigestible oligosaccharides. They are, however, fermented by a limited number of colonic bacteria. This could lead to changes in the colonic ecosystem in favor of some bacteria, such as bifidobacteria, which appear to be beneficial in some respects. FOS and other nondigestible oligosaccharides are referred to as bifidogenic factors.

Substances such as FOS that may promote the growth of beneficial bacteria in the colon are called prebiotics. Prebiotics are typically nondigestible oligosaccharides.

ACTIONS AND PHARMACOLOGY

ACTIONS

FOS may have anticarcinogenic, antimicrobial, hypolipidemic and hypoglycemic actions in some. They may also help improve mineral absorption and balance, and may have anti-osteoporotic and anti-osteopenic activities.

MECHANISM OF ACTION

The possible anticarcinogenic activity of FOS might be accounted for, in part, by the possible anticarcinogenic action of butyrate. Butyrate, along with other short-chain fatty acids, is produced by bacterial fermentation of FOS in the colon. Some studies suggest that butyrate may induce growth arrest and cell differentiation, and may also upregulate apoptosis, three activities that could be significant for antitumor activity. FOS may also aid in increasing the concentrations of calcium and magnesium in the colon. High concentrations of these cations in the colon may help control the rate of cell turnover. High concentrations of calcium in the colon may also lead to the formation of insoluble bile or salts of fatty acids. This might reduce the potential damaging effects of bile or fatty acids on colonocytes.

FOS may promote the growth of favorable bacterial populations, such as bifidobacteria, in the colon. Bifidobacteria may inhibit the growth of pathogenic bacteria, such as *Clostridium perfringens* and diarrheogenic strains of *Escherichia coli*.

FOS may lower serum triglyceride levels in some. The mechanism of this possible effect is unclear. Decreased hepatocyte triglyceride synthesis is a hypothetical possibility. FOS may also lower total cholesterol and LDL-cholesterol levels in some. Again, the mechanism of this possible effect is unclear. Propionate, a product of FOS fermentation in the colon, may inhibit HMG-CoA reductase, the rate-limiting step in cholesterol synthesis.

The possible effects of FOS on blood glucose may be explained in a few ways. FOS may delay gastric emptying and/or shorten small-intestinal tract transit time. Propionate may inhibit gluconeogenesis by its metabolic conversion to methylmalonyl-CoA and succinyl-CoA. These metabolites could inhibit pyruvate carboxylase. Propionate may also reduce plasma levels of free fatty acids. High levels of free fatty acids lower glucose utilization and induce insulin resistance. Propionate may enhance glycolysis via depletion of citrate in hepatocytes. Citrate is an allosteric inhibitor of phosphofructokinase.

FOS may bind/sequester such minerals as calcium and magnesium in the small intestine. The short-chain fatty acids formed from the bacterial fermentation of FOS may facilitate the colonic absorption of calcium and, possibly, also magnesium ions. This could be beneficial in preventing osteoporosis and osteopenia.

PHARMACOKINETICS

Little digestion of FOS occurs in the stomach and small intestine following ingestion of FOS. FOS are fermented in the colon by bifidobacteria and some other bacteria to produce the short-chain fatty acids (SCFA) acetate, propionate and butyrate; the gases hydrogen, hydrogen sulfide, carbon dioxide and methane; and lactate, pyruvate and succinate. Some acetate, propionate and butyrate is absorbed from the colon and transported by the circulation to various tissues where these SCFA undergo further metabolism. Many SCFA are metabolized by the colonocyes. Butyrate is an important respiratory fuel for the colonocytes.

Those with ileostomies may have a microbial population colonizing their ileums. In those cases, FOS could be fermented by some of the bacteria, much as they are in the colon.

INDICATIONS AND USAGE

Fructo-oligosaccharides appear to be of benefit in modulating the microbial ecology of the gut, boosting gastrointestinal immunity. FOS may also protect against colon cancer, and may have favorable lipid effects in some. FOS may also aid in calcium absorption.

RESEARCH SUMMARY

There is evidence that FOS can improve the microbial ecology of the gut and protect against some bacterial pathogens, particularly in the large intestine. FOS selectively stimulate the growth of bifidobacteria and also have many of the actions and benefits of dietary fibers.

A fermented milk product containing FOS significantly lowered LDL-cholesterol levels in male subjects with borderline elevated levels of serum total cholesterol. This double-blind, placebo-controlled study extended for three weeks. Other studies have credited FOS with lowering both cholesterol and triglyceride levels. FOS have been shown to lower hepatic lipogenesis. In one recent study, however, 15 grams of FOS daily for 20 days failed to favorably affect either blood glucose levels or serum lipid concentrations in patients with type 2 diabetes. More research is needed.

There is experimental evidence that FOS might inhibit colon cancer. In an animal model for both familial adenomatous polyposis and sporadic colon cancers, FOS were said to "dramatically" reduce the incidence of colon tumors.

FOS have also been shown to increase calcium absorption in animal studies.

CONTRAINDICATIONS, PRECAUTIONS, ADVERSE REACTIONS

CONTRAINDICATIONS

FOS are contraindicated in those who are hypersensitive to these substances. They are also contraindicated in those who are hypersensitive to inulins.

PRECAUTIONS

Those who develop gastrointestinal symptoms with the use of dietary fiber should exercise some caution in the use of FOS. Those with irritable bowel syndrome should exercise caution in the use of FOS. Those receiving whole body radiation or radiation to the gastrointestinal tract should avoid FOS supplements.

Those with lactose intolerance should exercise caution in the use of doses of FOS greater than 10 grams daily.

ADVERSE REACTIONS

Doses up to 10 grams daily are well tolerated. Higher doses may cause gastrointestinal symptoms. Doses greater than 30 grams daily can cause flatus. Doses greater than 40 grams daily can cause borborygmi and bloating. Doses greater than 50 grams daily can cause cramps and diarrhea. Some are more sensitive to FOS and may develop gastrointestinal symptoms at lower doses. Those with lactose intolerance have been reported to experience gastrointestinal symptoms at a dose of 25 grams.

DOSAGE AND ADMINISTRATION

FOS are available as nutritional supplements and in functional foods. Dosing is variable and ranges from 4 to 10 grams daily and sometimes higher. Those who use more than 10 grams daily should split the dosage throughout the day.

LITERATURE

Alles MS, de Roos NM, Bakx JC, et al. Consumption of fructo-oligosaccharides does not favorably affect blood glucose and serum lipid concentrations in patients with type 2 diabetes. *Am J Clin Nutr.* 1999; 69:64-69.

Bouhnik Y, Vahedi K, Achour L, et al. Short-chain fructo-oligosaccharide administration dose-dependently increases fecal bifidobacteria in healthy humans. *J Nutr.* 1999; 129:113-116.

Buddington RK, Williams CH, Chen SC, Witherly SA. Dietary supplement of neosugar alters the fecal flora and decreases activities of some reductive enzymes in human subjects. *Am J Clin Nutr.* 1996; 63:709-716.

Luo J, van Yperselle M, Rizkalla SW, et al. Chronic consumption of short-chain fructo-oligasaccharides does not affect basal hepatic glucose production or insulin resistance in type 2 diabetics. *J Nutr.* 2000; 130:1572-1577.

Ohta A, Baba S, Takizawa T, Adachi T. Effects of fructo-oligasaccharides on the absorption of magnesium in the magnesium-deficient rat model. *J Nutr Sci Vitaminol (Tokyo).* 1994; 40:171-180.

Ohta A, Motohashi Y, Sakai K, et al. Dietary fructo-oligasaccharides increase calcium absorption and levels of mucosal calbindin-D9K in the large intestine of gastrectomized rats. *Scand J Gastroenterol.* 1998; 33:1062-1068.

Ohta A, Ohtsuki M, Hosoro A, et al. Dietary fructo-oligasaccharides prevent osteopenia after gastrectomy. *J Nutr.* 1998; 128:106-110.

Oku T, Tokunaga T, Hosoya N. Nondigestibility of a new sweetener, "Neosugar," in the rat. *J Nutr.* 1984; 114:1574-1581.

Pierre F, Perrin P, Champ M, et al. Short-chain fructo-oligasaccharides reduce the occurrence of colon tumors and develop gut-associated lymphoid tissue in Min mice. *Cancer Res.* 1997; 57: 225-228.

Roberfroid MB, Delzenne NM. Dietary fructans. *Annu Rev Nutr.* 1998; 18:117-143.

Sahaafsma G, Meuling WJ, van Dokkum W, Bouley C. Effects of a milk product, fermented by *Lactobaccillus acidophilus* and with fructo-oligosaccharides added, on blood lipids in male volunteers. *Eur J Clin Nutr.* 1998; 52:436-440.

Teuri U, Vapaatalo H, Korpela R. Fructo-oligosaccharides and lactulose cause more symptoms in lactose maldigesters and subjects with pseudohypolactasia than in control lactose digesters. *Am J Clin Nutr.* 1999; 69:973-979.

Fucoxanthin

DESCRIPTION

Fucoxanthin is a marine carotenoid and a member of the carotenoid family of chemical substances. Fucoxanthin, like other carotenoids, is a natural fat-soluble pigment (brown, in the case of fucoxanthin) and is found in algae, including heterokonts and seaweeds, and in diatoms (phytoplankton). Fucoxanthin is also found in the edible brown seaweeds wakame (*Undaria pinnatifida*), hijiki (*Hijikia fusiformis*) and kombu (*Laminaria japonica*), as well as in the marine algae *Chrysophyceae*, *Prymneslophyceae*, *Bacillariophyceae*, *Prasinophyceae* and *Phaeophyceae*. Fucoxanthin and its metabolites are also typically found in sea organisms that feed on these carotenoids as conjugates. For example, fucoxanthin esters and fucoxanthinol esters are found in clams.

Fucoxanthin functions in algae as a light-harvesting pigment. It and chlorophyll are the two major light-harvesting pigments in brown algae and diatoms. Fucoxanthin exists in algae in the form of a fucoxanthin-chlorophyll a/c protein complex, which is associated, in the case of brown algae and diatoms, with photosystem II. The complex transfers light to chlorophyll a. The fucoxanthin protein complex shows homology to the chlorophyll a/b binding polypeptides of higher plants.

Fucoxanthin, as an antioxidant, protects algae against oxygen toxicity. Its possible protective roles as an antioxidant, as well as its possible anti-inflammatory and anticancer activities, have become of interest to researchers in the past decade. More recently, its possible activity as an anti-obesity agent has stimulated research on the carotenoid, mainly in Japan.

Fucoxanthin is chemically described as [(1S,3R)-3-hydroxy-4-[(3E,5E,7E,9E,11E,13E,15E)-18-[(1S,4S,6R)-4-hydroxy-2,2,6-trimethyl-7oxabicyclo[4.1.0]heptan-1-yl]-3,7,12, 16-tetramethyl-17-oxooctadeca-1,3,5,7,9,11,13,15-octaenylidene]-3,5, 5-trimethylcyclohexyl] acetate. It is also known as 3'-(Acetyloxy)-6',7'-didehydro-5,6-epoxy-5,5',6,6',7,8-hexahydro-3,5'-dihydroxy-8-oxo-beta,beta-carotene; (3'S,5'R,6'R)- 3'-acetoxy-5,6-epoxy-3,5'-dihydroxy-6',7'-didehydro-5,6,7,8,5',6'-hexahydro- β,β-carotene-8-one; and (3S,3'S,5R,5'R,6S,6'R)- 3'-(aacetyloxy)-6',7'-didehydro-5,6-epoxy-5,5',6,6',7,8-hexahydro-3,5'-dihydroxy-8-oxo-β,β-carotene. Its CAS registry number is 3351-86-8, its empirical formula is $C_{42}H_{58}O_6$, and its molecular weight is 658.91.

Fucoxanthin's allenic group (=CH=C=CH-) and 5,6 monoepoxide make fucoxanthin a unique chemical structure (see figure). Fucoxanthin is also classified as an epoxyxanthophyll or epoxide-containing xanthophyll. Fucoxanthan is represented by the following chemical structure.

Fucoxanthin

Fucoxanthinol is the deacetylated metabolite of fucoxanthin.

ACTIONS AND PHARMACOLOGY

ACTIONS

Fucoxanthin has antioxidant activity and may have anticancer, anti-inflammatory and antiobesity activities.

MECHANISM OF ACTION

Antioxidant activity: Fucoxanthin has demonstrated radical scavenging and singlet oxygen quenching activities. The quenching activity of fucoxanthin against the organic radicals 1,1-diphenyl-2-picrylhydrazyl (DPPH, a stable free radical), 12-doxylstearic acid (12DS), and the radical adduct of nitrobenzene with linoleic acid (NB-L) was studied using electron spin resonance (ESR). In the presence of fucoxanthin, the ESR signals for the DPPH, 12DS and NB-L radicals were significantly reduced. Fucoxanthin also has 2,2′–azinobis(3-ethylbenzothiazoline-6-sulfonic acid) (ATBS) radical, hydroxyl radical, superoxide anion and singlet oxygen scavenging activity.

Anticancer activity: Fucoxanthin has demonstrated a number of anticancer activities via different mechanisms.

Fucoxanthin was found to inhibit the growth of human hepatic HepG2 carcinoma cells. In 2007, cancer of the liver was the fourth most common cause of death from cancer. Most of the cases of hepatocellular cancer can be found in undeveloped countries. Fucoxanthin was shown to reduce the viability of HepG2 cells accompanied by the induction of cell cycle arrest during the G_0G_1 phase of the cell cycle. The cell cycle is the series of events that takes place in a cell leading to its replication. The cell cycle consists of four distinct phases G_1, S, G_2 and the M phase, where the cell divides forming two new cells. G_0 is the postmitotic phase prior to G_1. Two key classes of regulatory molecules—cyclins and cyclin-dependent kinases (CDKs)—acting in partnership, determine a cell's progress through the cell cycle. The retinoblastoma protein Rb, a tumor suppressor protein, prevents excessive growth by inhibiting the cell cycle when Rb is hypophosphorylated. The phosphorylation of Rb plays a crucial role in the progression of the G_1 phase

and the transition of G_1 to the S phase. Fucoxanthin was found to inhibit the phosphorylation of Rb. Further, the kinase activity of cyclin D when joined with its partner kinase CDK4 was suppressed by treatment with fucoxanthin. Fucoxanthin also induced activity of the ubiquitin-proteasome pathway leading to degradation of cyclin D and suppressed cyclin D mRNA. Thus, it appears that fucoxanthin caused the suppression of cyclin D via promotion of proteasomal degradation and repression of cyclin D, leading to cell cycle arrest. Incidentally, apoptosis was not observed in this case

Fucoxanthin reduced the viability of the human colon adenocarcinoma WiDr cell line accompanied by the induction of cell cycle arrest at the G_0G_1 phase of the cycle. In this case, apoptosis of the cells was also reported. In order to understand the possible mechanism of fucoxanthin's action, a number of factors that regulate the cell cycle were investigated, including the cyclins, the cyclin-dependent kinases (CDKs), the retinoblastoma protein Rb and p21, a key protein in cell cycle regulation. It was p21 that appeared to be affected by fucoxanthin. When p21 binds to the CDKs, it inhibits their activity. It appeared that fucoxanthin induced cell-cycle arrest at the G_0G_1 phase in human cancer cells via upregulation of the activity of p21.

Fucoxanthin was reported to reduce the viability of human prostate cancer cells via the induction of apoptosis. Apoptosis induction was characterized by DNA fragmentation, an increased percentage of hypodiploid cells and cleavages of procaspase-3 and PARP (poly(ADP-ribose) polymerase. Expression of Bax and Bcl-2 proteins, but not Bcl-X_L proteins, was reduced. The activation of caspase-3 by fucoxanthin was thought to be the major activity in the induction of apoptosis.

Fucoxanthin was found to induce apoptosis in human promyelocytic leukemia cells. Apoptosis in these cells was associated with loss of mitochondrial membrane potential, but not with an increase in reactive oxygen species. Fucoxanthin treatment caused cleavages of procapsase-3 and poly (ADP-ribose) polymerase, without any effect on the protein level of Bcl-2, Bcl-X_L or Bax. It was concluded that the fucoxanthin induction of apoptosis was likely due to mitochondrial membrane permeabilization and caspase-3 activation.

Anti-inflammatory activity: Endotoxin-induced uveitis (EIU) (induced by lipopolysaccharide [LPS]) is an acute, anterior segment intraocular inflammation (uveitis). Fucoxanthin was studied to see how it affected LPS-induced inflammation *in vitro* in a mouse macrophage cell line and *in vivo* in male Lewis rats. EIU was induced in the rats via footpad injection. Immediately following the LPS injection, varying doses of fucoxanthin were injected intravenously. Fucoxanthin suppressed the development of EIU in a dose-dependent fashion, and treatment with fucoxanthin decreased PGE_2 (prostaglandin E_2), NO (nitric oxide) and TNF (tumor necrosis factor)-alpha concentrations in the aqueous humor. On the *in vitro* side, mouse macrophage cells were pretreated with various doses of fucoxanthin for 24 hours, after which they were incubated with LPS for an additional 24 hours. The expression of COX (cyclooxygenase) and iNOS (inducible nitric oxide synthase) was significantly reduced compared with the untreated group. It was concluded that fucoxanthin suppressed the inflammatory response by blocking iNOS and COX protein expression. Significantly, the anti-inflammatory effect of fucoxanthin on the eyes was comparable with the effect of prednisolone in comparable doses.

Antiobesity activity: Obesity is a growing health problem worldwide, predisposing people to a wide variety of diseases, including type 2 diabetes, cardiovascular disease, musculoskeletal problems, certain cancers and a shortened lifespan. There is great interest in research circles in understanding the biochemistry of adipogenesis and the molecular events that underlie the differentiation of white versus brown adipocytes. Brown adipocytes, found in brown adipose tissue (BAT), express uncoupling protein 1 (UCP1) and have high energy expenditure potential. The attainment of brown adipocyte features in white adipocytes, found in white adipose tissue (WAT), is receiving a lot of recent attention. Some believe that the solution to this issue might be the holy grail of obesity research. The problem is that humans have very little BAT, and most of the fat in the body is stored in WAT.

Uncoupling proteins 1-3 (UCP1-3) belong to the mitochondrial anion carrier family. The first uncoupling protein discovered, UCP1 or thermogenin, is a thermogenic protein specifically expressed in brown adipocytes where it converts mitochondrial proton-motive force into heat. UCP1 catalyzes a proton leak in the inner mitochondrial membrane that can be activated by free fatty acids. Upon sympathetic stimulation of lipolysis in brown adipocytes, increased free fatty acid levels activate the proton leak catalyzed by UCP1. This UCP1-mediated proton leak serves for nonshivering thermogenesis in brown adipose tissue, either to defend normothermic body temperature in animals exposed to the cold or to combat excess food energy in response to diets of high caloric density.

Some Japanese researchers have been studying how fucoxanthin might fit into this puzzle. These researchers have been using rats and mice as test systems and, among other things, have found that fucoxanthin showed an antiobesity effect in rats via UCP1 expression in white adipose tissue (WAT). The researchers concluded that fucoxanthin upregulates the expression of UCP1 in WAT, which may contribute to reducing WAT weight—in rats. In another Japanese study, the investigators found that fucoxanthin and its deacetylated metabolite, fucoxanthinol, suppressed adipocyte differentiation in mouse 3T3-L1 cells. They concluded that this effect was probably mediated via the upregulation of peroxisome proliferator-activated receptor gamma (PPAR-gamma), which regulates adipogenic gene expression. It turned out also that the fucoxanthin metabolite, fucoxanthinol, had even greater suppressive effects than fucoxanthin on adipocyte differentiation. In still another study, the researchers reported that a dietary combination of fucoxanthin and fish oil attenuated the weight gain of white adipose tissue and decreased blood glucose in obese/diabetic KK-A^y mice. They reported that fucoxanthin decreased the blood glucose and plasma insulin concentration in KK-A^y mice, along with downregulating tumor necrosis factor (TNF)-alpha mRNA. Further, the combination of fucoxanthin and fish oil was more effective for attenuating the weight gain of WAT than fucoxanthin alone.

Further studies to elucidate the mechanism of this possible antiobesity effect of fucoxanthin and its metabolites are needed and warranted, as are clinical studies.

PHARMACOKINETICS

There is little information on the pharmacokinetics of fucoxanthin in humans. In one recent human study, fucoxanthin was found to be very poorly absorbed after oral intake, and the main form found in the plasma was the deacetylated metabolite of fucoxanthin, fucoxanthinol. This was consistent with an earlier study using Caco-2 human intestinal cells and mice. In that study, it was found that fucoxanthin was taken up by Caco-2 cells incubated with micellar fucoxanthin, and fucoxanthinol was found in the medium and cells, with its level increasing significantly in a time-dependent manner. No conjugated forms of fucoxanthin or fucoxanthinol were found in either the medium or the cells. In the animal study, fucoxanthinol was detected in the plasma of the mice one hour after intubation of fucoxanthin. These results strongly suggest that dietary fucoxanthin is incorporated as the deacetylated form, fucoxanthinol, from the digestive tract into the circulatory system of mammals. Further study of the pharmacokinetics of fucoxanthin, including absorption, distribution, metabolism and excretion is needed and warranted.

INDICATIONS AND USAGE

Preliminary *in vitro* and animal data suggest that the carotenoid fucoxanthin may have antiobesity, anticancer, antiangiogenic and anti-inflammatory properties.

RESEARCH SUMMARY

Fucoxanthin, a carotenoid found in some edible seaweeds, such as *Hijikia fusiformis* and *Undaria pinnatifida,* has recently excited some attention by exhibiting effects some hope presage a role for it in weight control. At present the data are very preliminary and are limited to in vitro and a few animal studies. Feeding rats and mice lipids derived from Undaria pinnatifida resulted in reduction of abdominal white adipose tissue weights. It was determined that a major active constituent of these lipids is fucoxanthin. The same research group subsequently showed that the carotenoid is able to suppress differentiation of precursor fat cells to fat cells in an in vitro cell line study. The researchers concluded that fucoxanthin might thus be able to inhibit weight gain through this process. In related recent research by some of the same researchers, a combination of fucoxanthin with fish oil was said to attenuate weight gain of white adipose tissue and concomitantly decrease blood glucose in obese/diabetic mice. In another study, also utilizing an obese/diabetic mouse model, fucoxanthin was reported to increase levels of docosahexaenoic acid (DHA, see DHA) in the livers of these animals. The researchers stated that enhanced DHA levels have been associated with reduced obesity and diabetes. More research is needed and warranted.

Several recent *in vitro* studies point to a possible role for fucoxanthin in cancer therapy. Fucoxanthin has demonstrated some test tube efficacy in a number of cancer cell lines, including prostate, colon, leukemia, hepatic and others. It has also shown some efficacy in animal models of cancer, inhibiting chemically induced mouse duodenal carcinogenesis, two-stage mouse skin cancer and spontaneous liver cancer in mice. Cell cycle arrest and induction of apoptosis have been observed in several of these studies. An antiangiogenic effect has been reported in another *in vitro* study, suggesting yet another possible anticancer mode of action. Again, much more study will be needed before any conclusions can be reached about a possible clinical anticancer role for this carotenoid.

Anti-inflammatory effects have also been reported by researchers working with fucoxanthin. In one study, an anti-inflammatory effect was observed in endotoxin-induced uveitis in rats. The eye inflammation was said to be reduced in a dose-dependent fashion, and the overall anti-inflammatory effect of the carotenoid was said to be equal to that of prednisolone when used in this context in similar doses. A number of inflammatory markers were significantly reduced by fucoxanthin. More research is needed and warranted.

CONTRAINDICATIONS, PRECAUTIONS, ADVERSE REACTIONS

CONTRAINDICATIONS

Fucoxanthin is contraindicated in those hypersensitive to any component of a fucoxanthin-containing product.

PRECAUTIONS

Pregnant women and nursing mothers should avoid fucoxanthin-containing supplements.

Those who wish to try fucoxanthin-containing supplements for the support of any health condition should first discuss its use with his or her physician.

Those who desire to obtain fucoxanthin from edible seaweed sources should be aware that seaweed contains iodine and that high intake of iodine could cause adverse events in some people. Moderate intake of edible seaweed, however, should not be a problem.

ADVERSE REACTIONS

No reports.

INTERACTIONS

DRUGS

Cholestyramine: Concomitant intake of cholestyramine and fucoxanthin may decrease the absorption of fucoxanthin.

Colestipol: Concomitant intake of colestipol and fucoxanthin may decrease the absorption of fucoxanthin.

Mineral oil: Concomitant intake of mineral oil and fucoxanthin may reduce the absorption of fucoxanthin.

Orlistat (Alli, Xenical): Orlistat may decrease the absorption of fucoxanthin.

NUTRITIONAL SUPPLEMENTS

Beta-carotene: Concomitant intake of beta-carotene and fucoxanthin may increase the absorption of fucoxanthin.

Medium-chain triglycerides: Concomitant intake of medium-chain triglycerides and fucoxanthin may enhance the absorption of fucoxanthin.

Pectin: Concomitant intake of pectin and fucoxanthin may decrease the absorption of fucoxanthin.

FOODS

Oils: Dietary oils, such as fish oils and olive oil, may enhance the absorption of fucoxanthin.

Olestra: Olestra may reduce the absorption of fucoxanthin.

HERBS

No known interactions.

OVERDOSAGE

There have been no reports of overdosage.

DOSAGE AND ADMINISTRATION

The optimal dose of fucoxanthin for the support of any health condition is not known.

Some fucoxanthin-containing dietary supplements are available. They typically contain five mg of fucoxanthin dissolved in oil.

LITERATURE

Asai A, Sugawara T, Ono H, et al. Biotransformation of fucoxanthinol into amarouciaxanthin A in mice and HepG2 cells: formation and cytotoxicity of fucoxanthin metabolites. *Drug Metab Dispos*. 2004;32(2):205-211.

Asai A, Yonekura L, Nagao A. Low bioavailability of dietary epoxyxanthophylls in humans. *Br J Nutr*. 2008;100(2):273-277.

Das SK, Hashimoto T, Kanazawa K. Growth inhibition of human hepatic carcinoma HepG2 cells by fucoxanthin is associated with down-regulation of cyclin D. *Biochim Biophys Acta*. 2008;1780(4):743-749.

Das SK, Hashimoto T, Shimizu K, et al. Fucoxanthin induces cell cycle arrest at G0/G1 phase in human colon carcinoma cells through up-regulation of p21WAF1/Cip1. *Biochim Biophys Acta*. 2005;1726(3):328-335.

Hosokawa M, Kudo M, Maeda H, et al. Fucoxanthin induces apoptosis and enhances the antiproliferative effect of the PPARgamma ligand, troglitazone, on colon cancer cells. *Biochim Biophys Acta*. 2004;1675(1-3):113-119.

Konishi I, Hosokawa M, Sashima T, et al. Halocynthiaxanthin and fucoxanthinol isolated from Halocynthia roretzi induce apoptosis in human leukemia, breast and colon cancer cells. *Comp Biochem Physiol C Toxicol Pharmacol*. 2006;142(1-2):53-59.

Kotake-Nara E, Asai A, Nagao A. Neoxanthin and fucoxanthin induce apoptosis in PC-3 human prostate cancer cells. *Cancer Lett*. 2005;220(1):75-84.

Kotake-Nara E, Terasaki M, Nagao A. Characterization of apoptosis induced by fucoxanthin in human promyelocytic leukemia cells. *Biosci Biotechnol Biochem*. 2005;69(1):224-227.

Maeda H, Hosokawa M, Sashima T, et al. Effect of medium-chain triacylglycerols on anti-obesity effect of fucoxanthin. *J Oleo Sci*. 2007;56(12):615-621.

Maeda H, Hosokawa M, Sashima T, et al. Fucoxanthin from edible seaweed, Undaria pinnatifida, shows antiobesity effect through UCP1 expression in white adipose tissues. *Biochem Biophys Res Commun*. 2005;332(2):392-397.

Maeda H, Hosokawa M, Sashima T, et al. Dietary combination of fucoxanthin and fish oil attenuates the weight gain of white adipose tissue and decreases blood glucose in obese/diabetic KK-Ay mice. *J Agric Food Chem*. 2007;55(19):7701-7706.

Maeda H, Hosokawa M, Sashima T, et al. Fucoxanthin and its metabolite, fucoxanthinol, suppress adipocyte differentiation in 3T3-L1 cells. *Int J Mol Med*. 2006;18(1):147-152.

Nishino H, Tsushima M, Matsuno T, et al. Anti-neoplastic effect of halocynthiaxanthin, a metabolite of fucoxanthin. *Anticancer Drugs*. 1992;3(5):493-497.

Nomura T, Kikuchi M, Kubodera A, et al. Proton-donative antioxidant activity of fucoxanthin with 1,1-diphenyl-2-picrylhydrazyl (DPPH). *Biochem Mol Biol Int*. 1997;42(2):361-370.

Okuzumi J, Takahashi T, Yamane T, et al. Inhibitory effects of fucoxanthin, a natural carotenoid, on N-ethyl-N'-nitro-N-nitrosoguanidine-induced mouse duodenal carcinogenesis. *Cancer Lett*. 1993;68(2-3):159-168.

Sachindra NM, Sato E, Maeda H, et al. Radical scavenging and singlet oxygen quenching activity of marine carotenoid fucoxanthin and its metabolites. *J Agric Food Chem*. 2007;55(21):8516-8522.

Shiratori K, Ohgami K, Ilieva I, et al. Effects of fucoxanthin on lipopolysaccharide-induced inflammation in vitro and in vivo. *Exp Eye Res*. 2005;81(4):422-428.

Sugawara T, Baskaran V, Tsuzuki W, et al. Brown algae fucoxanthin is hydrolyzed to fucoxanthinol during absorption by Caco-2 human intestinal cells and mice. *J Nutr*. 2002;132(5):946-951.

Sugawara T, Matsubara K, Akagi R, et al. Antiangiogenic activity of brown algae fucoxanthin and its deacetylated product, fucoxanthinol. *J Agric Food Chem*. 2006;54(26):9805-9810.

Terasaki M, Asai A, Zhang H, et al. A highly polar xanthophyll of 9'-cis-neoxanthin induces apoptosis in HCT116 human colon cancer cells through mitochondrial dysfunction. *Mol Cell Biochem*. 2007;300(1-2):227-237.

Tsukui T, Konno K, Hosokawa M, et al. Fucoxanthin and fucoxanthinol enhance the amount of docosahexaenoic acid in the liver of KKAy obese/diabetic mice. *J Agric Food Chem*. 2007;55(13):5025-5029.

Yan X, Chuda Y, Suzuki M, et al. Fucoxanthin as the major antioxidant in Hijikia fusiformis, a common edible seaweed. *Biosci Biotechnol Biochem*. 1999;63(3):605-607.

Yoshiko S, Hoyoku N. Fucoxanthin, a natural carotenoid, induces G1 arrest and GADD45 gene expression in human cancer cells. *In Vivo*. 2007;21(2):305-309.

Gamma-Butyrolactone (GBL)

> Products containing gamma-butyrolactone (GBL) or 1, 4 butanediol (BD) should not be used by anyone for supplementation.

DESCRIPTION

Gamma-butyrolactone or GBL is an organic oily liquid that is used as an intermediate in the synthesis of such substances as polyvinypyrrolidone and is also used as a solvent for polyacrylonitrile and cellulose acetate, among others. GBL is a constituent of paint removers, textile oils and drilling oils.

The reason GBL was introduced into the dietary supplement marketplace is because it is easily converted into gamma-hydroxybutyrate (GHB) after ingestion and is used as a prodrug of GHB (See Gamma-Hydroxybutyrate).

GBL is also known chemically as dihydro-2 (3H)-furanone; butyrolactone; 1,2-butanolide; 1,4-butanolide; gamma-hydroxybutyric acid lactone; 3-hydroxybutyric acid lactone and 4-hydroxybutanoic acid lactone. The chemical structure is as follows:

Gamma-Butyrolactone

GHB has been classified as a Schedule I substance and is illegal to use except for the treatment of narcolepsy, for which it is approved by the FDA (GHB is a Schedule III drug in that case), and in FDA-allowed clinical trials.

FDA has asked all GBL dietary supplement producers to recall their products.

Another organic solvent, 1,4 butanediol or BD, also gets converted to gamma-hydroxybutyrate upon ingestion. FDA has issued a warning regarding products that contain BD.

For more information on this substance, refer to the Gamma-Hydroxybutyrate (GHB) monograph.

LITERATURE

Centers for Disease Comtrol and Prevention. Adverse events associated with ingestion of gamma-butyrolactone-Minnesota, New Mexico, and Texas, 1998-1999. *MMWR Morb Mortal Wkly Rep.* 1999;48:137-140.

FDA. Warning on dietary supplements. *JAMA.* 1999;282:1218.

Lo Vecchio F, Curry SC, Bagnasco T. Butyrolactone-induced central nervous system depression after ingestion of RenewTrient, a "dietary supplement." *N Engl J Med.* 1998;339:847-848.

Poldrugo F, Snead OC 3d. 1, 4 Butanediol gamma-hydroxybutyric acid and ethanol. *Neuropharmacology.* 1984;23:109-113.

Ramburg-Schepens MO, Buffet M, Durak C, Mathieu-Nolf M. Gamma-butyrolactone poisoning and its similarities to gamma-hydroxybutyric acid: two cases. *Vet Hun Toxicol.* 1997;39:234-235.

Wood DM, Warren-Gash C, Ashraf T, et al. Medical and legal confusion surrounding gamma-hydroxybutyrate (GHB) and its precursors gamma-butyrolactone (GBL) and 1,4-butanediol (1,4BD). *QJM.* 2008;101(1):23-29.

Gamma-Hydroxybutyrate (GHB)

It is illegal to use or possess GHB except if enrolled in certain FDA-allowed clinical trials or for FDA-approved indications. GHB is a central nervous system depressant with abuse potential.

DESCRIPTION

Gamma-hydroxybutyrate or GHB was sold in the 1980s as a nutritional supplement. It was used mainly as a claimed aid to bodybuilding and sleep. In November 1990, FDA banned the OTC sale of GHB following reports of severe illness, including seizures and coma associated with use of GHB. In February 2000, the U.S. House of Representatives approved federal legislation making GHB illegal while allowing medical formulations to be available for clinical testing and potential medical use. Illicitly made GHB is now a Schedule I substance in company with heroin, LSD and cocaine. Medically formulated GHB, such as that developed and approved by the FDA for excessive daytime sleepiness and cataplexy in patients with narcolepsy, is classified as a Schedule III drug. GHB is the only drug to be on two drug schedules at once under U.S. law. GHB, marketed as Xyrem (sodium oxybate) by Jazz Pharmaceuticals, Inc. and prescribed for specific conditions, is on Schedule III. Schedule III drugs are considered safe when used properly and have a lower potential for abuse than do Schedule I and Schedule II drugs. A Schedule I drug is considered a highly dangerous and addictive drug.

Gamma-hydroxybutyrate is also known chemically as 4-hydroxybutyrate and oxybate and is represented by the following chemical formula:

$$HO-CH_2-CH_2-CH_2-COOH$$

Gamma-Hydroxybutyric acid (GHB)

It typically is in the form of sodium oxybate (sodium gamma-hydroxybutyrate or sodium 4-hydroxybutyrate). Other names used for GHB have been liquid ecstasy, liquid X, somatomax PM and Gamma-OH. Some of the effects of GHB are reported to be similar to the effects of 3,4-methylenedioxymethamphetamine or MDMA, more commonly known as ecstasy.

GHB is found naturally in animal tissues, including the brain, kidney, heart muscle and fat. It was synthesized in 1969 and used in Europe as an intravenous anesthetic agent. It was also found to be useful for narcolepsy and has been developed and approved for that use in the U.S.

ACTIONS AND PHARMACOLOGY

ACTIONS

GHB is a central nervous system depressant and has anesthetic and hypnotic actions. It also has activity against excessive daytime sleepiness and cataplexy. (Cataplexy is a condition characterized by weak or paralyzed muscles.)

MECHANISM OF ACTION

The precise mechanism of action of GHB is unclear. GHB is derived from the neurotransmitter gamma-aminobutyric acid (GABA) and is also converted to GABA. GHB is thought to function as an inhibitory chemical transmitter in the central nervous system. Further, it is thought that its central nervous system depressant effect is probably mediated through specific receptors for GHB as well as interaction with the GABA (B) receptor.

GHB is also thought to be a specific inhibitor of central dopamine release. And, under certain conditions, e.g. during sedation or anesthesia or in the presence of a high concentration of calcium, GHB may stimulate dopamine release.

GHB has been found to stimulate the release of growth hormone when administered intravenously in healthy male volunteers. The mechanism of this possible activity is unknown.

PHARMACOKINETICS

Following oral ingestion, GHB is rapidly absorbed from the gastrointestinal tract and transported by the portal circulation to the liver where most of it gets metabolized to carbon dioxide and water by first-pass metabolism pathways. A certain amount crosses the blood-brain barrier. Mean value for the terminal half life ranges from 20 to 23 minutes.

INDICATIONS AND USAGE

GHB is approved by the FDA for the treatment of narcolepsy. There are no indications for its use as a supplement. It is illegal to use it as a supplement.

RESEARCH SUMMARY

GHB has been approved by the FDA as an orphan drug for the treatment of narcolepsy, but banned by it as a supplement. There are, however, products being sold that contain gamma-butyrolactone (GBL) for which many claims are made. GBL is converted in the body to GHB. Claims for GBL include anti-depressive effects, sleep aid, growth-hormone releaser, sexual and athletic enhancers. None of these claims has been proved. Several cases of GBL toxicity have been reported, manifestations of which include bradycardia, hypothermia, central nervous system depression and uncontrolled movements. Use of any GBL/GHB products—excluding the approved drug form of GHB—is inadvisable and illegal.

CONTRAINDICATIONS, PRECAUTIONS, ADVERSE REACTIONS

CONTRAINDICATIONS

GHB is contraindicated in those with seizure disorders; those being treated with sedative hypnotic agents; those with bradycardia and other conditions associated with defects of cardiac conduction; those with cardiovascular disease, Cushing's syndrome, severe hypertension and hyperprolactinemia; and those with severe illness of any kind.

PRECAUTIONS

GHB is illegal to use except if enrolled in certain FDA-allowed clinical trials or for FDA-approved indications. The only indication that is presently approved by the FDA is for the treatment of narcolepsy. Gamma-butyrolactone (GBL) and 1,4 butanediol (BD) are chemicals that may be available. GBL and BD are metabolized to GHB in the body and should be avoided by all.

Under no conditions should GHB, GBL or BD be used with alcohol, benzodiazepines, skeletal muscle relaxants, opioids, antihistamines, barbiturates, anticonvulsants, major tranquilizers or protease inhibitors.

ADVERSE REACTIONS

The most common adverse events reported in patients participating in U.S. clinical trials of the effects of sodium oxybate (sodium gamma-hydroxybutyrate) for the treatment of narcolepsy are dizziness, nausea, headache and enuresis. In these trials, subjects were randomized to doses of 3, 6 or 9 grams daily, and the side effects appeared to be dose-related.

Other adverse effects reported in those taking GHB include vomiting, lightheadedness, confusion, abnormal muscle movements, bradycardia, drowsiness, incoordination, orthostatic hypotension, diarrhea, loss of bladder control, loss of consciousness, temporary amnesia, sleepwalking and seizure-like activity.

INTERACTIONS

GHB taken with any of the following drugs may lead to life-threatening situations: alcohol, anticonvulsants, benzodiazepines, antihistamines (particularly sedating antihistamines), skeletal muscle relaxants, major tranquilizers, opioids and protease inhibitors used for the treatment of HIV.

OVERDOSAGE

It is unclear whether GHB ingestion alone can be fatal (without co-ingesting other CNS depressant agents or other drugs). Symptoms of GHB overdosage include markedly decreased levels of consciousness, bradycardia, hypothermia, respiratory acidosis and emesis. Patients typically regain consciousness spontaneously within five hours of ingestion.

GHB ingestion in a patient taking the protease inhibitors ritonavir and saquinavir caused a near-fatal reaction. Co-ingestion of GHB and alcohol and other "recreational drugs" has been associated with low respiratory rates (at times requiring intubation), coma and death. Over 145 cases of GHB poisoning, including eight deaths, have been reported. Typically, those involved were using other CNS-depressant agents such as alcohol along with GHB. These reports include ingestions of substances such as gamma-butyrolactone (GB) and 1,4 butanediol, both of which are converted to GHB in the body.

DOSAGE AND ADMINISTRATION

It is illegal to use or possess GHB except if enrolled in certain FDA-allowed clinical trials or for the FDA-approved indication of narcolepsy.

LITERATURE

Centers for Disease Control and Prevention. Gamma-hydroxybutyrate use—New York and Texas, 1995-1996. *MMWR.* 1997;46:281-283.

Centers for Disease Control and Prevention. Multistate outbreak of poisonings associated with illicit use of gamma-hydroxybutyrate. *MMWR.* 1990;39:861-863.

Chin RL, Spores KA, Cullison B. Clinical course of gamma-hydroxybutyrate overdose. *Ann Emerg Med.* 1998;31:716-722.

FDA. Warning on dietary supplements. *JAMA.* 1999;282:1218.

Harrington RD, Woodward JA, Hooton TM, et al. Life-threatening interactions between HIV-I protease inhibitors and the illicit drugs MDMA and gamma-hydroxybutyrate. *Arch Intern Med.* 1999;159:2221-2224.

Lammers GL, Arends J, Declerck AC, et al. Gamma-hydroxybutyrate and narcolepsy: a double-blind, placebo-controlled study. *Sleep.* 1993;16:216-220.

Mamclak M, Scharf MB, Woods M. Treatment of narcolepsy with gamma-hydroxybutyrate. A review of clinical and sleep laboratory findings. *Sleep.* 1986;9(1 pt 2):285-289.

Takahara J, Yunoki S, Yakushiji W, et al. Stimulatory effects of gamma-hydroxybutyric acid on growth hormone and prolactin release in humans. *J Clin Endocrinol Metab.* 1977;44:1014-1017.

Tunnicliff G. Sites of action of gamma-hydroxybutyrate(GHB)-a neuroactive drug with abuse potential. *J Toxicol Clin Toxicol.* 1997;35:581-590.

Wood DM, Warren-Gash C, Ashraf T, et al. Medical and legal confusion surrounding gamma-hydroxybutyrate (GHB) and its precursors gamma-butyrolactone (GBL) and 1,4-butanediol (1,4BD). *QJM.* 2008;101(1):23-29.

Gamma-Linolenic Acid (GLA)

DESCRIPTION

Gamma-linolenic acid or GLA is an n-6 (omega-6) polyunsaturated fatty acid. It is comprised of 18 carbon atoms and three double bonds. GLA is an a11-cis n-6 polyunsaturated fatty acid also known as GLA, 18: 3n-6; 6,9,12-octadecatrienoic acid; (Z, Z, Z)- 6,9,12-octadecatrienoic acid; cis-6, cis-9, cis-12-octadecatrienoic acid, and gamolenic acid. The structural formula of GLA is:

GLA (gamma-linolenic acid)

GLA is found naturally to varying extents in the fatty acid fraction of some plant seed oils. In evening primrose seed oil, it is present in concentrations of 7 to 14% of total fatty acids; in borage seed oil, 20 to 27%; and in blackcurrant seed oil, 15 to 20%. GLA is also found in some fungal sources. GLA is produced naturally in the body as the delta 6-desaturase metabolite of the essential fatty acid linoleic acid. Under certain conditions, e.g. decreased activity of the delta-6 desaturase enzyme, GLA may become a conditionally essential fatty acid. GLA is present naturally in the form of triacylglycerols (TAGs). The stereospecificity of GLA varies among different oil sources. GLA is concentrated in the sn-3 position of evening primrose seed oil and blackcurrant seed oil and in the sn-2 position in borage seed oil. GLA is concentrated evenly in both the sn-2 and sn-3 positions of fungal oil.

ACTIONS AND PHARMACOLOGY

ACTIONS

GLA may have anti-inflammatory and antithrombotic actions. It may also have lipid-lowering activity.

MECHANISM OF ACTION

The anti-inflammatory and anti-aggregatory actions can be accounted for by reviewing its role in eicosanoid biosyntheses. GLA is a precursor in the synthesis of prostaglandin E_1 (PGE$_1$) as well as the series-3 prostaglandins. It also serves as a precursor in the synthesis of eicosapentaenoic acid (EPA). EPA is a precursor of the series-3 prostaglandins, the series-5 leukotrienes and the series-3 thromboxanes. These eicosanoids have anti-thrombogenic, anti-inflammatory and anti-atherogenic properties. PGE$_1$ inhibits platelet aggregation and has a vasodilation action. The incorporation of GLA and it metabolites in cell membranes may also play a role in the possible anti-inflammatory and anti-proliferative actions of GLA.

PHARMACOKINETICS

GLA-laden triacylglycerols (TAGs) following ingestion undergo hydrolysis via lipases to form monoglycerides and free fatty acids. Once formed, the monoglycerides and free fatty acids are absorbed by the enterocytes. In the enterocytes, a reacylation takes place reforming TAGs that are then assembled with phospholipids, cholesterol and apoproteins into chylomicrons. The chylomicrons are released into the lymphatics from whence they are transported to the systemic circulation. In the circulation, the chylomicrons are degraded by lipoprotein lipase and the fatty acids including GLA are distributed to various tissues in the body.

GLA is metabolized to the 20 carbon polyunsaturated fatty acid, dihomo-gamma-linolenic acid (DHLA) or eicosatrienoic acid (ETA), which is converted to prostaglandin E_1 (PGE_1). It is also metabolized to eicosapentaenoic acid (EPA). GLA and DHLA are normally not found in the free state in the cell to any appreciable degree but occur as components of phospholipids, neutral lipids and cholesterol esters, mainly in cell membranes. PGE_1 is metabolized to smaller prostaglandin remnants, which are primarily polar dicarboxylic acids. Most of the metabolites are excreted in the urine.

INDICATIONS AND USAGE

GLA appears to be effective in some cases of rheumatoid arthritis and may be indicated in some other inflammatory disorders, such as Sjogren's syndrome and ulcerative colitis. Possible other indications include diabetic neuropathy, acute respiratory distress syndrome, hypertension and elevated serum lipids. GLA has been used with some success in some cancers, principally cerebral gliomas. It has not proved useful for tardive dyskinesia, premenstrual syndrome or menopausal flushing. It may be indicated in some cases for atopic eczema and atopic dermatitis, particularly to help with itching, as well as for uremic skin conditions in hemodialysis patients. It should probably not be used in efforts to enhance immunity as it may be immunosuppressive.

RESEARCH SUMMARY

GLA, supplied in the form of evening primrose oil or borage seed oil, has been studied for many years for its possible effects in arthritis and other inflammatory processes. This is not surprising given its ability to modulate the pathways toward an anti-inflammatory state. It has been shown to suppress inflammation and reduce joint tissue injury in many animal models. Since an early double-blind study demonstrated significant improvement in sufferers of rheumatoid arthritis (RA) who received 540 milligrams of GLA per day for a year (relapsing when switched to placebo for three months), several other clinical studies have followed. These have yielded some encouraging results.

In a randomized double-blind, placebo-controlled study of RA sufferers, those receiving 1.4 grams of GLA in borage seed oil daily experienced significant relief. GLA reduced the number of tender joints 36% and the swollen joint count by 28%. Those on placebo experienced no significant improvement or declined in condition. The dose used in this study was much higher than in most other studies. Other recent studies similarly suggest that GLA is an effective treatment option for some with RA, particularly given its safety profile.

There is preliminary evidence that GLA might also be useful in Sjogren's syndrome and perhaps some other rheumatological disorder. It may be helpful for various dry-eye conditions. Recent animal work suggests GLA may enhance calcium absorption, reduce calcium excretion and increase calcium deposition in bone and thus play a therapeutic role in managing and preventing osteoporosis. A clinical pilot study noted encouraging results in elderly women given supplements of GLA, eicosapentaenoic acid (EPA) along with calcium carbonate. Those treated experienced increased lumbar and femoral bone mineral density over 36 months.

There is some evidence that prolonged use of GLA may result in reduced blood pressure in some hypertensive individuals, as well as fewer coronary events. These effects warrant further investigation.

There is some evidence that higher doses of GLA than typically used may improve blood lipids. In a small study, 17 subjects were assigned to two groups. One group of eight received 2 grams daily of GLA for six weeks, the other group received 500 milligrams daily for the same length of time. At the end of six weeks, the group that received 2 grams of GLA had a 37% lowering of their triglycerides and a 13% lowering of cholesterol. The lower dose showed no triglyceride or cholesterol-lowering activity. Unfortunately, there are no followup studies.

With respect to cancer, GLA has been shown to selectively kill 40 different human cancer cell lines in tissue culture without harm to normal cells. GLA appears to induce apoptotic death of tumor cells or, in various other ways, to suppress oncogene expression, at least in tissue culture. While the clinical use of GLA in cancer is only beginning, there is early encouraging news that it can help regress cerebral gliomas by 1 to 2 years. Other preliminary studies indicate GLA, alone or in combination with other substances, may be of some benefit in the treatment of pancreatic cancer, a finding that certainly warrants followup.

GLA's role in treating some skin disorders has focused primarily on atopic eczema, where the results continue to be mixed after years of study. In one of the best double-blind, multicenter studies to date, 160 patients with eczema of moderate severity were randomized to receive 500 milligrams of borage oil or placebo daily for a 24-week period. Various improvements were noted using GLA, and these reached statistical significance in one of the studies' subgroups. GLA has also been shown to have some efficacy in treating atopic dermatitis in both infant and adults, though here, too, results are mixed. GLA seems to have a positive effect on itching. One recent study showed that oral GLA supplementation can significantly relieve multiple uremic skin symptoms in hemodialysis patients.

GLA is being used to help ameliorate diabetic neuropathy with some encouraging results. In one multi-center randomized, double-blind, placebo-controlled study, those patients given 480 milligrams of GLA per day improved by all test parameters (at a level of statistical significance for 13 of the 16 parameters) over a one-year period. However, not all studies have been positive. There may be subgroups with diabetic neuropathy who could benefit from GLA. In a recent meta-analysis of treatments for tardive dyskinesia, no support was found for the use of GLA in this disorder. It has been suggested that GLA may be helpful in ulcerative colitis, but more research is needed to determine its role.

Treatment with GLA and EPA in the form of borage seed oil and fish oil significantly reduced the need for ventilatory support in 150 patients with acute respiratory distress syndrome. Patients thus treated were confined to intensive care an average of 12.8 days versus 17.5 days for controls.

Claims that GLA is useful in treating premenstrual syndrome (PMS) have not been supported by research findings, and GLA was found to be no better than placebo in preventing/treating menopausal flushing.

As an immune-modulator, GLA may primarily be an immune dampener rather than enhancer. Its ability to dampen some immune functions may make it useful in fighting some auto-immune disorders.

CONTRAINDICATIONS, PRECAUTIONS, ADVERSE REACTIONS

CONTRAINDICATIONS

Known hypersensitivity to a GLA-containing product.

PRECAUTIONS

GLA should not be used by pregnant women and nursing mothers unless recommended by a physician. Because of possible antithrombotic activity, those who take warfarin and hemophiliacs should exercise caution in its use. GLA should not be used before surgery.

ADVERSE REACTIONS

There have been no reports of serious adverse events in those taking GLA supplements. GLA is usually tolerated very well with no significant adverse effects.

INTERACTIONS

No interactions between GLA and aspirin, other NSAIDs, or herbs, such as *Allium sativum* (garlic) or *Ginkgo biloba* (Ginkgo), have been reported. Such interactions, if they were to occur, might be manifested by nosebleeds and/or in-

creased susceptibility to bruising. If this does occur, GLA intake should be lowered or stopped.

OVERDOSAGE

No overdosing has been reported.

DOSAGE AND ADMINISTRATION

There are several forms of GLA supplements. A concentrated form of GLA is available. GLA is also available as evening primrose oil, borage seed oil and blackcurrant seed oil. Doses tried for rheumatoid arthritis and other conditions range from about 360 milligrams to 2.8 grams daily in divided doses and usually with meals. Doses of up to 2 grams daily may be helpful in those with elevated triglycerides. The concentrations of GLA varies in the different oil preparations and, depending on the concentration, the number of capsules daily may be smaller or larger in order to make up the desired dose.

LITERATURE

Belch JJ, Ansell D, Madhok R, et al. Effects of altering dietary essential fatty acids on requirements for non-steroidal anti-inflammatory drugs in patients with rheumatoid arthritis: a double-blind, placebo-controlled study. *Ann Rheum Dis.* 1988; 47:96-104.

Berth-Jones J, Graham-Brown RA. Placebo-controlled trial of essential fatty acid supplementation in atopic dermatitis. *Lancet.* 1993; 341:1557-1560.

Chaintreuil J, Monnier L, Colette C, et al. Effects of dietary gamma-linolenate supplementation on serum lipids and platelet function in insulin-dependent diabetic patients. *Hum Nutr: Clin Nutr.* 1984; 38C:121-130.

Das UN, Prasad VV, Reddy DR. Local application of gamma-linolenic acid in the treatment of human gliomas. *Cancer Lett.* 1995; 94:147-155.

Fan YY, Chapkin RS. Importance of dietary gamma-linolenic acid in human health and nutrition. *J Nutr.* 1998; 128:1411-1414.

Gadek JE, De Michele SJ, Karlstad MD, et al. Effect of enteral feeding with eicosapentaenoic acid, gamma-linolenic acid, and antioxidants in patients with acute respiratory distress syndrome. Enteral nutrition in ARDS Study Group. *Crit Care Med.* 1999; 27:1409-1420.

Galli E, Picardo M, Chine L, et al. Analysis of polyunsaturated fatty acids in newborn sera: a screening tool for atopic dermatitis? *Int Arch Allergy Appl.* 1994; 82:422-423.

Henz BM, Jablonska S, Van De Kerkhof PC, et al. Double-blind, multicentre analysis of the efficacy of borage oil in patients with atopic eczema. *Br J Dermatol.* 1999; 149:685-688.

Horrobin DF, Morse PF. Evening primrose oil and atopic eczema. *Lancet.* 1995; 345: 260-261.

Hrelia S, Bordoni A, Biagi P, et al. gamma-Linoleic supplementation can affect cancer cell proliferation via modification of fatty acid composition. *Biochem Biophys Res Commun.* 1996; 14:441-447.

Huang Y-S, Mills DEM, eds. *Gamma-Linolenic Acid. Metabolism and its Roles in Nutrition and Medicine.* Champaign, IL: AOCS Press; 1996.

Keen H, Payan J, Allawi J. Treatment of diabetic neuropathy with gamma-linolenic acid. The gamma-Linolenic Acid Multicenter Trial Group. *Diabetes Care.* 1993; 16:8-16.

Kernoff PBA, Willis AL, Stone KJ, et al. Antithrombotic potential of di-homo-gamma-linolenic in man. *Brit Med J.* 1977; 2:1441.

Kruger MC, Coetzer H, de Winter R, et al. Calcium, gamma-linolenic acid and eicosapentaenoic acid supplementation in senile osteoporosis. *Aging (Milano).* 1998; 10: 385-394.

Morse PF, Horrobin DF, Manku MS, et al. Meta-analysis of placebo-controlled studies of the efficacy of gamma-linolenic acid in the treatment of atopic eczema. *Br J Dermatol.* 1989; 121:75-90.

Sim AK, Mc Craw AP. The activity of gamma-linolenate and dihomo-gamma linolenate methyl esters in non-human primates and in man. *Throm Res.* 1977; 10: 385-397.

Zurier RB, Rossett RG, Jacobson EW, et al. gamma-Linolenic acid treatment of rheumatoid arthritis. A randomized, placebo-controlled trial. *Arthritis Rheum.* 1996; 39: 1808-1817.

Gamma-Oryzanol

DESCRIPTION

Gamma-oryzanol, a phytosterol derived from rice bran oil, is comprised of a mixture of plant sterols esterified to the phenol, ferulic acid. Rice bran oil is the richest source of gamma-oryzanol, but it is also found in corn, barley and other food oils, and in rye and wheat bran. Phytosterols play a number of roles in plants, including in growth and development, for membrane fluidity and as antioxidants. Rice bran oil also contains tocotrienols, members of the vitamin E family. The gamma-oryzanol concentration of rice bran oil is variable. High gamma-oryzanol rice bran oil contains about 1% or 10 mg per gram. Crude rice bran oil contains about 1.5%. (See Phytosterols and Phytostanols.)

Gamma-oryzanol was first isolated by the Japanese in the 1950s and has been used by the Japanese as a medicine for the treatment of anxiety, menopausal symptoms, peptic ulcers, gastritis and elevated lipids. It is a popular substance among bodybuilders for its supposed anabolic effects. It is also often used in cosmetics as a sunscreen, demulcent, lightener and brightener.

Studies have shown that gamma-oryzanol has antioxidant, anti-inflammatory and lipid-lowering activities. However,

there are no credible studies demonstrating anabolic activity for this plant product.

Gamma-oryzanol is not just one substance, but a mixture of ferulic acid esters of ten triterpene alcohols: delta[7]-stigmastenyl ferulate, stigmasteryl ferulate, cycloartenyl ferulate, 24-methylenecycloartenyl ferulate, delta[7]-campestenylferulate, campesteryl ferulate, delta[7]-sitostenyl ferulate, sitosteryl ferulate, compestanyl ferulate and sitostanyl ferulate. Cycloartenyl ferulate, 24-methylenecycloartanyl ferulate, and campesteryl ferulate are the three major components of gamma-oryzanol. The fundamental structure of gamma-oryzanol is the ferulic acid aromatic nucleus esterified to cyclopentanoperihydrophenanthrene (see accompanying figures). The fundamental structure can be chemically described as (3beta)-9,19-cycloanost-24-en-3-ol-3-(4-hydroxy-3-methoxyphenyl)-propenoate. It is also called cycloartenyl ferulate. Its CAS Registry number is 21238-33-5, its empirical formula is $C_{40}H_{58}O_4$, and its molecular weight is 602.88. The chemical structures below are described within this monograph.

Oryzanol—Fundamental Structure

Ferulic Acid

ACTIONS AND PHARMACOLOGY

ACTIONS

Gamma-oryzanol may have anti-inflammatory, antioxidant and hypocholesterolemic activities.

MECHANISM OF ACTION

Anti-inflammatory activity: A number of studies have found that gamma-oryzanol has anti-inflammatory activity. In one study, gamma-oryzanol was shown to inhibit the activity of the proinflammatory transcription factor NF-kappaB in macrophages.

A recent study demonstrated anti-inflammatory effects of gamma-oryzanol in dextran sulfate sodium (DSS)-induced experimental colitis in mice. This is one of the animal models of inflammatory bowel disease (IBD), which includes ulcerative colitis and Crohn's disease, and is a widely used model for the study of the mechanisms of colonic inflammation and to evaluate candidate drugs for the treatment of IBD. This model exhibits a number of symptoms comparable to those of human ulcerative colitis, such as diarrhea, bloody stools, loss of weight, mucosal ulceration and shortening of the length of the colon. Gamma-oryzanol significantly suppressed DSS-induced colitis in the mice, improved their body weight and the consistency of their stools and decreased their intestinal bleeding. Prior to administration of gamma-oryzanol, elevations of the proinflammatory cytokines tumor necrosis factor-alpha (TNF-alpha), interleukin 1-beta (IL-1beta), interleukin-6 (IL-6) and others were noted in the DSS colitis tissue. Administration of gamma-oryzanol significantly inhibited the production of these cytokines. Gamma-oryzanol was also found to reduce COX-2 expression in DSS-induced colitis. One of the major transcription factors involved in proinflammatory gene regulation is NF-kappaB, and it was thought that this was the main target of the anti-inflammatory effect of gamma-oryzanol and that the anti-inflammatory effect on DSS colitis may be mediated, at least in part, by the inhibition of NF-kappaB via the scavenging of free radicals. Importantly, NF-kappaB activation is associated with free radical generation.

Clearly, gamma-oryzanol appears to have anti-inflammatory activity in the animal colitis model. However, the mechanism of action is not completely understood. Much clinical and experimental data suggest that chronic inflammation of the gut may be due to sustained oxidative stress. Ferulic acid, a metabolite of gamma-oryzanol, has potent antioxidant activity and has been demonstrated to reduce inducible nitric oxide synthase (iNOS), COX-2 and NF-kappaB p63 protein expression in the colonic mucosa of rats with colitis. Thus, ferulic acid seems a good candidate for the anti-inflammatory action of gamma-oryzanol in the above study. However, although ferulic acid did significantly inhibit inflammatory parameters of the DSS-induced colitis in the study, it seemed that the inhibition was not potent enough for it to be considered the only explanation of the anti-inflammatory effect of gamma-oryzanol. Much more study of the anti-inflammatory effect of gamma-oryzanol is needed and warranted.

Antioxidant activity: Gamma-oryzanol has been demonstrated to have a number of antioxidant activities, including scavenging of hydroxyl radicals, superoxide anion radicals and DPPH radicals (2,2,-diphenyl-1-picrylhydrazyl, a stable radical). It also inhibits lipid peroxidation initiated by the azo compound AMVN (2,2'-azobis [2,4-dimethylvaleronitrile]). It is thought that the antioxidant activity of gamma-oryzanol can be mainly attributed to its phenolic ferulic acid moiety/metabolite. Ferulic acid has potent antioxidant activity,

including all those mentioned above. Its antioxidant activity centers on its phenolic hydroxyl group, which donates electrons to quench radicals. Ferulic acid is also known to induce a robust cell stress response through the upregulation of cytoprotective enzymes, such as heme oxygenase-1, heat shock protein 70, extracellular signal-regulated kinase 1/2 and Akt (protein kinase B). In addition, ferulic acid has been shown to inhibit the expression and/or activity of cytotoxic enzymes, including inducible nitric oxide synthase (iNOS), caspases and cyclooxygenase-2 (COX-2). Ferulic acid is considered to be a hormetin, a substance that via mild stress-induced mechanisms stimulates protective mechanisms in cells resulting in biologically beneficial effects.

More research on the biological role of ferulic acid in gamma-oryzanol is needed and warranted.

Antilipidemic activity: Several animal studies over many years have found that gamma-oryzanol lowers total cholesterol and LDL-cholesterol levels. A few human studies have shown that as well. Phytosterols and phytostanols are known to lower total and LDL-cholesterol levels, and so it is not surprising that gamma-oryzanol may do so as well. The mechanism of the cholesterol-lowering activity of phytosterols is not completely understood. Phytosterols appear to inhibit the absorption of dietary cholesterol and the reabsorption (via the enterohepatic circulation) of endogenous cholesterol from the gastrointestinal tract. Consequently, the excretion of cholesterol in the feces leads to decreased serum levels of this sterol. Phytosterols do not appear to affect the absorption of bile acids.

The combination of a cholesterol-lowering phytostanol with an antioxidant and possible anti-inflammatory agent such as ferulic acid in one molecule makes gamma-oryzanol, which contains 10 different versions of this theme, an attractive substance that may help prevent atherogenesis. What is called for, though, are large, prospective, placebo-controlled and randomized clinical trials to investigate the possible lipid-lowering and antiatherogenic activities of gamma-oryzanol and to determine the optimal dosage of the substance for these possible effects.

PHARMACOKINETICS

The pharmacokinetics (PK) of gamma-oryzanol in humans is not complete. The PK below is a composite of a number of animal studies and a few human studies.

Supplemental gamma-oryzanol, following ingestion, undergoes hydrolysis in the small intestine, catalyzed by such enzymes as cholesteryl esterase to yield the various phytosterols comprising the substance, including beta-sitosterol, campesterol, and stigmasterol, and the polyphenol ferulic acid. The efficiency of absorption of the phytosterols is low and only about 5% or so of the various gamma-oryzanol phytosterols are absorbed from the intestinal lumen into the small intestine enterocytes. Prior to their absorption into the enterocytes, the phytosterols are incorporated into mixed micelles (mixtures of bile salts, lipids and sterols). A transporter called the Nieman Pick C1-like-1 (NPC1L1) sterol transporter channel is the transporter that is responsible for uptake of all sterols (phytosterols and cholesterol) into the enterocytes in the proximal small intestine. Parenthetically, the cholesterol-lowering drug ezetimibe works by inhibiting this transporter channel. Ezetimibe also inhibits the absorption of phytosterols. Most of the phytosterol portion in the enterocytes is expelled back into the enterocyte lumen via two sterolin pumps called ATP-binding cassette (ABC) half transporters ABCG5 and ABCG8A, which are expressed in the mucosal cells. The expelled portion of phytosterols is ultimately excreted in the feces. A portion of the absorbed phytosterols, which is incorporated into chylomicrons, makes its way to the liver. A portion of the phytosterols that makes its way to the liver becomes glucuronated. Both free and glucuronated phytosterols are secreted from the liver into the bile. Once again, this is accomplished by the above ATP-binding cassettes that are also found in the canalicular membrane. These secreted phytosterols ultimately have the same fate of being excreted in the feces. The low serum concentrations of phytosterols relative to cholesterol can be explained by decreased intestinal absorption and increased excretion of phytosterols into bile. For comparison, 50% to 60% of cholesterol is absorbed.

Sitosterolemia is a rare autosomal recessive disease, but a very serious one, marked by elevated levels of phytosterols—mainly sitosterol and campesterol, the most abundant phytosterols in the diet. However, any dietary phytosterol can be elevated in sitosterolemia. About 20% of the total sterols in the plasma is in the form of phytosterols; the remaining 80% comes from cholesterol. Those with sitosterolemia have arthralgias, tendon xanthomas and premature cardiovascular diseases. The defect in this disease is in either one or both of the genes that encode the ATP-binding cassettes, causing them to lose the ability to expel phytosterols.

The phenol ferulic acid has a high efficiency of absorption. About 60% of the ferulic acid derived from gamma-oryzanol enters the enterocytes of the small intestine by a yet unidentified mechanism. Some of the ferulic acid appears to get conjugated in the intestine and enters the portal circulation along with unconjugated ferulic acid. Some of the conjugated ferulic acid enters the hepatocytes and is secreted in the bile. The remaining ferulic acid enters the circulation and is distributed to various tissues of the body. Metabolites of ferulic acid, 3-hydroxyphenyl and 3-methoxy-4-hydroxy derivatives of phenyl propionic acid, hydracrylic acid and glycine conjugates are excreted in the urine. Some ferulic acid glucuronide is also found in the urine.

INDICATIONS AND USAGE

Gamma-oryzanol, a phytosterol constituent of rice bran oil, has antioxidative and anti-inflammatory effects. These effects, reportedly, may position this substance as an antiatherogenic agent and as a gastrointestinal protectant in some circumstances. Claims that it has anabolic effects are unsubstantiated. The idea that it might have favorable neuroendocrinological effects is poorly supported.

RESEARCH SUMMARY

First isolated in Japan in the early 1950s, gamma-oryzanol is an active component of rice bran oil (RBO). It is a mixture of ferulic acid esters of triterpene alcohols and sterols. RBO itself has been studied for some time for its possible lipid-lowering effects. These have been demonstrated in a variety of animal models and, to some extent, in humans. There have been fewer studies in this context using isolated gamma-oryzanol, which many have presumed is the most important component in terms of favorable lipid modulation. A review of the literature concluded that, despite flaws in many of the studies, both RBO and its constituent gamma-oryzanol significantly reduce lipid and some other cardiovascular risk factors in rats, rabbits and hamsters. They also cited a few small human trials in which gamma-oryzanol was given credit for lowering total cholesterol, LDL-cholesterol and increasing HDL-cholesterol. No significant adverse side effects were reported in any of these studies. While the data reviewed convinced the researchers that gamma-oryzanol shows promise in controlling hyperlipidemia, they stopped short of saying it has an established role in that context and called for more rigorous clinical investigation.

More recently, researchers reported that RBO and gamma-oryzanol reduced plasma lipid and lipoprotein cholesterol concentrations and aortic cholesterol ester accumulations more effectively in hamsters than did ferulic acid alone. In a study of hypercholesterolemic men, however, another group of researchers, while noting that RBO does, indeed, seem to exert significant favorable lipid-regulating effects, questioned the exact role the gamma-oryzanol component of RBO plays in this. They found that raising the level of the gamma-oryzanol content of the RBO did not increase the favorable effects. They pointed out, as well, that other constituents of the RBO can, independently, have favorable lipid-modulating actions. They hypothesized, however, that even if the increased quantities of gamma-oryzanol did not demonstrate increased lipid effects, its presence might nonetheless be useful for preventing oxidative degradation of other RBO components (such as unsaturated fatty acids, tocopherols and tocotrienols). This same group faulted most prior research on this issue as flawed in various ways. Clearly more research is needed to help determine whether gamma-oryzanol might emerge as a clinically useful substance in the prevention and treatment of heart disease.

Antiulcerogenic effects have been suggested for gamma-oryzanol in some preliminary *in vitro* and animal research. It has shown some indication of being able to reduce serum gastrin levels and was said to be slightly effective in another study as an inhibitor of histamine-stimulated acid secretion. RBO has been hypothesized to stimulate synthesis of prostaglandins, known inhibitors of gastric secretion. Dyspepsia symptoms were reportedly alleviated in human subjects using gamma-oryzanol in one dated study. Recently an experimentally induced colitis in mice was alleviated by gamma-oryzanol. In this study, the substance reportedly inhibited some proinflammatory factors, and the researchers concluded that it might have potential in treating inflammatory bowel disease (for example, ulcerative colitis and Crohn's disease). More research is needed and warranted.

Some bodybuilders and other athletes have used gamma-oryzanol for its claimed anabolic and performance-enhancing properties. These properties, however, have never been convincingly demonstrated. In fact, various animal studies indicate that, when injected, this substance induced anti-anabolic or catabolic activity. Others have reported that, contrary to some popular claims, it may lower, rather than elevate, testosterone levels. In a human study, using oral supplementation, weight-trained males were randomly divided into supplemented (500 mg/day) and control (placebo) groups. Both groups participated in a resistance exercise program over a period of some weeks. No differences were noted in performance levels between the two groups. Nor were any differences seen in a battery of hormone tests that included testosterone, cortisol, growth hormone and several others. Cardiovascular variables were also the same between the groups.

Some animal studies have noted various effects of gamma-oryzanol on anterior pituitary hormone secretion. In humans, a decrease in thyroid stimulating hormone was observed upon administration of the substance. It is hypothesized, on the basis of some further studies, that gamma-oryzanol may be able to increase levels of norepinephrine in the brain. The clinical relevance of these scattered data is unknown

CONTRAINDICATIONS, PRECAUTIONS, ADVERSE REACTIONS

CONTRAINDICATIONS

Gamma-oryzanol supplementation is contraindicated in those who are hypersensitive to any component of a gamma-oryzanol-containing dietary supplement. Gamma-oryzanol is also contraindicated in those with the rare genetic disorders sitosterolemia and cerebrotendinotic xanthomatosis.

PRECAUTIONS

Those who wish to use gamma-oryzanol supplements for any health condition should first discuss this with his or her physician.

Gamma-oryzanol supplements should be avoided by pregnant women and nursing mothers, because there are no long-term safety studies of this substance in these groups. There is no present information that high dietary intake of naturally occurring phytosterols, such as those consumed by vegetarian women, adversely affects pregnancy or lactation.

ADVERSE REACTIONS

Adverse reactions are rare and mainly mild gastrointestinal ones.

INTERACTIONS

DRUGS

Ezetimibe may inhibit the uptake of the phytosterols into the enterocytes of the small intestine.

Administration of an HMG-CoA reductase inhibitor (a "statin") along with gamma-oryzanol may have an additive effect on the lowering of total and LDL-cholesterol

Gamma-oryzanol was found to have no more than a slight inhibitory effect on cytochrome P450 activities in human liver microsomes, indicating that gamma-oryzanol would not be expected to cause clinically significant interactions with cytochrome P450-metabolized drugs.

NUTRITIONAL SUPPLEMENTS

Administration of the omega-3 long chain polyunsaturated acids DHA (docosahexaenoic acid) and EPA (eicosapentaenoic acid) along with gamma-oryzanol may produce a synergistic effect in lipid lowering.

HERBS

None known.

FOOD

None known.

OVERDOSAGE

No reports.

DOSAGE AND ADMINISTRATION

Gamma-oryzanol supplements are available in the form of capsules, tablets and liquid. Dosage ranges from 30 mg to 300 mg daily.

The gamma-oryzanol concentration of rice bran oil is variable. High gamma-oryzanol rice bran oil contains about 1%, or 10 milligrams per gram. A teaspoon of this oil (five milliliters) contains about 50 milligrams.

LITERATURE

Akiyama Y, Hori K, Hata K, et al. Screening of chemiluminescence constituents of cereals and DPPH radical scavenging activity of gamma-oryzanol. *Luminescence.* 2001;16(3):237-241.

Arai T. [Effect of gamma-oryzanol on indefinite complaints in the gastrointestinal symptoms in patients with chronic gastritis—studies on the endocrinological environment (author's transl)] [Article in Japanese.] *Horumon To Rinsho.* 1982;30(3):271-279.

Barone E, Calabrese V, Mancuso C. Ferulic acid and its therapeutic potential as a hormetin for age-related diseases. *Biogerontology.* Epub 2008 Jul 24.

Chen CW, Cheng HH. A rice bran oil diet increases LDL-receptor and HMG-CoA reductase mRNA expressions and insulin sensitivity in rats with streptozotocin/nicotinamide-induced type 2 diabetes. *J Nutr.* 2006;136(6):1472-1476.

Chotimarkorn C, Ushio H. The effect of trans-ferulic acid and gamma-oryzanol on ethanol-induced liver injury in C57BL mouse. *Phytomedicine.* Epub 2008 Apr 17.

Cicero AF, Gaddi A. Rice bran oil and gamma-oryzanol in the treatment of hyperlipoproteinaemias and other conditions. *Phytother Res.* 2001;15(4):277-289.

Fujiwara S, Sakurai S, Sugimoto I, et al. Absorption and metabolism of gamma-oryzanol in rats. *Chem Pharm Bull* (Tokyo). 1983;31(2):645-652.

Fujiwara S, Noumi K, Sugimoto I, et al. Mass fragmentographic determination of ferulic acid in plasma after oral administration of gamma-oryzanol. *Chem Pharm Bull* (Tokyo). 1982;30(3):973-979.

Hiraga Y, Nakata N, Jin H, et al. Effect of the rice bran-derived phytosterol cycloartenol ferulic acid ester on the central nervous system. *Arzneimittelforschung.* 1993;43(7):715-721.

Hiramatsu K, Tani T, Kimura Y, et al. Effect of gamma-oryzanol on atheroma formation in hypercholesterolemic rabbits. *Tokai J Exp Clin Med.* 1990;15(4):299-305.

Hirose M, Fukushima S, Imaida K, et al. Modifying effects of phytic acid and gamma-oryzanol on the promotion stage of rat carcinogenesis. *Anticancer Res.* 1999;19(5A):3665-3670.

Ichimaru Y, Moriyama M, Ichimaru M, et al. [Effects of gamma-oryzanol on gastric lesions and small intestinal propulsive activity in mice] [Article in Japanese.] *Nippon Yakurigaku Zasshi.* 1984;84(6):537-542.

Ieiri T, Kase N, Hashigami Y, et al. [Effects of gamma-oryzanol on the hypothalamo-pituitary axis in the rat] [Article in Japanese.] Nippon Naibunpi *Gakkai Zasshi.* 1982 Oct 20;58(10):1350-1356.

Ishihama A, Hamatsu Y, Ito T. On the effects of gamma-oryzanol upon anterior lobe of rat pituitary. *Yokohama Med Bull.* 1966;17(5):183-189.

Ishihara M. Effect of gamma-oryzanol on serum lipid peroxide level and clinical symptoms of patients with climacteric disturbances. *Asia Oceania J Obstet Gynaecol.* 1984;10(3):317-323.

Islam MS, Murata T, Fujisawa M, et al. Anti-inflammatory effects of phytosteryl ferulates in colitis induced by dextran sulphate sodium in mice. *Br J Pharmacol.* 2008;154(4):812-824.

Juliano C, Cossu M, Alamanni MC, et al. Antioxidant activity of gamma-oryzanol: mechanism of action and its effect on oxidative stability of pharmaceutical oils. *Int J Pharm.* 2005;299(1-2):146-154.

Miller A, Engel KH. Content of gamma-oryzanol and composition of steryl ferulates in brown rice (Oryza sativa L.) of European origin. *J Agric Food Chem.* 2006;54(21):8127-8133.

Mizuta K, Itaya K. [Effects of gamma-oryzanol and atropine on gastric secretion stimulated by insulin or 2-deoxy-D-glucose (author's transl)] [Article in Japanese.] *Nippon Yakurigaku Zasshi.* 1978;74(4):517-524.

Nakayama S, Manabe A, Suzuki J, et al. Comparative effects of two forms of gamma-oryzanol in different sterol compositions on hyperlipidemia induced by cholesterol diet in rats. *Jpn J Pharmacol.* 1987;44(2):135-143.

Nanua JN, McGregor JU, Godber JS. Influence of high-oryzanol rice bran oil on the oxidative stability of whole milk powder. *J Dairy Sci.* 2000;83(11):2426-2431.

Nyström L, Mäkinen M, Lampi AM, et al. Antioxidant activity of steryl ferulate extracts from rye and wheat bran. *J Agric Food Chem.* 2005;53(7):2503-2510.

Parrado J, Miramontes E, Jover M, et al. Prevention of brain protein and lipid oxidation elicited by a water-soluble oryzanol enzymatic extract derived from rice bran. *Eur J Nutr.* 2003;42(6):307-314.

Rong N, Ausman LM, Nicolosi RJ. Oryzanol decreases cholesterol absorption and aortic fatty streaks in hamsters. *Lipids.* 1997;32(3):303-309.

Rukmini C, Raghuram TC. Nutritional and biochemical aspects of the hypolipidemic action of rice bran oil: a review. *J Am Coll Nutr.* 1991;10(6):593-601.

Sakamoto K, Tabata T, Shirasaki K, et al. Effects of gamma-oryzanol and cycloartenol ferulic acid ester on cholesterol diet induced hyperlipidemia in rats. *Jpn J Pharmacol.* 1987;45(4):559-65.

Sasaki J, Takada Y, Handa K, et al. Effects of gamma-oryzanol on serum lipids and apolipoproteins in dyslipidemic schizophrenics receiving major tranquilizers. *Clin Ther.* 1990;12(3):263-8.

Scavariello EM, Arellano DB. [Gamma-oryzanol: an important component in rice brain oil] [Article in Spanish.] *Arch Latinoam Nutr.* 1998;48(1):7-12.

Seetharamaiah GS, Chandrasekhara N. Effect of oryzanol on cholesterol absorption & biliary & fecal bile acids in rats. *Indian J Med Res.* 1990;92:471-475.

Seetharamaiah GS, Krishnakantha TP, Chandrasekhara N. Influence of oryzanol on platelet aggregation in rats. *J Nutr Sci Vitaminol* (Tokyo). 1990;36(3):291-297.

Seetharamaiah GS, Chandrasekhara N. Effect of oryzanol on fructose induced hypertriglyceridaemia in rats. *Indian J Med Res*. 1988;88:278-81.

Shimomura Y, Kobayashi I, Maruto S, et al. Effect of gamma-oryzanol on serum TSH concentrations in primary hypothyroidism. *Endocrinol Jpn*. 1980;27(1):83-86.

Shinomiya M, Morisaki N, Matsuoka N, et al. Effects of gamma-oryzanol on lipid metabolism in rats fed high-cholesterol diet. *Tohoku J Exp Med*. 1983;141(2):191-197.

Srinivasan M, Sudheer AR, Menon VP. Ferulic Acid: therapeutic potential through its antioxidant property. *J Clin Biochem Nutr*. 2007;40(2):92-100.

Suh MH, Yoo SH, Chang PS, et al. Antioxidative activity of microencapsulated gamma-oryzanol on high cholesterol-fed rats. *J Agric Food Chem*. 2005;53(25):9747-9750.

Tamagawa M, Otaki Y, Takahashi T, et al. Carcinogenicity study of gamma-oryzanol in B6C3F1 mice. *Food Chem Toxicol*. 1992;30(1):49-56.

Tamagawa M, Shimizu Y, Takahashi T, et al. Carcinogenicity study of gamma-oryzanol in F344 rats. *Food Chem Toxicol*. 1992;30(1):41-48.

Umehara K, Shimokawa Y, Miyamoto G. Effect of gamma-oryzanol on cytochrome P450 activities in human liver microsomes. *Biol Pharm Bull*. 2004;27(7):1151-1153.

Wheeler KB, Garleb KA. Gamma oryzanol-plant sterol supplementation: metabolic, endocrine, and physiologic effects. *Int J Sport Nutr*. 1991;1(2):170-177.

Wilson TA, Nicolosi RJ, Woolfrey B, et al. Rice bran oil and oryzanol reduce plasma lipid and lipoprotein cholesterol concentrations and aortic cholesterol ester accumulation to a greater extent than ferulic acid in hypercholesterolemic hamsters. *J Nutr Biochem*. 2007;18(2):105-112.

Yamauchi J, Takahara J, Uneki T, et al. Inhibition of LH secretion by gamma-oryzanol in rat. *Horm Metab Res*. 1981;13(3):185.

Yasukawa K, Akihisa T, Kimura Y, et al. Inhibitory effect of cycloartenol ferulate, a component of rice bran, on tumor promotion in two-stage carcinogenesis in mouse skin. *Biol Pharm Bull*. 1998;21(10):1072-1076.

Zhang QH. [Effects of gamma-oryzanol on experimental coronary atherosclerosis in rats] [Article in Chinese.] *Zhonghua Xin Xue Guan Bing Za Zhi*. 1986;14(5):287-90, 319.

Gamma-Tocopherol

DESCRIPTION

Gamma-tocopherol is one of the four natural tocopherol homologues or isoforms, the others being alpha-, beta- and delta-tocopherol. Tocopherols and tocotrienols comprise the vitamin E family (See Vitamin E). Gamma-tocopherol is the principal tocopherol found in the lipid fraction of many seeds and nuts, including soybeans, corn and walnuts, and is the major tocopherol in the American diet. Because of the wide use of oils derived from these sources, gamma-tocopherol makes up approximately 65 to 70% of the total dietary intake of tocopherols, the other major dietary tocopherol being alpha-tocopherol.

Although gamma-tocopherol is the principal dietary tocopherol, plasma levels of this tocopherol average five times lower than alpha-tocopherol. Apparently, alpha-tocopherol is the only tocopherol maintained in human plasma. This situation is believed to be accounted for by the presence in the liver of alpha-tocopherol transfer protein (alpha-TTP). Alpha-TTP preferentially secretes alpha-tocopherol from the liver into the blood. This protein binds most strongly to alpha-tocopherol. Because alpha-tocopherol is the only tocopherol maintained in human plasma, the Food and Nutrition Board in their most recent report, and for the purpose of establishing RDAs for vitamin E, included only certain alpha-tocopherol forms in their definition of vitamin E activity.

Gamma-tocopherol is also known as d-gamma-tocopherol, RRR-gamma-tocopherol, 2R, 4'R, 8'R-gamma-tocopherol and 2, 7, 8-trimethyl-2 (4', 8', 12'-trimethyldecyl)-6-chromanol. It is abbreviated as gamma-TOH, gamma-T and gamma-TH. Gamma-tocopherol is a slightly viscous, pale yellow oil which is practically insoluble in water. Alpha-tocopherol differs from gamma-tocopherol by the presence of a methyl group in the 5 position of the chromanol ring. Gamma-tocopherol lacks this methyl group. Practically all supplemental RRR-alpha-tocopherol, commonly known as d-alpha-tocopherol, is produced from soybean oil-derived gamma-tocopherol by a chemical methylation. The structure is identical to natural d-alpha-tocopherol, but, since it is a semi-synthetic product, it is called natural-source alpha-tocopherol. In contrast to alpha-tocopherol, synthetic forms of gamma-tocopherol, such as *all rac*-gamma-tocopherol or dl-gamma-tocopherol, are not sold as nutritional supplements. Supplemental gamma-tocopherol is marketed as the free or unesterified form.

ACTIONS AND PHARMACOLOGY

ACTIONS

Gamma-tocopherol has antioxidant activity. It may also have anti-atherogenic, anti-apoptotic, antithrombotic, anticoagulant, anticarcinogenic and immunomodulatory actions.

MECHANISM OF ACTION

Gamma-tocopherol is a lipid soluble, chain-breaking, peroxyl radical scavenger. It can protect polyunsaturated fatty acids (PUFAs) within membrane phopholipids, as well as PUFAs within such plasma lipoproteins as low density lipoproteins (LDL), from oxidation. In this regard, gamma-tocopherol is considered to be a less-efficient scavenger of reactive oxygen species (ROS), such as peroxyl radicals, than alpha-tocopherol. This belief is based mainly on *in vitro* studies comparing the various tocopherol homologues.

A recent rat study demonstrated that both alpha-and gamma-tocopherol decreased arterial peroxidation and LDL oxidation and also increased endogenous superoxide dismutase activity. Interestingly, the effects of gamma-tocopherol were found to be more potent than those of alpha-tocopherol. The relative antioxidant activity of the various tocopherol homologous against ROS needs clarification.

It is clear, however, that gamma-tocopherol is a more effective scavenger of reactive nitrogen species (RNS) than is alpha-tocopherol. Gamma-tocopherol is more effective than alpha-tocopherol in inhibiting the oxidation of phopholipids by the RNS peroxynitrite. Peroxynitrite is formed by the reaction of nitric oxide with superoxide and may cause significant cellular damage by reacting with DNA and proteins, as well as with phospholipids. It is postulated by one group of investigators "that gamma-tocopherol acts *in vivo* as a trap for membrane-soluble electrophilic nitrogen oxides and other electrophilic mutagens, forming stable carbon-centered adducts through the nucleophilic 5-position, which is blocked in alpha-tocopherol." The chemical difference between alpha-tocopherol and gamma-tocopherol is the presence in alpha-tocopherol of a methyl group in the 5-position of the chromanol ring.

Gamma-tocopherol may have antiatherogenic activity. One study reported that those with coronary artery disease (CAD) have lower serum levels of gamma-tocopherol but not alpha-tocopherol, when compared with those without CAD. A few mechanisms have been postulated to account for the possible antiatherogenic activity of gamma-tocopherol. These include inhibition of LDL oxidation, inhibition of platelet aggregation and inhibition of apoptosis of coronary artery endothelial cells. Oxidized (ox)-LDL induces apoptosis of human coronary artery endothelial cells in culture, in part by activation of the NF-Kappa B signal transduction pathway. Gamma-tocopherol has been found in cell culture to inhibit ox-LDL-induced apoptosis of human coronary artery endothelial cells by inhibiting the activation of NF-Kappa B. In another study in human coronary smooth muscle cells, ox-LDL was found to mediate apoptosis of these cells, and both gamma- and alpha-tocopherol were found to inhibit this process. Both of these tocopherol homologues —alpha more so than gamma — were found to inhibit two of the pathways leading to apoptosis in these cells, the mitogen-activated protein kinase (MAPK) and Jun kinase pathways. Peroxynitrite is a potent mutagenic oxidant. It is formed during activation of phagocytes (polymorphonuclear leukocytes, monocytes and macrophages). Chronic inflammation in-

duced by these cells is thought to play a major role in the etiology of cancer and other degenerative disease. The possible anticarcinogenic activity of gamma-tocopherol may be accounted for, in part, by its peroxynitrite-scavenging activity.

Gamma-tocopherol, as well as the other tocopherol homologues, enhance both spontaneous and mitogen-stimulated lymphocyte proliferation. The mechanism of the possible immunomodulatory activity of gamma-tocopherol, as well as that of the other homologues, is unclear.

PHARMACOKINETICS

The efficiency of absorption of gamma-tocopherol, as is true for all the members of the vitamin E family, is low and variable. Absorption is lower on an empty stomach than with meals. Gamma-tocopherol is absorbed from the lumen of the small intestine into the enterocytes by passive diffusion. Prior to its absorption, gamma-tocopherol participates in micelle formation with dietary fats and products of lipid hydrolysis. This is aided by bile salts secreted by the liver. Gamma-tocopherol is secreted by the enterocytes into the lymphatics in the form of chylomicrons. Chylomicrons undergo metabolism in the circulation via lipoprotein lipase to form chylomicron remnants. During this process, some gamma-tocopherol is transferred to various tissues such as adipose tissue, muscle and possibly the brain. Chylomicron remnants can transfer it to LDL and very low density lipoproteins (VLDL). Chylomicron remnants can also acquire apolipoprotein E (apoE), which directs them to the liver for metabolism.

The chylomicron remnants are taken up by the liver. Gamma-tocopherol does not bind very well to hepatic alpha-tocopherol transfer protein (alpha-TTP). This is the protein that is involved in the secretion of alpha-tocopherol in VLDLs. It is for this reason, that even though gamma-tocopherol is the major dietary tocopherol in the American diet, (excluding alpha-tocopherol from nutritional supplements), alpha-tocopherol levels in plasma and most other tissues are about five-fold higher than gamma-tocopherol. Gamma-tocopherol is also more rapidly taken up and turned over in tissues, compared with alpha-tocopherol.

Reaction of gamma-tocopherol and peroxynitrite *in vitro* results in the formation of four major products: 2, 7, 8-trimethyl-2-(4, 8, 12-trimethyldecyl)-5-nitro-6-chromanol (NGT or tocoyellow), 2, 7, 8-trimethyl-2-(4, 8, 12-trimethyl-decyl)-5,6-chromaquinone (tocored) and two diastereomers of 8a-(hydroxy)-gamma-tocopherol.

About half of ingested and absorbed gamma-tocopherol is excreted in the urine, mainly as a glucuronide conjugate of 2, 7, 8-trimethyl-2-(2'-carboxyethyl)-6-hydroxychroman or gamma-CEHC. Fecal excretion is the main route of excretion of oral gamma-tocopherol. Fecal excretion substances includes non-absorbed gamma-tocopherol and gamma-tocopherol that may be excreted via the biliary route.

The gamma-tocopherol metabolite gamma-CEHC, also known as LLU (Loma Linda University)-alpha, is reported to have natriuretic activity. This is thought to be mediated by inhibition of a potassium channel in the apical membrane of the thick ascending limb of the kidney.

INDICATIONS AND USAGE

There is some evidence that both alpha- and gamma-tocopherol may have complementary antioxidant activities. There might thus be indications and uses of gamma-tocopherol that are distinct from those of alpha-tocopherol, or circumstances in which one works better than the other. In general, however, gamma-tocopherol is likely to have some or most of the same indications and uses as alpha-tocopherol (See Vitamin E), although it has not been as extensively studied as alpha-tocopherol. There is preliminary evidence that gamma-tocopherol may be more protective against cardiovascular disease than alpha-tocopherol. There is also some preliminary evidence that it could be more effective in preventing some cancers. On the other hand, there is one recent report that elevated blood levels of gamma-tocopherol may be associated with an increased incidence of knee osteoarthritis, especially in those who are black.

RESEARCH SUMMARY

Some studies have indicated that gamma-tocopherol is more potent than alpha-tocopherol in protecting against nitric-oxide initiated lipid peroxidation. This has been demonstrated in vitro and in animal experiments. Human data are more equivocal. Some studies have suggested that both tocopherols are required for optimal protection against reactive nitrogen species. Several researchers have thus suggested that gamma-tocopherol should be part of "standard" vitamin E supplements.

Recently, an *in vitro* study showed that gamma-tocopherol significantly reduced oxidized-LDL-induced apoptosis of human coronary artery endothelial cells. In a recent animal study, gamma-tocopherol, significantly more than alpha-tocopherol, was found to decrease platelet aggregation and to delay intra-arterial thrombus formation. Research continues.

There are some experimental data suggesting that gamma-tocopherol may, more effectively than alpha-tocopherol, prevent neoplastic transformation. Recently, gamma-tocopherol was shown to inhibit (more effectively than alpha-tocopherol) the growth of a human prostate cancer cell line.

There is one study in which an association has been made between high blood levels of gamma-tocopherol and increased incidence of knee osteoarthritis, especially in those

who are black. More research will have to be done before causality can be determined. Research is continuing.

CONTRAINDICATIONS, PRECAUTIONS, ADVERSE REACTIONS
CONTRAINDICATIONS
Gamma-tocopherol is contraindicated in those with known hypersensitivity to the substance.

PRECAUTIONS
Those on warfarin should be cautious in using high doses of gamma-tocopherol (doses greater than 100 milligrams daily) and, if they do so, they should have their INRs carefully monitored and their warfarin doses appropriately adjusted if indicated. Likewise, those with vitamin K deficiencies, such as those with liver failure, should be cautious in using high doses of gamma-tocopherol. Gamma-tocopherol should be used with caution in those with lesions with a propensity to bleed (e.g., bleeding peptic ulcers), those with a history of hemorrhagic stroke and those with inherited bleeding disorders (e.g., hemophilia).

High dose gamma-tocopherol supplementation should be stopped about one month before surgical procedures and may be resumed following recovery from the procedure. Those taking iron supplements should not take gamma-tocopherol concomitantly with the iron.

ADVERSE REACTIONS
Gamma-tocopherol has only recently been introduced into the nutritional supplement marketplace. No adverse reactions have been reported.

INTERACTIONS
DRUGS
Antiplatelet drugs, such as aspirin, dipyridamole, eptifibatide, clopidogrel, ticlopidine, tirofiban and abciximab: High doses of gamma-tocopherol may potentiate the effects of these antiplatelet drugs.

Cholestyramine: may decrease gamma-tocopherol absorption.
Colestipol: may decrease gamma-tocopherol absorption.
Isoniazid: may decrease gamma-tocopherol absorption.
Mineral oil: may decrease gamma-tocopherol absorption.
Neomycin: may impair utilization of gamma-tocopherol.
Orlistat: is likely to inhibit gamma-tocopherol absorption.
Sucralfate: may interfere with gamma-tocopherol absorption.
Warfarin: High dose (greater than 100 milligrams daily) gamma-tocopherol may enhance the anticoagulant response of warfarin. Monitor INRs and appropriately adjust dose of warfarin if necessary.

NUTRITIONAL SUPPLEMENTS
Alpha-tocopherol: Supplemental alpha-tocopherol may decrease plasma concentration of gamma-tocopherol.

Desiccated ox bile: may increase the absorption of gamma-tocopherol.

Iron: Most iron supplements contain the ferrous form of iron. This form can oxidize gamma-tocopherol, which is marketed in a free, unesterified form, to its pro-oxidant form, if taken concomitantly.

Medium-chain triglycerides: may enhance absorption of gamma-tocopherol if taken concomitantly.

Phytosterols and phytostanols, including beta-sitosterol and beta-sitostanol: may lower plasma gamma-tocopherol levels.

Plant phenolic compounds and flavonoids: may participate in redox cycling reactions and help maintain levels of reduced gamma-tocopherol.

Selenium: may function synergistically with gamma-tocopherol.

Vitamin C: may help maintain gamma-tocopherol in its reduced (antioxidant) form.

FOODS
Olestra: is likely to inhibit the absorptin of gamma-tocopherol. Although alpha-tocopherol is added to olestra, gamma-tocopherol is not.

HERBS
Some herbs, including garlic and ginkgo, possess antithrombotic activity. High doses of gamma-tocopherol used concomitantly with these herbs may enhance their antithrombotic activity.

OVERDOSAGE
There are no reports of gamma-tocopherol overdoses in the literature.

DOSAGE AND ADMINISTRATION
Presently marketed forms of gamma-tocopherol contain about 60% gamma-tocopherol along with smaller amounts of the other tocopherol homologues. The gamma-tocopherols, as well as the other tocopherols, are present in the free (unesterified) form. Typical doses are about 200 milligrams daily (as gamma-tocopherol).

LITERATURE
Brigelius-Flohe R, Traber MG. Vitamin E: function and metabolism. *FASEB J.* 1999; 13:1145-1155.

Christen S, Woodall AA, Shigenaga MK, et al. Gamma-tocopherol traps mutagenic electrophiles such as NOx and complements alpha-tocopherol: physiological implications. *Proc Natl Acad Sci USA.* 1997; 94:3217-3222.

Cooney RV, Harwood PJ, Franke AA, et al. Products of gamma-tocopherol reaction with NO2 their formation in rat insulinoma (RINm5f) cells. *Free Rad Biol Med.* 1995; 19:259-269.

Cooney RV, Franke AA Harwood PJ, et al. Gamma-tocopherol detoxification of nitrogen dioxide: superiority to alpha-tocopherol. *Proc Natl Acad Sci USA.* 1993; 90:1771-1775.

de Nigris F, Franconi F, Maida I, et al. Modulation by alpha- and gamma-tocopherol and oxidized low-density lipoprotein of apoptotic signaling in human coronary smooth muscle cells. *Biochem Pharmacol.* 2000; 59:1477-1487.

Handelman GJ, Machlin LJ, Fitch K, et al. Oral alpha-tocopherol supplements decrease plasma gamma-tocopherol levels in humans. *J Nutr.* 1985; 115:807-813.

Hoglen NC, Waller SC, Sipes IG, Liebler DC. Reactions of peroxynitrite with gamma-tocopherol. *Chem Res Toxicol.* 1997; 10:401-407.

Li D, Saldeen T, Mehta JL. Gamma-tocopherol decreases ox-LDL-mediated activation of nuclear factor-KappaB and apoptosis in human coronary artery endothelial cells. *Biochem Biophys Res Commun.* 1999; 259:157-161.

Li D, Saldeen T, Romero F, Mehta JL. Relative effects of alpha- and gamma-tocopherol on low-density lipoprotein oxidation and superoxide dismutase and nitric oxide synthase activity and protein expression in rats. *J Cardiovasc Pharmacol Ther.* 1999; 4:219-226.

Mc Intyre BS, Briski KP, Tirmenstein MA, et al. Antiproliferative and apoptotic effects of tocopherols and tocotrienols on normal mouse mammary epithelial cells. *Lipids.* 2000; 35:171-180.

Parker RS, Swanson JE. A novel 5[1]-carboxychroman metabolite of gamma-tocopherol secreted by HepG2 cells and excreted in human urine. *Biochem Biophys Res Commun.* 2000; 269:580-583.

Saldeen T, Li D, Mehta JL. Differential effects of alpha- and gamma-tocopherol on low-density lipoprotein oxidation, superoxide activity, platelet aggregation and arterial thrombogenesis. *J Am Coll Cardiol* 1999; 34:1208-1215.

Stone WL, Papas AM. Tocopherols and the etiology of colon cancer. *J Natl Cancer Inst.* 1997; 89:1006-1014.

Wechter WJ, Kantoci D, Murray ED Jr., et al. A new natriuretic factor: LLU-alpha. *Proc Natl Acad Sci USA.* 1996; 93:6002-6007.

Wolf G. Gamma-tocopherol: an efficient protector of lipids against nitric oxide-isolated peroxidative damage. *Nutr Rev.* 1997; 55:376-378.

Wu D, Meydani M, Beharka AA, et al. In vitro supplementation with different tocopherol homologues can affect the function of immune cells in olzd mice. *Free Rad Biol Med.* 2000; 28:643-651.

Yamashita K, Takeda N, Ikeda S. Effects of various tocopherol-containing diets on tocopherol secretion into bile. *Lipids.* 2000; 35:163-170.

Gelatin Hydrolysates

DESCRIPTION

Gelatin is a heterogeneous mixture of proteins derived from animal collagen by hydrolysis. It is not found naturally. It typically is obtained by boiling bovine, pig and ox skin and bones. Gelatin has many uses in the food and pharmaceutical industries. Nutritionally, it is an incomplete protein because it lacks L-tryptophan. It is used in foods as a stabilizer, thickener and texturizer. Pharmaceutically, it is used as an encapsulating agent. Gelatin capsules are widely used both in the pharmaceutical and nutritional supplement industries.

Recently, gelatin subjected to greater hydrolysis in order to produce water-soluble peptides of various molecular weights has entered the nutritional supplement marketplace for use in bone and joint health. The gelatin peptides are rich in the amino acids found in collagen, including L-proline, L-hydroxyproline and glycine. Gelatin and hydrolyzed collagen are similar (see Hydrolyzed Collagen).

ACTIONS AND PHARMACOLOGY

ACTIONS

Gelatin hydrolysates have putative activity against degenerative joint disease (DJD).

MECHANISM OF ACTION

The mechanism of the putative anti-arthritic activity of gelatin hydrolysates is a matter of speculation. Although the amino acids in gelatin hydrolysates are identical to those in collagen, it is unlikely that these amino acids would make a significant contribution to the synthesis of collagen in, for example, joint cartilage. L-hydroxyproline is not a genetic amino acid. Thus, it is not a precursor to protein synthesis but, rather, is formed post-translationally. Both glycine and L-proline are synthesized by the body, and it is unlikely that these amino acids in gelatin hydrolysates would play any role in the *de novo* synthesis of collagen. There is speculation that gelatin hydrolysates may contain certain oligopeptides, which may stimulate collagen synthesis. This is far from proven.

PHARMACOKINETICS

The digestion, absorption and metabolism of gelatin hydrolysates are similar to those that occur with dietary proteins and peptides.

INDICATIONS AND USAGE

Claims that gelatin can fight arthritis and help maintain healthy joint cartilage and bone are to date poorly supported.

RESEARCH SUMMARY

A mixture of gelatin, vitamin C and calcium has been promoted as an effective interventive in joint disease. Some preliminary studies supporting this claim need more rigorous follow-up.

CONTRAINDICATIONS, PRECAUTIONS, ADVERSE REACTIONS

CONTRAINDICATIONS

Known hypersensitivity to a gelatin hydrolysate-containing product.

PRECAUTIONS

Pregnant women and nursing mothers should avoid supplemental gelatin hydrolysates.

Those with renal failure or liver failure should exercise caution in the use of supplemental gelatin hydrolysates.

Those who use gelatin hydrolysates produced from bovine sources should only use products derived from raw materials (bovine skin and bone) classified as carrying no detectable infectivity. Bovine nervous system parts may carry the bovine spongiform encephalopathy (BSE) agent, the etiological agent of mad cow disease.

ADVERSE REACTIONS

No reports.

INTERACTIONS

There is one report of a collagen hydrolysate enhancing the effect of calcitonin in the treatment of osteoporosis.

DOSAGE AND ADMINISTRATION

Gelatin hydrolysates are available in powder form, usually in combination with other nutritional supplements, such as vitamin C and calcium. A typical dose is 10 grams daily. Gelatin hydrolysates are also available in capsules, usually in combination with other supplements, such as glucosamine, curcumin, chondroitin sulfate and willow bark.

LITERATURE

Adam M, Spacek P, Hulejova H, et al. [Postmenopausal osteoporosis. Treatment with calcitonin and a diet rich in collagen proteins.] [Article in Czech.] *Cas Lek Cesk*. 1996; 135:44-78.

Genistein

DESCRIPTION

Genistein belongs to the isoflavone class of flavonoids. It is also classified as a phytoestrogen. Phytoestrogens are plant-derived nonsteroidal compounds that possess estrogen-like biological activity. Genistein has been found to have both weak estrogenic and weak anti-estrogenic effects.

Genistein is the aglycone (aglucon) of genistin. The isoflavone is found naturally as the glycoside genistin and as the glycosides 6″-O-malonylgenistin and 6″-O-acetylgenistin. Genistein and its glycosides are mainly found in legumes, such as soybeans and chickpeas. Soybeans and soy foods are the major dietary sources of these substances. Nonfermented soy foods, such as tofu, contain higher levels of the genistein glycosides, while fermented soy foods, such as tempeh and miso, contain higher levels of the aglycone.

Genistein is a solid substance that is practically insoluble in water. Its molecular formula is $C_{15}H_{10}O_5$, and its molecular weight is 270.24 daltons. Genistein is also known as 5, 7-dihydroxy-3-   (4-hydroxyphenyl)-4H-1-benzopyran-4-one, and 4′, 5, 7-trihydroxyisoflavone. Genistin, which is the 7-beta glucoside of genistein, has greater water solubility than genistein. Genistein has the following structural formula:

Genistein

Genistein, when marketed as a nutritional supplement, is mainly present in the form of its glycoside genistin.

See also Soy Isoflavones.

ACTIONS AND PHARMACOLOGY

ACTIONS

Genistein may have estrogenic, antiestrogenic and nonestrogenic activities. It may also have antioxidant, anticarcinogenic, antiatherogenic, antiosteoporotic, antiperimenopausal hot flash and radioprotective activities.

MECHANISM OF ACTION

Genistein has weak estrogenic activity as measured in *in vivo* and *in vitro* assays. *In vivo*, its estrogenic activity is one-third that of glycitein and four times greater than that of daidzein.

Genistein has been found to have a number of antioxidant activities. It is a scavenger of reactive oxygen species and inhibits lipid peroxidation. It also inhibits superoxide anion generation by the enzyme xanthine oxidase. In addition, genistein, in animal experiments, has been found to increase the activities of the antioxidant enzymes superoxide dismutase, glutathione peroxidase, catalase and glutathione reductase.

Several mechanisms have been proposed for genistein's putative anticarcinogenic activity. These include upregulation of apoptosis, inhibition of angiogenesis, inhibition of DNA topoisomerase II and inhibition of protein tyrosine kinases. Genistein's weak estrogenic activity has been suggested as another mechanism for genistein's putative anti-prostate cancer activity. In addition to the above mechanisms, other mechanisms of genistein's putative anti-prostate cancer activity include inhibition of nuclear factor

(NF)-Kappa B in prostate cancer cells, downregulation of TGF (transforming growth factor)-beta, inhibition of EGF (epidermal growth factor)-stimulated growth, and induction of the *p21WAF1/CIP1* and *p16INK4a* tumor suppressor genes in prostate cancer cells by epigenetic mechanisms involving active chromatin modification. Regarding the latter action, genistein was found to increase acetylated histones 3,4, and H3/K4 at the *p21* and *p16* transcription start sites.

Dietary genistein has been demonstrated to inhibit metastasis of human prostate cancer cells in mice. Prostate cancer cell detachment and invasion represent early steps in the metastatic process. Genistein has been shown to inhibit both of these processes *in vitro*. These processes appear to be regulated by activation of focal adhesion kinase (FAK) and the p38 mitogen-activated protein kinase-heat shock protein 27 (HSP27) pathway; genistein has been shown to inhibit this pathway. The same group that reported on the *in vitro* studies recently reported on an animal model that they developed in order to study the antimetastatic potential of genistein *in vivo*. The animal model was comprised of four-week-old inbred male athymic BALB/c mice, in which were orthotopically implanted PC3-M human prostate cancer cells that formed lung micrometastasis in most of the mice. Dietary genistein was found to decrease human prostate cancer metastasis dose-dependently, corroborating the *in vitro* studies. Further research on the antimetastatic potential of genistein, including early clinical trials in men with prostate cancer, is in progress and certainly warranted.

Genistein's anti-estrogenic action may be another possible mechanism to explain its putative anti-breast cancer activity. In the final analysis, our understanding of the mechanism of genistein's putative anticarcinogenic activity is still in its early stages.

The possible anti-atherogenic activity of genistein may be attributed, in part, to its antioxidant activity. Genistein may have some lipid-lowering activity in some, but the mechanism of this is unclear. The weak estrogenic activity of genistein may also contribute to its possible anti-atherogenic action.

Genistein's weak estrogenic effect may help protect against osteoporosis by preventing bone resorption and promoting increased bone density. Genistein has been found to maintain trabecular bone tissue in rats. A recent randomized, double-blind, placebo-controlled trial involving 389 osteopenic, postmenopausal women reported that after three years of treatment, genistein exhibited a promising safety profile—genistein did not significantly change mammographic breast density or endometrial thickness—and positive effects on bone formation were found. The mechanism of genistein's possible anti-osteoporotic effect is unclear.

Soy isoflavones' weak estrogenic actions may also aid in reducing hot flash symptoms (see Indications and Usage).

Genistein treatment has been demonstrated to protect mice from ionizing radiation injury. It also has been shown to stimulate hematopoietic recovery and increase survival in irradiated mice. The mechanism of action of the radioprotective effect is not completely understood. Possibilities include genistein's antioxidant properties, immunostimulatory activity and its role in signal transduction pathways, where it is an inhibitor of topoisomerase, protein kinases and caspases involved in apoptotic pathways.

PHARMACOKINETICS

The pharmacokinetics of genistein in humans is complex and not well understood. The major dietary and supplemental form of genistein is the glycoside genistin. Some genistin may be hydrolyzed by hydrochloric acid in the stomach to genistein and some may be hydrolyzed by beta-glucosidases in food to genistein. Most of ingested genistin, however, is delivered to the large intestine intact. In the large intestine, bacterial beta-glucosidases hydrolyze genistin to genistein. Genistein is either absorbed or further metabolized in the large intestine to dihydrogenistein and 6'-hydroxy-O-desmethylangolensin. Genistein, which is absorbed from the large intestine and small intestine, is eventually transported to the liver. There, it undergoes conjugation with glucuronate and sulfate via hepatic phase II enzymes (UDP-glucuronosyltransferases and sulfotransferases). The glucuronide and sulfate conjugates of genistein are excreted in the urine and in the bile. The genistein conjugates may be deconjugated to release genistein, which may be reabsorbed via the enterohepatic circulation.

There is considerable individual variation in the absorption and metabolism of ingested genistin and genistein. There are some data suggesting that genistein may be more bioavailable than genistin. However, other data suggest that the extent of absorption of genistein is similar for the aglycone and the glucoside forms. There are little data available on the tissue distribution of genistein.

INDICATIONS AND USAGE

There is a growing body of *in vitro* and animal studies suggesting that genistein may be helpful in preventing and treating some cancers, principally breast and prostate cancers. The clinical studies that might support or refute claims that genistein has anti-atherogenic properties, and that it can be safely and effectively used as "natural" estrogen-replacement therapy, are in their early stages. There are, however, preliminary data suggesting that soy isoflavones, including genistein, may be helpful in some problems associated with menopause, including osteoporosis and "hot flashes." See Soy Isoflavones.

Epidemiological data have long suggested that dietary isoflavones may confer protection against various cancers, especially breast and prostate cancer. High dietary intake of soy products in parts of Asia significantly correlated with reduced incidence of both breast and prostate cancers. Epidemiological data have not been entirely consistent in this regard, but most studies suggest protective effects. Some studies have shown, moreover, that this protection is lost in the second generation of those Asians immigrating to the United States.

These data led to experimental animal studies demonstrating protective effects. In one study, genistein perinatally fed to rats significantly protected offspring from subsequent chemically induced mammary cancers. These researchers concluded that adequate perinatal exposure to genistein can confer permanent protective effects against breast cancer. They have further speculated that protective effects in humans, with respect to breast cancer specifically, may depend upon exposure to genistein early in life. More research is needed to clarify this issue.

A number of studies have shown that genistein can inhibit prostate cancer-cell growth *in vitro*. Some *in vitro* studies suggest that genistein may be both chemopreventive and therapeutic in prostate cancers regardless of androgen responsiveness. Clinical trials are needed.

A symptom that most perimenopausal women experience is the annoying feeling of intermittent intense heat, commonly known as a "hot flash." Hot flashes result from a vasomotor response to declining estrogen levels and can be very disruptive to one's life. While hormone replacement therapy (HRT) is an effective treatment for hot flashes, many women are concerned over potential adverse events of HRT. This concern became even greater following publication in 2002 of the results of The Women's Health Initiative (WHI) Estrogen plus Progestin Study, which was stopped on July 7, 2002 because of increased risk of breast cancer and cardiovascular disease in women taking active study pills, compared with those on placebo. Many women began using soy isoflavones, which some, but not all, studies suggested might help with hot flashes. A recent review of isoflavone-hot flash studies reported that studies that consistently reported a significant decrease in hot flash symptoms (intensity and frequency) all supplied more than 15 milligrams of the isoflavone genistein (calculated as aglycone equivalents) per treatment. Also see Soy Isoflavones.

CONTRAINDICATIONS, PRECAUTIONS, ADVERSE REACTIONS

CONTRAINDICATIONS

Genistein is contraindicated in those who are hypersensitive to any component of a genistin, or genistein-containing product.

PRECAUTIONS

Pregnant women and nursing mothers should avoid the use of genistein/genistin supplements pending long-term safety studies.

Men with prostate cancer should discuss the advisability of the use of genistein/genistin supplements with their physicians before deciding to use them.

Women with estrogen receptor-positive tumors should exercise caution in the use of genistein/genistin supplements and should only use them if they are recommended and monitored by a physician.

Women with estrogen receptor-positive breast cancer taking letrozole or tamoxifen should exercise caution in the use of genistein/genistin supplements and should only use them if they are recommended and monitored by a physician.

Those consuming soy isoflavones should ensure that they have an adequate intake of iodide. See Soy Isoflavones: Adverse Reactions.

INTERACTIONS

DRUGS

Letrozole. Letrozole is an aromatase inhibitor that is an approved drug for the adjuvant treatment of hormonally responsive breast cancer. Genistein may negate the inhibitory effect of letrozole. This is based on an animal study.

Tamoxifen. Tamoxifen is a selective estrogen response modulator (SERM) that is used in the treatment and prevention of estrogen receptor-positive breast cancer. Genistein may negate the inhibitory effect of tamoxifen. This is based on an animal study. However, another study found that genistein sensitized the inhibitory effect of tamoxifen on the growth of estrogen receptor-positive and HER-overexpressing human breast cancer cells.

DOSAGE AND ADMINISTRATION

Genistein is available in a few different isoflavone formulas. A standard soy isoflavone formula contains genistein mainly in the form of genistin, as well as daidzin and glycitin. The percentages of the various isoflavones present in this soy formula reflect the percentages of these substances as found in soybeans and are: genistin, about 50%; daidzin, about 38%; and glycitin, about 12%. A 50 mg dose of soy isoflavones—a typical daily dose—provides 25 mg of genistin, 19 mg of daidzin and about 6 mg of glycitin. Usually, 40% of the formula is comprised of soy isoflavones. Therefore, to get a dose of 50 mg of soy isoflavones, one needs 125 mg of the soy preparation.

Smaller amounts of genistein as the aglycone are available in some red clover preparations (see Biochanin A).

LITERATURE

Altavilla D, Crisafulli A, Marini H, et al. Cardiovascular effects of the phytoestrogen genistein. *Curr Med Chem Cardiovasc Hematol Agents.* 2004;2(2):179-186.

Barnes S. Effect of genistein on in vitro and in vivo models of cancer. *J Nutr.* 1995;125:777S-783S.

Barnes S, Peterson TG. Biochemical targets of the isoflavone genistein in tumor cell lines. *Proc Soc Exp Biol Med.* 1995;208:103-108.

Constantinou A, Huberman E. Genistein as an inducer of tumor cell differentiation: possible mechanisms of action. *Proc Soc Exp Biol Med.* 1995;208:109-115.

Dalu A, Haskell JF, Coward L, Lamartiniere CA. Genistein, a component of soy, inhibits the expression of the EGF and Erb B2/Neu receptors in the rat dorsolateral prostate. *The Prostate.* 1998;37:36-48.

D'Anna R, Cannata ML, Atteritano M, et al. Effects of the phytoestrogen genistein on hot flushes, endometrium, and vaginal epithelium in postmenopausal women: a 1-year randomized, double-blind, placebo-controlled study. *Menopause.* 2007;14(4):648-655.

Davis JN, Kucuk O, Sarkar FH. Genistein inhibits NF-Kappa B activation in prostate cancer cells. *Nutr Biochem.* 1999;35:167-174.

Davis JN, Muqim N, Bhuiyan M, et al. Inhibition of prostate specific antigen expression by genistein in prostate cancer cells. *Int J Oncol.* 2000;16:1091-1097.

Fotsis T, Pepper M, Adlercreutz H, et al. Genistein, a dietary-derived inhibitor of *in vitro* angiogenesis. *Proc Natl Acad Sci USA.* 1993;90:2690-2694.

Geller J, Sionit L, Partido C, et al. Genistein inhibits the growth of human-patient BPH and prostate cancer in histoculture. *The Prostate.* 1998;34:75-79.

Ju YH, Doerge DR, Allred KF, et al. Dietary genistein negates the inhibitory effect of tamoxifen on growth of estrogen-dependent human breast cancer (MCF-7) cells implanted in athymic mice. *Cancer Res.* 2002;62(9):2474-2477.

Ju YH, Doerge DR, Woodling KA, et al. Dietary Genistein Negates the Inhibitory Effect of Letrozole On The Growth Of Aromatase-expressing Estrogen-Dependent Human Breast Cancer Cells (MCF-7Ca) In Vivo. *Carcinogenesis.* Epub: 2008 Jul 16.

Kikuno N, Shiina H, Urakami S, et al. Genistein mediated histone acetylation and demethylation activates tumor suppressor genes in prostate cancer cells. *Int J Cancer.* 2008;123(3):552-560.

Lakshman M, Xu L, Ananthanarayanan V, et al. Dietary genistein inhibits metastasis of human prostate cancer in mice. *Cancer Res.* 2008;68(6):2024-2032.

Lamartiniere CA. Protection against breast cancer with genistein: a component of soy. *Amer J Clin Nutr.* 2000;71:1705S-1707S.

Landauer MR, Srinivasan V, Seed TM. Genistein treatment protects mice from ionizing radiation injury. *J Appl Toxicol.* 2003;23(6):379-385.

Mai Z, Blackburn GL, Zhou JR. Genistein sensitizes inhibitory effect of tamoxifen on the growth of estrogen receptor-positive and HER2-overexpressing human breast cancer cells. *Mol Carcinog.* 2007;46(7):534-542.

Majid S, Kikuno N, Nelles J, et al. Genistein induces the p21WAF1/CIP1 and p16INK4a tumor suppressor genes in prostate cancer cells by epigenetic mechanisms involving active chromatin modification. *Cancer Res.* 2008;68(8):2736-2744.

Marini H, Bitto A, Altavilla D, et al. Breast safety and efficacy of genistein aglycone for post-menopausal bone loss: a follow-up study. *J Clin Endocrinol Metab.* Epub: 2008 Sep 16.

Messina M, Redmond G. Effects of soy protein and soybean isoflavones on thyroid function in healthy adults and hypothyroid patients: a review of the relevant literature. *Thyroid.* 2006;16(3):249-258.

Wang TT, Sathyamoorthy N, Phang JM. Molecular effects of genistein on estrogen receptor mediated pathways. *Carcinogenesis.* 1996;17:271-275.

Wei H, Bowen R, Cai Q, et al. Antioxidant and antipromotional effects of the soybean isoflavone genistein. *Proc Soc Exp Biol Med.* 1995;208:124-130.

Williamson-Hughes PS, Flickinger BD, Messina MJ, et al. Isoflavone supplements containing predominantly genistein reduce hot flash symptoms: a critical review of published studies. *Menopause.* 2006;13(5):831-839.

Zhou Y, Mi MT. Genistein stimulates hematopoiesis and increases survival in irradiated mice. *J Radiat Res (Tokyo).* 2005;46(4):425-433.

Germanium

DESCRIPTION

Germanium is a metalloid element with atomic number 32 and atomic symbol Ge. Germanium is found in the earth's crust, in certain minerals and in living matter such as plants and the human body. Germanium is not an essential nutrient for humans.

A germanium-deficient diet fed to rats has been found to alter the mineral composition of bone and liver and decrease DNA in the tibia. Little more is known about the biologic role of this element.

Typical daily dietary intakes of germanium range from about 0.4 to 1.5 milligrams. Plant foods, such as wheat, vegetables, bran and leguminous seeds, are rich sources of germanium. Animal foods are low in germanium.

Some organic complexes of germanium are reported to inhibit tumor growth in animals. Some humans who con-

sumed high amounts of these organic germanium supplements, which were contaminated with germanium dioxide (which is nephrotoxic), died from renal failure.

The main nutritional supplement form of germanium is known as Ge-132, Germanium-132, germanium sesquioxide or bis-carboxyethyl germanium sesquioxide. This is a synthetic organic product. It has not been found naturally. Noteworthy is that many of the clinical trials studying the effect of germanium on subjects with various cancers used another synthetic germanium compound, spirogermanium or 8,8-diethyl-N,N-dimethyl-2-aza-8-germaspiro (4,5) decane-2-propranamine dihydrochloride. Spirogermanium has great toxicity, especially neurotoxicity. Spirogermanium is not sold as a nutritional supplement.

Topical products containing inorganic germanium are marketed in Japan for relief of pain and swelling.

ACTIONS AND PHARMACOLOGY
ACTIONS
Bis-carboxyethyl germanium sesquioxide, Ge-132, may have antiproliterative activity. Ge-132 may also have antioxidant activity.

MECHANISM OF ACTION
The mechanism of the possible antiproliferative activity is unknown. Ge-132 is not effective in cell culture. It is speculated that Ge-132's possible antiproliferative activity is due to immune enhancement. There are reports that Ge-132 stimulates natural killer (NK) cell and cytotoxic T lymphocyte activity, as well as increased production of interferon.

Ge-132 was reported to prevent paraquat-induced hepatic oxidant injury in mice. The mechanism of this possible antioxidant effect is unknown.

PHARMACOKINETICS
Reported studies indicate that about 30% of an ingested dose of Ge-132 is absorbed from the small intestine. Little metabolism of Ge-132 appears to occur, and the substance is mainly excreted by the kidneys.

INDICATIONS AND USAGE
There are no indications for the use of supplemental germanium. Some inorganic forms of germanium, such as germanium dioxide, have been shown to be severely toxic to the liver and kidneys, resulting in some fatalities. Some organic forms of germanium, notably germanium lactate citrate, have also been shown to be severely toxic. The risk of contamination in putatively non-toxic forms of supplemental germanium outweighs any possible benefits, none of which, in any case, is yet well established.

RESEARCH SUMMARY
The Food and Drug Administration reported in 1997 that at least 31 human cases linked intake of germanium products

with renal failure and, in some cases, death. Other adverse effects noted included anemia, muscle weakness and peripheral neuropathy. The total dose (not the daily dose) ingested in the cases reported on varied from 15 to more than 300 grams. Exposure varied from two to 36 months.

The Center For Food Safety and Applied Nutrition concluded: "Based on the evidence of persistent renal toxicity associated with germanium dioxide, the lack of conclusive findings of differential nephrotoxicity of organic germanium compounds, and the possibility of contamination of the organic germanium products with inorganic germanium, it is clear that germanium products present a potential human health hazard."

Some case histories are instructive. Based upon claims that germanium is an "anti-cancer" and "immunostimulatory" agent, a 25-year-old woman with stage II HIV disease consumed a total of 47 grams of germanium-lactate-citrate 18%. She developed severe renal insufficiency and hepatomegaly. A 55-year-old woman who consumed a similar amount of germanium compounds over a 19-month period was admitted to a hospital with general malaise, muscular weakness, anorexia and weight loss. She was found to have renal failure and muscular and nerve damage. Her decline soon ended in death. Other deaths have been reported in those who used germanium compounds as a general elixir, as well as in attempts to treat specific disorders.

A recent report described complete remission of pulmonary spindle cell carcinoma in a patient taking large doses of germanium sesquioxide. However, this would be considered pharmaceutical, not nutritional usage of this substance.

CONTRAINDICATIONS, PRECAUTIONS, ADVERSE REACTIONS

CONTRAINDICATIONS

Those with renal failure or those who are at risk for renal problems (for example, those with diabetes and those on potentially nephrotoxic drugs).

PRECAUTIONS

Because of the possibility of contamination of Ge-132 with germanium-containing compounds known to be toxic, including germanium dioxide and germanium lactate citrate, use of Ge-132 supplements requires extreme caution and is not recommended. Although pure Ge-132 has not yet been associated with renal failure, this possibility has not been ruled out.

Children, pregnant women, nursing mothers, those with renal failure and those with diabetes should absolutely avoid Ge-132 supplements. Also, those taking potentially nephrotoxic drugs should avoid Ge-132.

ADVERSE REACTIONS

Adverse reactions reported for those taking Ge-132—supposedly 100% pure—include nausea, diarrhea and skin eruptions. Germanium dioxide and germanium lactate citrate are nephrotoxic. Spirogermanium causes neurotoxicity and pulmonary toxicity.

Adverse effects reported for germanium dioxide and germanium lactate citrate, in addition to nephrotoxicity, include anemia, muscle weakness and peripheral neuropathy.

INTERACTIONS

There are no known interactions with Ge-132. There is always the possibility that Ge-132 might potentiate the nephrotoxicity of potentially nephrotoxic drugs.

OVERDOSAGE

Overdosage with pure Ge-132 has not been reported. However, overdosage with other forms of germanium has; in at least one case, multiple organ dysfunction, shock and death occurred.

DOSAGE AND ADMINISTRATION

No recommended dose. Germanium, in the form of Ge-132, also known as Germanium-132, germanium sesquioxide and bis-carboxyethyl germanium sesquioxide, is available as a nutritional supplement in capsules containing 30 to 150 milligrams. It is also available as a powder. Those who decide to use these supplements are cautioned to dose only under strict medical supervision and to be certain that the supplement (Ge-132) they are taking is 100% pure. Germanium may also be present in colloidal or liquid mineral preparations.

LITERATURE

Hess B, Raisin J, Zimmermann A, et al. Tubulointerstitial nephropathy persisting 20 months after discontinuation of chronic intake of germanium lactate citrate. *Am J Kidney Dis.* 1993; 21:548-552.

Kuebler JP, Tormey DC, Harper GR, et al. Phase II study of spirogermanium in advanced breast cancer. *Canc Treat Report.* 1984; 68:1515-1516.

Mainwaring MG, Poor C, Zander DS, Harman E. Complete remission of pulmonary spindle cell carcinoma after treatment with oral germanium sesquioxide. *Chest.* 2000; 117:591-593.

Nielsen FH. Ultratrace minerals. In: Shils ME, Olson JA, Shike M, Ross AC, eds. *Modern Nutrition in Health and Disease*, 9th ed. Baltimore MD: Williams and Wilkins; 1999:283-303.

Raisin J, Hess B, Blatter M, et al. [Toxicity of an organic germanium compound: deleterious consequences of a "natural remedy."] [Article in German.] *Schweiz Med Wochenschr.* 1992; 122:11-13.

Sanai T, Okuda S, Onoyama K, et al. Chronic tubulointerstitial changes induced by germanium dioxide in comparison with carboxyethylgermanium sesquioxide. *Kidney Int.* 1991; 40:882-890.

Schauss AG. Nephrotoxicity in humans by the ultratrace element germanium. *Ren Fail.* 1991; 13:1-4.

Shamir M, Sprung CL. [Fatal multiple organic system dysfunction associated with germanium metal used in complementary therapy.] [Article in Hebrew.] *Harefuah.* 1997; 133; 446-447, 502.

Takeuchi A, Yoshizawa N, Oshima S, et al. Nephrotoxicity of germanium compounds: report of a case and review of the literature. *Nephron.* 1992; 60:436-442.

Glandulars

DESCRIPTION

The term glandulars as used in the nutritional supplement marketplace refers to dried and ground-up raw animal glandular and nonglandular tissues or extracts of these tissues. The tissues include those from the following glands and organs: adrenal, thyroid, thymus, testis, ovary, pituitary, liver, pancreas, spleen, kidney, lung, heart, brain, uterus and prostate. Glandulars are believed by some to improve the function of the gland or organ from which the extract was produced. Most of these substances are derived from bovine sources; some are derived from ovine sources and some from porcine sources.

Glandulars and other tissue extracts have had roles in traditional medicine. At one time, extract of bone marrow was used as a hematinic agent for the treatment of iron-deficiency anemia. Desiccated thyroid is still used by many physicians in the management of hypothyroidism. Desiccated thyroid is the cleaned, dried and powdered thyroid gland, purified of fat and connective tissue; it is derived principally from hogs, but also from cows and sheep. Thymus extracts are being studied for their possible immunomodulatory activity.

ACTIONS AND PHARMACOLOGY

ACTIONS

The different glandulars and glandular extracts have various putative activities. Thymus and spleen extracts have putative immunomodulatory activities. Thyroid extracts have putative activity in managing hypothyroidism. Adrenal extracts have putative antiallergic and anti-inflammatory activities. Testis extracts have putative androgenic activity, and ovary extracts have putative estrogenic activity.

MECHANISM OF ACTION

For the most part, the various putative actions of the glandulars may be explained by the hormones and other factors that these tissue extracts contain. However, most of the glandulars marketed as nutritional supplements are unlikely to have physiologically meaningful levels of these bioactive substances. Some immune-modulatory substances have been isolated from thymus extracts as well as spleen extracts. Desiccated natural thyroid is available as a prescription drug for the management of hypothyroidism. The pharmaceutical preparation is standardized and contains both thyroxine and triiodothyronine. Thyroid extracts marketed as nutritional supplements are not allowed to have these hormones in them. Adrenal extracts may contain some cortisol. Cortisol does have anti-inflammatory and anti-allergic activities, but the amount of cortisol in the supplements is likely to be too low to have meaningful physiological activity. Testis extracts and ovary extracts contain testosterone and estrogen, respectively, but again, the amount of these hormones in the glandular supplements are unlikely to be physiologically significant.

PHARMACOKINETICS

The components of the various glandular supplements are digested, absorbed and metabolized by normal physiological processes.

INDICATIONS AND USAGE

Glandulars are said to have gland-restorative activity, immunomodulatory effects, androgenic and estrogenic properties and various rejuvenating qualities. A pharmaceutical thyroid preparation is used to treat hypothyroidism, but supplemental thyroid products are not useful for this purpose and should not be substituted for pharmaceutical therapy. Testis and ovary supplements, similarly, should not be substituted for androgen and estrogen therapies recommended by physicians. Claims, including antiallergy and anti-inflammatory claims, made for glandular supplements are not supported by credible evidence.

RESEARCH SUMMARY

There is no credible evidence showing that supplemental glandulars rejuvenate glands.

Most clinical trials, which have been few in number, have produced non-significant results using glandulars. Some have shown immunomodulatory effects, but these findings are inconclusive.

CONTRAINDICATIONS, PRECAUTIONS, ADVERSE REACTIONS

CONTRAINDICATIONS

Glandulars are contraindicated in those who are hypersensitive to any component of a glandular-containing supplement.

Supplemental testis extracts are contraindicated in those with cancer of the prostate or benign prostatic hypertrophy (BPH).

Supplemental ovary extracts are contraindicated in those with breast cancer, ovarian cancer and uterine cancer and in those at risk for these cancers.

PRECAUTIONS

Glandulars should be avoided by pregnant women, nursing mothers and children.

Glandulars marketed as nutritional supplements should never be used for estrogen replacement, androgen replacement, thyroid replacement or cortisol replacement.

DOSAGE AND ADMINISTRATION

No recommended doses.

LITERATURE

Kouttab NM, Prada M, Cazzola P. Thymodulin: biological properties and clinical applications. *Med Oncol Tumor Pharmacother.* 1989; 6:5-9.

Valesini G, Barnaba V, Benvenuto R, et al. A calf thymus acid lysate improves clinical symptoms and T-cell defects in the early stages of HIV inflection. Second report. *Eur J Cancer Clin Oncol.* 1987; 23:1915-1919.

Wysocki J, Wicrusz-Wysocka B, Wykratowicz A, Wysocki H. The influence of thymus extracts on the chemotaxis of polymorphonuclear neutrophils (PMN) from patients with insulin-dependent diabetes mellitus (IDD). *Thymus.* 1992; 20:63-67.

Also, see Liver Hydrolysate/Desiccated Liver.

Glucomannan

DESCRIPTION

Glucomannan is a hydrocolloidal polysaccharide comprised of D-glucose and D-mannose residues (hence, the name) bonded together in beta-1,4 linkages. Approximately 60% of the polysaccharide is made up of D-mannose and approximately 40%, of D-glucose. Some of the sugar residues in glucomannan are acetylated. The molecular weight of this slightly branched polysaccharide ranges from 200 kilodaltons to 2,000 kilodaltons.

Glucomannan, which is also classified as a soluble dietary fiber, is derived from konjac flour. Konjac flour itself is derived from the *Amorphophallus* species, plants which are related to the common philodendron house plant and which grow in only certain parts of the world, including some regions in China and Japan. One member of the *Amorphophallus* genus called *Amorphophallus konjac*, is also known as voodoo lilly, devil's tongue and konjac. Konjac flour, however is derived from the tubers of various species of *Amorphophallus*, and the term konjac is used generically for the various species, as well as for the flour from their tubers. In addition to being known as konjac, the plant is called ju ruo (pronounced in Chinese) by the Chinese people, and called konjaku or konnyaku by the Japanese.

Konjac flour has a long history of use in both China and Japan as a food substance and as a folk remedy. Glucomannan products are widely used in Japan and China as general health aids, topically, for skin care and as a thickening agent for foods, among other things. Glucomannan, sometimes called konjac mannan, is marketed in the United States as a dietary supplement. Polysaccharides containing D-mannose and D-glucose in similar proportions to that found in konjac flour are found in other organisms, such as certain yeasts. Yeast glucomannan is not marketed as a dietary supplement.

ACTIONS AND PHARMACOLOGY

ACTIONS

Glucomannan may have laxative activity. It may also have activity in the control of serum glucose and lipid levels. Glucomannan has putative bariatric activity.

MECHANISM OF ACTION

The laxative effect of glucomannan is thought to be due to the swelling of glucomannan with consequent increase in stool bulk.

Some studies indicate that glucomannan may improve glycemic control in Type 2 diabetics. The mechanism of this effect is unclear. Glucomannan may delay the absorption of carbohydrates by increasing gastric-emptying time and/or decreasing small intestinal transit time.

The mechanism of glucomannan's possible hypocholesterolemic activity is likewise, unclear. The polysaccharide may stimulate the conversion of cholesterol to bile acids, as well as the fecal excretion of bile acids. Glucomannan may also decrease the intestinal absorption of cholesterol.

The putative bariatric (weight reduction) effect of glucomannan is not well understood. The swelling of glucomannan that occurs when it absorbs water in the gastrointestinal tract may confer a feeling of satiety in some.

PHARMACOKINETICS

Following ingestion of glucomannan, very little of it is digested in the small intestine. Glucomannan is resistant to hydrolysis by the digestive enzymes. Significant degradation occurs in the large intestine via the action of colonic bacteria. Products of degradation in the large intestine, include formic acid, acetic acid, butyric acid, propionic acid, beta-1,4-D-mannobiose (4-O-beta-D-mannopyranosyl-D-mannopyranose), cellobiose (4-O-beta-D-glucopyranosyl-D-glucopyranose), 4-O-beta-D-glucopyr-anosyl-D-mannopyranose, glucose and mannose. There may be some absorption of these degradation products from the large intestine. Most of them are excreted in the feces, along with unchanged glucomannan. Butyrate is used as a respiratory fuel by the colonocytes.

INDICATIONS

Glucomannan has demonstrated some usefulness in the management of obesity, diabetes and constipation. It has some favorable effects on lipids.

RESEARCH SUMMARY

Some studies have demonstrated that glucomannan has some efficacy in the management of obesity. In an eight-week, double-blind study, 20 obese subjects received 1 gram of glucomannan or placebo daily. Subjects were instructed not to change eating or exercise habits. Glucomannan-supplemented subjects had a significant mean weight loss of 5.5 pounds. Serum cholesterol and LDL cholesterol were significantly reduced, as well, in the treated group.

In a double-blind trial, this one involving 60 children under age 15 with childhood obesity, there was a significant reduction in weight in both treated and placebo groups. Further, there was a concomitant significant reduction in alpha-lipoprotein and an increase in triglycerides in the treated group but not in the placebo group. However, in another controlled study of childhood obesity, excess weight and triglycerides were significantly decreased in treated subjects but not in controls.

In a 3-month study of severely obese patients, a hypocaloric diet therapy by itself was tested against the same hypocaloric diet in combination with 4 grams of glucomannan (in three doses) daily. The combination therapy resulted in more significant weight loss in relation to fatty mass alone, in an overall improvement in lipid status and carbohydrate tolerance and a greater adherence to the diet. The researchers concluded: "Due to the marked ability to satiate patients and the positive metabolic effects, glucomannan diet supplements have been found to be particularly efficacious and well tolerated even in the long-term treatment of severe obesity."

Glucomannan, given in a long-term feeding program to baboons, showed beneficial effects on glucose homeostasis. Subsequently, it was shown that 2.6-grams and 5.2-grams daily doses of glucomannan, added to a carbohydrate rich breakfast in eight patients with previous gastric surgery, improved their reactive hypoglycemia and decreased the postprandial rise in plasma insulin. Benefits were achieved without unpalatability and carbohydrate malabsorption.

In a recent randomized, placebo-controlled metabolic trial, glucomannan was found to improve metabolic control in high-risk Type 2 diabetic patients, as measured by glucose and lipid levels and blood pressure. More research is warranted.

Several studies have demonstrated that glucomannan is an effective treatment for many with chronic constipation. This has been demonstrated in double-blind, placebo-controlled and multicenter studies. One to 4 grams daily, in divided doses, are typically used in these studies of constipation.

CONTRAINDICATIONS, PRECAUTIONS, ADVERSE REACTIONS

CONTRAINDICATIONS

Glucomannan is contraindicated in those hypersensitive to any component of a glucomannan-containing product. It is also contraindicated in those with intestinal obstruction, difficulty in swallowing and esophageal narrowing.

PRECAUTIONS

Pregnant women and nursing mothers should avoid glucomannan supplements.

Glucomannan must be taken with adequate amounts of fluids. Inadequate fluid intake may cause glucomannan to swell and block the throat, esophagus or intestines.

Tablet forms of glucomannan should be avoided.

Glucomannan should not be taken before going to bed.

Type 2 diabetics who use glucomannan, may require adjustment of their antidiabetic medications.

ADVERSE REACTIONS

A few cases of esophageal obstruction have been reported with the use of glucomannan tablets. The most common adverse reactions are flatulence and abdominal distension. Diarrhea is occasionally reported.

INTERACTIONS

NUTRITIONAL SUPPLEMENTS

Fat-soluble vitamins (A, D, E, K): Concomitant intake of fat soluble vitamins and glucomannan may decrease the absorption of the fat-soluble vitamins.

FOODS

Glucomannan may decrease the absorption of fat-soluble vitamins found in foods.

OVERDOSAGE

Glucomannan overdosage has not been reported.

DOSAGE AND ADMINISTRATION

Glucomannan supplements are mainly available in capsules. Glucomannan powder is also available and there are glucomannan combination products.

Doses used range from one to four grams daily, taken in divided doses and with plenty of liquids.

LITERATURE

Arvill A, Bodin L. Effect of short-term ingestion of konjac glucomannan on serum cholesterol in healthy men. *Am J Clin Nutr.* 1995; 61:585-589.

Doi K, Matsuura M, Kawara A, et al. Influence of dietary fiber (konjac mannan) on absorption of vitamin B_{12} and vitamin E. *Tohoku J Exp Med*. 1983; 141 Suppl:677-681.

Henry DA, Mitchell AS, Aylward J, et al. Glucomannan and risk of oesophageal obstruction. *Br Med J*. 1986; 292:591-592.

Hopman WP, Houben PG, Speth PA, Lamers CB. Glucomannan prevents postprandial hypoglycemia in patients with previous gastric surgery. *Gut*. 188; 29:930-934.

Hou YH, Zhang LS, Zhou HM, et al. Influences of refined konjac meal on the levels of tissue lipids and the absorption of four minerals in rats. *Biomed Environ Sci*. 1990; 3:306-314.

Livieri C, Novazi F, Lorini R. [The use of highly purified glucomannan-based fibers in childhood obesity]. [Article in Italian]. *Pediatr Med Chir*. 1992; 14:195-198.

Matsuura Y. Degradation of konjac glucomannan by enzymes in human feces and formation of short-chain fatty acids by intestinal anaerobic bacteria. *J Nutr Sci Vitaminol (Tokyo)*. 1998; 44:423-436.

Melga P, Giusto M, Ciuchi E, et al. [Dietary fiber in the dietetic therapy of diabetes mellitus. Experimental data with purified glucomannans]. [Article in Italian]. *Riv Eur Sci Med Farmacol*. 1992; 14:367-373.

Passaretti S, Franzoni M, Comin U, et al. Action of glucomannans on complaints in patients affected with chronic constipation: a multicentric clinical evaluation. *Ital J Gastroenterol*. 1991; 23:421-425.

Staiano A, Simeone D, Del Giudice E, et al. Effect of the dietary fiber glucomannan on chronic constipation in neurologically impaired children. *J Pediatr*. 2000; 136:41-45.

Venter CS, Vorster HH, Van der Nest DG. Comparison between physiological effects of konjac-glucomannan can propionate in baboons fed "Western" diets. *J Nutr*. 1990; 120:1046-1053.

Vido L, Facchin P, Antonello I, et al. Childhood obesity treatment: double blinded trial on dietary fibres (glucomannan) versus placebo. *Padiatr Padol*. 1993; 28:133-136.

Vita PM, Restelli A, Caspani P, Klinger R. [Chronic use of glucomannan in the dietary treatment of severe obesity]. [Article in Italian]. *Minerva Med*. 1992; 83:135-139.

Vorster HH, De Jager J. The effect of the long-term ingestion of konjac-glucomannan on glucose tolerance and immunoreactive insulin values of baboons. *S Afr Med J*. 1984; 65:805-808.

Vuksan V, Jenkins DJ, Spadofora P, et al. Konjac-mannan (glucommanan) improves glycemia and other associated risk factors for coronary heart disease in Type 2 diabetes. A randomized controlled metabolic trial. *Diabetes Care*. 1999; 22:913-919.

Vuksan V, Sievenpiper JL, Owen R, et al. Beneficial effects of viscous Konjac-mannan in subjects with the insulin resistance syndrome. *Diabetes Care*. 2000; 23:9-14.

Walsh DE, Yaghoubian V, Behforooz A. Effect of glucomannan on obese patients: a clinical study. *Int J Obesity*. 1984; 8:289-293.

Glucosamine

DESCRIPTION

Glucosamine is an amino monosaccharide found in chitin, glycoproteins and glycosaminoglycans (formerly known as mucopolysaccharides) such as hyaluronic acid and heparan sulfate. Glucosamine is also known as 2-amino-2-deoxyglucose, 2-amino-2-deoxy-beta-D-glucopyranose and chitosamine. Glucosamine has the following chemical structure:

Glucosamine

Glucosamine is available commercially as a nutritional supplement in three forms: glucosamine hydrochloride or glucosamine HCl, glucosamine sulfate and N-acetylglucosamine.

At neutral as well as physiologic pH, the amino group in glucosamine is protonated, resulting in its having a positive charge. Salt forms of glucosamine contain negative anions to neutralize the charge. In the case of glucosamine hydrochloride, the anion is chloride, and in glucosamine sulfate the anion is sulfate. N-acetylglucosamine is a delivery form of glucosamine in which the amino group is acetylated, thus neutralizing its charge. To date, most of the clinical studies examining the effect of glucosamine on osteoarthritis have been performed with either the sulfate or the chloride salts of glucosamine. All three forms are water soluble.

The glucosamine used in supplements is typically derived from marine exoskeletons. Synthetic glucosamine is also available.

ACTIONS AND PHARMACOLOGY

ACTIONS

The actions of supplemental glucosamine have yet to be clarified. It may play a role in the promotion and maintenance of the structure and function of cartilage in the joints of the body. Glucosamine may also have anti-inflammatory properties.

MECHANISM OF ACTION

Until the specific actions of supplemental glucosamine are determined, the mechanism of action in relieving arthritic pain and in repair of cartilage is a matter of speculation. However, we do know a great deal about the biochemistry of the molecules in which glucosamine is found. Biochemically, glucosamine is involved in glycoprotein metabolism. Glycoproteins, known as proteoglycans, form the ground substance in the extra-cellular matrix of connective tissue. Proteoglycans are polyanionic substances of high-molecular weight and contain many different types of heteropolysaccharide side-chains covalently linked to a polypeptide-chain backbone. These polysaccharides make up to 95% of the proteoglycan structure. In fact, chemically, proteoglycans resemble polysaccharides more than they do proteins.

The polysaccharide groups in proteoglycans are called glycosaminoglycans or GAGs. GAGs include hyaluronic acid, chondroitin sulfate, dermatan sulfate, keratan sulfate, heparin and heparan sulfate. All of the GAGs contain derivatives of glucosamine or galactosamine.

Glucosamine derivatives are found in hyaluronic acid, keratan sulfate and heparan sulfate. Chondroitin sulfate contains derivatives of galactosamine.

The glucosamine-containing glycosaminoglycan hyaluronic acid is vital for the function of articular cartilage. GAG chains are fundamental components of aggrecan found in articular cartilage. Aggrecan confers upon articular cartilage shock-absorbing properties. It does this by providing cartilage with a swelling pressure that is restrained by the tensile forces of collagen fibers. This balance confers upon articular cartilage the deformable resilience vital to its function.

In the early stages of degenerative joint disease, aggrecan biosynthesis is increased. However, in later stages, aggrecan synthesis is decreased, leading eventually to the loss of cartilage resiliency and to most of the symptoms that accompany osteoarthritis.

During the progression of osteoarthritis, exogenous glucosamine may have a beneficial role. It is known that, *in vitro*, chondrocytes do synthesize more aggregan when the culture medium is supplemented with glucosamine. N-acetylglucosamine is found to be less effective in these *in vitro* studies. Glucosamine has also been found to have antioxidant activity and to be beneficial in animal models of experimental arthritis.

The counter anion of the glucosamine salt (i.e. chloride or sulfate) is unlikely to play any role in the action or pharmacokinetics of glucosamine. Further, the sulfate in glucosamine sulfate supplements should not be confused with the glucosamine sulfate found in such GAGs as keratan sulfate and heparan sulfate. In the case of the supplement, sulfate is the anion of the salt. In the case of the above GAGs, sulfate is present as an ester. Also, there is no glucosamine sulfate in chondroitin sulfate.

PHARMACOKINETICS

The pharmacokinetics of glucosamine is derived primarily from animal studies. About 90% of glucosamine administered orally as a glucosamine salt gets absorbed from the small intestine, and from there it is transported via the portal circulation to the liver. It appears that a significant fraction of the ingested glucosamine is catabolized by first-pass metabolism in the liver. Free glucosamine is not detected in the serum after oral intake, and it is not presently known how much of an ingested dose is taken up in the joints in humans. Some uptake in the articular cartilage is seen in animal studies.

INDICATIONS AND USAGE

Large recent studies have cast doubt on the claim that glucosamine may confer significant benefits in osteoarthritis, either alone or in combination with chondroitin sulfate (see Chondroitin Sulfate). Some believe, however, that the proper formulation of glucosamine may indeed confer significant benefits in some with osteoarthritis.

RESEARCH SUMMARY

Glucosamine alone and in combination with chondroitin sulfate has become one of the biggest sellers in the supplement supermarket, used by millions in an attempt to prevent and alleviate symptoms of arthritis and for bone/joint health generally. Some early studies indicated significant efficacy. Recently, however, large studies have emerged that call much of the prior positive evidence into some degree of question. Some contend, however, that when the "proper" form of glucosamine is used good results are obtained. Older studies are analyzed first below, followed by summaries of the more recent, less positive work and an explanation of the ensuing and ongoing controversy.

Two meta-analyses dating back some years reported that glucosamine is useful in the treatment of osteoarthritis. One of these meta-analyses included all double-blind, placebo-controlled trials that lasted four weeks or longer. This meta-analysis also included trials that studied the effects of chondroitin sulfate (see Chondroitin Sulfate). In all, there were 13 of these studies (six involving glucosamine and seven involving chondroitin sulfate).

All 13 studies found positive results in hip or knee osteoarthritis. The authors of the meta-analysis judged a trial positive if there was 25% or more improvement in the treatment group compared with placebo. The Levesque Index and global pain scores were used to assess improvement. Very significant improvement was associated with both glucosamine (39.5%) and chondroitin sulfate (40.2%), compared with placebo.

In another meta-analysis of nine randomized, controlled trials of glucosamine, glucosamine was significantly superior to placebo in seven of the studies and was superior to ibuprofen and equal to ibuprofen in the other two studies.

A long-term, randomized placebo-controlled trial of glucosamine sulfate's effects on osteoarthritis ended with the conclusion that the supplement halts progression of structural joint damage and reduces symptoms of those with osteoarthritis of the knee. The study involved 212 patients 50 years or older who received 1500 milligrams of glucosamine sulfate daily or placebo.

Radiographic evidence, at a three-year follow-up, showed joint space narrowing–the prime indicator of arthritic joint damage–in the placebo group consistent with what has been documented to be typical in untreated osteoarthritis. The glucosamine-supplemented subjects, on the other hand, showed only a non-significant increase in joint space at the same three-year follow-up.

In another study there was an apparent synergistic effect using glucosamine and chondroitin together. The combination was more effective than either substance alone in inhibiting progression of degenerative cartilage lesions in an experimental study.

The idea that glucosamine might be effective in osteoarthritis was based, in part, on the following: Glucosamine is crucial for the construction of glycosaminoglycans (GAGs) in articular cartilage. Reduced GAG content in osteoarthritic cartilage matrix corresponds with the severity of osteoarthritis. Oral glucosamine appears to be capable of prompting the chondrocytes to secrete more GAGs. This knowledge, derived from animal and *in vitro* studies, has prompted clinical trials of glucosamine in osteoarthritis.

In contrast with the positive findings of past years, recent research has yielded generally, but not entirely, negative results, surprising many researchers. The Glucosamine/chondroitin Arthritis Intervention Trial (GAIT) was a randomized, double-blind, placebo and active comparator (celecoxib) controlled trial of 1,583 individuals with symptomatic osteoarthritis of the knee. Those randomized to receive the drug celecoxib had significant reduction in knee pain, compared with placebo. The glucosamine/chondroitin group, however, fared no better than those on placebo. This National Institutes of Health-funded study involved 16 participating clinics. Some subjects were randomized to receive only glucosamine hydrochloride (500 mg three times daily), only chondroitin sulfate (400 mg three times daily), combination chondroitin/glucosamine (in the same dosages)

or 200 mg celecoxib daily. Study agents were mandated to be of pharmaceutical grade, since previous inquiries have confirmed that both glucosamine and chondroitin products are not infrequently at variance with labeling, i.e., are inconsistent in content and potency, especially from one product to another.

The study, though overall negative, was not wholly without positive findings. In one subgroup of patients with moderate-to-severe knee pain at entry, some benefit was seen in those receiving the combination chondroitin/glucosamine supplement. An improvement in knee joint swelling that reached statistical significance was noted in those taking chondroitin sulfate alone. Notable was the very high placebo-response level in this study, a finding that has plagued other studies of these substances in osteoarthritis patients. Such findings are believed by some to make detection of positive responses more difficult. Nonetheless, the statistical robustness of the major negative finding was of high magnitude, imparting a high level of confidence in its accuracy. A *post hoc* analysis of the chondroitin sulfate subjects in whom knee swelling relief was statistically confirmed indicated that the best results were obtained in those with relatively milder symptoms and baseline radiographic changes.

An editorial accompanying the GAIT study in *The New England Journal of Medicine* said it was unfortunate that the inquiry did not use glucosamine sulfate instead of glucosamine hydrochloride, since several other studies had previously shown that the hydrochloride was not efficacious, whereas some other data seemed to indicate that the sulfate was. Nevertheless, the editorialist found the GAIT findings compelling and concluded: "On the basis of the results from GAIT, it seems prudent to tell our patients with symptomatic osteoarthritis of the knee that neither glucosamine hydrochloride nor chondroitin sulfate alone has been shown to be more efficacious than placebo for the treatment of knee pain." The editorialist further recommended that if individuals use glucosamine that they use glucosamine sulfate, rather than glucosamine hydrochloride and that they consider using a combination glucosamine sulfate and chondroitin sulfate for the possible additive effect. The editorial stated that there is no evidence that these substances can have any preventive effects in healthy persons or in persons with knee pain but normal radiographs. Three months of treatment was said to be adequate to test the substances for possible efficacy at the doses typically recommended.

This editorial pointed out that it was not surprising that glucosamine hydrochloride was not effective, given the results of recent systematic reviews and meta-analyses. These showed that when either glucosamine hydrochloride from any source or glucosamine sulfate *not* manufactured by Rottapharm, maker of the only glucosamine product approved as a drug in Europe, were used no positive effects were found in knee osteoarthritis. By contrast, when the Rottapharm glucosamine sulfate was compared with placebo in seven randomized trials, the glucosamine was significantly better than placebo in reducing pain and/or improving function. (In three other trials, however, the Rottapharm product was no better than placebo.)

One group of researchers has taken the position that even the data involving the Rottapharm product cannot be relied upon, attributing differences in results variable in terms of glucosamine forms, products, dosages and trial designs to industry involvement and funding. An editorial in *Arthritis & Rheumatism* recently took exception to that conclusion. It pointed to the pharmaceutical status of the Rottapharm glucosamine sulfate product, the general consistency of well-designed studies using the product and the fact that the European League Against Rheumatism has assigned its highest ratings to the glucosamine sulfate data involving the product. The editorial argued that industry participation in studies has been shown to improve, rather than degrade, design quality in many cases. The editorial pointed out that, since the Rottapharm product is an approved drug in all European Union countries and in another 50 countries worldwide and not simply another largely unregulated supplement, as they said was implied in the meta-analysis, it was appropriate and usual for the pharmaceutical originator of the product to be involved in and funding the studies. The editorial also noted that a panel of researchers expert in this field recently concluded that the Rottapharm product may, indeed, be superior to others, based upon, among other things, a finding that the Rottapharm product produces higher plasma concentrations of glucosamine than do other products, such as those used in the GAIT study. The levels seen with the Rottapharm product were said to exhibit a strong correlation with synovial fluid levels in a range demonstrated *in vitro* to inhibit interleukin-1-induced gene expression. This mechanism, the editorialist observed, has replaced the older hypothesis of direct stimulation of glycoaminoglycan synthesis "that may contribute only marginally, if at all, to the overall effect, unless through the availability of sulfate ions."

Authors of the critical meta-analysis were faulted in this editorial for failing to "apply the principles of a sound systematic review ... but instead put together different efficacy outcomes and trial designs by mixing 4-week studies with 3-year trials, intramuscular/intra-articular administration with oral ones, and low-quality small studies reported in the early 1980s with high-quality studies reported in 2007." The editorial concluded that while industry interference in trial outcomes must always be guarded against, there was no direct evidence of that in these trials,

and that conflicts of interest "by declared independent investigators, including financial (e.g., grants) and non-financial aspects, may be at least as much a cause for concern" in any/all research.

More recently still, an editorial in *The Annals of Internal Medicine* declared that "the jury is still out" on glucosamine sulfate's possible favorable role in osteoarthritis. After 40 years of investigation, the definitive studies related to this issue still remain to be done. They are needed and warranted.

CONTRAINDICATIONS, PRECAUTIONS, ADVERSE REACTIONS

CONTRAINDICATIONS
Known hypersensitivity to a glucosamine-containing product.

WARNINGS AND PRECAUTIONS
Glucosamine may increase insulin resistance. Glucosamine increases insulin resistance in normal and experimentally diabetic animals. In these animals, intravenous glucosamine significantly decreases the rate of glucose uptake in skeletal muscle. In animals given oral glucosamine, this is not observed.

Those with type 2 diabetes and those who are overweight and have problems with glucose tolerance should have their blood sugars carefully monitored if they use glucosamine supplements. Because of insufficient safety data, children, pregnant women and nursing mothers should avoid using glucosamine.

ADVERSE REACTIONS
Side effects that have been reported are mainly mild gastrointestinal complaints such as heartburn, epigastric distress and diarrhea. No allergic reactions have been reported including sulfa-allergic reactions to glucosamine sulfate.

INTERACTIONS
Glucosamine may increase insulin resistance and consequently affect glucose tolerance. Diabetics who, under medical advisement, decide to use glucosamine supplements will need to monitor their blood glucose and may need to adjust the doses of the medications they take to control blood glucose. This needs to be done under medical supervision. No other drug, nutritional supplement, food or herb interaction is known.

OVERDOSAGE
None known.

DOSAGE AND ADMINISTRATION
The three forms of glucosamine available commercially are glucosamine hydrochloride, glucosamine sulfate and N-acetyl glucosamine. The usual dose used by those with osteoarthritis is 1,500 mg daily in divided doses. These three forms of glucosamine are available in 500 mg capsules.

The amount of glucosamine base varies with the supplemental form. Pure glucosamine hydrochloride is about 83% in glucosamine base, pure glucosamine sulfate is about 65% in glucosamine base, and pure N-acetyl glucosamine, about 75% in glucosamine base. It is important that all clinical studies standardize the glucosamine dose of the form used to glucosamine base.

Supplements are available containing glucosamine and low-molecular-weight chondroitin sulfate. (See Chondroitin Sulfate.)

It usually takes several weeks of supplementation before effects, if any, are noted.

LITERATURE

Bijlsma JW, Lafeber FP. Glucosamine sulfate in osteoarthritis: the jury is still out. *Ann Intern Med.* 2008;148(4):315-316.

Bruyere O, Pavelka K, Rovati LC, et al. Total joint replacement after glucosamine sulphate treatment in knee osteoarthritis: results of a mean 8-year observation of patients from two previous 3-year, randomised, placebo-controlled trials. *Osteoarthritis Cartilage.* 2008;16(2):254-260.

Bruyere O, Reginster JY. Glucosamine and chondroitin sulfate as therapeutic agents for knee and hip osteoarthritis. *Drugs Aging.* 2007;24(7):573-580.

Clegg DO, Reda DJ, Harris CL, et al. Glucosamine, chondroitin sulfate, and the two in combination for painful knee osteoarthritis. *N Engl J Med.* 2006;354(8):795-808.

Deal CL, Moskowitz RW. Nutraceuticals as therapeutic agents in osteoarthritis. The role of glucosamine, chondroitin sulfate, and collagen hydrolysate. *Rheum Dis Clin North Am.* 1999;25:379-395.

Distler J, Anguelouch A. Evidence-based practice: review of clinical evidence on the efficacy of glucosamine and chondroitin in the treatment of osteoarthritis. *J Am Acad Nurse Pract.* 2006;18(10):487-493.

Drovanti A, Bignamini AA, Rovati AL. Therapeutic activity of oral glucosamine sulfate in osteoarthritis, a placebo-controlled double-blind investigation. *Clin Ther.* 1980;3:260-272.

Felson DT. Glucosamine sulfate might have no effect on pain or structural changes associated with osteoarthritis. *Nat Clin Pract Rheumatol.* 2008;4(10):518-519.

Hochberg MC. Nutritional supplements for knee osteoarthritis—still no resolution. *N Engl J Med.* 2006;354(8):858-60.

Houpt JB, McMillan R, Wein C, et al. Effect of glucosamine hydrochloride in the treatment of pain of osteoarthritis of the knee. *J Rheumatol.* 1999;26:2423-2430.

Leffler CT, Philippi AF, Leffler SG, et al. Glucosamine, chondroitin, and manganese ascorbate for degenerative joint disease of the knee or low back: a randomized double-blind, placebo-controlled pilot study. *Mil Med.* 1999;64:85-91.

McAlindon TE, LaValley MP, Gulin JP, et al. Glucosamine and chondroitin for treatment of osteoarthritis: a systematic quality assessment and meta-analysis. *JAMA.* 2000;283(11):1469-1475.

McClain DA, Crook, ED. Hexosamines and insulin resistance. *Diabetes.* 1996; 45:l003-l006.

Nelson JL, Robergs RA. Exploring the potential ergogenic effects of glycerol hyperhydration. *Sports Med.* 2007;37(11):981-1000.

Noack W, Fischer, M., Forster, KK, et al. Glucosamine sulfate in osteoarthritis of the knee. *Osteoarthritis Cartilage.* 1994;2:51-59.

Poolsup N, Suthisisang C, Channark P, et al. Glucosamine long-term treatment and the progression of knee osteoarthritis: systematic review of randomized controlled trials. *Ann Pharmacother.* 2005;39(6):1080-1087.

Pujalte JM, Llavore EP, Ylescupidez FR. Double-blind evaluation of oral glucosamine sulfate in the basic treatment of osteoarthritis. *Curr Med Res Opin.* 1980;7:110-114.

Reginster JY. The efficacy of glucosamine sulfate in osteoarthritis: financial and nonfinancial conflict of interest. *Arthritis Rheum.* 2007;56(7):2105-2110.

Reginster JY, Bruyere O, Neuprez A. Current role of glucosamine in the treatment of osteoarthritis. *Rheumatology* (Oxford). 2007;46(5):731-735.

Reginster JY, Deroisy R, Rovati LC, et al. Long-term effects of glucosamine sulphate on osteoarthritis progression: a randomised, placebo-controlled clinical trial. *Lancet.* 2001;357(9252):251-256.

Reichelt A, Forster K, Fisher M, et al. Efficacy and safety of intramuscular glucosamine sulfate in osteoarthritis of the knee. A randomized, placebo-controlled, double-blind study. *Arzneimittelforschung.* 1999;44:75-80.

Richy F, Bruyere O, Ethgen O, et al. Structural and symptomatic efficacy of glucosamine and chondroitin in knee osteoarthritis: a comprehensive meta-analysis. *Arch Intern Med.* 2003;163(13):1514-1522.

Rozendaal RM, Koes BW, van Osch GJ, et al. Effect of glucosamine sulfate on hip osteoarthritis: a randomized trial. *Ann Intern Med.* 2008;148(4):268-277.

Setnikar I, Giacchetti C, Zanolo G. Pharmacokinetics of glucosamine in the dog and in man. *Arzneimittelforschung.* 1986;36:729-735.

Setnikar I, Palumbo R, Canali S, et al. Pharmacokinetics of glucosamine in man. *Arzneimittelforschung.*1993;43:1109-1113.

Sutton L, Rapport L, Lockwood B. Glucosamine: con or cure? Part I. *Nutrition.* 2002;18(6):534-536.

Sutton L, Rapport L, Lockwood B. Glucosamine: con or cure? Part II. *Nutrition.* 2002;18(7-8):693.

Towheed TE, Anastassiades TP. Glucosamine and chondroitin for treating symptoms of osteoarthritis. Evidence is widely touted but incomplete. *JAMA.* 2000;283:1483-1484.

Towheed TE, Anastassiades TP. Glucosamine therapy for osteoarthritis. Editorial. *JRheumatol* 1999;26:2294-2297.

Vlad SC, LaValley MP, McAlindon TE, et al. Glucosamine for pain in osteoarthritis: why do trial results differ? *Arthritis Rheum.* 2007;56(7):2267-2277.

Glutamine Peptides

DESCRIPTION

Glutamine peptides refer to certain dipeptides used in total parenteral nutrition (TPN) as delivery forms of L-glutamine. The term also refers to peptides containing L-glutamine, which are found in some nutritional supplements, particularly those marketed as sports and fitness products.

L-glutamine depletion is a typical feature of such metabolic stress conditions as trauma (including surgical trauma), infection, sepsis, cancer and severe burns. The metabolic response to these conditions is characterized by catabolism and negative nitrogen balance. Under these conditions, L-glutamine, which is normally manufactured by the body (mainly in skeletal muscles) in sufficient quantities to satisfy physiological demands, is required exogenously. Under these conditions, L-glutamine becomes an essential amino acid and must be supplied to the body in order to prevent breakdown of muscle tissue, immune dysfunction and compromise of the gut mucosal barrier function with consequent bacterial translocation into the body. L-glutamine is arguably the most needed amino acid and, indeed, one of the most needed nutrients under these circumstances.

Until recently, L-glutamine was lacking from TPN. The reason for this is because L-glutamine is not very soluble in water—one gram dissolves in 20.8 ml of water at 30 degrees Celsius—and L-glutamine is unstable in solution. The problem has been solved by the synthesis of glutamine-containing dipeptides, which are very soluble in water and stable in solution.

Two synthetic glutamine-containing dipeptides that may be used in TPN are L-alanyl-L-glutamine (Ala-Gln) and glycyl-L-glutamine (Gly-Gln). The molecular weight of Ala-Gln is 217.24 daltons, and L-glutamine comprises 67% of the dipeptide. L-glutamine comprises 72% of Gly-Gln, and its molecular weight is 203.22 daltons.

ACTIONS AND PHARMACOLOGY

ACTIONS

Glutamine peptides may have immunomodulatory, anticatabolic/anabolic, gut mucosal barrier-protective and antioxidant actions.

MECHANISM OF ACTION

The glutamine dipeptides, Ala-Gln and Gly-Gln, have demonstrated immunomodulatory, anticatabolic/anabolic, gastrointestinal mucosal protective and antioxidant activities when used in TPN. These activities have not yet been demonstrated with glutamine peptides marketed as nutritional supplements for fitness purposes. The mechanism of the immunomodulatory action of the glutamine dipeptides is unclear. The mechanism may in part be due to the ability of L-glutamine to ameliorate the negative effects of TPN on the immune system. Also, L-glutamine is the preferred respiratory fuel for lymphocytes and appears to be required to support the proliferation of mitogen-stimulated lymphocytes, as well as the production of interleukin-2 (IL-2) and interferon-gamma (IFN-gamma). It also appears to be required for the maintenance of lymphokine-activated killer cells (LAK). It can also enhance phagocytosis by neutrophils and monocytes.

The anticatabolic/anabolic action of the glutamine dipeptides can be explained by their effect in sparing skeletal muscle L-glutamine stores. Most of the L-glutamine in the body is synthesized in skeletal muscle, where it is also stored. Under conditions of metabolic stress, skeletal muscle can be depleted of its L-glutamine, which is used for metabolic activities of other tissue/cells, such as enterocytes and lymphocytes.

The gastrointestinal mucosal-protective effect of the glutamine dipeptides can be explained in a few ways. L-glutamine is the preferred respiratory fuel for enterocytes and colonocytes. Maintaining the bioenergetics of these cells is fundamental to maintaining the integrity of the intestine. In addition, L-glutamine helps maintain secretory IgA, which functions primarily by preventing the attachment of bacteria to mucosal cells. L-glutamine may inhibit translocation of Gram-negative bacteria from the intestine into the body.

Metabolic stress goes hand in hand with oxidative stress. L-glutamine can help in ameliorating oxidative stress by serving as precursor to glutathione.

PHARMACOKINETICS

Glutamine dipeptides in TPN are transported via the circulation to the various tissues of the body, where they are taken up by cells and metabolized. Ala-Gln is first metabolized to L-alanine and L-glutamine, while Gly-Gln is metabolized to glycine and L-glutamine. L-glutamine participates in various metabolic activities, including the production of L-glutamate and other amino acids, glutathione, energy, proteins, pyrimidine and purine nucleotides and amino sugars. L-glutamine is eliminated by glomerular filtration and is almost completely reabsorbed by the renal tubules.

Most of the glutamine dipeptides administered orally or enterally are absorbed intact from the lumen of the small intestine into the enterocytes. A portion of the glutamine dipeptides gets metabolized within the enterocytes. That which is not metabolized enters the portal circulation from whence it is transported to the liver. Again, some metabolism takes place in the liver, and that portion not metabolized enters the systemic circulation and is distributed to various tissues of the body.

INDICATIONS AND USAGE

Like glutamine itself (see Glutamine), the dipeptide forms added to TPN are credited with helping in the recovery of trauma, surgical and other critically ill patients. There is as yet no credible evidence that oral use of glutamine peptide supplements has anabolic or ergogenic effects in those who are not metabolically compromised.

RESEARCH SUMMARY

Studies have shown that glutamine and glutamine dipeptides exert similar metabolic effects. The dipeptides themselves are now being used in clinical nutrition.

In one recent, double-blind, randomized, controlled study, duration of hospital stay was significantly reduced in patients who had undergone major abdominal surgery and who had received glutamine dipeptides via TPN over a five-day period. Mean cumulative nitrogen balance was significantly better in these patients, as was immune function, as measured by lymphocyte counts and generation of cysteinyl leukotrienes by polymorphonuclear neutrophils, a measure of neutrophil function.

CONTRAINDICATIONS, PRECAUTIONS, ADVERSE REACTIONS

CONTRAINDICATIONS

Glutamine peptides are contraindicated in those hypersensitive to any component of a glutamine peptide-containing product.

PRECAUTIONS

The use of glutamine dipeptides in TPN must be done under medical supervision.

Those with renal and liver failure should exercise caution in the use of glutamine peptide supplements.

Pregnant women and nursing mothers should avoid the use of oral glutamine peptide supplements unless prescribed by their physicians.

ADVERSE REACTIONS

There are rare reports of constipation and bloating with high dose glutamine peptides in TPN.

INTERACTIONS

DRUGS

See L-Glutamine.

OVERDOSAGE

No reports of overdosage.

DOSAGE AND ADMINISTRATION

The use of glutamine dipeptides in TPN is relatively recent. The two synthetic dipeptides used are L-alanyl -L-glutamine and glycyl-L-glutamine. Doses suggested (given as L-glutamine) are 12 grams daily for surgical trauma and about 25 grams daily for severe trauma and infections.

Those who use oral glutamine peptide supplements for fitness or sports purposes use 1.5 to 4.5 grams (as L-glutamine) daily.

LITERATURE

Decker-Baumann C, Buhl K, Frohmuller S, et al. Reduction of chemotherapy-induced side-effects by parenteral glutamine supplementation in patients with metastatic colorectal cancer. *Eur J Cancer.* 1999; 35:202-207.

Furst P, Pogan K, Stehle P. Glutamine dipeptides in clinical nutrition. *Nutrition.* 1997; 13:731-737.

Khan J, Iiboshi Y, Cui L, et al. Alanyl-glutamine-supplemented parenteral nutrition increases luminal mucus gel and decreases permeability in the rat small intestine. *J Parenter Enteral Nutr.* 1999; 23:24-31.

Li YS, L. JS, Jiang JW, et al. Glycyl-glutamine-enriched long-term total parenteral nutrition attenuates bacterial translocation following small bowel transplantation in the pig. *J Surg Res.* 1999; 82:106-111.

Minami H, Morse EL, Adibi SA. Characteristics and mechanism of glutamine-dipeptide absorption in human intestine. *Gastroenterology.* 1992; 103:3-11.

Morlion BJ, Stehle P, Wachtler P, et al. Total parenteral nutrition with glutamine dipeptide after major abdominal surgery: a randomized, double-blind, controlled-study. *Ann Surg.* 1998; 227:302-308.

Schroder J, Kahlke V, Fandrich F, et al. Glutamine dipeptide-supplemented parenteral nutrition reverses gut mucosal structure and interleukin-6 release of rat intestinal mononuclear cells after hemorrhagic shock. *Shock.* 1998; 10:26-31.

Glutathione

DESCRIPTION

The term glutathione is typically used as a collective term to refer to the tripeptide L-gamma-glutamyl-L-cysteinylglycine in both its reduced and dimeric forms. Monomeric glutathione is also known as reduced glutathione and its dimer is also known as oxidized glutathione, glutathione disulfide and diglutathione. In this monograph, reduced glutathione will be called glutathione— this is its common usage by biochemists—and the glutathione dimer will be referred to as glutathione disulfide.

Glutathione is widely found in all forms of life and plays an essential role in the health of organisms, particularly aerobic organisms. In animals, including humans, and in plants, glutathione is the predominant non-protein thiol and functions as a redox buffer, keeping with its own SH groups those of proteins in a reduced condition, among other antioxidant activities. Glutathione has the following structural formula:

Glutathione

Glutathione is present in tissues in concentrations as high as one millimolar. Cysteine, the business residue of glutathione, neither has the solubility nor activity of glutathione at physiological pH. It appears that nature has built the cysteine molecule into the glutathione tripeptide to make the amino acid more soluble and allow it to have redox buffering activity in a living tissue environment. Glutathione also plays roles in catalysis, metabolism, signal transduction, gene expression and apoptosis. It is a cofactor for glutathione S-transferases, enzymes which are involved in the detoxification of xenobiotics, including carcinogenic genotoxicants, and for the glutathione peroxidases, crucial selenium-containing antioxidant enzymes (see Selenium). It is also involved in the regeneration of ascorbate from its oxidized form, dehydroascorbate (see Vitamin C). There are undoubtedly roles of glutathione that are still to be discovered.

Glutathione is present in the diet in amounts usually less than 100 milligrams daily, and it does not appear that much of the oral intake is absorbed from the intestine into the blood (see Pharmacokinetics). Glutathione is not an essential nutrient since it can be synthesized from the amino acids L-cysteine, L-glutamate and glycine. It is synthesized in two ATP-dependent steps: first, gamma-glutamylcysteine is synthesized from L-glutamate and cysteine via the enzyme gamma-glutamylcysteine synthetase—the rate limiting step— and second, glycine is added to the C-terminal of gamma-glutamylcysteine via the enzyme glutathione synthetase. The liver is the principal site of glutathione synthesis. In healthy tissue, more than 90% of the total glutathione pool is in the reduced form and less than 10% exists in the disulfide form. The enzyme glutathione disulfide reductase is the principal enzyme that maintains glutathione in its reduced form. This latter enzyme uses as its cofactor NADPH (reduced nicotinamide adenine dinucleotide phosphate). NADPH is generated by the oxidative reaction in the pentose phosphate pathway.

The consequences of a functional glutathione deficiency, which results in tissue oxidative stress, can be seen in some pathological conditions. For example, those with glucose 6-phosphate dehydrogenase deficiency produce lower amounts of NADPH and hence, lower amounts of reduced glutathione. This condition is characterized by a hemolytic anemia. Conditions causing chronic glutathione deficiency all result in hemolytic anemia, among other pathological consequences. Oxidative stress caused by glutathione deficiency results in fragile erythrocyte membranes. Malaria-causing organisms (*Plasmodia* species) do not like to feed on these sick erythrocytes. That is about the only good news regarding this situation. Chronic functional glutathione deficiency is also associated with immune disorders, an increased incidence of malignancies, and in the case of HIV disease, probably accelerated pathogenesis of the disease. Acute manifestations of functional glutathione deficiency can be seen in those who have taken an overdosage of acetaminophen. This results in depletion of glutathione in the hepatocytes, leading to liver failure and death, if not promptly treated.

Glutathione is an orphan drug for the treatment of AIDS-associated cachexia. It is thought that this disorder is due, in part, to oxidatively-stressed and damaged enterocytes. There is some evidence that although orally administered glutathione may not be absorbed into the blood from the small intestine to any significant extent, that it may be absorbed into the enterocytes where it may help repair damaged cells. Glutathione in one form or another is the subject of some medicinal chemistry research and some clinical trials. For example, an aerosolized form of glutathione is being studied in AIDS and cystic fibrosis patients. Glutathione, the principal antioxidant of the deep lung, appears to be diminished in those with AIDS. Prodrugs of gamma-L-glutamyl-L-cysteine are being evaluated as anticataract agents.

Glutathione (reduced) is known chemically as N-(N-L-gamma-glutamyl-L-cysteinyl)glycine and is abbreviated as GSH. Its molecular formula is $C_{10}H_{17}N_3O_6S$ and its molecular weight is 307.33 daltons. Glutathione disulfide is also known as L-gamma-glutamyl-L-cysteinyl-glycine disulfide and is abbreviated as GSSG. Its molecular formula is $C_{20}H_{32}N_6O_{12}S_2$.

The marketed glutathione dietary supplement products are obtained from yeast fermentation, as is the orphan drug. L-Cysteine and N-acetylcysteine are precursors of glutathione and are also available as dietary supplements (see L-Cysteine and N-Acetylcysteine).

ACTIONS AND PHARMACOLOGY

ACTIONS

Glutathione has antioxidant activity. It may have detoxification, and immunomodulatory activities, and may have beneficial effects on sperm motility and in the protection against noise-induced hearing loss.

MECHANISM OF ACTION

Glutathione is the principal intracellular nonprotein thiol and plays a major role in the maintenance of the intracellular redox state. It may be thought of as an intracellular redox buffer. Glutathione is a nucleophilic scavenger and an electron donor via the sulfhydryl group of its business residue, cysteine. Its reducing ability maintains molecules such as ascorbate and proteins in their reduced state. Glutathione is also the cofactor for the selenium-containing glutathione peroxidases (see Selenium), which are major antioxidant enzymes. These enzymes detoxify peroxides, such as hydrogen peroxide and other peroxides. Another antioxidant activity of glutathione is the maintenance of the antioxidant/reducing agent ascorbate in its reduced state. This is accomplished via glutathione-dependent dehydroascorbate reductase which is comprised of glutaredoxin and protein isomerase reductase. Glutathione may also react with the reactive nitrogen species peroxynitrite to form *S*-nitrosoglutathione.

Glutathione S-transferases (GSTs) consist of a family of multifunctional enzymes that metabolize a wide variety of electrophilic compounds via glutathione conjunction. GSTs are involved in the detoxification of xenobiotic compounds and in the protection against such degenerative diseases as cancer. The mechanism of these enzymes involves a nucleophilic attack by glutathione on an electrophilic substrate. The resulting glutathione conjugates that form are more soluble than the original substrates and thus more easily exported from the cell. The release of glutathione-S-conjugates from cells is an ATP-dependent process mediated by membrane glycoproteins belonging to the multidrug-resistance protein (MRP) family. Proteins of the MRP family are essential for the transport of glutathione S-conjugates into the extracellular space. They are also known as glutathionine-S-conjugate pumps.

Absorption of orally administered glutathione has been observed in some animals (mice, rats, guinea pigs). Oral glutathione has been demonstrated to reverse age-associated decline in immune responsiveness in mice. In one study, glutathione was found to enhance T-cell mediated responsiveness, including delayed-type hypersensitivity (DTH). The mechanism of this effect was ascribed to the antioxidant activity of glutathione.

Parenterally administered glutathione was found to improve sperm motility in a small human trial. Again, the effect was thought to be due to the antioxidant activity of this substance.

Noise-induced hearing loss is thought to be due to oxidative stress. Intraperitoneal administration of glutathione to guinea pigs was found to protect against noise-induced hearing loss and once more, the antioxidant activity of glutathione was thought to account for this effect.

PHARMACOKINETICS

The pharmacokinetics of oral glutathionine in humans are not well understood. It appears that in some animals (mice, rats, guinea pigs), serum glutathione levels do increase following its oral administration. Most human studies of glutathione have not found this to be the case. It appears that oral glutathione is hydrolyzed in the intestine via the intestinal gamma-glutamyl transferase enzyme. A small amount of orally administered glutathione may reach the portal circulation, but apparently this is also rapidly metabolized by hepatic gamma-glutamyltransferase. Thus, most studies have not observed a significant increase in circulating glutathione following its oral administration. However, there is an occasional study that does show an increase in circulating glutathione after oral administration. Further, there is some evidence that glutathione may be absorbed into the enterocytes following ingestion, but may not be released by these cells into the circulation. Research is needed to resolve the issue of glutathione absorption.

INDICATIONS AND USAGE

Though glutathione is undoubtedly a potent antioxidant, indications for its use as a supplement are not yet well established. There is preliminary evidence that it might eventually prove to be useful in the management of some cancers, atherosclerosis, diabetes, lung disorders, noise-induced hearing loss, male infertility and to help prevent or ameliorate various toxicities. It may also have some anti-viral activity. Glutathione is an orphan drug for the treatment of AIDS-associated cachexia.

RESEARCH SUMMARY

The use of glutathione in cancer treatment has been two-fold. It has been investigated as an antitumor agent in its own right and as a chemoprotectant used to diminish the toxicities of some cancer drugs. In one animal study, glutathione produced significant regression of aflatoxin-induced liver cancers and significantly enhanced survival. All rats exposed to aflatoxin but not given glutathione died within 24 months of exposure to the carcinogen, but 81% of the glutathione-treated animals were still alive at the end of the 24 months. The researchers concluded that the glutathione-effect noted in this study "strongly suggests that this antioxidant merits further investigation as a potential antitumor agent in humans."

Human cancer studies, so far, have utilized glutathione in a secondary role—principally to protect against the toxicity of cisplatin. Its role in this regard has been found effective in several studies wherein it has been demonstrated to diminish cisplatin-induced nephrotoxicity and neurotoxicity.

Early research indicates that exogenous glutathione may significantly inhibit platelet aggregation and improve other hemostatic and hemorheological factors in atherosclerotic patients. In other preliminary clinical work, glutathione has been found to help preserve renal function in patients who had coronary artery bypass operations.

A glutathione aerosol preparation has been helpful in reversing the oxidant-antioxidant imbalance in idiopathic pulmonary fibrosis, and it has helped suppress lung epithelial surface inflammatory cell-derived oxidants in patients with cystic fibrosis. Similar aerosol treatment has been given to HIV patients to augment deficient glutathione levels of the lower respiratory tract with the idea of improving host defense in these immuno-compromised individuals. More research is needed.

Glutathione has also been shown to enhance insulin secretion in elderly subjects with impaired glucose tolerance. There are some further preliminary indications that glutathione might be helpful in some with diabetes, but more research is needed before any meaningful conclusions can be made.

In a double-blind, placebo-controlled study, injected gluta-thione demonstrated a significant positive effects on sperm motility and morphology in infertile men. And, finally, in another study that needs followup, glutathione exhibited significant *in vitro* inhibition of herpes simplex virus type 1 replication. It appears that the mechanism of this effect is due to glutathione's redox-modulating active. Some viral infections, including HIV infection, result in oxidative stress which may be a major mechanism of their pathogenesis, Modulating oxidative stress could be an antiviral maneuver.

CONTRAINDICATIONS, PRECAUTIONS, ADVERSE REACTIONS

CONTRAINDICATIONS

Glutathione is contraindicated in those hypersensitive to any component of a glutathione-containing product.

PRECAUTIONS

Pregnant women and nursing mothers should avoid the use of supplementary glutathione.

Glutathione is an orphan drug for the treatment of AIDS-associated cachexia. Its use for this indication must be medically supervised.

ADVERSE REACTIONS

Oral doses of up to 600 milligrams daily are well tolerated. There are no reports of adverse reactions.

INTERACTIONS

DRUGS

Cisplatin: Glutathione, administered parenterally, may ame-liorate some of the adverse reactions of cisplatin.

OVERDOSAGE

There have been no reports of glutathione overdosage in the literature.

DOSAGE AND ADMINISTRATION

Glutathione is available as a single ingredient dietary supplement or in combination products. Dosage ranges from 50 to 600 milligrams daily.

LITERATURE

Anderson ME, Luo JL. Glutathione therapy: from prodrugs to genes. *Semin Liver Dis*. 1998; 18:415-424.

Aw TW, Wierzbicka G, Jones DP. Oral glutathione increases tissue glutathione in vivo. *Chem Biol Interact*. 1991; 80:89-97.

Bains JS, Shaw CA. Neurodegenerative disorders in humans: the role of glutathione in oxidative stress-mediated neuronal death. *Brain Res Brain Res Rev*. 1997; 25:335-358.

Borok Z, Buhl R, Grimes GJ, et al. Effect of glutathione aerosol on oxidant-antioxidant imbalance in ideopathic pulmonary fibrosis. *Lancet*. 1991; 338:215-216.

Broquist HP. Buthionine sulfoximine, an experimental tool to induce glutathionine deficiency: elucidation of glutathionine and ascorbate in their role as antioxidants. *Nutr Rev*. 1992; 50:110-111.

Brown LA, Bai C, Jones DP. Glutathione protection in aveolar type II cells from fetal and neonatal rabbits. *Am J Physiol*. 1992; 262:L305-L312.

Cascinu S, Cordella L, Del Ferro E, et al. Neuroprotective effect of reduced glutathione on cisplatin-based chemotherapy in advanced gastric cancer: a randomized double-blind placebo-controlled study. *J Clin Oncol*. 1995; 13:26-32.

Cheung P-Y, Wang W, Schulz R. Glutathione protects against ischemia-perfusion injury by detoxifying peroxynitrite. *J Mol Cell Cardiol*. 2000; 32:1669-1678.

De Mattia G, Bravi MC, Laurenti O, et al. Influence of reduced glutathione infusion on glucose metabolism in patients with non-insulin-dependent diabetes mellitus. *Metabolism*. 1998; 47:993-997.

Exner R, Wessner B, Manhart N, Roth E. Therapeutic potential of glutathione. *Wien Klin Wochenschr*. 2000; 112:610-616.

Favilli F, Marraccini P, Iantomasi T, Vincenzini MT. Effect of orally administered glutathione levels in osme organs of rats: role of specific transporters. *Br J Nutr*. 1997; 78:293-300.

Flagg EW, Coates RJ, Eley JW, et al. Dietary glutathione intake in humans and the relationship between intake and plasma total glutathionine level. *Nutr Canc.* 1994; 21:33-46.

Furukawa T, Meydani SN, Blumberg JB. Reversal of age-associated decline in immune responsiveness by dietary glutathione supplementation in mice. *Mech Ageing Dev.* 1987; 38:107-117.

Griffith OW. Biologic and pharmacologic regulation of mammalian glutathione synthesis. *Free Rad Biol Med.* 1999; 27:922-935.

Hagen TM, Jones DP. Transepithelial transport of glutathione in vascularly perfused small intestine of rat. *Am J Physiol.* 1987; 252(5 Pt 1):G607-G613.

Hagen TM, Wierzbicka GT, Sillau AH, et al. Bioavailability of dietary glutathione: effect on plasma concentration. *Am J Physiol.* 1990; 259(4 Pt 1):G524-G529.

Hayes JD, McLellan LI. Glutathione and glutathione-dependent enzymes represent a co-ordinately regulated defence against oxidative stress. *Free Rad Res.* 1999; 31:273-300.

Hayes JD, Strange RC. Glutathione S-transferase polymorphisms and their biological consequences. *Pharmacology.* 2000; 61:154-166.

Hercbergs A, Brok-Simoni F, Holtzman F, et al. Erythrocyte glutathione and tumor response to chemotherapy. *Lancet.* 1992; 339:1074-1076.

Holroyd KJ, Buhl R, Borok Z, et al. Correction of glutathione deficiency in the lower respiratory tract of HIV seropositive individuals by glutathione aerosol treatment. *Thorax.* 1993; 48:985-989.

Hwang C, Sinskey AJ, Lodish HF. Oxidized redox state of glutathione in the endoplasmic reticulum. *Science.* 1992; 257:1496-1502.

Janaky R, Ogita K, Pasqualotta BA, et al. Glutathione and signal transduction in the mammalian CNS. *J Neurochem.* 1999; 73:889-902.

Lash LH, Hagen TM, Jones DP. Exogenous glutathione protects intestinal epithelial cells from oxidative injury. *Proc Natl Acad Sci USA.* 1986; 83:4641-4645.

Lenzi A, Culasso F, Gandini L, et al. Placebo-controlled, double-blind, cross-over trial of glutathione therapy in male infertility. *Hum Reprod.* 1993; 8:1657-1662.

Lenzi A, Picardo M, Gandini L, et al. Glutathione treatment of dyspermia: effect on the lipoperoxidation process. *Hum Reprod.* 1994; 9:2044-2050.

Loguercio C, Di Pierro M. The role of glutathione in the gastrointestinal tract: a review. *Ital J Gastroenterol Hepatol.* 1999; 31:401-407.

Lyons J, Rauh-Pfeiffer A, Yu YM, et al. Blood glutathione synthesis rates in healthy adults receiving a sulfur amino acid-free diet. *Proc Natl Acad Sci USA.* 2000; 97:5071-5076.

Martensson J, Jain A, Meister A. Glutathione is required for intestinal function. *Proc Natl Acad Sci USA.* 1990; 87:1715-1719.

Meister A. On the antioxidant effects of ascorbic acid and glutathionine. *Biochem Pharmacol.* 1992; 44:1905-1915.

Murphy ME, Scholich H, Sies H. Protection by glutathione and other thiol compounds against the loss of protein thiols and tocopherol homologs during microsomal lipid peroxidation. *Eur J Biochem.* 1992; 210:139-146.

Nagasawa HT, Cohen JF, Holleschau AM, Rathbun WB. Augmentation of human and rat lenticular glutathione in vitro by prodrugs of gamma-L-glutamyl-L-cysteine. *J Med Chem.* 1996; 39:1676-1681.

Novi AM. Regression of aflatoxin B$_1$-induced hepatocellular carcinomas by reduced glutathione. *Science.* 1981; 212:541-542.

Ohinataab Y, Yamasobac T, Schachta J, Millera JM. Glutathione limits noise-induced hearing loss. *Hear Res.* 2000; 146:28-34.

Palamara AT, Perno C-F, Ciriolo MR, et al. Evidence for antiviral activity of glutathione: in vitro inhibition of herpes simplex virus type 1 replication. *Antiviral Res.* 1995; 27:237-253.

Paolisso G, Giugliano D, Pizza G, et al. Glutathione infusion potentiates glucose-induced insulin secretion in aged patients with impaired glucose tolerance. *Diabetes Care.* 1992; 15:1-7.

Roum JH, Borok Z, McElvaney NG, et al. Glutathione aerosol suppresses lung epithelial surface inflammatory cell-derived oxidants in cystic fibrosis. *J Appl Physiol.* 1999; 87:438-443.

Samiec PS, Drews-Botsch C, Flagg EW, et al. Glutathione in human plasma: decline in association with aging, age-related macular degeneration, and diabetes. *Free Radic Biol Med.* 1998; 24:699-704.

Schmidinger M, Budinsky AC, Wenzel C, et al. Glutathione in the prevention of cisplatin induced toxicities. A prospectively randomized pilot trial in patients with head and neck cancer and non small cell lung cancer. *Wien Klin Wochenschr.* 2000; 112:617-623.

Shaw CA, ed. *Glutathione in the Nervous System.* London: Taylor and Francis; 1998.

Sies H. Glutathione and its role in cellular functions. *Free Rad Biol Med.* 1999; 27:916-921.

Smyth JF, Bowman A, Perren T, et al. Glutathione reduces the toxicity and improves quality of life of women diagnosed with ovarian cancer treated with cisplatin: results of a double-blind, randomized trial. *Ann Oncol.* 1997; 8:569-573.

Sternberg P Jr, Davidson PC, Jones DP, et al. Protection of retinal pigment epithelium from oxidative injury by glutathione and precursors. *Invest Opthalmol Vis Sci.* 1993; 34:3661-3668.

Witschi A, Reddy S, Stofer B, Lauterburg BH. The systemic availability of oral glutathione. *Eur J Clin Pharmacol.* 1992; 43:667-669.

Glycerol

DESCRIPTION

Glycerol is one of the most common alcohols found in human metabolism. It is a 3-carbon molecule containing three hydroxyl groups. Its molecular formula is $C_3H_8O_3$, and its molecular weight is 92.09 daltons. A syrupy liquid with a sweet taste, glycerol is about 0.6 times as sweet as cane sugar. Glycerol is also known as glycerin, glycerine, 1,2,3-propanetriol and trihydroxypropane. The structural formula for glycerol is:

Glycerol

Glycerol is the backbone of triacylglycerols (triglycerides or neutral fats) and phospholipids. These substances are present in most life forms, and dietary intake of glycerol comes mainly from these molecules in animal and plant products. Glycerol is also used as a sweetener in syrup, liquor and some foods.

Glycerol has had diverse uses in medicine. It has moisturizing and lubricating properties and can increase serum osmolality. It is given orally to reduce intraocular pressure and vitreous volume in eye surgery and is used as an adjunct in the management of acute glaucoma. Glycerol may also be used topically to reduce corneal edema, which may be of use in eye examinations. Glycerol has also been used (intravenously or orally) for the management of cerebral edema secondary to acute stroke, to lower intracranial pressure and to improve rehydration during acute gastrointestinal disease. It is a hyperosmotic laxative and may be used rectally in suppositories. It is used as a cerumenolytic and as a demulcent in cough preparations.

Oral glycerol by itself may have dehydrating activity. However, if ingested with added fluid, it may increase total body water. This is known as glycerol hyperhydration, and glycerol is used by some athletes to improve thermoregulation and endurance during exercise or exposure to hot environments.

ACTIONS AND PHARMACOLOGY

ACTIONS

Supplemental glycerol has putative hyperhydration and athletic performance-enhancing activities.

MECHANISM OF ACTION

The main effect of glycerol itself results from its dehydrating activity. For example, oral glycerol can increase serum osmolality, thus drawing fluid from other parts of the body. This is the mechanism, at least in part, for its ocular hypotensive effect in the treatment of acute glaucoma. Therefore, it seems paradoxical to talk about glycerol's hyperhydration effect. However, in combination with ample water, it may be more hydrating than water alone, at least for some. The mechanism of this effect and how it may relate to enhanced athletic performance is still highly unclear.

PHARMACOKINETICS

Following ingestion, glycerol is efficiently absorbed and rapidly metabolized. It is absorbed from the lumen of the small intestine into the enterocytes and from those cells into the portal circulation, from whence it is transported to the liver. In the hepatocytes, much of glycerol is phosphorylated via the enzyme glycerol kinase to produce L-glycerol 3-phophate. ATP is necessary for this reaction.

Some L-glycerol 3-phosphate reacts with fatty acyl CoA molecules to ultimately form triglycerides (triacylglycerols) and phospholipids. Most L-glycerol 3-phosphate undergoes oxidation to dihydroxyacetone phosphate, catalyzed either by cytosolic glycerol 3-phosphate dehydrogenase, an enzyme that requires NAD+ as electron receptor, or by mitochondrial glycerol 3-phosphate dehydrogenase. The coupling of the two glycerol 3-phosphate dehydrogenases leads to the passage of electrons from NADH to enter the mitochondrial electron transfer chain for the production of ATP. This transfer of electrons from cytosolic NADH to the mitochondrial electron transport chain is known as the glycerol phosphate shuttle. Dihydroxyacetone phosphate can either move in the direction of further oxidation to finally yield carbon dioxide, water and ATP or be converted to glyceraldehyde 3-phosphate and move in the direction of glucose and glycogen synthesis.

Glycerol not metabolized in the liver is transported to various tissues and undergoes metabolism. Similar reactions to those discussed above occur in the kidney.

Glycerol is eliminated in the kidney by filtration and, in concentrations up to 0.15 mg/ml, undergoes complete tubular reabsorption. In higher concentration, glycerol begins to appear in the urine and induces an osmotic diuresis.

The elimination half-life of glycerol is from 30 to 45 minutes.

INDICATIONS AND USAGE

Glycerol may be useful for improving hydration and, thus, exercise endurance in some, but research results related to this putative benefit are mixed. There is no evidence that glycerol helps with weight loss. Intravenous glycerol is helpful in some with acute ischemic cerebral infarct. Oral glycerol has been useful in preventing some of the neurologic and audiologic sequellae of childhood bacterial meningitis.

RESEARCH SUMMARY

Pre-exercise administration of glycerol significantly improved cycling endurance time in two double-blind, randomized, cross-over trials. Mean heart rate was also reduced in glycerol-supplemented subjects.

Pre-exercise administration of glycerol in another study, however, failed to affect exercise performance in a group of triathletes. Results of animal work have been similarly mixed. A recent review of the potential ergogenic effects of glycerol hyperhydration concluded that "although some investigators have indicated positive effects of glycerol hyperhydration on fluid retention, thermoregulation, cardiovascular responses and performance, others have shown no advantage to glycerol ingestion." What is clear, however, these reviewers asserted, is that "glycerol has the capacity to enhance fluid retention. This may provide a performance advantage when compared with fellow athletes who may experience a decrement in performance sooner rather than later." They have called for better-designed studies. Glycerol did not increase weight loss in a placebo-controlled trial.

Intravenous administration of glycerol in subjects with acute ischemic cerebral infarct has resulted in significantly fewer neurological deficits in one study. Several other trials demonstrating similar benefits have been double-blind, randomized trials, but some of these benefits have been transient.

Glycerol-treated infants and children with bacterial meningitis had less severe hearing impairment and fewer neurologic deficits than did controls. Oral administration of glycerol was utilized.

CONTRAINDICATIONS, PRECAUTIONS, ADVERSE REACTIONS

CONTRAINDICATIONS

Supplemental glycerol is contraindicated in those with severe dehydration, anuria, congestive heart failure and pulmonary edema. It is also contraindicated in those who are hypersensitive to glycerol.

PRECAUTIONS

Glycerol supplementation should be avoided by pregnant women and nursing mothers.

Those with cardiac, renal or hepatic problems should avoid supplemental glycerol, as should those with diabetes and those with hemolytic anemia.

Anyone using oral glycerol for supplementation must drink plenty of fluid concomitantly. See Dosing and Administration.

Those using glycerol need to be aware that contact of glycerol with strong oxidizing agents, such as potassium permanganate, potassium chlorate or chromium trioxide, may produce an explosion.

ADVERSE REACTIONS

There are rare reports of cardiac dysrhythmias occurring with oral glycerol use and one report of hypertension occurring. Other adverse reactions include headache, dizziness, confusion and amnesia (in elderly subjects) and hyperglycemia. Hyperosmolarity, which occurs with oral glycerol, is usually clinically significant only in those with type 2 diabetes. Those with type 2 diabetes may develop nonketotic hyperosmolar hyperglycemia.

The most frequent adverse reactions are gastrointestinal and include nausea and vomiting, bloating and diarrhea.

DOSAGE AND ADMINISTRATION

The doses are variable in those who use glycerol for hydration purposes and for possible exercise performance enhancement. Some use 2 to 4 tablespoons of glycerol in water, orange juice or a sports drink. The ratio of fluids to glycerol is about 20 to 1. This is taken approximately 2.5 hours prior to exercise. The volume of a tablespoon is 15 ml, and one ml of glycerol weighs 1.25 grams. The energy value of glycerol is about 4 kcal or 4 Cal per gram. Pharmaceutical grade glycerol is used.

LITERATURE

Inder WJ, Swanney MP, Donald RA, et al. The effect of glycerol and desmopressin on exercise performance and hydration in triathletes. *Med Sci Sports Exerc.* 1998;30:1263-1269.

Montner P, Stark DM, Riedesel ML, et al. Pre-exercise glycerol hydration improves cycling endurance time. *Int J Sports Med.* 1996;17:27-33.

Nelson JL, Robergs RA. Exploring the potential ergogenic effects of glycerol hyperhydration. *Sports Med.* 2007;37(11):981-1000.

Robergs RA, Griffin SE. Glycerol. Biochemistry, pharmacokinetics and clinical and practical applications. *Sports Med.* 1998;26:145-167.

Wagner DR. Hyperhydrating with glycerol: implications for athletic performance. *J Am Diet Assoc.* 1999;99:207-212.

Glycine

DESCRIPTION

Glycine is a protein amino acid found in the protein of all life forms. It is the simplest amino acid in the body and the only protein amino acid that does not have chirality. Although most glycine is found in proteins, free glycine is found in body fluids as well as in plants. The normal diet contributes approximately 2 grams of glycine daily.

Glycine is not considered an essential amino acid, i.e., the cells in the body can synthesize sufficient amounts of glycine to meet physiological requirements. However, glycine is of major importance in the synthesis of proteins, peptides, purines, adenosine triphosphate (ATP), nucleic acids, porphyrins, hemoglobin, glutathione, creatine, bile salts, one-carbon fragments, glucose, glycogen, and L-serine and other amino acids. Glycine is also a neurotransmitter in the central nervous system (CNS). Glycine and gamma-aminobutyric acid (GABA) are the major inhibitory neurotransmitters in the CNS. Recently, a glycine-gated chloride channel has been identified in neurophils that can attenuate increases in intracellular calcium ions and diminish oxidant damage mediated by these white blood cells. Thus, glycine may be a novel antioxidant.

Glycine is also known as amino acetic acid, aminoethanolic acid, glycocoll, glycinium and sucre de gelatine. Its IUPAC abbreviation is Gly and its one-letter abbreviation, used when spelling out protein structures, is G. It is a neutral amino acid. Glycine is a solid water-soluble substance that has a sweetish taste. Its structural formula is:

Glycine

ACTIONS AND PHARMACOLOGY
ACTIONS
Supplemental glycine may have antispastic activity. Very early findings suggest it may also have antipsychotic activity as well as antioxidant and anti-inflammatory activities.

MECHANISM OF ACTION
In the CNS, there exist strychnine-sensitive glycine binding sites as well as strychnine-insensitive glycine binding sites. The strychnine-insensitive glycine-binding site is located on the NMDA receptor complex. The strychnine-sensitive glycine receptor complex is comprised of a chloride channel and is a member of the ligand-gated ion channel superfamily. The putative antispastic activity of supplemental glycine could be mediated by glycine's binding to strychnine-sensitive binding sites in the spinal cord. This would result in increased chloride conductance and consequent enhancement of inhibitory neurotransmission.

The ability of glycine to potentiate NMDA receptor-mediated neurotransmission raised the possibility of its use in the management of neuroleptic-resistant negative symptoms in schizophrenia.

Animal studies indicate that supplemental glycine protects against endotoxin-induced lethality, hypoxia-reperfusion injury after liver transplantation, and D-galactosamine-mediated liver injury. Neutrophils are thought to participate in these pathologic processes via invasion of tissue and releasing such reactive oxygen species as superoxide. *In vitro* studies have shown that neutrophils contain a glycine-gated chloride channel that can attenuate increases in intracellular calcium and diminish neutrophil oxidant production. This research is early-stage, but suggests that supplementary glycine may turn out to be useful in processes where neutrophil infiltration contributes to toxicity, such as ARDS.

PHARMACOKINETICS
Following ingestion of glycine, the amino acid is absorbed from the small intestine via an active transport mechanism. From the small intestine, glycine is transported to the liver by means of the portal circulation where a portion enters into one of several metabolic pathways. Glycine not metabolized in the liver enters the systemic circulation and is distributed to various tissues in the body. Glycine readily crosses the blood-brain barrier.

INDICATIONS AND USAGE
Glycine may be indicated to help alleviate the symptoms of spasticity. An indication for potentiating some anti-convulsant drugs and preventing some seizures could emerge, as could an indication for its use in managing schizophrenia. Research in progress also suggests usefulness in some cancers. There is no evidence to support use of glycine as an ergogenic aid, and it is too early to say whether it can play any useful role in lipid metabolism. There are no well-designed clinical trials to support its use in benign prostate hypertrophy.

RESEARCH SUMMARY
Glycine first attracted interest in the medical research community for its reputed ability to dampen reflex excitability in the CNS. A pilot study of its effects on severe chronic leg spasticity (most of the subjects were suffering from chronic multiple sclerosis) yielded improvement in spasticity and mobility of the lower limbs, rated at about 25% overall. The dose used was 1 gram daily for six months to a year. All patients noted some benefits, and no adverse events were recorded. Other researchers have since reported that glycine can potentiate some but not all anticonvulsant drugs in some animal models. It has also been shown to prevent some experimentally produced seizures.

The effects of oral glycine (200 mg/kg/day) were tested in two siblings suffering from 3-phosphoglycerate dehydrogenase deficiency, an inborn error of L-serine biosynthesis. A significant amount of glycine is made from L-serine. Among the features of this disorder are intractable seizures. L-serine in doses up to 500 mg/kg/day failed to control the seizures, but oral glycine completely stopped them, and electroencephalographic abnormalities resolved after six months of treatment.

High-dose glycine may be beneficial in the management of enduring negative symptoms of schizophrenia. Twenty-two treatment-resistant schizophrenic patients participated in a double-blind, placebo-controlled, six-week, crossover treatment trial with 0.8 grams per kilogram daily of glycine added to their ongoing antipsychotic medication. Glycine intake ranged from 40 to 90 grams daily. Only mild gastrointestinal side effects (nausea and vomiting) were reported in one patient taking glycine. Patients taking glycine experienced significantly diminished negative symptoms. Followup studies are planned.

Recent animal studies suggest that glycine may have some anti-cancer properties. In one recent study, 51 weeks of glycine supplementation did not stop early foci formation of cancer but reduced formation of small liver tumors by 23%, medium-sized tumors by 64% and large tumors by nearly 80% in rats given an agent that is a peroxisome proliferator and liver carcinogen.

In another recent study, dietary glycine inhibited B16 melanoma tumors in mice. Glycine-supplemented mice had tumors that were 50 to 70% smaller in size than those in controls. The protective mechanism in this case appeared to be inhibition of angiogenesis effected by suppressed endothelial-cell proliferation. Tumors in mice fed glycine had 70% fewer arteries than were present in the tumors of controls.

Whether very preliminary data suggesting some positive effects of glycine on lipid metabolism will be mirrored in human research remains to be seen.

Partly because glycine is a precursor of creatine, some have assumed that it might have some of the same ergogenic potential that has been claimed for creatine. This, so far, has not been demonstrated. Glycine is claimed to be beneficial for benign prostatic hypertrophy based on a dated clinical study that has never been confirmed.

CONTRAINDICATIONS, PRECAUTIONS, ADVERSE REACTIONS

CONTRAINDICATIONS

Glycine supplementation is contraindicated in those hypersensitive to any component of the preparation. It is also contraindicated in those who are anuric (some glycine gets converted to ammonia).

PRECAUTIONS

Glycine supplementation should be avoided by pregnant women and nursing mothers. Because of some conversion of glycine to ammonia, those with hepatic impairment should avoid glycine supplementation unless prescribed.

ADVERSE REACTIONS

Doses of 1 gram daily are very well tolerated. Mild gastrointestinal symptoms are infrequently noted. In one study doses of 90 grams daily were also well tolerated.

INTERACTIONS

Antispastic drugs. Theoretically, supplemental glycine might have additive effects when used in conjunction with baclofen, diazepam, dantrolene sodium and tizanidine.

No other drug, nutritional supplement, food or herb interactions are known.

OVERDOSAGE

There are no reports of overdosage in humans. The majority of mice receiving 3 to 4.5 grams per kilogram by intravenous infusion experienced bradycardia, prolongation of the PQ interval, QRS duration and death.

DOSAGE AND ADMINISTRATION

Glycine is available in 500 milligram tablets and capsules. Those who supplement use up to 1 gram daily in divided doses. Doses used for management of schizophrenia have ranged from 40 to 90 grams daily.

LITERATURE

Barbeau A. Preliminary study of glycine administration in patients with spasticity. *Neurol.* 1974; 24:392.

de Kooning JT, Duran M, Dorling L, et al. Beneficial effects of L-serine and glycine in the management of seizures in 3-phosphoglycerate dehydrogenase deficiency. *Ann Neurol.* 1998; 44:261-265.

Heresco-Levy U, Javitt DC, Ermilov M, et al. Efficacy of high-dose glycine in the treatment of enduring negative symptoms of schizophrenia. *Arch Gen Psychiatry.* 1999; 56:29-36.

Olsson J, Hahn RG. Glycine toxicity after high-dose i.v. infusion of 1.59 % glycine in the mouse. *Br J Anaest.* 1999; 82:250-254.

Rose ML, Cattley RC, Dunn C, et al. Dietary glycine prevents the development of liver tumors caused by the peroxisome proliferator WY-14, 643. *Carcinogenesis.* 1999; 20:2075-2081.

Rose ML, Madren J, Bunzendahl H, Thurman RG. Dietary glycine inhibits the growth of B16 melanoma tumors in mice. *Carcinogenesis.* 1999; 20:793-798

Simpson RK Jr, Gondo M, Robertson CS, Goodman JC. The influence of glycine and related compounds on spinal cord injury-related spasticity. *Neurochem Res.* 1995; 20:1203-1210.

Simpson RK Jr, Robertson CS, Goodman JC. The role of glycine in spinal shock. 1996; 19:215-224.

Smith JE, Hall PV, Galvin MR, et al. Effects of glycine administration on canine experimental spinal spasticity and the levels of glycine, glutamate, and aspartate in the lumbar spinal cord. *Neurosurg.* 1979; 4:153-156.

Toth E, Lajtha A. Glycine potentiates the action of some anticonvulsant drugs in some seizure models. *Neurochem Res.* 1984; 9:1711-1718.

Wheeler M, Stachlewitz RT, Yamashina S, et al. Glycine-gated channels in neutrophils attenuate calcium influx and superoxide production. FASEB J. 2000; 14:476-484.

Wheeler MD, Ikejema K, Mol Life Sci. Enomoto N, et al. Glycine: a new anti-inflammatory immunonutrient. *Cell Mol Life Sci.*1999; 56:843-856.

Yagasaki K, Funabiki R. Effects of dietary supplemented amino acids on endogenous hypercholesterolemia in rats. *J Nutr Sci Vitaminol.* 1990; 36 Suppl 12:S165-S168.

Glycitein

DESCRIPTION

Glycitein belongs to the isoflavone class of flavonoids. It is also classified as a phytoestrogen since it is a plant-derived nonsteroidal compound that possesses estrogen-like biological activity. Glycitein has been found to have weak estrogenic activity.

Glycitein is the aglycone of glycitin. The isoflavone is found naturally as the glycoside (glucoside) glycitin and as the glycosides 6″-0-malonylglycitin and 6″-0-acetylglycitin. Glycitein and its glycosides are mainly found in legumes, such as soybeans and chickpeas. Soybeans and soy foods are the major dietary sources of these substances. Glycitein glycosides are the least abundant of the isoflavones in soybeans and soy foods, where they comprise about 5 to 10% of the total isoflavones. However, in soy germ, glycitein glycosides comprise about 40% of the isoflavones.

Glycitein is a solid substance that is virtually insoluble in water. Glycitein is also known as 7-hydroxy-6-methoxy-3-(4-hydroxyphenyl)- 4H-1-benzopyran-4-one and 4′, 7-dihydroxy-6-methoxyisoflavone.

Glycitein, when marketed as a nutritional supplement, is mainly present in the form of its beta-glucoside, glycitin.

See also Soy Isoflavones.

ACTIONS AND PHARMACOLOGY

ACTIONS

Glycitein may have estrogenic and antiestrogenic activities. It may also have antioxidant, anticarcinogenic, anti-atherogenic and neuroprotective activities.

MECHANISM OF ACTION

Of all the soy isoflavones, glycitein has been the least studied. Glycitein has weak estrogenic activity as measured in *in vivo* and *in vitro* assays. *In vivo*, its estrogenic activity is the highest of the soy isoflavones: three times greater than that of genistein and 12 times greater than that of daidzein.

Glycitein's antioxidant activity has been demonstrated by its ability to scavenge hydroxyl radicals generated via the Fenton reaction, superoxide anion radicals generated via the xanthine/xanthine oxidase reaction and peroxynitrite radicals generated via the reaction of superoxide anions with nitric oxide.

Observational studies have shown an inverse relation between soy consumption and risk of prostate cancer. However, the specific cellular mechanisms responsible for this putative anticancer activity are not clear. Signaling cascades are involved in cellular growth, proliferation and differentiation. The extracellular signal-regulated kinase (ERK1/2) signaling cascade is necessary for the survival, growth and development of normal prostate epithelium. The role of ERK1/2 signaling in prostate carcinogenesis is unclear. Glycitein was demonstrated to activate ERK1/2 via vascular endothelial growth factor receptor (VEGFR) signaling in nontumorigenic (RWPE-1) prostate epithelial cells. Of the three soy isoflavones (genistein, daidzein and glycitein) and equol, glycitein was the most potent activator of ERK1/2 and glycitein decreased RWPE-1 cell proliferation by approximately 40%. The ability of isoflavones, and in particular glycitein, to modulate the ERK1/2 signaling cascade via VEGFR signaling in the prostate may be responsible, in part, for the possible anticancer activity of soy.

Glycitein was found to protect against beta amyloid-induced toxicity and oxidative stress in transgenic *Caenorhabditis elegans* (*C. elegans*). Alzheimer's disease is characterized by the presence of amyloid beta peptide aggregation and increased oxidative stress, both causing neuronal injury and neuronal death. In order to better understand the possible neuroprotective mechanisms of soy isoflavones, several experiments were performed using a transgenic *C. elegans* model expressing the human amyloid-beta peptide. Among the three soy isoflavones tested—genistein, daidzein and glycitein—only glycitein alleviated beta amyloid (Abeta) expression-induced paralysis in the transgenic *C. elegans* model. The activity of glycitein correlated with a reduced level of the reactive oxygen species hydrogen peroxide in the transgenic *C. elegans*. Further, the transgenic *C. elegans* treated with glycitein exhibited reduced formation of beta-amyloid. One can conclude from this study that glycitein may suppress Abeta toxicity via combined antioxidant activity and inhibition of Abeta deposition. Further research on the possible neuroprotective activity of glycitein is needed and warranted.

PHARMACOKINETICS

Little is known about the pharmacokinetics of glycitein in humans. Studies show that, following ingestion of soy isoflavones, glycitein is found in the plasma, indicating that it is absorbed to some extent. A recent paper reported on the *in vitro* and *in vivo* metabolism of glycitein. The *in vitro* phase I metabolism of glycitein using rat liver microsomes, human liver microsomes and human fecal flora showed glycitein to be converted into six metabolites with 8-hydroxy-glycitein and 6-hydroxy-daidzein being the major products. Intestinal metabolism led to four metabolites with 6-hydroxy-daidzein as the main product. The *in vivo* metabolism of glycitein resulted in the formation of three oxidative and two bacterial metabolites; the demethylation product 6-hydroxy-daidzein was the major *in vivo* metabolite. This study demonstrated that glycitein is a substrate for cytochrome P450 enzymes as well as human intestinal microflora *in vitro* and *in vivo*. Significantly, only a small amount of the oxidative and bacterial metabolites of glycitein were found in rat urine and feces, providing evidence that glycitein may be a stable molecule. Further research on the pharmacokinetics and pharmacodynamics of glycitein is needed and warranted.

See Genistein and Daidzein.

INDICATIONS AND USAGE

Though not as studied as genistein and daidzein, two other soy isoflavones, glycitein presumably has some of the same anticancer effects. It may also have some of the benefits observed in the use of soy isoflavones, with respect to atherogenesis and problems associated with menopause, including "hot flashes" and osteoporosis. It also appears to possess neuroprotective activity and may play a role in neurodegenerative disorders.

See Soy Isoflavones, Genistein and Daidzein.

RESEARCH SUMMARY

Because glycitein is found only in small amounts in soybeans, glycitein research has lagged far behind research on genistein and daidzein, two other soy isoflavones. Recently, however, research has shown that 40% of the plant estrogens in soy germ is glycitein. Its estrogenicity, which is higher than that of daidzein and genistein, coupled with another recent finding that glycitein may be more readily absorbed in the body, has resulted in increased interest in this isoflavone. More research is underway.

CONTRAINDICATIONS, PRECAUTIONS, ADVERSE REACTIONS

CONTRAINDICATIONS

Glycitein is contraindicated in those who are hypersensitive to any component of a glycitein or glycitin-containing product.

PRECAUTIONS

Pregnant women and nursing mothers should avoid the use of glycitein/glycitin-containing supplements pending long-term safety studies.

Men with prostate cancer should discuss the advisability of the use of glycitein/glycitin-containing supplements with their physicians before deciding to use them.

Women with estrogen receptor-positive tumors should exercise caution in the use of glycitein/glycitin-containing supplements and should use them only if they are recommended and monitored by a physician.

DOSAGE AND ADMINISTRATION

Glycitein is available in a few different formulations. A standard soy isoflavone formula contains glycitein principally in the form of glycitin, as well as genistin and daidzin with much smaller amounts of the aglycones glycitein, genistein and daidzein. The percentage of the soy isoflavones present in such a supplement reflect the percentages of these substances in soybeans and are: glycitin, about 12%; genistin, about 50%; and daidzin, about 38%. A 50-milligram dose of the soy isoflavone supplement—a typical daily dose—delivers about 6 mg of glycitin, 25 mg of genistin and 19 mg of daidzin. Usually 40% of the supplement is comprised of soy isoflavones. Therefore, to get a dose of 50 mg of soy isoflavones, which includes 6 mg of glycitin, 125 mg of the soy supplement are required.

Soy isoflavone supplements derived from soy germ are richer in glycitin. Typically, about 40% of a soy germ isoflavone supplement is comprised of glycitin, about 50% of daidzin and about 10% of genistin.

LITERATURE

Clubbs EA, Bomser JA. Glycitein activates extracellular signal-regulated kinase via vascular endothelial growth factor receptor signaling in nontumorigenic (RWPE-1) prostate epithelial cells. *J Nutr Biochem.* 2007;18(8):525-532.

Gutierrez-Zepeda A, Santell R, Wu Z, et al. Soy isoflavone glycitein protects against beta amyloid-induced toxicity and oxidative stress in transgenic Caenorhabditis elegans. *BMC Neurosci.* 2005;6:54.

Lee SO, Renouf M, Ye Z, et al. Isoflavone glycitein diminished plasma cholesterol in female golden Syrian hamsters. *J Agric Food Chem.* 2007;55(26):11063-11067.

Rüfer CE, Maul R, Donauer E, et al. In vitro and in vivo metabolism of the soy isoflavone glycitein. *Mol Nutr Food Res.* 2007;51(7):813-823.

Simons AL, Renouf M, Hendrich S, et al. Metabolism of glycitein (7,4'-dihydroxy-6-methoxy-isoflavone) by human gut microflora. *J Agric Food Chem.* 2005;53(22):8519-8525.

Song TT, Hendrich S, Murphy PA. Estrogenic activity of glycitein, a soy isoflavone. *J Agric Food Chem.* 1999; 47:1607-1610.

Zhang Y, Wang G-J, Song TT, et al. Urinary disposition of the soybean isoflavones daidzein, genistein and glycitein differs among humans with moderate fecal isoflavone degradation activity. *J Nutr.* 1999; 129:957-962.

For additional references, see Soy Isoflavones.

Grape Seed Proanthocyanidins

DESCRIPTION

Grape seed proanthocyanidins refer to procyanidin mixtures extracted from grape (*Vitis vinifera*) seeds. Procyanidins are derivatives of the flavan-3-ol class of flavonoids. This class includes (+)-catechin, commonly referred to as catechin, and (-)-epicatechin, commonly referred to as epicatechin. Procyanidins are dimers and oligomers of catechin and epicatechin and their gallic acid esters. Procyanidins are widely distributed in the plant kingdom and, in addition to being found in grape seeds, are found in cocoa and chocolate, apples, peanuts, almonds, cranberries, blueberries and in the bark of pines, among other plant sources.

Grape seed proanthocyanidins are mainly comprised of dimers, trimers and tetramers of catechin and epicatechin and their gallates. They also contain smaller amounts of pentamers, hexamers and heptamers of these flavan-3-ols and their gallates. The procyanidin dimers and oligomers are also known as oligomeric procyanidins (OPCs) and procyanidolic oligomers or PCOs. Grape seed proanthocyanidins comprise approximately 60 to 70% of the polyphenol content of grapes. The procyanidins are colorless in their pure state.

See also Cocoa Flavonoids and Pycnogenol.

ACTIONS AND PHARMACOLOGY

ACTIONS

Grape seed proanthocyanidins have antioxidant activity. They may also have anti-inflammatory, anticarcinogenic and anti-atherogenic activities.

MECHANISM OF ACTION

Grape seed proanthocyanidins have been found to have a number of antioxidant activities in the laboratory. These include scavenging of hydroxyl and peroxyl radicals, and inhibition of the oxidation of low-density lipoprotein (LDL). The inhibitory potential related to lipid peroxidation appears to increase with the degree of polymerization of the molecules. That is, grape seed proanthocyanidins with a greater number of catechin and epicatechin units appear to have more potent inhibitory activity than those with fewer catechin and epicatechin units. Further, the position of linkage between inter-flavan units also appears to influence lipid peroxidation inhibitory activity. Procyanidin isomers with a 4-6 inter-flavan linkage appear to show stronger inhibitory activity than those with a 4-8 linkage. Finally, the presence of a gallate group also appears to affect the inhibitory activity of the procyanidins with respect to lipid peroxidation. A procyanidin dimer with a gallate group linked at the 3-hydroxy position appears to show much greater inhibition of lipid peroxidation than a dimer without such a group.

Grape seed proanthocyanidins have shown anti-inflammatory, anticarcinogenic and anti-atherogenic activities, again in the laboratory. These activities are thought to be due, in large part, to the antioxidant activities of these molecules. These proanthocyanidins have been found to be cytotoxic for some human cancer lines in culture. Upregulation of apoptosis by the proanthocyanidins in these cancer lines is another possible mechanism for their possible anticarcinogenic activity.

PHARMACOKINETICS

Little is known about the pharmacokinetics of grape seed proanthocyanidins in humans. It appears that they do, at least in part, get absorbed. However, the extent of absorption appears to vary widely, not only among the various components of the grape seed proanthocyanidins, but also among subjects.

INDICATIONS AND USAGE

Experimental data suggest that grape seed proanthocyanidins may have anticancer activity, that they protect against some forms of lipid peroxidation and that they may be cardioprotective, hepatoprotective and capillary protective. They appear to have anti-inflammatory activity. Claims that they are useful in the treatment of arthritis, varicose veins, diabetic retinopathy and some allergies are largely based upon anecdotal testimony; clinical trials are lacking.

RESEARCH SUMMARY

Antitumor-promoting activity, described as highly significant, has been observed in animals treated with topical grape seed proanthocyanidins. Skin tumor incidence, multiplicity and volume were all significantly inhibited. These effects were attributed to inhibition of epidermal lipid peroxidation. Higher doses resulted in greater degrees of cancer inhibition.

An extract of grape seed proanthocyanidins has significantly inhibited human breast cancer, lung cancer and gastric adenocarcinoma cells *in vitro*. The extract did not inhibit neoplastic K562 myelogenous leukemic cells. In the same experiment, the extract enhanced growth and viability of normal human gastric mucosal cells and J774A.1 murine macrophage cells. These promising preliminary findings warrant more research.

Grape seed proanthocyanidins have been shown to significantly inhibit the peroxidation of polyunsaturated fatty acids and some other lipids in animal and *in vitro* studies. Some experimental data suggest that these effects might help protect capillaries, heart, brain and liver tissues in some circumstances. In one study, a grape seed proanthocyanidin extract more potently protected brain and hepatic tissues from the damage of experimentally induced reactive oxygen species damage than did other antioxidants (vitamin C, vitamin E succinate and beta-carotene). In other *in vitro* experiments, grape seed proanthocyanidins have strongly inhibited reactive oxygen species activities implicated in microvascular injury.

Acetaminophen-induced programmed and unprogrammed liver-cell death was dramatically prevented and reduced in mice treated with a grape seed proanthocyanidin extract. Exposure to the extract for seven days prior to acetaminophen administration was notably more effective than pretreatment for three days. The extract significantly counteracted acetaminophen-promoted apoptotic DNA fragmentation.

In another animal model, grape seed proanthocyanidins were shown to increase resistance to myocardial ischemia reperfusion injury. And in a recent experiment utilizing cholesterol-fed rabbits, an extract of grape seed proanthocyanidins significantly attenuated the development of aortic atherosclerosis compared with controls that did not receive the extract.

CONTRAINDICATIONS, PRECAUTIONS, ADVERSE REACTIONS

CONTRAINDICATIONS

Grape seed proanthocyanidins are contraindicated in those with a known hypersensitivity to any of the ingredients in a grape seed proanthocyanidin-containing product.

PRECAUTIONS

Grape seed proanthocyanidin supplementation should be avoided by pregnant women and nursing mothers.

DOSAGE AND ADMINISTRATION

Grape seed proanthocyanidins are available in products called grape seed extracts. These products contain grape seed procyanidins as well as catechin and epicatechin. Typical doses are 50 to 100 mg daily. Products called OPCs or PCOs (procyanidolic oligomers) are typically grape seed extracts.

LITERATURE

Bagchi D, Garg A, Krohn RL, et al. Protective effects of grape seed proanthocyanidins and selected antioxidants against TPA-induced hepatic and brain lipid peroxidation and DNA fragmentation, and peritoneal macrophage activation in mice. *Gen Pharmacol.* 1998; 30:771-776.

Gabetta B, Fuzzati N, Griffini A, et al. Characterization of proanthocyanidins from grape seeds. *Fitoterapia.* 2000; 71:162-175.

Sato M, Maulik G, Ray PS, et al. Cardioprotective effects of grape seed proanthocyanidins against ischemic reperfusion injury. *J Mol Cell Cardiol.* 1999; 31:1289-1297.

Yamakoshi J, Kataoka S, Koga T, Ariga T. Proanthocyanidin-rich extract from grape seed attenuates the development of aortic atherosclerosis in cholesterol-fed rabbis. *Atherosclerosis.* 1999; 142:139-149.

Ye X, Krohn RL, Liu W, et al. The cytotoxic effects of a novel IH636 grape seed proanthocyanidin extract on cultured human cancer cells. *Mol Cell Biochem.* 1999; 196:99-108.

Zhao J, Wang J, Chen Y, Agarwal R. Anti-tumor-promoting activity of a polyphenolic fraction isolated from grape seed in the mouse skin two-stage initiation-promotion protocol and identification of procyanidin B5-3' -gallate as the most effective antioxidant constituent. *Carcinogenesis.* 1999; 20:1737-1745.

Green Tea Catechins

DESCRIPTION

Catechins belong to the flavan-3-ol class of flavonoids. Green tea catechins are the flavan-3-ols found in green tea leaves (*Camellia sinensis*). The major four catechins in green tea leaves are (-)-epigallocatechin gallate (EGCG), (-)-epicatechin gallate (ECG), (-)-epigallocatechin (EGC) and (-)-epicatechin (EC). They are all polyphenolic substances. Black tea leaves have a much lower content of these catechins. That's because black tea leaves undergo extensive fermentation, during which the majority of the catechins are enzymatically oxidized to the major pigments of black tea leaves, theaflavin and thearubigen.

The green tea catechins make up approximately 30% of the dry weight of green tea leaves. Of the catechins, EGCG is the most abundant one in green tea leaves. Green tea, an aqueous infusion of green tea leaves, has been a popular beverage in China and Japan for centuries. In these countries, it is thought that green tea has a number of health-promoting benefits, and it is used in the management of various disorders. Epidemiological studies suggest that green tea may have cancer chemopreventive, as well as anti-atherogenic, properties.

The possible health benefits of green tea are attributed to the catechins. These polyphenolic substances are antioxidants. EGCG appears to be the most potent antioxidant of all the green tea catechins.

ACTIONS AND PHARMACOLOGY

ACTIONS

Green tea catechins have antioxidant activity. They may also have anticarcinogenic, anti-inflammatory, anti-atherogenic, thermogenic and antimicrobial activities.

MECHANISM OF ACTION

Green tea catechins have been found to have a number of antioxidant activities, including scavenging of such reactive oxygen species as superoxide, hydroxyl and peroxyl radicals, inhibition of lipid peroxidation, inhibition of 2'-deoxyguanosine oxidation in DNA to 8-hydroxy-2'-deoxyguanosine and inhibition of the oxidation of low-density lipoproteins. EGCG appears to have the greatest antioxidant activity of all the green tea catechins and, in some studies, it has been found to be a more potent antioxidant than ascorbate and reduced glutathione.

The possible anticarcinogenic activity of the green tea catechins may be accounted for by a number of different mechanisms. Much of the research has been done with EGCG, and it appears that, just as EGCG appears to be the most potent antioxidant of the green tea catechins, it also may have the greatest possible anticarcinogenic activity. EGCG and also EGC and ECG have been found to induce apoptosis in some tumor cell lines. EGCG has been shown to inhibit angiogenesis. EGCG and ECG have been demonstrated to inhibit tyrosine phosphorylation of the receptor tyrosine kinase PDGF-Rbeta (platelet-derived growth factor receptor-beta) and its downstream signaling pathway and, consequently, to inhibit transformation of human glioblastoma cells. Interestingly, only the green tea catechins possessing the gallate group in their structure had this activity. Green tea catechins have also been found to upregulate the synthesis of some hepatic phase II enzymes that are involved in the detoxication (detoxification) of some xenobiotics, including chemical carcinogens.

In addition to their possible activity in preventing malignant transformation and inhibiting tumor growth, the green tea catechins may have antimetastatic potential. In this regard, EGCG has been found to inhibit the proteolytic enzyme urokinase. Urokinase is an enzyme that cancer cells may use in order to invade normal tissue and form metastases. EGCG and ECG have been demonstrated to inhibit metalloproteinase- -2(MMP-2) (also known as gelatinase A) and metalloproteinase-9(MMP-9) (also known as gelatinase B). These enzymes also appear to play an important role in tumor invasion and metastases. Finally, EGCG has been found to downregulate the expression of the androgen receptor in human prostate cancer cells in culture, consequently inhibiting androgen action. This and its inhibition of 5-alpha reductase may account for EGCG's antiproliferative effect on cultured human prostate cancer cells.

The possible anti-inflammatory activity of the green tea catechins may, in large part, be accounted for by their antioxidant actions. EGCG has been found to inhibit the activity of the transcription factors AP-1 and NF-kappa B, both of which may mediate many inflammatory processes and both of which may be activated by reactive oxygen species. EGCG's antioxidant activity may itself mediate this inhibition.

Again, a few different mechanisms may come into play in the possible anti-atherogenic activity of the green tea catechins. PDGF-R beta, which was discussed above, may also be involved in smooth muscle proliferation. Smooth muscle proliferation is involved in the pathogenic process of atherosclerosis. EGCG and ECG have been shown to inhibit tyrosine phosphorylation of PDGF-Rbeta and its downstream signaling pathway and, consequently, the proliferation of smooth muscle.

The inhibition of the oxidation of low-density lipoproteins is another possible anti-atherogenic mechanism. The green tea catechins may also have antithrombotic activity and may aid in lowering total cholesterol and LDL-cholesterol levels. The antithrombotic effect appears to be at the platelet level. These catechins have been found to inhibit ADP- and collagen-induced platelet aggregation in rats. Coagulation parameters were not affected. The mechanism of the possible cholesterol-lowering effect is unclear. It is thought that the green tea catechins may stimulate the secretion of bile salts and the fecal excretion of cholesterol.

The green tea catechins have been found to promote thermogenesis. The proposed mechanism for this is inhibition of the enzyme catechol-O-methyl-transferase. This enzyme inactivates norepinephrine.

The mechanism of the possible antimicrobial activity of the green tea catechins is unclear.

PHARMACOKINETICS

The pharmacokinetics of the green tea catechins in humans remain incompletely understood. They are absorbed from the gastrointestinal tract following ingestion, and blood levels of the various catechins have been measured. However, the extent of their absorption, as well as of their distribution, metabolism and excretion, is unclear. A recent human study indicates that the green tea catechins are mainly found in blood in the protein-rich fraction of plasma and in high-density lipoproteins. They are also found in low-density lipoproteins (LDL), but it is unclear if they are present in sufficient amounts in LDL to enhance its resistance to oxidation. Another recent human study has detected two catechin metabolites in the urine following ingestion of green tea. These metabolites are (-)-5(3', 4', 5'-trihydroxy-phenyl)-gamma-valerolactone and (-)-5-(3', 4'-dihydroxyphenyl)-gamma-valerolactone. They appear to be produced by intestinal microorganisms with EGC and EC as the precursors of the above metabolites, respectively. These metabolites were also detected in the plasma and the feces. Human pharmacokinetic studies of the green tea catechins are needed in order to better understand their possible beneficial health effects.

INDICATIONS AND USAGE

Green tea catechins may have anticarcinogenic, anti-athero-sclerotic, anti-inflammatory and antimicrobial activities. It has been suggested that their reported thermogenic effects might be helpful in controlling body weight. There is the suggestion in one recent study that green tea catechins might be helpful in sleep apnea. They may also be bone protective, skin protective, oral/dental protective and neuroprotective, as well as prove to be of some benefit in some patients with diabetes.

RESEARCH SUMMARY

Though epidemiological data are mixed with respect to the effects of green tea consumption on the incidence of cancer, the predominant data suggest that green tea confers protective effects against many cancers. The incidence of prostate cancer, for example, is the lowest in the world in China, a country with high green tea consumption. Esophageal cancer risk has been found to be reduced by 60% in those who consume two to three cups of green tea daily in China. And smokers in Japan are reportedly less likely to develop lung cancer if they regularly consume green tea.

A prospective cohort study of 8,552 Japanese found a significant inverse relationship between green tea consumption and cancer incidence. Females consuming more than 10 cups of green tea daily had the most notable protection, compared with those consuming less than three cups per day.

Green tea consumption has also been associated with a better outcome in some with breast cancer. Higher intakes of green tea (mean: 8 cups/day), compared with lower intakes (mean: 2 cups/day), are associated with a significantly reduced recurrence rate and a longer disease-free period, particularly among premenopausal women with histologically classified stage I and II breast cancer. Stage III cancer patients did not appear to benefit from green tea consumption. Among the specific green tea-related benefits noted in the stage I and II patients were decreased numbers of axillary lymph node metastases.

Preliminary associations have now been made between higher green tea consumption and reduced levels of breast, prostate, stomach, pancreas, colon and lung cancers.

Additionally, both green tea generally, and green tea catechins specifically, have shown efficacy in combating several cancers in animal models of carcinogenesis and *in vitro* tests. Epigallocatechin-3-gallate (EGCG) especially has shown marked anti-cancer effects against breast, colon, prostate, pancreatic, skin, bladder, lung, stomach, ovarian, leukemic and liver cancer, among others. EGCG has been shown to induce apoptosis in several of these cancer types while leaving normal cells unaffected. EGCG has also been shown to inhibit urokinase, a proteolytic enzyme often required for cancer growth. Further, angiogenesis has been shown to be significantly inhibited by EGCG. Recently, EGCG demonstrated an ability to inhibit androgen activity in an androgen-responsive prostate cell line.

Green tea and its catechins have protected against a broad range of chemically induced cancers in *in vitro* and animal studies. Those effects have been reported in all stages of some cancers. Additionally, green tea has been reported to enhance the activity of some anti-cancer drugs. It has increased concentrations of doxorubicin, for example, in some cancer cells without also increasing doxorubicin concentrations in normal cells.

A recent review stated that "today, green tea is accepted as a cancer preventive on the basis of numerous *in vitro, in vivo* and epidemiological studies." The reviewers note that the Chemopreventive Branch of the National Cancer Institutes has launched a project to develop tea compounds for cancer chemopreventive human trials. Another recent review similarly found the preventive effects of green tea in cancer "widely supported by results from epidemiological, cell culture, animal and clinical studies," observing that tea polyphenols "potently" induce apoptotic cell death and cell cycle arrest in tumor cells while entirely sparing normal cells. They welcomed the launching of recent Phase I and II clinical trials in humans. It is hoped that these more ambitious trials will shed further light on the extent to which the green tea compounds can be of benefit in human cancers.

The incidence of cardiovascular disease in China is about 80% lower than in developed countries. High consumption of green tea in China has been associated with this notable decreased risk of cardiovascular disease. Numerous epidemiological studies have associated higher intakes of green tea with decreased risk of atherogenesis in Japan and elsewhere. *In vitro* and animal studies have shown that green tea and its catechins, especially EGCG, can help prevent oxidation of LDL-cholesterol. Recently, a human study demonstrated that EGCG inhibits phospholipid hydroperoxidation in plasma. Mixed results have been reported on the ability of green tea to significantly reduce LDL-cholesterol oxidation in humans. One recent study produced results suggesting that daily consumption of seven to eight cups of green tea might reduce LDL-cholesterol oxidation to an extent possibly sufficient to reduce the risk of cardiovascular disease. In *in vitro* and animal studies green tea and its catechins have reduced total cholesterol and LDL-cholesterol levels, have exhibited anti-thrombotic effects and have inhibited the proliferation of smooth muscle, activities that further suggest anti-atherogenic properties.

The Chinese have long believed that green tea has hypotensive effects. Epidemiological evidence is mixed on this score. Some of it reveals a slight reduction in blood pressure associated with higher levels of tea intake. Another group of researchers detected a stronger effect of moderate-strength green or oolong tea consumption on reducing blood pressure in the Chinese population. One group of researchers demonstrated that both black and green tea polyphenols attenuate blood pressure increases in stroke-prone, spontaneously hypertensive rats. Aortic atherosclerosis evaluated via X-ray measurement of calcified deposits in the abdominal aorta was inhibited in older individuals who consumed more than four cups of black tea daily. Drinking more than 10 cups of green tea daily has been associated in another study with significant reduction of cardiovascular disease risk in both men and women. An inverse relationship between green tea consumption and heart attack has also been reported. An analysis of seven studies reported an 11% decrease in myocardial infarction being associated with an increase in green tea consumption of three cups per day. Endothelial dysfunction linked to cardiovascular impairment has been inhibited in some studies with green tea compounds. In one study, higher plasma catechin concentration was associated with improved flow-mediated dilation, which is blunted in coronary heart disease patients.

Green tea and its constituents have exhibited a variety of anti-inflammatory effects, raising hopes that they might be helpful in treating some forms of arthritis, dermatosis, gout and other inflammatory conditions. In an animal model of inflammatory polyarthritis with similarities to human rheumatoid arthritis, green tea polyphenols, in three experiments, significantly reduced the incidence of arthritis (33 to 50%), compared with controls (84 to 100%). Inflammatory cytokines, tumor necrosis factor and interferon-gamma and RA-specific immunoglobulin-G were all reduced in the animals given the green tea polyphenols.

These polyphenols, administered orally and topically, have also protected against chemical- and solar-induced skin inflammations in animal experiments. Significant protection against UVB-radiation was reported in one experiment utilizing hairless mice. Oral feeding was more effective than topical application in this case.

A green tea extract was tested to see if it could help reduce the risk of cutaneous squamous cell carcinoma and melanoma in subjects whose psoriasis and some other skin diseases were being treated with a combination of psoralens and exposure to ultraviolet A radiation. While this combination treatment has been shown to be very effective, it has also been shown to significantly increase skin cancer risk. In the recent study alluded to above, a green tea extract, given pre- and post-treatment, significantly prevented the DNA damage and inflammatory processes associated with the combination treatment in animals and in human subjects.

Further experimentation continues to confirm that green tea polyphenols, applied topically and, to some extent, taken orally, protect to a degree against UV radiation-induced cancers in a variety of animals. A recent review concluded: "The *in vitro* and *in vivo* animal and human studies have suggested that green tea polyphenols are photoprotective in nature and can be used as pharmacological agents for the prevention of solar UVB light-induced skin disorders including photoaging, melanoma and non-melanoma skin cancers."

Another recent study reached the conclusion that green tea extracts increase energy expenditure and fat oxidation in humans. These thermogenic effects were said to go beyond green tea's thermogenic caffeine effects and to be synergistic with them. Compared with placebo, 90 mg of EGCG and 50 mg of caffeine produced a significant 4% increase in 24-hour energy expenditure and a significant decrease in 24-hour respiratory quotient in healthy men. Supplementation with 50 mg of caffeine alone did not have significant thermogenic effects.

The researchers concluded that "green tea has thermogenic properties and promotes fat oxidation beyond that explained by its caffeine content per se. The green tea extract may play a role in the control of body composition via sympathetic activation of thermogenesis, fat oxidation, or both."

One recent review found that green tea and green tea extracts have inhibited adipogenesis in cell lines, animals and humans. An obesity-preventive effect, these researchers concluded, is widely supported by a variety of studies spanning a decade. Further research, however, will be needed to firmly establish this in humans.

There is some epidemiological and laboratory data that suggest a green tea catechin effect favorable to insulin sensitivity. Rats given green tea instead of water for 12 weeks had lower fasting plasma levels of glucose, insulin, triglycerides and free fatty acids than did control rats given water instead of tea. There is some further experimental data suggesting that EGCG may rehabilitate damaged *beta* cells, which produce insulin. Whether it can benefit some with diabetes can only be determined through further study.

Experimental animal studies and some human data indicated that green tea devoid of sugar may help inhibit dental caries.

One study has shown benefit even when green tea is combined with sugar. Rats fed a cariogenic diet were significantly protected by green tea polyphenols from caries development. A recent study showed that green tea catechins can reduce periodontal breakdown induced by the proteinase activity of *Porphyromonas gingivalis*. Another study indicates that green tea inhibits human salivary amylase and thus reduces the cariogenic potential of starch-containing foods. Additionally, both black and green tea are sources of fluoride, which may help prevent tooth loss and protect against oral cancer. Green tea is now considered a functional food for oral health and is included in some toothpastes.

There is *in vitro* evidence that green tea and its catechins have some antiviral and other antimicrobial activities. Recently, various green tea catechins were shown to inhibit extracellular release of vero toxin from enterohemorrhagic *Escherichia coli*.

Other research has shown that the influenza virus, in its early stages of infectivity, is adversely affected by green tea and green tea compounds. So is the herpes simplex virus. Green tea has been shown to inhibit some types of *Salmonella*, and has been useful in fighting some intestinal infective agents without causing an imbalance in intestinal flora. Green tea catechins inhibit *Helicobacter pylori* and have shown effectiveness against *Candida albicans*, both alone and in combination with low-dose antimycotics.

An association has been made between green tea consumption and increased bone mineral density. In some preliminary studies, it was shown to be protective against hip fracture, independent of smoking status, hormone replacement therapy, coffee drinking and the addition of milk to tea. Studies with bone cells show a green-tea proliferative effect.

Recent studies support the idea that green tea catechins might have some neuroprotective effects and could possibly be of benefit in neurodegenerative diseases, including Alzheimer's disease. The neuroprotective effects of theanine are being studied. More research is needed before green tea compounds can definitively be said to have meaningful clinical neuroprotective effects.

A recent sleep study in rodents produced results suggestive of a possible role for green tea compounds in sleep apnea. In this study, green tea polyphenols reduced the neural susceptibility to intermittent hypoxia during sleep in the rodents. Further research is needed and warranted.

In conclusion, one group of reviewers recently stated: "Since green tea beneficial health effects are being increasingly proved, it could be advisable to encourage the regular consumption of this widely available, tasty and inexpensive beverage."

CONTRAINDICATIONS, PRECAUTIONS, ADVERSE REACTIONS

CONTRAINDICATIONS

Green tea catechin supplementation is contraindicated in those who are hypersensitive to any component of a green tea catechin-containing preparation.

PRECAUTIONS

Pregnant women and nursing mothers should avoid green tea catechin supplementation pending long-term safety studies. Catechins may decrease platelet aggregation. Those taking drugs affecting platelet aggregation, such as aspirin, those taking warfarin and those with either genetic or acquired bleeding tendencies should exercise caution in the use of green tea catechin supplements.

Green tea catechin supplementation should be stopped before any surgical procedure.

ADVERSE REACTIONS
None known.

INTERACTIONS
DRUGS

Platelet active drugs: Green tea catechins may enhance the effect of these drugs.

Caffeine: Green tea catechins and caffeine may have a synergistic effect in enhancing thermogenesis. Green tea catechins may inhibit catechol-O-methyl-transferase, an enzyme that metabolizes norepinephrine. Caffeine may inhibit cyclic AMP phosphodiesterase, an enzyme that metabolizes norepinephrine-induced cyclic AMP.

Chemotherapeutic agents: Animal studies suggest that green tea catechins may enhance the effects of chemotherapeutic agents such as doxorubicin and that they may ameliorate some of their toxicity. There is no human data on this.

OVERDOSAGE
There are no reports of overdosage.

DOSAGE AND ADMINISTRATION
Green tea catechin supplements in a number of green tea extract formulas are available. EGCG is the principal catechin in these supplements. Typical doses are 125 mg to 250 mg daily (of the catechins). There are a number of green tea food products available.

LITERATURE
Adhami VM, Siddiqui IA, Ahmad N, et al. Oral consumption of green tea polyphenols inhibits insulin-like growth factor-I-induced signaling in an autochthonous mouse model of prostate cancer. *Cancer Res.* 2004;64(23):8715-8722.

Ahmad N, Mukhtar H. Green tea polyphenols and cancer: biologic mechanisms and practical implications. *Nutr Rev.* 1999;57:78-83.

Babu PV, Liu D. Green tea catechins and cardiovascular health: an update. *Curr Med Chem.* 2008;15(18):1840-1850.

Basu A, Lucas EA. Mechanisms and effects of green tea on cardiovascular health. *Nutr Rev.* 2007;65(8 Pt 1):361-375.

Bettuzzi S, Brausi M, Rizzi F, et al. Chemoprevention of human prostate cancer by oral administration of green tea catechins in volunteers with high-grade prostate intraepithelial neoplasia: a preliminary report from a one-year proof-of-principle study. *Cancer Res.* 2006;66(2):1234-1240.

Bettuzzi S, Rizzi F, Belloni L. Clinical relevance of the inhibitory effect of green tea catechins (GtCs) on prostate cancer progression in combination with molecular profiling of catechin-resistant tumors: an integrated view. *Pol J Vet Sci.* 2007;10(1):57-60.

Burckhardt IC, Gozal D, Dayyat E, et al. Green tea catechin polyphenols attenuate behavioral and oxidative responses to intermittent hypoxia. *Am J Respir Crit Care Med.* 2008;177(10):1135-1141.

Cabrera C, Artacho R, Giménez R. Beneficial effects of green tea–a review. *J Am Coll Nutr.* 2006;25(2):79-99.

Cao Y, Cao R. Angiogenesis inhibited by drinking tea. *Nature.* 1999;398:381.

Chen D, Milacic V, Chen MS, et al. Tea polyphenols, their biological effects and potential molecular targets. Histol Histopathol. 2008;23(4):487-496.

Crespy V, Williamson G. A review of the health effects of green tea catechins in in vivo animal models. *J Nutr.* 2004;134(12 Suppl):3431S-3440S.

Demeule M, Brossard M, Pagé, M, et al. Matrix metalloproteinase inhibition by green tea catechins. *Biochim Biophys Acta.* 2000;1478:51-60.

Dulloo AG, Duret C, Rohrer D, et al. Efficacy of a green tea extract rich in catechin polyphenols and caffeine in increasing 24-h energy expenditure and fat oxidation in humans. *Am J Clin Nutr.* 1999;70:1040-1045.

Dulloo AG, Seydoux J, Girardier L, et al. Green tea and thermogenesis: interactions between catechin-polyphenols, caffeine and sympathetic activity. *Int J Obes Relat Metab Disord.* 2000;24:252-258.

Gupta S, Ahmad N, Mukhtar H. Prostate cancer chemoprevention by green tea. *Semin Urol Oncol.* 1999;17:70-76.

Haqqi TM, Anthony DD, Gupta S, et al. Prevention of collagen-induced arthritis in mice by a polyphenolic fraction from green tea. *Proc Natl Acad Sci USA.* 1999;96:4524-4529.

Haque AM, Hashimoto M, Katakura M, et al. Green tea catechins prevent cognitive deficits caused by Abeta1-40 in rats. *J Nutr Biochem.* 2008;19(9):619-626.

Jankun J, Selman SH, Swiercz R, Skrzypczak-Jankun E. Why drinking green tea could prevent cancer. *Nature.* 1997;387:561.

Kang WS, Lim IH, Yuk DY, et al. Antithrombotic activities of green tea catechins and (-)-epigallocatechin gallate. *Throm Res.* 1999;96:229-237.

Khan N, Afaq F, Saleem M, et al. Targeting multiple signaling pathways by green tea polyphenol (-)-epigallocatechin-3-gallate. *Cancer Res.* 2006;66(5):2500-2505.

Koo MW, Cho CH. Pharmacological effects of green tea on the gastrointestinal system. *Eur J Pharmacol.* 2004;500(1-3):177-185.

Koo SI, Noh SK. Green tea as inhibitor of the intestinal absorption of lipids: potential mechanism for its lipid-lowering effect. *J Nutr Biochem.* 2007;18(3):179-183.

L'Allemain G. [Multiple actions of EGCG, the main component of green tea]. [Article in French]. *Bull Cancer.* 1999;86:721-724.

Li C, Lee M-J, Sheng S, et al. Structural identification of two metabolites of catechins and their kinetics in human urine and blood after tea ingestion. *Chem Res Toxicol.* 2000;13:177-184.

Miura Y, Chiba T, Miura S, et al. Green tea polyphenols (flavan 3-ols) prevent oxidative modification of low density lipoproteins: an ex vivo study in humans. *J Nutr Biochem.* 2000;11:216-222.

Moon HS, Lee HG, Choi YJ, et al. Proposed mechanisms of (-)-epigallocatechin-3-gallate for anti-obesity. *Chem Biol Interact.* 2007;167(2):85-98.

Moyers SB, Kumar NB. Green tea polyphenols and cancer chemoprevention: multiple mechanisms and endpoints for phase II trials. *Nutr Rev.* 2004;62(5):204-211.

Mukhtar H, Katiyar SK, Agarwal R. Green tea and skin—anticarcinogenic effects. *JInvest Dermatol.* 1994;102:3-7.

Nagle DG, Ferreira D, Zhou YD. Epigallocatechin-3-gallate (EGCG): chemical and biomedical perspectives. *Phytochemistry.* 2006;67(17):1849-1855.

Nakagawa K, Ninomiya M, Okubo T, et al. Tea catechin supplementation increases antioxidant capacity and prevents phospholipid hydroperoxidation in plasma of humans. *JAgric Food Chem.* 1999;47:3967-3973.

Okushio K, Suzuki M, Matsumoto N, et al. Identification of (-)-epicatechin metabolites and their metabolic fate in the rat. *Drug Metab Disp.* 1999;27:309-316.

Sachinidis A, Seul C, Seewald S, et al. Green tea compounds inhibit tyrosine phosphorylation of PDGF beta-receptor and transformation of A172 human glioblastoma. *FEBS Lett.* 2000;471:51-55.

Shi X, Ye J, Leonard SS, et al. Antioxidant properties of (-)-epicatechin-3-gallate and its inhibition of Cr (VI)-induced DNA damage and Cr (IV)- or TPA-stimulated NF-Kappa B activation. *Mol Cell Biochem.* 2000;206:125-132.

Suganuma M, Okabe S, Sueoka N, et al. Green tea and cancer chemoprevention. *Mutation Res.* 1999;428:339-344.

Sugita-Konishi Y, Hara-Kudo Y, Amano F, et al. Epigallocatechin gallate and gallocatechin gallate in green tea catechins inhibit extracellular release of Vero toxin from enterohemorrhagic Escherichia coli. O157:H7. *Biochem Biophys Acta*. 1999;1472:42-50.

Sutherland BA, Rahman RM, Appleton I. Mechanisms of action of green tea catechins, with a focus on ischemia-induced neurodegeneration. *J Nutr Biochem*. 2006;17(5):291-306.

Wolfram S, Wang Y, Thielecke F. Anti-obesity effects of green tea: from bedside to bench. *Mol Nutr Food Res*. 2006;50(2):176-187.

Yang TTC, Koo MWL. Inhibitory effect of Chinese green tea on endothelial cell-induced LDL oxidation. *Atherosclerosis*. 2000;148:67-73.

Zaveri NT. Green tea and its polyphenolic catechins: medicinal uses in cancer and noncancer applications. *Life Sci*. 2006;78(18):2073-2080.

Hemp Seed Oil

DESCRIPTION

Hemp seed oil is derived from the seeds of the plant *Cannabis sativa*. Hemp seed oil is a relatively rich source of alpha-linolenic acid (ALA) and is one of the few plant seed oils containing more than small amounts of gamma-linolenic acid (GLA). ALA concentrations in hemp seed oil range from approximately 15% to 25%. GLA concentration ranges from approximately 1% to 6%. The most abundant fatty acid in hemp seed oil is linoleic acid, which comprises approximately 50% to 70% of the fatty acid content.

Hemp seed and hemp seed oil normally do not contain significant quantities of tetrahydrocannabinol or any of the other psychoactive substances produced by *Cannabis sativa*. However, trace amounts of these substances have been reported in some batches of the oil. This is most likely due to contamination of the seed by adherent resin or other plant residues.

ALA, GLA, linoleic acid and all fatty acids in hemp seed oil are present in the form of triglycerides or neutral fats.

ACTIONS AND PHARMACOLOGY

ACTIONS

Hemp seed oil has putative antithrombotic and anti-inflammatory activities.

MECHANISM OF ACTION

Antithrombotic and anti-inflammatory activities have not been demonstrated with hemp seed oil. Therefore, any proposed mechanism of actions is entirely speculative. Hemp seed oil is relatively rich in ALA, which may be metabolized to eicosapentaenoic acid (EPA). EPA is a precursor of the anti-inflammatory and antithrombotic eicosanoids. ALA metabolites may also inhibit the production of some pro-inflammatory eicosanoids, as well as some of the pro-inflammatory cytokines.

GLA is a precursor in the synthesis of prostaglandin E_1 (PGE_1), which inhibits platelet aggregation and has vasodilatory activity.

PHARMACOKINETICS

There are no reported pharmacokinetic studies of hemp seed oil. However, much is known about the physiology and biochemistry of edible oils, and certain assumptions can be made. ALA- and GLA-laden triglycerides in hemp seed oil are probably absorbed from the small intestine, aided by bile salts. During the process, there is some deacylation of the fatty acids of the triglycerides. Reacylation takes place within the mucosal cells of the small intestine, and the ALA- and GLA-laden triglycerides enter the lymph system in the form of chylomicrons. ALA- and GLA-laden chylomicrons are transported from the lymph into the blood, where ALA and GLA are then carried in lipid particles to the various cells of the body. They then get metabolized to EPA, PGE_1 and various eicosanoids.

INDICATIONS AND USAGE

It has been claimed that hemp seed oil inhibits platelet aggregation, favorably affects lipids and reduces the risk of heart attack. Other claims include usefulness in arthritis, autoimmune disorders and inflammation, in general. There is no research that supports any of these claims.

RESEARCH SUMMARY

There is no published research showing benefit (or lack of benefit) from the use of hemp seed oil. To the extent that it is a source of alpha-linolenic acid, as well as gamma-linolenic acid, it may have some of the benefits of those substances.

CONTRAINDICATIONS, PRECAUTIONS, ADVERSE REACTIONS

CONTRAINDICATIONS

Known hypersensitivity to a hemp seed oil-containing product.

PRECAUTIONS

Pregnant women and nursing mothers should avoid supplemental hemp seed oil. Because of possible antithrombotic activity of hemp seed oil, those with hemophilia and those taking warfarin should be cautious. Likewise, hemp seed oil should be halted in those having surgical procedures. Hemp seed oil is abundant in linoleic acid. Some laboratory studies suggest linoleic acid may stimulate the growth of prostate cancer and breast cancer cells. It is unclear if this has relevance to those with prostate or breast cancer. However, to be on the safe side, those with prostate or breast cancer should be cautious about using this substance. Cannabinoids have been found in certain batches of hemp seed oil.

ADVERSE REACTIONS

Hemp seed oil may cause mild gastrointestinal symptoms, such as nausea and diarrhea.

INTERACTIONS

DRUGS

Interactions may occur between hemp seed oil, ALA and its metabolites, and aspirin and other NSAIDs. Such interactions, if they were to occur, might be manifested by nosebleeds and increased susceptibility to bruising. If this occurs, consideration should be given to lowering or stopping intake. Such interaction may also occur between hemp seed oil and warfarin.

NUTRITIONAL SUPPLEMENTS

Interactions may occur if hemp seed oil is used with such nutritional supplements as fish oils, which have possible antithrombotic activity.

HERBS

Interactions may occur between hemp seed oil, ALA and its metabolites, and such herbs as garlic (*Allium sativum*) and ginkgo (*Ginkgo biloba*). Such interactions might be manifested by nosebleeds and easy bruising.

OVERDOSAGE

There are no reports of hemp seed overdosage.

DOSAGE AND ADMINISTRATION

Hemp seed oil comes in capsules and bottles of oil. The ALA content ranges from 15 to 25%. Three to 4 grams of ALA is approximately equivalent to the 0.3 grams, which one would derive from a fish-rich diet. Since hemp seed oil is easily oxidized, it is important that it contain an antioxidant, such as vitamin E.

LITERATURE

Costantino A, Schwartz RH, Kaplan P. Hemp oil ingestion causes positive urine tests for delta 9-tetrahydrocannabinol carboxylic acid. *J Anal Toxicol.* 1997; 21:482-485.

Deferne J-D, Pate DW. Hemp seed oil: a source of valuable essential fatty acids. *J Int Hemp Assoc.* 1996; 3:4-7.

Lehman T, Sager F, Brenneisen R. Excretion of cannabinoids in urine after ingestion of cannabis seed oil. *J Anal Toxicol.* 1997; 21:373-375.

Rose DP. Effects of dietary fatty acids on breast and prostate cancers: evidence from *in vitro* experiments and animal studies. *Am J Clin Nutr.* 1997; 66:1513S-1522S.

Rose DP, Connolly JM. Effects of fatty acids and eicosanoid synthesis inhibitors in the growth of two human prostate cancer cell lines. *Prostate.* 1991; 18:243-254.

Rose DP, Connolly JM. Stimulation of growth of human breast cancer cell lines in culture by linoleic acid. *Biochem Biophys Res Commun.* 1989; 164:277-283.

Struempler RE, Nelson G, Urry FM. A positive cannabinoids workplace drug test following the ingestion of commercially available hemp seed oil. *J Anal Toxicol.* 1997; 21:283-285.

Hesperetin

DESCRIPTION

Hesperetin belongs to the flavanone class of flavonoids. Hesperetin, in the form of its glycoside hesperidin, is the predominant flavonoid in lemons and oranges.

Hesperetin is a solid substance that is poorly soluble in water. Its molecular formula is $C_{16}H_{14}O_6$, and its molecular weight is 302.28 daltons. It is also known as 3',5,7-trihydroxy-4'-methoxyflavanone and (S)-2,3- dihydro-5,7-dihydroxy-2-(3-hydroxy-4-methoxyphenyl)-4-*H*-1-benzopyran-4-one. Hesperetin is the aglycone (aglucon) of hesperedin. Hesperetin has the following structural formula:

Hesperetin

ACTIONS AND PHARMACOLOGY

ACTIONS

Hesperetin may have antioxidant, anti-inflammatory, anti-allergic, hypolipidemic, vasoprotective and anticarcinogenic actions.

MECHANISM OF ACTION

Hesperetin is a phenolic antioxidant. It may scavenge such reactive oxygen species as superoxide anions and may protect against peroxidation.

Hesperetin's possible anti-inflammatory activity may be accounted for by its interference with the metabolism of arachidonic acid and histamine release. There is evidence that hesperetin inhibits phospholipase A_2, lipoxygenase and cyclo-oxygenase. Hesperetin may inhibit histamine release from mast cells.

Hesperetin may reduce plasma cholesterol levels by inhibition of 3-hydroxy-3-methylglutaryl coenzyme A (HMG-CoA) reductase as well as acylcoenzyme A: cholesterol acyltransferase (ACAT). Inhibition of these enzymes has been demonstrated in rats fed a high-cholesterol diet.

The mechanism of hesperetin's possible vasoprotective action is unclear. Hesperetin has been shown to decrease microvascular permeability. It may protect endothelial cells from hypoxia by stimulating certain mitochondrial enzymes such as succinate dehydrogenase.

The mechanism of hesperetin's possible anticarcinogenic action is also unclear. It may be accounted for, in part, by hesperetin's possible antioxidant activity. Other possibilities include inhibition of polyamine biosynthesis and inhibition of lipoxygenase and cyclo-oxygenase.

PHARMACOKINETICS

Hesperetin is typically administered as hesperidin. See Hesperidin.

INDICATIONS AND USAGE

Hesperetin may be helpful in lowering cholesterol and, possibly, otherwise favorably affecting lipids. *In vitro* and animal research also suggests the possibility that hesperetin might have some anticancer effects and that it might have some anti-aromatase activity, as well as activity against *Helicobacter pylori*. More research will be required before hesperetin is indicated for any of these situations.

RESEARCH SUMMARY

Like hesperidin, hesperetin has shown some favorable effects on lipids, but, unlike hesperidin, this research has so far been confined to *in vitro* and animal studies. In the best-designed of the animal studies to date, hesperetin significantly lowered plasma cholesterol levels (but not triglyceride levels) in rats fed a high-cholesterol diet.

No conclusions can yet be drawn from early animal work that suggests hesperetin-induced anticancer effects. Similarly, isolated studies showing anti-aromatase and anti-*Helicobacter pylori* activity *in vitro* need follow-up.

CONTRAINDICATIONS, PRECAUTIONS, ADVERSE REACTIONS

See Hesperidin.

DOSAGE AND ADMINISTRATION

Hesperetin is typically administered as hesperidin. See Hesperidin.

LITERATURE

Ameer B, Weitraub RA, Johnson JV, et al. Flavanone absorption after naringinin, hesperidin and citrus administration. *Clin Pharmacol Ther.* 1996; 60:34-40.

Bae EA, Han MJ, Kim DH. In vitro anti-Helicobacter pylori activity of some flavonoids and their metabolites. *Planta Med.* 1999; 65:442-443.

Borradaile NM, Carroll KK, Kurowaska EM. Regulation of HepG2 cell apolipoprotein B metabolism by the citrus flavanones hesperetin and naringenin. *Lipids.* 1999; 34:591-598.

Choi JS, Park KV, Moon SH, et al. Antimutagenic effect of plant flavonoids in the Salmonella assay system. *Arch Pharm Res.* 1994; 17:71-75.

Franke AA, Cooney RV, Custer LJ, et al. Inhibition of neoplastic transformation and bioavailability of dietary flavonoid agents. *Adv Exp Med Biol.* 1998; 439:237-248.

Jeong HJ, Shin YG, Kim IH, Pezzuto JM. Inhibition of aromatase activity by flavonoids. *Arch Pharm Res.* 1999; 22:309-312.

Lee S-H, Jeong T-S, Park YB, et al. Hypocholesterolemic effect of hesperetin mediated by inhibition of 3-hydroxy-3-methylglutaryl coenzyme A reductase and acyl coenzyme A: cholesterol acyltransferase in rats fed high-cholesterol diet. *Nutr Res.* 1999; 19:1245-1258.

Hesperidin

DESCRIPTION

The flavonoid hesperidin is a flavanone glycoside (glucoside) comprised of the flavanone (a class of flavonoids) hesperitin and the disaccharide rutinose. Hesperidin is the predominant flavonoid in lemons and oranges. The peel and membranous parts of these fruits have the highest hesperidin concentrations. Therefore, orange juice containing pulp is richer in the flavonoid than that without pulp. Sweet oranges (*Citrus sinensis*) and tangelos are the richest dietary sources of hesperidin. Hesperidin is classified as a citrus bioflavonoid.

Hesperidin, in combination with a flavone glycoside called diosmin, is used in Europe for the treatment of venous insufficiency and hemorrhoids. Hesperidin, rutin and other flavonoids thought to reduce capillary permeability and to have anti-inflammatory action were collectively known as vitamin P. These substances, however, are not vitamins and are no longer referred to, except in older literature, as vitamin P.

Hesperidin is a solid substance with low solubility in water. It is, however, much more soluble in water than its aglycone hesperetin. Hesperidin's molecular formula is $C_{28}H_{34}O_{15}$, and its molecular weight is 610.57 daltons.

The disaccharide of hesperidin, rutinose, is comprised of the sugars rhamnose (6-deoxy-L-mannose) and glucose. Hesperidin is also known as hesperetin 7-rhamnoglucoside, hesperetin-7-rutinoside and (S)-7-[[6-0-(6-deoxy-alpha-L-mannopyranosyl)-beta-D-glucopyranosyl] oxy]-2, 3-dihydro-5-hydroxy-2-(3-hydroxy-4-methoxyphenyl)-4*H*-1-benzopyran-4-one. Hesperidin is represented by the following chemical structure:

Hesperidin

ACTIONS AND PHARMACOLOGY

ACTIONS

Hesperidin may have antioxidant, anti-inflammatory, anti-allergic, hypolipidemic, vasoprotective and anticarcinogenic actions.

MECHANISM OF ACTION

Although some studies indicate that hesperidin has antioxidant activity *in vivo*, others do not demonstrate antioxidant activity *in vitro*.

The possible anti-inflammatory action of hesperidin is probably due to the possible anti-inflammatory action of its aglycone hesperetin. Hesperetin appears to interfere with the metabolism of arachidonic acid as well as with histamine release. Hesperetin appears to inhibit phospholipase A2, lipoxygenase and cyclo-oxygenase. There is evidence that hesperetin inhibits histamine release from mast cells, which would account for the possible anti-allergic activity of hesperidin.

Again, the possible hypolipidemic effect of hesperidin is probably due to hesperetin's possible action in lipid lowering. Hesperetin may reduce plasma cholesterol levels by inhibition of 3-hydroxy-3-methylglutaryl coenzyme A (HMG CoA) reductase, as well as acyl coenzyme A: cholesterol acytransferase (ACAT). Inhibition of these enzymes by hesperetin has been demonstrated in rats fed a high cholesterol diet.

The mechanism of hesperidin's possible vasoprotective action is unclear. Animal studies have shown that hesperidin decreases microvascular permeability. Hesperidin, itself or via hesperetin, may protect endothelial cells from hypoxia by stimulating certain mitochondrial enzymes, such as succinate dehydrogenase.

The mechanism of hesperidin's possible anticarcinogenic action is also unclear. One explanation may be the inhibition of polyamine synthesis. Inhibition of lipoxygenase and cyclo-oxygenase is another possibility.

PHARMACOKINETICS

There is not much known about the pharmacokinetics of hesperidin in humans. It is unclear if hesperidin itself is absorbed from the intestine intact as a glycoside. The aglycone hesperetin is detected in the serum following ingestion and may be formed prior to or following absorption. Hesperetin may undergo glucuronidation in the wall of the intestine, as well as in the liver. Hesperetin is detected in the urine within three hours after ingestion of hesperidin. Urinary excretion appears to be the major route of excretion of the aglycone. Not much more is known about the metabolism of hesperidin.

INDICATIONS AND USAGE

Hesperidin has demonstrated some ability to favorably affect lipids and to treat some vascular disorders in humans. Other claims made for hesperidin are based on *in vitro* and animal studies. These include claims that hesperidin is useful in cancer and immune disorders. There are also claims that hesperidin is an anti-allergen and anti-inflammatory agent based on results from animal experiments.

RESEARCH SUMMARY

In several animal studies, hesperidin has significantly increased HDL-cholesterol while lowering total lipid and triglyceride plasma levels. A recent clinical trial tested the effects of hesperidin-rich orange juice in 25 subjects with elevated cholesterol levels. Subjects drank one glass of orange juice daily for four weeks, two glasses daily for four weeks and three glasses daily for four weeks. By the third phase of the study, HDL levels in these subjects increased 21% and the LDL/HDL ratio dropped 16%. Folate levels significantly increased. This was interpreted as a positive result, as well, since folate has been shown to cause declines in levels of homocysteine which, at high levels, is believed to increase the risk of heart disease.

These positive effects, attributed by the researchers to the hesperidin content of orange juice, persisted throughout a five-week washout period that followed the conclusion of testing. During that period, subjects were asked not to drink any juice.

Hesperidin has demonstrated antihypertensive and diuretic effects in both normotensive rats and spontaneously hypertensive rats. It has also shown some ability to protect against ischemia-reperfusion tissue damage in some animal models.

In combination with micronized diosmin, hesperidin has significantly improved acute internal hemorrhoids of pregnancy in a clinical open trial.

Anticancer, antimutagenic and immune-modulating effects have been seen with the use of hesperidin in numerous *in vitro* and animal studies. Among the cancers investigated in these studies are esophageal, colon, urinary bladder and skin cancers. In one study that compared the cancer-inhibiting effects of a number of dietary flavonoids and bioflavonoids, hesperidin, hesperetin and catechin were said to be the most potent. More research is needed.

Similarly, more research is warranted to see whether preliminary animal studies suggesting that hesperidin may have significant antiallergenic and anti-inflammatory effects will have clinical relevance.

CONTRAINDICATIONS, PRECAUTIONS, ADVERSE REACTIONS

CONTRAINDICATIONS

Hesperidin is contraindicated in those who are hypersensitive to hesperidin or any component of an hesperidin-containing product.

PRECAUTIONS

Pregnant women and nursing mothers should avoid use of supplemental hesperidin at doses higher than may be found in some multivitamin preparations (about 20 mg) unless such use is recommended by a physician.

ADVERSE REACTIONS

Supplemental hesperidin is usually well tolerated. Adverse reactions include gastrointestinal ones, such as nausea.

INTERACTIONS

NUTRITIONAL SUPPLEMENTS

Vitamin C: The interaction between flavonoids, such as hesperidin and hesperetin, and vitamin C is unclear. It has been believed for some time that flavonoids work synergistically with vitamin C, enhancing the absorption of the vitamin and preventing its oxidation. However, recent research indicates that flavonoids, such as hesperetin, may actually inhibit the uptake of vitamin C into cells. More research is needed to clarify this issue.

OVERDOSAGE

There are no reports of overdosage.

DOSAGE AND ADMINISTRATION

Hesperidin is present in such nutritional supplements as vitamin C with bioflavonoids. Typical dose in these products is about 20 mg. Hesperidin is available in hesperidin-complex supplements. Doses for this type of supplement are usually 500 mg to 2 grams daily. In Europe, hesperidin is available for the management of venous insufficiency and hemorrhoids in a combination product with diosmin. A 500-mg dose of this combination product is comprised of 50 mg of hesperidin and 450 mg of diosmin. Dose for this mixed flavonoid product, for the above conditions, is 1 to 3 grams daily. Another flavonoid, hesperidin methyl chalcone, is often marketed in formulations with hesperidin. This is a different flavonoid, and very few studies have been performed using it. A good source of hesperidin is orange juice containing pulp.

LITERATURE

Ameer B, Weintraub RA, Johnson JV, et al. Flavanone absorption after naringin, hesperidin, and citrus administration. *Clin Pharmacol Ther.* 1996; 60:34-40.

Berkarda B, Koyuncu H, Soybir GT, Baykut F. Inhibitory effect of hesperidin on tumor initiation and promotion in mouse skin. *Res Exp Med. (Berl).* 1998; 198:93-99.

Bok SH, Lee SH, Park YB, et al. Plasma and hepatic cholesterol and hepatic activities of 3-hydroxy-3-methyl-glutaryl-CoA reductase and acyl CoA: cholesterol transferase are lower in rats fed citrus peel extract or a mixture of citrus bioflavonoids. *J Nutr.* 1999; 129:1182-1185.

Emin JA, Oliveira AB, Lapa AJ. Pharmacological evaluation of the anti-inflammatory activity of a citrus bioflavonoid, hesperidin, and the isoflavonoids duartin and claussequinone in rats and mice. *J Pharm Pharmacol.* 1994; 46:118-122.

Galati EM, Monforte MT, Kirjavainen S, et al. Biological effects of hesperidin, a citrus flavonoid (Note I): anti-inflammatory and analgesic activity. *Farmaco.* 1994; 40:709-712.

Galati EM, Trovato A, Kirjavainen S, et al. Biological effects of hesperidin, a citrus flavonoid. (Note III): antihypertensive and diuretic activity in rat. *Farmaco.* 1996; 51:219-221.

Koyuncu H, Berkarda B, Baykut F, et al. Preventive effect of hesperidin against inflammation in CD-1 mouse skin caused by tumor promoter. *Anticancer Res.* 1999; 19(4B):3237-3241.

Matsuda H, Yano M, Kubo M, et al. [Pharmacological study on citrus fruits. II. Anti-allergic effect of fruit of Citrus unshiu MARKOVICH (2). On flavonoid components.] [Article in Japanese.] *Yakugaku Zasshi.* 1991; 111:193-198.

Miyake Y, Yamamoto K, Tsujihara N, Osawa T. Protective effects of lemon bioflavonoids on oxidative stress in diabetic rats. *Lipids.* 1998; 33:689-695.

Montforte MT, Trovato A, Kirjavainen S, et al. Biological effects of hesperidin, a citrus flavonoid. (Note II): hypolipidemic activity on experimental hypercholesterolemia in rat. *Farmaco.* 1995; 50:595-599.

Tanaka T, Makita H, Kawabata K, et al. Chemoprevention of azoxymethane-induced rat colon carcinogenesis by the naturally occurring flavonoids, diosmin and hesperidin. *Carcinogenesis.* 1997; 18:957-965.

Hexacosanol

DESCRIPTION

Hexacosanol is a 26-carbon, long-chain, saturated primary alcohol. Along with other long-chain alcohols, such as docosanol, octacosanol and triacontanol, it belongs to a family of organic compounds called fatty alcohols. It is a component of vegetable waxes and is found in wheat germ oil, rice bran oil and wool wax, among other things.

Hexacosanol has also been isolated from the plant *Hygrophilia erecta*, a medicinal herb that grows in India and Vietnam.

Hexacosanol is also known as 1-hexacosanol, n-hexacosanol and ceryl alcohol.

ACTIONS AND PHARMACOLOGY

ACTIONS

Hexacosanol may have neuroprotective activity and neurotrophic activity, and it may increase phagocytic activity of macrophages.

MECHANISM OF ACTION

Hexacosanol has been shown to attenuate the degeneration of cholinergic neurons after injury, to possess neurotrophic activities on cultured neurons and to increase the phagocytic activity of mice macrophages. It has also been found to increase the regeneration of both sensory and motor axons in the sciatic nerve of the mouse *in vivo*. The mechanism of these actions is unknown.

PHARMACOKINETICS

Little is known about the pharmacokinetics of hexacosanol in humans. It is likely, as in the case of its close relative, octacosanol, that absorption of this fatty alcohol is variable and poor. There are no published reports regarding its distribution, metabolism and excretion. Again, in comparison with octacosanol, it is likely that bile is the main route of excretion.

INDICATIONS AND USAGE

Hexacosanol has demonstrated significant neuroprotective effects in preliminary *in vitro* and *in vivo* studies. *In vitro* and *in vivo* animal studies have demonstrated that hexacosanol can inhibit glucose-stimulated insulin secretion. It has also been shown to stimulate phagocytosis in cultured macrophages.

RESEARCH SUMMARY

Hexacosanol has shown an ability to promote the maturation of central neurons in culture. It significantly increased both neurite outgrowth and the number of collaterals. It was said to strikingly enhance biochemical differentiation of cultured neurons.

In a subsequent *in vitro* study, hexacosanol strongly attenuated degeneration of cholinergic neurons. The researchers described this as the first report of an *in vivo* neurotrophic influence exerted by an exogenously administered long-chain fatty alcohol and concluded that "the low dosage needed and the peripheral administration of this compound may be of great advantage in the reduction of cell loss in some neurodegenerative disorders like Alzheimer's disease or stroke."

Still more recent studies have further confirmed the neurotrophic properties of hexacosanol. In one of these studies

conducted in an animal model, injected hexacosanol significantly protected the pyramidal neurons of the hippocampus from the neurotoxic substance kainic acid. It was estimated that hexacosanol spared 72% of the toxin-exposed neurons.

Hexacosanol also significantly inhibited the increased locomotor activity normally associated with exposure to kainic acid. Some researchers have stated: "The peripheral administration of hexacosanol may lead to a significant breakthrough in the treatment of excitotoxin-related human diseases."

In yet another *in vivo* study, hexacosanol was tested to see whether it has nerve-regeneration effects. Mice with crushed sciatic nerves, given injected hexacosanol, exhibited a 40% increase in the regeneration rate of sensory fibers compared with controls. There was significant recovery of neuromuscular function, as measured by quantitative electromyography and sensorimotor tests, in the hexacosanol-treated animals. Research is ongoing.

Hexacosanol has also shown an ability to inhibit glucose-stimulated insulin secretion, in both *in vitro* and *in vivo* animal studies. These studies have suggested a direct hexacosanol effect on islets of Langerhans. This activity may prevent insulin resistance.

And, finally, a preliminary study has demonstrated that hexacosanol can increase the phagocytosis activity of cultured macrophages. More research is warranted.

CONTRAINDICATIONS, PRECAUTIONS, ADVERSE REACTIONS

CONTRAINDICATIONS

Known hypersensitivity to a hexacosanol-containing product.

PRECAUTIONS

Because of lack of long-term safety studies, children, pregnant women and nursing mothers should avoid supplemental hexacosanol.

ADVERSE REACTIONS

None known.

OVERDOSAGE

No reports of overdosage.

DOSAGE AND ADMINISTRATION

Hexacosanol is available as a nutritional supplement, typically in combination with other long-chain fatty alcohols, such as octacosanol. Doses used are 500 to 1250 micrograms daily.

LITERATURE

Azzouz M, Kenel PF, Warter J-M, et al. Enhancement of mouse sciatic nerve regeneration by the long-chain fatty acid, n-hexacosanol. *Exp Neurol*. 1996; 138:189-197.

Borg J. The neurotrophic factor, n-hexacosanol, reduces the neuronal damage induced by the neurotoxin, kainic acid. *J Neurosci Res.* 1991; 29:62-67.

Borg J, Kesslak PJ, Cotman CW. Peripheral administration of a long-chain fatty alcohol promotes septal cholinergic neurons survival after fimbria-fornix transection. *Brain Res.* 1990; 518:295-298.

Borg J, Toazara J, Hietter H, et al. Neurotrophic effect of naturally occurring long-chain fatty alcohols on cultured CNS neurons. *FEBS Lett.* 1987; 213:406-410.

Damge C, Hillaire-Buys D, Koenig M, et al. Effect of n-hexacosanol on insulin secretion in the rat. *Eur J Pharmacol.* 1995; 274:133-139.

Moosbrugger I, Bischoff P, Beck JP, et al. Studies on the immunological effects of fatty alcohols—I. Effects of n-hexacosanol on murine macrophages in culture. *Int J Immunopharmacol.* 1992; 14:292-302.

Human Growth Hormone and Secretagogues

DESCRIPTION

Human growth hormone (HGH) is a heterogenous mixture of polypeptides secreted by the anterior pituitary gland. The principal form of HGH is a polypeptide containing 191 amino acids with a molecular weight of 215,000 daltons. This form of HGH is produced by recombinant DNA technology and is marketed for the treatment of short stature in growth hormone(GH)-deficient children and adolescents. Recombinant HGH or somatropin is also used for the treatment of GH deficiency in adults, short stature in association with renal insufficiency, AIDS-related wasting and short stature associated with Turner's Syndrome. In all of these cases, GH must be administered parenterally since it has very poor oral bioavailability.

GH is the primary hormone responsible for growth in humans, as well as other mammals, and it helps regulate such metabolic processes as anabolism and lipolysis. Normal human aging is associated with decreased GH secretion. Mean GH level in those over the age of 60 is about half of that in young adults. The reduction in GH levels with aging is believed to contribute to age-related decreases in muscle mass and strength and decreased lipolysis.

The effects of GH are largely mediated via IGF-1 (insulin-like growth factor 1). IGF-1 is a mitogen and may promote some cancers, including prostate, breast and colorectal cancers. Clearly, long-term safety studies, as well as efficacy studies, are essential to evaluate the role, if any, of GH replacement in the aging population.

The release of GH from somatotroph cells of the anterior pituitary gland is a complex process involving multiple regulators. The hypothalamic peptide GHRH (growth hormone-releasing hormone) acts on the somatotrophs to release GH, while the inhibitory peptide somatostatin blocks GH release. In addition, GH release appears to be influenced by a third, separate mechanism, as well—a growth hormone secretagogue pathway. GH secretagogues, abbreviated GHSs, can be amino acids, such as L-arginine, small peptides and nonpeptides. Further, neurotransmitters, such as acetylcholine, dopamine and norepinephrine, and neuropeptides, such as opioid peptides, are also involved in the control of GH secretion.

Recently, HGH has entered the dietary supplement marketplace, as have IGF-1 (see Insulin-Growth Factor 1) and several so-called GH secretagogues or releasers. The substances being marketed as GH secretagogues or releasers include the amino acids L-arginine, L-glutamine, L-ornithine, glycine, L-dopa, as well as such substances as ornithine alpha-ketoglutarate (see Ornithine Alpha-Ketoglutarate) and the herbs *Macuna pruriens* and *Tribulus terrestris*.

ACTIONS AND PHARMACOLOGY

ACTIONS

Supplemental HGH and secretagogues or releasers have putative anabolic and lipolytic activities, as well as putative "anti-aging" activity.

MECHANISM OF ACTION

The mechanism of the putative actions of supplemental HGH and secretagogues or releasers is unknown. The actions of endogenous GH and parenteral GH are thought to be mediated via the anabolic hormone IGF-1 and by interaction with specific GH receptors that are widely distributed in body tissues.

PHARMACOKINETICS

Orally administered GH has very poor bioavailability. It is claimed that GH is significantly absorbed from the oral mucosa if delivered by a spray. There is no substantiation for this. It is likely that orally administered GH is digested in the small intestine to the amino acids that comprise the molecule.

INDICATIONS AND USAGE

There are no indications for the non-pharmaceutical use of HGH in any form. Claims that it is an anti-aging substance, that it enhances athletic and sexual performance, that it promotes joint health, is a sleep aid and an immune enhancer, that it has antidiabetic and antiatherosclerotic effects, and is a neuroprotector, are unsupported by credible evidence. Injected HGH may reduce fat and increase lean body mass in some, but serious side effects may attend the use of HGH for this purpose. There is preliminary evidence that injected HGH may be of benefit in some with Crohn's disease and that it might be helpful in treating dilated cardiomyopathy. There is some fear that high doses of HGH might promote some cancers.

RESEARCH SUMMARY

Recombinant human growth hormone, given parenterally to men aged 61 to 81, reportedly resulted in significant improvements in lean body mass, muscle tone, skin thickness and density of lumbar vertebrae. Significant loss of adipose tissue was also reported. The researchers concluded that "the effects of six months of human growth hormone treatment on lean body mass and adipose tissue were equivalent in magnitude to the changes incurred during 10 to 20 years of aging."

Subsequent studies also demonstrated some positive effects of HGH replacement therapy on body composition in those over 60. Some serious side effects were also noted, however, including arthralgias of both small and large joints, insulin resistance leading to higher serum fasting glucose levels, fluid retention in the lower extremities, carpal tunnel syndrome, gynecomastia and headaches. Due to the prevalence of some of these side effects, the researchers who conducted the first human trial reduced the dosage of HGH they had been using by half.

In a preliminary study, recombinant human growth hormone, given parenterally for three months to patients with idiopathic dilated cardiomyopathy, was reported to increase myocardial mass and reduce the size of the left ventricular chamber. These changes were associated with improved clinical status.

Recently, in another preliminary study, injected HGH was said to be beneficial in some with Crohn's disease. Improvement was measured by scores on the Crohn's Disease Activity Index over a four-month period.

There is no credible evidence that oral HGH has any health benefit.

CONTRAINDICATIONS, PRECAUTIONS, ADVERSE REACTIONS

(For information on the pharmaceutical use of somatropin, see *Physicians' Desk Reference*.)

CONTRAINDICATIONS

Supplemental human growth hormone is contraindicated in those with any evidence of active malignancy. It is also contraindicated in those who are hypersensitive to any component of an HGH-containing product.

PRECAUTIONS

Pregnant women and nursing mothers should avoid the use of HGH-containing supplements.

Adolescents should avoid the use of supplemental HGH.

Those with diabetes should avoid the use of supplemental HGH.

Oral forms of HGH are not meant to be used parenterally and should never be used in such a manner.

ADVERSE REACTIONS

None known for HGH-containing supplements.

INTERACTIONS

None known for HGH-containing supplements.

DOSAGE AND ADMINISTRATION

Oral recombinant human growth hormone is available and marketed as a dietary supplement, typically in the form of an oral spray. There are no recommended doses.

LITERATURE

Bengtsson B-Å, Eden S, Lonn L, et al. Treatment of adults with growth hormone deficiency with recombinant human GH. *J Clin Endocrinol Metab*. 1993; 76:309-317.

Cohn L, Feller AG, Draper MW, Rudman IW, Rudman D. Carpal tunnel syndrome and gynaecomastia during growth hormone treatment of elderly men with low circulating IGF-1 concentrations. *Clin Endocrinol*. 1993; 39:417-425.

Fazio S, Sabatini D, Capaldo B, et al. A preliminary study of growth hormone in the treatment of dilated cardiomyopathy. 1996; 334:809-814.

Marcus R, Hoffman AR. Growth hormone as therapy for older men and women. *Annu Rev Pharmacol Toxicol*. 1998; 38:45-61.

Rudman D, Feller AG, Nagraj HS, et al. Effects of human growth hormone in men over 60 years old. *N Engl J Med*. 1990; 323:1-6.

Huperzine A

DESCRIPTION

Huperzine A is a plant alkaloid derived from the Chinese club moss plant, *Huperzia serrata*, which is a member of the *Lycopodium* species. *Huperzia serrata* has been used in Chinese folk medicine for the treatment of fevers and inflammation.

Huperzine A has been found to have acetylcholinesterase activity. Huperzine B, also derived from *Huperzia serrata*, is a much less potent acetylcholinesterase inhibitor. Natural huperzine A is a chiral molecule also called L-huperzine A or (-)-huperzine A. Synthetic huperzine A is a racemic mixture called (±)-huperzine A. Huperzine A is also known as HUP, hup A and selagine. In Chinese medicine, the extract of *Huperzia serrata* is known as Chien Tseng Ta and shuangyiping. Huperzine A derivatives are being developed for pharmaceutical application.

ACTIONS AND PHARMACOLOGY

ACTIONS

Huperzine A may have cognition-enhancing activity in some.

MECHANISM OF ACTION

Alzheimer's disease is a neurodegenerative disorder associated with neuritic plaques that affect the cerebral cortex, amygdala and hippocampus. There is also neurotransmission damage in the brain. One of the major functional deficits in Alzheimer's disease is a hypofunction of cholinergic neurons. This leads to the cholinergic hypothesis of Alzheimer's disease and the rationale for strategies to increase acetylcholine in the brains of Alzheimer's disease patients. Two FDA-approved drugs for the treatment of Alzheimer's disease, tacrine and donepezil, are acetylcholinesterase inhibitors.

Huperzine A is also an acetylcholinesterase inhibitor and has been found to increase acetylcholine levels in the rat brain following its administration. It also increases norepinephrine and dopamine, but not serotonin levels. The natural L or (-)-huperzine A is approximately three times more potent than the racemic or ($\pm$)-huperzine A *in vitro*.

PHARMACOKINETICS

There are limited pharmacokinetic studies with huperzine A. It appears that huperzine A is rapidly absorbed from the gastrointestinal tract and transported to the liver via the portal circulation. Some first-pass metabolism takes place in the liver, and huperzine A and its metabolites are distributed widely in the body, including to the brain. Following ingestion, the time to reach peak blood level is approximately 80 minutes.

INDICATIONS AND USAGE

Huperzine A has potent pharmacological effects and, particularly since long-term safety has not been determined, it should only be used with medical supervision. It may have some effectiveness in Alzheimer's disease and age-related memory impairment. It has been used to treat fever and some inflammatory disorders, but there is no credible scientific evidence to support these uses.

RESEARCH SUMMARY

Numerous studies, most of them from China, suggest that huperzine A may be as effective as the drugs tacrine and donepezil in Alzheimer's disease. This is not so surprising since *in vitro* and animal model tests have demonstrated that huperzine A effectively inhibits acetylcholinesterase, an enzyme that catalyzes acetylcholine breakdown. Tacrine and donepezil work in the same way to conserve acetylcholine in the brain—the mode by which they presumptively improve memory and cognition in those with Alzheimer's and age-related cognitive impairment. Huperzine A may prove superior to tacrine (dose-limited due to its hepatotoxicity) if long-range studies, yet to be conducted, demonstrate its safety.

In one double-blind, randomized study, huperzine A, in injectable form, was tested against a saline control in 56 patients with multi-infarct dementia or senile dementia and in 104 patients with senile and pre-senile simple memory disorders. Huperzine A produced significant positive effects as measured by the Wechsler Memory Scale. Dizziness was experienced by a few of the huperzine A-treated patients.

In another study, this one multicenter, double-blind, placebo-controlled and randomized, 50 subjects with Alzheimer's disease were given huperzine A or placebo for eight weeks. Significant improvement was noted in 58 percent of the patients in terms of memory, cognitive and behavioral functions. Research is ongoing.

CONTRAINDICATIONS, PRECAUTIONS, ADVERSE REACTIONS

CONTRAINDICATIONS

Known hypersensitivity to a huperzine A-containing product.

PRECAUTIONS

Huperzine A should be avoided by children, pregnant women and nursing mothers.

Because of possible adverse effects in those with seizure disorders, cardiac arrhythmias and asthma, those with these disorders should avoid huperzine A. Those with irritable bowel disease, inflammatory bowel disease and malabsorption syndromes should avoid huperzine A.

ADVERSE REACTIONS

Adverse effects reported with huperzine A include gastrointestinal effects, such as nausea and diarrhea, sweating, blurred vision, fasciculations and dizziness. Possible adverse effects include vomiting, cramping, bronchospasm, bradycardia, arrhythmias, seizures, urinary incontinence, increased urination and hypersalivation.

INTERACTIONS

DRUGS

Acetylcholinesterase Inhibitors: Use of huperzine A along with the acetylcholinesterase inhibitors donepezil or tacrine may produce additive effects, including additive adverse effects. Other acetylcholinesterase inhibitors include neostigmine, physostigmine and pyridostigmine, and use of these agents along with huperzine A may produce additive effects, including additive adverse effects.

Cholinergic Drugs: Use of huperzine A along with cholinergic drugs, such as bethanechol, may produce additive effects, including additive adverse effects.

NUTRITIONAL SUPPLEMENTS

Use of huperzine A with choline, phosphatidylcholine, CDP-choline and L-alpha-glycerylphosphorylcholine hypothetically might produce additive effects, including additive adverse effects.

OVERDOSAGE

There are no reports of overdosage with huperzine A.

DOSAGE AND ADMINISTRATION

There are various forms of huperzine A available, including extracts of *Huperzia serrata*, natural (-)-huperzine A and synthetic racemic (±)-huperzine A. Natural (-)-huperzine A is approximately three times more potent than the synthetic racemic mixture. The doses of natural (-)-huperzine A used in clinical studies ranged from 60 micrograms to 200 micrograms daily. Huperzine A should only be used with a physician's recommendation and monitoring.

LITERATURE

Cheng DH, Tang XC. Comparative studies of huperzine A, E-2020 and tacrine on behavior and cholinesterase activities. *Pharmacol Biochem Behav*. 1998; 60:377-386.

Cheng DH, Ren H, Tang XC. Huperzine A, a novel promising acetylcholinesterase inhibitor. *Neuroreport*. 1996; 8:97-101.

Quian BC, Wang M, Zhou ZF, et al. Pharmacokinetics of tablet huperzine A in six volunteers. *Chung Kuo Yao Li Hsueh Pao*. 1995; 16:396-398.

Tang XC, Kindel GH, Kozikowski AP, Hanin I. Comparison of the effects of natural and synethetic huperzine A on rat brain cholinergic function in vitro and in vivo. *J Ethnopharmacol*. 1994; 44:147-155.

Xiong ZQ, Tang XC. Effect of huperzine A, a novel acetylcholinesterase inhibitor, on radial maze performance in rats. *Pharmacol Biochem Behav*. 1995; 51:415-419.

Xu SS, Gao ZX, Weng Z, et al. Efficacy of tablet huperzine-A on memory, cognition and behavior in Alzheimer's disease. *Chung Kuo Yao Li Hsueh Pao*. 1995; 16:391-395.

Ye JW, Cai JX, Wang LM, Tang XC. Improving effects of huperzine A on spatial working memory in aged monkeys and young adult monkeys with experimental cognitive impairment. *J Pharmacol Exp Ther*. 1999; 288:814-819.

Zhang RW, Tang XC, Han YY, et al. Drug evaluation of huperzine A in the treatment of senile memory disorders. [Article in Chinese] *Chung Kuo Yao Li Hsueh Pao*. 1991; 12:250-252.

Hydrolyzed Collagen

DESCRIPTION

Hydrolyzed collagen refers to enzymatically or chemically processed collagen, which is mainly derived from bovine, ox and pig skin and bone. Hydrolyzed collagen consists of water-soluble peptides of various molecular weights. These peptides are rich in the amino acids found in collagen, including glycine, L-proline and L-hydroxyproline. Nutri-

tional supplements containing hydrolyzed collagen are marketed for bone and joint health purposes. Hydrolyzed collagen and gelatin hydrolysates are similar. See Gelatin.

ACTIONS AND PHARMACOLOGY

ACTIONS

Hydrolyzed collagen has putative activity against degenerative joint disease (DJD). It also may have antiulcer activity.

MECHANISM OF ACTION

The mechanism of the putative anti-arthritic activity of hydrolyzed collagen is a matter of speculation. It is claimed that the amino acids of hydrolyzed collagen contribute to the synthesis of new collagen and new cartilage in joints. If this were the case, then hydrolyzed cartilage would be a disease-modifying substance. The amino acids in hydrolyzed collagen may contribute to joint collagen synthesis. However, if they did, it is unlikely that this contribution would be significant. L-hydroxyproline is not a genetic amino acid. It is formed in collagen post-translationally. Therefore, L-hydroxyproline in hydrolyzed collagen would not contribute to collagen synthesis. Further, both glycine and L-proline are synthesized by the body, and it is entirely unclear how any glycine or L-proline in hydrolyzed collagen would make any significant contribution to collagen synthesis in joints. There is speculation that some oligopeptides that may be found in hydrolyzed collagen might have a stimulatory effect on collagen synthesis. There is some preliminary evidence that collagen hydrolysates may stimulate proliferation of chondrocytes, adipocytes and elements of the extracellular matrix.

PHARMACOKINETICS

The digestion, absorption and metabolism of hydrolyzed collagen are typically slower than that of other dietary proteins and peptides. The reason for this is that the peptides formed from collagen contain a high quantity of L-proline and L-hydroxyproline. Proline and L-hydroxyproline form bonds with other amino acids that are significantly more resistant to enzymatic hydrolysis in the small intestine.

INDICATIONS AND USAGE

It is claimed that hydrolyzed collagen is useful in counteracting degenerative joint diseases. There is some preliminary evidence to support this claim. Hydrolyzed collagen may have antiulcer activity.

RESEARCH SUMMARY

Some preliminary research suggests that hydrolyzed collagen may have effects that could be beneficial in some with degenerative joint diseases. A recent 24-week study (prospective, randomized, placebo-controlled, double-blind) on the use of collagen hydrolysates in athletes with activity-related joint pain was found to show significant improvement of joint pain in the athletes treated with the collagen hydrolysates (10 grams/day). A rat study reported that collagen hydrolysates provided beneficial effects on bone metabolism, especially in the calcium-deficient condition.

Pig collagen hydrolysate and beef collagen hydrolysate were found to protect rat stomach mucosa against ulcerative lesions caused by ethanol. Some Russian scientists have been interested in the peptides that are produced via hydrolysis of collagen. They have named these peptides glyprolines because they are rich in the amino acids L-proline and glycine. They report that a glyproline with the sequence L-proline-glycine-L-proline has the highest antiulcer activity of all the glyprolines.

CONTRAINDICATIONS, PRECAUTIONS, ADVERSE REACTIONS

CONTRAINDICATIONS

Hydrolyzed collagen is contraindicated in those who are hypersensitive to any component of a hydrolyzed collagen-containing product.

PRECAUTIONS

Pregnant women and nursing mothers should avoid the use of supplemental hydrolyzed collagen.

Those with renal failure or liver failure should exercise caution in the use of hydrolyzed collagen.

Those who use hydrolyzed collagen produced from bovine sources should be sure that the products are derived from raw materials (bovine skin and bone) classified as carrying no detectable infectivity. Bovine nervous system parts may carry the bovine spongiform encephalopathy (BSE) organism, the etiological agent of mad cow disease.

INTERACTIONS

There is one report of hydrolyzed collagen enhancing the effect of calcitonin in the treatment of osteoporosis.

DOSAGE AND ADMINISTRATION

Hydrolyzed collagen is available in powder form by itself or in combination with other nutritional supplements, including glucosamine and chondroitin sulfate. A typical dose is 10 grams daily.

LITERATURE

Adam M, Spacek P, Hulejova H, et al: [Postmenopausal osteoporosis. Treatment with calcitonin and a diet rich in collagen proteins]. [Article in Czech]. *Cas Lek Cesk*. 1996;135:74-78.

Bello AE, Oesser S. Collagen hydrolysate for the treatment of osteoarthritis and other joint disorders: a review of the literature. *Curr Med Res Opin*. 2006;22(11):2221-2232.

Castro GA, Sgarbieri VC, Carvalho JE, et al. Protective effect of collagen derivates on the ulcerative lesions caused by oral administration of ethanol. *J Med Food*. 2007;10(1):154-158.

Clark KL, Sebastianelli W, Flechsenhar KR, et al. 24-Week study on the use of collagen hydrolysate as a dietary supplement in athletes with activity-related joint pain. *Curr Med Res Opin*. 2008;24(5):1485-1496.

Koepff P, Muller A, Scheiber R, et al. Agents for the treatment of arthroses. United States Patent Number 4,804,745. Feb. 14, 1989.

Lee SK, Posthauer ME, Dorner B, et al. Pressure ulcer healing with a concentrated, fortified, collagen protein hydrolysate supplement: a randomized controlled trial. *Adv Skin Wound Care*. 2006;19(2):92-96.

Olson GB, Savage S, Olson J. The effects of collagen hydrolysat on symptoms of chronic fibromyalgia and temporomandibular joint pain. *Cranio*. 2000;18(2):135-141.

Wu J, Fujioka M, Sugimoto K, et al. Assessment of effectiveness of oral administration of collagen peptide on bone metabolism in growing and mature rats. *J Bone Miner Metab*. 2004;22(6):547-553.

Hydroxycitric Acid

DESCRIPTION

(-) - Hydroxycitric acid, commonly called hydroxycitric acid, is found in the fruits of the genus *Garcinia*. Supplemental hydroxycitric acid is typically an extract of the rinds of *Garcinia cambogia* fruit, also called Brindle berry. Fruit of this plant has long been used in India as a condiment, and the dried rind is used as a flavoring agent. The dried fruit rind is also used in Indian folk medicine for gastrointestinal complaints and rheumatism. Hydroxycitric acid is the principal acid in the fruits of *Garcinia cambogia* and makes up to 16% of the content of the dried fruit.

Hydroxycitric acid, in addition to being called (-)- hydroxycitric acid, is also known as hydroxycitrate, (-) — threo-hydroxycitric acid and 4S-hydroxycitric acid. It is abbreviated as (-)-HCA and sometimes as HCA. It is a different substance than either citric acid or isocitric acid, which are key intermediates in the tricarboxylic acid or Krebs cycle. The terms for the acid and anion forms, hydroxycitric acid and hydroxycitrate, respectively, are used interchangeably. However, the anion form is the form that occurs under biological conditions.

ACTIONS AND PHARMACOLOGY

ACTIONS

Hydroxycitric acid is a putative antiobesity agent.

MECHANISM OF ACTION

Hydroxycitric acid is a competitive inhibitor of the enzyme adenosine triphosphate-citrate (*pro-3S*) — lyase or ATP citrate lyase. In the cytosol, ATP citrate lyase catalyzes the conversion of citrate and coenzyme A to oxaloacetate and acetyl coenzyme A (acetyl CoA). Acetyl CoA is used in the synthesis of fatty acids, cholesterol and triglycerides and also in the synthesis of acetylcholine in the central nervous system.

Oxaloacetate may enter the gluconeogenic pathway, which can lead to the production of glucose and glycogen. It is believed that the putative antiobesity effect of hydroxycitric acid is due to suppression of fatty acid and fat synthesis. In addition, hydroxycitric acid is thought to suppress food intake via an anorectic effect. This is believed to be accounted for by hydroxycitric acid's stimulation of liver gluconeogenesis.

PHARMACOKINETICS

There is little reported on the pharmacokinetics of hydroxycitric acid in humans. Animal studies indicate that it is absorbed via the gastrointestinal tract and transported to the liver and other body tissues. There are no reports indicating if the marketed hydroxycitric acid is transported into liver cells in humans.

INDICATIONS AND USAGE

Claims are made that hydroxycitric acid is an effective weight-loss agent. These claims are not presently supported by well-controlled studies.

RESEARCH SUMMARY

A suggestion from animal work that hydroxycitric acid might be an effective antiobesity agent has not been confirmed in human studies. A recent well-controlled trial of hydroxycitric acid failed to produce any significant weight loss compared with placebo. This was a 12-week double-blind study in which overweight subjects were randomized to receive 1500 milligrams of hydroxycitric acid daily or placebo.

In another recent study, also conducted double-blind, placebo-controlled and randomized, researchers sought to see whether hydroxycitric acid supplementation could increase fat oxidation in human subject. The researchers found no significant effect.

CONTRAINDICATIONS, PRECAUTIONS, ADVERSE REACTIONS

CONTRAINDICATIONS

Known hypersensitivity to a hydroxycitric acid-containing product.

PRECAUTIONS

Pregnant women and nursing mothers should avoid hydroxycitric acid supplements. Because of the theoretical possibility that hydroxycitric acid might affect the formation of acetylcholine in the brain, those with dementia syndromes, including Alzheimer's disease, should avoid hydroxycitric acid. Those with diabetes should be cautious about using hydroxycitric acid.

ADVERSE REACTIONS

In a 12-week weight loss study comparing hydroxycitric acid, 1500 milligrams daily, against a placebo, the number of reported adverse reactions was not significantly different between the placebo group and hydroxycitric acid groups.

OVERDOSAGE

There are no reports of overdosage.

DOSAGE AND ADMINISTRATION

Hydroxycitric acid is available in *Garcinia cambogia* extracts. Some products contain hydroxycitric acid in the lactone form, which has not shown activity in animal models. There are products available that are free of the lactone form. Typical doses are about 1500 milligrams (as hydroxycitric acid) daily.

LITERATURE

Conte AA. A non-prescription alternative in weight reduction therapy. *Am J Bariatr Med*. 1993; Summer:17-19.

Greenwood MR, Cleary MP, Gruen R, et al. Effect of (-)-hydroxycitrate on development of obesity in the Zucker obese rat. *Am J Physiol*. 1981; 240:E72-E78.

Heymsfield SB, Allison DB, Vasseli JR, et al. *Garcinia cambogia* (hydroxycitric acid) as a potential antiobesity agent: a randomized controlled trial. *JAMA*. 1998; 280:1596-1600.

Kriketos AD, Thompson HR, Greene H, Hill JO. (-)-Hydroxycitric acid does not affect energy expenditure and substrate oxidation in adult males in a post-absorptive state. *Int J Obes Relat Metab Disord*. 1999; 23:867-873.

Hydroxyethylrutosides

DESCRIPTION

Hydroxyethylrutosides (HR) refer to a mixture of semi-synthetic derivatives of the flavonoid rutin. Rutin is a naturally occurring flavonol glycoside comprised of the flavonol quercetin and the disaccharide rutinose (see Rutin). Hydroxyethylrutosides are comprised of the mono-, di-, tri- and tetrahydroxyethyl derivatives of rutin and are prepared by the hydroxyethylation of the phenolic groups of rutin.

Formulations, mainly consisting of the trihydroxyethyl derivative of rutin, are used in Europe, Mexico and other Latin American countries for the treatment of such venous disorders as varicose veins and hemorrhoids. The generic name for these formulations is troxerutin.

Trihydroxyethylrutoside, the principal flavonoid in troxerutin, is also known as 7, 3', 4'-tris [O- (2-hydroxyethyl)]rutin, trioxyethylrutin and 2- [3, 4-bis (2-hydroxyethoxy) phenyl]-3 [[6-O-(6-deoxy-alpha-L-mannopyranosyl)-beta-D-glucopyranosyl]oxy] -5-hydroxy-7- (2-hydroxyethoxy) -4*H*-1-benzopyran-4-one. It is a solid, yellow substance that is soluble in water. Its molecular formula is $C_{33}H_{42}O_{19}$, and its molecular weight is 742.69 daltons.

ACTIONS AND PHARMACOLOGY

ACTIONS
Hydroxyethylrutosides may have venoprotective, vasoprotective and antioxidant actions.

MECHANISM OF ACTION
The mechanisms of the possible veno- and vasoprotective actions of HR are not clear. During blood stasis, such as occurs during venous insufficiency, hypoxic conditions can activate endothelial cells. The activation of endothelial cells may result in phospholipase A2 activation, leading to the release of inflammatory mediators, neutrophil adhesiveness to the endothelium with subsequent release of superoxide anions and leukotriene B4, and depletion of ATP. At least *in vitro*, HR appear to inhibit some of these processes, such as the activation of phospholipase A2 and the recruitment and activation of neutrophils. HR may have reactive oxygen and nitrogen species scavenging activity, which could also contribute to the possible protective effects. It is unclear, however, what the active forms of HR are *in vivo*.

PHARMACOKINETICS
There is little known about the pharmacokinetics of HR in humans. Radioactive labeling studies indicate that HR are absorbed from the intestine following absorption and that the major route of HR excretion is via the biliary-enteric route. However, it is unclear how much HR are absorbed intact—that is, as the glycosides—and it is also unclear what the metabolic fate of HR is following absorption.

INDICATIONS AND USAGE
Hydroxyethylrutosides have demonstrated significant efficacy in the treatment of venous insufficiency and related disorders. There is preliminary evidence that HR might be useful in some with Meniere's disease.

RESEARCH SUMMARY
A meta-analysis of randomized, placebo-controlled trials using HR in the treatment of chronic venous insufficiency found improvement in HR-treated subjects, compared with placebo, as measured by significant disappearance of the following symptoms: pain, cramps, tired legs, swelling and restless legs.

In another review of the therapeutic efficacy of HR, the substance was found to show "promise as a useful additional option for the management of edema and other symptoms of chronic venous insufficiency." Positive effects were confirmed in venous insufficiency associated with pregnancy and lymphoedema. Reductions in retinal vascular permeability have been seen in HR-treated patients with diabetic retinopathy, and HR have been shown, in other studies, to be efficacious in treating some women with hemorrhoids of pregnancy.

Finally, there is a double-blind, placebo-controlled, cross-over study showing significant, positive HR effects in the treatment of subjects with well-defined Meniere's disease. Dose in this trial was 2 grams of HR daily for three months. Side effects were few.

CONTRAINDICATIONS, PRECAUTIONS, ADVERSE REACTIONS

CONTRAINDICATIONS
Hydroxyethylrutosides are contraindicated in those hypersensitive to any component of an HR-containing product.

PRECAUTIONS
HR should be avoided by pregnant women and nursing mothers unless they are prescribed by physicians.

ADVERSE REACTIONS
HR are generally well tolerated. Gastrointestinal side effects, such as nausea, are occasionally reported.

DOSAGE AND ADMINISTRATION
Troxerutin (trihydroxyethylrutoside) is available is some combination products. It is used in Europe and Latin American countries in the management of varicose veins and hemorrhoids. Doses used for these conditions range from 500 mg to 2 grams daily.

LITERATURE

Janssens D, Michiels C, Arnould T, Remacle J. Effects of hydroxyethylrutosides on hypoxia-induced activation of human endothelial cells *in vitro*. *Br J Pharmacol*. 1996; 118:599-604.

MacLennan WJ, Wilson J, Rattenhuber V, et al. Hydroxyethylrutosides in elderly patients with chronic venous insufficiency: its efficacy and tolerability. *Gerontology*. 1994; 40:45-52.

Moses M, Ranacher G, Wilmot TJ, Golden GJ. A double-blind clinical trial of hydroxyethylrutosides in Meniere's disease. *J Laryngol Otol*. 1984; 98:265-272.

Poynard T, Valterio C. Meta-analysis of hydroxyethylrutosides in the treatment of chronic venous insufficiency. *Vasa*. 1994; 23:244-250.

Wadworth AN, Faulds D. Hydroxyethylrutosides. A review of its pharmacology, and therapeutic efficacy in venous insufficiency and related disorders. *Drugs*. 1992; 44: 1013-1032.

Hydroxytyrosol

DESCRIPTION
Olive oil is the principal fat component in the Mediterranean diet and its consumption has been associated with a lower incidence of coronary heart disease (CHD), some cancers, including prostate, breast and colorectal cancer, and other

chronic degenerative diseases. The specific substances in olive oil that appear to confer these health benefits, include the polyphenolic compounds oleuropein aglycone and hydroxytyrosol.

Several studies have found that hydroxytyrosol has a number of health-promoting activities, including antioxidant activity, anti-inflammatory activity, antithrombotic activity and anti-cancer activity.

Hydroxytrosol found in olive oil is largely responsible for its high stability. It is also found in the olive pulp, olive mill wastewaters and as a metabolite of the neurotransmitter dopamine in our brains, where it is more commonly known as 3,4-dihydroxyphenylthanol. It is also found in red wine.

Hydroxytyrosol is mainly formed from the hydrolysis of the secoiridoid oleuropein aglycone, which itself is derived from the glycoside oleuropein. (See Oleuropein.)

Olive oil production involves crushing olives (*Olea europaea*), including the pits, to produce a thick paste. During the procedure, the crushed olives are continuously washed with water, a process called malaxation. The paste is then mechanically pressed to squeeze out the oil content. In addition to providing olive oil, the pressing also squeezes out the paste's water content. The washing and pressing steps produce a large amount of olive mill wastewater. Olive mill wastewater produced during olive oil extraction is a black liquid effluent comprising vegetation water, washing and treatment water and some of the olive pulp and residual oil. Large amounts of the wastewater are produced each year in the Mediterranean region. The good news is that the olive mill wastewaters are a major source of the olive phenolic hydroxytyrosol. The bad news is that the olive mill wastewaters can cause major disposal problems and heavy environmental impact.

The olive pit and the pulp are rich in water-soluble phenolic compounds. These compounds are extracted from olives during malaxation, according to partition coefficients, and end up in the vegetation water, which explains why oleuropein and its derivatives, including hydroxytyrosol produced in olive pulp, can be found in abundance in vegetation waters. A number of other phenolics, such as tyrosol and its derivatives, are also abundant in vegetation waters.

Most of the hydroxytyrosol-containing dietary supplements are produced by a proprietary variation of the above method, eliminating the pits and adding citric acid in order to convert oleuropein to hydroxytyrosol and to stabilize the vegetation water to prevent fermentation, among other modifications.

The types of phenols in extra virgin olive oil are different from those of the olive fruit. The olives mainly contain the polar glycosides oleuropein and ligstroside. Oleuropein is the ester of elenoic acid with 3,4'-dihydroxyphenylethanol (hydroxytyrosol), and ligstroside is the ester of elenoic acid with 4-hydoxyphenylethanol (tyrosol). Oleuropein and ligstroside are the parent compounds of the less polar oleuropein- and ligstroside-aglycones (eg, oleocanthal). Oleuropein and ligstroside-aglycones are formed during ripening by removal of the glucose moiety from the oleuropein- and ligstroside-glycosides via beta-glucosidase. Those aglycones and their various derivatives are the most abundant phenols in olive oil.

Hydroxytyrosol is chemically described as 4-(2-hydroxyethyl)-1,2-benzendiol. It is also called 3,4-dihydroxyphenylethanol, 2-(3,4-dihydroxyphenyl)ethanol, beta-3,4-dihydroxyphenylethyl alcohol and 3-hydroxytyrosol. Its empirical formula is $C_8H_{10}O_3$, its molecular weight is 154.16 and its CAS Registration number is 10597-60-1. Hydroxytyrosol is represented by the following chemical structure.

Hydroxytyrosol

Hydroxytyrosol is sometimes abbreviated as DOPET (for 3,4-dihydroxyphenylethanol). The solubility of hydroxytyrosol in water is 5 grams/100 millilter at 25°C.

ACTIONS AND PHARMACOLOGY

ACTIONS

Hydroxytyrosol has antioxidant activity. It may also have anticancer, anti-inflammatory, antimicrobial, antithrombotic and retinoprotective activities.

MECHANISM OF ACTION

Anticancer activity: Certain studies have found that hydroxytyrosol might have anticancer effects.

Hydroxytyrosol demonstrated a potent inhibitory activity on DNA synthesis in HL60 human promyelocytic leukemia cells. It also induced apoptosis, or programmed cell death, in these cells. Further, it inhibited the progression of the cell cycle in synchronized HL60 cells, causing the cells to accumulate in the G_0/G_1 phase of the cell cycle after 25 hours of treatment. It also induced differentiation of the cells. Among the different proteins involved in the regulation of the cell cycle, hydroxytyrosol reduced the level of cyclin-dependent kinase (CDK)6 and increased that of cyclin D3. With regard to the CDK inhibitors, p15 was not affected by the treatment; however, the expression of p21WAF1/Cip1 and p27Kip1 was increased at both translation (protein) and transcription (messenger RNA) levels. Thus, hydroxytyrosol may affect the expression of genes involved in the regulation of tumor cell proliferation and differentiation. The exact mechanism of action of these effects is unclear. Studies are ongoing.

Another group reported that hydroxytyrosol induces apoptosis in HL60 human promyelocytic leukemia cells. They found that apoptosis of the cells was a consequence of a rapid cytochrome c release—which precedes caspase 8 activation—from intermembrane mitochondrial space. They also found that hydroxytyrosol induced apoptosis in normal resting and activated peripheral blood lymphocytes. Hydroxytyrosol did not induce apoptosis in two colorectal cell lines—HT-29 and CaCo2. The researchers concluded that the downregulation of the immune response might explain the possible anti-inflammatory and chemopreventive effects of olive oil at the intestinal level. They further speculated that the downregulation of lymphocytic proliferation without any effect on intestinal cells might be useful in helping in the treatment of chronic inflammatory bowel pathologies, such as Crohn's disease. In addition, they thought that the possibility of inducing apoptosis in quiescent lymphocytes might be important in the treatment of indolent hematological tumors (chronic leukemias, low grade lymphomas, etc.) which are characterized by a slow growth rate, an increase of malignant cell survival and strong resistance to traditional chemotherapeutic intervention. Interesting ideas, but they require much study.

Anti-inflammatory activity: Hydroxytyrosol was demonstrated to reduce the production of the cytokine tumor necrosis factor alpha (TNF-alpha) in lipopolysaccharide (LPS)-treated BALB/c mice, an animal model of inflammation. Similar anti-inflammatory activity was also shown in the THP-1 human monocyte cell line. There are a couple of reports of hydroxytyrosol inhibiting the proinflammatory 5-lipoxygenase (5-LOX) enzyme. The inhibition of 5-LOX interferes with eicosanoid metabolism, thereby reducing leukotriene B4 production in leukocytes. The exact mechanism of action of the possible anti-inflammatory effect of hydroxytyrosol is unclear.

Antimicrobial activity: Hydroxytyrosol has been found to have antibacterial activity against both gram-negative and gram-positive strains of bacteria, including *Salmonella* sp., *Vibrio* sp. and *Staphylococcus aureus*. It has also been shown to inhibit various mycoplasma strains, including *Mycoplasma hominis*, *Mycoplasma pneumoniae* and *Mycoplasma fermentans*. The antimicrobial effect of plant secondary metabolites, such as the olive phenolics, is the plant's defense against microbes that might injure them

Phenols have long been known to have antimicrobial activity, including antibacterial, antiviral and antifungal activities. The antimicrobial action of phenols is related to their ability to denature proteins, and they are generally classified as surface-acting agents. They act by causing leakage of cytoplasmic constituents. High concentrations precipitate proteins, while lower concentrations inactivate enzymes. However, the specific antimicrobial mechanism of action of hydroxytyrosol is not completely known.

Continued research in this area is necessary in order to determine the role hydroxytyrosol might have in the treatment and prevention of bacterial and other microbial infections in humans.

Antioxidant activity: Hydroxytyrosol has potent antioxidant-activity. Its ORAC (oxygen radical absorbance capacity), one method of determining antioxidant capacity of a food or a chemical substance, is one of the highest known for a natural antioxidant. The ORAC assay uses fluorescein as a fluorescent probe in order to provide a measure of the scavenging capacity of antioxidants against the peroxyl radical. In addition to possessing scavenging activity against peroxyl radicals, it possesses scavenging activity against a wide range of radicals, including hydroxyl, peroxynitrite and superoxide anion radicals.

Hydroxytyrosol also inhibits the oxidation of LDL (low density lipoprotein), *in vitro* and *in vivo*. Oxidized LDL is thought to be crucial in the pathogenesis of atherosclerosis. However, in one study where inhibition of LDL oxidation was not seen *ex vivo*, the author questioned the importance of hydroxytyrosol as a possible antiatherogenic agent. Hydroxytyrosol was demonstrated to efficiently protect against the oxidative stress-induced impairment of the nitric oxide radical (NO·) response of isolated rat aorta. Under physiological conditions, NO is of pivotal importance in the regulation of vascular tone. The lipophilic hydroperoxide cumene hydroperoxide (CHP) was used to induce oxidative stress in the rat aorta. CHP is used as a model compound for lipid hydroperoxides (LOOH), which are formed in the process of lipid peroxidation during oxidative stress. The formation of hydroxyl radicals by hemolytic cleavage of LOOH induces oxidative stress. The hydroxyl radical is one of the most reactive species known. The potent hydroxyl radical scavenging activity of hydroxytyrosol is attributed to its catechol moiety.

In another rat study, hydroxytyrosol was found to reduce the consequences of sidestream smoke-induced oxidative stress. In the study, urinary levels of the F2 isoprostane, 8-isoprostaglandin F_{2alpha} (8-iso-PGF$_{2alpha}$), were used to monitor oxidative stress. The F2 isoprostanes are a family of prostaglandin F_{2alpha} isomers that are produced from arachidonic acid via free radical-catalyzed mechanisms. Exposure of rats to passive smoking increased the urinary excretion of

8-iso-PGF$_{2alpha}$, and treatment of the rats with hydroxytyrosol completely prevented the increase of the F2 isoprostane in rats exposed to passive smoking-induced oxidative stress.

Other antioxidant activities of hydroxytyrosol include protection of colon tumor cells and human erythrocytes from the cytotoxic effects and oxidant damage caused by treatment with hydrogen peroxide, suppressing peroxynitrite-dependent nitration of tyrosine, and, in particular, protecting the cells from peroxynitrite-induced DNA damage.

Antithrombotic activity: A few studies suggest that hydroxytyrosol possesses antithrombotic activity.

Hydroxytyrosol demonstrated an *in vitro* anti-aggregatory effect in human platelet-rich plasma. The anti-aggregatory effect of the polyphenol was accompanied by decreased serum concentration of thromboxane B2 (TXB$_2$) and the eicosanoid 12-hydroxyeicosatetraenoic acid (12-HETE), which play important roles in platelet aggregation.

In a human study, hydroxytyrosol, in the form of a hydroxytyrosol-rich olive oil wastewater extract, was found to lower serum TXB$_2$ in patients with uncomplicated type 1 diabetes, leading to an anti-aggregatory platelet effect.

Inhibition of platelet aggregation by hydroxytyrosol was again found in a recent study that examined a few olive oil phenols, their effect on platelet aggregation and the role cyclic adenosine monophosphate phosphodiesterase (cAMP-PDE) inhibition may play in the effect. Hydroxytyrosol was found to inhibit platelet aggregation, but in contrast to oleuropein aglycone, which turned out to be a more potent inhibitor of platelet aggregation, hydroxytyrosol did not inhibit cAMP-PDE, while oleuropein aglycone did.

Further research on the possible antithrombotic effect of hydroxytyrosol and its mechanism of action is needed and warranted.

Retinoprotective activity: The human cell line ARPE-19 is a cellular model of smoking- and age-related macular degeneration. Smoking is considered a risk factor for the development of this chronic degenerative disease. It is thought that the chemical in cigarette smoke, acrolein, which is a major component of the gas phase cigarette smoke and also a product of lipid peroxidation, may be largely responsible for the risk. Exposure of the retinal pigment epithelial cells to acrolein for a period of 24 hours caused significant loss of cell viability, oxidative damage to proteins and DNA, decrease in cellular antioxidants and in antioxidant enzymes, inactivation of the cellular protective Keap1/Nrf2 pathway and mitochondrial dysfunction. Pretreatment with hydroxytyrosol dose-dependently protected the retinal pigment epithelial cells from acrolein-induced oxidative damage and

mitochondrial dysfunction. Studies of hydroxytyrosol in age-related macular degeneration are indicated and warranted.

PHARMACOKINETICS

The pharmacokinetics (PK) of hydroxytyrosol in humans is limited. Following ingestion, hydroxytyrosol is efficiently absorbed from the lumen of the small intestine into the enterocytes via passive diffusion. From the enterocytes, hydroxytyrosol enters the portal circulation, which takes it to the liver from whence it enters the systemic circulation. The systemic circulation transports hydroxytyrosol to the various tissues of the body. Hydroxytyrosol appears to cross the blood-brain barrier to enter the brain where it can mix with hydroxytyrosol that is produced from the catabolism of dopamine. The major metabolites of hydroxytyrosol in humans are 4-hydroxy-3-methoxyphenylethanol, also called homovanillyl alcohol, produced from hydroxytyrosol via the enzyme catechol-O-methyltransferase (COMT), 4-hydroxy-3-methoxyphenylacetic acid (homovanillic acid) and the glucuronide conjugates of hydroxytyrosol. Most of the ingested hydroxytyrosol is ultimately excreted in the urine as the glucuronide conjugate. The above metabolites and some unconjugated hydroxytyrosol are also found in the urine. Glucuronidation of hydroxytyrosol appears to occur in both the small intestine and in the liver.

Further PK studies on hydroxytyrosol in humans are needed in order to fill in all the details on its ADME (absorption, distribution, metabolism and excretion).

INDICATIONS AND USAGE

Hydroxytyrosol, a polyphenol abundant in olive oil, appears to have significant antioxidative, anti-inflammatory and antithrombotic activities which, in turn, may confer upon it neuroprotective, retinoprotective and cardioprotective effects. It could be helpful in some of the complications of diabetes, shows emerging promise as an anticancer agent and is reported, in one study, to have antimycoplasmal activity.

RESEARCH SUMMARY

The Mediterranean diet, characterized by a significant use of olive oil as the primary source of fat, has long been associated, in epidemiology, with reduced cardiovascular risk. The hydroxytyrosol polyphenol component of olive oil (found also in red wine) has been shown, in both *in vitro* and *in vivo* studies, to have antiatherogenic activity. The exact mechanism of action, in this context, is unknown, but in one study of cholesterol-fed rats, hydroxytyrosol demonstrated antioxidant and lipid-lowering effects. Serum levels of total cholesterol, triglycerides and LDL-cholesterol were all significantly reduced in these animals when administered hydroxytyrosol. Serum levels of HDL-cholesterol were increased significantly. In another study, the olive polyphenol significantly protected against impaired nitric oxide response of isolated rat aorta induced by oxidative stress. A diminished response leads to elevated blood pressure, a major risk factor for cardiovascular disease. Among other things, hydroxytyrosol demonstrated in this study that it is an efficient scavenger of hydroxyl radicals. In other studies it has similarly effectively scavenged peroxynitrite and super-oxide radicals, also implicated in cardiovascular and other disease processes. In still other investigations, hydroxytyrosol has demonstrated an anti-aggregating platelet activity, suggesting that it can help prevent some thrombotic conditions. In one study, five type 1 diabetic subjects were given 25 mg of the polyphenol the first day and then 12.5 mg per day the following three days. Platelet function was improved in ways that suggested an antithrombotic effect in these atherogenic-prone subjects. In contrast with these generally positive findings, however, there are data showing that even high daily intake of olive oil itself cannot raise plasma levels of olive phenols sufficient to significantly prevent LDL-cholesterol oxidization in animals, including humans. More research is needed and warranted to determine whether hydroxytyrosol supplements can be clinically efficacious.

In another study of hydroxytyrosol's antioxidative activity, the substance was said to protect retinal pigment epithelial cells from experimentally induced oxidative stress and mitochondrial dysfunction. The researchers concluded that hydroxytryrosol might prove an effective agent in reducing and/or preventing smoking-induced or age-related retinal pigment epithelial degeneration (such as age-associated macular degeneration). Again, more research is required. Passive smoking-induced oxidative stress was significantly reduced in rats administered hydroxytyrosol. And mice brain cells were protected from oxidative stress in another study employing the polyphenol.

Several recent studies suggest an additional role for hydroxytyrosol in some cancers. Following up on evidence that olive oil itself has anti-inflammatory and chemopreventive effects, researchers have examined the role of hydroxytyrosol in various cancer cell lines. In one of these cells lines the polyphenol demonstrated anti-inflammatory, antioxidative, antiproliferative and apoptotic effects. Similar positive effects were seen in human leukemia and colon adenocarcinoma cells. Recently, hydroxytyrosol has been demonstrated to favorably effect the expression of genes involved in the regulation of tumor cell proliferation and differentiation. This promising research warrants further follow-up.

Finally, there is one study indicating that the olive polyphenol has activity against several strains of mycoplasma. This study grew out of the observation that some of the other components of olive have previously demonstrated some antibacterial and antifungal activity. Hydroxytyrosol itself has previously shown some efficacy against various bacterial strains. Again, further study is needed and warranted.

CONTRAINDICATIONS, PRECAUTIONS, ADVERSE REACTIONS

CONTRAINDICATIONS
Hydroxytyrosol supplements are contraindicated in those hypersensitive to any component of a hydroxytyrosol-containing product. Hypersensitivity to hydroxytyrosol is probably very rare.

PRECAUTIONS
Those who wish to use hydroxytyrosol supplements for a health condition should first discuss this with his or her physician.

Because of the possible antithrombotic effect of hydroxytyrosol, hemophiliacs and those taking warfarin (Coumadin) should exercise caution in its use. Hydroxytyrosol-containing supplements should be stopped a few days before any surgery and can be resumed following the surgery.

Because of lack of long-term studies on the safety of hydroxytyrosol-containing dietary supplements, pregnant females and nursing mothers should be cautious in their use.

ADVERSE REACTIONS
No reports.

INTERACTIONS
No reports.

OVERDOSAGE
There are no reports of overdosage.

DOSAGE AND ADMINISTRATION
Hydroxytyrosol-containing dietary supplements are available in capsules and in liquid form. Doses higher than those recommended on the label should generally not be exceeded.

LITERATURE
Bitler CM, Viale TM, Damaj B, et al. Hydrolyzed olive vegetation water in mice has anti-inflammatory activity. *J Nutr.* 2005;135(6):1475-1479.

Christian MS, Sharper VA, Hoberman AM, et al. The toxicity profile of hydrolyzed aqueous olive pulp extract. *Drug Chem Toxicol.* 2004;27(4):309-330.

D'Angelo S, Manna C, Migliardi V, et al Pharmacokinetics and metabolism of hydroxytyrosol, a natural antioxidant from olive oil. *Drug Metab Dispos.* 2001;29(11):1492-1498.

Fabiani R, Rosignoli P, De Bartolomeo A, et al. Oxidative DNA damage is prevented by extracts of olive oil, hydroxytyrosol, and other olive phenolic compounds in human blood mononuclear cells and HL60 cells. *J Nutr.* 2008;138(8):1411-1416.

Fabiani R, Rosignoli P, De Bartolomeo A, et al. Inhibition of cell cycle progression by hydroxytyrosol is associated with upregulation of cyclin-dependent protein kinase inhibitors p21(WAF1/Cip1) and p27(Kip1) and with induction of differentiation in HL60 cells. *J Nutr.* 2008;138(1):42-48.

Fabiani R, De Bartolomeo A, Rosignoli P, et al. Cancer chemoprevention by hydroxytyrosol isolated from virgin olive oil through G1 cell cycle arrest and apoptosis. *Eur J Cancer Prev.* 2002;11(4):351-358.

Furneri PM, Piperno A, Sajia A, et al. Antimycoplasmal activity of hydroxytyrosol. *Antimicrob Agents Chemother.* 2004;48(12):4892-4894.

Jemai H, Fki I, Bouaziz M, et al. Lipid-lowering and antioxidant effects of hydroxytyrosol and its triacetylated derivative recovered from olive tree leaves in cholesterol-fed rats. *J Agric Food Chem.* 2008 Apr 23;56(8):2630-2636.

Léger CL, Carbonneau MA, Michel F, et al. A thromboxane effect of a hydroxytyrosol-rich olive oil wastewater extract in patients with uncomplicated type I diabetes. *Eur J Clin Nutr.* 2005;59(5):727-730.

Liu Z, Sun L, Zhu L, et al. Hydroxytyrosol protects retinal pigment epithelial cells from acrolein-induced oxidative stress and mitochondrial dysfunction. *J Neurochem* 2007; 103: 2690-2700.

Paiva-Martins F, Pinto M. Isolation and characterization of a new hydroxytyrosol derivative from olive (Olea europaea) leaves. *J Agric Food Chem.* 2008;56(14):5582-5588.

Ragione FD, Cucciolla V, Borriello A, et al. Hydroxytyrosol, a natural molecule occurring in olive oil, induces cytochrome c-dependent apoptosis. *Biochem Biophys Res Commun.* 2000;278(3):733-739.

Rietjens SJ, Bast A, Haenen GR. New insights into controversies on the antioxidant potential of the olive oil antioxidant hydroxytyrosol. *J Agric Food Chem.* 2007;55(18):7609-7614.

Rietjens SJ, Bast A, de Vente J, et al. The olive oil antioxidant hydroxytyrosol efficiently protects against the oxidative stress-induced impairment of the NObullet response of isolated rat aorta. *Am J Physiol Heart Circ Physiol.* 2007;292(4):H1931-1936.

Romero C, Brenes M, García P, et al. Hydroxytyrosol 4-beta-D-glucoside, an important phenolic compound in olive fruits and derived products. J Agric Food Chem. 2002;50(13):3835-3839.

Schaffer S, Podstawa M, Visioli F, et al. Hydroxytyrosol-rich olive mill wastewater extract protects brain cells in vitro and ex vivo. *J Agric Food* Chem. 2007;55(13):5043-5049.

Schmitt CA, Handler N, Heiss EH, et al. No evidence for modulation of endothelial nitric oxide synthase by the olive oil polyphenol hydroxytyrosol in human endothelial cells. *Atherosclerosis.* 2007;195(1):e58-64.

Soni MG, Burdock GA, Christian MS, et al. Safety assessment of aqueous olive pulp extract as an antioxidant or antimicrobial agent in foods. *Food Chem Toxicol.* 2006;44(7):903-915.

Tuck KL, Hayball PJ. Major phenolic compounds in olive oil: metabolism and health effects. *J Nutr Biochem.* 2002;13(11):636-644.

Visioli F, Caruso D, Plasmati E, et al. Hydroxytyrosol, as a component of olive mill waste water, is dose- dependently absorbed and increases the antioxidant capacity of rat plasma. *Free Radic Res.* 2001;34(3):301-305.

Visioli F, Galli C, Plasmati E, et al. Olive phenol hydroxytyrosol prevents passive smoking-induced oxidative stress. *Circulation.* 2000;102(18):2169-2171.

Weinbrenner T, Fitó M, Farré Albaladejo M, et al. Bioavailability of phenolic compounds from olive oil and oxidative/antioxidant status at postprandial state in healthy humans. *Drugs Exp Clin Res.* 2004;30(5-6):207-212.

Indole-3-Carbinol

DESCRIPTION

Indole-3-carbinol or I3C is a breakdown product of the glucosinolate glucobrassicin, also known as indole-3-gluco-sinolate. Glucosinolates are beta-thioglucoside N-hydroxy-sulfates, which are primarily found in cruciferous vegetables (cabbage, broccoli sprouts, brussels sprouts, cauliflower, bok choy and kale).

Indole-3-carbinol may have cancer chemopreventive activity. Glucosinolates themselves have minimal anticancer activity. Indole-3-carbinol is produced from indole-3-gluco-sinolate via the action of the enzyme myrosinase (thiogluco-side glucohydrolase), an enzyme which is present in cruciferous vegetables and activated upon maceration of the vegetables.

The possible anticancer activity of substances such as I3C was recognized by the Roman statesman, Cato the Elder (234-149 BC), who in his treatise on medicine wrote: "If a cancerous ulcer appears upon the breasts, apply a crushed cabbage leaf and it will make it well." Crushing a cabbage leaf would convert indole-3-glucosinolate to I3C, among other reactions.

ACTIONS AND PHARMACOLOGY

ACTIONS

Indole-3-carbinol may modulate estrogen metabolism. It may also have anticarcinogenic, antioxidant and anti-atherogenic activities.

MECHANISM OF ACTION

The estrogen metabolites 16 alpha-hydroxyestrone and 4-hydroxyestrone have been demonstrated to be carcinogens and are thought to be responsible for the possible carcino-genic effects of estrogen. On the other hand, the estrogen metabolite 2-hydroxyestrone has been found to be protective against several types of cancer, including breast cancer. Indole-3-carbinol has been shown to increase the ratio of 2-hydroxyestrone to 16 alpha-hydroxyestrone and also to inhibit the 4-hydroxylation of estradiol. Indole-3-carbinol increases 2-hydroxylation of estrogens via induction of cytochrome P4501A1 (CYP1A1). Indole-3-carbinol is converted by stomach acid to diindolymethane (DIM) and indole (3,2,b) carbazole (ICZ). DIM and ICZ have similar activities regarding estrogen metabolism.

Regarding its possible anticarcinogenic effects, indole-3-carbinol has been shown to modulate the activities of both Phase I enzymes, such as cytochrome P4501A1, -1A2, -2B1, -2B2, -3A1 and -3A2, and Phase II enzymes, such as glutathione S-transferase (GST), quinone reductase and uridine glucuronide transferase. Indole-3-carbinol modulates the metabolism of carcinogens, such as benzo(a)pyrene, aflatoxin B_1 and 4-(methylnitrosoamino)-1-(3-pyridyl)-1-butanone (NNK). Indole-3-carbinol has also been shown to upregulate apoptosis in some cancer cell lines.

As mentioned above, indole-3-carbinol induces the synthesis of 2-hydroxyestrone. 2-hydroxyestrone has been found to inhibit the oxidation of low-density lipoprotein. This indicates that indole-3-carbinol has indirect antioxidant activity. 2-hydroxyestrone also appears to inhibit smooth muscle proliferation. Inhibition of smooth muscle proliferation and inhibition of the oxidation of LDL could account for the possible anti-atherogenic activity of indole-3-carbinol.

PHARMACOKINETICS
There is much unknown about the pharmacokinetics of indole-3-carbinol in humans. It is converted to DIM and ICZ by stomach acid, and DIM and ICZ are absorbed from the gastrointestinal tract. The extent of absorption of I3C, DIM and ICZ, as well as their distribution, metabolism and excretion, are currently being studied.

INDICATIONS AND USAGE
I3C may have anticarcinogenic effects and, possibly, some anti-atherogenic activity. It may be useful in inhibiting the formation of papillomatosis cysts caused by the human papilloma virus (HPV). Claims that it helps build muscle are unsubstantiated.

RESEARCH SUMMARY
I3C has significantly reduced the number of tumor-bearing animals and the number of tumors per animal, compared with controls, in an animal model of spontaneous mammary tumorogenesis. I3C, administered after carcinogen initiation, also significantly inhibited chemically induced mammary tumors.

Aflatoxin-induced tumors in fish were inhibited by I3C when given before exposure to aflatoxin. On the other hand, I3C appeared to promote aflatoxin-induced tumor activity when given after initiation with aflatoxin in these animals. In a rat study, however, I3C had inhibitory effects on aflatoxin-induced tumor formation when given both before and after aflatoxin exposure. More research on this issue is needed. Still other animal studies have demonstrated that I3C exerted protective effects of various types against cancers of the endometrium, lung, tongue, colon and liver.

Cell culture work has shown that HPV proliferation was inhibited by the action of I3C. Subsequently, it was shown that feeding I3C to nude mice significantly inhibited the formation of papillomatous cysts. This, in turn, led to a human study in which I3C again significantly inhibited the formation of these lesions—this time in children.

There is preliminary evidence from *in vitro* studies that I3C-induced metabolites can inhibit oxidation of LDL-cholesterol and that they can also inhibit smooth muscle cell proliferation.

CONTRAINDICATIONS, PRECAUTIONS, ADVERSE REACTIONS
CONTRAINDICATIONS
Indole-3-carbinol is contraindicated in those hypersensitive to this substance or to any component of an indole-3-carbinol-containing product.

PRECAUTIONS
Pregnant women and nursing mothers should avoid indole-3-carbinol supplements pending long-term safety studies. Those with cancer should confer with their physician before deciding to use indole-3-carbinol.

INTERACTIONS
DRUGS
Antacids, H2 blockers, proton-pump inhibitors: The conversion of indole-3-carbinol to DIM and ICZ requires stomach acid. It is unclear if indole-3-carbinol itself would have all the possible activities mentioned above if it were not converted to DIM and ICZ.

Tamoxifen: Indole-3-carbinol may be synergistic with tamoxifen in protecting against breast cancer.

DOSAGE AND ADMINISTRATION
Indole-3-carbinol is available as a stand-alone supplement and in combination products. Dosage ranges from 200 mg to 800 mg daily.

Indole-3-carbinol, as well as diindolylmethane, are available in combination formulas used by some body builders.

LITERATURE
Albert-Puleo M. Physiological effects of cabbage with reference to its potential as a dietary cancer-inhibitor and its use in ancient medicine. *J Ethnopharm.* 1983; 9:261-272.

Bailey GS, Hendricks JD, Shelton DW, et al. Enhancement of carcinogenesis by the natural anti-carcinogen indole-3-carbinol. *J Natl Cancer Inst.* 1987; 78:931-934.

Bradlow HL, Michnovicz JJ, Wong GYC, et al. Long term responses of women to indole-3-carbinol or a high fiber diet. *Cancer Epidemiol Biomarkers Prev.* 1994; 3:591-595.

Bradlow HL, Sepkovic DW, Telang NT, Osborne MP. Multifunctional aspects of the action of indole-3-carbinol as an antitumor agent. *Ann NY Acad Sci.* 1999; 889:204-213.

Cover CM, Hsieh SJ, Cram EJ, et al. Indole-3-carbinol and tamoxifen cooperate to arrest the cell cycle of MCF-7 human breast cancer cells. *Cancer Res.* 1999; 59:1244-1251.

Grubbs CJ, Steele VE, Casebolt T, et al. Chemoprevention of chemically-induced mammary carcinogenesis by indole-3-carbinol. *Anticancer Res.* 1995; 15:709-716.

He Y-H, Freisen MD, Ruch RJ, Schut HAJ. Indole-3-carbinol as a chemopreventive agent in 2-amino-1-methyl-6-phenylimidazo [4,5-*b*] pyridine (PhIP) carcinogenesis: inhibition of PhIP-DNA adduct formation, acceleration of PhIP metabolism, and induction of cytochrome P450 in female F344 rats. *Food Chem Toxicol.* 2000; 38:15-23.

Kim DJ, Han BS, Ahn B, et al. Enhancement by indole-3-carbinol of liver and thyroid gland neoplastic development in a rat medium-term multiorgan carcinogenesis model. *Carcinogenesis.* 1997; 18:377-381.

Michnovicz JJ, Bradlow HL. Induction of estradiol metabolism by dietary indole-3-carbinol in humans. *J Natl Cancer Inst.* 1990; 50:947-950.

Niwa T, Swaneck G, Bradlow HL. Alterations in estradiol metabolism in MCF-7 cells induced by treatment with indole-3-carbinol and related compounds. *Steroids.* 1994; 59:523-527.

Wong GYC, Bradlow HL, Sepkovic DW, et al. A dose-ranging study of indole-3-carbinol for breast cancer prevention. *J Cell Biol.* 1988; 28:111-116.

Zeligs MA. Diet and estrogen status: the cruciferous connection. *J Med Food.* 1998; 1:67-82.

Inosine

DESCRIPTION

Inosine is a purine ribonucleoside widely found in plants, animals and other forms of living matter. It is comprised of the purine base hypoxanthine and the sugar D-ribose. The structural formula is:

Inosine

Inosine, in the form of its nucleotide, inosine 5′-monophosphate (inosinate), is the precursor of adenosine monophosphate (AMP) and guanosine monophosphate (GMP) in the *de novo* biosynthesis of purine nucleotides. It is also an intermediate in the so-called salvage pathway of purine nucleotide synthesis, and it is an intermediate in the degradation of purines and purine nucleosides to the purine end-product, uric acid. Inosine is also found as a minor nucleoside in transfer RNA.

Disodium inosinate is commonly used in foods for flavor enhancement and comprises a significant proportion of the dietary intake of inosine. Inosine itself has been used as a pharmaceutical agent. Some time ago, Trophicardyl was used in France for the treatment of cardiovascular conditions, including ischemia, cardiomyopathy and arrythmias. The active drug was inosine. In Russia, Riboxin, again inosine, was and is still used for the treatment of similar disorders. Inosine pranobex (Isoprinosine), a delivery form of inosine, is an orphan drug indicated for the treatment of subacute sclerosing panencephalitis. This drug is also thought to have immunomodulatory activity.

Inosine is also known as hypoxanthine riboside, 9-beta-D-ribofuranosylhypoxanthine and hypoxanthosine. It is abbreviated I.

ACTIONS AND PHARMACOLOGY

ACTIONS

Inosine may have neuroprotective, cardioprotective, anti-inflammatory and immunomodulatory activities.

MECHANISM OF ACTION

Inosine has been found to have potent axon-promoting effects *in vivo* following unilateral transection of the corticospinal tract of rats. The mechanism of this action is unclear. Possibilities include serving as an agonist of a nerve growth factor-activated protein kinase (N-Kinase), conversion to cyclic nucleotides that enable advancing nerve endings to overcome the inhibitory effects of myelin, stimulation of differentiation in rat sympathetic neurons, augmentation of nerve growth factor-induced neuritogenesis and promotion of the survival of astrocytes, among others.

The mechanism of inosine's possible cardioprotective effect is similarly unclear. Inosine has been reported to have a positive inotropic effect and also to have mild coronary vasodilation activity. Exogenous inosine may contribute to the high-energy phosphate pool of cardiac muscle cells and favorably affect bioenergetics generally. Inosine has also been reported to enhance the myocardial uptake of carbohydrates relative to free fatty acids as well as glycolysis.

In cell culture studies, inosine has been found to inhibit the production, in immunostimulated macrophages and spleen cells, of the proinflammatory cytokines, tumor necrosis factor (TNF)-alpha, interleukin (IL)-1, interleukin (IL)-12, macrophage-inflammatory protein-1 alpha and interferon (IFN)-gamma. It also suppressed proinflammatory cytokine production and mortality in a mouse endotoxemic model. These actions might account for the possible immunomodulatory, anti-inflammatory and anti-ischemic actions of inosine.

PHARMACOKINETICS

Ingested inosine is absorbed from the small intestine, from whence it is transported via the portal circulation to the liver. In the liver, inosine may be catabolized by a series of reactions culminating in the production of uric acid and also may be metabolized to adenine- and guanine-containing nucleotides. Inosine not metabolized in the liver is transported via the systemic circulation and distributed to various tissues of the body, where it is metabolized in similar fashion as in the liver. Uric acid, the purine end-product of inosine catabolism, is excreted in the urine.

INDICATIONS AND USAGE

The primary popular claim made for inosine, that it enhances exercise and athletic performance, is refuted by the available research data. There is some preliminary evidence that inosine may have some neurorestorative, anti-inflammatory, immunomodulatory and cardioprotective effects.

RESEARCH SUMMARY

In a double-blind, placebo-controlled, cross-over study of nine highly trained endurance runners, 6 grams daily of inosine failed to demonstrate any benefit in various exercise tests, including a three-mile treadmill run. By one of the measures used, placebo was significantly superior to inosine.

In another placebo-controlled study, inosine again failed to confer any advantage over placebo in 10 competitive male cyclists, as measured by tests of aerobic and anaerobic cycling performance. Here too, inosine was actually inferior to placebo under some test conditions, suggesting, the researchers concluded, that it might have an ergolytic effect.

Preliminary research has suggested that inosine can suppress proinflammatory cytokine production and mortality in a mouse endotoxemic model and that it has some cardioprotective effects in an animal model of ischemic heart. This was associated with an observed inosine-linked increase in glycolytic activity and improved energy production.

Inosine has also recently shown neurorestorative effects in the rat corticospinal tract after injury. It had previously been shown to induce axon outgrowth from primary neurons in culture. The more recent *in vivo* study encouraged the researchers to hope that inosine "might help to restore essential circuitry after injury to the central nervous system." More research is needed.

CONTRAINDICATIONS, PRECAUTIONS, ADVERSE REACTIONS

CONTRAINDICATIONS

Supplemental inosine is contraindicated in those with a history of gouty arthritis with acute attacks. Known hypersensitivity to an inosine-containing product.

PRECAUTIONS

Pregnant women and nursing mothers should avoid supplemental inosine.

Those with a history of hyperuricemia should be extremely cautious about use of inosine.

ADVERSE REACTIONS

Mild gastrointestinal symptoms, such as abdominal discomfort and nausea, have occasionally been reported.

OVERDOSAGE

No reports of overdosage.

DOSAGE AND ADMINISTRATION

No typical doses. Doses of 5 to 10 grams daily were used in the above-reported studies of the effects of inosine on athletic performance.

LITERATURE

Benowitz LI, Goldberg DE, Madsen JR, et al. Inosine stimulates extensive axon collateral growth in the rat corticospinal tract after injury. *Proc Natl Acad Sci.* 1999; 96:13486-13490.

Hasko G, Kuhel DG, Nemeth ZH, et al. Inosine inhibits inflammatory cytokine production by a posttranscriptional mechanism and protects against endotoxin-induced shock. *J Immunol.* 2000; 164:1013-1019.

Korotkov AA, Zhorzholiani TD, Chkheidze LG, Shalamberidze DN. [Effect of inosine after early infusion of contrykal and heparin in various hemodynamic types of acute myocardial ischemia.] [Article in Russian.] *Kardiologiia.* 1998; 28:91-94.

Lewandowski ED, Johnston DL, Roberts R. Effects of inosine on glycolysis and contracture during myocardial ischemia. *Cir Res.* 1991; 68:578-587.

Mc Naughton L, Dalton B, Tarr J. Inosine supplementation has no effect on aerobic or anaerobic cycling performance. *Int J Sports Nutr.* 1999; 9:333-334.

Milano S, Dieli M, Millott S, et al. Effect of isoprinosine on IL-3, IFN-gamma and IL-4 production *in vivo* and *in vitro*. *Int J Immunopharmacol.* 1991; 13:1013-1018

Renoux G, Renoux M, Guillaumin J-M. Isoprinosine as an immunopotentiator. *J Immunopharmacol.* 1979; 1:337-356.

Starling RD, Trappe TA, Short KR, et al. Effect of inosine supplementation on aerobic and anaerobic cycling performance. *Med Sci Sports Exerc.* 1996; 28:1193-1198.

Williams MH, Kreider RB, Hunter DW, et al. Effect of inosine supplementation on 3-mile treadmill run performance and VO_2 peak. *Med Sci Sports Exec.* 1990; 22:517-522.

Zimmer HG. Effect of inosine on cardiac adenine nucleotide metabolism in rats. *Adv Myocardiol.* 1985; 6:173-183.

Inositol Hexaphosphate

DESCRIPTION

Inositol hexaphosphate, also known as phytate, is a component of most cereal grains and seeds, occurring in conjunction with plant fiber, and is a source of *myo*-inositol in the diet. Inositol hexaphosphate is responsible for storing more than 80 percent of the total phosphate in cereals and legumes. Phytate has strong chelating power for doubly charged metal ions, such as magnesium, calcium and zinc. Some studies suggest that phytate may slow tumor growth rates.

Inositol hexaphosphate, in addition to being known as phytate, is known as *myo*-inositol hexaphosphate, and *myo*-inositol 1,2,3,4,5,6-hexakisphosphate. Inositol hexaphosphate is abbreviated as $InsP_6$ and sometimes as IP-6. The structural formula is:

Inositol hexaphosphate

ACTIONS AND PHARMACOLOGY

ACTIONS

Inositol hexaphosphate is a putative antiproliferative agent and may have antioxidant activity.

MECHANISM OF ACTION

Some speculate that inositol hexaphosphate's possible antiproliferative activity is due to its chelating divalent cations which may be important for tumor growth. Others speculate that inositol hexaphosphate, along with inositol, are metabolized to inositol triphosphates, which are believed to be involved in cell signaling and regulating cell growth, and that this may underlie its possible effects. Chelation by inositol hexaphosphate of ferrous cations could inhibit the Fenton reaction, a reaction which generates reactive oxygen species. Enhancement of natural killer cell activity is offered as still another speculative mechanism.

PHARMACOKINETICS

It is unclear how much inositol hexaphosphate is absorbed in humans following ingestion. Inositol hexaphosphate may, in part, be hydrolyzed to *myo*-inositol. (See *myo*-inositol.)

INDICATIONS AND USAGE

There is preliminary evidence that inositol hexaphosphate may eventually find some use in the treatment of some cancers.

RESEARCH SUMMARY

A few studies performed *in vitro* and in animal models suggest that inositol hexaphosphate inhibits some cancers, specifically epithelial cancers, including breast and colon cancers. It has also significantly inhibited human rhabdomyosarcoma in an animal model. More research is needed to see whether this substance can play a role in the clinical treatment of some cancers. There is some epidemiologic data suggesting that dietary phytate may have chemopreventive activity.

CONTRAINDICATIONS, PRECAUTIONS, ADVERSE REACTIONS

CONTRAINDICATIONS

Known hypersensitivity to an inositol hexaphosphate-containing product.

PRECAUTIONS

Supplemental inositol hexaphosphate should be avoided by pregnant women and nursing mothers, due to lack of long-term safety studies.

ADVERSE REACTIONS

No significant adverse effects were noted in one report on the use of a daily dose of 8.8 grams of inositol hexaphosphate taken for several months.

INTERACTIONS

Inositol hexaphosphate may form chelates with divalent cations such as calcium, magnesium, manganese, zinc, copper and iron found in foods, if taken with foods or nutritional supplements containing these elements. It may also interact with food proteins.

OVERDOSAGE

No reports of overdosage.

DOSAGE AND ADMINISTRATION

None recommended.

LITERATURE

Graf E, Eaton JW. Antioxidant function of phytic acid. *Free Rad Biol Med.* 1990; 8:61-69.

Jariwalla RJ, Sabin R, Lawson S, Herman ZS. Lowering of serum cholesterol and triglycerides and modulation by dietary phytates. *J Appl Nutr.* 1990; 42:18-28.

Jariwalla RJ, Sabin R, Lawson S, et al. Effect of dietary phytic acid (phytate) on the incidence and growth rate of tumors promoted in Fisher rats by magnesium supplement. *Nutr Res.* 1988; 8:813-827.

Porres JM, Stahl CH, Cheng W-H, et al. Dietary intrinsic phytate protects colon from lipid peroxidation in pigs with a moderately high dietary iron intake. *Proc Soc Exp Biol Med.* 1999; 221:80-86.

Shamsuddin AM. Inositol phosphates have novel anticancer function. *J Nutr.* 1995; 125:725S-732S.

Shamsuddin AM. Reduction of cell proliferation and enhancement of NK-cell activity. 1992. United States Patent Number 5,082,833.

Vucenik I, Kalebic T, Tantivejkulk, Shamsuddin A. Novel anticancer function of inositol hexaphosphate. Inhibition of human rhabdomyosarcoma *in vitro* and *in vivo*. *Anticanc Res.* 1998; 18:1377-1384.

Inositol Nicotinate

DESCRIPTION

Inositol nicotinate is a delivery form of nicotinic acid that has been used in Europe and Japan for the treatment of hyperlipidemias, peripheral vascular disorders, including Raynaud's disease, intermittent claudication, Buerger's disease (thromboangiitis obliterans), and necrobiosis lipoidica, a disorder marked by shiny leg lesions due to atrophy of the skin. Inositol nicotinate is marketed in the United States as a nutritional supplement. The flushing reaction ("niacin flush") which occurs in those taking immediate-release or crystalline nicotinic acid, is usually not as severe with inositol nicotinate.

Inositol nicotinate is also known as inositol niacinate, *myo*-inositol hexa-3-pyridinecarboxylic acid, hexanicotinoyl inositol, *meso*-inositol hexanicotinate, inositol hexanicotinate, inositol hexaniacinate and hexanicotinyl *cis*-1,2,3,5-*trans*-4,6-cyclohexane. Its molecular formula is $C_{42}H_{30}N_6O_{12}$ and its molecular weight is 810.73 daltons. Each molecule of inositol nicotinate contains six molecules of nicotinic acid esterified to one molecule of *myo*-inositol. By weight,

approximately 80% of inositol nicotinate is nicotinic acid and 20% is *myo*-inositol. The chemical structure of inositol nicotinate is represented as follows:

Inositol Nicotinate

ACTIONS AND PHARMACOLOGY

ACTIONS

Inositol nicotinate may have antihyperlipidemic activity. It may also have activity in the management of certain peripheral vascular diseases, such Raynaud's disease and intermittent claudication.

MECHANISM OF ACTION

The possible antihyperlipidemic activity of inositol nicotinate is accounted for by its metabolic conversion to nicotinic acid. See monograph on Niacin (Nicotinic Acid) for a discussion of the possible mechanisms of the antihyperlipidemic activity of nicotinic acid.

Inositol nicotinate has shown some activity in some with Raynaud's disease and intermittent claudication. Features of Raynaud's disease include intense vasoconstriction or vasospasm and platelet aggregation. The mechanism of inositol nicotinate's possible activity in Raynaud's disease is unknown. Nicotinic acid, the principal metabolite of inositol nicotinate, can cause vasodilation of cutaneous vessels. This results in increased blood flow principally to the face, neck and chest and is responsible for the so called niacin-flush. The vasodilatory activity of nicotinic acid is thought to be prostaglandin-mediated. However, the vasodilatory effect of nicotinic acid is transitory and unlikely to play a significant role in the possible activity of inositol nicotinate in Raynaud's disease.

Intermittent claudication results from occlusive arterial disease of the lower limbs and is characterized by pain, which develops during exercise and which disappears at rest. The pain is due to ischemia resulting from the obstruction or vasoconstriction of peripheral arteries. Inositol nicotinate may help some with this disorder. Again, the possible activity of inositol nicotinate is most likely mediated via its metabolite nicotinic acid. The mechanism of this possible effect is not understood. Hypothetical possibilities include nicotinic acid's hypolipidemic activity, its possible fibrinogen-lowering activity and, less likely, nicotinic acid's transient vasodilatory activity.

PHARMACOKINETICS

The pharmacokinetics of inositol nicotinate are not completely known. The molecule, at least in part, is absorbed from the small intestine intact. Metabolism of inositol nicotinate to *myo*-inositol and nicotinic acid appears to occur principally in the blood. Serum nicotinic acid levels appear to reach peak serum levels approximately 10 hours following ingestion of inositol nicotinate. Inositol nicotinate may be considered as a sustained-release form of nicotinic acid. See monographs on Niacin (Nicotinic Acid) and *Myo*-Inositol for discussions of the pharmacokinetics of these substances.

INDICATIONS AND USAGE

Inositol nicotinate has uses similar to those of nicotinic acid (see monograph on Niacin [Nicotinic Acid]). It has shown some promise in the treatment of hyperlipidemia, Raynaud's disease, intermittent claudication and other peripheral vascular diseases. Its use in dermatological conditions is too preliminary to support conclusions.

RESEARCH SUMMARY

Much of the research that applies to nicotinic acid applies to inositol nicotinate (see monograph on Niacin [Nicotinic Acid]). Inositol nicotinate is sometimes used for the treatment of Raynaud's disease. In one double-blind, placebo-controlled trial, 23 patients with primary Raynaud's disease were randomized to receive placebo or 4 grams of inositol hexanicotinate daily during cold weather. The treated subjects had significantly fewer and shorter vasospasm attacks than did the controls.

CONTRAINDICATIONS, PRECAUTIONS, ADVERSE REACTIONS

CONTRAINDICATIONS

Inositol nicotinate is contraindicated in those hypersensitive to any component of an inositol nicotinate-containing product. It is also contraindicated in those with hepatic dysfunction, unexplained elevations of serum aminotransferases (transaminases), active peptic ulcer disease and arterial bleeding.

PRECAUTIONS

Pregnant women and nursing mothers should avoid the use of inositol nicotinate.

The use of inositol nicotinate as an antihyperlipidemic agent or for the management of peripheral vascular disorders such as Raynaud's disease and intermittent claudication, or for any medical condition requires medical supervision.

Those with diabetes, gout, renal dysfunction and cardiovascular disease (especially acute myocardial infarction and unstable angina) should exercise caution in the use of inositol nicotinate, as should those with a past history of hepatobiliary disease, jaundice, peptic ulcer disease or gastritis.

Inositol nicotinate should not be substituted for equivalent doses of immediate-release (regular crystalline) nicotinic acid. Cases of severe hepatic toxicity, including fulminant hepatic necrosis, have occurred in those who have substituted sustained-release nicotinic acid products for immediate-release nicotinic acid at equivalent doses. Even though this has not been reported for inositol nicotinate, since inositol nicotinate behaves as a sustained-release form of nicotinic acid, this situation is theoretically possible. Those who switch from immediate-release nicotinic acid to inositol nicotinate, should start off, under medical supervision, with low doses of inositol nicotinate and the dose should be slowly increased to obtain the desired therapeutic response.

Inositol nicotinate, at high doses, may adversely affect glucose tolerance. Diabetics who use inositol nicotinate for lipid lowering, should have their serum glucose levels carefully monitored and the dose of their antidiabetic medications adjusted as necessary.

ADVERSE REACTIONS

Adverse reactions of high-dose nicotinic acid include flushing, pruritis, dizziness, palpitations, impaired glucose tolerance, elevated uric acid levels and liver dysfunction. Inositol nicotinate appears to be a well-tolerated delivery form of nicotinic acid. It has only recently been introduced into the United States marketplace. However, few adverse reactions have been reported in Europe where the product has been in use for about three decades.

INTERACTIONS

See Niacin (Nicotinic Acid).

OVERDOSAGE

There have been no reported overdoses involving inositol nicotinate reported in the literature.

DOSAGE AND ADMINISTRATION

Inositol nicotinamide is available as a single ingredient product or in combination with other nutritional supplements. Dosage used has ranged from 500 milligrams to 4 grams daily taken with meals. Doses higher than 4 grams are rarely used.

LITERATURE

Head KA. Inositol hexanicotinate: a safer alternative to niacin. *Alt Med Rev.* 1996; 1:176-184.

Holti G. An experimentally controlled evaluation of the effect of inositol nicotinate upon the digital blood flow of patients with Raynaud's phenomenon. *J Int Med Res*. 1979; 7:473-483.

O'Hara J, Jolly PN, Nicol CG. The therapeutic efficacy of inositol nicotinate (Hexopal) in intermittent claudication: a controlled trial. *Br J Clin Pract*. 1988; 42:377-383.

Ring EF, Bacon PA. Quantitative thermographic assessment of inositol nicotinate therapy in Reynaud's phenomena. *J Int Med Res*. 1977; 5:217-222.

Sunderland GT, Belch JJ, Sturrock RD, et al. A double blind randomized placebo controlled trial of hexopal in primary Reynaud's disease. *Clin Rheumatol*. 1988; 7:46-49.

Insulin-Like Growth Factor 1 (IGF-1)

DESCRIPTION

Insulin-like growth factor-1 (IGF-1) is a single-chain polypeptide of 70 amino acids. It is a trophic factor that circulates at high levels in the blood-stream and mediates many, if not most, of the effects of growth hormone. Although the main source of IGF-1 in the serum is the liver, many other tissues synthesize it and are sensitive to its trophic action. IGF-1 was called somatomedin in the older literature. IGF-1 and insulin have similar three-dimensional structures.

IGF-1 appears to influence neuronal structure and functions throughout the life span. It has been shown to have the ability to preserve nerve cell function and promote nerve growth in experimental studies. Because of these properties, recombinant human IGF-1 is in clinical trials for the treatment of amyotrophic lateral sclerosis (ALS).

Recently, recombinant human IGF-1 has entered the dietary supplement marketplace, as have recombinant human growth hormone and several so-called growth hormone secretagogues or releasers.

ACTIONS AND PHARMACOLOGY

ACTIONS

Supplemental IGF-1 has putative anabolic and lipolytic activities.

MECHANISM OF ACTION

The mechanism of the putative actions of supplemental IGF-1 is unknown.

PHARMACOKINETICS

Orally administered IGF-1 has very poor bioavailability. There is no credible evidence that IGF-1 is absorbed from the oral mucosa if administered as a spray. It is likely that orally administered IGF-1 is digested in the small intestine to the amino acids that comprise the molecule.

INDICATIONS AND USAGE

Claims for supplemental IGF-1 are sweeping and include antiaging, promotion of lean muscle mass, enhanced athletic and sexual performance, joint protection, antidiabetic and antiatherosclerotic effects, sleep aid, immune enhancer, neuroprotector and much more. There is no credible evidence to support these claims for oral IGF-1. High levels of IGF-1 have been associated with elevated risk of several cancers, especially prostate cancer.

RESEARCH SUMMARY

There is no research to support the use of IGF-1 as a nutritional supplement, whether in oral or injected form. There is research showing associations between high levels of circulating IGF-1 and several cancers.

Claims that IGF-1 supplements significantly increase lean muscle mass are unsubstantiated. Use of IGF-1 in doses far higher than those used by most bodybuilders failed to produce more than very modest anabolic effects in AIDS patients. It is possible that some clinical indications, but not supplemental indications, will emerge from experimental work currently underway with IGF-1. There is a hint in some of this work that IGF-1 might, for example, have some neuroprotective and neurorestorative effects in some conditions.

CONTRAINDICATIONS, PRECAUTIONS, ADVERSE REACTIONS

CONTRAINDICATIONS

Supplemental IGF-1 is contraindicated in those with any evidence of active malignancy. It is also contraindicated in those who are hypersensitive to any component of an IGF-1-containing product.

PRECAUTIONS

Pregnant women and nursing mothers should avoid the use of supplemental IGF-1-containing products.

Adolescents should avoid the use of supplemental IGF-1-containing products.

Supplemental IGF-1 is not meant to be used parenterally and should never be used in such a manner.

ADVERSE REACTIONS

None known for supplemental IGF-1-containing supplements.

INTERACTIONS

There are no known interactions for supplemental IGF-1-containing supplements.

OVERDOSAGE

No reports for supplemental IGF-1-containing supplements.

DOSAGE AND ADMINISTRATION

Supplemental IGF-1 is available and marketed as a dietary supplement, typically in the form of an oral spray. There are no recommended doses.

LITERATURE

Carro E, Nuñez A, Busiguina S, Torres-Aleman I. Circulating insulin-like growth factor 1 mediates effects of exercise on the brain. *J Neurosci*. 2000; 20:2926-2933.

Chan JM, Stampfer MJ, Giovanucci E, et al. Plasma insulin-like growth factor 1 and prostate cancer risk: a prospective study. *Science*. 1998; 279:563-566.

Giovannucci E, Pollak MN, Platz EA, et al. A prospective study of plasma insulin-like growth factor-1 and binding protein-3 and risk of colorectal neoplasia in women. *Cancer Epidemiol Biomarkers Prev*. 2000; 9:345-349.

Hankinson SE, Willett WC, Colditz GA, et al. Circulating concentrations of insulin-like growth factor-1 and risk of breast cancer. *Lancet*. 1998; 351:1393-1396.

Le Roith D. Insulin-like growth factors. *N Engl J Med*. 1997; 336:633-640.

Lewis ME, Neff NT, Contreras PC, et al. Insulin-like growth factor-1: potential for treatment of motor neuronal disorders. *Exp Neurol*. 1993; 124:73-88.

Magee BA, Shooter GK, Wallace JC, Francis GL. Insulin-like growth factor 1 and its binding proteins: a study of the binding interface using B-domain analogues. *Biochem*. 1999; 38:15863-15870.

Mantzoros CS, Tzonou A, Signorello LB, et al. Insulin-like growth factor 1 in relation to prostate cancer and benign prostate hyperplasia. *Brit J Cancer*. 1997; 76:1115-1118.

Niblock MM, Brunso-Bechtold J, Riddle DR. Insulin-like growth factor 1 stimulates dendritic growth in primary somatosensory cortex. *J Neurosci*. 2000; 20:4165-4176.

Inulins

DESCRIPTION

Inulins refer to a group of naturally occurring fructose-containing oligosaccharides. They belong to a class of carbohydrates known as fructans. Fructans, in addition to inulins, include another group of naturally occurring fructose-containing oligosaccharides called levans. Inulins are usually of plant origin, while levans are found in fungi and bacteria. Inulins are mainly comprised of fructose units and typically have a terminal glucose. The bond between fructose units in inulins is a beta-(2-1) glycosidic linkage. Plant inulins contain 2 to 150 fructose units. The smallest inulin is called 1-kestose and is composed of two residues of fructose and one of glucose. Inulins are naturally synthesized from sucrose.

Chemically, inulins with a terminal glucose are known as alpha-D-glucopyranosyl-[beta-D-fructofuranosyl](n-1)-D-fructofuranosides, which is abbreviated GpyFn. Inulins without glucose are beta-D-fructopyranosyl-[D-fructofuranosyl](n-1)-D-fructofuranosides, abbreviated as FpyFn. Lower case n refers to the number of fructose residues in inulin; py is the abbreviation for pyranosyl. The basic structural formula follows:

Inulin

n or m equal the number of fructose units

G = glucose, F = fructose

Inulins are present in onions, leeks, garlic, bananas, asparagus and artichokes, among other vegetables and fruits. Because of their sweet taste and their texture, inulins are added to various foods. Inulin intake in the U.S. ranges from 1 to 4 grams daily. It is higher in the European diet.

Inulins are only slightly digested in the small intestine. They are, however, fermented by a limited number of colonic bacteria. This could lead to changes in the colonic ecosystem in favor of some bacteria, such as bifidobacteria, which may have health benefits. Inulins are considered to be bifidogenic factors. Their energy content is about half that of digestible carbohydrates or about 1 to 2 kcal/grams.

Substances such as inulins that promote the growth of beneficial bacteria in the colon are called prebiotics. Prebiotics are typically nondigestible oligosaccharides.

Inulins are marketed as nutritional supplements and functional foods. The sources of these inulins are roots of chicory (*Cichorium intybus*) and Jerusalem artichokes (*Helianthus tuberosus*). Oligofructose refers to the partial enzymatic hydrolysate of inulins. Fructooligosacchrides usually refer to synthetic short-chain fructans. The average chain length in inulins is 10.

ACTIONS AND PHARMACOLOGY

ACTIONS

Inulins may have antitumor, antimicrobial, hypolipidemic and hypoglycemic actions. They may also help to improve mineral absorption and balance and may have antiosteoporotic activity.

MECHANISM OF ACTION

The possible antitumor activity of inulins, particularly with respect to colon cancer, might be accounted for, in part, by the possible antitumor action of butyrate. Butyrate, the anion of the short-chain fatty acid butyric acid, is produced by bacterial fermentation of inulins in the colon. Some studies suggest that butyrate may induce growth arrest and cell differentiation and upregulate apoptosis, three activities that could be significant for antitumor activity. Inulins may also aid in increasing the concentrations of calcium and magnesium in the colon. High concentrations of these cations in the colon may help control the rate of cell turnover. High concentrations of calcium may also lead to the formation of insoluble bile or salts of fatty acids. This might reduce the potential damaging effects of bile or fatty acids on colonocytes.

Inulins may promote the growth of favorable bacterial populations, such as bifidobacteria, in the colon. Bifidobacteria may inhibit the growth of pathogenic bacteria, such as *Clostridium perfringens* and diarrheogenic strains of *Escherichia coli*.

Inulins have been found to lower serum triglycerides in rats, and there is some indication that they may lower serum triglycerides in some humans, as well. The mechanism of this possible effect is unclear. It is speculated that the possible triglyceride-lowering effect is due to decreased triglyceride synthesis in the liver. Inulins may lower cholesterol levels in some type 2 diabetics. There is less evidence that inulins lower cholesterol in those with hypercholesterolemia who do not have diabetes. Propionate, a product of inulin fermentation in the colon, may inhibit hydroxymethylglutaryl-CoA (HMG-CoA) reductase, the rate-limiting step in cholesterol biosynthesis.

The possible beneficial effects of inulins on blood glucose—there is some evidence that inulins may lower fasting blood sugar in type 2 diabetics—may be explained as follows: Inulins may delay gastric emptying and/or shorten small-intestinal transit time. Propionate may inhibit gluconeogenesis. It may do this by its metabolic conversion to methylmalonyl-CoA and succinyl CoA, metabolites that may inhibit pyruvate carboxylase. Propionate may reduce plasma levels of free fatty acids. High levels of plasma free fatty acids lower glucose utilization and induce insulin resistance. Propionate may also enhance glycolysis via depletion of citrate in hepatocytes. Citrate is an allosteric inhibitor of phosphofructokinase.

Inulins, similar to dietary fiber, may bind/sequester such minerals as calcium and magnesium in the small intestine. The short-chain fatty acids (acetate, propionate, butyrate) formed from the bacterial fermentation of inulins in the intestinal tract may facilitate the colonic absorption of calcium and possibly also magnesium ions. This could be beneficial in preventing osteoporosis and osteopenia.

PHARMACOKINETICS

Little digestion of inulins takes place in the stomach and small intestine following ingestion of inulins. Inulins are fermented in the colon by bifidobacteria and some other bacteria to produce the short-chain fatty acids acetate, propionate and butyrate; the gases hydrogen, hydrogen sulfide, carbon dioxide and methane; and lactate, pyruvate and succinate. Acetate, propionate and butyrate that are not metabolized in colonocytes are absorbed from the colon and transported via the portal circulation to the liver. These short-chain fatty acids are extensively metabolized in hepatocytes. Acetate, propionate and butyrate that are not metabolized in hepatocyes are transported by the circulation to various tissues, where they undergo further metabolism. Butyrate is an important respiratory fuel for the colonocytes and is metabolized in them to carbon dioxide and water. Energy, in the form of ATP, is produced from the catabolism of butyrate.

Those with ileostomies may have a microbial population colonizing their ileums. In those cases, inulins could be fermented by some of the bacteria in similar fashion to the way they are fermented in the colon.

INDICATIONS AND USAGE

Inulins, like some other prebiotic substances, may help protect against colorectal cancer and some infectious bowel diseases. They may also have lipid-lowering effects. Animal research is suggestive of these benefits, but human research is in short supply.

RESEARCH SUMMARY

There is the suggestion from animal research that inulins may help prevent colon carcinogenesis by stimulating growth of bifidobacteria. In experiments with rats, dietary administration of inulins inhibited the development of colonic aberrant crypt foci, putative preneoplastic lesions that are believed to give rise to colonic adenomas and carcinomas. Oligofructose, a partial enzymatic hydrolysate of inulins, also inhibited these crypt foci but not as effectively as inulins.

Recently, 12 healthy male volunteers ate a breakfast cereal containing 18% inulin for several weeks. At the end of the trial, plasma total cholesterol and triacylglycerol levels were significantly decreased.

CONTRAINDICATIONS, PRECAUTIONS, ADVERSE REACTIONS

CONTRAINDICATIONS

Inulins are contraindicated in those who are hypersensitive to these substances.

PRECAUTIONS

Those who develop gastrointestinal symptoms with the use of dietary fiber should exercise caution in the use of inulins. Those with irritable bowel syndrome should exercise caution in the use of inulins. Those receiving whole body-radiation or radiation to the gastrointestinal tract should avoid supplementation with inulins.

ADVERSE REACTIONS

Doses up to 10 grams daily are well tolerated. Higher doses may cause such gastrointestinal symptoms as flatulence, bloating and diarrhea.

Occasional allergic reactions have been reported.

INTERACTIONS

NUTRITIONAL SUPPLEMENTS

Inulins may enhance the colonic absorption of calcium and magnesium supplements if used concomitantly with them.

Probiotics: The possible beneficial effects of inulins may be enhanced if used in combination with probiotics.

FOODS

Inulins may enhance the colonic absorption of calcium and magnesium in foods.

OVERDOSAGE

No reports of overdosage.

DOSAGE AND ADMINISTRATION

Inulins are available in tablets, powder and functional foods. Dosing is variable and ranges from 4 to 10 grams daily. Those who use more than 10 grams daily should split the dosage throughout the day. Doses higher than 30 grams daily may cause significant gastrointestinal discomfort.

LITERATURE

Brighenti F, Casiraghi MC, Canzi E, Ferrari A. Effect of consumption of a ready-to-eat breakfast cereal containing inulin on the intestinal milieu and blood lipids in healthy male volunteers. *Eur J Clin Nutr.* 1999; 53:726-733.

Menne E, Guggenbuhl N, Roberfroid M. Fn-type chicory inulin hydrolysate has a prebiotic effect in humans. *J Nutr.* 2000; 130:1197-1199.

Reddy BS, Hamid R, Rao CV. Effect of dietary oligofructose and inulin on colonic preneoplastic aberrant crypt foci inhibition. *Carcinogenesis.* 1997; 18:1371-1374.

Roberfroid MB, Delzenne NM. Dietary fructans. *Annu Rev Nutr.* 1998; 18:117-143.

Roberfroid MB, Van Loo JA, Gibson GR. The bifidogenic nature of chicory inulin and its hydrolysis products. *J Nutr.* 1998; 128:11-19.

Williams CM. Effects of inulin on lipid parameters in humans. *J Nutr.* 1999; 129(7 Suppl):1471S-1473S.

Iodine

DESCRIPTION

Iodine, consumed principally as its iodide salts, is an essential trace element which is vital to the function of the thyroid gland. It is an essential component of thyroid hormones, which are required for normal development and metabolism. The fact that trace element composition of foods is very much dependent on geography was first recognized with respect to iodine. Iodine is present in low amounts in the earth's crust and thus in its soil. It is plentiful in the oceans and is found in sea animals and sea plants, such as seaweeds. Iodine is a non-metallic element belonging to the halogen group. Its atomic number is 53, and its atomic mass is 126.90 daltons. Its atomic symbol is I. The terms iodine and iodide are frequently used interchangeably.

The thyroid hormones are iodine-containing substances and they do not function without iodine. Approximately 80% of the body's iodine pool, or about 15 milligrams in adults, is present in the thyroid gland. Moderate deficiency of iodine may result in a goiter. Severe iodine deficiency may result in endemic myxedema among adults and in endemic cretinism among infants. Iodine deficiency results in decreased production of the thyroid hormones thyroxine or T_4 and triiodothyronine or T_3. The fall in the level of T_4 leads to increased thyroid stimulating hormone (TSH) output from the pituitary gland, resulting in an increase in the size of the thyroid gland which can lead to the formation of a goiter. In addition to causing goiters, iodine deficiency may result in a wide spectrum of effects on growth and development, particularly on brain development. Iodine deficiency is the most common cause of preventable mental deficit in the world.

In the early 1900s and prior to that, iodine deficiency and endemic goiter were very common in the United States. In the early 1920s, it was demonstrated in school children in Ohio that endemic goiter could be prevented and reduced by administration of small amounts of iodine in the form of iodide. Shortly afterwards, mass prophylaxis of endemic goiter with iodized salt was introduced in the United States and Switzerland, leading to a sharp fall in the incidence of goiter, as well as cretinism. Goiter, myxedema and other iodine deficiency disorders (IDD), including cretinism, still continue to be major public health problems on the global level. Approximately 20% of the world's population is iodine-deficient and at risk for IDD.

In addition to iodized salt, rich sources of iodine include fish and sea vegetables (seaweeds). Iodine is also available in animal products, such as eggs, milk, meat and poultry. In industrialized countries, most animal feeds are enriched with iodine.

ACTIONS AND PHARMACOLOGY

ACTIONS
Iodine's major action is its precursor role in the formation of thyroid hormones. Iodine may also be protective against radioactive iodine and consequent thyroid cancer. Iodine is used therapeutically for the treatment of certain hyperthyroid conditions and thyroid storm. The radionuclide ^{123}I is used for thyroid imaging and ^{131}I is used therapeutically for radioactive ablation of benign overactive thyroid and of locally invasive or metastatic thyroid cancer.

MECHANISM OF ACTION
Iodine in the form of iodide is preferentially taken up by the thyroid gland. Iodide is accumulated in the thyroid by means of an active iodide transport mechanism which is catalyzed by a sodium/iodide symporter, which mediates the sodium/potassium ATPase-dependent coupling of inward iodide and sodium fluxes. The thyroid gland is not the only organ capable of iodide uptake. However, the thyroid is the only organ known to organify iodide. Iodide is released by the thyroid cells into the colloid follicle phase, and there it is oxidized by hydrogen peroxide formed from the thyroid peroxidase system. Iodine reacts with tyrosine residues in thyroglobulin to form thyroxine (T_4 and triiodothyronine (T_3. The formation of T_4 and T_3 takes place post-translationally. The iodinated thyroglobulin is absorbed back into the thyroid cells where proteolytic enzymes break it down. The thyroid hormones T_4 and T_3 are released into the circulation and distributed to the various tissues of the body.

Potassium iodide may be used following radiation exposure from a nuclear reactor accident. Pharmacological doses of iodide block uptake by the thyroid of radioactive isotopes, particularly ^{131}I, thus minimizing the risk of radiation-induced thyroid cancer.

PHARMACOKINETICS
Iodine in the form of iodide is rapidly and efficiently absorbed from the small intestine following ingestion. A large fraction of absorbed iodine is taken up by the thyroid gland via the sodium/iodide symporter. In addition to the thyroid gland, active iodide occurs in the salivary glands, the gastric mucosa and in the lactating mammary gland. The nonlactating mammary gland does not accumulate iodide.

Recently, it has been reported that accumulation of iodide via a sodium/iodide symporter appears to occur in human breast cancer tissue. The major route of excretion of excess iodine is by the kidneys.

INDICATIONS AND USAGE
Apart from its use in iodine-deficiency disorders and for certain hyperthyroid conditions and thyroid storm, iodine is used as an expectorant and has demonstrated some ability to protect against the toxic effects of radioactive materials. It has also shown some preliminary efficacy in the treatment of sarcoidosis and has ameliorated some of the symptoms of fibrocystic disease of the breast. There are some preliminary reports that iodine is helpful in the treatment of erythematous dermatoses. Recently, some researchers have expressed concern that those on vegetarian diets may be at increased risk of iodine deficiency. Similarly, those on salt-restricted diets in general may be at the same or greater increased risk.

RESEARCH SUMMARY
There are reports that potassium iodide is a useful expectorant in chronic obstructive pulmonary disease including bronchitis, emphysema and asthma. It has been used in some studies of these conditions at doses of 300 to 1,000 milligrams two or three times daily. While somewhat effective, potassium iodide is not often used in this context due to the availability of more effective and safer expectorants.

Potassium iodide can effectively reduce thyroid uptake of radioiodine by 90% to 99% when administered immediately after exposure. Dosage used for this purpose has been reported at 130 milligrams per day. A 50% reduction in uptake of radioiodine has been achieved when potassium iodide was administered three to four hours after exposure to radiation. Limited benefit was seen when therapy began between four and twelve hours post-exposure. Potassium iodide has not protected against other radioactive substances.

The World Health Organization (WHO) has recommended that communities near nuclear reactors stockpile potassium iodides. Some credit Poland's prompt and widespread use of potassium iodide after the 1986 Chernobyl nuclear reactor disaster with the fact that Poland did not experience a significant increase in the incidence of childhood thyroid cancers, while fallout areas in Ukraine, Belarus and Russia (where potassium iodide was not widely used) have experienced large increases in these cancers.

Treatment with elemental iodine for four months has reportedly produced significant relief from symptoms of fibrocystic breast disease in one study. Upon discontinuing iodine, women in this study suffered a recurrence of pain and soreness. Some subsequent studies have also reported significant benefit from supplementation with other iodine-containing compounds used to treat this condition. Sodium iodide exhibited marked efficacy but was accompanied by a high rate of side effects. In one analysis of three clinical studies, molecular iodine was found to be the most beneficial in the treatment of fibrocystic breast disease.

There is one case report in which 300 milligrams of potassium iodide three times daily was of significant benefit in subjects with sarcoidosis. Pain and swelling in the arthritic ankle largely disappeared within 48 hours after initiation of treatment, and there was rapid regression of erythema nodosum on the leg.

Some others have reported benefit from 200 milligrams of potassium iodide three times daily in subjects with erythema nodosum. Best response has been seen when given soon after onset in patients with positive C-reactive protein reactions. There is also very preliminary evidence that the same doses of potassium iodide may be helpful in some with erythema multiforme and nodular vasculitis. More research is needed to confirm these findings.

Recently, some researchers have concluded that vegetarians, especially "strict" vegetarians who exclude all animal products from their diets, may be at increased risk of iodine deficiency. Both strict vegan diets and lactovegetarian diets that exclude seaweed and iodized salt provide very low iodine, according to the findings of one recent study. Non-vegetarian diets that exclude iodized salt and naturally rich sources of iodine, especially fish and seafood, also deliver very little iodine.

Urinary excretion studies have suggested that there has been a decline in iodide intake in several populations tested, e.g., school children in Switzerland and blood donors in New Zealand. Some have attributed this to the growing popularity of salt-restriction in diet generally. Some European populations have also recently been reported to exhibit overt and borderline iodine deficiencies.

One researcher has concluded that "the subclinical effects of low iodine intake and the physiological significance of low iodine excretion need to be studied further."

CONTRAINDICATIONS, PRECAUTIONS, ADVERSE REACTIONS

CONTRAINDICATIONS

Iodide and iodine are contraindicated in those hypersensitive to iodide- and iodine-containing products.

PRECAUTIONS

Pregnant women and nursing mothers should avoid intakes of iodine (iodide) greater than RDA amounts. These amounts are 220 micrograms daily for pregnant women and 290 micrograms daily for nursing mothers. Use of iodide doses much higher than 220 micrograms daily by pregnant women may cause fetal damage. Use by nursing mothers of iodide doses much greater than 290 micrograms daily may cause rash and thyroid suppression in the infant.

Older people with nodular goiters are at risk of developing hyperthyroidism from use of potassium iodide and iodized salt.

Potassium iodide and iodized salt may exacerbate symptoms in some with autoimmune thyroiditis.

Children with cystic fibrosis appear to have an exaggerated susceptibility to the goitrogenic effect of high doses of iodide.

ADVERSE REACTIONS

Doses of iodide up to 1,000 micrograms daily are generally well tolerated. Pharmacological doses of iodide have caused a number of adverse reactions. The adverse reactions include hypersensitivity reactions, flare-up of adolescent acne, rashes, arrhythmias, central nervous system effects (confusion, numbness, tingling, weakness in the hands or feet), hypothyroidism, hyperthyroidism (Jod-Basedow phenomenon), parotitis (iodide mumps), thyroid adenoma and small bowel lesions.

Manifestations of hypersensitivity reactions include angioedema, symptoms resembling serum sickness (fever, arthralgia, eosinophilia, lymphadenopathy), cutaneous and mucosal hemorrhages, urticaria, thrombotic thrombocytopenia purpura (TTP) and fatal periarteritis. Nonspecific small bowel lesions manifested by stenosis with or without ulcerations have been associated with the use of enteric-coated potassium iodide. These lesions may cause hemorrhage, obstruction, perforation and death.

Chronic intake of pharmacological doses of iodides can lead to iodism. Iodism is characterized by frontal headache, pulmonary edema, coryza, eye irritation, skin eruptions, gastric disturbances and inflammation of the tonsils, larynx, pharynx and submaxillary and parotid glands.

The most common adverse effect of salt iodization is the development of iodine-induced hyperthyroidism (IIH). IIH affects mainly older people with nodular goiter. Another possibility is the exacerbation of autoimmune thyroiditis. Theoretically, salt iodization can induce hypothyroidism by acute blockage of the synthesis and secretion of thyroid hormones. Hypothyroidism, however, has not been reported with salt iodization. Also, allergic responses to salt iodization are rare. IIH may develop when iodine deficiency increases thyrocyte proliferation and mutation rates. This can lead to the development of hyperfunctioning autonomous nodules in the thyroid gland and hyperthyroidism following iodine supplementation. A recent study reported transient hyperthyroidism in one out of 32 young adults with goiter and hypothyroidism after receiving 200 micrograms daily of iodine.

INTERACTIONS

DRUGS

Antithyroid Drugs: Concomitant use of antithyroid drugs and iodide may potentiate the hypothyroid effect of iodides.

Lithium: Concomitant use of pharmacological doses of potassium iodide and lithium may result in hypothyroidism.

Warfarin: Concomitant use of pharmacological doses of potassium iodide (for hyperthyroidism) and warfarin may decrease the anticoagulant effectiveness of warfarin.

NUTRITIONAL SUPPLEMENTS

Selenium: Intake of selenium and iodide may have synergistic activity in the treatment of Kashin-Beck disease, an osteoarthropathy (see Selenium).

FOODS

Certain foods contain substances which are metabolized to 5-vinyloxazolidine-2-thione and thiocyanate. 5-Vinyloxazolidine-2-thione and thiocyanate may compete with iodide and negatively affect the iodine status of the thyroid gland and may cause hypothyroidism. These food substances are called goitrogens and are found in foods such as cassava and such cruciferous foods as cabbage, Brussels sprouts, broccoli, cauliflower and rutabaga. Certain flavonoids may have goitrogenic activity. C-gluosylflavones such as vitexin, which are found in millet, have been found to inhibit thyroid peroxidase activity. The soybean isoflavones genistein and daidzein have also been found to inhibit thyroid peroxidase.

OVERDOSAGE

The administration of pharmacological doses of potassium iodide to those with impaired renal function may lead to serious hyperkalemia.

DOSAGE AND ADMINISTRATION

Potassium iodide is available as a nutritional supplement, typically in combination products. Doses are usually 150 micrograms daily for adults.

Approximately 77% of potassium iodide is comprised of iodide.

Iodine is commonly available in iodized salt. Iodine content in iodized salt ranges from 20 to 40 milligrams per kilogram or 20 to 40 micrograms per gram. Kosher salt typically does not contain iodine. Chefs in many of the better restaurants prefer using kosher salt to iodized salt.

Iodized oil is used in some countries as a dietary iodine source.

The median intake of iodine from food in the United States is approximately 240 to 300 micrograms/day for men and 190 to 210 micrograms/day for women.

Dietary Reference Intakes (DRI) for iodine by age group (micrograms/day) are as follows:

Infants	Adequate Intake (AI)
0-6 months	110
7-12 months	130

Children	Recommended Daily Allowance (RDA)
1-3 years	90
4-8 years	90

Boys	
9-13 years	120
14-18 years	150

Girls	
9-13 years	120
14-18 years	150

Men	
19-30 years	150
31-50 years	150
51-70 years	150
Older than 70 years	150

Women	
19-30 years	150
31-50 years	150
51-70 years	150
Older than 70 years	150

Pregnancy	
14-18 years	220
19-30 years	220
31-50 years	220

Lactation	
14-18 years	290
19-30 years	290
31-50 years	290

The following summarizes the Tolerable Upper Intake Level (UL) for various age groups and conditions:

Infants	
0-6 months	ND
7-12 months	ND

Children	
1-3 years	200
4-8 years	300
9-13 years	600

Adolescents
14-18 years   900

Adults
19 years and older   1,100

Pregnancy
14-18 years   900
19 years and older   1,100

Lactation
14-18 years   900
19 years and older   1,100

UL = Tolerable Upper Intake Level
ND = Not Determinable

The DV (Daily Value) for iodine, which is used for determining percentage of nutrient daily values on nutritional supplement and food labels, is 150 micrograms. The basis for the DV for iodine is the 1973 U.S. RDA.

The World Health Organization's (WHO) recommendations are slightly different and are:

Age (years) or status	Intake (micrograms/ day)
0 to 1	50
1 to 6	90
7 to 12	120
Greater than 12	150
Pregnancy	200
Lactation	200

LITERATURE

Carrasco N. Iodide transport in the thyroid gland. *Biochim Biophys Acta.* 1993;1154:65-82.

Caserio RJ, Eaglstein WH, Allen CM. Treatment of granuloma annulare with potassium iodide (letter). *J Am Acad Dermatol.* 1984;10:294.

Crocker DG. Nuclear reactor accidents—the use of KI as a blocking agent against radioiodine uptake in the thyroid—a review. *Health Physics.* 1984;46:1265-1279.

Davidsson L. Are vegetarians an 'at risk group' for iodine deficiency? *Br J Nutr.* 1999;81:3-4.

Delange F. Risks and benefits of iodine supplementation. *Lancet.* 1998;351:923-924.

Ghent WR, Eskin BA, Low DA, et al. Iodine replacement in fibrocystic disease of the breast. *Can J Surg.* 1993;36:453-460.

Graham N, Hogan DB, Simpson D. Potassium iodide in the treatment of sarcoidosis (letter). *Can Med Assoc J.* 1981;124:124-127.

Hetzel BS. Iodine and neuropsychological development. *J Nutr.* 2000;130:493S-495S.

Hetzel BS, Clugston GA. Iodine. In: Shils ME, Olson JA, Shike M, Ross CA. *Modern Nutrition in Health and Disease,* 9th ed. Baltimore, MD: Williams and Wilkens;1999:253-264.

Horio T, Danno K, Okamoto H, et al. Potassium iodide in erythema nodosum and other erythematous dermatoses. *J Am Acad Dermatol.* 1983;9:77-81.

Horio T, Imamura S, Danno K, et al. Potassium iodide in the treatment of erythema nodosum and nodular vasculitis. *Arch Dermatol.* 1981;117:29-31.

Institute of Medicine, Food and Nutrition Board. Dietary Reference Intakes for vitamin A, vitamin K, arsenic, boron, chromium, copper, iodine, iron, manganese, molybdenum, nickel, silicon, vanadium, and zinc. Washington, DC: National Academy Press, 2001.

Kahaly G, Dienes HP, Beyer J, et al. Randomized, double-blind, placebo-controlled trial of low dose iodide in endemic goiter. *J Clin Endocrinol Metab.* 1997;82:4049-4053.

La Rosa GL, Lupo L, Giuffrida D, et al. Levothyroxine and potassium iodide are both effective in treating benign solitary solid cold nodules of the thyroid. *Ann Intern Med.* 1995;122:1-8.

Moreno-Reyes R, Suetens C, Mathieu F, et al. Kashin-Beck osteoarthropathy in rural Tibet in relation to selenium and iodide status. *N Engl J Med.* 1998;339:1112-1120.

Nauman J, Wolff J. Iodide prophylaxis in Poland after the Chernobyl reactor accident: benefits and risks. *Am J Med.* 1993;94:524-532.

Remer T, Neubert A, Manz F. Increased risk of iodine deficiency with vegetarian's nutrition. *Br J Nutr.* 1999;81:45-49.

Tazebay UH, Wapnir IL, Levy O, et al. The mammary gland iodide transporter is expressed during lactation and in breast cancer. *Nature Med.* 2000;6:871-878.

Tonglet R, Bourdoux P, Minga T, et al. Efficacy of low oral doses of iodized oil in the control of iodine deficiency in Zaire. *N Engl J Med.* 1992;326:236-241.

Ipriflavone

DESCRIPTION

Ipriflavone is a synthetic derivative of the plant isoflavone, genistein. Genistein is mainly found in soya in the form of genistin but also found in other plant sources, as well, in lower amounts. Ipriflavone occurs in trace amounts in some soy sauces. Although ipriflavone is sometimes classified as a phytoestrogen, it has no direct estrogenic activity. Ipriflavone does not activate any of the estrogen receptors. It does appear to have a favorable impact on bone density, and ipriflavone has been approved for the treatment of involutional osteoporosis in some European countries and in Japan.

The structural formula of ipriflavone is:

Ipriflavone

Ipriflavone is also known as 7-isopropoxy-3-phenyl-4H-1-benzopyran-4-one; 7-(1-methylethoxy)-3-phenyl-4H-1-ben-zopyran-4-one; 7-isopropoxy-3-phenylchromone and 7-isopropoxyisoflavone. Ipriflavone is abbreviated as IP. It is a solid substance that has poor solubility in water.

ACTIONS AND PHARMACOLOGY

ACTIONS

Ipriflavone may have a beneficial action on bone density.

MECHANISM OF ACTION

Osteoporosis is the consequence of an imbalance between osteoclastic and osteoblastic activity, coupled with an increased rate of bone turnover that occurs with menopause. Osteoclasts are the bone-resorbing cells, and osteoblasts are the bone-forming cells. In osteoporosis, a net loss of bone mass occurs due to either excessive-bone-resorbing activity of osteoclasts or impaired bone-forming activity of osteoblasts.

In vitro and animal studies suggest ipriflavone inhibits osteoclastic bone resorption and that it may also stimulate bone formation. Ipriflavone does not possess any estrogenic activity. The mechanism of action of ipriflavone on osteo-casts and their precursor cells is not well understood. There is some evidence that ipriflavone may stimulate osteoblast activity by down-regulation of endothelin receptors. Iprifla-vone may also reduce the ability of endothelin-1 to inhibit mineralization. Ipriflavone was found to be effective in preventing bone loss in ovariectomized rats. Ipriflavone, in contrast to estradiol, did not lower ovariectomized-induced rise in serum alkaline phosphatase or insulin-like growth factor-1 (IGF-1) and IGF-1 binding protein (IGFBP-3) concentrations.

PHARMACOKINETICS

Ipriflavone is absorbed from the small intestine; from there it enters the portal circulation. Greater absorption is obtained with food, and lipid-containing foods especially enhance its absorption. Ipriflavone is metabolized in the liver. The two major metabolites are 7-hydroxy-ipriflavone and 7-(1-car-boxy-ethoxy)-isoflavone. Ipriflavone and its metabolites are distributed to the various tissues of the body via the systemic circulation.

In the blood, ipriflavone and its metabolites are bound to albumin. Elimination of ipriflavone and its metabolites is mainly by the urinary route. A smaller fraction of ingested ipriflavone is eliminated in the feces.

INDICATIONS AND USAGE

Ipriflavone may be indicated to help prevent and reduce bone resorption in osteoporosis. It may also help relieve bone pain associated with osteoporosis. There is some evidence that it can help correct some lipid disturbances associated with estrogen deficiency. Because ipriflavone does not have direct estrogenic effects, it may be suitable for use in aging men with bone loss, as well as in women. It has been suggested that ipriflavone might help prevent or reduce bone loss in men who have prostate cancer and are receiving androgen-reducing therapies.

RESEARCH SUMMARY

Ipriflavone is a currently approved drug indicated for the treatment and prevention of osteoporosis in Japan, Italy, Hungary and some other countries. It is available as a supplement in the United States. Its efficacy is increased when it is combined with calcium and other supplements that help diminish bone loss associated with menopause and aging. It is also sometimes combined with low-dose estrogen preparations.

Ipriflavone's efficacy in osteoporosis is well established by the results of numerous clinical studies, as well as studies involving many animal models. Many carefully controlled studies demonstrate that oral doses of 200 milligrams of ipriflavone three times a day (often combined with one gram of oral calcium daily) can have significant effects, increasing bone mineral density, reducing bone pain and diminishing the incidence of bone fractures—usually in post-menopausal women. Significant improvements in mobility have also been observed. Some studies have continued for as long as two years without incidence of significant side-effects.

Ipriflavone may exert its beneficial effects by inhibiting formation of the osteoclasts that are involved in bone resorption and by promoting the activity of the osteoblasts involved in building new bone. Its lack of direct estrogenic effects may make it a useful alternative in some cases to standard therapies and may, in particular, make it a useful therapy in men with bone loss associated with aging or androgen-limiting therapies (such as those sometimes used in the treatment of prostate cancer). More study is needed to determine ipriflavone's efficacy in this context.

CONTRAINDICATIONS, PRECAUTIONS, ADVERSE REACTIONS

CONTRAINDICATIONS

Known hypersensitivity to an ipriflavone-containing product.

PRECAUTIONS

Because of lack of long-term safety studies, ipriflavone should be avoided by pregnant women and nursing mothers. Those taking theophylline should be aware of an interaction with ipriflavone causing higher theophylline levels.

ADVERSE REACTIONS

Mild gastrointestinal side effects such as nausea have been reported.

INTERACTIONS

DRUGS

Theophylline: Ipriflavone is reported to inhibit the metabolism and elimination of theophylline. Both ipriflavone and its metabolite 7-hydroxy-isoflavone inhibit CYP (cytochrome P450) 1A2 and also CYP2C9. Inhibition of cytochrome P450 metabolism of theophylline produces higher serum levels of theophylline per given theophylline dose and, therefore, those on theophylline who also take ipriflavone must have their serum theophylline levels carefully monitored in order to avoid any toxic effects of elevated theophylline levels.

Tolbutamide: Ipriflavone and 7-hydroxy-ipriflavone inhibit tolbutamide hydroxylase activity. Consequently, use of ipriflavone may be expected to give higher levels of tolbutamide when the two are administered concurrently.

Nifedipine: 7-hydroxy-ipriflavone inhibits nifedipine oxidase activity. Consequently, use of ipriflavone may be expected to give higher levels of nifedipine in those using these products together.

Estrogen: Ipriflavone may add to the effects of estrogen.

SERM's: Ipriflavone may add to the effects of selective estrogen receptor modulators (SERMs).

Calcitonin: Ipriflavone may add to the effects of calcitonin.

Biophosphonates: Ipriflavone may add to the effects of and biophosphonates in the management of osteoporosis.

NUTRITIONAL SUPPLEMENTS

Ipriflavone may add to the effects of vitamins D and K, calcium, fluoride and boron in the management of osteoporosis.

OVERDOSAGE

There are no reports of ipriflavone overdosage.

DOSAGE AND ADMINISTRATION

The typical dose for use in the management of osteoporosis is 200 milligrams taken twice or three times daily.

LITERATURE

Agnusedi D, Crepaldi G. Isaia G, et al. A double blind, placebo-controlled trial of ipriflavone for prevention of postmenopausal spinal bone loss. *Calcif Tissue Int.* 1997; 61:142-147.

Agnusdei D, Bufalino L. Efficacy of ipriflavone in established osteoporosis and long-term safety. *Calif Tissue Int.* 1997; 61 Suppl 1:S23-S27.

Albanese CV, Cudd A, Argentino L, et al. Ipriflavone directly inhibits osteoclastic activity. *Biochem Biophys Res Communi.* 1994; 199:930-936.

Arjmandi BH, Birnbaum RS, Barengolts E, Kakreja SC. The synthetic phytoestrogen, ipriflavone, and estrogen prevent bone loss by different mechanisms. *Calcif Tissue Int.* 2000; 66:61-65.

Ferene L, Istvan S. Pharmacokinetics of ipriflavone. *Acta Pharm Hung.* 1995; 66:219-222.

Gennari C, Agnusdei D, Crepaldi G, et al. Effect of ipriflavone-a synthetic derivative of natural isoflavones-on bone mass loss in the early years after menopause. *Menopause.* 1998; 5:9-15.

Hagiwara H, Naruse M, Adachi C, et al. Ipriflavone down-regulates endothelin receptor levels during differentiation of rat calvarial osteoblast-like cells. *J Biochem.* 1999; 126:168-173.

Head, KA. Ipriflavone: an important bone-building isoflavone. *Altern Med Rev.* 1999; 4:10-22.

Kitatani K, Morii H. Ipriflavone. *Nippon Rinsho.* 1998; 56:1537-1543.

Melis GB, Paoletti AM, Cagnacci A, et al. Lack of any estrogenic effect of ipriflavone in postmenopausal women. *J Endocrinol Invest.* 1992; 15:755-761.

Monostory K, Vereczkey L, Levai F, Szatmari I. Ipriflavone as an inhibitor of human P450 enzymes. *Br J Pharmacol.* 1998; 123:605-610.

Reginster JY. Ipriflavone: pharmacological properties and usefulness in postmenopausal osteoporosis. *Bone Miner.* 1993; 23:223-232.

Sato M, Grese TA, Dodge JA, et al. Emerging therapies for the prevention or treatment of postmenopausal osteoporosis. *J Med Chem.* 1999; 42:1-24.

Schreiber MD, Rebar RW. Isoflavones and postmenopausal bone health: a viable alternative to estrogen therapy? *Menopause.* 1999; 6:233-241.

Iron

DESCRIPTION

Iron is an essential trace mineral in human nutrition. It is involved in the entire process of respiration, including oxygen transport and electron transport. The principal goal of respiration is the production of biologic energy. Iron-deficiency, which can lead to a microcytic, hypochromic anemia, is the most common nutritional disorder in the world. Approximately 25% of the world's population is iron-deficient. Even iron-deficiency states which do not lead to anemia may have global effects on human health. On the other hand, iron overload disorders, which can lead to cirrhosis, coronary heart disease and congestive heart failure, among other things, are also a public health concern.

Iron is a transition metal with atomic number 26 and an atomic mass of 55.85 daltons. Its chemical symbol is Fe. Physiologically, iron exists in one of two oxidation states: ferrous (II) iron or ferric (III) iron.

The function and synthesis of hemoglobin, which carries most of the oxygen in the blood, is dependent on iron. Basic to the electron transport reactions that produce energy in the mitochondria of cells is the combining of oxygen with hydrogen to form water. The reaction occurs by means of a flow of electrons, derived from the oxidation of foodstuffs, across electron-carrier proteins called cytochromes, and via the final combination of these electrons with oxygen to produce water. The final enzyme in the electron transport chain is cytochrome oxidase. The cytochromes and cytochrome oxidase rely on iron for their production and function. Iron is also involved in the production of myoglobin, L-carnitine and aconitase, all of which are involved in energy production in the body. In addition to its fundamental roles in energy production, iron is involved in DNA synthesis and iron may also play roles in normal brain development and in immune function. Iron is also involved in the synthesis of collagen and in the synthesis of serotonin, dopamine and norepinephrine.

Although iron is clearly essential for a wide range of vital biological processes, it is also a potentially toxic substance. The shift back and forth between its two oxidation states— ferrous (II) and ferric (III)—via single electron-transfer reactions is the property that makes iron such an essential component of the cytochromes in the electron transport chain. However, this redox property also contributes to its potential toxicity. Redox cycling between ferrous (II) and ferric (III) can generate the highly reactive oxygen species hydroxyl radicals, which can damage lipids, DNA and proteins. The symptoms of the iron overload disorder hereditary hemochromatosis are due to iron toxicity.

The best dietary sources of iron are green vegetables, legumes and meat. Milk products, snack foods and soft drinks are not good sources of iron. Much of the iron ingested in the American diet in the form of bread and cereals is not well absorbed. The average dietary intake of iron in the United States ranges from 10 to 20 milligrams daily. Many, including adolescents and pregnant and lactating women, may be at risk for iron deficiency.

ACTIONS AND PHARMACOLOGY
ACTIONS
The major activity of supplemental iron is in the prevention and treatment of iron deficiency anemia. Iron has putative immune-enhancing, anticarcinogenic and cognition-enhancing activities.

MECHANISM OF ACTION
Iron is necessary for the production of hemoglobin. Iron-deficiency can lead to decreased production of hemoglobin and a microcytic, hypochromic anemia.

Under experimental conditions, iron-deficient subjects were found to have certain abnormalities in cell-mediated immunity and in the ability of neutrophils to kill different bacteria. The mechanism of those possible immune effects of iron is unknown. On the other hand, free iron may stimulate the growth of pathogenic bacteria.

Iron-deficiency has been associated with the Plummer-Vinson syndrome. In this condition, there is difficulty swallowing solid food because of a thin, web-like membrane that grows across the upper passageway of the esophagus. Those with Plummer-Vinson syndrome are at increased risk of cancer of the esophagus and stomach. Iron supplementation can prevent this syndrome. There is no other human evidence that iron has anticarcinogenic activity. The mechanism of iron's action in the Plummer-Vinson syndrome is unknown.

Some studies have suggested that children and adolescents with iron-deficiency may also have learning problems and that iron supplementation may increase cognitive skills in some children and adolescents with iron deficiency. The possible role of iron in these cases may be accounted for, in part, by iron's role in neurotransmitter synthesis, particularly in the synthesis of dopamine. Iron deficient rats have been reported to have phenylketonuria and disturbed brain function. It has been suggested that iron-deficiency in the rats resulted in altered phenylalanine metabolism producing phenylketonuria. Phenylketonuria has not been reported in iron-deficient humans.

PHARMACOKINETICS
The absorption of iron from the gastrointestinal tract is highly regulated. In fact, iron homeostasis is maintained by regulating its absorption, since the body does not have a regulated mechanism to excrete excess iron. Much remains unknown about its absorption, as well as the pharmacokinetics of iron in humans, in general. Dietary iron sources include heme iron, elemental iron which is used in food fortification, dietary ferric iron and iron salts used for supplementation. The discussion will begin with the iron salts.

The efficiency of absorption depends on the salt form, the amount administered, the dosing regimen and the size of iron stores. Subjects with normal iron stores absorb 10% to 35% of an iron dose. Those who are iron deficient may absorb up to 95% of an iron dose. Ingested inorganic iron is solubilized and ionized by the acid gastric juice. Iron supplements are mainly in the ferrous form (Fe II). Iron supplements that may be in the ferric form (Fe III) are reduced to the ferrous form. Absorption of iron may occur at any level of the small intestine but is most efficient in the duodenum. Iron is taken up by one of a few proteins on the luminal surface of the mucosal epithelium of the small intestine. Possible iron-binding proteins include a beta$_3$-integrin, the Hfe protein which functions together with beta-microglobulin and Nramp2 or divalent metal ion transporter1 (DMT1). Each of these proteins is a transmembrane protein. It is unclear how they operate in the transport of iron into the enterocytes. Nramp2 (DMT1) is a member of a class of proteins called natural resistance-associated macrophage proteins.

Within the enterocyte, iron—still in the ferrous form—is transferred to the cytosolic proteins mobilferrin and paraferritin. Paraferritin transports iron to the serosal surface of the enterocyte from whence it enters the portal circulation. As it enters the portal circulation, ferrous (Fe II) iron is oxidized to ferric (Fe III) iron by the copper-containing protein ceruloplasmin. Ferric iron bound to transferrin is carried in the portal circulation to the liver and then to all of the tissues of the body.

Transferrin, the principal iron transporter in the blood and other body fluids, distributes ferric (Fe III) iron throughout the body, principally to the red blood cell precursors in the bone marrow for hemoglobin synthesis. Approximately 70% to 90% of transferrin-bound iron is taken up by the erythropoietic cells of bone marrow for hemoglobin synthesis. Smaller amounts are delivered to other cells for the formation of cytochromes, cytochrome oxidase, myoglobin, or for other iron-requiring enzymes. Transferrin binds to a transferrin receptor located on the cell membrane forming an iron-transferrin-transferrin receptor complex which enters the cell by endocytosis. Within the cell, iron is released into the cytosol. Within the cytosol of the erythroblast, iron is transported by an unknown mechanism to mitochondria where it is inserted into protoporphyrin to form heme.

Iron in excess of need is stored principally as ferritin in the reticuloendothelial system of liver, spleen, bone marrow and other organs. Iron is released from ferritin in the form of ferrous (Fe II) iron and enters the plasma where it is oxidized by ceruloplasmin to ferric (Fe III) iron and taken up and transported in the plasma by transferrin.

Iron loss occurs principally through nonspecific mechanisms, including exfoliation of intestinal cells, urinary and biliary secretions and menstruation. Pre-menopausal women normally lose iron via menstrual bleeding. Iron losses can occur from gastrointestinal bleeding, bleeding from trauma, including surgical procedures, and from uterine bleeding in post-menopausal women on hormone replacement therapy. The body has a limited capacity to excrete iron. Very little iron is excreted by the kidneys or via the biliary route. Some iron losses occur through sloughing of skin and mucosal cells.

The absorption of heme iron is not well understood. To be absorbed, iron contained in heme proteins must first be freed by digestion of the protein to yield heme. Heme is absorbed from the small intestine by an unknown mechanism. Within the enterocytes, iron is freed from protoporphyrin by the enzyme heme oxygenase which converts the porphyrin ring to bilirubin and also yields ferric (III) iron and carbon monoxide. Ferric (III) iron binds to paraferritin which releases ferric iron from the serosal side of the cell into the circulation where it binds to transferrin. The remaining pharmacokinetics is as described above.

Dietary ferric (III) iron is solubilized and ionized by acid gastric juice. Some fraction of dietary ferric iron is reduced in the stomach. Some binds to mucin and is transported to the small intestine. Mucin protects ferric (III) iron against precipitation at the alkaline pH of the small intestine. The enzyme ferric reductase, which resides in the brush border of the duodenum, is capable of converting ferric iron to the ferrous form, which may be transported into the enterocytes by such iron-transport proteins as Nramp2, also known as divalent metal ion transporter1 (DMT1). The remaining pharmacokinetics of dietary ferric iron is as described above.

Iron-fortified cereals contain so-called reduced iron. This is finely powdered metallic iron and is generally poorly assimilated. It must first be oxidized to ferric (III) iron and then reduced to ferrous (II) iron in the stomach and small intestine before it can be absorbed.

Carbonyl iron or iron pentacarbonyl (diiron enneacarbonyl) is another nutritional supplement form of iron. Carbonyl iron requires stomach acid for its absorption.

In the treatment of iron deficiency anemia, an increase in the reticulocyte count is seen in three to four days and peaks in seven to ten days. The hemoglobin values may increase at a rate of 1.5 to 2.2 grams per deciliter per week for the first two weeks, followed by 0.7 to 1.6 grams per deciliter per week until normal values are achieved.

INDICATIONS AND USAGE

Apart from its use in preventing and treating iron-deficiency anemia, iron has been used with some success in reducing the frequency of breath-holding spells (BHS) in children. It is helpful in Plummer-Vinson syndrome and, in that context, may help prevent cancer of the esophagus and stomach in those with this syndrome. There is the suggestion in some research that iron might diminish learning problems and enhance cognition in some children and adolescents with iron deficiency. It may have some favorable effects on immunity and exercise performance—but, again, these benefits are most likely largely limited to those with frank or borderline iron deficiency. Iron's efficacy in malaria appears to be limited to improving iron status; it has no apparent effect on parasite rate or density. There is very preliminary evidence that it may have some modest, indirect beneficial effects in promotion of weight loss. Unrecognized iron deficiency may be significant in patients with critical illnesses, generally, according to findings of one recent study. In recent years, several research efforts have suggested that excess iron levels pose health risks for some groups.

RESEARCH SUMMARY

The frequency of breath-holding spells (BHS) diminished significantly in children with this disorder given iron 5 mg/kg/day for 16 weeks, compared with controls. Some 88% of those given iron had complete or partial responses compared with 6% in the placebo group. In a more recent study, 63 of 91 children with BHS had concomitant iron deficiency anemia. Complete or partial remission from BHS was achieved in children receiving 6 mg/kg/day for three months. Controls had a 21% partial or complete rate of remission.

Iron supplementation has been useful in preventing Plummer-Vinson syndrome characterized by difficulty in swallowing due to a membrane that grows across the upper esophagus. This condition is associated with an increased incidence of esophageal and gastric cancers. There is no other credible evidence that supplemental iron has other anticarcinogenic effects.

Iron deficiency anemia is associated, in some instances, with emotional, social and learning disorders in children and adolescents. Iron supplementation has improved these conditions in some studies. Iron deficiency in the absence of anemia can also cause some of these same problems and can be helped with iron supplementation, another study suggests.

Some researchers have reported that up to 25% of adolescent girls in the United States are iron deficient. In one study, the effects of iron supplements were tested in adolescent girls with non-anemia iron deficiency to see if they might improve cognition. This was a double-blind, placebo-controlled trial. Subjects were randomized to receive 650 milligrams of iron twice daily or placebo for eight weeks. Those with iron supplementation were reported to perform significantly better than those in the placebo group on tests related to verbal learning and memory.

Iron deficiency is known to diminish various aspects of immune function. Adequate levels help maintain cellular immunity and help to protect against some infections. Cell-mediated immune response may be impaired when iron deficiency negatively impacts the iron-requiring enzyme called ribonculeotide reductase, an enzyme that appears to be essential for the proper function of the T-lymphocyte arm of immunity. Resistance to candida, herpes simplex virus and some other pathogens appears to be reduced in those with poor iron status. On the other hand, excess iron may predispose individuals to some infections.

Claims that iron boosts energy and enhances exercise performance may be true—provided the claim is limited to those who are iron deficient. Muscle weakness and decreased exercise tolerance can occur in those who are iron deficient but not necessarily suffering from iron-deficiency anemia. Iron deficiency without anemia is not uncommon among some endurance athletes (e.g., long-distance runners), more among women than men.

Supplemental iron has been reported to be of some benefit in women on very-low calorie weight reduction diets. In one study, obese women on these diets lost more (but not significantly greater) weight when given supplemental iron. The researchers concluded: "The greater recovery of thyroid hormone levels may have maintained metabolic rates to allow for greater weight loss." Some follow-up may be warranted.

Iron deficiency may be more widespread than generally believed. One recent study reported the presence of functional iron deficiency in 35% of 51 consecutive adult patients presenting to the general intensive care unit of a teaching hospital over a six-week period. Patients with massive hemorrhage or exchange transfusion in the two weeks before admission, those who were pregnant or lactating, those older than 80 years, those with hematological malignant disorders and those with bone marrow depression were excluded. Patients with functional iron deficiency had longer stays in intensive care than did those without iron deficiency (mean length of stay 7.6 days versus 3.3 days, respectively).

On the other hand, there is also evidence that some population subsets may be getting too much iron, some of it through supplementation. One group has estimated that up to one million people in the United States may have hemochromatosis, a hereditary disorder characterized by excess intestinal absorption of iron. Early symptoms include fatigue and joint pain. Fatal complications can include diabetes, cancer, heart disease and cirrhosis of the liver. One recent study found that stroke victims who have elevated levels of iron are significantly more likely to experience more severe neurological damage than are those with normal iron levels. Research is ongoing.

CONTRAINDICATIONS

Iron supplements are contraindicated in those with hemochromatosis and hemosiderosis.

Iron supplements are contraindicated in those who are hypersensitive to any component of an iron-containing supplement.

PRECAUTIONS

Iron supplements should not be used for the treatment of anemias other than iron deficiency anemia.

Treatment of iron deficiency anemia must only be undertaken under medical supervision.

Those with elevated serum ferritin levels should be extremely cautious in the use of iron supplements.

Pregnant women and nursing mothers should not use supplemental doses of iron higher than RDA amounts (30 and 15 milligrams daily, respectively) unless higher doses are recommended by their physicians.

Iron supplements can be highly toxic or lethal to small children. Those who use iron supplements should use childproof bottles and keep the bottles away from children.

Iron supplements should be used with extreme caution in those with chronic liver failure, alcoholic cirrhosis, chronic alcoholism and pancreatic insufficiency.

Carbonyl iron requires adequate stomach acid for absorption. Therefore, carbonyl iron should be taken with food and should not be used with antacids.

Iron should be used with caution in those with a history of gastritis, peptic ulcer disease or gastrointestinal bleeding.

ADVERSE REACTIONS

The most common side effects are gastrointestinal ones and include nausea, vomiting, bloating and other abdominal discomfort, black stools, diarrhea, constipation and anorexia.

Temporary staining of teeth occurs from iron-containing liquids.

INTERACTIONS

DRUGS

Acid Pump Inhibitors: (lansoprazole, omeprazole, pantoprazole, rabeprazole): Use of acid pump inhibitors may suppress the absorption of carbonyl iron.

Antacids: Aluminum-or magnesium-containing antacids may decrease the absorption of iron if used concomitantly.

Bisphosphonates (alendronate, etidronate, risedronate): Concomitant use of a bisphosphonate and a ferrous (II) iron supplement may decrease the absorption of the bisphosphonate.

H_2 Blockers (cimetidine, famotidine, nizatidine, ranitidine): Use of H_2 blockers may suppress the absorption of carbonyl iron.

Levodopa: Concomitant intake of levodopa and iron may reduce absorption of levodopa.

Levothyroxine: Concomitant intake of levothyroxine and iron may decrease the absorption of levothyroxine.

Penicillamine: Concomitant intake of iron and penicillamine may decrease the absorption of penicillamine.

Quinolones (ciprofloxacin, gatifloxacin, levofloxacin, lomefloxacin, moxifloxacin, norfloxacin, ofloxacin, sparfloxacin, trovafloxacin): Concomitant use of a quinolone and iron may decrease the absorption of the quinolone and iron.

Tetracyclines (doxycycline, minocycline, tetracycline): Concomitant intake of a tetracycline and iron may decrease the absorption of both the tetracycline and iron.

NUTRITIONAL SUPPLEMENTS

Beta-carotene: Beta-carotene may enhance the absorption of iron if they are taken concomitantly.

Calcium: Calcium carbonate may decrease absorption of iron if used concomitantly.

Copper: Intake of iron supplements may decrease the copper status of tissues.

Inositol Hexaphosphate: Concomitant intake of inositol hexaphosphate and iron may depress the absorption of iron.

L-Cysteine: Concomitant intake of L-cysteine and iron may increase the absorption of iron.

Magnesium: Concomitant intake of magnesium and iron may decrease the absorption of iron.

N-Acetyl-L-Cysteine: Concomitant intake of N-acetyl-L-cysteine and iron may increase the absorption of iron.

Tocotrienols: Concomitant intake of tocotrienols—which are typically used in their nonesterified forms—and iron may cause oxidation of the tocotrienols.

Vanadium: Concomitant intake of vanadium and iron may decrease the absorption of iron.

Vitamin C: Concomitant intake of vitamin C and iron may enhance the absorption of iron.

Vitamin E (alpha-tocopherol, gamma-tocopherol, mixed tocopherols): Concomitant intake of non-esterified tocopherols and iron may cause oxidation of the tocopherols.

Zinc: Concomitant intake of zinc and iron may decrease the absorption of iron.

FOODS

Cysteine-containing Proteins: Foods rich in cysteine-containing proteins (e.g. animal muscle tissue) may increase the absorption of iron if ingested concomitantly.

Oxalic Acid: Concomitant intake of iron with foods rich in oxalic acid (spinach, sweet potatoes, rhubarb and beans) may decrease the absorption of iron.

Phytic Acid: Concomitant intake of iron with foods rich in phytic acid (unleavened bread, raw beans, seeds, nuts and grains and soy isolates) may decrease the absorption of iron.

Teas: Concomitant intake of tea and iron may cause decreased absorption of iron. This is attributed to the tannins in tea.

LABORATORY TESTS

Guaic assay: Earlier studies reported a high false positive rate for guaic assay for occult blood in those receiving iron supplements. However, more recent data indicate that iron supplementation has no significant effect on guaic or other tests for occult blood.

OVERDOSAGE

Acute iron overdosage can be divided into four stages. In the first stage, which occurs up to six hours after ingestion, the principal symptoms are vomiting and diarrhea. Other symptoms include hypotension, tachycardia and CNS depression ranging from lethargy to coma. The second phase may occur at 6-24 hours after ingestion and is characterized by a temporary remission. In the third phase, gastrointestinal symptoms recur accompanied by shock, metabolic acidosis, coma, hepatic necrosis and jaundice, hypoglycemia, renal failure and pulmonary edema. The fourth phase may occur several weeks after ingestion and is characterized by gastrointestinal obstruction and liver damage.

In a young child, 75 milligrams per kilogram is considered extremely dangerous. A dose of 30 milligrams per kilogram can lead to symptoms of toxicity. Estimates of a lethal dosage range from 180 milligrams per kilogram and upwards. A peak serum iron concentration of five micrograms or more per ml is associated with moderate to severe poisoning in many.

DOSAGE AND ADMINISTRATION

There are several forms used for iron supplementation. They include ferrous sulfate, ferrous fumarate, ferrous gluconate, ferrous ascorbate and carbonyl iron.

The approximate amount of the above forms required to supply 60 milligrams of elemental iron are:

ferrous ascorbate	437 mg
ferrous fumarate	183 mg
ferrous gluconate	518 mg
ferrous sulfate	186 mg
carbonyl iron	300 mg

Iron replacement therapy for adults is 2-3 mg/kg daily in three divided doses. This must be done under a physician's supervision.

Iron is present in some combination supplements at doses of 10 to 18 milligrams daily.

Dietary Reference Intakes (DRI) for iron by age group:

DRI values (milligrams/day)

Infants	Adequate Intake (AI)
0-6 months	0.27
7-12 months	11

Children	Recommended Daily Allowance (RDA)
1-3 years	7
4-8 years	10

Boys	
9-13 years	8
14-18 years	11

Girls	
9-13 years	8
14-18 years	15

Men	
19-30 years	8
31-50 years	8
51-70 years	8
Older than 70 years	8

Women	
19-30 years	18
31-50 years	18
51-70 years	8
Older than 70 years	8

Pregnancy	
14-18 years	27
19-30 years	27
31-50 years	27

Lactation	
14-18 years	10
19-30 years	9
31-50 years	9

The following summarizes the Tolerable Upper Intake Level (UL) for various age groups and conditions:

Infants
0-6 months	40
7-12 months	40

Children (UL)
1-3 years	40
4-8 years	40
9-13 years	40

Adolescents
14-18 years	45

Adults
19 years and older	45

Pregnancy
14-18 years	45
19 years and older	45

Lactation
14-18 years	45
19 years and older	45

UL = Tolerable Upper Intake Level. The UL represents total intake from food and supplements.

The DV (Daily Value) for iron, which is used for determining percentage of nutrient daily values on nutritional supplement and food labels, is 18 mg. The basis for the DV for iron is the 1973 U.S. RDA.

LITERATURE

Adish AA, Esrey SA, Gyorkos TW, et al. Effect of consumption of food cooked in iron pots on iron status and growth of young children: a randomised trial. *Lancet.* 1999;353:712-716.

Anderson GJ. Control of iron absorption. *J Gastroenterol Hepatol.* 1996;11:1030-1032.

Andrews NC. Disorders of iron metabolism. *N Engl J Med.* 1999;341:1986-1995.

Andrews NC, Fleming MD, Gunshin H. Iron transport across biological membranes. *Nutr Rev.* 1999;57:114-123.

Baer D. Hereditary iron overload and African Americans (editorial). *Am J Med.* 1996;101:5-8.

Beard JL. Iron requirements in adolescent females. *J Nutr.* 2000;130(2S Suppl):440S-442S.

Beguin Y, Huebers HA, Josephson B, et al. Transferrin receptors in rat plasma. *Proc Natl Acad Sci USA.* 1988;85:637-640.

Bellamy MC, Gedney JA. Unrecognized iron deficiency in critical illness. *Lancet.* 1998;352:1903.

Beutler E, Larsh SE, Gurney CW. Iron therapy in chronically fatigued nonanemic women: a double-blind study. *Ann Intern Med.* 1960;52:378-394.

Bruner AB, Joffe A, Duggan A, et al. Randomised study of cognitive effects of iron supplementation in non-anaemic iron-deficient adolescent girls. *Lancet.* 1996;348:992-997.

Dallman PR. Iron deficiency and the immune response. *Am J Clin Nutr.* 1987;46:329-334.

de Valk B, Marx JJM. Iron, atherosclerosis, and ischemic heart disease. *Arch Int Med.* 1999;159:1542-1548.

Fairbanks VF. Iron in medicine and nutrition. In: Shils ME, Olson JA, Shike M, Ross AC, eds. *Modern Nutrition in Health and Disease.* Baltimore, MD: Williams and Wilkins; 1999:193-221.

Feder JN, Gnirke A, Thomas W, et al. A novel MHC class I like gene is mutated in patients with hereditary hemochromatosis. *Nat Genet.* 1996;13:399-408.

Finch CA, Huebers H. Perspectives in iron metabolism. *N Engl J Med.* 1982;306:1520-1528.

Garcia-Casal MN, Leets I, Layrisse M. Beta-carotene and inhibitors of iron absorption modify iron uptake by Caco-2 cells. *J Nutr.* 2000;130:5-9.

Harris ED. The iron-copper connection: the link to ceruloplasmin grows stronger. *Nutr Rev.* 1995;53:170-173.

Huebers HA, Beguin Y, Pootrakul P, et al. Intact transferrin receptors in human plasma and their relation to erythropoiesis. *Blood.* 1990;75:102-107.

Institute of Medicine, Food and Nutrition Board. Dietary Reference Intakes for vitamin A, vitamin K, arsenic, boron, chromium, copper, iodine, iron, manganese, molybdenum, nickel, silicon, vanadium, and zinc. Washington, DC: National Academy Press, 2001.

Kurz KM, Galloway R. Improving adolescent iron status before childbearing. *J Nutr.* 2000;130:(2S Suppl):437S-439S.

Lehto P, Kivisto KT, Neuvonen PJ. The effect of ferrous sulfate on the absorption of norfloxacin, ciprofloxacin and ofloxacin. *B J Clin Pharmacol.* 1994;37:82-85.

Mendler MH, Turlin B, Moirand R, et al. Insulin resistance-associated hepatic iron overload. *Gastroenterology.* 1999;117:1155-1163.

Moirand R, Mortaji AM, Loréal O, et al. A new syndrome of liver iron overload with normal transferrin saturation. *Lancet.* 1997;349:95-97.

Morse AC, Beard JL, Jones BC. A genetic development model of iron deficiency: biological aspects. *Proc Soc Exp Biol Med.* 1999;220:147-152.

Neuvonen PJ, Turakka H. Inhibitory effect of various iron salts on the absorption of tetracycline in man. *Eur J Clin Pharmacol.* 1974;7:357-360.

Oski FA. Iron deficiency in infancy and childhood. *N Engl J Med.* 1993;329:190-193.

Pigeon C, Turlin B, Iancu TC, et al. Carbonyl-iron supplementation induces hepatocyte nuclear changes in BALB/CJ male mice. *J Hepatol.* 1999;30:926-934.

Salonen JT, Nyyssönen K, Korpela H, et al. High stored iron levels are associated with excess risk of myocardial infarction in Eastern Finnish men. *Circulation*. 1992;86:803-811.

Scrimshaw NS, San Giovanni JP. Synergism of nutrition, infection, and immunity: an overview. *Am J Clin N*. 1997;66:464S-477S.

Smith MA, Harris PLR, Sayre LM, et al. Iron accumulation in Alzheimer disease is a source of redox-generated free radicals. *Proc Acad Sci USA*. 1997;94:9866-9868.

Wessling-Resnick M. Iron transport. *Annu Rev Nutr*. 2000;20:120-151.

Wienk KJH, Marx JJM, Beynen AC. The concept of iron bioavailability and its assessment (review). *Eur J Nutr*. 1999;38:51-75.

Wurapa RK, Gordeuk VR, Brittenham GM, et al. Primary iron overload in African Americans. *Am J Med*. 1996;101:9-18.

Kombucha

DESCRIPTION

Kombucha, also known as the Manchurian or Kargasok mushroom, is not a mushroom but a symbiotic mixture of bacteria, including *Acetobacter xylinum*, *Acetobacter ketogenum* and *Pichia fermentans*, and various yeasts. The yeasts are usually of the genera *Saccharomyces*, *Brettanomyces* and *Zygosaccharomyces*. Kombucha is used as a tea and is prepared by incubating it in sugared black or green tea. The tea is mildly effervescent and has a cider-like acid taste.

Anecdotes abound regarding kombucha's ability to treat a wide spectrum of disorders, including AIDS and baldness. A few years ago, a media stir was created when it was reported that a patient with far-advanced AIDS made a "miraculous" recovery after drinking Kombucha tea. What wasn't reported was that the patient had begun a new FDA-allowed experimental therapy at the same time.

Kombucha tea is prepared by the user, and it is possible for the home-brewed version to become contaminated with pathogenic bacteria or fungi.

ACTIONS AND PHARMACOLOGY

ACTIONS
Kombucha has putative "cure-all" activity.

MECHANISM OF ACTION
Kombucha tea may have some antibiotic activity.

PHARMACOKINETICS
There are no reports on the pharmacokinetics of kombucha, and it is unlikely that any pharmacokinetic studies have been performed.

INDICATIONS AND USAGE

Claims have been made that kombucha tea cures everything from AIDS to baldness, flatulence and cancer. There is no credible evidence that it is effective in preventing or treating any disorder, and its use has been associated with significant toxicity in some cases. Its use in immuno-compromised individuals is particularly inadvisable.

RESEARCH SUMMARY

There is no credible research that supports the use of kombucha for any purpose. Its use has been associated with occasional allergic reactions, jaundice, nausea, vomiting, and head and neck pain. The Iowa Department of Public Health recommended against its use when two cases of severe unexplained illness (one of which ended in death) were reported in two individuals who had been consuming kombucha tea daily for two months. Two cases of symptomatic lead poisoning were reported in individuals who drank kombucha tea brewed in a ceramic pot. It was hypothesized that the tea elicited lead from the glaze pigment of the pot.

A recent case report noted that a 53-year-old Asian man with no significant past medical history presented in the emergency room with a 2-month history of progressive muscle weakness. A month prior to symptom manifestation he had begun consuming kombucha in milk. He was diagnosed with a myositis associated with pleural effusions, pericardial effusion and "mechanic's hands," characterized by darkened hyperkeratotic changes on the palmar aspect of the fingers as well as on the palms. Those examining and treating the man believed the probable cause to be the kombucha.

A recent review of clinical evidence concluded that kombucha's unsubstantiated benefits do not outweigh its documented risks. No efficacy for kombucha was found, yet multiple cases of kombucha toxicity were cited. The reviewer concluded: "The potential for harm seems considerable." The recommendation remains the same: be cautious about the use of kombucha for any purpose.

CONTRAINDICATIONS, PRECAUTIONS, ADVERSE REACTIONS

CONTRAINDICATIONS
Kombucha is contraindicated in those who are hypersensitive to any component of the preparation.

PRECAUTIONS
Children, pregnant women, nursing mothers, the elderly and those with compromised immune systems should avoid the use of kombucha.

Kombucha may contain antibiotic substances and, theoretically, could cause antibiotic resistance.

Those who use kombucha should be extremely careful in its preparation in order to avoid contamination with pathogenic bacteria and or fungi. The tea should not be prepared or stored in ceramic or lead containers, as lead can leach into the tea.

ADVERSE REACTIONS

Those who drink more than 4 ounces daily of kombucha tea frequently experience nausea, vomiting and headaches. There have been reports of allergic reactions, jaundice, and head and neck pain. There are reports of two women with unexplained metabolic acidosis following use of kombucha tea. One died. However, it was unclear whether the kombucha tea had any role in causing the metabolic acidosis. Another 115 people who made tea from the same batch of kombucha had no adverse reactions. There are a few reports of elevated serum liver tests and a report of lead poisoning from drinking kombucha tea prepared in a ceramic pot. A case of cutaneous anthrax associated with kombucha has been reported, possibly secondary to contamination of the tea during its preparation.

OVERDOSAGE

There are no reported cases of overdosage with kombucha.

DOSAGE AND ADMINISTRATION

There is no typical dosage and no recommended dosage.

LITERATURE

Currier RW, Goddard J, Buehler K, et al. Unexplained severe illness possibly associated with consumption of Kombucha tea—Iowa, 1995. *MMWR Morb Mort Wkly Rep.* 1995;44:892-893,899-900.

Derk CT, Sandorfi N, Curtis MT. A case of anti-Jo1 myositis with pleural effusions and pericardial tamponade developing after exposure to a fermented Kombucha beverage. *Clin Rheumatol.* 2004;23(4):355-357.

Ernst E. Kombucha: a systematic review of the clinical evidence. *Forsch Komplementarmed Klass Naturheilkd.* 2003;10(2):85-87.

Greenwalt CJ, Steinkraus KH, Ledford RA. Kombucha, the fermented tea: microbiology, composition, and claimed health effects. *J Food Prot.* 2000;63(7):976-981.

Hauser SP, [Dr. Sklenar's Kombucha mushroom infusion—a biological cancer therapy. Documentation No. 18.] [Article in German.] *Schweiz Rundsch Med Prax.* 1990;79:243-246.

Mayser P, Fromme S, Leitzmann C, et al. The yeast spectrum of the "tea fungus Kombucha." *Mycoses.* 1995;38:289-295.

Phan TG, Estell J, Duggin G, et al. Lead poisoning from drinking Kombucha tea brewed in a ceramic pot. *Med J Aust.* 1998;169:644-646.

Sadjadi J. Cutaneous anthrax associated with the Kombucha "mushroom" in Iran. *JAMA.* 1998;280:1567-1568.

Srinivasan R, Smolinske S, Greenbaum D. Probable gastrointestinal toxicity of Kombucha tea: is this beverage healthy or harmful? *J Gen Int Med.* 1997;12:643-644.

Teoh AL, Heard G, Cox J. Yeast ecology of Kombucha fermentation. *Int J Food Microbiol.* 2004;95(2):119-126.

L-Alpha-Glycerylphosphorylcholine (Alpha-GPC)

DESCRIPTION

L-alpha-glycerylphosphorylcholine is a substance derived from soy lecithin. It is phosphatidylcholine without the two fatty acid chains contained within the phosphatidylcholine structure. Although it is popularly referred to as a phospholipid, it is not. It is a phospholipid-derived substance.

Alpha-GPC has the following structural formula:

L-alpha-glycerylphosphorylcholine

L-alpha-glycerylphosphorylcholine is either abbreviated as alpha-GPC or GPC. It is also known as choline alfoscerate; choline-glycerophosphate, and choline-hydroxide, (R)-2,3-dihydroxypropyl hydrogen phosphate, inner salt. Alpha-GPC is believed to be a delivery form of choline (see Choline).

ACTIONS AND PHARMACOLOGY

ACTIONS

Alpha-GPC is a putative cognition enhancer and a putative growth hormone secretagogue.

MECHANISM OF ACTION

The actions of supplemental alpha-GPC are speculative and, therefore, any proposed mechanism of action is likewise speculative. Alpha-GPC is a delivery form of choline, and choline can be metabolized to acetylcholine. Some with Alzheimer's disease may suffer from a cholinergic defect, and, theoretically, a delivery form of choline may positively affect some with cognition disorders in which there exists a cholinergic deficit. In a similar speculative vein, it is known that cholinergic potentiation may modulate the growth hormone (GH) response to the hypothalamic hormone GHRH or growth hormone releasing hormone. Again, if alpha-GPC is a significant precursor of acetylcholine, it may have a GH secretagogue effect.

PHARMACOKINETICS

Some pharmacokinetic data are available from animal studies. Human pharmacokinetic data are lacking. It is unclear as to how much of an ingested dose of alpha-GPC gets into the brain or, for that matter, how much choline from a dose of ingested alpha-GPC gets to the brain.

INDICATIONS AND USAGE

It has been claimed that alpha-GPC is indicated for situations in which increased human growth hormone secretion is desirable and for the treatment of cognitive disorders. Evidence is insufficient to warrant support for either of these claimed indications at this time.

RESEARCH SUMMARY

The claim has been made that this putative acetylcholine precursor encourages the body to secrete increased levels of human growth hormone. There is some preliminary evidence that this is so, but whether this has any therapeutic significance remains to be seen. Safety data are also lacking. Claims that alpha-GPC is helpful in the treatment of cognitive disorders in the elderly are based upon scant and preliminary findings which, nonetheless, may warrant further investigation.

CONTRAINDICATIONS, PRECAUTIONS, ADVERSE REACTIONS

CONTRAINDICATIONS

Alpha-GPC is contraindicated in those who are hypersensitive to any component of the preparation.

PRECAUTIONS

Because of lack of long-term safety data, children, pregnant women and nursing mothers should avoid use of alpha-GPC.

ADVERSE REACTIONS

To date, no adverse reactions have been reported.

INTERACTIONS

There are no known drug, nutritional supplement, food or herb interactions.

OVERDOSAGE

There are no reports of overdosing.

DOSAGE AND ADMINISTRATION

Those who use alpha-GPC take 500 milligrams to 1 gram daily. About 40% of alpha-GPC is choline.

LITERATURE

Amenta F, Del Valle M, Vega JA, Zaccheo D. Age-related structural changes in the rat cerebellar cortex: effect of choline alfoscerate treatment. *Mech Ageing Dev.* 1991; 61: 173-186.

Amenta F, Ferrante F, Vega JA, Zaccheo D. Long term choline alfoscerate treatment counters age-dependent microanatomical changes in rat brain. *Prog Neuropsychopharmacol Biol Psychiatry.* 1994; 18:915-924.

Ceda GP. Ceresini G. Denti L, et al. Alpha-glycerylphosphorylcholine administration increases the GH responses to GHRH of young and elderly subjects. *Horm Metab Res.* 1992; 24:119-121.

Ricci A, Bronzetti E, Vega JA, Amenta F. Oral choline alfoscerate counteracts age-dependent loss of mossy fibres in the rat hippocampus. *Mech Ageing Dev.* 1992; 66: 81-91.

L-Arginine

DESCRIPTION

L-arginine is a protein amino acid present in the proteins of all life forms. It is classified as a semi-essential or conditionally essential amino acid. This means that under normal circumstances the body can synthesize sufficient L-arginine to meet physiological demands. There are, however, conditions where the body cannot. L-arginine is essential for young children and for those with certain rare genetic disorders in which synthesis of the amino acid is impaired. Some stress conditions that put an increased demand on the body for the synthesis of L-arginine include trauma (including surgical trauma), sepsis and burns. Under these conditions, L-arginine becomes essential, and it is then very important to ensure adequate dietary intake of the amino acid to meet the increased physiological demands created by these situations.

L-arginine, even when it is not an essential amino acid as defined above, is a vital one. In addition to participating in protein synthesis, it plays a number of other roles in the body. These include the detoxification of ammonia formed during the nitrogen catabolism of amino acids via the formation of urea. In addition, L-arginine is a precursor in the formation of nitric oxide, creatine, polyamines, L-glutamate, L-proline, agmatin (a possible neurotransmitter in the brain) and the arginine-containing tetrapeptide tuftsin, believed to be an immunomodulator. L-arginine is a glycogenic amino acid; it can be converted to D-glucose and glycogen if needed by the body or it can be catabolized to produce biological energy.

L-arginine, when administered in high doses, stimulates pituitary release of growth hormone and prolactin and pancreatic release of glucagon and insulin. Intravenous L-arginine may be used as an aid in the evaluation of problems with growth and stature that may be due to growth hormone deficiency. Intravenous arginine hydrochloride may be used as a fourth-line agent in the treatment of severe metabolic alkalosis. L-arginine is also used as an immunonutrient in enteral and parenteral nutrition to help improve the immune status in those suffering from sepsis, burns and trauma.

L-arginine is predominately synthesized in the kidney. It is a key intermediate in the Krebs-Henseleit urea cycle. L-ornithine and L-citrulline are precursors in the synthesis of L-arginine, and L-arginine is converted to urea and L-ornithine via the enzyme arginase. The portion of L-arginine that is not converted to urea enters the circulation, and is distributed to the various tissues and metabolized as discussed above. A much smaller amount of L-arginine is produced in the liver.

The typical dietary intake of L-arginine is 3.5 to 5 grams daily. Most dietary L-arginine comes from plant and animal proteins. Small amounts of free L-arginine are found in vegetable juices and fermented foods, such as miso and yogurt. Soy protein and other plant proteins are richer in L-arginine than are animal proteins, which are richer in lysine. It is thought that the possible hypocholesterolemic effect of soy protein is due, at least in part, to the higher L-arginine content in this protein.

L-arginine is a basic amino acid with the molecular formula $C_6H_{14}N_4O_2$ and with a molecular weight of 174.20 daltons. It has 3 pKs: $pK_1=2.18$, $pK_2=9.09$ and $pK_3=13.2$. Therefore, it carries a positive charge at physiological pH. The stereoisomer of L-arginine, D-arginine, does not have any biological activity, as far as we know. L-arginine is also known as 2-amino-5-guanidinovaleric acid and (S)-2-amino-5-[(aminoiminomethyl)amino] pentaenoic acid. Its one-letter abbreviation is R. It is also abbreviated as Arg. The terms L-arginine and arginine are frequently used interchangeably. The structural formula of L-arginine is as follows:

L-arginine

ACTIONS AND PHARMACOLOGY

ACTIONS

Supplemental L-arginine may have anti-atherogenic, antioxidant and immunomodulatory actions. It may also have wound-repair activity.

MECHANISM OF ACTION

Many of supplemental L-arginine's activities, including its possible anti-atherogenic actions, may be accounted for by its role as the precursor to nitric oxide or NO. NO is produced by all tissues of the body and plays very important roles in the cardiovascular system, immune system and nervous system. NO is formed from L-arginine via the enzyme nitric oxide synthase or synthetase (NOS), and the effects of NO are mainly mediated by 3,'5'-cyclic guanylate

or cyclic GMP. NO activates the enzyme guanylate cyclase, which catalyzes the synthesis of cyclic GMP from guanosine triphosphate or GTP. Cyclic GMP is converted to guanylic acid via the enzyme cyclic GMP phosphodiesterase.

NOS is a heme-containing enzyme with some sequences similar to cytochrome P-450 reductase. Several isoforms of NOS exist, two of which are constitutive and one of which is inducible by immunological stimuli. The constitutive NOS found in the vascular endothelium is designated eNOS and that present in the brain, spinal cord and peripheral nervous system is designated nNOS. The form of NOS induced by immunological or inflammatory stimuli is known as iNOS. iNOS may be expressed constitutively in select tissues such as lung epithelium.

All the nitric oxide synthases use NADPH (reduced nicotinamide adenine dinucleotide phosphate) and oxygen (O_2) as cosubstrates, as well as the cofactors FAD (flavin adenine dinucleotide), FMN (flavin mononucleotide), tetrahydrobiopterin and heme. Interestingly, ascorbic acid appears to enhance NOS activity by increasing intracellular tetrahydrobiopterin. eNOS and nNOS synthesize NO in response to an increased concentration of calcium ions or in some cases in response to calcium-independent stimuli, such as shear stress.

In vitro studies of NOS indicate that the Km of the enzyme for L-arginine is in the micromolar range. The concentration of L-arginine in endothelial cells, as well as in other cells, and in plasma is in the millimolar range. What this means is that, under physiological conditions, NOS is saturated with its L-arginine substrate. In other words, L-arginine would not be expected to be rate-limiting for the enzyme, and it would not appear that supraphysiological levels of L-arginine—which could occur with oral supplementation of the amino acid—would make any difference with regard to NO production. The reaction would appear to have reached its maximum level. However, *in vivo* studies have demonstrated that, under certain conditions, e.g. hypercholesterolemia, supplemental L-arginine could enhance endothelial-dependent vasodilation and NO production.

The discordance between the *in vivo* results—increased NO production under certain conditions—and the *in vitro* enzyme studies described above is known as the "arginine paradox." There are a few explanations for the "arginine paradox." NOS may be inhibited by asymmetric dimethylarginine or ADMA, which is known to be elevated in hypercholesterolemia and which increases mononuclear cell (monocyte and T-lymphocyte) adhesiveness in hypercholesterolemics. ADMA is formed by post-translational methylation of L-arginine residues in proteins and is released from the proteins following their hydrolysis. The "arginine paradox" may be explained in part by increasing levels of L-arginine overcoming the inhibition of NOS by ADMA. In addition to hypercholesterolemia, elevated levels of ADMA are associated with hypertension, diabetes, preeclampsia, smoking and aging. Elevation of ADMA may be due to altered metabolism of this substance by dimethylarginine dimethylaminohydrolase or DDAH. DDAH is the major enzyme involved in ADMA catabolism. Decreased levels of DDAH have been found in diabetic and hypercholesterolemic animal models.

Other explanations of the "arginine paradox" include the presence of other inhibitors of NOS yet to be discovered, impaired transport of L-arginine into or within endothelial cells and impaired regeneration of L-arginine from L-citrulline. There is another interesting possibility. A non-enzymatic pathway by which NO may be produced has recently been described. Endothelial dysfunction is associated with increased oxidative stress resulting in increased formation of such reactive oxygen species as hydrogen peroxide and superoxide anions. Further, during conditions of oxidative stress, enzymatic synthesis of NO may decrease, and NO reacts with superoxide anions to form the reactive nitrogen species peroxynitrite. Under these conditions, L-arginine can essentially scavenge hydrogen peroxide and superoxide to form NO non-enzymatically. Interestingly, in this non-enzymatic reaction, L-arginine, as well as the non-biological D-arginine, can both form NO.

NO formed from supplemental L-arginine can play a major role in the possible anti-atherogenic activity of L-arginine. NO inhibits mononuclear cell adhesion, platelet aggregation, proliferation of vascular smooth muscle, production of some reactive oxygen species, such as superoxide anions, and promotion of endothelium-dependent dilation. Leukocyte adhesion, platelet aggregation, smooth muscle proliferation, endothelial dysfunction and oxidative stress are all part of the process of atherogenesis. L-arginine may also have anti-atherogenic activity independent of its role in the enzymatic formation of NO.

L-arginine may itself have antioxidant activity. L-arginine has been found to inhibit the oxidation of low-density lipoproteins (LDL) to oxidized LDL (oxLDL). The oxidation of LDL to oxLDL is believed to be a pivotal early step in atherogenesis. L-arginine may also scavenge superoxide anions and hydrogen peroxide (see above), as well as inhibit lipid peroxidation.

L-arginine has been shown to have immunomodulatory activity. For example, in human breast cancer, supplementation with this amino acid has been reported to increase the quantity and cytotoxic activity of natural killer (NK) cells and lymphokine-activated-killer (LAK) cells. L-arginine is considered an immunonutrient and is added to enteral and parenteral feedings for burn, sepsis and trauma patients. The mechanism of L-arginine's possible immunomodulating activity is not entirely clear. It may, at least in part, be again due to L-arginine's role in the production of NO. Production of NO, with consequent decrease of the cyclic AMP/cyclic GMP ratio in NK cells, would favor the production of interleukin-1, which is known to activate NK cells and may directly enhance NK cell cytotoxicity. L-arginine is also a precursor in the synthesis of the tetrapeptide tuftsin, which itself appears to have immunomodulatory activity. Tuftsin's activity appears to depend on two of the four amino acids present in its structure, L-arginine and L-proline. L-arginine also participates in the synthesis of L-proline.

L-arginine's possible activity in wound repair may be due to its precursor role in the formation of L-ornithine and, ultimately, L-proline. L-proline is a key element in collagen biosynthesis.

PHARMACOKINETICS
Following ingestion, L-arginine is absorbed from the lumen of the small intestine into the enterocytes. Absorption is efficient and occurs by an active transport mechanism. Some metabolism of L-arginine takes place in the enterocytes. L-arginine not metabolized in the enterocytes enters the portal circulation from whence it is transported to the liver, where again some portion of the amino acid is metabolized. L-arginine not metabolized in the liver enters the systemic circulation, where it is distributed to the various tissues of the body. L-arginine participates in various metabolic activities, including the production of proteins, D-glucose, glycogen, L-ornithine, urea, nitric oxide, L-glutamate, creatine, polyamines, L-proline, agmatin and tuftsin. L-arginine is eliminated by glomerular filtration and is almost completely reabsorbed by the renal tubules. L-arginine produces peak plasma levels approximately one to two hours after oral administration.

INDICATIONS AND USAGE
L-arginine shows promise in the treatment and prevention of cardiovascular disease (including atherosclerosis, hypertension, hyperlipidemia and angina pectoris), in the treatment of some forms of male infertility and some kidney disorders and it is helpful in accelerating wound healing in some circumstances. It has demonstrated some positive immune-modulating and anticancer effects. There is preliminary evidence that it could be helpful in some men with erectile dysfunction and in some others with migraine, liver disease and primary ciliary dyskinesia. There is conflicting but mostly negative evidence related to claims that it can improve exercise performance and promote lean muscle mass.

RESEARCH SUMMARY

Numerous *in vitro* experiments have shown that L-arginine has effects on endothelial cells that could be expected to inhibit cardiovascular disease. Inferences have been drawn from these studies suggesting that L-arginine, through its nitric oxide activity, especially in the endothelial cells of the blood vessels, inhibits vasoconstriction, thrombolytic activity, cell proliferation, inflammation and other activities that promote cardiovascular disease.

Some of the promise of these *in vitro* studies has been realized in animal and clinical studies. In hypercholesterolemic animal models, L-arginine helps normalize lipids and vasodilatory response, inhibits platelet aggregation and formation of intimal lesions. Further, it has been seen in some of these animal studies to cause pre-existing lesions to regress.

Similarly, L-arginine has had significant positive effects in hypercholesterolemic and hypertensive humans. It has also been helpful in those with angina pectoris. In a recent long-term study, supplemental L-arginine, given for six months, resulted in significant improvement in coronary small-vessel endothelial function associated with a decrease in plasma endothelin concentrations.

In a double-blind, placebo-controlled study of 22 subjects with stable angina, supplemental L-arginine (1 gram twice daily) significantly improved exercise capacity. L-arginine supplementation resulted in a 70% reduction in angina attacks in another study.

In other studies, L-arginine was credited with significantly reducing lipid peroxidation in patients with diabetes mellitus. Conflicting results were produced by two studies related to L-arginine's effects on vasomotor response in smokers. In one of these studies, L-arginine significantly reversed abnormal myocardial blood flow response to a cold pressor test; in the other small study, no significant positive effect was seen.

The treatment of oligospermia with L-arginine was first reported many years ago. In one of these early studies, 178 men with oligospermia were given 4 grams of L-arginine daily. Severe oligospermia was diagnosed in 93 of these subjects. Treatment ceased in subjects who showed no improvement after two months. A 100% increase in sperm count was achieved in 42 cases, resulting in 15 pregnancies. There was marked increase in sperm number and motility in an additional 69 patients, resulting in another 13 pregnancies.

Subsequent studies have shown that L-arginine improves sperm count and motility. A recent small study credited L-arginine with producing pregnancies, but larger clinical trials are needed to confirm the efficacy seen in the early work.

L-arginine is of benefit in some kidney diseases and shows some promise in interstitial cystitis. It helps improve kidney function in some diabetic animal models and prevents chronic renal failure in others. A recent study indicated that L-arginine facilitates renal vasodilatation and natriuresis in renal transplant patients. There was also the suggestion in this study that L-arginine counteracts the antinatriuretic effect of cyclosporin.

Several studies have found that L-arginine benefits some with interstitial cystitis. Other studies, however, have not reported benefit. It appears that L-arginine can decrease pain and urgency in some subsets of interstial cystitis patients, but more research is needed to confirm this.

L-arginine has long been used following trauma and during sepsis. Studies have shown that L-arginine improves nitrogen balance and thus reduces protein catabolism. Animal studies have shown that L-arginine can be of significant benefit after severe burn injury, increasing survival, improving cardiac function and preventing bacterial translocation. Intravenous L-arginine has been helpful in some human traumas, helping to speed healing while inhibiting post-injury wasting and weight loss.

L-arginine shows many effects on immune function both *in vitro* and *in vivo*. In various animal studies, L-arginine has, reportedly, improved host immunity in a variety of conditions through its effects on the thymus and T-lymphocytes. It has also been reported to reduce the incidence of chemically induced tumors and to reduce the size of pre-existing tumors. It has significantly inhibited metastatic spread of some cancers in animal work.

In human work, oral L-arginine has increased the responsiveness of some immune components and has decreased the number and percent of T suppressor/cytotoxic cells (CD8) in healthy human volunteers. In a clinical trial involving patients undergoing abdominal surgery, intravenous L-arginine diminished postoperative reduction in the mitogenic responses of peripheral blood lymphocytes to ConA and PHA. Enhancement of these same responses was reported in a study in which L-arginine was given to HIV patients. L-arginine supplementation in this study, did not, however, alter T-lymphocyte subsets or ratios.

In a more recent study of L-arginine's effects in HIV-infected subjects, supplementation for six months (7.4 grams daily) failed to produce any improvement in immunological parameters measured, but body weight increased in L-arginine-supplemented subjects.

In healthy human volunteers, administering 30 grams of L-arginine daily for three days resulted in enhanced natural-killer (NK) and lymphokine-activated-killer (LAK) cell activity. A mean rise of 91% in NK cell activity and a mean rise of 58% in LAK cell activity were observed. The researchers concluded: "The substantial enhancement of human NK and LAK cell activity by large doses of L-arginine could be useful in many immunosuppressed states, including malignant disease, AIDS and HIV infection, in which depressed NK cell activity is an important component of the disease process."

Supplementation with L-arginine has significantly increased the quantity and cytotoxic activity of NK cells and lympho-kine-activated cells in patients with breast cancer in one study. Research is ongoing.

There is recent, preliminary evidence that oral L-arginine can help some men with erectile dysfunction. In a double-blind, placebo-controlled study, 50 men with this disorder were randomized to receive 5 grams of L-arginine daily or placebo for six weeks. Nine of 29 L-arginine-supplemented subjects and two of 17 controls reported significant subjective improvement in erectile function. All nine of the L-arginine responders had low urinary levels of stable metabolites of nitric oxide at baseline. These levels doubled by the end of the study. More research is needed.

In another recent study, L-arginine was found to be helpful in subjects suffering from primary ciliary dyskinesia, a genetic disorder characterized by impaired cilia motility and abnormally low levels of nasal nitric oxide. L-arginine, in combination with ibuprofen, also proved helpful in significantly reducing migraine pain intensity compared with placebo in another recent, preliminary, multi-center study of 40 migraine patients.

Research related to L-arginine's claimed hepatoprotective effects is dated. The data, however, looked promising and deserve follow-up.

Claims that L-arginine enhances exercise performance and promotes development of lean body mass while burning fat in healthy individuals are poorly supported. Weight gain was decreased in obese mice fed L-arginine, but there are no human data to support anti-obesity claims for L-arginine.

There are hypothetical reasons to believe that L-arginine, popular with some body builders, might have ergogenic/anabolic effects but, so far, these effects have not been demonstrated. High dose oral L-arginine has, however, been shown to induce release of growth hormone and prolactin but, again, no studies have been conducted to see whether this could have any meaningful ergogenic or anabolic effect.

CONTRAINDICATIONS, PRECAUTIONS, ADVERSE REACTIONS

CONTRAINDICATIONS

Supplemental L-arginine is contraindicated in those with the rare genetic disorder argininemia. It is also contraindicated in those hypersensitive to any component of an arginine-containing preparation.

PRECAUTIONS

Because of absence of long-term safety studies, and because of the possibility of growth hormone stimulation, pregnant women and nursing mothers should avoid L-arginine supplementation.

Those with renal or hepatic failure should exercise caution in the use of supplemental L-arginine.

Proteins of the herpes simplex virus are rich in L-arginine, and there are a few reports (mainly anecdotal) of those taking supplemental L-arginine who have had recurrences of oral herpes lesions. Although it is unlikely that those with a history of herpes simplex virus infection will have recurrences if they use L-arginine supplements, they should nevertheless be aware of this possibility.

ADVERSE REACTIONS

Oral supplementation with L-arginine at doses up to 15 grams daily are generally well tolerated. The most common adverse reactions of higher doses — from 15 to 30 grams daily — are nausea, abdominal cramps and diarrhea. Some may experience these symptoms at lower doses.

INTERACTIONS

DRUGS

Cyclosporine: L-arginine may counteract the antinaturetic effect of cyclosporin.

Ibuprofen: L-arginine may increase the absorption of ibuprofen if taken concomitantly.

Organic nitrates: L-arginine supplements theoretically may potentiate the effects of organic nitrates if taken concomitantly.

Sildenafil citrate: Theoretically, L-arginine supplements taken concomitantly with sildenafil citrate, may potentiate the effects of the drug.

HERBS

Yohimbe: L-Arginine, if used concomitantly, may enhance the effect of yohimbe.

DOSAGE AND ADMINISTRATION

L-arginine is available in tablet, capsule and powder form and as L-arginine hydrochloride and free base L-arginine. It is also available in medical foods as an aid in the enhancement of immune function.

Various doses are used. For cardiovascular health reasons, doses from 8 to 21 grams daily have been used in divided doses. To help aid with sperm quantity and quality, doses of 10 to 20 grams daily have been used in divided doses. Doses of 5 grams daily have been used for erectile dysfunction. Doses of 1.5 to 2.4 grams daily have been used for interstitial cystitis.

LITERATURE

Adams MR, McCredie R, Jessup W, et al. Oral L-arginine improves endothelium-dependent dilatation and reduces monocyte adhesion to endothelial cells in young men with coronary artery disease. *Atherosclerosis*. 1997; 129:261-269.

Andres A, Morales JM, Praga M, et al. L-arginine reverses the antinatriuretic effect of cyclosporin in renal transplant patients. *Nephrol Dial Transplant*. 1997; 12:1437-1440.

Barbul A. Arginine: biochemistry, physiology, and therapeutic implications. *JPEN*. 1986; 10:227-238.

Barbul A, Sisto DA, Wasserkrug HL, Efron G. Arginine stimulates lymphocyte immune response in healthy human beings. *Surgery*. 1981; 90:244-251.

Bode-Boger SM, Boger RH, Galland A, et al. L-arginine-induced vasodilation in healthy humans: pharmacokinetic-pharmacodynamic relationship. *Br J Clin Pharmacol*. 1998; 46:489-497.

Brandes RP, Brandes S, Boger RH, et al. L-Arginine supplementation in hypercholesterolemic rabbits normalizes leukocyte adhesion to non-endothelial matrix. *Life Sci*. 2000; 66:1519-1524.

Cartledge JJ, Davies A-M, Eardley I. A randomized double-blind placebo-controlled crossover trial of the efficacy of L-arginine in the treatment of interstitial cystitis. *BJU Int*. 2000; 85:421-426.

Chan JS, Boger RH, Bode-Boger SM. Et al. Asymmetric dimethylarginine increases mononuclear cell adhesiveness in hypercholesterolemic humans. *Arterioscler Thromb Vasc Biol*. 2000; 20:1040-1046.

Chen J, Wollman Y, Chernichovsky T, et al. Effect of oral administration of high-dose nitric oxide donor L-arginine in men with organic erectile dysfunction: results of a double-blind, randomized, placebo-controlled study. *BJU Int*. 1999; 83:269-273.

Clarkson P, Adams MR, Powe AJ, et al. Oral L-arginine improves endothelium-dependent dilation in hypercholesterolemic young adults. *J Clin Invest*. 1996; 97:1989-1994.

Cooke JP. Singer AH, Tsao P, et al. Antiatherogenic effects of L-arginine in the hypercholesterolemic rabbit. *J Clin Invest*. 1992; 90:1168-1172.

Griffith RS, DeLong DC, Nelson JD. Relation of arginine-lysine antagonism to herpes simplex growth in tissue culture. *Chemotherapy*. 1981; 27:209-213.

Hambrecht R, Hilbrich L, Erbs S, et al. Correction of endothelial dysfunction in chronic heart failure: additional effects of exercise training and oral L-arginine supplementation. *J Am Coll Cardiol*. 2000; 35:701-713.

Horton JW, White J, Maass D, Sanders B. Arginine in burn injury improves cardiac performance and prevents bacterial translocation. *J Appl Physiol*. 1998; 84:695-702.

Isidori A, Lo Monaco A, Cappa M. A study of growth hormone release in man after oral administration of amino acids. *Current Med Res Opinion*. 1981; 7:475-481.

Kapuler AM, Gurusiddiah S. The amino acids precursory to proteins are primary human food: proline, glutamine, and arginine found free in the juices of common vegetables and herbs. *J Med Food*. 1998; 1:97-115.

Korting GE, Smith SD, Wheeler MA, et al. A randomized double-blind trial of oral L-arginine for treatment of interstitial cystitis. *J Urol*. 1999; 161:558-565.

Lerman A, Burnett JC Jr, Higano ST, et al. Long-term L-arginine supplementation improves small-vessel coronary endothelial function in humans. *Circulation*. 1998; 97:2123-2128.

Loukides S, Kharitonov S, Wodehouse T, et al. Effect of arginine on mucocilliary function in primary ciliary dyskinesia. *Lancet*. 1998; 352:371-372.

Lubec B, Hayn M, Kitzmü ller E, et al. L-arginine reduces lipid peroxidation in patients with diabetes mellitus. *Free Rad Biol Med*. 1997; 22:355-357.

Mantha SV. Mediation of L-arginine-induced retardation of hypercholesterolemic atherosclerosis in rabbits by antioxidant mechanisms. *Nutr Res*. 1999; 10:1529-1539.

Nagase S, Takemura K, Ueda A, et al. A novel nonenzymatic pathway for the generation of nitric oxide by the reaction of hydrogen peroxide and D- or L-arginine. *Biochem Biophys Res Commun*. 1997; 233:150-153.

Narita I, Border WA, Ketteler M, et al. L-arginine may mediate the therapeutic effects of low protein diets. *Proc Natl Acad Sci USA*. 1995; 92:4552-4556.

Park KGM, Hayes PD, Garlick PJ et al. Stimulation of lymphocyte natural cytotoxicity by L-arginine. *Lancet*. 1991; 337:645-646.

Reis DJ, Regunathan S. Is agmatine a novel neurotransmitter in brain? *Trends Pharmacol Sci*. 2000; 21:187-193.

Sandrini G, Franchini S, Lanfranchi S, et al. Effectiveness of ibuprofen-arginine in the treatment of acute migraine headaches. *Int J Clin Pharmacol Res*. 1998; 18:145-150.

Schachter A, Goldman JA, Zuckerman Z. Treatment of oligospermia with the amino acid arginine. *J Urology*. 1973; 110:311-313.

Scibona M, Meschini P, Capparelli S, et al. [L-arginine and male infertility]. [Article in Italian]. *Minerva Urol Nefrol*. 1994; 46:251-253.

Tangphao O, Grossman M, Chalon S, et al. Pharmacokinetics of intravenous and oral L-arginine in normal volunteers. *Br J Clin Pharmacol*. 1999; 47:261-266.

Tentolouris C, Tousoulis D, Davies GJ, et al. Serum cholesterol level, cigarette smoking, and vasomotor responses to L-arginine in narrowed epicardial coronary arteries. *Amer J Cardiol.* 2000; 85:500-503.

Wascher TC, Posch K, Wallner S, et al. Vascular effects of L-arginine: anything beyond a substrate for the NO-synthase? *Biochem Biophys Res Commun.* 1997; 234:35-38.

L-Aspartate

DESCRIPTION

L-aspartate is a protein amino acid naturally found in all life forms. L-aspartate is a dicarboxylic amino acid. Although most L-aspartate is in proteins, small amounts of free L-aspartate are found in body fluids and in plants. The normal diet contains about 2 grams of L-aspartate daily. L-aspartate is also in the alternative dipeptide sweetener aspartame; the amount of L-aspartate from the sweetener is a small fraction of total L-aspartate consumed.

L-aspartate is considered a non-essential amino acid, meaning that, under normal physiological conditions, sufficient amounts of the amino acid are synthesized in the body to meet the body's requirements. L-aspartate is formed by the transamination of the Krebs cycle intermediate oxaloacetate. The amino acid serves as a precursor for synthesis of proteins, oligopeptides, purines, pyrimidines, nucleic acids and L-arginine. L-aspartate is a glycogenic amino acid, and it can also promote energy production via its metabolism in the Krebs cycle. These latter activities were the rationale for the claim that supplemental aspartate has an anti-fatigue effect on skeletal muscle, a claim that was never confirmed.

L-aspartate is also known as L-amino succinate. Its IUPAC abbreviation is Asp. Its one-letter abbreviation, used when spelling out protein structures, is D. It is a solid, with an acid form that is slightly soluble in water, and with salt forms that are more water-soluble. Available salts include magnesium, calcium, potassium, zinc and combinations thereof. L-aspartate is used interchangeably with the term aspartic acid. The biological form of this substance, however, is the anion of aspartic acid, L-aspartate. Aspartic acid has the following chemical structure:

Aspartic acid

ACTIONS AND PHARMACOLOGY

ACTIONS

L-aspartate salts are delivery forms for cations such as magnesium, potassium, calcium and zinc.

MECHANISM OF ACTION

L-aspartates can form salts with cations such as magnesium, potassium, calcium and zinc.

PHARMACOKINETICS

Following ingestion, L-aspartate is absorbed from the small intestine by an active transport process. Following absorption, L-aspartate enters the portal circulation and from there is transported to the liver, where much of it is metabolized to protein, purines, pyrimidines and L-arginine, and is catabolized as well. L-aspartate is not metabolized in the liver; it enters the systemic circulation, which distributes it to various tissues of the body. The cations associated with L-aspartate independently interact with various substances in the body and participate in various physiological processes.

INDICATIONS AND USAGE

There is no support for the claim that aspartates are exercise performance enhancers, i.e. ergogenic aids.

RESEARCH SUMMARY

There are claims that L-aspartate is a special type of mineral transporter for cations, such as magnesium, into cells. Magnesium aspartate has not been found to be more biologically effective when compared with other magnesium salts.

There are also claims that L-aspartate has ergogenic effects, that it enhances performance in both prolonged exercise and short intensive exercise. It is hypothesized that L-aspartate, especially the potassium magnesium aspartate salt, spares stores of muscle glycogen and/or promotes a faster rate of glycogen resynthesis during exercise. It has also been hypothesized that L-aspartate can enhance short intensive exercise by serving as a substrate for energy production in the Krebs cycle and for stimulating the purine nucleotide cycle.

An animal study using injected aspartate failed to find any evidence of a glycogen-sparing effect or any ergogenic effects whatsoever. A more recent double-blind human study of male weight trainers similarly found aspartate supplementation to have no effect, and another study of the effect of aspartate on short intensive exercise again found no effect.

CONTRAINDICATIONS, PRECAUTIONS, ADVERSE REACTIONS

CONTRAINDICATIONS

L-aspartate supplementation is contraindicated in those hypersensitive to any component of the preparation.

PRECAUTIONS

Because of lack of long-term safety studies, L-aspartate salts should be avoided by children, pregnant women and lactating women.

ADVERSE REACTIONS

Mild gastrointestinal side effects including diarrhea have been reported.

INTERACTIONS

No drug, nutritional supplement, food or herb interactions are known.

OVERDOSAGE

Overdosage has not been reported.

DOSAGE AND ADMINISTRATION

L-aspartate salts of potassium, magnesium, calcium and zinc are available, as well as mixed salts of magnesium potassium aspartate and calcium magnesium aspartate. See Calcium, Magnesium, Potassium and Zinc for dose recommendations of these minerals.

LITERATURE

Bac P, Pages N, Herrenknecht CLA, Teste JF. Inhibition of mouse-killing behavior in magnesium-deficient rats: effect of pharmacological doses of magnesium pidolate, magnesium aspartate, magnesium lactate, magnesium gluconate and magnesium chloride. *Magnes Res.* 1995; 8:37-45.

de Haan A, van Doorn JE, Westra HG. Effects of potassium + magnesium aspartate on muscle metabolism and force development during short static exercise. *Int J Sports Med.* 1985; 6:44-49.

Hagan RD, Upton SJ, Duncan JJ, et al. Absence of effect of potassium- magnesium aspartate on physiologic responses to prolonged work in aerobically trained men. *Int J Sports Med.* 1982; 3:177-181.

Hicks JT. Treatment of fatigue in general practice: a double-blind study. *Clinical Medicine.* 1964; 71:85-90.

Maughan RJ, Sadler DJ. The effects of oral administration of salts of aspartic acid on the metabolic response to prolonged exhausting exercise in man. *Int J Sports Med.* 1983; 4:119-123.

Trudeau F, Murphy R. Effects of potassium-aspartate salt administration on glycogen use in the rat during a swimming stress. *Physiol Behav.* 1993; 54:7-12.

Tuttle JL, Potteiger JA, Evans BW, Ozmun JC. Effects of acute potassium-magnesium aspartate supplementation on ammonia concentrations during and after resistance training. *Int J Sport Nutr.* 1995; 5:102-109.

L-Carnitine

DESCRIPTION

L-carnitine, an amino acid derivative, is found in nearly all cells of the body. L-carnitine transports long-chain fatty acids across the inner mitochondrial membranes in the mitochondria, where they are processed by beta-oxidation to produce biological energy in the form of adenosine triphosphate or ATP.

L-carnitine is known chemically as (R)-3-carboxy-2-hydroxy-N,N,N-trimethyl-1-propanaminium hydroxide, inner salt; beta-hydroxy-gamma-N,N,N-trimethylaminobutyrate; gamma-amino-beta-hydroxybutyric acid trimethylbetaine; (3-carboxy-2-hydroxypropyl) trimethylammonium hydroxide, inner salt; gamma-trimethyl-beta-hydroxybutyrobetaine, and 3-hydroxy-4-(trimethylammonio) butanoate. L-carnitine is also known as levocarnitine and was formerly called vitamin BT. L-carnitine is a quarternary amine and belongs to the same chemical family as choline and is soluble in water. L-carnitine is represented by the following chemical structure:

$$CH_3\text{---}\underset{\underset{CH_3}{|}}{\overset{\overset{CH_3}{|}}{N^+}}\text{---}CH_2\text{---}\underset{\overset{HO\quad H}{|}}{C}\text{---}CH_2\text{---}\overset{\overset{O}{\|}}{C}\text{---}O^-$$

L-Carnitine

L-carnitine occurs naturally in animal products. Generally, only very small amounts of it are found in plants, with few exceptions, such as avocado and some fermented soy products, e.g. tempeh. L-carnitine is a chiral molecule. Its stereoisomer D-carnitine does not have the biological activity of L-carnitine and may even antagonize L-carnitine in its biological roles.

L-carnitine is synthesized in the human body, chiefly in the liver and kidneys, from the essential amino acids L-lysine and L-methionine. Niacin, vitamins B_6 and C, and iron are involved in its biosynthesis. L-carnitine is described as a conditionally essential nutrient. This refers to certain conditions where exogenous L-carnitine may be required, such as in long-term parenteral nutrition, those on valproic acid therapy and possibly for the elderly.

L-carnitine is available in a few forms. Oral L-carnitine is available as a nutritional supplement and as a prescribed orphan drug treatment for primary and secondary L-carnitine deficiencies. Intravenous L-carnitine (levocarnitine) is available as a prescription orphan drug for the treatment of primary and secondary L-carnitine deficiencies. Acetyl-L-carnitine, another delivery form of both L-carnitine and acetyl groups, is available as a nutritional supplement. Another delivery form of L-carnitine, proprionyl-L-carnitine, is available in Europe but not at present in the U.S.

ACTIONS AND PHARMACOLOGY

ACTIONS

Supplemental L-carnitine may have cardioprotective activity in addition to beneficially affecting cardiac function. It may have a triglyceride-lowering effect in some as well as help to elevate HDL-cholesterol levels. L-carnitine may also have antioxidant properties.

Acetyl-L-carnitine may have neuroprotective activity. It may also aid in the treatment of age-related cholinergic deficits, such as those found in dementia disorder, including Alzheimer's disease (see Acetyl-L-carnitine).

MECHANISM OF ACTION

There are at least two major functions of L-carnitine. All tissues except the brain use long-chain fatty acids for bioenergy production. In cardiac and skeletal muscle, a major contribution of bioenergy comes from the beta-oxidation of long-chain fatty acids. Long-chain fatty acids require L-carnitine to transport them across the inner membranes of the mitochondria, wherein their metabolism produces bioenergy. Following the delivery of long-chain fatty acids into other mitochondria, L-carnitine, either by itself or esterified to an acyl group, recrosses the mitochondrial membrane to allow for continual use in this shuttle process.

Another function of L-carnitine is to remove short-chain and medium-chain fatty acids from the mitochondria in order to maintain coenzyme A levels in these organelles. These fatty acids accumulate as a result of normal and abnormal metabolism. This mechanism prevents the build-up in the mitochondria of short-chain and medium-chain fatty acids that may interfere with the bioenergy-producing process vital to the normal function of the cell.

Two types of L-carnitine deficiency states exist: primary systemic carnitine deficiency (SCD) and secondary carnitine deficiency syndromes. SCD is an autosomal recessive disorder characterized by progressive cardiomyopathy, skeletal myopathy, hypoglycemia and hyperammonemia. SCD appears to be due, in part, to loss of function of the transporter protein called OCT N2, which helps carry L-carnitine into cells. Patients with SCD have low L-carnitine levels in liver and skeletal muscle and variable concentrations of L-carnitine in the serum. Treatment with large doses of L-carnitine either orally or intravenously is sometimes beneficial in this rare genetic disorder.

Secondary L-carnitine deficiency disorders include a large number of entities. Some of these are genetic defects of metabolism such as methylmalonic aciduria, cytochrome C oxidase deficiency, fatty acyl-coenzyme A dehydrogenase deficiency, including long-chain and medium-chain deficiency, isovaleric acidemia, glutaric aciduria and propionic acidemia.

The mechanism of L-carnitine deficiency in these disorders is unclear. Some hypothesize that an accumulation of short-chain and medium-chain fatty acyl CoA molecules occurs in the mitochondria because insufficient L-carnitine is available to expel them. This accumulation would disturb the bioenergy-producing processes of the mitochondria. Symptoms of secondary muscle L-carnitine deficiency, not surprisingly, include muscle weakness and fatigue.

Secondary L-carnitine deficiency may also be found secondary to other conditions such as chronic renal failure treated by hemodialysis, cirrhosis with cachexia, chronic severe myopathies, myxedema, hypopituitarism, adrenal insufficiency, hyperammonemia associated with valproic acid therapy, valproate-induced Reye's syndrome, advanced AIDS and pregnancy. It may also be seen in those with HIV who are being treated with the nucleoside analogues didanosine (ddI), zalcitabine (ddC) and stavudine (d4T). In addition, it may occur in premature infants receiving parenteral nutrition. There is some preliminary evidence that secondary L-carnitine deficiency may also be associated with aging.

L-carnitine may possess antioxidant properties. A disturbance in long-chain fatty acid oxidation in mitochondria and/or the accumulation of small-chain and medium-chain fatty acyl CoA molecules in the mitochondria might be expected to increase oxidative stress. There is some evidence that proprionyl-L-carnitine, a delivery form of L-carnitine, might protect the ischemic heart from reperfusion injury via an antioxidant effect.

PHARMACOKINETICS

About 60 to 75% of L-carnitine from food is absorbed. The percentage absorbed from supplements appears to be lower. In one study only 20% of a 2-gram dose of L-carnitine was found to be absorbed following ingestion. Most of an ingested dose of L-carnitine is absorbed by the small intestine, apparently by facilitative diffusion and active transport. Following the administration of a dose of L-carnitine of 1,980 milligrams twice daily, the maximum plasma concentration level (C_{max}) was 80 nanomoles per milliliter, and the time to maximum concentration (T_{max}) occurred at 3.3 hours. The bioavailability of oral L-carnitine is about 15%. L-carnitine is not bound to plasma protein or albumin.

Five normal adult male volunteers, administered a dose of [^{3}H-methyl]-L-carnitine following 15 days of a high-carnitine diet and additional L-carnitine supplement, excreted 58 to 65% of administered radioactive dose in 5 to 11 days in the urine and feces. Maximum concentration of [^{3}H-methyl]-L-carnitine in serum occurred from 2.0 to 4.5 hours after radioactive L-carnitine administration. Major metabolites found were trimethyl N-oxide, primarily in urine (8% to 49% of the administered dose) and [^{3} H]-gamma-butyrobetaine, primarily in feces (0.44% to 45% of the administered dose). Fecal excretion of total L-carnitine was less then 1% of total L-carnitine excretion. After attainment of steady state following four days of oral administration of about 2,000 milligrams twice a day of L-carnitine, urinary excretion of L-carnitine was about 9% of the orally administered dose. Approximately 95% of filtered L-carnitine is reabsorbed in healthy humans. Hypothyroidism decreases the urinary excretion of L-carnitine, while hyperthyroidism increases it.

Following absorption from the intestine, about 25% of L-carnitine may be acylated in the intestinal mucosa. Orally administered L-carnitine and its acylated metabolite are distributed to most tissues of the body. Uptake of L-carnitine into cells is thought to occur by facilitative diffusion and, in some cases, by active transport. Most of the body's stores of L-carnitine are found in cardiac and skeletal muscle.

INDICATIONS AND USAGE

The strongest evidence for the use of supplemental L-carnitine may be in the management of cardiac ischemia and peripheral arterial disease. It may also more generally be indicated for cardioprotection. It lowers triglyceride levels and increases levels of HDL-cholesterol in some. It is used with some benefit in those with primary and secondary carnitine deficiency syndromes. There is less evidence to support arguments that carnitine is indicated in liver, kidney and immune disorders or in diabetes and Alzheimer's disease. There is little evidence that supplemental L-carnitine boosts energy, increases athletic performance or inhibits obesity. There is no support for the claim that healthy vegetarians require L-carnitine supplementation.

RESEARCH SUMMARY

Favorable results have been reported for many years with regard to the use of L-carnitine in the treatment of various forms of cardiovascular disease. The walking capacity of patients with intermittent claudication was significantly improved in one double-blind, cross-over study of patients receiving oral L-carnitine. The data in this study suggests that L-carnitine enhances pyruvate utilization and oxidative phosphorylation efficiency in the skeletal muscle of the ischemic leg.

In a more recent, multicenter study, propionyl-L-carnitine was compared with placebo in the treatment of those with peripheral arterial disease of the legs. The study of 162 patients receiving propionyl-L-carnitine and 166 patients receiving placebo continued for one year. Walking ability and quality of life were evaluated at regular intervals. Those initially presenting with the most severe disability (able to walk no more than 250 meters) exhibited significant improvement, increasing walking distance by 98 meters compared with 54 meters in the placebo group. Those able to walk more than 250 meters at baseline also improved, versus placebo, but not at a level of statistical significance.

Supplemental L-carnitine has been helpful in some rare primary genetic L-carnitine deficiency syndromes, as well as in more common secondary L-carnitine deficiency syndromes (see pharmacology). It has been estimated that about 40% of those with the myopathies associated with the secondary deficiency syndromes respond to dietary L-carnitine, evidenced by enhanced muscle strength and reduced myoglobinuria.

An indirect role for supplemental L-carnitine in some forms of liver disease is suggested, because hepatic disease impairs the last stage of L-carnitine synthesis resulting in L-carnitine deficiencies in heart and skeletal muscle. Preliminary work suggests that L-carnitine can reduce fat deposits in some fatty livers. Research is ongoing.

The kidney is also an important locus of carnitine synthesis. Chronic kidney disease may eventually be an indication for L-carnitine supplementation, but more research is needed to demonstrate this. There is some evidence that dialysis patients can benefit from L-carnitine supplementation since dialysis removes the low-molecular-weight L-carnitine.

There is no evidence that L-carnitine will prevent diabetes, although abnormal carnitine metabolism is associated with diabetes. Ongoing research may demonstrate some benefit from L-carnitine supplementation. Animal model work in diabetes has shown improved myocardial function with administration of parenteral L-carnitine.

The claim that L-carnitine may have beneficial effects in Alzheimer's disease is unproved. Acetyl-L-carnitine, a derivative of L-carnitine and a delivery form of the substance, on the other hand, has shown some very preliminary benefit in this regard (see Acetyl-L-Carnitine). Investigation of L-carnitine may have some positive impact on some immune disorders, including AIDS. In a study of 20 patients with advanced AIDS, subjects were randomly assigned to receive either placebo or 6 grams of L-carnitine daily. At baseline, L-carnitine concentrations in the peripheral blood mononuclear cells (PBMC) of the AIDS patients were found to be lower than in healthy controls, even though the AIDS patients had normal serum concentrations of L-carnitine.

The study continued for two weeks. It demonstrated a significant trend toward restoration of normal intracellular L-carnitine levels. This increase in cellular L-carnitine was strongly associated with improved lymphocyte proliferative responsiveness to mitogens. The researchers suggested that

"L-carnitine supplementation could have a role as a complementary therapy for HIV-infected individuals." The study also noted a significant decrease in the triglyceride levels of those patients receiving L-carnitine supplements. More research is clearly warranted.

L-carnitine effects on immunity are suggested, as well, from animal model work. Reductions in circulating cytokines and tumor necrosis factor have been observed.

There is little convincing evidence that L-carnitine supplements have any significant impact on physical performance or obesity. There is no support for the claim that vegetarians, including strict vegetarians, require L-carnitine supplementation. There is no evidence of carnitine deficiency in this population. Plasma carnitine concentrations in strict vegetarians are only an insignificant 10% lower than in omnivores.

CONTRAINDICATIONS, PRECAUTIONS, ADVERSE REACTIONS

CONTRAINDICATIONS

Known hypersensitivity to an L-carnitine-containing product.

PRECAUTIONS

Standard assays for mutagenicity indicate that L-carnitine is not mutagenic.

Reproductive studies have been performed in rats and rabbits at doses up to 3.8 times the human doses used for the treatment of primary and secondary L-carnitine deficiency on the basis of surface area and have revealed no evidence of impaired fertility or harm to the fetus due to L-carnitine. However, there are no adequate and well-controlled studies in pregnant women. Because animal reproduction studies are not always predictive of human response, supplemental L-carnitine should be used by pregnant women only if clearly indicated and only under medical supervision. It is not known whether L-carnitine is excreted in human milk. Supplemental L-carnitine is not advised for nursing mothers. Those with seizure disorders should only use L-carnitine under medical advisement and supervision.

ADVERSE REACTIONS

Mild gastrointestinal symptoms have been reported in those taking oral L-carnitine, including transient nausea and vomiting, abdominal cramps and diarrhea. Mild myasthenia has been reported in uremic patients taking the racemic mixture D,L-carnitine. There are no reports of mild myasthenia in uremic patients receiving L-carnitine. Supplemental L-carnitine is generally well tolerated.

Although the incidence is low, seizures have been reported to occur in those with or without pre-existing seizure disorders receiving either oral or intravenous L-carnitine. In those with pre-existing seizure activity, an increase in seizure frequency and/or severity has been reported.

INTERACTIONS

Therapy with valproic acid, the nucleoside analogues didanosine (ddI), zalcitabine (ddC) and stavudine (d4T) may produce secondary L-carnitine deficiencies. So might the pivalic acid-containing antibiotics, pivampicillin, pivmecillinam and pivcephalexin. These antibiotics are used in Europe.

Choline supplementation may lead to increased L-carnitine retention. Vitamin C deficiency may lead to secondary L-carnitine deficiency.

OVERDOSAGE

There have been no reports of toxicity from L-carnitine overdosage. The oral LD_{50} of L-carnitine in mice is 19.2 grams per kilogram.

DOSAGE AND ADMINISTRATION

L-carnitine is available in a few forms. Oral L-carnitine is available as a nutritional supplement and as a prescribed treatment for primary and secondary L-carnitine deficiencies. Intravenous L-carnitine is available as a prescription drug for the treatment of primary and secondary L-carnitine deficiencies. Acetyl-L-carnitine is available as a nutritional supplement. Propionyl-L-carnitine is available in Europe but not currently in the United States. DL-carnitine should be avoided. The available salts of L-carnitine are L-carnitine HC1, L-carnitine tartrate and L-carnitine fumarate.

Those who take supplemental L-carnitine for cardiovascular health (and most other possible indications) take 500 milligrams to 2 grams daily. The higher amounts are taken in divided doses. The doses are taken with or without food.

See Physician's Desk Reference for dosage and administration of levocarnitine in the treatment of primary and secondary L-carnitine deficiencies. See Acetyl-L-carnitine for dosage of this supplement.

LITERATURE

Bohles H, Richter K, Wagner-Thiesson E, Schafer H. Decreased serum carnitine in valproate induced Reye syndrome. *Eur J Pediatr.* 1982; 139:185-186.

Bohmer T, Rynding A, Solberg HE. Carnitine levels in human serum in health and disease. *Clin Chim Acta.* 1974; 57:55-61.

Borum PR. Carnitine. A*nn Rev Nutr.* 1983; 3:233-259.

Brevetti G, Diehm C, Lambert D. European multicenter study on propionyl-L-carnitine in intermittent claudication. *J Am Coll Cardiol.* 1999; 35:1618-1624.

Brevetti G, Chiarello M, Ferulano G, et al. Increases in walking distance in patients with peripheral vascular disease: a double-blind, cross-over study. *Circul.* 1988; 77:767-773.

Brooks H, Goldberg L, Holland R, et al. Carnitine-induced effects on cardiac and peripheral hemodynamics. *J Clin Pharmacol.* 1977; 17:561-578.

Christiansen R, Bremer J. Active transport of butyrobetaine and carnitine into isolated liver cells. *Biochem Biophys Acta*. 1977; 448:562-577.

de Simone C, Famularo G, Tzantzoglov S, et al. Carnitine depletion in peripheral blood mononuclear cells from patients with AIDS: effect of L-carnitine. *AIDS*. 1994; 8:655-660.

Famularo G, Moretti S, Marcellini S, et al. Acetyl-carnitine deficiency in AIDS patients with neurotoxicity on treatment with antiretroviral nucleoside analogues. *AIDS*. 1997; 11:185-190.

Lindstedt S, Lindstedt G. Distribution and excretion of carnitine $^{14}CO_2$ in the rat. *Acta Chim Scand*. 1961; 15:701-702.

Maebashi M, Kawamura N, Sato M, et al. Lipid-lowering effects of carnitine in patients with type-IV hypolipoproteinaemia. *Lancet*. 1978; 2:805-807.

Marzo A, Arrigoni Martelli E, Mancinelli A, et al. Protein binding of L-carnitine family components. *Eur J Drug Met Pharmacokin* Special Issue III. 1992; 364-368.

Nezu J, Tamai I, Oku A, et al. Primary systemic carnitine deficiency is caused by mutations in a gene encoding sodium ion-dependent carnitine transporter. *Nat Gen*. 1999; 21:91-94.

Opie LH. Role of carnitine in fatty acid metabolism of normal and ischemic myocardium. *Am Heart J*. 1979; 97:375-388.

Levocarnitine. *Physicians' Desk Reference*. 54 ed. Montvale, NJ; Medical Economics Company. 2000:2957-2959.

Pola P, Savi L Grilli M, et al. Carnitine in the therapy of dyslipidemic patients. *Curr Therapeu Res*. 1980; 27:208-216.

Prockup LD, Engel WK, Shug AL. Nearly fatal muscle carnitine deficiency with full recovery after replacement therapy. *Neurol*. 1983; 33:1629-1631.

Rebouche CJ. Carnitine. In: Shils ME, Olson JA, Shike M, Ross AC, eds. Modern Nutrition in Health and Disease. 9th ed. Baltimore, MD: Williams & Wilkins; 1999:505-512.

Rebouche CJ. Carnitine function and requirements during the life cycle. FAS*EB J*. 1992; 6:3379-3386.

Rebouche CJ, Engel AG. Carnitine metabolism and deficiency syndromes. *Mayo Clin Proc*. 1983; 58:533-540.

Rebouche CJ, Paulson DJ. Carnitine metabolism and function in humans. *Ann Rev Nutr*. 1986; 6:41-68.

Rossi CS, Siliprandi N. Effects of carnitine on serum HDL-cholesterol: report of two cases. *Johns Hopkins Medical J*. 1982; 150:51-54.

Sachan DS, Rhew TH, Ruark RA. Ameliorating effects of carnitine on alcohol-induced fatty liver. *Am J Clin Nutr*. 1984; 39:738-744.

Triggs WJ, Bohan TP, Shen-Nan L, Wilmore J. Valproate-induced coma with ketosis and carnitine insufficiency. *Arch Neurol*. 1990; 47 006031-1133.

Vacha GM, Giorcelli G, Siliprandi N, Corsi G. Favorable effects of L-carnitine treatment on hypertriglyceridemia in hemodialysis patients: decisive role of low levels of high-density lipoprotein-cholesterol. *Am J Clin Nutr*. 1983; 38:532-540.

L-Citrulline

DESCRIPTION

L-citrulline is an alpha-amino acid that is present in all mammals, including humans, in plants, and, in fact, in small amounts in almost every living organism. One of the richest plant sources of L-citrulline is watermelon (*Citrullus vulgaris* Schrader), from which the amino acid was first isolated and from which its name is derived. L-citrulline is also present at high levels in other members of the cucurbitaceae family, including cucumbers, pumpkins, muskmelons, bitter melons, squashes, gourds, dishrag gourds, wax gourds, honeydews, cantaloupes and luffas. It is also found in high concentration in young walnut seedlings, and in negligible amounts in the kernels and sap of Japanese white birch. L-citrulline can also be obtained via tryptic digestion of casein.

L-citrulline is classified as a nonessential amino acid, which is defined as an amino acid that the body can synthesize in sufficient quantities for all its biochemical and physiological needs. There are, however, conditions in which the body cannot manufacture an adequate amount. L-citrulline is then required in the diet. One such condition is short bowel syndrome. The gut is the main site of L-citrulline production in the body. Short bowel syndrome is a malabsorption disorder caused by the surgical resection of the small intestine. Thus, the main site of L-citrulline production is greatly diminished, and, as a consequence of reduced plasma L-citrulline levels, plasma L-arginine levels are also reduced (L-citrulline is the major precursor of L-arginine). In this condition, both L-citrulline and L-arginine become essential amino acids and must be supplied in the diet. In that regard, L-citrulline and L-arginine are better thought of as conditionally essential or semi-essential amino acids.

There are other conditions where dietary L-citrulline needs to be supplied. L-citrulline is a key intermediate in the urea cycle. A human being is a ureotelic organism, meaning that humans excrete excess nitrogen in the form of urea and do so via the urea cycle, a metabolic cycle which is operative in the liver and composed of five biochemical steps. Certain genetic inborn errors of urea metabolism exist in which either excessive amounts of L-citrulline are produced or very small amounts of L-citrulline are produced. In either case, rather than urea being produced, excess amounts of ammonia are produced. This can be handled just fine by an ammonotelic bony fish but can be life-threatening for humans. Fortunately, the inborn errors of metabolism of the urea cycle are rare. The first step in the urea cycle is the reaction of ammonia and bicarbonate fueled by adenosine triphosphate (ATP) and catalyzed by the enzyme carbamoyl phosphate synthetase (CPS) to produce carbamoyl phosphate. The second metabolic step of the cycle is the reaction of carbamoyl phosphate and L-ornithine to produce L-citrulline, catalyzed by the enzyme ornithine transcarbamylase (OTC). Deficiencies of either of these two enzymes lead to low serum levels of L-citrulline and are treated with oral L-citrulline.

L-citrulline is also classified as a nonprotein amino acid. What this means is that L-citrulline cannot be incorporated into proteins during the process of translation, which is the transfer of genetic information into proteins. Each protein amino acid has its own trinucleotide codon. L-citrulline does not have its own trinucleotide codon. However, L-citrulline is found in some proteins; when this occurs, it is due to a post-translational modification of those proteins. The proteins so modified are called citrullinated proteins.

It is only relatively recently that L-citrulline has raised interest in the scientific community. For years, it was thought of as just an intermediate in the urea cycle. However, that began to change in the 1980s when it was demonstrated that there is a continuous release of L-citrulline from the small intestine into the circulation, which is mainly taken up by the kidneys and metabolized into L-arginine (See L-Arginine). With the discovery of L-arginine's role as a precursor in the production of nitric oxide (NO) and the importance of NO in the cardiovascular system, the nervous system and the immune system, the close link between L-citrulline and L-arginine has raised considerable interest in the scientific community. Most recently, there is some evidence that this nonprotein amino acid may play a major role in the regulation of protein synthesis.

The empirical formula of L-citrulline is $C_6H_{13}N_3O_3$, and its molecular weight is 175.19. It is described chemically as 2-amino-5-(carbamoylamino) pentanoic acid, and its CAS Registry number is 372-75-8. L-citrulline is also known as citrulline, N^5-(aminocarbonyl)-L ornithine, delta-ureidonorvaline, alpha-amino-delta-ureidovaleric acid and by the three letter abbreviation CIT. L-citrulline is very soluble in water. Although L-citrulline is an L-amino acid, it is usually referred to as just citrulline. L-citrulline is represented by the following chemical structure.

L-citrulline

ACTIONS AND PHARMACOLOGY
ACTIONS
L-citrulline has antioxidant activity. It may have antihypertensive activity and, under certain conditions, it has putative anabolic activity.

MECHANISM OF ACTION
Antioxidant activity: L-citrulline operates as a secondary metabolite in some plants. Secondary metabolites protect plants against various stress situations. One interesting activity that L-citrulline possesses is the protection of watermelons, specifically watermelon leaves, against the ravages of drought conditions.

Plants are susceptible to stress and injury from pests, fungi and weeds. Drought is one of the major abiotic stresses affecting plant productivity. Under drought conditions, the generation and proliferation of reactive oxygen species, including hydroxyl radicals, increases and results in oxidative damage to plant cells, affecting their nucleic acids, proteins, carbohydrates and lipids. Plant cells have a number of antioxidant defense mechanisms against oxidative stress, including small antioxidant molecules and antioxidant enzymes. However, under drought conditions, the stress of the drought may overwhelm all of those defense mechanisms.

It is noteworthy that wild watermelon plants that inhabit the Kalahari Desert in Botswana exhibit very high drought tolerance. Even when exposed to prolonged drought in strong sunlight, the photosynthetic apparatus of the plants remains intact. It turns out that drought stress induces massive accumulation of L-citrulline in the watermelon leaves. Even the regular watermelon that we eat has been found to possess significant amounts of L-citrulline in its flesh and rind. In fact, the explorer David Livingston thought that watermelon originated in the Kalahari Desert. However, the concentrations of L-citrulline in the Kalahari watermelons and watermelon leaves are much higher than they are in the watermelons that we eat. Studies have shown L-citrulline to be an extremely potent scavenger—arguably the most potent scavenger—of hydroxyl radicals and it has been demonstrated to protect DNA and metabolic enzymes against oxidative stress. The exact mechanism of L-citrulline's protective effect against oxidative stress and the various chemical reactions that take place between L-citrulline and hydroxyl radicals need further study. Interestingly, L-arginine itself appears to have some detrimental effects in the watermelon, and it is thought that the wild watermelon plant has evolved regulatory mechanisms for accumulating L-citrulline preferentially rather than L-arginine. On the other hand, it has been found that watermelon consumption increases plasma L-arginine concentration in adults, and that appears to be a good thing.

Antihypertensive activity: The vascular endothelial bioavailability of nitric oxide (NO) is the major factor in the regulation of vascular tone. Normal blood pressure requires a relaxed vascular tone. When the bioavailability of endothelial NO decreases, for example when the blood vessel is under oxidative stress, the result is blood vessel constriction, which leads to hypertension. The signaling molecule NO regulates vascular tone by increasing intracellular cGMP (cyclic-guanosine monophosphate), which activates cGMP-dependent protein kinase 1 (PKG1).

As discussed above, L-arginine is the precursor of NO, including endothelial NO (eNO). One might speculate that increasing L-arginine in the body would yield increased amounts of NO, including eNO, which would lead to blood vessel relaxation and decreased blood pressure. Supplemental L-arginine has been used in a number of studies to improve eNO-mediated vasodilation. The results have been generally disappointing, and it is thought that, in part, this is because of the catabolism of L-arginine in the liver and the small intestine via arginase enzymes. In contrast, supplemental L-citrulline is readily absorbed, is not catabolized in either the liver or the small intestine and winds up being converted to L-arginine.

A recent study looked at the effect of supplemental L-citrulline on the production of L-arginine, urinary cGMP and nitrate excretion rates (measures for cGMP and NO production), the ratio of plasma L-arginine over asymmetric dimethylarginine (ADMA), an endogenous inhibitor of NO synthase (L-arginine/ADMA ratio), pharmacokinetic parameters (C_{max}, T_{max}, C_{min}, AUC) and flow-mediated vasodilation (FMD). The study was a double-blind, randomized, placebo-controlled cross-over study with 20 healthy, normotensive subjects who received six different dosing regimes of placebo, L-citrulline and L-arginine. The study lasted seven days. This study wasn't meant to determine if L-citrulline has antitensive activity, but to establish a model for a study that might give us that answer.

The results of the study were as follows: L-citrulline dose-dependently increased AUC (area under the curve) and C_{max} (maximum concentration) of plasma L-arginine more effectively than L-arginine. The highest dose of L-citrulline (3 grams twice a day) increased the C_{min} (minimum concentration) of plasma L-arginine and significantly improved the L-arginine/ADMA ratio, indicating decreased inhibition of NOS—a good thing. Further, urinary cGMP and urinary nitrate both were significantly increased—also a good thing. However, the FMD data showed no difference from baseline with any treatment—not such a good thing. However, pooled analysis of all FMD data revealed a correlation between the increase of L-arginine/ADMA ratio and improvement of FMD—better than nothing. The authors of the study concluded that supplemental L-citrulline raises plasma L-arginine concentration and augments NO-dependent signaling in a dose-dependent manner. Not much more can be concluded from this study. The volunteers were healthy and normotensive. Larger prospective clinical studies with longer treatment periods to investigate the effects of supplemental L-citrulline on endothelial function in those with endothelial dysfunction and vascular disease (including hypertension, hypercholesterolemia, coronary artery disease and peripheral artery disease) are necessary and warranted.

The spontaneous hypertensive rat (SHR) is an animal model for essential hypertension. As discussed above, the vascular bioavailability of endothelial nitric oxide (eNO) is the major determinant of vascular tone and blood pressure. Low eNO vascular bioavailability is associated with vascular constriction and the development of hypertension. It was found that low levels of NO in the kidneys of female SHRs during nephrogenesis precede hypertension in the animals (prehypertension). In these female offspring, the gene expression of arginosuccinate synthase, which is involved in renal L-arginine synthesis and the gene expression of the renal cationic amino acid Y-transporter, which is involved in L-arginine reabsorption, were both decreased in 2-day and 2-week SHRs compared with normotensive control rats. In addition, 2-week-old female SHRs had much less NO in their kidneys but not in their hearts. Maternal supplementation with L-citrulline was found to increase renal NO in the female pup SHRs at 2 weeks and persistently ameliorated the development of hypertension. In the male pup SHR offspring, hypertension developed at 20 weeks. The mechanism of action of the antihypertensive effects of L-citrulline is not clear.

Anabolic activity (putative): There are a number of studies showing that under certain conditions, dietary L-citrulline may have protein anabolic activity. L-citrulline was demonstrated to modulate muscle protein metabolism in old malnourished rats. Protein energy malnutrition is not uncommon in the elderly, particularly those who have poor or no support from family and/or friends. One hypothesis is that the poor response to nutrition with advancing age might be related to splanchnic sequestration of amino acids, meaning that fewer amino acids reach the systemic circulation. L-citrulline, unlike L-arginine, is not taken up and metabolized by the liver and may offer a means to increase nitrogen balance and improve nutritional status. In a study of old malnourished rats, it was found that L-citrulline supplementation led to higher protein synthesis overall and higher protein content in the muscles. A standard diet did not have any effect on protein synthesis or on protein content in the muscles. The exact mechanism of this possible anabolic effect is unclear.

In another study, a group of rats underwent massive intestinal resection. L-citrulline was found to increase L-arginine levels and improve nitrogen balance in these animals. The fact that L-citrulline is not taken up and metabolized by the liver may also have something to do with restoring nitrogen balance in this situation.

In these two different situations—old malnourished rats and rats having undergone massive intestinal resection—L-citrulline was found to have a dramatic effect on nitrogen balance and protein status. Recently, it has been found that L-citrulline may also stimulate muscle protein synthesis. The mechanism of action of this effect is unclear, but there are some thoughts about it—the effect may be due to L-citrulline's ability to generate L-arginine or to stimulate insulin and/or growth hormone secretion, or L-citrulline may be a vehicle to bring nitrogen to the muscles. The last two possibilities would be indirect actions of L-citrulline. However, L-citrulline may have direct action in stimulating protein synthesis in muscles. Some recent studies appear to suggest the possibility of direct action. If that is indeed the case, L-citrulline may play a major role in protein homeostasis. Are there any examples of amino acids that can directly stimulate protein synthesis and that may even possess signaling activities? L-leucine is the one that comes to mind and, interestingly, neither L-leucine nor L-citrulline is metabolized in the liver. Much research in this important area is needed and certainly warranted.

PHARMACOKINETICS

This section on the pharmacokinetics (PK) of L-citrulline begins with the various biochemical reactions that L-citrulline participates in either as reactant or product.

L-citrulline from L-arginine via nitric oxide synthase:

The nitric oxide synthase (NOS) reaction converts L-arginine to NO and L-citrulline. The reaction has L-arginine, NADPH and oxygen as reactants and NO, L-citrulline and NADP as products. There are three forms (isoforms) of nitric oxide synthase—a neuronal type called nNOS, an endothelial type called eNOS and an inducible form called iNOS.

L-citrulline formation in the enterocytes of the small intestine from L-glutamine and L-arginine:

The small intestine is the main source of L-citrulline production in humans and the major precursor of L-citrulline is the amino acid L-glutamine. Nearly 90% of the circulating L-citrulline arises from L-glutamine. The contribution of L-arginine to L-citrulline synthesis accounts for approximately 10% of the circulating L-citrulline. L-glutamine is converted to L-glutamate via glutaminase. L-glutamate is converted to L-ornithine via ornithine aminotransferase. L-ornithine is converted to L-citrulline via ornithine carbamoyltransferase.

L-citrulline is transported to the kidneys where it is converted to L-arginine via arginosuccinate synthase and arginosuccinate lyase.

L-citrulline can also be synthesized in the small intestine from L-arginine because the enterocytes possess the two enzymes—arginase II and ornithine carbamoyl transferase—needed for L-citrulline synthesis. However, the activity of the two enzymes that catabolize L-citrulline—arginosuccinate synthase and arginosuccinate lyase—is very low in the small intestine. Therefore, L-citrulline cannot be used *in situ* (the small intestine) to produce L-arginine and is released as such into the circulation. Importantly, L-citrulline is not taken up by the liver, but is mainly taken up by the kidneys. Since the kidney possesses arginosuccinate synthase and arginosuccinate lyase activity but not the other enzymes of the urea cycle, L-arginine is released, and 75% of L-citrulline produced in the small intestine is taken up by the kidneys, where it is converted into L-arginine. The intestinal synthesis rate of L-citrulline formation is the crucial regulatory event in renal L-arginine synthesis. The arginine-citrulline-arginine interorgan cycle can be seen as a means to protect dietary L-arginine from excessive liver degradation, since L-arginine is catabolized in the liver by arginase, and to correctly adapt the rate of urea formation according to protein intake, since L-arginine is a major positive urea formation regulator. (L-arginine is the activator of N-acetyl-glutamate, which in turn activates carbamoyl phosphate synthetase). L-glutamine is the second major substrate regulating the rate of urea formation; the ammonia derived from L-glutamine metabolism upregulates liver glutaminase. L-citrulline may be seen as a means to sustain protein homeostasis, particularly when the intake of protein is low. In the condition of low protein intake, ornithine carbamoyl-tranferase expression in the liver increases, thus promoting the formation of L-citrulline and thereby allowing the downregulation of the formation of urea in the liver.

L-citrulline formation in the urea cycle (in the liver):

The liver and the small intestine are the two organs that play a major role in the metabolism of L-arginine. Since the activity of arginase is very high in the liver, most of the L-arginine that reaches the liver is converted into urea.

The urea cycle, also known as the Krebs-Henseleit cycle, is operative in the liver and consists of five reactions—two in the mitochondria and three in the cytosol. The major role of the urea cycle is the detoxification of ammonia, the end product of nitrogen metabolism. Bony fish can excrete ammonia directly, but humans need to convert ammonia to urea. The first step in the urea cycle is the conversion of ammonia and carbon dioxide to carbamoyl phosphate catalyzed by the enzyme carbamoyl phosphate synthetase.

Carbamoyl phosphate then reacts with L-ornithine to produce L-citrulline catalyzed by the enzyme ornithine transcarbamoylase. The first two reactions take place in the mitochondria; the remaining three in the cytosol. L-citrulline then reacts with aspartate to form arginosuccinate catalyzed by the enzyme arginosuccinate synthase. Arginosuccinate is then converted to L-arginine and fumarate, catalyzed by the enzyme arginosuccinase, and, finally, L-arginine is converted to L-ornithine and urea, catalyzed by the enzyme arginase. The cycle continues.

It is clear from all of these reactions that the biochemistry of L-arginine is very closely tied to the biochemistry of L-citrulline. It also appears that L-arginine may not be the best supplement form of L-arginine since it gets broken down in the liver via the enzyme arginase and also a fairly large proportion of dietary L-arginine is extracted during a first-pass splanchnic extraction and degraded by the intestine via the enzyme arginase to yield L-ornithine and L-proline. Could L-citrulline be a better delivery form of L-arginine than L-arginine itself? The Pharmacokinetics (PK) of L-citrulline that follows addresses this.

Pharmacokinetics of L-citrulline:

The PK of L-citrulline in humans is not complete, but much is known. Following ingestion, L-citrulline is absorbed from the lumen of the small intestine into the enterocytes. Rat studies and studies in Caco-2 cells, a model of human enterocytes, have demonstrated that L-citrulline absorption involves a sodium-dependent active transport mechanism. Absorption of L-citrulline appears to be efficient. L-citrulline is released from the enterocytes into the circulation, and approximately 83% of the circulating L-citrulline is taken up by the kidneys where most of it is converted to L-arginine via arginosuccinate synthase and arginosuccinate lyase. This occurs in the cells of the proximal tubules of the kidneys. In contrast to L-arginine, L-citrulline bypasses first-pass splanchnic extraction and reaches the kidneys completely intact. The L-arginine produced from L-citrulline and L-citrulline itself are absorbed and reabsorbed, respectively, by the renal tubules. Less than 1% of an oral dose of L-citrulline is excreted in urine.

L-arginine released in the bloodstream is distributed to the various tissues of the body where it can be utilized for protein synthesis, urea synthesis, NO production and other biochemical reactions. (See L-Arginine.) Interestingly and importantly, some studies have shown that the C_{max} (maximum concentration in the plasma) of L-arginine when subjects are administered L-citrulline is significantly higher than the C_{max} of L-arginine when subjects are given an equivalent dose of supplemental L-arginine. As mentioned above, L-arginine undergoes significant catabolism in the liver via arginase, and in the small intestine, again, via arginase. Supplemental L-citrulline is neither catabolized in the liver nor in the small intestine, remaining chemically intact. Thus, it turns out that supplemental L-citrulline appears to be a better delivery form of L-arginine than is L-arginine itself. It may also be concluded that oral L-citrulline can be used to enhance the availability of L-citrulline and L-arginine in the systemic bloodstream, without enhancing urea excretion, and thus may improve nitrogen balance *in vivo* in humans.

INDICATIONS AND USAGE

L-citrulline, a nonprotein amino acid precursor of L-arginine, may be helpful in treating/preventing hypertension, metabolic syndrome and cardiovascular disease, generally. It may also be useful in sustaining/improving protein metabolism in some intestinal diseases, such as short-bowel syndrome. It has long been used to treat some inherited urea cycle disorders. Some consider it a safer way of utilizing L-arginine, a conditionally essential amino acid, and that it might thus serve as a substitute supplement in disorders related to L-arginine deficiency. There is no convincing evidence to support the claim that L-citrulline may enhance athletic performance or be helpful in erectile dysfunction. It may, however, play some positive role in muscle protein metabolism. The suggestion that it might be effective in some autoimmune disorders, such as rheumatoid arthritis, psoriasis and multiple sclerosis remains entirely hypothetical.

RESEARCH SUMMARY

L-citrulline is found only in very small amounts in most foods. One rich source of it, however, is watermelon, and watermelon feeding studies (in animals) have shown that three cups of watermelon juice daily can boost plasma L-arginine levels by 12 per cent and six cups daily can boost those levels by 22 percent. (One would expect variations in this result, however, depending upon the strain and relative maturity of the watermelons used.) The prospect of using L-citrulline to boost L-arginine levels in the body has excited attention recently because, unlike L-arginine itself, L-citrulline is not taken up and largely metabolized by the liver, a process that yields urea. Thus it may be a safer vehicle for boosting L-arginine in the body than through the use of L-arginine itself.

The importance of this is considerable since L-arginine's essentiality is well established in some circumstances: in mammals, including humans; in infants; in adults with burns and other trauma; in individuals with renal failure; and in those with massive small bowel resection, as well as some other disorders of the gut. One group of researchers has recently concluded that L-citrulline should now be viewed as a potential, safer approach to providing oral, enteral and parenteral nutrition in gut-compromised patients.

An L-citrulline-rich diet has significantly combated protein-energy malnutrition in a rat model of short bowel-syndrome. This is to be expected since the primary site of L-citrulline production in the body is significantly reduced in massive intestinal resection. Short-bowel syndrome leaves the body short of this amino acid and thus of its frequently essential descendant, L-arginine. Some other animal studies suggest that L-citrulline may have some protein anabolic effect. In one study of old, undernourished rats, supplementation with the amino acid improved nitrogen balance and muscle protein synthesis. Whether this effect can be found in older human, undernourished and malnourished patients needs to be investigated. The mechanism by which this amino acid may aid nutrition could equally apply in some cases of nutritive deficit related to cancer, type 2 diabetes, trauma and some other diseases/disorders.

The idea that L-citrulline might be useful as an athletic performance enhancer was not confirmed in a study of young male and female volunteers subjected to incremental treadmill challenges. Test subjects were given three to nine grams of the substance prior to testing and compared with placebo controls. Contrary to expectations there was actually a reduction in time to exhaustion among those taking the amino acid during a 24-hour period prior to challenge. This was a small study from which no meaningful conclusions can be drawn.

At least as significant as its potential role in the gut is the potential for L-citrulline to be of benefit in cardiovascular health. The recycling of L-citrulline to L-arginine plays a crucial role in the production of nitric oxide (NO) in endothelial cells. As a vital vasorelaxant, NO production is of importance in maintaining cardiovascular health. Impaired NO production results in the endothelial dysfunction that is associated with atherosclerosis, lipid disorders, hypertension, diabetes and other indicators of heart disease and the metabolic syndrome. Once again, because of problems inherent in L-arginine availability and safety in the body, L-citrulline is viewed as the better way to treat conditions associated with L-arginine deficiencies.

L-citrulline was found to inhibit the progression of atherosclerosis experimentally induced via a high-cholesterol diet in rabbits. The researchers concluded that the amino acid achieved this result through antioxidative and NO-boosting actions. The regression of lesions in these animals given the amino acid orally for 12 weeks was said to be dramatic. In another animal study, maternal supplementation with L-citrulline increased renal nitric oxide and exerted long-lasting antihypertensive effects in young, spontaneously hypertensive rats. The rat dams were supplemented with the amino acid during pregnancy and lactation. The antihypertensive effects observed persisted in the offspring for several weeks. In yet another animal study, the metabolic syndrome was significantly ameliorated in an animal model of noninsulin-dependent diabetes mellitus (the Zucker diabetic fatty rat). Supplementation was in the form of watermelon juice, which the authors suggested may be a useful functional food. Reduced serum concentration of cardiovascular risk factors and improved glycemic control were noted in this study. Clearly research in this context needs to be extended into the clinical domain.

There is some very preliminary evidence that L-citrulline may have immunomodulating effects that could be favorable, possibly through enhancement of T-lymphocytes. Enhanced NO production by macrophages should, additionally, it is suggested, help resist a number of infectious agents. A role in autoimmune disorders has also been proposed, possibly mediated through the amino acid's presence in myelin protein, but this remains hypothetical.

Recently, watermelon was touted in the press as a possible "natural Viagra." Other researchers, however, cast doubt on the idea that eating watermelon, even in very large quantities, would be sufficient to have any meaningful impact on erectile dysfunction.

CONTRAINDICATIONS, PRECAUTIONS, ADVERSE REACTIONS

CONTRAINDICATIONS
Supplemental L-citrulline is contraindicated in those hypersensitive to any component of an L-citrulline-containing dietary supplement.

PRECAUTIONS
The use of L-citrulline supplements for any health condition should be discussed with ones physician.

Because of an absence of long-term safety studies, pregnant women and nursing mothers should avoid L-citrulline supplements. There is no precaution for eating foods containing L-citrulline, including watermelon.

ADVERSE REACTIONS
Oral supplementation with L-citrulline at doses up to 15 grams daily is generally well tolerated. Gastrointestinal symptoms, including diarrhea, might be expected with very high doses.

INTERACTIONS

DRUGS
No known interactions.

NUTRITIONAL SUPPLEMENTS
No known interactions.

FOODS
No known interactions.

HERBS
No known interactions.

OVERDOSAGE
No reports.

DOSAGE AND ADMINISTRATION
L-citrulline dietary supplements are available. A typical dose is three grams a day. Optimal doses are not known.

Watermelon is a rich source of L-citrulline.

L-citrulline concentrations in seeded watermelons range from 0.5 to 3.6 mg per gram fresh weight, with an average of 1.8 mg per gram fresh weight.

L-citrulline concentrations in seedless watermelons range from 0.7 to 3.5 mg per gram fresh weight with an average of 2.4 mg per gram fresh weight.

LITERATURE

Akashi K, Miyake C, Yokota A. Citrulline, a novel compatible solute in drought-tolerant wild watermelon leaves, is an efficient hydroxyl radical scavenger. *FEBS Lett*. 2001;508(3):438-442.

Barroso A, Oliveira L, Campesatto-Mella E, et al. L-citrulline inhibits [3H]acetylcholine release from rat motor nerve terminals by increasing adenosine outflow and activation of A1 receptors. *Br J Pharmacol*. 2007;151(4):541-550.

Berning C, Bieger I, Pauli S, et al. Investigation of citrullinemia type I variants by in vitro expression studies. *Hum Mutat*. 2008;29(10):1222-1227.

Collins JK, Wu G, Perkins-Veazie P, et al. Watermelon consumption increases plasma arginine concentrations in adults. *Nutrition*. 2007;23(3):261-266.

Curis E, Crenn P, Cynober L. Citrulline and the gut. *Curr Opin Clin Nutr Metab Care*. 2007;10(5):620-626.

Curis E, Nicolis I, Moinard C, et al. Almost all about citrulline in mammals. *Amino Acids*. 2005;29(3):177-205.

Cynober L. Pharmacokinetics of arginine and related amino acids. *J Nutr*. 2007;137(6 Suppl 2):1646S-1649S.

Flam BR, Eichler DC, Solomonson LP. Endothelial nitric oxide production is tightly coupled to the citrulline-NO cycle. *Nitric Oxide*. 2007;17(3-4):115-121.

Hayashi T, Juliet PA, Matsui-Hirai H, et al. L-citrulline and l-arginine supplementation retards the progression of high-cholesterol-diet-induced atherosclerosis in rabbits. *Proc Natl Acad Sci U S A*. 2005;102(38):13681-13686.

Herbers AH, Blijlevens NM, Donnelly JP, et al. Bacteraemia coincides with low citrulline concentrations after high-dose melphalan in autologous HSCT recipients. *Bone Marrow Transplant*. 2008;42(5):345-349.

Hickner RC, Tanner CJ, Evans CA, et al. L-citrulline reduces time to exhaustion and insulin response to a graded exercise test. *Med Sci Sports Exerc*. 2006;38(4):660-666.

Ko JM, Kim GH, Kim JH, et al. Six cases of citrin deficiency in Korea. *Int J Mol Med*. 2007;20(6):809-815.

Koeners MP, van Faassen EE, Wesseling S, et al. Maternal supplementation with citrulline increases renal nitric oxide in young spontaneously hypertensive rats and has long-term antihypertensive effects. *Hypertension*. 2007;50(6):1077-1084.

Koga T, Zhang WY, Gotoh T, et al. Induction of citrulline-nitric oxide (NO) cycle enzymes and NO production in immunostimulated rat RPE-J cells. *Exp Eye Res*. 2003;76(1):15-21.

Ligthart-Melis GC, van de Poll MC, Boelens PG, et al. Glutamine is an important precursor for de novo synthesis of arginine in humans. *Am J Clin Nutr*. 2008;87(5):1282-1289.

Mandel H, Levy N, Izkovitch S, et al. Elevated plasma citrulline and arginine due to consumption of Citrullus vulgaris (watermelon). *J Inherit Metab Dis*. 2005;28(4):467-472.

Miceli E, Poggi N, Missanelli A, et al. Is serum citrulline measurement clinically useful in coeliac disease? *Intern Emerg Med*. 2008;3(3):233-236.

Moinard C, Nicolis I, Neveux N, et al. Dose-ranging effects of citrulline administration on plasma amino acids and hormonal patterns in healthy subjects: the Citrudose pharmacokinetic study. *Br J Nutr*. 2008;99(4):855-862.

Moinard C, Cynober L. Citrulline: a new player in the control of nitrogen homeostasis. *J Nutr*. 2007;137(6 Suppl 2):1621S-1625S.

Osowska S, Duchemann T, Walrand S, et al. Citrulline modulates muscle protein metabolism in old malnourished rats. *Am J Physiol Endocrinol Metab*. 2006;291(3):E582-E586.

Osowska S, Moinard C, Neveux N, et al. Citrulline increases arginine pools and restores nitrogen balance after massive intestinal resection. *Gut*. 2004;53(12):1781-1786.

Rimando AM, Perkins-Veazie PM. Determination of citrulline in watermelon rind. *J Chromatogr A*. 2005;1078(1-2):196-200.

Romero MJ, Platt DH, Caldwell RB, et al. Therapeutic use of citrulline in cardiovascular disease. *Cardiovasc Drug Rev*. 2006;24(3-4):275-290.

Rougé C, Des Robert C, Robins A, et al. Manipulation of citrulline availability in humans. *Am J Physiol Gastrointest Liver Physiol*. 2007;293(5):G1061-G1067.

Sato M. [Citrullination, a novel post-translational modification of histone] [Article in Japanese.] *Seikagaku*. 2007;79(7):686-690.

Schellekens GA, de Jong BA, van den Hoogen FH, et al. Citrulline is an essential constituent of antigenic determinants recognized by rheumatoid arthritis-specific autoantibodies. *J Clin Invest*. 1998;101(1):273-281.

Schwedhelm E, Maas R, Freese R, et al. Pharmacokinetic and pharmacodynamic properties of oral L-citrulline and L-arginine:

impact on nitric oxide metabolism. *Br J Clin Pharmacol.* 2008;65(1):51-59.

Suzuki A, Yamada R, Yamamoto K. Citrullination by peptidylarginine deiminase in rheumatoid arthritis. *Ann N Y Acad Sci.* 2007;1108:323-339.

Takahara K, Akashi K, Yokota A. Purification and characterization of glutamate N-acetyltransferase involved in citrulline accumulation in wild watermelon. *FEBS J.* 2005;272(20):5353-5364.

Van de Poll MC, Ligthart-Melis GC, Boelens PG, et al. Intestinal and hepatic metabolism of glutamine and citrulline in humans. *J Physiol.* 2007;581(Pt 2):819-827.

Van Gaalen F, Ioan-Facsinay A, Huizinga TW, et al. The devil in the details: the emerging role of anticitrulline autoimmunity in rheumatoid arthritis. *J Immunol.* 2005;175(9):5575-5580.

Wu G, Collins JK, Perkins-Veazie P, et al. Dietary supplementation with watermelon pomace juice enhances arginine availability and ameliorates the metabolic syndrome in Zucker diabetic fatty rats. *J Nutr.* 2007;137(12):2680-2685.

L-Cysteine

DESCRIPTION

L-cysteine is a protein amino acid naturally present in the proteins of life forms. L-cysteine is a sulfur amino acid and contains a sulfhydryl group. Although most cysteine is found in proteins, small amounts of free cysteine are found in body fluids and in plants. The normal diet contributes approximately 1 gram of L-cysteine daily.

L-cysteine is considered a nonessential amino acid, meaning that, under normal physiologic conditions, sufficient amounts of this amino acid are formed from the dietary essential amino acid L-methionine and the nonessential amino acid L-serine via a transsulfuration reaction. L-cysteine is a conditionally essential amino acid under certain circumstances, for example, for preterm infants.

L-cysteine serves as a precursor for synthesis of proteins, glutathione, taurine, coenzyme A and inorganic sulfate. Glutathionine itself has a number of biochemical functions, including maintenance of normal cellular redox state. Certain conditions, e.g. an acetaminophen overdose, can deplete hepatic glutathione, and this can be life-threatening. The antidote to an acetaminophen overdose is L-cysteine, in the delivery form of N-acetylcysteine. The L-cysteine derived from N-acetylcysteine helps to restore hepatic glutathione.

L-cysteine is also known as L-2-amino-3-mercaptopropanoic acid, 2-amino-3-mercaptopropanoic acid, beta-mercaptoalanine, 2-amino-3 mercaptopropionic acid and alpha-amino-beta-thiolpropionic acid. L-cysteine is represented by the following chemical structure:

L-cysteine

Its IUPAC abbreviation is Cys, and its one-letter abbreviation, used when spelling out protein structures, is C. L-cysteine is a white, solid substance that is soluble in water. It is hygroscopic and slowly decomposes and oxidizes. In solution, it undergoes oxidation to L-cystine, which is a dimer of L-cysteine. N-acetylcysteine is a preferred delivery form of L-cysteine because of greater stability and possible higher absorbability. (See N-Acetylcysteine).

ACTIONS AND PHARMACOLOGY

ACTIONS

The most significant action of supplemental L-cysteine is as a redox modulator.

MECHANISM OF ACTION

Certain conditions, e.g. an acetaminophen overdose, deplete hepatic glutathione and subject the tissues to oxidative stress resulting in loss of cellular integrity. L-cysteine serves as a major precursor for synthesis of glutathione.

PHARMACOKINETICS

Following ingestion, some L-cysteine is oxidized to L-cystine, and both L-cysteine and L-cystine are absorbed from the small intestine by active-transport processes. L-cysteine absorption is largely sodium-dependent, while L-cystine is absorbed by a sodium-independent transport system. Following absorption, L-cysteine enters the portal circulation, which distributes it to the liver. There, much of it is metabolized to protein, glutathione, taurine and sulfate. L-cysteine, which does not get metabolized by the liver, enters the systemic circulation which distributes it to various tissues of the body.

INDICATIONS AND USAGE

It has been claimed that L-cysteine has anti-inflammatory properties, that it can protect against various toxins, and that it might be helpful in osteoarthritis and rheumatoid arthritis. More research will have to be done before L-cysteine can be indicated for any of these conditions. Research to date has mostly been in animal models.

RESEARCH SUMMARY

There is some evidence from animal studies that cysteine can help ensure adequate glutathione synthesis during and after inflammatory challenge, thus helping to "ameliorate," in the words of one research group, "adverse effects of oxidative damage induced by disease or drugs."

Cysteine-supplemented mice and guinea pigs have enjoyed significantly extended life spans, and other animals, challenged with various toxins, have, when pre-supplemented with cysteine, survived considerably longer than non-supplemented controls. In one of these studies, 90% of control rats given large doses of acetaldehyde died. But other rats first given a combination of vitamins C and B, along with cysteine, and then exposed to the same dose of acetaldehyde, all survived. Cysteine's protective mechanisms could relate to its own antioxidant properties, its promotion of glutathione (a major antioxidant) or even, it has been hypothesized, to some ability to participate in DNA repair.

There is inconclusive evidence that cysteine could play a positive role in the treatment of osteoarthritis and rheumatoid arthritis.

CONTRAINDICATIONS, PRECAUTIONS, ADVERSE REACTIONS
CONTRAINDICATIONS
L-cysteine supplementation is contraindicated in those hypersensitive to any component of the preparation.

PRECAUTIONS
Because of lack of long-term safety studies, L-cysteine supplementation should be avoided by children, pregnant women and nursing mothers.

Although the incidence of cystine renal stones is low, they do occur. Those who form renal stones, particularly cystine stones, should avoid L-cysteine supplements.

L-cysteine, like other sulfhydryl-containing substances, could produce a false-positive result in the nitroprusside test for ketone bodies used in diabetes.

ADVERSE REACTIONS
With typical doses of 1 to 1.5 grams daily, the most commonly reported side effects have been gastrointestinal, such as nausea. There are rare reports of cystine renal stone formation.

INTERACTIONS
NUTRITIONAL SUPPLEMENTS
Zinc: L-cysteine complexes with zinc and may increase the absorption of zinc.

Vitamin C: Ascorbic acid may inhibit the oxidation of L-cysteine to L-cystine.

OVERDOSAGE
There are no reports of overdosage in those taking L-cysteine supplements. However, large doses of L-cysteine are neuroexcitotoxic in several species. Single injections of L-cysteine (0.6-1.5 g/kg) into 4-day-old pups resulted in massive damage to cortical neurons, permanent retinal dystrophy, atrophy of the brain and hyperactivity.

DOSAGE AND ADMINISTRATION
The usual supplemental dosage of L-cysteine is 500 milligrams to 1.5 grams daily. Those who supplement with L-cysteine should drink at least six to eight glasses of water daily in order to prevent cystine renal stones. Some studies indicate that an intake of 3 to 5 grams daily of vitamin C may prevent cystine stones. However, high-dose vitamin C itself may contribute to renal stones in some (see Vitamin C).

Another delivery form of L-cysteine is N-acetylcysteine (see N-Acetylcysteine).

LITERATURE
Anderson R, Lukey PT, Theron AJ, Dippenaar U. Ascorbate and cysteine-mediated selective neutralization of extracellular oxidants during N-formyl peptide activation of human phagocytes. *Agents Actions.* 1987;20:77-86.

Anderson R, Theron AJ, Ras GJ. Regulation by the antioxidants ascorbate, cysteine, and dapsone of the increased extracellular and intracellular generation of reactive oxidants by activated phagocytes from cigarette smokers. *Am Rev Respir Dis.* 1987; 135:1027-1032

Asper R, Schmucki O. Cystinuric therapy by ascorbic acid. *Urol Int.* 1982;37:91-109.

Campbell NR, Reade PC, Radden BG. Effect of cysteine on the survival of mice with transplanted malignant lymphoma. *Nature.* 1974;251:158-159.

Csako G. False-positive results for ketone with the drug mensa and other free-sulfhydryl compounds. *Clin Chem.* 1987;33(2 pt 1):289-292.

Fettman MJ, Valerius KD, Ogilvie GK. Effects of dietary cysteine on blood sulfur amino acid, glutathione, and malondialdehyde concentrations in cats. *Am J Vet Res.* 1999;60:328-333.

Oeriu S, Vachitu E. The effect of the administration of compounds which contain sulfhydryl groups on the survival rate of mice, rats and guinea pigs. *Journ Geront.* 1965;20;47.

Stipanuk MH. Homocysteine, cysteine and taurine. In: Shils ME, Olson JA, Shike M, Ross AC, eds. *Modern Nutrition in Health and Disease.* Ninth edition. Baltimore, MD: Williams & Wilkins; 1999:543-558.

L-Glutamine

DESCRIPTION
L-glutamine is a protein amino acid found in proteins of all life forms. It is classified as a semi-essential or conditionally essential amino acid. This means that under normal circumstances the body can synthesize sufficient L-glutamine to meet physiological demands. However, there are conditions

where the body cannot do so. Recently, L-glutamine has come to be regarded as one of the most important of the amino acids when the body is subjected to such metabolic stress situations as trauma (including surgical trauma), cancer, sepsis and burns. Under such conditions, L-glutamine becomes an essential amino acid, and it is therefore very important to ensure adequate intakes of the amino acid in order to meet the increased physiological demands created by these situations.

L-glutamine is the most abundant amino acid in the body, and plasma glutamine levels are the highest of any amino acid. L-glutamine is predominantly synthesized and stored in skeletal muscle. The amino acid L-glutamate is metabolized to L-glutamine in a reaction catalyzed by the enzyme glutamine synthase, a reaction which, in addition to L-glutamate, requires ammonia, ATP and magnesium.

L-glutamine is a very versatile amino acid and participates in many reactions in the body. It is important in the regulation of acid-base balance. L-glutamine allows the kidneys to excrete an acid load, protecting the body against acidosis. This is accomplished by the production of ammonia, which binds hydrogen ions, to produce ammonium cations that are excreted in the urine along with chloride anions. Bicarbonate ions are simultaneously released into the bloodstream. L-glutamine helps protect the body against ammonia toxicity by transporting ammonia, in the form of L-glutamine's amide group, from peripheral tissues to visceral organs, where it can be excreted as ammonium by the kidneys or converted to urea by the liver.

The amide group can also participate in other metabolic activities, as can the amino group of L-glutamine. L-glutamine serves as the most important nitrogen shuttle, supplying nitrogen for metabolic purposes (from glutamine-producing tissues, such as skeletal muscle) to glutamine-consuming tissues.

L-glutamine participates in the formation of purine and pyrimidine nucleotides, amino sugars (such as glucosamine), L-glutamate and other amino acids, nicotinamide adenine dinucleotide and glutathione. It also participates in protein synthesis, energy production and, if necessary, the production of D-glucose and glycogen. Importantly, L-glutamine can serve as the primary respiratory substrate for the production of energy in enterocytes and lymphocytes. L-glutamine is considered an immunonutrient, and supplemental L-glutamine is used in medical foods for such stress situations as trauma, cancer, infections and burns.

The typical dietary intake of L-glutamine is 5 to 10 grams daily. Most dietary L-glutamine comes from animal and plant proteins. Small amounts of free L-glutamine are found in vegetable juices and fermented foods, such as miso and yogurt. L-glutamine is the amide of L-glutamic acid. Its molecular formula is $C_5H_{10}N_2O_3$, and its molecular weight is 146.15 daltons. The structural formula is:

L-glutamine

L-glutamine is also known as 2-aminoglutaramic acid, levoglutamide, (S)-2, 5-diamino-5-oxopentaenoic acid and glutamic acid 5-amide. Its one-letter abbreviation is Q, and it is also abbreviated as Gln. The terms L-glutamine and glutamine are used interchangeably. D-glutamine, the stereoisomer of L-glutamine, does not have, as far as is known, biological activity. L-glutamine is not very soluble in water, and aqueous solutions are unstable at temperatures of 22 to 24 degrees Celsius. For these reasons, the more soluble and more stable glutamine dipeptides are used as delivery forms of L-glutamine in total parenteral nutrition (TPN) solutions. See Glutamine Peptides.

ACTIONS AND PHARMACOLOGY

ACTIONS

Supplemental L-glutamine may have immunomodulatory, anticatabolic/anabolic and gastrointestinal mucosal-protective actions. It may also have antioxidant activity.

MECHANISM OF ACTION

Supplemental L-glutamine's possible immunomodulatory role may be accounted for in a number of ways. L-glutamine appears to play a major role in protecting the integrity of the gastrointestinal tract and, in particular, the large intestine. During catabolic states, the integrity of the intestinal mucosa may be compromised with consequent increased intestinal permeability and translocation of Gram-negative bacteria from the large intestine into the body. The demand for L-glutamine by the intestine, as well as by cells such as lymphocytes, appears to be much greater than that supplied by skeletal muscle, the major storage tissue for L-glutamine. L-glutamine is the preferred respiratory fuel for enterocytes, colonocytes and lymphocytes. Therefore, supplying supplemental L-glutamine under these conditions may do a number of things. For one, it may reverse the catabolic state by sparing skeletal muscle L-glutamine. It also may inhibit translocation of Gram-negative bacteria from the large intestine. L-glutamine helps maintain secretory IgA, which functions primarily by preventing the attachment of bacteria to mucosal cells.

L-glutamine appears to be required to support the proliferation of mitogen-stimulated lymphocytes, as well as the production of interleukin-2 (IL-2) and interferon-gamma (IFN-gamma). It is also required for the maintenance of lymphokine-activated killer cells (LAK). L-glutamine can enhance phagocytosis by neutrophils and monocytes. It can lead to an increased synthesis of glutathione in the intestine, which may also play a role in maintaining the integrity of the intestinal mucosa by ameliorating oxidative stress.

The exact mechanism of the possible immunomodulatory action of supplemental L-glutamine, however, remains unclear. It is conceivable that the major effect of L-glutamine occurs at the level of the intestine. Perhaps enteral L-glutamine acts directly on intestine-associated lymphoid tissue and stimulates overall immune function by that mechanism, without passing beyond the splanchnic bed.

The anticatabolic/anabolic activity of supplemental L-glutamine can be explained by its effect in sparing skeletal muscle L-glutamine stores.

PHARMACOKINETICS

Following ingestion, L-glutamine is absorbed from the lumen of the small intestine into the enterocytes. Absorption is efficient and occurs by an active transport mechanism. Some metabolism of the amino acid takes place in the enterocytes. L-glutamine that is not metabolized in the enterocytes enters the portal circulation from whence it is transported to the liver, where again some portion of the amino acid is metabolized. L-glutamine not metabolized in the liver enters the systemic circulation, where it is distributed to the various tissues of the body. L-glutamine participates in various metabolic activities, including the formation of L-glutamate catalyzed by the enzyme glutaminase. It also participates in the synthesis of proteins, glutathione, pyrimidine and purine nucleotides and amino sugars. The transport of L-glutamine into cells is via an active process. L-glutamine is eliminated by glomerular filtration and is almost completely reabsorbed by the renal tables.

INDICATIONS AND USAGE

Glutamine has been shown to be beneficial when administered in the form of glutamine peptides via TPN in some patients with varying forms of catabolic stress, e.g., some cancer, transplantation, intensive-care, surgical and immune-suppressed patients. Benefits from enteral glutamine supplementation are generally less pronounced, but preliminary significant results have been reported with the use of oral glutamine in very-low-birth-weight infants and in some major trauma patients in whom glutamine seems to strengthen immunity, particularly in the gastrointestinal tract. Glutamine may help protect against some of the side effects of cancer chemotherapy and radiotherapy.

There is little concurring evidence that glutamine is an effective ergogenic aid, but there is some suggestion that it might help protect against exercise-induced immune impairment. Some dated research suggesting that glutamine might help curb alcohol craving has not been followed up. Claims that it helps prevent neurodegenerative disorders or that it modulates mood have not been substantiated.

RESEARCH SUMMARY

Several well-designed studies have demonstrated that the addition of glutamine to TPN helps decrease intestinal permeability and mucosal and villous atrophy in the small intestine. Inhibition of intestinal permeability is believed to decrease microbial translocation and thus reduce infective opportunities in the gut. Increased intestinal permeability has been associated with a number of traumas, illnesses and some surgeries.

Studies have shown worthwhile reductions in length of hospital stay attributed to glutamine-supplemented TPN in bone-marrow transplantation patients and in those who had resection for colon or rectal cancer. In another study, mortality was significantly better in intensive-care patients who received TPN supplemented with glutamine than in those whose TPN did not include glutamine.

In addition, glutamine in TPN has been credited with improving nutritional status in some critically ill patients, including cancer patients. And it appears to allow for more aggressive radiotherapy and chemotherapy by protecting against some of the side effects of those treatments.

Enteral glutamine has also demonstrated positive results. In a recent placebo-controlled study, oral glutamine significantly decreased the severity and duration of painful oral mucositis (stomatitis) in autologous bone-marrow transplantation patients. It was similarly helpful in alleviating radiation-induced oral mucositis in a recent randomized pilot trial. Very-low-birth-weight infants orally supplemented with glutamine between days 3 and 30 of life had far less hospital-acquired sepsis than controls (11% versus 30%) and had better tolerance to enteral feedings.

In a placebo-controlled study examining infectious morbidity in multiple trauma patients, oral glutamine was credited with significantly reducing the incidence of pneumonia, sepsis and bacteremia. In another recent randomized study of critically ill patients, supplementation with oral glutamine was said to have significant hospital cost benefits, reducing cost per survivor by 30%.

While claims that glutamine is an effective ergogenic aid are poorly supported, there is some evidence that the substance can help protect against some of the immune impairment that is sometimes seen in exercise "overtraining." Lower resting levels of plasma glutamine have been observed in some athletes suffering from overtraining syndrome, characterized, in part, by transient immunosuppression. In a few preliminary studies, oral glutamine supplementation appears to improve some measures of immunity and to decrease post-exercise infection. Results are not consistent, however, and more research is needed.

Some dated research suggesting that oral glutamine might help curb alcohol craving has not been followed up. One study demonstrated a significant decrease in voluntary alcohol consumption in rats supplemented with glutamine. A subsequent small, uncontrolled study focused on a group of subjects with extensive history of alcoholism. Considerable improvement was noted. More research is needed.

CONTRAINDICATIONS, PRECAUTIONS, ADVERSE REACTIONS

CONTRAINDICATIONS

Supplemental L-glutamine is contraindicated in those hypersensitive to any component of a glutamine-containing product.

PRECAUTIONS

Pregnant women and nursing mothers should avoid supplemental L-glutamine unless prescribed by a physician.

Those with renal or hepatic failure should exercise caution in the use of supplemental L-glutamine.

ADVERSE REACTIONS

Doses of L-glutamine up to 21 grams daily appear to be well tolerated. Reported adverse reactions are mainly gastrointestinal and not common. They include constipation and bloating. There is one older report of two hypomanic patients whose manic symptoms were exacerbated following the use of 2 to 4 grams daily of L-glutamine. The symptoms resolved when the L-glutamine was stopped. These patients were not rechallenged, nor are there any other reports of this nature.

INTERACTIONS

DRUGS

Human growth hormone: Concomitant use of L-glutamine and human growth hormone may enhance nutrient absorption in those with severe short bowel syndrome. L-glutamine has orphan drug status for this indication.

Indomethacin: Concomitant use of L-glutamine and indomethacin may ameliorate increased intestinal permeability caused by indomethacin. The reported dose used for L-glutamine was 21 grams daily taken in divided doses three times a day. Further, misoprostol is reported to have a synergistic effect with this combination in ameliorating intestinal permeability.

Methotrexate: There is one report that methotrexate may decrease the possible effectiveness of supplemental L-glutamine for chemotherapy-induced mucositis. In another report, nine patients with breast cancer were reported to have decreased symptoms of methotrexate-related toxicity when given supplemental L-glutamine at a dose of 0.5 gram/kilogram/day.

Paclitaxel: In one report, L-glutamine at a dose of 10 grams three times daily, given 24 hours after receiving paclitaxel, appeared to prevent the development of myalgia and arthralgia, adverse reactions of paclitaxel.

DOSAGE AND ADMINISTRATION

L-glutamine is available in capsules, tablets and powder form. It is also available in medical foods for oral and enteral nutrition use and in a dipeptide form for parenteral nutrition use. (See Glutamine Peptides.) Typical doses for those with cancer, AIDS, trauma, burns, infections and other stress-related conditions range from 4 to 21 grams daily. Those who take L-glutamine for these indications must be under medical supervision.

Those with chemotherapy- or radiation-induced stomatitis have taken doses of 2 to 4 grams twice daily or 2 grams four times daily. This was done by dissolving a given amount of L-glutamine in water or normal saline — one gram dissolves in 20.8 ml of water at 30 degrees Celsius — and using it as a swish and swallow. Again, this must be performed under medical supervision. Since L-glutamine is unstable in water, fresh solutions should be prepared daily.

Those who use supplemental L-glutamine as a possible ergogenic aid use between 1.5 to 4.5 grams daily, taken between meals.

LITERATURE

Abcouwer SF, Souba WW. Glutamine and arginine. In: Shils ME, Olson JA, Shike M, Ross AC, eds. *Modern Nutrition in Health and Disease.* 9th ed. Baltimore, MD: Williams and Wilkins. 1999:559-569.

Anderson PM, Ramsay NK, Shu XO, et al. Effect of low-dose oral glutamine on painful stomatitis during bone marrow transplantation. *Bone Marrow Transplant.* 1998;22:339-344.

Anderson PM, Schroeder G, Skubitz KM. Oral glutamine reduces the duration and severity of stomatitis after cytotoxic cancer chemotherapy. *Cancer.* 1998;83:1433-1439.

Antonio J, Street C. Glutamine: a potentially useful supplement for athletes. *Can J Appl Physiol.* 1999;24:1-14.

Bulus N, Cersosimo E, Ghishan F, Abumrad NN. Physiologic importance of glutamine. *Metabolism.* 1989;38(Suppl1):1-5.

Byrne TA, Morrissey TB, Nattakom TV, et al. Growth hormone, glutamine, and a modified diet enhance nutrient absorption in patients with severe short bowel syndrome. *J Parenter Enteral Nutr.* 1995;19:296-302.

Cao Y, Feng Z, Hoos A, Klimberg VS. Glutamine enhances gut glutathione production. *J Parenter Enteral Nutr.* 1998;22:224-247.

Furukawa S, Saito H, Inoue T, et al. Supplemental glutamine augments phagocytosis and reactive oxygen intermediate production by neutrophils and monocytes from postoperative patients *in vitro. Nutrition.* 2000;16:323-329.

Furukawa S, Saito H, Ming-Tsan L, et al. Enteral administration of glutamine in purulent peritonitis. *Nutrition.* 1999;15:29-31.

Haub MD, Potteiger JA, Nau KL, et al. Acute L-glutamine ingestion does not improve maximal effort exercise. *J Sports Med Phys Fitness.* 1998;38:240-244.

Hond ED, Peeters M, Hiele M, et al. Effect of glutamine on the intestinal permeability changes induced by indomethacin in humans. *Aliment Pharmacol Ther.* 1999;13:679-685.

Houdijk, APJ, Rijnsburger ER, Jansen J, et al. Randomized trial of glutamine-enriched enteral nutrition on infectious morbidity in patients with multiple trauma. *Lancet.* 1998;352:772-776.

Huang EY, Leung SW, Wang CJ, et al. Oral glutamine to alleviate radiation-induced oral mucositis: a pilot randomized trial. *Int J Rad Oncol Biol Phys.* 2000;46:535-539.

Ito A, Higashiguchi T. Effects of glutamine administration on liver regeneration following hepatectomy. *Nutrition.* 1999;15:23-28.

Lacey JM, Wilmore DW. Is glutamine a conditionally essential amino acid? *Nutr Rev.* 1990;48:297-309.

Mebane AH. L-Glutamine and mania. *Am J Psychiatry.* 1984;141:1302-1303.

Neu J, Roig JC, Meetze WH, et al. Enteral glutamine supplementation for very low birth weight infants decreases mortality. *J Pediatr.* 1997;131:691-699.

Noyer CM, Simon D, Borczuk A, et al. A double-blind placebo-controlled pilot study of glutamine therapy for abnormal intestinal permeability in patients with AIDS. *Am J Gastroenterol.* 1998;93:972-975.

Rogers LL, Pelton RB, Williams RJ. Voluntary alcohol consumption of rats following administration of glutamine. *J Biol Chem.* 1955;214:503-506.

Rohde T, MacLean DA, Klarlund Pedersen B. Glutamine, lymphocyte proliferation and cytokine production. *Scan J Immunol.* 1996;44:648-650.

Rohde T, MacLean DA, Pedersen BK. Effect of glutamine supplementation on changes in the immune system induced by repeated exercise. *Med Sci Sports Exerc.* 1998;30:856-862.

Sacks GS. Glutamine supplementation in catabolic patients. *Ann Pharmacother.* 1999;33:348-354.

Wilmore DW, Schloerb PR, Ziegler TR. Glutamine in the support of patients following bone marrow transplantation. *Curr Opin Clin Nutr Metab Care.* 1999;2:323-327.

Windmueller HG, Spaeth AF. Identification of ketone bodies and glutamine as the major respiratory fuels *in vivo* for postabsorptive rat small intestine. *J Biol Chem.* 1978;253:69-76.

Ziegler TR, Benfell K, Smith RJ, et al. Safety and metabolic effects of L-glutamine administration in humans. *J Parenter Enteral Nutr.* 1990;14:137S-146S.

L-Histidine

DESCRIPTION

L-histidine is a protein amino acid that is found in the proteins of all life forms. Although most L-histidine is found in proteins, a small amount of free L-histidine does exist in plants and fermented foods. The naturally occurring dipeptides found in muscle, carnosine and anserine are both comprised of L-histidine and beta-alanine.

L-histidine is one of the 10 essential amino acids for infants. It has never been clear if L-histidine is an essential amino acid for adults. At the very least, it is a conditional essential amino acid for adults. That is, even though L-histidine is synthesized in adult human tissues, sufficient quantities may not be made to meet the physiological requirements imposed by certain stress or disease situations.

L-histidine is a solid water-soluble substance. Chemically, it is called (S)-alpha-amino-1H-imidazole-4-propanoic acid; alpha-amino-4 (or 5)-imidazolepropionic acid; L-2-amino-3-(1H-imidazol-4yl) propionic acid, and glyoxaline-5-alanine. Its IUPAC abbreviation is His, and its one-letter abbreviation is H. L-histidine is classified as a basic amino acid. L-histidine has the following structural formula:

L-Histidine

ACTIONS AND PHARMACOLOGY

ACTIONS

The actions of supplemental L-histidine are entirely unclear. It may have some immunomodulatory as well as antioxidant activity.

MECHANISM OF ACTION

Since the actions of supplemental L-histidine are unclear, any postulated mechanism is entirely speculative. However, some facts are known about L-histidine and some of its metabolites, such as histamine and trans-urocanic acid, which suggest that supplemental L-histidine may one day be shown to have immunomodulatory and/or antioxidant activities. Low free histidine has been found in the serum of some rheumatoid arthritis patients. Serum concentrations of other amino acids have been found to be normal in these patients. L-histidine is an excellent chelating agent for such metals as copper, iron and zinc. Copper and iron participate in a reaction (Fenton reaction) that generates potent reactive oxygen species that could be destructive to tissues, including joints.

L-histidine is the obligate precursor of histamine, which is produced via the decarboxylation of the amino acid. In experimental animals, tissue histamine levels increase as the amount of dietary L-histidine increases. It is likely that this would be the case in humans as well. Histamine is known to possess immunomodulatory and antioxidant activity. Suppressor T cells have H_2 receptors, and histamine activates them. Promotion of suppressor T cell activity could be beneficial in rheumatoid arthritis. Further, histamine has been shown to down-regulate the production of reactive oxygen species in phagocytic cells, such as monocytes, by binding to the H_2 receptors on these cells. Decreased reactive oxygen species production by phagocytes could play antioxidant, anti-inflammatory and immunomodulatory roles in such diseases as rheumatoid arthritis.

This latter mechanism is the rationale for the use of histamine itself in several clinical trials studying histamine for the treatment of certain types of cancer and viral diseases. In these trials, down-regulation by histamine of reactive oxygen species formation appears to inhibit the suppression of natural killer (NK) cells and cytotoxic T lymphocytes, allowing these cells to be more effective in attacking cancer cells and virally infected cells.

PHARMACOKINETICS

L-histidine is absorbed from the small intestine via an active transport mechanism requiring the presence of sodium. From the small intestine, L-histidine is transported to the liver by means of the portal circulation, where some is metabolized and from whence some enters the systemic circulation to be distributed to various tissues in the body.

L-histidine is metabolized in several different ways. It is a substrate for protein synthesis; decarboxylation produces histamine; it is converted to trans-urocanate in the skin; it forms the dipeptides carnosine and anserine in muscle; it is a precursor of the thiol antioxidant, L-ergothioneine; and it forms alpha-ketoglutarate.

INDICATIONS AND USAGE

L-histidine may be indicated for use in some with rheumatoid arthritis. It is not indicated for treatment of anemia or uremia or for lowering serum cholesterol.

RESEARCH SUMMARY

It has been reported that rheumatoid arthritis (RA) sufferers have abnormally low blood levels of this amino acid. In a pilot study, RA patients received up to 6 grams of supplemental histidine daily and were said to benefit with as little as 1 gram daily. A subsequent study with 4.5 grams daily in some with more active and prolonged disease found much less benefit—but still enough to warrant further research.

CONTRAINDICATIONS, PRECAUTIONS, ADVERSE REACTIONS

CONTRAINDICATIONS

L-histidine supplementation is contraindicated in anyone hypersensitive to any component of the preparation.

PRECAUTIONS

L-histidine supplements should be avoided by children, pregnant women and nursing mothers. Those with allergies or peptic ulcer disease should only use L-histidine supplements under strict medical supervision. Although there are no reports of adverse events in these groups, increased histamine production from L-histidine might negatively affect those with these conditions.

ADVERSE REACTIONS

Mild gastrointestinal side effects have been reported. L-histidine is generally well tolerated.

INTERACTIONS

Medroxyprogesterone Acetate: L-histidine was observed to enhance (in tissue culture) the effect of medroxyprogesterone acetate in reducing the number of human breast cancer cells that were in the S phase.

H_1 and H_2 Blockers: Although not reported, L-histidine, via its metabolism to histamine, might decrease the efficacy of H_1 and H_2 blockers.

No other drug, nutritional supplement, food or herb interaction are known.

OVERDOSAGE

None reported.

DOSAGE AND ADMINISTRATION

Tablets and capsules typically are available in 500 milligram to 1000 milligram dosages. Dosages have ranged from 500 milligrams to 4.5 grams daily.

LITERATURE

Blumenkrantz MJ, Shapiro DJ, Swendseid ME, Kopple JD. Histidine supplementation for treatment of anaemia of uraemia. *Br Med J.* 1975; 2(5970):530-533.

Gerber DA. Decreased concentration of free histidine in serum in rheumatoid arthritis, an isolated amino acid abnormality not associated with generalized hypoaminoacidemia. *J Rheumatol.* 1975; 2:384-392.

Gerber DA. Low free serum histidine concentration in rheumatoid arthritis. A measure of disease activity. *J Clin Invest.* 1975; 55:1124-1173.

Gerber DA, Sklar JE, Niedwiadowiez J. Lack of effect of oral L-histidine on the serum cholesterol in human subjects. *Am J Clin Nutr.* 1971; 24:1382-1383.

Gerber DA, Tanenbaum L, Ahrens M. Free serum histidine levels in patients with rheumatoid arthritis and control subjects following an oral load of free L-histidine. *Metabolism.* 1976; 25:655-657.

Ghezzo F, Racca S, Conti G, et al. L-histidine medroxyprogesterone acetate interaction modulates human breast cancer cell growth and progestin receptor expression in vitro. *Pharmacy Res.* 1997; 35:119-122.

Griswold DE, Alessi S, Badger AM, et al. Inhibitions of T suppressor cell expression by histamine type 2 (H$_2$) receptor antagonists. *J Immunol.* 1984; 132:3054-3057.

Hellstrand K, Dalgren C, Hermodsson S. Histaminergic regulation of NK cells. Role of monocyte-derived reactive oxygen metabolites. *J Immunol.* 1994; 153:4940-4947.

Lee NS, Fitzpatrick D, Meier E, Fisher H. Influence of dietary histidine on tissue histamine concentration, histidine decorboxylase and histamine methyltransferase activity in the rat. *Agents Actions.* 1981; 11:307-311.

Pinals RS, Harris ED, Burnett JB, Gerber DA. Treatment of rheumatoid arthritis with L-histidine: a randomized, placebo-controlled, double-blind trial. *J Rheumatol.* 1977; 4:414-419.

L-Lysine

DESCRIPTION

L-lysine is protein amino acid. It is classified as an essential amino acid for humans and therefore must be supplied in the diet. Certain proteins, such as those found in meat, poultry and milk are rich in L-lysine. Proteins found in grains, cereals and their products are typically low in L-lysine. For example, wheat is low in L-lysine; wheat germ, however, is rich in L-lysine. Small amounts of free L-lysine are found in vegetables, vegetable juices and in such fermented foods as miso and yogurt.

L-lysine's popularity as a nutritional supplement arose as a result of some studies suggesting that the amino acid may decrease the recurrence rate of some infected with herpes simplex virus.

L-lysine is a basic amino acid and carries a positive charge at physiological pH. It is a solid substance that is very soluble in water. L-lysine has three pKa's: pKa$_1$=2.20, pKa$_2$=8.90 and pKa$_3$=10.28. L-lysine is marketed as a nutritional substance, either as L-lysine monohydrochloride or as the free base, L-lysine. The molecular weight of L-lysine is 146.19 daltons, its molecular formula is $C_6H_{14}N_2O_2$, and its structural formula is:

L-lysine

L-lysine is also known as (S)- 2, 6, -diaminohexanoic acid and alpha, epsilon-diaminocaproic acid It is abbreviated as Lys or by its one letter abbreviation, K. L-lysine and lysine are frequently used interchangeably. The D-stereoisomer (D-lysine) is not biologically active.

ACTIONS AND PHARMACOLOGY

ACTIONS

Supplemental L-lysine has putative anti-herpes simplex virus activity. There is preliminary research suggesting that it may have some anti-osteoporotic activity.

MECHANISM OF ACTION

Proteins of the herpes simplex virus are rich in L-arginine, and tissue culture studies indicate an enhancing effect on viral replication when the amino acid ratio of L-arginine to L-lysine is high in the tissue culture media. When the ratio of L-lysine to L-arginine is high, viral replication and the cytopathogenicity of herpes simplex virus have been found to be inhibited.

L-lysine may facilitate the absorption of calcium from the small intestine.

PHARMACOKINETICS

Following ingestion, L-lysine is absorbed from the lumen of the small intestine into the enterocytes by an active transport process. Some metabolism of L-lysine takes place within the enterocytes. That which is not metabolized is transported to the liver via the portal circulation. In the liver, L-lysine, along with other amino acids, participates in protein biosynthesis. Some is metabolized to L-alpha-aminoadipic acid semialdehyde, which is further metabolized to acetoacetyl-CoA. The intermediate in this pathway is saccharopine. L-lysine does not participate in transamination. It is the exception to the general rule that the first step in catabolism of an amino acid is the removal of its alpha-amino group by transamination to form the respective alpha-keto acid. L-lysine is both a glycogenic and a ketogenic amino acid. It can participate in the formation of D-glucose and glycogen, as well as lipids. It can also participate in the production of energy.

L-lysine that is not metabolized in the liver is transported to the various tissues of the body, where it is involved in reactions similar to those described above. L-hydroxylysine, found in collagen and elastin, is formed post-translationally.

INDICATIONS AND USAGE

Lysine may reduce the recurrence rate of herpes simplex virus (HSV) infections and/or reduce their severity in some, though research results have been mixed with respect to this putative benefit. Very preliminary research indicates a possible role for lysine in the prevention and treatment of osteoporosis.

RESEARCH SUMMARY

A number of clinical studies have found that lysine is useful in preventing and sometimes shortening outbreaks of herpes simplex infections. A few studies have found no effect. *In vitro* and animal studies have also found evidence of lysine's anti-herpetic effects.

In a double-blind, placebo-controlled, multicenter trial of oral lysine, the treatment group received 1000 mg of lysine three times daily (3000 mg daily) for six months. During that period, the treated subjects had an average of 2.4 fewer HSV infections, and their symptoms were significantly less severe and healing times significantly reduced.

In another randomized, double-blind, cross-over study, a daily dose of 1248 mg (but not 624 mg) of lysine was found to decrease the recurrence rate of HSV in non-immunocompromised subjects. In this study, the 1248 mg dosage did not shorten healing time.

There is one study suggesting that supplemental lysine can both enhance intestinal absorption and improve renal conservation of absorbed calcium and that it might thus be helpful in osteoporosis. Further research is needed.

CONTRAINDICATIONS, PRECAUTIONS, ADVERSE REACTIONS

CONTRAINDICATIONS

L-lysine supplementation is contraindicated in those with the rare genetic disorder hyperlysinemia/hyperlysinuria.

PRECAUTIONS

Pregnant women and nursing mothers should only consider using supplemental L-lysine if their diets are low in this amino acid. They should avoid supplemental L-lysine for other reasons.

Proteins such as casein, which are high in L-lysine relative to L-arginine, are associated with elevated cholesterol levels. Those with hypercholesterolemia who are interested in taking supplemental L-lysine should be aware of this.

Those with hepatic or renal failure should exercise caution in the use of supplemental L-lysine.

ADVERSE REACTIONS

Doses up to 3 grams daily are generally well tolerated. Very high doses—greater than 10 to 15 grams daily—may cause gastrointestinal symptoms, such as nausea, abdominal cramps and diarrhea.

There is one report of Fanconi's syndrome and tubulointestinal nephritis in a 44-year old woman associated with the use of supplemental L-lysine.

INTERACTIONS

NUTRITIONAL SUPPLEMENTS

Concomitant use of calcium supplements and L-lysine may increase calcium absorption. This is based on a very preliminary study that needs follow-up.

OVERDOSAGE

There are no reports of overdosage with L-lysine.

DOSAGE AND ADMINISTRATION

Typical dosage used for possible prevention of herpes simplex virus recurrence is 500 mg to 3 grams daily. The average dose is 1 gram daily. Higher doses are split throughout the day.

LITERATURE

Civitelli R, Villareal DT, Agnusedei D, et al. Dietary L-lysine and calcium metabolism in humans. *Nutrition.* 1992; 8:400-405.

Di Giovanna JJ, Blank H. Failure of lysine in frequently recurrent herpes simplex infection. Treatment and prophylaxis. *Arch Dermatol.* 1984; 120:48-51.

Flondin NW. The metabolic roles, pharmacology, and toxicology of lysine. *J Am Coll Nutr.* 1997; 16:7-21.

Griffith RS, De Long DC, Nelson JD. Relation of L-arginine—lysine antagonism to herpes simplex growth in tissue culture. *Chemotherapy.* 1981; 27:209-213.

Griffith RS, Walsh DE, Myrmel KH, et al. Success of L-lysine therapy in frequently recurrent herpes simplex infection. Treatment and prophylaxis. *Dermatologica.* 1987; 175:183-190.

Lo JC, Chertow GM, Rennke H, Seifter JL. Fanconi's syndrome and tubulointestinal nephritis in association with L-lysine ingestion. *Am J Kidney Dis.* 1996; 28:614-617.

McCune MA, Perry HO, Muller SA, O'Fallon WM. Treatment of recurrent herpes simplex infections with L-lysine monohydrochloride. *Cutis.* 1984; 34:366-373.

Rajamohan T, Kurup PA. Lysine: arginine ratio of a protein influences cholesterol metabolism: Part 1—studies on sesame protein having low lysine: arginine ratio. *Indian J Exp Biol.* 1997; 35:1218-1223.

Thein DJ, Hurt WC. Lysine as a prophylactic agent in the treatment of recurrent herpes simplex labialis. *Oral Surg Oral Med Oral Pathol.* 1984; 58:659-666.

L-Methionine

DESCRIPTION

L-methionine is a protein amino acid. It is classified as an essential amino acid for humans and therefore must be supplied in the diet. According to the Food and Agriculture Organization of the United Nations (FAO) and World Health Organization (WHO), recommended daily L-methionine intake is 13 mg per kg or about one gram daily for adults. Actual intake is higher. This is principally derived from dietary proteins. Rich sources of L-methionine include cheeses, eggs, fish, meat and poultry. L-methionine is also found in fruits and vegetables, but not as abundantly. Small amounts of free L-methionine occur in vegetables, vegetable juices and fermented foods.

In addition to its role as a precursor in protein synthesis, L-methionine participates in a wide range of biochemical reactions, including the production of S-adenosylmethionine (SAM or SAMe), L-cysteine, glutathione, taurine and sulfate. SAM itself, as a methyl donor (see SAMe), is involved in the synthesis of creatine, epinephrine, melatonin and the polyamines spermine and spermidine, among several other substances.

L-methionine is also a glycogenic amino acid and may participate in the formation of D-glucose and glycogen. The ability of L-methionine to reduce the liver-toxic effects of such hepatotoxins as acetaminophen and methotrexate has led to the suggestion that methionine should be added to acetaminophen products. However, there is some recent research suggesting that elevated L-methionine intake may promote intestinal carcinogenesis. This is unclear. Further, one of the metabolites of L-methionine, L-homocysteine, has been implicated as a significant factor in coronary heart disease and other vascular diseases.

L-methionine is a sulfur-containing amino acid that is minimally soluble in water. Its molecular formula is $C_5H_{11}NO_2S$, and its molecular weight is 149.21 daltons. L-methionine is also known as 2-amino-4-(methylthio)butyric acid, alpha-amino-gamma-methylmercaptobutyric acid, (S)-2-amino-4-(methylthio)butanoic acid and gamma-methyl-thio-alpha-aminobutyric acid. It is abbreviated as Met and its one-letter abbreviation is M. The terms L-methionine and methionine are used interchangeably. The D-stereoisomer, D-methionine, does not possess biological activity with regard to protein synthesis and the biochemical reactions mentioned above. However, D-methionine, as well as L-methionine, may possess antioxidant activity. L-methionine is represented by the following chemical structure:

L-methionine

ACTIONS AND PHARMACOLOGY

ACTIONS

L-methionine may protect against the toxic effects of hepatotoxins, such as acetaminophen. Methionine may have antioxidant activity.

MECHANISM OF ACTION

The mechanism of the possible anti-hepatotoxic activity of L-methionine is not entirely clear. It is thought that metabolism of high doses of acetaminophen in the liver lead to decreased levels of hepatic glutathione and increased oxidative stress. L-methionine is a precursor to L-cysteine. L-cysteine itself may have antioxidant activity. L-cysteine is also a precursor to the antioxidant glutathione. Antioxidant activity of L-methionine and metabolites of L-methionine appear to account for its possible anti-hepatotoxic activity. Recent research suggests that methionine itself has free-radical scavenging activity by virtue of its sulfur, as well as its chelating ability.

PHARMACOKINETICS

Following ingestion, L-methionine is absorbed from the lumen of the small intestine into the enterocytes by an active transport process. Some metabolism of L-methionine takes place within the enterocytes. That which is not metabolized is transported to the liver via the portal circulation. In the liver, L-methionine, along with other amino acids, participates in protein biosynthesis. It may also participate in a wide variety of metabolic reactions, including the formation of SAMe, L-homocysteine, L-cysteine, taurine and sulfate. It can also be metabolized to produce D-glucose and glycogen. L-methionine not metabolized in the liver is transported to the various tissues of the body where it is involved in reactions similar to those described above.

INDICATIONS AND USAGE

There are no indications for the use of supplemental methionine unless specifically recommended by a physician. It is effective as an antidote in some cases of acetaminophen poisoning. But, because some research suggests that it may promote some cancers, its use as a supplement is inadvisable.

RESEARCH SUMMARY

When given within 10 hours of acetaminophen poisoning, oral methionine has been found to be as effective as N-acetylcysteine in preventing severe liver damage and death. There is preliminary evidence that methionine might also help protect against some of the adverse side effects of methotrexate and gentamicin, among others.

On the other hand, high intake of methionine can lead to increased levels of the oxidant homocysteine. There is some fear that high intake of dietary methionine can promote some cancers, and there is some very preliminary experimental data to support that fear. There is also some epidemiological data suggesting a link between increased dietary methionine and increased risk of gastric cancer. More research is needed.

CONTRAINDICATIONS, PRECAUTIONS, ADVERSE REACTIONS

CONTRAINDICATIONS

L-methionine is contraindicated in those with the genetic disorder homocystinuria. It is also contraindicated in those who are hypersensitive to any component of a methionine-containing product.

PRECAUTIONS

L-methionine supplements should be avoided by pregnant women and nursing mothers unless they are prescribed by a physician.

L-methionine supplementation should be avoided by those with neoplastic disease. It should also be avoided by those with elevated homocysteine levels and used with caution in those with coronary heart disease.

Supplemental L-methionine should be used with great caution in those with schizophrenia and those with hepatic and renal failure. In any case, L-methionine supplements should only be used if recommended and monitored by a physician.

ADVERSE REACTIONS

Doses of L-methionine of up to 250 mg daily are generally well tolerated. Higher doses may cause nausea, vomiting and headache. Healthy adults taking 8 grams of L-methionine daily for four days were found to have reduced serum folate levels and leucocytosis. Healthy adults taking 13.9 grams of L-methionine daily for five days were found to have changes in serum pH and potassium and increased urinary calcium excretion. Schizophrenic patients given 10 to 20 grams of L-methionine daily for two weeks developed functional psychoses. Single doses of 8 grams precipitated encephalopathy in patients with cirrhosis.

INTERACTIONS

DRUGS

Acetaminophen and methotrexate: L-methionine may decrease hepatic toxicity in those with acetaminophen overdosage or in those taking methotrexate. Theoretically, it may decrease hepatic toxicity in the case of other potential hepatotoxic drugs, as well.

Gentamicin: Methionine may protect against the ototoxic effects of gentamicin.

NUTRITIONAL SUPPLEMENTS

Dietary supplementation with L-methionine was found to decrease glycine levels when given to healthy women on a low-protein diet.

High L-methionine intake in a diet high in salt and nitrites/ nitrates may increase the risk of stomach cancer.

OVERDOSAGE

There are no reports of overdosage.

DOSAGE AND ADMINISTRATION

L-methionine supplements should only be taken with a physician's recommendation.

LITERATURE

Bellone J, Farello G, Bartoletta E, et al. Methionine potentiates both basal and GHRH-induced GH secretion in children. *Clin Endocrinol (Oxf).* 1997; 47:61-64.

Breillot F, Hadida F, Echinard-Darin P, et al. Decreased rat rhabdomyosarcoma pulmonary metastases in response to low methionine diet. *Anticanc Res.* 1986; 76:6299-639.

Duranton B, Freund JN, Galluser M, et al. Promotion of intestinal carcinogenesis by dietary methionine. *Carcinogenesis.* 1999; 20:493-497.

Hladovec J, Sommerova Z, Pisarikova A. Homocysteinemia and endothelial damage after methionine load. *Thrombo Res.* 1997; 88:361-364.

Jones AL, Hayes PC, Proudfoot AT, Vale JA, Prescott LF, Krenzelok EP. Should methionine be added to every paracetamol tablet? *BMJ.* 1997; 315:301-304.

Kroger H, Hauschild A, Ohde M, et al. Nicotinamide and methionine reduce the liver toxic effects of methotrexate. *Gen Pharmacol.* 1999; 33:203-206.

La Vecchia C, Negri E, Franceschi S, Decarli A. Case-control study on influence of methionine, nitrite, and salt on gastric carcinogenesis in northern Italy. *Nutr Canc.* 1997; 27:65-68.

Meakins TS, Persaud C, Jackson AA. Dietary supplementation with L-methionine impairs the utilization of urea-nitrogen and increases 5-L-oxoprolinuria in normal women consuming a low protein diet. *J Nutr* 1998; 128:720-727.

Sha S-H, Schacht J. Antioxidants attenuate gentamicin-induced free radical formation *in vitro* and ototoxicity *in vivo*: D-methionine is a potential protectant. *Hearing Res.* 2000; 142:34-40.

Vale JA, Meredith TJ, Goulding R. Treatment of acetaminophen poisoning. The use of oral methionine. *Arch Int Med.* 1981; 141(3 Spec No):394-396.

L-Ornithine

DESCRIPTION

L-Ornithine is a nonprotein amino acid. It is used in the body in the biosynthesis of L-arginine, L-proline and polyamines. L-Ornithine is a basic amino acid, positively charged at physiological pH. It is also known as alpha,delta-diaminovaleric acid and 2,5-diaminopentanoic acid. The molecular formula of L-ornithine is $C_5H_{12}N_2O_2$, and its molecular weight is 132.16 daltons. The structural formula is:

L-Ornithine

L-Ornithine is used as a nutritional supplement principally for its putative anabolic activity. There is little evidence to support this use. However, a derivative of L-ornithine called ornithine alpha-ketoglutarate or OKG (see Ornithine Alpha-Ketoglutarate) may, under certain conditions, have immunomodulatory and anticatabolic and/or anabolic actions.

ACTIONS AND PHARMACOLOGY

ACTIONS

L-Ornithine has putative anabolic, immunomodulatory and wound-healing activities.

MECHANISM OF ACTION

L-Ornithine may at very high doses—around 30 grams—stimulate the pituitary release of growth hormone by virtue of its metabolism to L-arginine (see L-Arginine).

Burn injury and other traumas affect the status of L-arginine in the various tissues of the body. *De novo* synthesis of L-arginine during these conditions is probably not sufficient for normal immune function, nor for normal protein synthesis. Under these conditions, L-ornithine may have immunomodulatory and wound-healing activities, again, by virtue of its metabolism to L-arginine.

PHARMACOKINETICS

Following ingestion, L-ornithine is absorbed from the small intestine via a sodium-dependent active transport process. The transport system for L-ornithine is shared with L-arginine, L-lysine and L-cystine. L-ornithine is transported via the portal circulation to the liver where it undergoes extensive metabolism to L-arginine, polyamines and proline, among other metabolites. L-Ornithine that is not metabolized in the liver is distributed by the systemic circulation to the various cells of the body.

INDICATIONS AND USAGE

It is claimed that ornithine has anabolic effects and improves athletic performance, that it has wound-healing effects and is immuno-enhancing. There is little support for these claims. There is at least preliminary evidence, however, that the better-studied ornithine alpha-ketoglutarate may have some of these activities. Inasmuch as ornithine is metabolized to arginine, which also demonstrates some of these effects, it is possible that ornithine, when more thoroughly studied, might exhibit some similar effects. See Arginine and Ornithine Alpha-Ketoglutarate.

RESEARCH SUMMARY

In one double-blind, placebo-controlled study, a combination of 1 gram of arginine and 1 gram of ornithine daily, used in conjunction with a high-intensity strength-training program over a five-week period, increased total strength and lean body mass in adult males, compared with controls. Most trials using ornithine alone, however, have reported no significant anabolic effects. Most of these studies have failed to show that ornithine supplementation has any significant effect on insulin secretion or human growth hormone levels in bodybuilders. There is apparently only one study reporting that ornithine increased growth hormone levels in bodybuilders, and this study used a very high dose of the supplement (13 grams daily). Numerous gastrointestinal side effects were associated with this dosage.

CONTRAINDICATIONS, PRECAUTIONS, ADVERSE REACTIONS

CONTRAINDICATIONS

L-Ornithine is contraindicated in those with a deficiency of ornithine-delta-aminotransferase. This is a genetic disorder resulting in gyrate atrophy of the choroid and retina and progressive blinding chorioretinal degeneration. It is rare.

L-Ornithine is also contraindicated in those hypersensitive to any component of an ornithine-containing supplement.

PRECAUTIONS

Pregnant women and nursing mothers should avoid L-ornithine supplementation.

ADVERSE REACTIONS

Doses higher than 10 grams daily may cause such gastrointestinal symptoms as nausea, abdominal cramps and diarrhea.

DOSAGE AND ADMINISTRATION

Those who use L-ornithine take doses of 500 milligrams to 2 grams, usually before bedtime and on an empty stomach. Some combine L-ornithine with similar doses of L-arginine.

LITERATURE

Barbul A. Arginine: biochemistry, physiology, and therapeutic implications. *J Parenter Enteral Nutr.* 1986; 10:227-238.

Bucci L, Hickson JF Jr, et al. Ornithine ingestion and growth hormone release in bodybuilders. *Nutr Res.* 1990; 10:239-245.

Bucci LR, Hickson JF Jr, Wolinsky I, Pivarnik JM. Ornithine supplementation and insulin release in bodybuilders. *Int J Sport Nut.* 1992; 2:289-291.

DeBandt J-P, Coudray-Lucas C, Lioret N, et al. A randomized controlled trial of the influence of the mode of enteral ornithine alpha-ketoglutarate administration in burn patients. *J Nutr.* 1998; 128:563-569.

Elam RP, Hardin DH, Sutton RA, Hagen L. Effects of arginine and ornithine on strength, lean body mass and urinary hydroxyproline in adult males. *J Sports Med Phys Fitness.* 1989; 29:52-56.

Fogelholm GM, Naveri HK, Kiilavuori KT, Harkoner MH. Low-dose amino acid supplementation: no effects on serum human growth hormone and insulin in male weightlifters. *Int J Sport Nutr.* 1993; 3:290-297.

Iwasaki K, Mano K, Ishihara M, et al. Effects of ornithine or arginine administration on serum amino acid levels. *Biochem Int.* 1987; 14:971-976.

Jeevanandam M, Holaday NJ, Petersen SR. Ornithine alpha-ketoglutarate (OKG) supplementation is more effective than its component salts in traumatized rats. *J Nutr.* 1996; 126:2141-2150.

Lambert MI, Hefer JA, Millar RP, Macfarlane PW. Failure of commercial oral amino acid supplements to increase serum growth hormone concentrations in male body builders. *Int J Sport Med.* 1993; 3:298-305.

Torre PM, Ronnenberg AG, Hartman WJ, Prior RL. Supplemental arginine and ornithine do not affect splenocyte proliferation in surgically treated rats. *J Parenter Enteral Nut.* 1993; 17:532-536.

L-Phenylalanine

DESCRIPTION

L-phenylalanine is a protein amino acid. It is classified as an essential amino acid because the body requires a dietary source of the amino acid to meet its physiological demands. L-phenylalanine is found in proteins of all life forms. Dietary sources of the amino acid are principally derived from animal and vegetable proteins. Vegetables and juices contain small amounts of the free amino acid. The free amino acid is also found in fermented foods such as yogurt and miso. The alternative sweetener aspartame is a dipeptide of L-phenylalanine, as is the methyl ester, and L-aspartic acid.

In addition to being involved in protein synthesis, L-phenylalanine is the precursor of L-tyrosine. The conversion of L-phenylalanine to L-tyrosine is via the enzyme L-phenylalanine hydroxylase. It is this enzyme that is virtually absent in those with the inborn error of metabolism phenylketonuria (PKU). L-tyrosine produced from L-phenylalanine is a precursor in the synthesis of the neurotransmitters norepinephrine and dopamine, among other reactions. L-phenylalanine is marketed as a nutritional supplement and used by some for its putative antidepressant activity.

L-phenylalanine is also known as beta-phenylalanine, alpha-aminohydrocinnamic acid, (S)-2-amino-3- phenylpropanoic acid and alpha-amino-beta-phenylpropionic acid. It is abbreviated as either Phe or by its one-letter abbreviation F. The molecular formula of L-phenylalanine is $C_9H_{11}NO_2$, and its molecular weight is 165.19 daltons. L-phenylalanine is an aromatic amino acid with the following structural formula:

L-phenylalanine

ACTIONS AND PHARMACOLOGY

ACTIONS

L-phenylalanine has putative antidepressant activity. It may also, when used in conjunction with UVA irradiation, have antivitiligo activity.

MECHANISM OF ACTION

The mechanism of L-phenylalanine's putative antidepressant activity may be accounted for by its precursor role in the synthesis of the neurotransmitters norepinephrine and dopamine. Elevated brain norepinephrine and dopamine levels are thought to be associated with antidepressant effects.

The mechanism of L-phenylalanine's possible antivitiligo activity is not well understood. It is thought that L-phenylalanine may stimulate the production of melanin in the affected skin.

PHARMACOKINETICS

Following ingestion, L-phenylalanine is absorbed from the small intestine by a sodium dependent active transport process. L-phenylalanine is transported from the small intestine to the liver via the portal circulation. In the liver, L-phenylalanine is involved in a number of biochemical reactions, including protein synthesis, the formation of L-tyrosine and oxidative catabolic reactions. L-phenylalanine that is not metabolized in the liver is distributed via the systemic circulation to the various tissues of the body, where it undergoes metabolic reactions similar to those that take place in the liver.

INDICATIONS AND USAGE

L-phenylalanine may be helpful in some with depression. It may also be useful in the treatment of vitiligo. There is some evidence that L-phenylalanine may exacerbate tardive dyskinesia in some schizophrenic patients and in some who have used neuroleptic drugs.

RESEARCH SUMMARY

Both oral and intravenous administration of L-deprenyl and L-phenylalanine in doses of 5 to 10 milligrams and 250 milligrams per day, respectively, demonstrated significant antidepressant effects in 155 unipolar depressed patients. In another preliminary study, L-phenylalanine was said to have mood-elevating effects in 31 of 40 depressed subjects. Followup is needed.

Several clinical studies have shown that L-phenylalanine may be helpful in the treatment of vitiligo in both children and adults. L-phenylalanine, in doses up to 100 mg/kg/day significantly improved vitiligo in 200 subjects when combined with UVA/sunlight. Best results were achieved in early-stage disease, but significant repigmentation occurred in some with later-stage disease who used the supplement/ sunlight combination for prolonged periods. Another study confirmed these effects but found that no added benefit was derived from doses exceeding 50 mg/kg/day.

Recently, other researchers have reported on their six-year experience in treating vitiligo with L-phenylalanine in combination with daily sun exposure. Subjects treated by these researchers received oral L-phenylalanine 50 or 100 mg/kg/day plus topical 10% phenylalanine gel daily. The total average improvement rate was rated at 83.1%, but the improvement rate limited to those judged to have good response was 56.7%, with a 90.3% rate for the face, 42.8% for the trunk and 37.1% for the limbs. This uncontrolled, retrospective study involved 193 patients, male and female, children and adults, with evolving vitiligo of various types. There was no statistically significant difference in response rates between those who received 50 mg/kg/day versus those receiving 100 mg/kg/day or between children and adults.

On the negative side, there is a report that a loading dose of 100 mg/kg of L-phenylalanine exacerbated symptoms of tardive dyskinesia in some neuroleptic-treated depressives. In another study, the same L-phenylalanine challenge exacerbated tardive dyskinesia symptoms in schizophrenic subjects.

CONTRAINDICATIONS, PRECAUTIONS, ADVERSE REACTIONS

CONTRAINDICATIONS

L-phenylalanine is contraindicated in those with phenylketonuria. It is also contraindicated in those taking non-selective monoamine oxidase (MAO) inhibitors. L-phenylalanine is contraindicated in those hypersensitive to any component of an L-phenylalanine-containing supplement.

PRECAUTIONS

Pregnant women and nursing mothers should avoid supplementation with L-phenylalanine.

Tardive dyskinesia has been reported to be exacerbated after ingestion of L-phenylalanine by schizophrenics. Therefore, those with schizophrenia should exercise extreme caution in the use of supplemental L-phenylalanine.

Use of L-phenylalanine for vitiligo must be done under medical supervision.

Those with hypertension should exercise caution in the use of L-phenylalanine.

ADVERSE REACTIONS

L-phenylalanine will exacerbate symptoms of phenylketonuria if used by phenylketonurics. L-phenylalanine was reported to exacerbate tardive dyskinesia when used by some with schizophrenia.

INTERACTIONS

DRUGS

Non-selective monoamine oxidase (MAO) inhibitors: including phenelzine sulfate, tranylcypromine sulfate and pargyline HC1 — Concomitant use of L-phenylalanine and non-selective MAO inhibitors may cause hypertension.

Selegiline: L-phenylalanine and the selective MAO inhibitor selegiline may have synergistic antidepressant activity if used concomitantly.

Neuroleptic Drugs: L-phenylalanine may potentiate the tardive dyskinesia side reactions of neuroleptic drugs if used concomitantly with them.

OVERDOSAGE

There are no reports of Phenylalanine overdosage in the literature.

DOSAGE AND ADMINISTRATION

L-phenylalanine supplements as well as DL-phenylalanine (see DL-Phenylalanine) supplements are available in the nutritional supplement marketplace. Those who use L-phenylalanine supplements typically use 500 milligrams to 1.5 grams daily.

LITERATURE

Birkmayer W, Riederer P, Linauer W, Knoll J. L-deprenyl plus L-phenylalanine in the treatment of depression. *J Neural Transm.* 1984; 59:81-87.

Camacho F, Mazuecos J. Treatment of vitiligo with oral and topical phenylalanine: 6 years of experience. *Arch Dermatol.* 1999; 135:216-217.

Gardos G, Cole JO, Matthews JD, et al. The acute effects of a loading dose of phenylalanine in unipolar depressed patients with and without tardive dyskinesia. *Neuropsychopharmacology.* 1992; 6:241-247.

Gibbs J, Falasco JD, McHugh PR. Cholecystokinin-decreased food intake in rhesus monkeys. *Am J Physiol.* 1976; 230:15-18.

Kostiuk PG, Martyniuk AE. [Possible molecular mechanisms of brain dysfunction in phenylketonuria.] [Article in Russian.] *Patol Fiziol Eksp Ter.* 1992; Jul-Aug(4):34-36.

Kuiters GR, Hup JM, Siddiqui AH, Cormane RH. Oral phenylalanine loading and sunlight as source of UVA irradiation in vitiligo on the Caribbean island of Curacao. *J Trop Med Hyg.* 1986; 89:149-155.

Mosnik DM, Spring B, Rogers K, Baruah S. Tardive dyskinesia exacerbated after ingestion of phenylalanine by schizophrenic patients. *Neuropsycopharmacology.* 1997; 16:136-146.

Sabelli HC, Fawcett J, Gusovsky F, et al. Clinical studies on the phenylalanine hypothesis of affective disorder: urine and blood phenylacetic acid and phenylalanine dietary supplements. *J Clin Psychiatry.* 1986; 47:66-70.

Schulpis CH, Antoniou C, Michas T, Starigos J. Phenylalanine plus ultraviolet light: preliminary report of a promising treatment for childhood vitiligo. *Pediatr Dermatol.* 1989; 6:332-335.

Siddiqui AH, Stolk LM, Bhaggoe R, et al. L-phenylalanine and UVA irradiation in the treatment of vitiligo. *Dermatology.* 1994; 188:215-218.

Zhao G. [Inherited metabolic aberration of phenylalanine in the family members of patients with essential hypertension and stroke]. [Article in Chinese]. *Chung Hua I Hsueh Tsa Chih.* 1991; 71:388-390.

L-Theanine

DESCRIPTION

L-theanine is a non-protein amino acid mainly found naturally in the green tea plant (*Camellia sinensis*). It is also found naturally in only one other known source, the edible mushroom *Boletus badius*, commonly known as the Bay bolete. L-theanine is the predominant amino acid in green tea and makes up 50% of the total free amino acids in the plant. The amino acid constitutes between 1% and 2% of the dry weight of green tea leaves. L-theanine is considered the main component responsible for the taste of green tea, which in Japanese is called umami. Umami, which was first described by a Japanese scientist over a hundred years ago, is now considered one of the five basic tastes: sweet, salty, sour, bitter and umami. Umami is the Japanese term for savory. L-theanine has been marketed in Japan for several years as a nutritional supplement for mood modulation and entered the United States dietary supplement marketplace a few years ago.

L-theanine is a derivative of L-glutamic acid. It is a water-soluble solid substance with the molecular formula $C_7H_{14}O_3N$ and a molecular weight of 160.19 daltons. L-theanine is also known as gamma-ethylamino-L-glutamic acid, gamma-glutamylethylamide, r-glutamylethylamide, L-glutamic acid gamma-ethylamide and L-N-ethylglutamine. The chemical structure is:

L-theanine

ACTIONS AND PHARMACOLOGY

ACTIONS

L-theanine may have activity in modulating the metabolism of cancer chemotherapeutic agents and ameliorating their side effects. It may also have mood-modulating activity and neuroprotective and immunoprotective effects.

MECHANISM OF ACTION

In animal tumor models, L-theanine has been found to increase the antitumor activity of some anthracyline agents (doxorubicin, idarubicin) and to ameliorate some of the side effects of these agents. It appears that L-theanine inhibits the efflux of these agents from tumor cells, increasing the inhibitory concentration of the drugs in the target cells. At the same time, L-theanine appears to decrease the oxidative stress caused by these agents on normal cells. Most of the side effects of these agents are due to oxidative stress. The mechanism by which L-theanine inhibits the efflux of such cancer chemotherapeutic agents as doxorubicin is unclear. L-theanine appears to have modest antioxidant activity, and this may explain, in part, L-theanine's ability to ameliorate some of the side effects of the chemotherapeutic agents. Further, L-theanine, by an unclear mechanism, appears to inhibit the influx of chemotherapeutic normal cells.

The mechanism of L-theanine's possible mood-modulating activity is also unclear. The amino acid might affect the metabolism and the release of some neurotransmitters in the brain, such as dopamine.

Human gamma-delta T cells are known to mediate innate immunity to microbes through T cell receptor-dependent recognition of unprocessed antigens with conserved molecular patterns. The nonpeptide alkylamine antigens are shared by bacteria fungi, parasites, tumor cells and edible plant substances, including mushrooms, apples and green tea. It has been shown that L-theanine, a precursor of the nonpeptide antigen ethylamine, primed peripheral blood gamma-delta T cells to mediate a memory response on reexposure to ethylamine and to secrete interferon (IFN)-gamma in response to bacteria. Such priming may enhance innate immunity to bacteria and tumor cells and may account for some of the health benefits of green tea.

PHARMACOKINETICS

Little is known about the pharmacokinetics of L-theanine in humans. From animal studies, it appears that L-theanine is absorbed from the small intestine via a sodium-coupled active transport process and appears to cross the blood-brain barrier. It has been found in rat studies that the D-enantiomer of theanine may decrease the absorption of L-theanine, the L-enantiomer. It is unclear if D-theanine possesses any of the actions found with L-theanine. Not much is known beyond that. However, research is ongoing.

INDICATIONS AND USAGE

L-theanine has exhibited anticancer effects and an ability to favorably modulate the activity of some anticancer drugs in *in vitro* and animal experiments. It has also demonstrated hypotensive effects in animal work. It has inhibited LDL-cholesterol oxidation in preliminary *in vitro* tests. It was recently reported to enhance learning ability in animals and to induce relaxation in human subjects, possibly through its effects on serotonin, dopamine and other neurotransmitters. It has also been shown to inhibit caffeine stimulation in another preliminary animal study. It demonstrates some neuroprotective and immunoprotective effects.

RESEARCH SUMMARY

L-theanine has been shown to enhance the anticancer activity of doxorubicin and idarubicin in *in vitro* and animal studies. In an *in vitro* study, L-theanine increased doxorubicin's inhibition of Ehrlich ascites carcinoma more than two-fold and increased nearly three-fold the concentration of doxorubicin in the tumor compared with treatment with doxorubicin alone.

Subsequently, L-theanine, in combination with doxorubicin, was shown to significantly reduce tumor weight (to 62% of the control level) in M5076 ovarian sarcoma-bearing mice. The doxorubicin dose used in this combination was ineffective by itself in inhibiting tumor growth. L-theanine was reported to increase doxorubicin concentration in the tumor by two- to seven-fold while simultaneously decreasing doxorubicin concentrations in normal tissues.

A combination of L-theanine and doxorubicin significantly inhibited both primary ovarian sarcoma and hepatic metastasis of the tumor. L-theanine was credited in this study with enhancing the activity of doxorubicin.

In another study, L-theanine was used in conjunction with idarubicin, an anthracycline derivative used clinically to treat acute myelocytic leukemia. The use of idarubicin has been limited due to the frequency with which it produces severe leukopenia. Combined with idarubicin in the treatment of P388 leukemia-bearing mice, L-theanine significantly inhibited suppression of bone marrow cells and leukopenia, while simultaneously enhancing the antitumor activity of idarubicin.

L-theanine, in combination with doxorubicin, was further shown to have the ability to significantly inhibit even doxorubicin-resistant leukemia in mice.

In an *in vitro* test, L-theanine showed some ability to inhibit LDL peroxidation. The polyphenol component of a green-tea extract was more potent in this regard than the L-theanine component. The caffeine component, on the other hand, was less effective than L-theanine.

L-theanine has also exhibited hypotensive effects in spontaneously hypertensive rats but not in Wistar kyoto rats. Recently, L-theanine, at certain doses, was shown to inhibit caffeine stimulation, measured by electroencephalography in rats.

L-theanine, previously shown to penetrate the blood-brain barrier through the leucine-preferring transport system, has been demonstrated to produce significant increases in serotonin and/or dopamine concentrations in the brain, principally in the striatum, hypothalamus and hippocampus.

These findings led to recent studies investigating the possibility that L-theanine might enhance learning ability, induce relaxation and relieve emotional stress. Memory and learning ability were said to be improved in young male Wistar rats given 180 mg of L-theanine daily for four months. Performance was assessed using a test for learning ability and passive and active avoidance tests for memory.

In another recent study, rats fed L-theanine for three weeks *ad libitum* showed some signs of improved memory and learning. In a double-blind, randomized, placebo-controlled trial, the cognitive mood effects of L-theanine (250 mg) and caffeine (150 mg) were investigated both in isolation and in combination. The combination was found to improve some measures of mood and cognition. The mental effects of L-theanine were tested in a small group of volunteers divided into two groups defined as "high-anxiety" and "low-anxiety" groups. The volunteers were females aged 18 to 22. Their level of anxiety was assessed by a manifest anxiety scale. Subjects received water, 50 mg of L-theanine or 200 mg of L-theanine solution once a week. Brain waves were measured 60 minutes after administration. The 200 mg dose (dissolved in 100 ml of water) resulted in significantly greater production of alpha waves than was observed in subjects receiving water. Greatest production was consistently seen about 40 minutes after L-theanine intake. The effect was dose-dependent. The researchers regarded the significantly increased production of alpha-brain wave activity as an index of increased relaxation. More rigorous follow-up is needed.

A neuroprotective effect of L-theanine was observed in mice following middle cerebral artery occlusion. Size of cerebral infarct was reduced.

Recently, L-theanine was credited with enhancement of peripheral blood T cells, boosting immunologic memory. More research is indicated.

CONTRAINDICATIONS, PRECAUTIONS, ADVERSE REACTIONS

CONTRAINDICATIONS
L-theanine is contraindicated in those who are hypersensitive to any component of an L-theanine-containing product.

PRECAUTIONS
Pregnant women and nursing mothers should avoid L-theanine supplements. Use of L-theanine supplements concomitantly with cancer chemotherapeutic agents must be done under medical supervision.

ADVERSE REACTIONS
There are no known adverse reactions.

INTERACTIONS

DRUGS
Doxorubicin and Idarubicin: L-theanine may enhance the antitumor effects of these drugs and may ameliorate some of their side effects.

DOSAGE AND ADMINISTRATION
L-theanine supplements have been available in Japan for some time for promotion of relaxation and modulation of mood. Doses used are between 50 and 200 mg, as necessary. L-theanine supplements are now available in the United States.

L-theanine is also available in some green tea preparations. The amino acid constitutes between 1% and 2% of the dry weight of green tea leaves. Two to three cups of green tea contain approximately 30-50 milligrams of the amino acid. Matcha, a variety of fine, powdered green tea used in the Japanese tea ceremony, has a higher amount of L-theanine when compared to other green tea varieties.

LITERATURE

Bryan J. Psychological effects of dietary components of tea: caffeine and L-theanine. *Nutr Rev.* 2008;66(2):82-90.

Bukowski JF, Percival SS. L-theanine intervention enhances human gammadeltaT lymphocyte function. *Nutr Rev.* 2008;66(2):96-102.

Desai MJ, Gill MS, Hsu WH, et al. Pharmacokinetics of theanine enantiomers in rats. *Chirality.* 2005;17(3):154-162.

Egashira N, Hayakawa K, Mishima K, et al. Neuroprotective effect of gamma-glutamylethylamide (theanine) on cerebral infarction in mice. *Neurosci Lett.* 2004;363(1):58-61.

Egashira N, Hayakawa K, Osajima M, et al. Involvement of GABA(A) receptors in the neuroprotective effect of theanine on focal cerebral ischemia in mice. *J Pharmacol Sci.* 2007;105(2):211-214.

Egashira N, Ishigami N, Pu F, et al. Theanine prevents memory impairment induced by repeated cerebral ischemia in rats. *Phytother Res.* 2008;22(1):65-68.

Eschenauer G, Sweet BV. Pharmacology and therapeutic uses of theanine. *Am J Health Syst Pharm.* 2006;63(1):26,28-30.

Haskell CF, Kennedy DO, Milne AL, et al. The effects of L-theanine, caffeine and their combination on cognition and mood. *Biol Psychol.* 2008;77(2):113-122.

Juneja LR, Chu D-C, Okubo T, et al. L-Theanine—a unique amino acid of green tea and its relaxation effect in humans. *Trends Food Sci Tech.* 1999;10:199-204.

Kakuda T. Neuroprotective effects of the green tea components theanine and catechins. *Biol Pharm Bull.* 2002;25(12):1513-1518.

Kakuda T, Nozawa A, Unno T, et al. Inhibiting effects of theanine on caffeine stimulation evaluated by EEG in the rat. *Biosci Biotechnol Biochem.* 2000;64:287-293.

Kamath AB, Wang L, Das H, et al. Antigens in tea-beverage prime human Vgamma 2Vdelta 2 T cells in vitro and in vivo for memory and nonmemory antibacterial cytokine responses. *Proc Natl Acad Sci USA.* 2003;100(10):6009-6014.

Kimura K, Ozeki M, Juneja LR, et al. L-Theanine reduces psychological and physiological stress responses. *Biol Psychol.* 2007;74(1):39-45.

Kitaoka S, Hayashi H, Yokogoshi H, et al. Transmural potential changes associated with the in vitro absorption of theanine in the guinea pig intestine. *Biosci Biotechnol Biochem.* 1996;60:1768-1771.

Nathan PJ, Lu K, Gray M, et al. The neuropharmacology of L-theanine(N-ethyl-L-glutamine): a possible neuroprotective and cognitive enhancing agent. *J Herb Pharmacother.* 2006;6(2):21-30.

Owen GN, Parnell H, De Bruin EA, et al. The combined effects of L-theanine and caffeine on cognitive performance and mood. *Nutr Neurosci.* 2008;11(4):193-198.

Sadzuka Y, Inoue C, Hirooka S, et al. Effects of theanine on alcohol metabolism and hepatic toxicity. *Biol Pharm Bull.* 2005;28(9):1702-1706.

Sadzuka Y, Sugiyama T, Miyagishima A, et al. The effects of theanine, as a novel biochemical modulator, on the antitumor activity of adriamycin. *Cancer Lett.* 1996;105:203-209.

Sadzuka Y, Sugiyama T, Sonobe T. Efficacies of tea components on doxorubicin induced antitumor activity and reversal of multidrug resistance. *Toxicology Lett.* 2000;113:155-162.

Sugiyama T, Sadzuka Y. Combination of theanine with doxorubicin inhibits hepatic metastasis of M5076 ovarian sarcoma. *Clin Cancer Res.* 1999;5:413-416.

Sugiyama T, Sadzuka Y. Enhancing effects of green tea components on the antitumor activity of adriamycin against M5076 ovarian carcinoma. *Cancer Lett.* 1998;133:19-26.

Sugiyama T, Sadzuka Y. Theanine, a specific glutamate derivative in green tea, reduces the adverse reactions of doxorubicin by changing the glutathione level. *Cancer Lett.* 2004;212(2):177-184.

Sugiyama T, Sadzuka Y, Sonobe T. Theanine, a major amino acid in green tea, inhibits leukopenia and enhances antitumor activity induce by idarubicin. *Proc Am Assoc Cancer Res.* 1999;40:10(Abstract 63).

Yamada T, Terashima T, Honma H, et al. Effects of theanine, a unique amino acid in tea leaves, on memory in a rat behavioral test. *Biosci Biotechnol Biochem.* 2008;72(5):1356-1359.

Yamada T, Terashima T, Kawano S, et al. Theanine, gamma-glutamylethylamide, a unique amino acid in tea leaves, modulates neurotransmitter concentrations in the brain striatum interstitium in conscious rats. *Amino Acids.* Epub: 2008 Jan 15.

Yokogoshi H, Kato Y, Sagesaka YM, et al. Reduction effect of theanine on blood pressure and brain 5-hydroxyindoles in spontaneous hypertensive rats. *Biosci Biotechnol Biochem.* 1995;59:615-618.

Yokogoshi H, Kobayashi M. Hypotensive effect of gamma-glutamylmethylamide in spontaneously hypertensive rats. *Life Sci.* 1998;62:1065-1068.

Yokogoshi H, Kobayashi M, Mochizuki M, et al. Effect of theanine, r-glutamylethylamide on brain monoamines and striatal dopamine release in conscious rats. *Neurochem Res.* 1998;23:667-673.

L-Tryptophan

DESCRIPTION

L-tryptophan is one of the eight essential amino acids for humans (10 for children). It is the least abundant essential amino acid. An essential amino acid is an amino acid that the body can not make, or if it can, it does not make it in sufficient amounts for all of its biological needs (for example, L-histidine and L-arginine for children). L-tryptophan is a protein amino acid, meaning that it is a building block of proteins. L-tryptophan also has other important functions. It is the precursor of the neurotransmitter serotonin, the pineal gland hormone melatonin (see Melatonin), the possible neuroprotectant kynurenic acid, vitamin B_3 (niacin or nicotinic acid and niacinamide or nicotinamide), and the coenzymes NADH (nicotinamide adenine dinucleotide) and NADPH (nicotinamide adenine dinucleotide phosphate).

A deficiency of niacin and/or L-tryptophan causes pellagra, which is characterized by the three Ds of dermatitis, diarrhea and dementia and, if untreated for some time, a fourth D,

death. Pellagra is a vitamin B_3 deficiency disease caused by dietary lack of niacin and protein, especially proteins containing the essential amino acid L-tryptophan. Because L-tryptophan can be converted into niacin, foods with L-tryptophan but without niacin, such as milk, prevent pellagra. However, if dietary L-tryptophan is diverted into the production of protein, niacin deficiency may still exist, leading to pellagra.

By the end of the 1980s, some millions of people, mainly women and mainly in the United States, were using supplemental L-tryptophan for a variety of reasons—premenstrual syndrome (PMS), sleep disorders, anxiety, depression, fibromyalgia, seasonal affective disorder (SAD) and chronic pain syndromes. Supplemental L-tryptophan was also used as an adjunct in the treatment of cocaine, amphetamine, alcohol and other drug abuse and for jet lag. In the context of the intensive care unit, some physicians used it as a sedative to help relax their intensive care unit patients with a substance that was less likely to suppress their respiration than a pharmaceutical sedative might. The physicians thought that this was particularly useful for those patients who had compromised respiration to begin with.

In fact, there were even some clinical studies that appeared to support some of the above uses of L-tryptophan.

In the fall of 1989, L-tryptophan supplementation was to see its darkest days. In October 1989, Dr. Philip Herzman and his colleagues in New Mexico met to compare notes on three female patients with unusual clinical presentations involving myalgia (muscle pain), weakness, oral ulcers, abdominal pain, skin rash and a striking increase in eosinophils (a subset of white blood cells) in their blood. These physicians recognized that all three patients developed these symptoms after using supplemental L-tryptophan, and they thought that the supplemental L-tryptophan might have caused the problem. They reported the illnesses and their suspected association of the illnesses to supplemental L-tryptophan to the New Mexico Health and Environment Department and the CDC (Centers for Disease Control and Prevention). The New Mexico Health and Environmental Department discovered several similar cases, almost all of which involved supplemental L-tryptophan. As awareness of the problem grew—the CDC notified all state health departments about a health problem possibly due to ingestion of supplemental L-tryptophan—a number of cases were reported from other states. In November 1989, the CDC proposed the name of eosinophilia-myalgia syndrome, or EMS, for the disease, since all the presumptive cases had both eosinophilia (elevation of eosinophils in their blood) and severe myalgia (muscle pain). Since trichinosis also causes eosinophilia and myalgia, the initial CDC surveillance definition of an EMS case required serological testing or a muscle biopsy to rule out trichinosis. However, since the clinical presentation of EMS was sufficiently distinct from trichinosis, the initial requirement of negative testing for trichinosis was dropped from the surveillance definition.

The association between use of supplemental L-tryptophan and EMS was a strong one and on November 11, 1989, the FDA issued a nationwide warning advising consumers to discontinue the use of L-tryptophan supplements and subsequently requested a nationwide recall of all L-tryptophan products sold over-the-counter. With the removal of L-tryptophan supplements from the marketplace, the number of reported new cases of EMS dropped rapidly. As of June 1993, 1,511 cases of EMS had been reported to the CDC, including 37 deaths. Although the preponderance of EMS cases came from the United States, 97 cases were reported from Germany, 24 from France, 16 from Canada, three each from Switzerland and Belgium, two each from the UK, and Japan and one each from Spain and Australia. In the United States, 84% of the cases were women and 97% non-Hispanic white, and the highest incidence of EMS cases was in the Western states. In terms of risk factors, the number one risk factor for EMS was the use of L-tryptophan supplements. The dose of supplemental L-tryptophan and the age of the user were also considered risk factors for EMS. Older users of L-tryptophan were more likely to develop EMS than younger users and the risk of developing EMS increased with larger doses of L-tryptophan. A 50% attack rate was demonstrated in those who ingested more than four grams of L-tryptophan on a regular basis, suggesting that the EMS agent was a toxicant.

The hunt for possible toxicants and contaminants in the suspected L-tryptophan supplements that could be identified as causing EMS immediately began, but, although some suspects were identified, none was positively identified that could have caused EMS.

In 1991, the FDA banned L-tryptophan supplements from sale in the U.S. In 2001, the FDA loosened the restriction on the marketing of L-tryptophan supplements, but did ban its importation except under certain circumstances. As of May 2, 2005, the FDA completely cancelled the import ban alert for L-tryptophan. Following this, L-tryptophan supplements began again appearing on the nutritional supplement marketplace, including in health food stores, compounding pharmacies and over the Internet, where they continue to be found.

L-tryptophan is chemically described as (2*S*)-2-amino-3-(1*H*-indol-3-yl)propanoic acid.

It is also known as (*S*)-alpha-amino-1*H*-indole-3-propanoic acid and 2-amino-3-indolylpropanoic acid. It is abbreviated as Trp or by its one-letter designation W. Its empirical formula is $C_{11}H_{12}N_2O_2$, its molecular weight is 204.22 and

its CAS Registry Number is 73-23-3. The minimum daily requirement for L-tryptophan is said to be 0.25 grams daily for males and 0.15 grams for females. The average Western diet contains about one to three grams daily. L-tryptophan is represented by the following chemical structure.

L-Tryptophan

ACTIONS AND PHARMACOLOGY

ACTIONS

L-tryptophan may have antidepressant activity, activity against premenstrual syndrome (PMS) and sleep-promoting activity.

MECHANISM OF ACTION

Antidepressant activity: A Cochrane Collaboration meta-analysis concluded that although a number of studies were performed to determine if L-tryptophan and 5-hydroxytryptophan (5-HT, see 5-Hydroxytryptophan) possessed antidepressant activity, only a few were of sufficient quality to be reliable. However, those few did suggest that both L-tryptophan and 5-hydroxytryptophan were better than placebo at alleviating depression. The authors also stated that "further studies are needed to evaluate the efficacy and safety of 5-HT and tryptophan before their widespread use can be recommended." The possible antidepressant effect is accounted for by the conversion of L-tryptophan and 5-hydroxytryptophan to the neurotransmitter serotonin.

In a double-bind placebo-controlled trial of L-tryptophan combined with the selective serotonin reuptake inhibitor (SSRI) fluoxetine, it was found that combining 20 milligrams of fluoxetine with two to four grams of L-tryptophan daily for a group diagnosed with major depressive disorder produced a more rapid antidepressant effect when compared with those patients who just used fluoxetine alone. The tryptophan group also seemed to have a protective effect on slow-wave sleep. The four gram per day dose of L-tryptophan, but not the two gram per day dose, produced daytime drowsiness. Again, the mechanism of action of the L-tryptophan was most likely due to its conversion to the neurotransmitter serotonin in the brain.

The mechanism of the possible antidepressant activity of L-tryptophan is accounted for by its conversion to the neurotransmitter serotonin, which plays a central role in the affective state. Antidepressants may work by either binding to one or more of the family of serotonin 5-HT receptors (5-

HT1—5-HT7) or by inhibiting the reuptake of serotonin. The tricyclic antidepressants may work, in part, by binding to the serotonin 5-HT6 receptor, a member of the G protein superfamily, which is positively coupled to an adenylate cyclase second-messenger system. The selective serotonin reuptake inhibitors (SSRIs) selectively inhibit the reuptake of serotonin.

Anti-premenstrual syndrome (PMS) activity: Prior to the recall of L-tryptophan in 1989, L-tryptophan supplementation was used by many women for relief of PMS symptoms. A number of studies lent some support to this use. One placebo-controlled clinical trial of L-tryptophan in PMS showed that increasing serotonin levels during the late luteal phase of the menstrual cycle via administration of L-tryptophan had a beneficial effect in patients with PMS.

Sleep-promoting activity: Over the course of more than 40 years, a number of studies have suggested that L-tryptophan reduces sleep latency, produces an increase in rated subjective sleepiness and a decrease in total wakefulness and/or increase in sleep time. The best results have been in those with mild insomnia. It is thought that the sleep-promoting effect of L-tryptophan is accounted for by its conversion to the neurohormone melatonin.

A recent study determined the effect of L-tryptophan intake on age-related changes in the activity-rest circadian rhythms and c-fos expression of ring doves with aging. C-fos is a cellular proto-oncogene. Neuroscientists measure expression of c-fos as an indirect marker of neuronal activity because c-fos is often expressed when neurons fire action potentials. The suprachiasmatic nucleus (SCN) is a bilateral region of the brain, located in the hypothalamus, which is responsible for controlling endogenous circadian rhythms. The hormonal and neuronal activities it generates regulate many different bodily functions over a 24-hour period. Both L-tryptophan and melatonin, a metabolite of L-tryptophan made in the pineal gland, reduced the nocturnal activity of all ring doves. However, only the highest doses were effective in the old ring doves. Sleep parameters, calculated from the activity data, indicated worsened sleep quality in old animals, but it was improved with the treatments. In addition, the expression of c-fos in the suprachiasmatic nucleus was reduced after both treatments.

The suprachiasmatic nucleus appears to be the target for the observed nocturnal effects of L-tryptophan and melatonin. Further, this supports the use of L-tryptophan to reverse the disturbances of the circadian activity-rest cycle related with aging.

PHARMACOKINETICS
Following ingestion, L-tryptophan is absorbed from the small intestine by a sodium-dependent active transport process. L-tryptophan is transported from the small intestine to the liver via the portal circulation. In the liver, L-tryptophan is involved in a number of biochemical reactions, including protein synthesis and oxidative catabolic reactions. L-tryptophan that is not metabolized in the liver is distributed via the systemic circulation to the various organs and tissues of the body where it undergoes metabolic reactions similar to those that take place in the liver. L-tryptophan can cross the blood-brain barrier via an active transport mechanism. L-tryptophan is the precursor of serotonin (5-hydroxytyramine, or 5-HT), melatonin, kynurenine, nicotinic acid and nicotinamide adenine dinucleotide (NAD). Within the CNS, greater than 95% of L-tryptophan is catabolized through the kynurenine (KYN) pathway, resulting, among other things, in the production of neuroactive intermediates, which can be neurotoxic or neuroprotective.

L-tryptophan is converted into serotonin in two steps, the first via the enzyme tryptophan hydroxylase to 5-hydroxytryptophan (5-HTP) and the second via vitamin B_6-dependent L-aromatic amino acid decarboxylase to serotonin, or 5-HT. Serotonin is subsequently metabolized to 5-hydroxyindole acetaldehyde, which is rapidly metabolized to 5-hydroxyindoleacetic acid (5-HIAA) via the enzyme monoamine oxidase (MAO).

The uptake of the serotonin precursor L-tryptophan into the brain depends on nutrients that influence the availability of L-tryptophan by changing the ratio of plasma L-tryptophan to the sum of the other large neutral amino acids (LNAAs). The LNAAs are L-valine, L-leucine, L-isoleucine, L-phenylalanine and L-tyrosine. The ratio of L-tryptophan to the LNAAs is increased by foods such as carbohydrates and the whey protein alpha-lactalbumin. An increase in the plasma L-tryptophan to LNAA ratio is considered to be an indirect indication of increased availability of brain serotonin.

L-tryptophan is converted into melatonin in four steps—the first via the enzyme tryptophan hydroxylase to 5-hydroxytryptophan and the second via vitamin B_6-dependent L-aromatic amino acid decarboxylase to serotonin. Serotonin is then metabolized to N-acetylserotonin via serotonin N-acetyltransferase and finally to melatonin via the enzyme hydroxyindole-O-methyltransferase, using S-adenosylmethionine (SAMe) as the methyl donor.

L-tryptophan is converted into niacin in six steps: L-tryptophan to kynurenine via tryptophan pyrrolase, kynurenine to 3-hydroxykynurenine, 3-hydroxykynurenine to 3-hydroxyanthranlic acid, 3-hydroxyanthranilic acid to carboxymuconic aldehyde intermediate, carboxymuconic aldehyde intermediate to quinolinic acid and quinolinic acid to nicotinic acid. Carboxymuconic aldehyde intermediate is also converted to picolinic acid.

The kynurenine pathway is the major pathway of L-tryptophan catabolism. It is also responsible for the biosynthesis of the coenzyme nicotinamide adenine dinucleotide, or NAD. 95% of L-tryptophan ingested from the diet is metabolized via the kynurenine pathway, while only a small amount is converted into 5-hydroxytryptamine, or serotonin.

There has been increasing interest in the kynurenine pathway over the last few years for a several reasons. A number of important physiological functions have been associated with this pathway, including behavior and thermoregulation; it is implicated in a number of different neurological disorders, including Alzheimer's disease, Huntington's disease, Parkinson's disease, cognitive decline, cerebral ischemia, convulsive disorders, HIV/AIDS dementia and schizophrenia. The kynurenine pathway possesses neuroactive metabolites with different biological properties, including prooxidant and antioxidant activities, and proinflammatory and anti-inflammatory activities. It also appears to be involved in neuroprotection, immune regulation and tumor inhibition. Clearly, this is an extremely complex pathway with a wide range of effects, both negative and positive, and much study of it is needed and certainly warranted.

In the liver, the indole ring of L-tryptophan is oxidatively excised via the enzyme tryptophan 2,3-dioxygenase (TDO) to produce N-formyl kynurenine. In the brain and peripheral tissues, the enzyme responsible for this reaction is indolamine 2,3-dioxygenase (IDO), which requires superoxide anions for its activity. Therefore, IDO requires enzymatic systems that generate oxidative species. IDO is inhibited by superoxide dismutase (SOD) and nitric oxide (NO). Significantly, IDO may itself act as an antioxidant. The next step in the kynurenine pathway is the degradation of N-formyl kynurenine to L-kynurenine via the enzyme kynurenine formamidase. L-kynurenine can serve as a substrate for the enzyme kynurenase, which converts it to anthranilic acid, kynurenine 3-hydroxylase, which converts it to 3-hydroxykynurenine and kynurenine aminotranferases, which are responsible for the irreversible transamination of L-kynurenine to kynurenic acid.

The kynurenine pathway then proceeds to the formation of quinolinic acid via a few steps, starting with the hydroxylation of L-kynurenine to 3-hydroxykynurenine catalyzed by kynurenine 3-hydroxylase, followed by the conversion of 3-hydroxykynurenine to 3-hydroxyanthranilic acid. 3-hydroxyanthranilate dioxygenase then opens the ring of 3-hydroxyanthranilic acid to produce 2-amino-3-carboxymuconate-semialdehyde, which is rapidly transformed into quinolinic acid. Quinolinic acid is metabolized to nicotinic acid dinucleotide (NAD) via quinolate phosphoribosyl tranferase.

Urinary metabolites of tryptophan include 3-hydroxykynurenine, xanthurenic acid and 5-hydroxyindoleacetic acid (5-HIAA). The major metabolite of L-tryptophan found in the feces is skatole (3-methylindloe).

INDICATIONS AND USAGE

L-tryptophan, an essential amino acid and precursor of the neurotransmitter serotonin, though previously banned by the FDA, is again available as a nutritional supplement. Once possibly associated with a deadly autoimmune disorder called eosinophilia-myalgia syndrome (EMS), the FDA banned most of it from sale in the United States in 1991. The possible association with EMS, however, was never conclusively proved, and some researchers questioned the data linking the amino acid with EMS. Subsequently, in 2001, the FDA relaxed restrictions on marketing the substance (though at the time it continued to prohibit its importations from other countries). It did so, however, with reservations at the time, stating: "Based on the scientific evidence that is available at the present time, we cannot determine with certainty that the occurrence of EMS in susceptible persons consuming L-tryptophan supplements derives from the content of L-tryptophan, an impurity contained in the L-tryptophan, or a combination of the two in association with other, as yet unknown, external factors." As of May 2, 2005, the FDA completely cancelled the import alert.

Claims for L-tryptophan (found, for example, in meats, dairy products, various seeds, some grains, bananas, mangoes, dried dates, spirulina, some nuts and in protein-based foods generally), include antidepressant, sedative, hypnotic, anti-insomnia effects. It is said to have mood-modulating properties capable of ameliorating some of the symptoms of premenstrual syndrome and seasonal affective disorder. It has also been suggested that it might be helpful in more serious mental disturbances, including schizophrenia and bipolar disorder, and that it could have some ability to attenuate amphetamine abuse. It has also been claimed that it has anti-inflammatory effects.

RESEARCH SUMMARY

When a 1989 EMS outbreak resulting in 37 deaths and some 1,500 cases of permanent disability was linked by some to consumption of L-tryptophan supplements, the FDA soon acted to largely restrict the marketing and importation of the amino acid. Some claimed that there was evidence that the tryptophan that caused the problem was produced by one Japanese manufacturer. Additionally, a group of researchers reported that they found an impurity in the tryptophan produced by that manufacturer and they concluded that this was the most likely cause of the EMS outbreak, not the tryptophan itself. Further confounding the situation, however, were other reports that the problem could not conclusively be linked to the Japanese manufacturer and that EMS had been associated with use of L-tryptophan both prior to and after the 1989 incident. Some others reported that excessive use of the amino acid, rather than any contaminant, might be the culprit, arguing that excess use results in metabolites that lead to impaired histamine metabolism, compromised histamine degradation and excessive histamine activity, which, in turn, they claim, can contribute to or cause EMS. However, none of that was ever proved. Hence the FDA eventually relaxed its restrictions on the marketing and importation of the amino acid.

As a number of researchers have noted over the years, L-tryptophan, as the precursor to serotonin synthesis, is a plausible candidate as a "natural" antidepressant. It is, in fact, licensed as an approved antidepressant in several countries. Generally, however, its efficacy as an antidepressant has been demonstrated in an adjunctive role with other established antidepressants, notably monoamine oxidative inhibitors. Evidence for its ability to combat depression on its own is not as clearly established. Clinical studies to date involving L-tryptophan and 5-hydroxytryptophan (5-HTP), which derives from the amino acid and crosses the blood-brain barrier and is converted to serotonin in the dopaminergic and serotonergic neurons, have yielded mixed results with respect to depression. Given its availability in the neurons just mentioned, it would be expected to have an antidepressant effect in some individuals and, in fact, it does in some studies, does not in some others and has a weak effect in still others. Some studies have found evidence that convinced their authors that the amino acid has effects similar to widely used serotonergic antidepressants.

A review of the literature recently led another group of researchers to conclude, however, that the data, so far, is inconclusive. Additionally, because the amino acid is not entirely clear of the EMS cloud, even at this late date, these authors clearly found the use of the substance unappealing. They did, however, state that large, well-designed, placebo-controlled studies are indicated. It should be mentioned in passing that one dated paper suggested that L-tryptophan might be more effective than lithium carbonate alone in the treatment of bipolar and schizophrenic patients. Follow-up is lacking and no conclusions can be drawn.

Claims that L-tryptophan might be a useful sleep aid, combating insomnia, are based on a few studies. One of these, dating back almost 40 years, described supplementation with the amino acid in seven patients suffering insomnia. It was claimed that they enjoyed increases in total sleep. Another dated paper, this one a review of several studies of the amino acid related to sleep, concluded that L-tryptophan has clinical hypnotic value. The studies upon which this review was based, however, were small and mostly poorly controlled, and the observed effects were often weak in terms of increased total sleep. Data were better in support of the claim of reduced sleep latency (time to fall asleep). The best effects, according to another reviewer, have been seen in normal (non-insomnia) subjects who have trouble initially falling asleep (latency) and in those with mild insomnia. Reduction in sleep latency has been achieved in these studies with, typically, doses of 1 to 15 grams of the amino acid. The sedative effect of L-tryptophan is attributed by some to either direct central serotonergic activation or to an indirect increase in melatonin levels or both.

L-tryptophan's relationship to melatonin (it is a melatonin precursor) has recently been studied on another front. Several studies have demonstrated that melatonin has some positive effects on animal models of ulcerative colitis, experimental pancreatitis and septic shock owing to its ability to favorably modulate a number of inflammatory factors. One recent study using a mouse contact hypersensitivity model reported a positive L-tryptophan effect reportedly achieved by promoting the production of the anti-inflammatory cytokine interleuken-10.

The possible role of L-tryptophan in the premenstrual syndrome (PMS) has been periodically investigated for some time. Some early research suggested a relationship between mood and other cyclical PMS changes and tryptophan metabolism. More recently, a pilot study of 13 patients diagnosed with late luteal phase dysphoric disorder (premenstrual depression) were treated with 6 grams daily of the amino acid with reported good results: significant amelioration of symptoms (depression, irritability, insomnia, carbohydrate craving). A prior study using only 1.5 grams of the amino acid daily had shown no positive result. Hence, these researchers stressed the need for the higher dosage used in their study. In a more rigorous follow-up study, the same group administered 6 grams of L-tryptophan to 37 patients with the same disorder and compared them with 34 matched controls who received placebo in a double-blind fashion. Treatments were administered for 17 days from time of ovulation to the third day of menstruation in each of three consecutive menstrual cycles. Again, the amino acid produced positive results based, it was said, upon its ability to increase serotonin synthesis during the late luteal phase of the menstrual cycle.

In a small open study, L-tryptophan was as effective as light therapy in vanquishing the symptoms of seasonal affective disorder (SAD). The amino acid was thought to be more durable than light in terms of treating SAD, in that relapse seemed to occur more slowly after withdrawal of L-tryptophan than it did after withdrawal of the light therapy.

Dietary tryptophan attenuated amphetamine self-administration in the rat in yet another study.

Given the various positive results achieved with this amino acid, research is clearly needed to definitively determine whether it is implicated in any way in EMS. If it is not, then clearly far more research is needed and warranted to follow up on these positive results in disparate, significant (and, in some cases, currently very difficult-to-treat) disorders. In this regard, it is worth noting that a prescription-only tryptophan product has been available since 1985 with, one group of researchers has stated, no cases of EMS reported.

CONTRAINDICATIONS, PRECAUTIONS, ADVERSE REACTIONS

CONTRAINDICATIONS
Supplemental L-tryptophan is contraindicated in those hypersensitive to any component of an L-tryptophan-containing supplement.

PRECAUTIONS
Those who are interested in the use of L-tryptophan for any health condition should first discuss its use with his or her physician.

L-tryptophan should be avoided during or within 2 weeks after discontinuing the use of monoamine oxidase inhibitors (MAOIs).

Those with cataracts should be cautious in the use of L-tryptophan. Animal data suggest that photo-oxidation of L-tryptophan and some of its metabolites, particularly the metabolites found in the kynurenine pathway, may be involved in cataract formation. However, cataracts secondary to L-tryptophan use have not been reported in humans.

Those with bladder cancer should be cautious in the use of L-tryptophan. Some, but not all, animal studies have shown a relationship between L-tryptophan supplementation and bladder cancer. (There are no human reports of bladder cancer associated with the use of supplementary L-tryptophan.) It is thought that the risk for bladder cancer may be linked to a disorder of the metabolism of L-tryptophan that may be corrected by the administration of vitamin B_6.

Those with diabetes or a family history of diabetes should be cautious in the use of L-tryptophan. The L-tryptophan metabolite xanthurenic acid has been found to have a diabetogenic effect in animals. There are no human reports of diabetes associated with the use of supplemental L-tryptophan.

L-tryptophan should not be used concurrently with any antidepressant, including selective serotonin reuptake inhibitors (SSRIs), tricyclic antidepressants or monoamine oxidase inhibitors (MAOIs). Concurrent use of L-tryptophan with any of these antidepressants may increase the risk of adverse reactions.

L-tryptophan should not be used concurrently with serotonin 5-HT1 receptor agonists, including naratriptan, sumatriptan, almotriptan, frovatriptan and zolmitriptan. Such use may increase the risk of adverse reactions.

L-tryptophan should be avoided by pregnant women and nursing mothers.

ADVERSE REACTIONS
Eosinophilia-myalgia syndrome (EMS). See Description and Research Summary above.

L-tryptophan in doses below five grams daily may cause daytime drowsiness, dizziness and dry mouth. Higher doses of L-tryptophan may cause nausea, anorexia and headache, as well as dizziness and daytime drowsiness.

INTERACTIONS

DRUGS
5-HT1 receptor agonists (naratriptan, sumatriptan, almotriptan, frovatriptan, zolmitriptan): Concurrent use of L-tryptophan with a 5-HT1 agonist may increase the risk of adverse reactions.

Monoamine oxidase inhibitors (MAOIs, eg, isocarboxazid, phenelzine sulfate, tranylcypromine): Concurrent use of L-tryptophan with an MAOI (type A) may increase the risk of adverse reactions.

Selective serotonin reuptake inhibitors (SSRIs, such as citalopram, escitalopram, fluvoxamine maleate, fluoxetine, paroxetine, sertraline, venlafaxine): Concurrent use of L-tryptophan with an SSRI may potentiate the antidepressant effect of the SSRI and may also increase the risk of adverse reactions.

Lithium: Clinical observations suggest the possibility that the combination of L-tryptophan and lithium may reduce the need for the higher, more toxic doses of lithium necessary to control bipolar affective disorders.

NUTRITIONAL SUPPLEMENTS
None known.

FOODS
Alpha-lactalbumin, carbohydrates, whey protein: May increase the brain availability of L-tryptophan.

HERBS
None known.

OVERDOSAGE
No reports in humans.

DOSAGE AND ADMINISTRATION
Those who wish to use L-tryptophan should only use the highest quality and purity grade L-tryptophan, preferably pharmaceutical grade and 99% to 100% pure, and should

make sure the L-tryptophan is manufactured by a trusted and respected company under the highest quality control conditions.

Dosage should be discussed with one's physician.

LITERATURE

Ardis T, Cahir M, Elliott J, et al. Effect of acute tryptophan depletion on noradrenaline and dopamine in the rat brain. *J Psychopharmacol*. Epub: 2008 Jun 18.

Ball HJ, Yuasa HJ, Austin CJ, et al. Indoleamine 2,3-dioxygenase-2; a new enzyme in the kynurenine pathway. *Int J Biochem Cell Biol*. Epub: 2008 Jan 11.

Baloh RW, Dietz J, Spooner JW. Myoclonus and ocular oscillations induced by L-tryptophan. *Ann Neurol*. 1982;11(1):95-97.

Barry S, Clarke G, Scully P, et al. Kynurenine pathway in psychosis: evidence of increased tryptophan degradation. *J Psychopharmacol*. Epub: 2008 Jun 18.

Blackburn WD Jr. Eosinophilia myalgia syndrome. *Semin Arthritis Rheum*. 1997;26(6):788-793.

Bowen DJ, Spring B, Fox E. Tryptophan and high-carbohydrate diets as adjuncts to smoking cessation therapy. *J Behav Med*. 1991;14(2):97-110.

Brewerton TD, Reus VI. Lithium carbonate and L-tryptophan in the treatment of bipolar and schizoaffective disorders. *Am J Psychiatry*. 1983;140(6):757-760.

Bryan GT. The role of urinary tryptophan metabolites in the etiology of bladder cancer. *Am J Clin Nutr*. 1971;24(7):841-847.

Chen CN, Kalucy RS, Hartmann MK, et al. Plasma tryptophan and sleep. *Br Med J*. 1974;4(5944):564-566.

Feksa LR, Latini A, Rech VC, et al. Tryptophan administration induces oxidative stress in brain cortex of rats. *Metab Brain Dis*. 2008;23(2):221-233.

Feksa LR, Latini A, Rech VC, et al. Promotion of oxidative stress by L-tryptophan in cerebral cortex of rats. *Neurochem Int*. 2006;49(1):87-93.

FDA/CFSAN. Food and Drug Administration web site. Information Paper on L-tryptophan and 5-hydroxy-L-tryptophan. Available at: http://www.cfsan.fda.gov/~dms/ds-tryp1.html. Accessed August 1, 2008

Garau C, Aparicio S, Rial RV, et al. Age related changes in the activity-rest circadian rhythms and c-fos expression of ring doves with aging. Effects of tryptophan intake. *Exp Gerontol*. 2006;41(4):430-438.

Gillin JC, Kaplan JA, Wyatt RJ. Clinical effects of tryptophan in chronic schizophrenic patients. *Biol Psychiatry*. 1976;11(5):635-639.

Guillemin GJ, Cullen KM, Lim CK, et al. Characterization of the kynurenine pathway in human neurons. *J Neurosci*. 2007;27(47):12884-12892.

Hartmann E. Effects of L-tryptophan on sleepiness and on sleep. *J Psychiatr Res*. 1982-1983;17(2):107-113.

Hartmann E. L-Tryptophan: effects on sleep. *Monogr Neural Sci*. 1976;3:26-32.

Hartmann E. Editorial: L-tryptophan: a possible natural hypnotic substance. *JAMA*. 1974;230(12):1680-1681.

Hartmann E. L-tryptophan as a physiological hypnotic. *Lancet*. 1971;1(7703):807.

Hartmann E. L-tryptophan: a rational hypnotic with clinical potential. *Am J Psychiatry*. 1977;134(4):366-370.

Hartmann E. L-tryptophane: an effective hypnotic. *Curr Psychiatr Ther*. 1977;17:165-169.

Hartmann E, Chung R. Sleep-inducing effects of L-tryptophan. *J Pharm Pharmacol*. 1972;24(3):252-253.

Hartmann E, Chung R, Chien CP. L-Tryptophane and sleep. *Psychopharmacologia*. 1971;19(2):114-127.

Hartmann E, Cravens J, List S. Hypnotic effects of L-tryptophan. *Arch Gen Psychiatry*. 1974;31(3):394-397.

Hartmann E, Elion R. The insomnia of 'sleeping in a strange place': effects of l-tryptophane. *Psychopharmacology* (Berl). 1977;53(2):131-133.

Hartmann E, Lindsley JG, Spinweber C. Chronic insomnia: effects of tryptophan, flurazepam, secobarbital, and placebo. *Psychopharmacology* (Berl). 1983;80(2):138-42.

Hartmann E, Spinweber CL. Sleep induced by L-tryptophan. Effect of dosages within the normal dietary intake. *J Nerv Ment Dis*. 1979;167(8):497-499.

Hartmann EL. Effect of L-tryptophan and other amino acids on sleep. *Nutr Rev*. 1986;44 Suppl:70-73.

Hartmann EL. L-tryptophan and sleep. *Adv Biosci*. 1978;21:75-84.

Hrboticky N, Leiter LA, Anderson GH. Menstrual cycle effects on the metabolism of tryptophan loads. *Am J Clin Nutr*. 1989;50(1):46-52.

Ishihara A, Hashimoto Y, Tanaka C, et al. The tryptophan pathway is involved in the defense responses of rice against pathogenic infection via serotonin production. *Plant J*. 2008;54(3):481-495.

Kilbourne EM, Philen RM, Kamb ML, et al. Tryptophan produced by Showa Denko and epidemic eosinophilia-myalgia syndrome. *J Rheumatol Suppl*. 1996;46:81-88; discussion 89-91.

King RB. Pain and tryptophan. *J Neurosurg*. 1980;53(5):731.

Klarskov K, Johnson KL, Benson LM, et al. Structural characterization of a case-implicated contaminant, 'Peak X,' in commercial preparations of 5-hydroxytryptophan. *J Rheumatol*. 2003;30(1):89-95.

Klarskov K, Johnson KL, Benson LM, et al. Eosinophilia-myalgia syndrome case-associated contaminants in commercially available 5-hydroxytryptophan. *Adv Exp Med Biol*. 1999;467:461-468.

Kuhn E, Rysánek K, Brodan V, et al. Changes in blood tryptophan level during sleep deprivation. *Experientia*. 1976;32(9):1117-1118.

Kujundzić RN, Lowenthal JW. The role of tryptophan metabolism in iNOS transcription and nitric oxide production by chicken macrophage cells upon treatment with interferon gamma. *Immunol Lett*. 2008;115(2):153-159.

Levitan RD, Shen JH, Jindal R, et al. Preliminary randomized double-blind placebo-controlled trial of tryptophan combined with fluoxetine to treat major depressive disorder: antidepressant and hypnotic effects. *J Psychiatry Neurosci*. 2000;25(4):337-346. Erratum in: *J Psychiatry Neurosci*. 2000;25(5):439.

Lyness WH. Effect of L-tryptophan pretreatment on d-amphetamine self administration. *Subst Alcohol Actions Misuse*. 1983;4(4):305-312.

Majewska M, Zajac K, Zemelka M, et al. Influence of melatonin and its precursor L-tryptophan on Th1 dependent contact hypersensitivity. *J Physiol Pharmacol*. 2007;58 Suppl 6:125-132.

Markus CR. Dietary Amino Acids and Brain Serotonin Function; Implications for Stress-Related Affective Changes. *Neuromolecular Med*. Epub: 2008 May 31.

Markus CR. Effects of carbohydrates on brain tryptophan availability and stress performance. *Biol Psychol*. 2007;76(1-2):83-90.

Markus CR, Jonkman LM, Lammers JH, et al. Evening intake of alpha-lactalbumin increases plasma tryptophan availability and improves morning alertness and brain measures of attention. *Am J Clin Nutr*. 2005;81(5):1026-1033.

Markus CR, Sierksma A, Verbeek C, et al. Moderate whisky consumption in combination with an evening meal reduces tryptophan availability to the brain but does not influence performance in healthy volunteers. *Br J Nutr*. 2004;92(6):995-1000.

Markus CR, Olivier B, de Haan EH. Whey protein rich in alpha-lactalbumin increases the ratio of plasma tryptophan to the sum of the other large neutral amino acids and improves cognitive performance in stress-vulnerable subjects. *Am J Clin Nutr*. 2002;75(6):1051-1056.

Mayeno AN, Gleich GJ. Eosinophilia-myalgia syndrome and tryptophan production: a cautionary tale. *Trends Biotechnol*. 1994 Sep;12(9):346-352.

Mayeno AN, Lin F, Foote CS, et al. Characterization of 'peak E,' a novel amino acid associated with eosinophilia-myalgia syndrome. *Science*. 1990;250(4988):1707-1708.

Miller EM, Nieburg HA. L-tryptophan in the treatment of levodopa induced psychiatric disorders. *Dis Nerv Syst*. 1974;35(1):20-23.

Miura H, Ozaki N, Shirokawa T, et al. Changes in brain tryptophan metabolism elicited by ageing, social environment, and psychological stress in mice. *Stress*. 2008;11(2):160-169.

Moja EA, Mendelson WB, Stoff DM, et al. Reduction of REM sleep by a tryptophan-free amino acid diet. *Life Sci*. 1979;24(16):1467-1470.

Owe-Young R, Webster NL, Mukhtar M, et al. Kynurenine pathway metabolism in human blood-brain-barrier cells: implications for immune tolerance and neurotoxicity. *J Neurochem*. 2008;105(4):1346-1357.

Paredes SD, Barriga C, Rodríguez AB. Melatonin and tryptophan as therapeutic agents against the impairment of the sleep-wake cycle and immunosenescence due to aging in Streptopelia risoria. *Neuro Endocrinol Lett*. 2007;28(6):757-760.

Peyrot F, Ducrocq C. Potential role of tryptophan derivatives in stress responses characterized by the generation of reactive oxygen and nitrogen species. *J Pineal Res*. 2008;45(3):235-246.

Raju TN, Kanth VR, Reddy PU. Influence of kynurenines in pathogenesis of cataract formation in tryptophan-deficient regimen in Wistar rats. *Indian J Exp Biol*. 2007;45(6):543-548.

Riedel WJ, Klaassen T, Deutz NE, et al. Tryptophan depletion in normal volunteers produces selective impairment in memory consolidation. *Psychopharmacology* (Berl). 1999;141(4):362-369.

Romani L, Fallarino F, De Luca A, et al. Defective tryptophan catabolism underlies inflammation in mouse chronic granulomatous disease. *Nature*. 2008;451(7175):211-215.

Saleem DM, Haider S, Khan MM, et al. Role of tryptophan in the pathogenesis of hepatic encephalopathy. *J Pak Med Assoc*. 2008;58(2):68-70.

Schmitt JA, Jorissen BL, Dye L, et al. Memory function in women with premenstrual complaints and the effect of serotonergic stimulation by acute administration of an alpha-lactalbumin protein. *J Psychopharmacol*. 2005;19(4):375-384.

Schmidt HS. L-tryptophan in the treatment of impaired respiration in sleep. *Bull Eur Physiopathol Respir*. 1983;19(6):625-629.

Schneider-Helmert D. [Treatment of sleep disorders with L-tryptophan. Uses of interval therapy in severe insomnia and hypnotic dependence] [Article in German.] *Fortschr Med*. 1987;105(6):113-116.

Schneider-Helmert D, Spinweber CL. Evaluation of L-tryptophan for treatment of insomnia: a review. *Psychopharmacology* (Berl). 1986;89(1):1-7.

Seltzer S. Pain relief by dietary manipulation and tryptophan supplements. *J Endod*. 1985;11(10):449-453.

Seltzer S, Stoch R, Marcus R, et al. Alteration of human pain thresholds by nutritional manipulation and L-tryptophan supplementation. *Pain*. 1982;13(4):385-393.

Seltzer S, Dewart D, Pollack RL, et al. The effects of dietary tryptophan on chronic maxillofacial pain and experimental pain tolerance. *J Psychiatr Res*. 1982-1983;17(2):181-186.

Shaw DM. L-tryptophan in depression. *Lancet*. 1970;1(7656):1111.

Shaw K, Turner J, Del Mar C. Are tryptophan and 5-hydroxytryptophan effective treatments for depression? A meta-analysis. *Aust N Z J Psychiatry*. 2002;36(4):488491.

Shaw K, Turner J, Del Mar C. Tryptophan and 5-hydroxytryptophan for depression. *Cochrane Database Syst Rev*. 2002;(1):CD003198.

Shaw K, Turner J, Del Mar C. Tryptophan and 5-hydroxytryptophan for depression. *Cochrane Database Syst Rev*. 2001;(3):CD003198. Update in: *CochraneDatabase Syst Rev*. 2002;(1):CD003198.

Shpeen SE, Morse DR, Furst ML. The effect of tryptophan on postoperative endodontic pain. *Oral Surg Oral Med Oral Pathol*. 1984;58(4):446-449.

Silver RM. Pathophysiology of the eosinophilia-myalgia syndrome. J Rheumatol Suppl. 1996;46:26-36.

Simat TJ, Kleeberg KK, Müller B, et al. Synthesis, formation, and occurrence of contaminants in biotechnologically manufactured L-tryptophan. *Adv Exp Med Biol*. 1999;467:469-480.

Smith FL, Yu DS, Smith DG, et al. Dietary tryptophan supplements attenuate amphetamine self-administration in the rat. Pharmacol Biochem Behav. 1986;25(4):849-855.

Spinweber CL. L-tryptophan administered to chronic sleep-onset insomniacs: late-appearing reduction of sleep latency. *Psychopharmacology* (Berl). 1986;90(2):151-155.

Steinberg S, Annable L, Young SN, et al. A placebo-controlled clinical trial of L-tryptophan in premenstrual dysphoria. *Biol Psychiatry*. 1999;45(3):313-320.

Winokur A, Lindberg ND, Lucki I, et al. Hormonal and behavioral effects associated with intravenous L-tryptophan administration. *Psychopharmacology* (Berl). 1986;88(2):213-219.

Wyatt RJ, Engelman K, Kupfer DJ, et al. Effects of L-tryptophan (a natural sedative) on human sleep. *Lancet*. 1970;2(7678):842-846.

Yoshida O, Brown RR, Bryan GT. A possible role of urinary metabolites of tryptophan in the heterotopic recurrence of bladder cancer in man. *Am J Clin Nutr*. 1971;24(7):848-851.

Yoshida O, Brown RR, Bryan GT. Relationship between tryptophan metabolism and heterotopic recurrences of human urinary bladder tumors. *Cancer*. 1970;25(4):773-780.

L-Tyrosine

DESCRIPTION

L-tyrosine is a protein amino acid. It is classified as a conditionally essential amino acid.

Under most circumstances, the body can synthesize sufficient L-tyrosine, principally from L-phenylalanine, to meet its physiological demands. However, there are conditions where the body requires a dietary source of the amino acid for its physiological demands. For example, L-tyrosine is an essential amino acid for those with phenylketonuria. L-tyrosine is found in proteins of all life forms. Dietary sources of L-tyrosine are principally derived from animal and vegetable proteins. Vegetables and juices contain small amounts of the free amino acid. The free amino acid is also found in fermented foods such as yogurt and miso.

In addition to being involved in protein synthesis, L-tyrosine is a precursor for the synthesis of the catecholamines epinephrine, norepinephrine and dopamine, the thyroid hormones thyroxine and triiodothyronine, and the pigment melanin.

L-tyrosine is also known as beta- (para-hydroxyphenyl) alanine, alpha-amino-para-hydroxyhydrocinnamic acid and (S)- alpha-amino-4-hydroxybenzenepropanoic acid. It is abbreviated as either Tyr of by its one-letter abbreviation Y. The molecular formula of L-tyrosine is $C_9H_{10}NO_3$, and its molecular weight is 181.19 daltons. L-tyrosine is an aromatic amino acid with the following structural formula:

L-tyrosine

ACTIONS AND PHARMACOLOGY

ACTIONS

L-tyrosine has putative antidepressant activity.

MECHANISM OF ACTION

The mechanism of L-tyrosine's putative antidepressant activity may be accounted for by the precursor role of L-tyrosine in the synthesis of the neurotransmitters norepinephrine and dopamine. Elevated brain norepinephrine and dopamine levels are thought to be associated with antidepressant effects.

PHARMACOKINETICS

Following ingestion, L-tyrosine is absorbed from the small intestine by a sodium-dependent active transport process. L-tyrosine is transported from the small intestine to the liver via the portal circulation. In the liver, L-tyrosine is involved in a number of biochemical reactions, including protein synthesis and oxidative catabolic reactions. L-tyrosine that is not metabolized in the liver is distributed via the systemic circulation to the various tissues of the body.

INDICATIONS AND USAGE

Results are mixed, but largely negative, with respect to claims that tyrosine is an effective antidepressant. Claims that it can alleviate some of the mental and physical symptoms of environmental stress are based on preliminary evidence. Further claims that tyrosine is useful in narcolepsy and attention deficit disorder have been refuted by some studies. Another study found that tyrosine supplementation did not improve neuropsychological performance in subjects with phenylketonuria. Claims that tyrosine is helpful in alleviating symptoms of premenstrual syndrome (PMS) and drug withdrawal are largely anecdotal and unconfirmed. There is no evidence tyrosine has any effect on dementia, Alzheimer's disease or Parkinson's disease.

RESEARCH SUMMARY

Two small, early studies suggested that tyrosine might have useful antidepressant effects. A subsequent follow-up with more subjects and conducted in a randomized, double-blind fashion failed to find any significant antidepressant activity, compared with placebo, in subjects with major depression. The dose used was 100 mg/kg/day of tyrosine for four weeks.

One study has concluded that tyrosine can protect against some forms of environmental stress. Subjects were given a 100 mg/kg dose of tyrosine and then exposed for 4.5 hours to cold and hypoxia in this double-blind, placebo-controlled crossover study. Tyrosine was reported to significantly decrease adverse symptoms, including mood and performance impairment. Follow-up is needed.

In another double-blind, placebo-controlled trial, tyrosine had no significant effect on subjects with narcolepsy and associated cataplexy. Dose used was 9 grams daily for four weeks. Similarly, tyrosine failed to produce lasting, significant improvement in subjects with attention deficit disorder. In this small, open study, tyrosine seemed to improve this condition after two weeks of supplementation, but this improvement was not sustained.

Recently, tyrosine was tested to see if it could improve the neuropsychological test performances of individuals with phenylketonuria. This was a randomized, double-blind, placebo-controlled crossover study. Maximum dosage used was 100 to 150 mg/kg/day. The supplementation increased plasma tyrosine concentrations. Higher tyrosine levels correlated at baseline with improved performance on the neuropsychological tests, yet higher concentrations achieved through supplementation in this trial did not enhance test scores.

CONTRAINDICATIONS, PRECAUTIONS, ADVERSE REACTIONS

CONTRAINDICATIONS

L-tyrosine is contraindicated in those with the inborn errors of metabolism alkaptonuria and tyrosinemia type I and type II. It is also contraindicated in those taking non-selective monoamine oxidase (MAO) inhibitors. L-tyrosine is con-traindicated in those hypersensitive to any component of an L-tyrosine-containing supplement.

PRECAUTIONS

Pregnant women and nursing mothers should avoid supplementation with L-tyrosine.

Those with hypertension should exercise caution in the use of L-tyrosine.

Those with melanoma should avoid L-tyrosine supplements.

ADVERSE REACTIONS

L-tyrosine is generally well tolerated. There are some reports of those taking supplemental L-tyrosine experiencing insomnia and nervousness.

INTERACTIONS

DRUGS

Non-selective MAO inhibitors: including phenelzine sulfate, tranylcypromine sulfate and pargyline HC1—Concomitant use of L-tyrosine and non-selective MAO inhibitors may cause hypertension.

DOSAGE AND ADMINISTRATION

Those who use supplemental L-tyrosine typically take 500 to 1500 mg daily.

LITERATURE

Banderet LE, Lieberman HR. Treatment with tyrosine, a neurotransmitter precursor, reduces environmental stress in humans. *Brain Res Bull*. 1989; 22:759-762.

Elwes RD, Crewes H, Chesterman LP, et al. Treatment of narcolepsy with L-tyrosine: double-blind, placebo-controlled trial. *Lancet*. 1989; 2(8671):1067-1069.

Gelenberg AJ, Gibson CJ. Tyrosine for the treatment of depression. *Nutr Health*. 1984; 3:163-173.

Gelenberg AJ, Wojcik JD, Falk WE, et al. Tyrosine for depression: a double-blind trial. *J Affect Disord*. 1990; 19:125-132.

Gelenberg AJ, Wojcik JD, Gibson CJ, Wurtman RJ. Tyrosine for depression. *J Psychiatr Res*. 1982-83; 17:175-180.

Reimherr FW, Wender PH, Wood DR, Ward M. An open trial of L-tyrosine in the treatment of attention deficit disorder, residual type. *Am J Psychiatry*. 1987; 144:1071-1073.

Smith ML, Hanley WB, Clarke JTR, et al. Randomised controlled trial of tyrosine supplementation on neuropsychological performance in phenylketonuria. *Arch Dis Child*. 1998; 78:116-121.

Young SN. Behavioral effects of dietary neurotransmitter precursors: basic and clinical aspects. *Neurosci Biobehav Rev*. 1996; 20:313-323.

Lactoferrin

DESCRIPTION

Lactoferrin is a glycoprotein that belongs to the iron transporter or transferrin family. It was originally isolated from bovine milk, where it is found as a minor protein component of whey proteins (see Whey Proteins). Lactoferrin contains 703 amino acids and has a molecular weight of 80 kilodaltons. In addition to its presence in milk, it is also found in exocrine secretions of mammals and is released from neutrophil granules during inflammation.

Lactoferrin is considered a multifunctional or multi-tasking protein. It appears to play several biological roles. Owing to its iron-binding properties, lactoferrin is thought to play a role in iron uptake by the intestinal mucosa of the suckling neonate. That is, it appears to be the source of iron for breast-fed infants. It also appears to have antibacterial, antiviral, antifungal, anti-inflammatory, antioxidant and immunomodulatory activities.

Three isoforms of lactoferrin have been isolated: lactoferrin-alpha, lactoferrin-beta and lactoferrin-gamma. Lactoferrin-beta and lactoferrin-gamma have RNase activity, whereas lactoferrin-alpha does not. Receptors for lactoferrin are found in monocytes, lymphocytes, neutrophils, intestinal tissue and on certain bacteria. Lactoferrin is abbreviated LF and Lf. Bovine lactoferrin is abbreviated bLF.

Bovine lactoferrin, derived from whey proteins, is marketed as a nutritional supplement. Supplemental lactoferrin typically contains low amounts of iron.

ACTIONS AND PHARMACOLOGY

ACTIONS

Supplemental lactoferrin may have antimicrobial, immunomodulatory, antioxidant and anti-inflammatory actions.

MECHANISM OF ACTION

The possible antibacterial activity of supplemental lactoferrin might be accounted for, in part, by its ability to strongly bind iron. Iron is essential to support the growth of pathogenic bacteria. Lactoferrin may also inhibit the attachment of bacteria to the intestinal wall. A breakdown product of lactoferrin is the peptide lactoferricin. Lactoferricin, classified as a bioactive peptide, may also have antibacterial, as well as antiviral, activity. The possible antiviral activity of supplemental lactoferrin may be due to its inhibition of virus-cell fusion and viral entry into cells.

A few mechanisms are proposed for lactoferrin's possible immunomodulatory activity. Lactoferrin may promote the growth and differentiation of T lymphocytes. Lactoferrin appears to bind uniquely in the region of major histocompatability (MHC) proteins and the CD4 and CD8 determinants on T4 (helper) and T8 (suppressor) lymphocytes; it bears sequence homologies with the MHC Class II determinant. Lactoferrin also appears to play a role in the regulation of cytokines and lymphokines, such as tumor necrosis (TNF)-alpha and interleukin (IL)-6. Lactoferrin's possible antioxidant activity may also contribute to its possible immunomodulatory activity.

Lactoferrin's possible antioxidant activity can also be accounted for by its ability to strongly bind iron. Free iron is a major contributor to the generation of reactive oxygen species via the Fenton reaction.

Lactoferrin's possible anti-inflammatory action may be accounted for by its possible antioxidant and immunomodulatory activities.

PHARMACOKINETICS

Little is known of the pharmacokinetics of oral lactoferrin. Lactoferrin appears much more resistant to proteolytic action than most dietary proteins. Lactoferrin is digested in the intestine to the bioactive peptide lactoferricin. Most of the possible actions of oral lactoferrin may be confined to the gut. There is some preliminary evidence that lactoferrin and lactoferricin may be absorbed, in part, from the lumen of the small intestine into enterocytes and that these molecules enter other cells as well. However, this is unclear.

INDICATIONS AND USAGE

There is some preliminary evidence from *in vitro* and animal research that supplemental lactoferrin may have some immune-enhancing effects. There is no evidence that it is effective as a treatment or preventive in any form of cancer. Neither is there any credible evidence to support claims that it helps those with fatigue or allergy.

RESEARCH SUMMARY

A number of *in vitro* and animal studies have shown that lactoferrin has various bactericidal and fungicidal effects. It has exhibited significant activity against *Escherichia coli*, *Proteus mirabilis*, *Staphyloccocus aureus*, *Candida albicans* and other pathogens in these studies. *In vitro*, lactoferrin has similarly shown some significant activity against HIV, herpes simplex virus type 1, hepatitis C virus, cytomegalovirus and some other viruses.

Human studies, however, are almost entirely lacking. One small, recent study showed that oral lactoferrin reduced the duration and severity of bacterial infection in five neutropenic patients receiving chemotherapy for acute myelogenous leukemia, compared with nine matched controls. More research is needed.

CONTRAINDICATIONS, PRECAUTIONS, ADVERSE REACTIONS

CONTRAINDICATIONS

Supplemental lactoferrin is contraindicated in those with hypersensitivity to any component of a lactoferrin-containing product.

PRECAUTIONS

Pregnant women and nursing mothers should avoid using lactoferrin supplements.

INTERACTIONS

Some in vitro studies suggest that lactoferrin acts synergistically with antifungal agents.

DOSAGE AND ADMINISTRATION

Oral lactoferrin dosed at 40 mg daily has been used in a couple of clinical trials of the substance. Those who supplement with lactoferrin typically take 250 mg daily. Lactoferrin is also found in whey protein supplements.

LITERATURE

Adamik B, Zimecki M, Wlaszczyk A, et al. Lactoferrin effects on the *in vitro* immune response in critically ill patients. *Arch Immunol Ther Exp (Warcz)*. 1998; 46:169-176.

Baveye S, Elass E, Mazurier J, et al. Lactoferrin: a multifunctional glycoprotein involved in the modulation of the inflammatory process. *Clin Chem Lab Med*. 1999; 37:281-286.

Britigan BE, Serody JS, Cohen MS. The role of lactoferrin as an anti-inflammatory molecule. *Adv Exp Med Biol*. 1994; 357:143-156.

Ikeda M, Nozak A, Sugiyama K, et al. Characterization of antiviral activity of lactoferrin against hepatitis C virus infection in human cultured cells. *Virus Res*. 2000; 66:51-63.

Levay PF, Viljoen M. Lactoferrin: a general review. *Haemtologica*. 1995; 80:252-267.

Lonnerdal B, Iyer S. Lactoferrin: molecular structure and biological function. *Annu Rev Nutr*. 1995; 15:93-110.

Swart PJ, Kuipers EM, Smit C, et al. Lactoferrin. Antiviral activity of lactoferrin. *Adv Exp Med Biol*. 1998; 443:205-213.

Trumpler U, Straub PW, Rosenmund A. Antibacterial prophylaxis with lactoferrin in neutropenic patients. *Eur J Clin Microbiol Infect Dis*. 1989; 8:310-313.

Vorland LH. Lactoferrin: a multifunctional glycoprotein. *APMIS*. 1999; 107:971-981.

Vorland LH, Ulvatne H, Andersen J, et al. Antibacterial effects of lactoferricin B. *Scand J Infect Dis*. 1999; 31:179-184.

Zimecki M, Wlaszczyk A, Cheneau P, et al. Immunoregulatory effects of a nutritional preparation containing bovine lactoferrin taken orally by healthy individuals. *Arch Immunol Ther Exp (Warcz)*. 1998; 46:231-240.

Lactotripeptides

DESCRIPTION

In a general sense, the term lactotripeptides refers to peptides derived from milk, which are comprised of chains of three amino acids. In the early 1990s, Japanese researchers isolated two tripeptides from fermented milk and, subsequently, directly from casein, a major milk protein, which were found to have an antihypertensive effect. They named the two tripeptides, collectively, lactotripeptides. One of the two lactotripeptides contains the amino acid sequence L-isoleucine-L-proline-L-proline (L-isoleucyl-L-prolyl-L-proline, Ile-Pro-Pro, IPP; CAS number 26001-32-1). The other lactotripeptide contains the amino acid sequence L-valine-L-proline-L-proline (L-valyl-L-prolyl-L-proline, Val-Pro-Pro, VPP; CAS number 58872-39-2). IPP's molecular weight is 325.3 and its empirical formula is $C_{16}H_{27}N_3O_4$. VPP's molecular weight is 311.4 and its empirical formula is $C_{15}H_{25}N_3O_4$.

L-valyl-L-prolyl-L-proline

L-isoleucyl-L-prolyl-L-proline

In the 1990s lactotripeptides were found to have blood pressure-lowering activity, first in an experimental animal model for hypertension and later in humans with hypertension, as well as prehypertension. Approximately 18 human clinical trials, mostly in Japan, but a few in the United States, have shown some degree of blood pressure-lowering by lactotripeptides. A recent meta-analysis provided evidence that lactotripeptides (VPP and IPP) have hypotensive effects in prehypertensive and hypertensive subjects. Interestingly, some cultures have held the belief that milk from various animals, including cows, goats, camels and yaks, has positive effects on blood pressure, stroke and cardiovascular disease.

Lactotripeptides are produced in two different ways. One delivery form of lactotripeptides is a fermented milk beverage. The milk is fermented with *Lactobacillus helviticus* and *Saccharomyces cerevisiae* and lactotripeptides are produced in this process via a *Lactobacillus helviticus* cell wall-associated proteinase. The other process of producing lactotripeptides is by enzymatic cleavage of the milk protein casein by a protease derived from the filamentous fungus, *Aspergillus oryzae*. The VPP and IPP produced by this enzymatic treatment are formulated into pills (tablets and capsules). The lactotripeptide milk beverage and the lactotripeptide tablets are approved by the Japanese government as FOSHU (foods for specific health use). Tablets and capsules containing lactotripeptides are now marketed in the United States.

ACTIONS AND PHARMACOLOGY

ACTIONS

Lactotripeptides have a blood pressure-lowering effect, may beneficially affect endothelial integrity and may improve bone mass and structure and decrease fracture risk.

MECHANISM OF ACTION

Both VPP and IPP inhibit angiotensin I-converting enzyme (ACE) *in vitro*. VPP and IPP also cause a lowering of both systolic and diastolic blood pressure in spontaneous hypertensive rats (SHRs), a major animal model for hypertension. It is thought that the blood pressure-lowering effect of lactotripeptides in SHRs is due to inhibition of ACE, resulting in decreased production of the vasoconstrictor angiotensin II and increased amounts of the vasodilator bradykinin.

The renin angiotensin system (RAS) is central to the regulation of the cardiovascular system as well as to blood pressure regulation. A brief review of RAS is as follows: Renin, a protein with enzymatic activity that is made in the kidneys, converts angiotensinogen, a protein made in the liver, to angiotensin I (AngI), a decapeptide. AngI is converted to angiotensin II (AngII), an octapeptide, by the angiotensin I-converting enzyme (ACE). Additionally, in the kinin-kallikrein system, ACE converts the vasodilatory nonapeptide bradykinin to an inactive heptapeptide. ACE possesses two catalytic domains—the C-domain that catalyzes the conversion of AngI to AngII and the N-domain that catalyzes the conversion of bradykinin to the heptapeptide. Vasoconstriction and elevated blood pressure occur when AngII binds to angiotensin II receptor type 1 (AT$_1$), a G protein coupled receptor. Inhibition of ACE leads to decreased amounts of AngII, resulting in vasodilation and decreased blood pressure. In addition, inhibition of ACE prevents the inactivation of bradykinin, allowing this nonapeptide to act in its vasodilatory role, contributing to lower blood pressure.

A recent placebo-controlled, double-blind crossover human clinical study in males with mild hypertension who were treated with lactotripeptides for one week did not note any change in either systolic or diastolic blood pressure between those treated with VPP and IPP and those administered placebo. This was not unexpected, since it typically takes more than a week to observe a blood pressure change from lactotripeptides. However, it was found in this trial that lactotripeptides improved vascular endothelial function independent of blood pressure-lowering effects. To determine vascular endothelial function, reactive hyperemia of the left upper forearm was measured using plethysmography as an index of vascular endothelial function. Possible mechanisms by which VPP and IPP improve vascular endothelial dysfunction are as follows: Vascular tone is key to blood pressure control and endothelial bioavailability of nitric oxide (NO) is key to vascular tone. Vascular tone is regulated by NO, which causes vascular relaxation by increasing intracellular cGMP (cyclic-guanosine monophosphate) and activating cGMP-dependent protein kinase 1 (PKG1). ACE activation leads to production of AngII, which binds to its receptor, causing vasoconstriction and possible activation of the enzyme nicotinamide adenine dinucleotide phosphate-oxidase (NADPH-oxidase). NADPH-oxidase catalyzes the production of superoxide radicals that can react with endothelial nitric oxide, forming peroxynitrite and decreasing the endothelial bioavailability of endothelial NO, thus causing vasoconstriction. Inhibition of ACE decreases the production of AngII and prevents the inactivation of bradykinin, resulting in vasodilatation and increased endothelial bioavailability of NO. This mechanism can result in improved vascular endothelial function, even in the absence of blood pressure changes.

VPP and IPP, but especially IPP, were found to stimulate gene expression of osteoblasts differentiated from human mesenchymal stem cells *in vitro*. IPP was found to upregulate parathyroid hormone-related protein (PTHrP), bone morphogenic protein (BMP-5), and cAMP response element binding (CREB) protein, and downregulate vitamin D receptor (VDR) and caspase-8, a calcium-dependent cysteine protease, which plays an essential role in apoptosis (programmed cell death). The specific mechanism of action of lactotripeptides in the stimulation of osteoblasts is unclear; nor is it clear if lactotripeptides stimulate osteoblasts *in vivo*.

PHARMACOKINETICS

Proline is commonly classified as an amino acid. However, it is actually an imino acid, and bonds between proline and other amino acids in peptides are not amide bonds, but imide bonds. Imide bonds are much more resistant to enzymatic hydrolysis than are amide bonds, the usual bond between amino acids in peptides. Following oral intake of lactotripeptides, VPP and IPP reach the small intestine intact. The efficiency of absorption of tripeptides from the intestine is low, although not nearly as low as peptides containing more than three amino acids. Following absorption, VPP and IPP are transported into the portal circulation where they are distributed in the plasma to various tissues, including the aorta and the lungs. Further research on the pharmacokinetics of lactotripeptides is warranted in order to have a more complete picture of the pharmacokinetics of these substances.

INDICATIONS AND USAGE

The lactotripeptides show promise in the control of blood pressure and may promote bone mass and help reduce risk of fracture.

RESEARCH SUMMARY

Numerous animal and human studies, as well as *in vitro* studies, attest to the merits of lactotripeptides in controlling blood pressure. One such study, conducted double-blind and placebo-controlled, placed 144 human subjects on a regimen of lactotripeptides administered in the form of a drink that was taken with breakfast daily over a period of 18 weeks. This test drink contained 1.47 mg of valine-proline-proline (VPP) and 1.6 mg of isoleucine-proline-proline (IPP). Both IPP and VPP had previously been shown, in various other experiments, to be among the more effective peptides in terms of their effects on blood pressure in both animal models and in human trials. All of the subjects had either high-normal blood pressure (prehypertension) or mild hypertension. The subjects were matched with controls who received a placebo drink that contained no lactotripeptides.

The experimental subjects experienced significantly reduced blood pressure, both systolic and diastolic, compared with the control subjects. Moreover, once lactotripeptides were withdrawn at the end of the study, follow-up observations showed that the experimentals continued to enjoy lower systolic blood pressure for four weeks. Lactotripeptides have been demonstrated to act in ways similar to the so-called ACE-inhibiting drugs, which act on the angiotensin-I-converting enzyme implicated in hypertension. But unlike the ACE-inhibiting drugs, lactotripeptides, once discontinued, do not result in the rebound phenomenon that leads to rapid, abnormal increase in blood pressure, at least in some of the clinical trials.

Though the study discussed above utilized a beverage as the delivery form, some others have used lactotripeptide pills (available in a number of places, including the United States). One study divided 131 volunteers with high-normal blood pressure or mild hypertension into four groups given two tablets daily containing either no lactotripeptides (the controls) or doses of VPP and IPP in the amounts of 1.8 mg, 2.5 mg and 3.6 mg. Dose-dependent reductions in systolic blood pressure at levels of statistical significance were observed in all three groups that received pills containing the active ingredients. When compared with the controls, however, only the group that received the highest dosage achieved a statistically significant difference.

In February 2008, a study of the effect of lactotripeptides on Dutch hypertensive subjects, conducted in the Netherlands, reported no significant effect on blood pressure. However, the rather large systolic blood pressure drop during the run-in period of the study (approximately 9 mmHg for both the treatment and placebo groups) was much larger than typically observed in prior clinical studies, suggesting that a longer run-in period might have been necessary in the study in order to have given a more accurate picture of the blood pressure changes. The authors of the paper concluded: "More well-conducted trials in different populations are needed to see whether supplementation with dairy peptides could have a place in the treatment of mild hypertension."

A few months later, in June 2008, another study (double-blind, randomized crossover design) conducted again in the Netherlands on Dutch subjects with high-normal blood pressure to mild hypertension, reported that lactotripeptides demonstrated a modest sustained fall in daytime office systolic blood pressure after the first dosing of lactotripeptides.

A meta-analysis on the effect of lactotripeptides on blood pressure in prehypertensive and hypertensive subjects was recently published. The authors of the meta-analysis scanned the Medline, PubMed, Embase, Science Citation Index, and Cochrane Controlled Trials Register databases and identified 12 high-quality, randomized controlled trials that matched their inclusion criteria. The trials were conducted in Japan and Finland and included 623 subjects. The pooled data from the trials demonstrated that lactotripeptides were associated with a 4.8 mmHg reduction in systolic blood pressure and a 2.2 mmHg drop in diastolic blood pressure. Interestingly, the authors found that the hypotensive effects became more obvious as the intervention lengthened. They concluded:

"Our analysis provided evidence that milk-derived IPP and VPP have a hypotensive effect in prehypertensive and hypertensive subjects."

Given that the lactotripetides are not associated with any significant side effects and given that recent findings demonstrate that even small increases in blood pressure significantly increase risk of stroke and coronary heart disease, lactotripetides may become a valuable addition to the non-drug armamentarium being used to combat hypertension: reduced sodium consumption, weight reduction, reduced alcohol intake, a diet rich in fruits and vegetables, low-fat dairy products, reduced intake of saturated and total fats and regular exercise.

Evidence is emerging that lactotripeptides may be helpful in promoting better bone health. One recent study suggested that long term supplementation with lactotripeptides can enhance osteoblast function, resulting in increased bone formation and mineralization. This was an *in vitro* experiment, and the researchers acknowledged that *in vivo* effects might differ. Further research is indicated.

CONTRAINDICATIONS, PRECAUTIONS, ADVERSE REACTIONS

CONTRAINDICATIONS

Known hypersensitivity to a lactotripeptide-containing product.

PRECAUTIONS

Lactotripeptides are not meant for primary treatment of hypertension. They are meant to promote, support and maintain healthy blood pressure. Those who might want to consider the use of lactotripeptides are those with prehypertension (defined as a systolic blood pressure of 120 to 139 mmHg and/or a diastolic blood pressure of 80 to 90 mmHg), those already on antihypertensive medications who still have not reached their target blood pressure goals and want to add a mild, possible blood pressure-lowering agent before adding another drug, and those recently diagnosed with mild hypertension or borderline hypertension who would like to see if they can get their blood pressure down with non-pharmacological treatments, including diet and exercise, before starting pharmacological treatment. Use of lactotripeptides to manage hypertension should always be discussed with ones physician.

ADVERSE REACTIONS

There have been no reports of adverse events in those taking lactotripeptides either as a sour milk beverage or in pill form. Specifically, there are no reports of ACE inhibitor-induced cough or of angioedema.

INTERACTIONS

No interactions between lactotripeptides with dietary supplements, pharmaceuticals or foods have been reported.

OVERDOSAGE

None reported.

DOSAGE AND ADMINISTRATION

Two pill forms of lactotripeptides are available in the United States: capsules and tablets. The tablets contain 5 mg of VPP and IPP in 3 tablets and the recommended dose is 3 tablets daily. The capsules contain 5 mg of VPP and IPP in 2 capsules and the recommended dose is two capsules daily. The optimal doses are not known. Doses up to 150 mg daily have been used without reported side effects.

A sour milk beverage containing similar doses of lactotripeptides is available in Japan.

The lactotripeptide capsules and tablets contain no lactose or casein.

LITERATURE
Bernard BK, Nakamura Y, Bando I, et al. Studies of the toxicological potential of tripeptides (L-valyl-L-prolyl-L-proline and L-isoleucyl-L-prolyl-L-proline): II. Introduction. *Int J Toxicol.* 2005;24 Suppl 4:5-11.

Engberink MF, Schouten EG, Kok FJ, et al. Lactotripeptides show no effect on human blood pressure: results from a double-blind randomized controlled trial. *Hypertension.* 2008;51(2):399-405.

Foltz M, Meynen EE, Bianco V, et al. Angiotensin converting enzyme inhibitory peptides from a lactotripeptide-enriched milk beverage are absorbed intact into the circulation. *J Nutr.* 2007;137(4):953-958.

Hata Y, Yamamoto M, Ohni M, et al. A placebo-controlled study of the effect of sour milk on blood pressure in hypertensive subjects. *Am J Clin Nutr.* 1996;64(5):767-771.

Hirota T, Ohki K, Kawagishi R, et al. Casein hydrolysate containing the antihypertensive tripeptides Val-Pro-Pro and Ile-Pro-Pro improves vascular endothelial function independent of blood pressure-lowering effects: contribution of the inhibitory action of angiotensin-converting enzyme. *Hypertens Res.* 2007;30(6):489-496.

Huttunen MM, Pekkinen M, Ahlström ME, et al. Long-term effects of tripeptide Ile-Pro-Pro on osteoblast differentiation in vitro. *J Nutr Biochem.* 2008;19(10):708-715.

Huttunen MM, Pekkinen M, Ahlström ME, et al. Effects of bioactive peptides isoleucine-proline-proline (IPP), valine-proline-proline (VPP) and leucine-lysine-proline (LKP) on gene expression of osteoblasts differentiated from human mesenchymal stem cells. *Br J Nutr.* 2007;98(4):780-788.

Maeno M, Yamamoto N, Takano T. Identification of an antihypertensive peptide from casein hydrolysate produced by a proteinase from Lactobacillus helveticus CP790. *J Dairy Sci.* 1996;79(8):1316-1321.

Masuda O, Nakamura Y, Takano T. Antihypertensive peptides are present in aorta after oral administration of sour milk containing these peptides to spontaneously hypertensive rats. *J Nutr.* 1996;126(12):3063-3068.

Mizuno S, Matsuura K, Gotou T, et al. Antihypertensive effect of casein hydrolysate in a placebo-controlled study in subjects with high-normal blood pressure and mild hypertension. *Br J Nutr.* 2005;94(1):84-91.

Mizushima S, Ohshige K, Watanabe J, et al. Randomized controlled trial of sour milk on blood pressure in borderline hypertensive men. *Am J Hypertens.* 2004;17(8):701-706.

Mizuno S, Nishimura S, Matsuura K, et al. Release of short and proline-rich antihypertensive peptides from casein hydrolysate with an Aspergillus oryzae protease. *J Dairy Sci.* 2004;87(10):3183-3188.

Nakamura Y, Masuda O, Takano T. Decrease of tissue angiotensin I-converting enzyme activity upon feeding sour milk in spontaneously hypertensive rats. *Biosci Biotechnol Biochem.* 1996;60(3):488-489.

Nakamura Y, Yamamoto N, Sakai K, et al. Purification and characterization of angiotensin I-converting enzyme inhibitors from sour milk. *J Dairy Sci.* 1995;78(4):777-783.

Nakamura Y, Yamamoto N, Sakai K, et al. Antihypertensive effect of sour milk and peptides isolated from it that are inhibitors to angiotensin I-converting enzyme. *J Dairy Sci.* 1995;78(6):1253-1257.

Ohsawa K, Satsu H, Ohki K, et al. Producibility and digestibility of antihypertensive beta-casein tripeptides, Val-Pro-Pro and Ile-Pro-Pro, in the gastrointestinal tract: analyses using an in vitro model of mammalian gastrointestinal digestion. *J Agric Food Chem.* 2008;56(3):854-858.

Sano J, Ohki K, Higuchi T, et al. Effect of casein hydrolysate, prepared with protease derived from Aspergillus oryzae, on subjects with high-normal blood pressure or mild hypertension. *J Med Food.* 2005;8(4):423-430.

van der Zander K, Jäkel M, Bianco V, et al. Fermented lactotripeptides-containing milk lowers daytime blood pressure in high normal-to-mild hypertensive subjects. *J Hum Hypertens.* Epub: 2008 Jun 5.

van Platerink CJ, Janssen HG, Horsten R, et al. Quantification of ACE inhibiting peptides in human plasma using high performance liquid chromatography-mass spectrometry. *J Chromatogr B Analyt Technol Biomed Life Sci.* 2006;2;830(1):151-157.

Ward HA, Chapelais G, Kuhnle GG, et al. Breast cancer risk in relation to urinary and serum biomarkers of phytoestrogen exposure in the EPIC-Norfolk study. *Breast Cancer Res.* 2008;10(2):R32.

Xu JY, Qin LQ, Wang PY, et al. Effect of milk tripeptides on blood pressure: A meta-analysis of randomized controlled trials. *Nutrition.* 2008;24(10):933-940.

Yamamoto N. Antihypertensive peptides derived from food proteins. *Biopolymers.* 1997;43(2):129-34. Erratum in: *Biopolymers* 1997;43(5):401-402.

Yamamoto N, Akino A, Takano T. Antihypertensive effect of the peptides derived from casein by an extracellular proteinase from Lactobacillus helveticus CP790. *J Dairy Sci.* 1994;77(4):917-922.

Yamamoto N, Akino A, Takano T. Purification and specificity of a cell-wall-associated proteinase from Lactobacillus helveticus CP790. *J Biochem.* 1993;114(5):740-745.

Yamamoto N, Maeno M, Takano T. Purification and characterization of an antihypertensive peptide from a yogurt-like product fermented by Lactobacillus helveticus CPN4. *J Dairy Sci.* 1999;82(7):1388-1393.

Yamamoto N, Takano T. Antihypertensive peptides derived from milk proteins. *Nahrung.* 1999;43(3):159-164.

Lactulose

DESCRIPTION

Lactulose is a semisynthetic disaccharide comprised of the sugars D-lactose and D-fructose. It is not found naturally. The sugars are joined by a beta glycosidic linkage making it resistant to hydrolysis by human digestive enzymes. There is no disaccharidase in the microvillus membrane of small intestine enterocytes that can hydrolyze lactulose; nor is the disaccharide absorbed from the small intestine. Lactulose is, however, fermented by a limited number of colonic bacteria. This can lead to changes in the colonic ecosystem in favor of some bacteria, such as lactobacilli and bifidobacteria, which may confer some health benefits.

Lactulose is used in the treatment of constipation and hepatic encephalopathy. The efficacy of lactulose in these conditions is based on its fermentation in the colon by certain bacteria and the increase of the biomass of these bacteria in the colon. The products of fermentation are mainly organic acids, such as lactic acid and small-chain fatty acids, which, by exerting a local osmotic effect in the colon, result in increased fecal bulk and stimulation of peristalsis. The higher doses used for hepatic encephalopathy lower the colonic pH, and ammonia, in the form of ammonium ions, is used by the bacteria for amino acid and protein synthesis. This lowers the serum ammonia levels and improves mental function.

The stimulation of the growth of bacteria, such as bifido-bacteria, may have other health benefits, such as protection against cancer of the colon. Lactulose is referred to as a bifidogenic factor. Substances such as lactulose that promote the growth of beneficial bacteria in the colon are called prebiotics. Prebiotics are typically nondigestible oligosac-charides. In addition to its uses in treatment of hepatic encephalopathy and constipation, lactulose is used in Japan in functional foods and as a nutritional supplement. These uses of lactulose are being explored in the United States, as well.

Lactulose is a solid substance that is very soluble in water and has a sweet taste. It is sweeter than lactose but not as sweet as fructose. Lactulose is also known as 4-O-beta-D-galactopyranosyl-D-fructofuranose. Its molecular formula is $C_{12}H_{22}O_{11}$, and its molecular weight is 342.30 daltons. The structural formula is:

Lactulose

ACTIONS AND PHARMACOLOGY

ACTIONS

Therapeutically, lactulose has laxative and ammonia-detoxifying actions.

Supplemental lactulose may have antitumor, antimicrobial, hypolipidemic and hypoglycemic actions in some. It may also help improve mineral absorption and balance, and may have antiosteoporotic activity.

MECHANISM OF ACTION

The possible antitumor activity of lactulose might be accounted for, in part, by the possible antitumor action of butyrate. Butyrate, along with other short-chain fatty acids, is produced by bacterial fermentation of lactulose in the colon. Some studies suggest that butyrate may induce growth arrest and cell differentiation and may also upregulate apoptosis, three activities that could be significant for possible antitumor activity. Lactulose may also aid in increasing the concentrations of calcium and magnesium in the colon. High concentrations of these cations in the colon may help control the rate of cell turnover. High concentrations of calcium in the colon may also lead to the formation of insoluble bile or salts of fatty acids. This might reduce the potential damaging effects of bile or fatty acids on colonocytes.

Lactulose may promote the growth of favorable bacterial populations, such as bifidobacteria, in the colon. Bifidobacteria may inhibit the growth of pathogenic bacteria, such as *Clostridium perfringens* and diarrheogenic *Escherichia coli*.

Lactulose may aid in lowering serum triglycerides in some. The mechanism of this possible effect is unclear. Decreased hepatocyte *de novo* synthesis of triglycerides is one hypothetical possibility. Lactulose may also lower total cholesterol and LDL-cholesterol levels in some. Again, the mechanism of this possible effect is unclear. Propionate, a product of lactulose fermentation in the colon, may inhibit HMG-CoA reductase, the rate-limiting step in cholesterol synthesis.

The possible effects of lactulose on blood glucose may be explained in a few ways. Lactulose may delay gastric emptying and/or shorten small-intestinal tract transit time. This may be via the short-chain fatty acids produced from lactulose in the colon. Short-chain fatty acids may be involved in the so-called "ileocolonic brake," which refers to the inhibition of gastric emptying by nutrients reaching the ileo-colonic junction. Short-chain fatty acids may also stimulate contractions of the ileum and shorten ileal emptying. In addition, propionate may inhibit gluconeogenesis by its metabolic conversion to methylmalonyl-CoA and succinyl-CoA. These metabolites could inhibit pyruvate carboxylase. Propionate may also reduce plasma levels of free fatty acids. High levels of free fatty acids lower glucose utilization and induce insulin resistance. Finally, propionate may enhance glycolysis via depletion of citrate in hepatocytes. Citrate is an allosteric inhibitor of phosphofructokinase.

Lactulose may bind/sequester such minerals as calcium and magnesium in the small intestine. The short-chain fatty acids formed from the bacterial fermentation of lactulose may facilitate the colonic absorption of calcium and, possibly, also magnesium ions. This could be beneficial in preventing osteoporosis and osteopenia.

PHARMACOKINETICS

Following ingestion, lactulose reaches the colon with very little digestion or absorption taking place in the stomach or small intestine. Lactulose is fermented by bifidobacteria, lactobacilli and some other bacteria in the colon to produce the short-chain fatty acids acetate, propionate and butyrate; the gases hydrogen, hydrogen sulfide, carbon dioxide and methane; and lactate, pyruvate, succinate and formate. Acetate, propionate and butyrate that are not metabolized in colonocyes are absorbed from the colon and transported via the portal circulation to the liver. These short-chain fatty acids are extensively metabolized in hepatocytes. Acetate, propionate and butyrate that are not metabolized in hepatocytes are transported by the circulation to various tissues, where they undergo further metabolism. Butyrate is an important respiratory fuel for the colonocytes. Lactulose is completely metabolized in the colon, and no lactulose is excreted in the feces.

Those with ileostomies may have a microbial flora colonizing their ileums. In those cases, lactulose could be fermented by some of the bacteria in a fashion similar to their fermentation in the colon.

INDICATIONS AND USAGE

Lactulose is used to treat constipation and hepatic encephalopathy. Preliminary research suggests that it might protect against a number of intestinal pathogens, that it might be helpful in the treatment of some inflammatory bowel diseases and that it could help prevent colorectal cancers. There is additional preliminary evidence suggesting that it could be of benefit in osteoporosis, diabetes mellitus and renal failure.

RESEARCH SUMMARY

Lactulose has proved effective in the treatment of some with chronic constipation, helping to restore normal peristalsis and defecation rhythm, softening stools and diminishing pain and other symptoms of dyspeptic disorders.

Lactulose is used with good results in some with compensated liver disease; lactulose has been shown in various studies to increase protein tolerance and help prevent hepatic encephalopathy.

Lactulose has helped protect against *Salmonella* infection and has shown activity against a number of other intestinal pathogens. It has reduced the incidence of bacterial translocation from the gut to mesenteric lymph nodes in rats with obstructive jaundice. It has also prevented bacterial translocation in animal models of surgical trauma. Other experiments suggest that lactulose might be helpful in idiopathic, as well as infectious inflammatory bowel diseases.

Lactulose has suppressed experimentally induced colonic aberrant crypt foci in rats and has helped protect colonic mucosa against a known colon carcinogen.

There is some early but promising clinical work. In one controlled study, patients who had undergone endoscopic removal of colorectal polyps were given antioxidant vitamins or lactulose to see if these substances could reduce the recurrence rate of adenomatous polyps. Over the course of this five-year study, polyps recurred in 5.7% of those taking the vitamins (A, C and E) and in 14.7% of those taking lactulose, compared with a recurrence rate of 35.9% in untreated controls. There were 209 subjects in the study.

Lactulose has also been shown to significantly stimulate calcium absorption in postmenopausal women, though the research has not yet been done to see whether it slows the rate of bone loss in aging subjects. There is, in addition, preliminary research suggesting that lactulose might improve glucose tolerance and have other effects on carbohydrate metabolism that could be of benefit in those with diabetes mellitus.

Finally, there is the suggestion in other preliminary research that lactulose might be helpful in the treatment of chronic renal failure. Lactulose has been shown to promote fecal excretion of water, sodium, potassium, amonium, urea, creatine and hydronium ions.

CONTRAINDICATIONS, PRECAUTIONS, ADVERSE REACTIONS

CONTRAINDICATIONS

Some lactulose preparations contain galactose. Therefore, lactulose is contraindicated in those who require a low galactose diet. Lactulose is also contraindicated in those who are hypersensitive to any component of a lactulose-containing preparation.

PRECAUTIONS

In the United States, lactulose is a prescription drug. Its use requires medical supervision. Its use as a dietary supplement is considered experimental.

Those who develop gastrointestinal symptoms (flatus, bloating, diarrhea) with the use of dietary fiber should exercise caution in the use of lactulose.

Those with lactose intolerance should exercise caution in the use of lactulose.

One of the metabolites of lactulose is hydrogen gas. Hypothetically, this represents a potential hazard for those using lactulose who may be required to undergo electrocautery procedures during proctoscopy or colonoscopy. Accumulation of hydrogen gas in significant amounts in the presence of an electric spark may result in an explosion. Therefore, those undergoing these procedures should stop lactulose intake at least a week before the procedure.

Pregnant women and nursing mothers should avoid lactulose.

ADVERSE REACTIONS

Laxative doses are typically 20 to 40 grams daily. Doses up to 10 grams daily are usually well tolerated. Some may be more sensitive to the possible gastrointestinal side effects of lactulose. The adverse reactions are mainly gastrointestinal and include flatus and abdominal cramps. Doses of greater than 13 grams daily can cause diarrhea. Also, nausea and vomiting have been reported following the higher doses. Some find the taste of lactulose to be disagreeable.

INTERACTIONS

DRUGS

Concomitant use of nonabsorbable antacids with lactulose may inhibit the desired lactulose-induced drop in colonic pH which might affect laxative activity and activity in the treatment of hepatic encephalopathy.

NUTRITIONAL SUPPLEMENTS

The concomitant use of such probiotics as *Bifidobacterium longum* and lactulose may enhance the possible health benefits of lactulose.

Lactulose may enhance the colonic absorption of calcium and magnesium supplements if used concomitantly.

FOODS

Lactulose may enhance the colonic absorption of calcium and magnesium in foods.

OVERDOSAGE

There have been no reports of overdosage.

DOSAGE AND ADMINISTRATION

Lactulose is available in some functional foods and nutritional supplements in Japan. Its use in the U.S. for supplemental purposes is still experimental. Supplemental doses used in Japan are about 2 to 5 grams daily. Doses higher than 10 grams daily are likely to cause gastrointestinal side effects (flatus, abdominal cramping, diarrhea). Doses of 10 to 20 grams daily and up to 40 grams daily are used to treat constipation. Doses from 60 to 120 grams daily are used to treat hepatic encephalopathy. Pharmaceutical lactulose is available in solutions and in the form of a crystalline powder. Lactulose is a prescription drug in the U.S. for pharmaceutical uses.

LITERATURE

Bianchi G, Ronchi M, Marchesini G. Effects of lactulose on carbohydrate metabolism and diabetes mellitus. *Scand J Gastroenterol Suppl.* 1997; 222:62-64.

Challa A, Rao JR, Chawan CB, Shackelford L. *Bifidobacterium longum* and lactulose suppress azoxymethane-induced colonic aberrant crypt foci in rats. *Carcinogenesis.* 1997; 18:517-521.

Clausen MR, Mortensen PB. Lactulose, disaccharides and colonic flora. Clinical consequences. *Drugs.* 1997; 53:930-942.

Gardiner KR, Erwin PJ, Anderson NH, et al. Lactulose as an antiendotoxin in experimental colitis. *Br J Surg.* 1995; 82:469-472.

Horsmans Y, Solbreux PM, Daenens C, et al. Lactulose improves psychomotor testing in cirrhotic patients with subclinical encephalopathy. *Aliment Pharmacol Ther.* 1997; 11:165-170.

Huchzermeyer H, Schumann C. Lactulose — a multifaceted substance. *Z Gastroenterol.* 1997; 35:945-955.

Ozcelik MF, Eroglu C, Pekmezci S, et al. The role of lactulose in the prevention of bacterial translocation in surgical trauma. *Acta Chir Belg.* 1996; 96:44-48.

Physicians' Desk Reference. 62nd edition. Montvale, NJ. Thomson Healthcare Inc.; 2008.

Ponz de Leon M, Roncucci L. Chemoprevention of colorectal tumors: role of lactulose and of other agents. *Scan J Gastroenterol Suppl.* 1997; 222:72-75.

Rowland IR, Bearne CA, Fischer R, Pool-Zobel BL. The effect of lactulose on DNA damage induced by DMH in the colon of human flora-associated rats. *Nutr Cancer.* 1996; 26:37-47.

Salminen S, Salminen E. Lactulose, lactic acid bacteria, intestinal microecology and mucosal protection. *Scand J Gastroenterol Suppl.* 1997; 222:45-48.

Teuri U, Vapaatalo H, Korpela R. Fructooligosaccharides and lactulose cause more symptoms in lactose maldigesters and subjects with pseudohypolactasia than in control lactose digesters. *Am J Clin Nutr.* 1999; 69:973-979.

Van den Heuvel EG, Muijs T, Van Dokkum W, Schaafsma G. Lactulose stimulates calcium absorption in postmenopausal women. *J Bone Miner Res.* 1999; 14:1211-1216.

Larch Arabinogalactan

DESCRIPTION

Larch arabinogalactan refers to a polysaccharide derived from wood of the Western larch or *Larix occidentalis*. Arabinogalactans occur in other types of larch, but that which is marketed for supplemental usage comes from the Western larch. Larch arabinogalactan is not one substance but a mixture of several different arabinogalactans with molecular weights as low as 3,000 daltons and as high as 100,000 daltons.

Arabinogalactans are water-soluble polysaccharides widely found in plants, fungi and bacteria. They are comprised of D-galactose and L-arabinose residues in the form of a beta-D-(1-3)-galactan main chain with side chains made up of galactose and arabinose units of various lengths. Galactan itself is a polymer of galactose.

In plants, arabinogalactans occur as arabinogalactan proteins. These proteins are proteoglycans involved in plant growth and development; they may also be involved in signal transduction in plants.

Dietary intake of arabinogalactans comes from carrots, radishes, tomatoes, pears and wheat, among other plant foods. Gum arabic, a commonly used food additive, is composed of highly branched arabinogalactan. Arabinogalactans are also found in such herbs as *Echinacea* spp. and such edible mushrooms as *Ganoderma lucidum*. Arabinogalactans are thought to contribute to the possible immune-enhancing activities of echinacea and ganoderma.

Larch arabinogalactan is considered a nondigestible soluble dietary fiber. It is also thought to stimulate the colonic growth of such bacteria as bifidobacteria and lactobacilli. These bacteria may confer certain health benefits. Substances that stimulate the growth of bifidobacteria are called bifidogenic factors. Substances that promote the colonic growth of beneficial bacteria are called prebiotics.

ACTIONS AND PHARMACOLOGY

ACTIONS

Larch arabinogalactan may have immune-enhancing activity.

MECHANISM OF ACTION

Larch arabinogalactan has shown some immune-enhancing activity in the laboratory, particularly with regard to the stimulation of human natural killer cell cytotoxicity.

The mechanism of the possible immune-enhancing activity is not known.

PHARMACOKINETICS

Little is reported on the pharmacokinetics of larch arabinogalactan in humans. It appears that there is little digestion of the polysaccharide in the stomach and small intestine. Like similar substances, it is most likely fermented in the colon to produce the short-chain fatty acids acetate, propionate and butyrate; the gases hydrogen, hydrogen sulfide, carbon dioxide and methane; and lactate, pyruvate and succinate. This requires corroboration by human studies.

INDICATIONS AND USAGE

Larch arabinogalactan exhibits immune-enhancing properties in animal and *in vitro* studies.

RESEARCH SUMMARY

Larch arabinogalactan has enhanced natural killer (NK) cell cytotoxicity and has also enhanced the function of some other immune-system components in experimental studies. It has inhibited the metastasis of tumor cells to the liver in the laboratory. Human trials are needed.

CONTRAINDICATIONS, PRECAUTIONS, ADVERSE REACTIONS

CONTRAINDICATIONS

Larch arabinogalactan is contraindicated in those hypersensitive to any component of a larch arabinogalactan-containing preparation.

PRECAUTIONS

Since larch arabinogalactan contains galactose and since the pharmacokinetics of the polysaccharide in humans has not been clarified, those who require a low galactose diet should avoid the substance.

Pregnant women and nursing mothers should avoid larch arabinogalactan supplements, pending long-term safety studies.

Those with lactose intolerance should exercise caution in the use of supplemental larch arabinogalactan.

ADVERSE REACTIONS

Doses of up to 10 grams daily appear to be well tolerated. There are no reports of adverse reactions. However, as with similar products, it would be expected that at higher doses (e.g., greater than 30 grams daily) gastrointestinal side effects, such as flatus, abdominal cramps and diarrhea, would be likely to occur in some.

INTERACTIONS

No known interactions with drugs, nutritional supplements, foods or herbs.

OVERDOSAGE

There are no reports of overdosage.

DOSAGE AND ADMINISTRATION

Larch arabinogalactan is available in capsules, powder and combination products marketed as nutritional supplements. Dosage is variable and ranges from 1 to 3 grams daily and sometimes higher.

LITERATURE

Hauer J, Anderer FA. Mechanism of stimulation of human natural killer cytotoxicity by arabinogalactan from *Larix occidentalis. Cancer Immunol Immunother.* 1993; 36:237-244.

He Y, Li.R, Chen Q, et al. [Chemical studies of immunologically active polysaccharides of Ganoderma lucidum (Leyss.ex Fr.) Karst.] [Article in Chinese.] *Chung Kuo Chung Yao Tsa Chih.* 1992; 17:226-228,256.

Kelly GS. Larch arabinogalactan: clinical relevance of a novel immune—enhancing polysaccharide. *Altern Med Rev.* 1999; 4:96-103.

Odonmazig P, Ebringerova A, Machova E, Alfodi J. Structural and molecular properties of the arabinogalactan isolated from Mongolian larchwood (*Larix dahurica* L). *Carbohydr Res.* 1994; 252:317-324.

Ponder GR, Richards GN. Arabinogalactan from Western larch. Part III: alkaline degredation revisited, with novel conclusions on molecular structure. *Carbohydrate Polymers.* 1997; 34:251-261.

Lithium

DESCRIPTION

Lithium is the lightest element of the alkali-metal group and the lightest metal. Its atomic number is 3 and its symbol Li. Lithium is a very reactive metal and is found naturally as lithium salts. Lithium is best known for its pharmaceutical use in the treatment of bipolar disorder or manic-depressive illness. Lithium is not currently considered an essential nutrient for humans. However, certain lithium deficiency states have been reported in some animals. Rats fed diets low in lithium were found to have depressed fertility, birth weight, litter size and weaning weight. Goats fed diets deficient in lithium were reported to have depressed fertility, birth weight and life span, as well as altered activity of several liver and blood enzymes. At least for rats and goats, lithium may serve an essential nutrient role.

Lithium is present in the human diet in ultratrace quantities and is found in some natural mineral waters. The typical daily dietary intake of lithium is approximately 200 to 600 micrograms. Fish, processed meat, milk, milk products, eggs, potatoes and vegetables are rich sources of this mineral. It has been suggested that lithium, at low-dosage levels, has a generally beneficial effect on human behavior. This suggestion was based on a report that associated higher incidence of violent crimes with low-lithium drinking water.

Lithium carbonate and lithium citrate are the pharmaceutical forms used for the treatment of bipolar affective disorder. Lithium gamma-linolenic acid is in clinical studies for the treatment of certain types of cancer. Lithium succinate is used in the United Kingdom as a topical treatment for seborrheic dermatitis.

For information on the pharmaceutical use of lithium for the treatment of manic-depressive illness, refer to the *hysicians' Desk Reference*. For information on lithium interactions, refer to the *PDR Guide to Drug Side Effects, and Indications*.

ACTIONS AND PHARMACOLOGY
ACTIONS
None known for dietary lithium.

INDICATIONS AND USAGE
There are no indications for the supplemental use of lithium. Suggestions that it might be useful in treating alcoholism, cancer or immune disorders are unfounded. Its use in treating manic-depressive illness requires strict medical supervision. There is very little safety margin between therapeutic and toxic doses.

RESEARCH SUMMARY
There is no credible research to support the supplemental or medically unsupervised use of lithium for any purpose.

CONTRAINDICATIONS, PRECAUTIONS, ADVERSE REACTIONS
CONTRAINDICATIONS
There are no indications for the supplemental use of lithium.

OVERDOSAGE
None known for dietary lithium. See *Physicians' Desk Reference* for pharmaceutical lithium.

DOSAGE AND ADMINISTRATION
No recommended dosage. Lithium may be found in colloidal minerals and some mineral waters.

LITERATURE
Nielsen FH. Ultratrace minerals. In: Shils ME, Olson JA, Shike M, Ross AC, eds. *Modern Nutrition in Health and Disease*. 9th ed. Baltimore, MD: Williams and Wilkins; 1999: 283-303.

Pickett EE, O'Dell BL. Evidence for dietary essentiality of lithium in the rat. *Biol Trace Elem Res*. 1992; 34:299-319.

Schrauzer GN, Shrestha KP. Lithium in drinking water and the incidence of crimes, suicides and arrests related to drug addictions. *Biol Trace Elem Res*. 1990; 25:105-113.

Lithium Gamma-Linolenic Acid (Li-GLA)

DESCRIPTION
Lithium gamma-linolenic acid is the lithium salt of the 18-carbon, n-6 polyunsaturated fatty acid gamma-linolenic acid or GLA. (See GLA.) Lithium gamma-linolenic acid, abbreviated Li-GLA, was developed to enhance the water solubility of GLA.

Lithium gamma-linolenic acid, in addition to being known as Li-GLA, is known as lithium gammalinolenate.

ACTIONS AND PHARMACOLOGY
ACTIONS
Li-GLA has putative cytotoxic activity against cells chronically infected with HIV-1 and putative antiproliferative activity in tumor cells.

MECHANISM OF ACTION
The mechanism of the putative actions of Li-GLA are speculative. It is hypothesized that the antiproliferative activity in tumor cells is due to the generation, from Li-GLA, of reactive oxygen species, which damage the tumor cells. Likewise, it is speculated that such reactive oxygen species are cytotoxic to cells chronically infected with HIV-1.

PHARMACOKINETICS
Studies of Li-GLA on pancreatic cancer patients have used intravenous infusions of the substance. Little information is available on the pharmacokinetics of oral Li-GLA.

INDICATIONS AND USAGE
Li-GLA has shown activity against HIV infected T-cells. It also has shown antiproliferative activity in tumor cells.

RESEARCH SUMMARY
Li-GLA has been reported, in preliminary research, to have selective cell-killing effects in human T-lymphoblastoid cells chronically infected with HIV. This *in vitro* work needs follow-up.

Li-GLA inhibits the growth of pancreatic cancer cells *in vitro*. It has also been reported to prolong the survival of those with pancreatic cancer. Follow-up with randomized prospective studies is needed to determine if Li-GLA might have any role to play in the management of pancreatic cancer or any other type of cancer.

CONTRAINDICATIONS, PRECAUTIONS, ADVERSE REACTIONS

CONTRAINDICATIONS

Known hypersensitivity to a lithium gamma-linolenic acid-containing product.

PRECAUTIONS

Li-GLA should not be used by pregnant women or nursing mothers unless recommended by a physician. Li-GLA should not be used before surgery. Lithium gamma-linolenic acid should not be used unless prescribed and monitored by a physician.

ADVERSE REACTIONS

Li-GLA has mainly been used in clinical studies administered intravenously. There is little experience with oral Li-GLA.

INTERACTIONS

No interactions between Li-GLA and warfarin, aspirin, other NSAIDs or herbs, such as *Allium sativum* (garlic) or *Ginkgo biloba,* have been reported. Such interactions, if they were to occur, might be manifested by nosebleeds and/or increased susceptibility to bruising. If this does occur, Li-GLA intake should be lowered or stopped.

OVERDOSAGE

There have been no reports of overdosage in the literature.

DOSAGE AND ADMINISTRATION

Oral Li-GLA is presently not available.

LITERATURE

Botha JH, Robinson KM, Leary WP. The response of human carcinoma cell lines to gamma-linolenic acid with special reference to the effects of agents which influence prostaglandin and thromboxane syntheses. *Prostaglandins Leukot Med.* 1985; 19:63-77.

de Antueno R, Elliot M, Ells G, et al. *In vivo* and *in vitro* biotransformation of the lithium salt of gamma-linolenic acid by three human carcinomas. *Br J Cancer.* 1997; 75:1812-1818.

Fearon KC, Falconer JS, Ross JA, et al. An open-label phase I/II dose escalation study of the treatment of pancreatic cancer using lithium gammalinolenate. *Anticancer Res.* 1996; 16; 867-874.

Ferguson PJ. Synergistic cytotoxicity between gamma-linolenic acid and the flavonoid naringenin against a human oral squamous carcinoma cell line (Meeting abstract). *Proc Annu Meet Am Assoc Cancer Res.* 1997; 38:A2148.

Ilc K, Ferrero JM, Fischel JL, et al. Cytotoxic effects of two gamma linolenic salts (lithium gammalinolenate or meglumine gammalinolenate) alone or associated with a nitrosourea: an experimental study on human glioblastoma cell lines. *Anticancer Drugs.* 1999; 10:413-417.

Kairemo KJ, Jekunen AP, Korppi-Tommola ET, Pyrhonen SO. The effect of lithium gamma-linolenate therapy of pancreatic cancer on perfusion in liver and pancreatic tissues. *Pancreas.* 1998; 16:105-106.

Kinchington D, Randall S, Winther M, Horrobin D. Lithium gamma-linolenate-induced cytotoxicity against cells chronically infected with HIV-1. *FEBS Lett.* 1993; 330:219-221.

Ravichandran D, Cooper A, Johnson CD. Effect of lithium gamma-linoenate on the growth of experimental human pancreatic carcinoma. *Br J Surg.* 1998; 85:1201-1205.

Ravichandran D, Cooper A, Johnson CD. Growth inhibitory effect of lithium gammalinolenate on pancreatic cancer cell lines: the influence of albumin and iron. *Eur J Cancer.* 1998; 34:188-192.

Seegers JC, Lotterling ML, Panzer A, et al. Comparative anti-mitotic effects of lithium gamma-linolenate, gamma-linolenic acid and arachidonic acid, on transformed and embryonic dells. *Prostaglandins Leukot Essent Fatty Acids.* 1998; 59:285-291.

Liver Hydrolysate/ Desiccated Liver

DESCRIPTION

Liver hydrolysate and desiccated liver have been marketed as nutritional supplements for over a century. They are principally used as a source of heme iron (see Iron).

Liver hydrolysate is typically prepared from bovine liver by partial enzymatic hydrolysis and processed to remove most of the fat and cholesterol. Desiccated liver is typically prepared by a freeze-drying process and retains fat and cholesterol. Liver hydrolysate is also known as liver extract and liquid liver extract.

ACTIONS AND PHARMACOLOGY

ACTIONS

Liver hydrolysate and desiccated liver may have hematinic activity. Liver hydrolysate has putative hepatoprotective activity.

MECHANISM OF ACTION

Hematinic activity refers to the ability of a substance to improve the quality of the blood, including the hemoglobin level and the number of erythrocytes. Liver hydrolysate and desiccated liver contain heme iron, an absorbable form of iron, which may promote the production of hemoglobin.

The putative hepatoprotective activity of liver hydrolysate is unknown.

PHARMACOKINETICS

The components of liver hydrolysate and desiccated liver are digested, absorbed and metabolized by normal physiological processes.

INDICATIONS AND USAGE

Claims are made that liver supplements improve fat metabolism, impart energy, help damaged tissues regenerate and protect the liver. There is no credible evidence to support any of these claims.

RESEARCH SUMMARY

There are no credible studies supporting the use of liver supplements.

CONTRAINDICATIONS, PRECAUTIONS, ADVERSE REACTIONS

CONTRAINDICATIONS

Liver hydrolysate and desiccated liver are contraindicated in those who are hypersensitive to any component of a liver hydrolysate- or desiccated liver-containing supplement.

PRECAUTIONS

Liver hydrolysate and desiccated liver supplements should be avoided by pregnant women, nursing mothers and children.

Those with hemochromatosis, sickle cell anemia, sideoblastic anemia and thalassemia should be extremely cautious in the use of liver hydrolysate and desiccated liver supplements.

Those who receive frequent blood transfusions and those with chronic liver failure should be extremely cautious in the use of liver hydrolysate and desiccated liver supplements.

The treatment of iron-deficiency anemia should be under the advice and supervision of a physician. Liver hydrolysate and desiccated liver are not standard treatments for iron-deficiency anemia.

ADVERSE REACTIONS

No reports.

INTERACTIONS

DRUGS

Heme iron is unlikely to have the types of drug interactions that iron salts do (see Iron).

NUTRITIONAL SUPPLEMENTS

Heme iron in liver hydrolysate and desiccated liver may be additive to the effects of iron supplements.

DOSAGE AND ADMINISTRATION

There are several forms of liver hydrolysate and desiccated liver that are marketed as nutritional supplements. There are no typical doses of these supplements.

LITERATURE

Fujisawa K. Therapeutic effects of liver hydrolysate preparation on chronic hepatitis: a double-blind, controlled study. *Asian Med J.* 1984; 26:497-526.

Ohbayashi A, Akioka T, Tasaki H. A study of effects of liver hydrolysate on hepatic circulation. *J Therapy.* 1972; 54:1582-1585.

Washizuka M, Hiraga Y, Furuichi H, et al. [Effect of liver hydrolysate on ethanol- and acetaldehyde- induced deficiencies]. [Article in Japanese]. *Nippon Yakurigaku Zasshi.* 1998; 111:117-125.

Lutein and Zeaxanthin

DESCRIPTION

Lutein and zeaxanthin are members of the carotenoid family, a family best known for another one of its members, beta-carotene (see Beta-Carotene). They are natural fat-soluble yellowish pigments found in some plants, algae and photosynthetic bacteria. They serve as accessory light-gathering pigments and to protect these organisms against the toxic effects of ultra-violet radiation and oxygen. They also appear to protect humans against phototoxic damage. Lutein and zeaxanthin are found in the macula of the human retina, as well as the human crystalline lens. They are thought to play a role in protection against age-related macular degeneration (ARMD) and age-related cataract formation. They may also be protective against some forms of cancer. These two carotenoids are sometimes referred to as macular yellow, retinal carotenoids or macular pigment.

Food sources of lutein and zeaxanthin, include corn, egg yolks and green vegetables and fruits, such as broccoli, green beans, green peas, brussels sprouts, cabbage, kale, collard greens, spinach, lettuce, kiwi and honeydew. Lutein and zeaxanthin are also found in nettles, algae and the petals of many yellow flowers. In green vegetables, fruits and egg yolk, lutein and zeaxanthin exist in non-esterified forms. They also occur in plants in the form of mono-or diesters of fatty acids. For example, lutein and zeaxanthin dipalmitates, dimyristates and monomyristates are found in the petals of the marigold flower (*Tagetes erecta*). Many of the marketed lutein nutritional supplements contain lutein esters, with much smaller amounts of zeaxanthin esters, which are derived from the dried petals of marigold flowers.

Lutein dipalmitate is found in the plant *Helenium autumnale* L. Compositae. It is also known as helenien and it is used in France for the treatment of visual disorders. Zeaxanthin in its fatty acid ester forms, is the principal carotenoid found in the plant *Lycium chinese* Mill. *Lycium chinese* Mill, also known as Chinese boxthorn, is used in traditional Chinese medicine for the treatment of a number of disorders, including visual problems.

Lutein and zeaxanthin belong to the xanthophyll class of carotenoids, also known as oxycarotenoids. The xanthophylls, which in addition to lutein and zeaxanthin, include alpha-and beta-cryptoxanthin, contain hydroxyl groups. This makes them more polar than carotenoids, such as beta-carotene and lycopene, which do not contain oxygen. Although lutein and zeaxanthin have identical chemical formulas and are isomers, they are not stereoisomers, as is sometimes believed. They are both polyisoprenoids containing 40 carbon atoms and cyclic structures at each end of their conjugated chains. Also, they both occur naturally as *all-trans* (*all-E*) geometric isomers. The principal difference between them is in the location of a double bond in one of the end rings. This difference gives lutein three chiral centers rather than the two that are found in zeaxanthin. The chemical structures are illustrated below.

Lutein

Zeaxanthin

Owing to its three chiral centers, there are 2^3 or 8 stereoisomers of lutein. The principal natural stereoisomer of lutein is (3R,3′R,6′R)-lutein. Lutein is also known as xanthophyll (also, the group name of the oxygen-containing carotenoids), vegetable lutein, vegetable luteol and beta, epsilon-carotene-3,3′diol. The molecular formula of lutein is $C_{40}H_{56}O_2$ and its molecular weight is 568.88 daltons. The chemical name of the principal natural stereoisomer of lutein is (3R,3′R,6′R)-beta,epsilon-carotene-3,3′-diol.

Zeaxanthin has two chiral centers and therefore, 2^2 or 4 stereoisomeric forms. One chiral center is the number 3 atom in the left end ring, while the other chiral center is the number 3′ carbon in the right end ring. One stereoisomer is (3R,3′R)-zeaxanthin; another is (3S-3′S)-zeaxanthin. The third stereoisomer is (3R,3′S)-zeaxanthin, and the fourth, (3S,3′R)-zeaxanthin. However, since zeaxanthin, in contrast to lutein, is a symmetric molecule, the (3R,3′S)-and (3S,3′R)-stereoisomers are identical. Therefore, zeaxanthin has only three stereoisomeric forms. The (3R,3′S)-or (3S,3′R)-stereoisomer is called *meso*-zeaxanthin.

The principal natural form of zeaxanthin is (3R,3′R)-zeaxanthin. (3R,3′R)-and *meso*-zeaxanthin are found in the macula of the retina, with much smaller amounts of the (3S,3′S)-stereoisomer. It is thought that *meso*-zeaxanthin in the macula is formed from (3R,3′R,6′R)-lutein. Zeaxanthin is also known as beta, beta-carotene-3,3′-diol, *all-trans*-beta-carotene-3,3′-diol, (3R,3′R)-dihydroxy-beta-carotene (the principal natural stereoisomer), zeaxanthol and anchovyxanthin. Its molecular formula is $C_{40}H_{56}O_2$ and its molecular weight is 568.88 daltons. Zeaxanthin is the principal pigment of yellow corn *zea mays* L, from which its name is derived. It is also produced by certain bacteria, such as *Flavobacterium multivorum*, which are yellow in color.

Chicken egg yolks are a rich food source of lutein and zeaxanthin. The average amount of lutein in chicken egg yolk is approximately 290 micrograms per yolk, and the average amount of zeaxanthin, approximately 210 micrograms per yolk. Lutein-containing plant extracts, which are mainly derived from marigolds, are widely fed to chickens in order to give their egg yolks and skin a deeper yellow color. However, the downside of obtaining lutein and zeaxanthin via consuming egg yolks, is a possible elevation of LDL-cholesterol.

ACTIONS AND PHARMACOLOGY

ACTIONS
Lutein and zeaxanthin may be ophthalmoprotective.

MECHANISM OF ACTION
Lutein and zeaxanthin, which are naturally present in the macula of the human retina, filter out potentially phototoxic blue light and near-ultraviolet radiation from the macula. The protective effect is due in part, to the reactive oxygen species quenching ability of these carotenoids. Further, lutein and zeaxanthin are more stable to decomposition by pro-oxidants than are other carotenoids such as beta-carotene and lycopene. Zeaxanthin is the predominant pigment in the fovea, the region at the center of the macula. The quantity of zeaxanthin gradually decreases and the quantity of lutein increases in the region surrounding the fovea, and lutein is the predominant pigment at the outermost periphery of the macula. Zeaxanthin, which is fully conjugated (lutein is not), may offer somewhat better protection than lutein against phototoxic damage caused by blue and near-ultraviolet light radiation.

Lutein and Zeaxanthin, which are the only two carotenoids that have been identified in the human lens, may be protective against age-related increases in lens density and cataract formation. Again, the possible protection afforded by these carotenoids may be accounted for, in part, by their reactive oxygen species scavenging abilities.

PHARMACOKINETICS
Lutein and zeaxanthin exist in several forms. Nutritional supplement forms are comprised of these carotenoids either in their free (non-esterified) forms or in the form of fatty acid esters. Lutein and zeaxanthin exist in a matrix in foods. In the case of the chicken egg yolk, the matrix is comprised of lipids (cholesterol, phospholipid, triglycerides). The carotenoids are dispersed in the matrix along with fat-soluble

nutrients, including vitamins A, D and E. In the case of plants, lutein and zeaxanthin are associated with chloroplasts or chromoplasts.

The efficiency of absorption of lutein and zeaxanthin is variable, but overall appears to be greater than that of beta-carotene. Esterified forms of these carotenoids may be more efficiently absorbed when administered with high-fat meals (about 36 grams), than with low-fat meals (about 3 grams). Lutein and zeaxanthin esters are hydrolyzed in the small intestine via esterases and lipases. Lutein and zeaxanthin that are derived from supplements or released from the matrices of foods, are either solubilized in the lipid core of micelles (formed from bile salts and dietary lipids) in the lumen of the small intestine, or form clathrate complexes with conjugated bile salts. Micelles and possibly clathrate complexes deliver lutein and zeaxanthin to the enterocytes.

Lutein and zeaxanthin are released from the enterocytes into the lymphatics in the form of chylomicrons. They are transported by the lymphatics to the general circulation via the thoracic duct. In the circulation, lipoprotein lipase hydrolyzes much of the triglycerides in the chylomicrons, resulting in the formation of chylomicron remnants. Chylomicron remnants retain apolipoproteins E and B48 on their surfaces and are mainly taken up by the hepatocytes and to a smaller degree by other tissues. Within hepatocytes, lutein and zeaxanthin are incorporated into lipoproteins. Lutein and zeaxanthin appear to be released into the blood mainly in the form of high-density lipoproteins (HDL) and, to a lesser extent, in the form of very-low density lipoprotein (VLDL). Lutein and zeaxanthin are transported in the plasma predominantly in the form of HDL.

Lutein and zeaxanthin are mainly accumulated in the macula of the retina, where they bind to the retinal protein tuberlin. Zeaxanthin is specifically concentrated in the macula, especially in the fovea. Lutein is distributed throughout the retina.

The form of lutein in the plasma is (3R,3′R,6′R)-lutein. Zeaxanthin found in plasma is predominantly (3R,3′R)-zeaxanthin. Lutein appears to undergo some metabolism in the retina to *meso*-zeaxanthin.

INDICATIONS AND USAGE
Lutein and zeaxanthin show some promise of protecting against macular degeneration and may reduce the risk of cataracts in some.

RESEARCH SUMMARY
Epidemiological data have found a relationship between low plasma concentrations of the carotenoids, lutein and zeaxanthin, and risk of developing age-related macular degeneration (AMD). Laboratory evidence has suggested that supplemental lutein and/or zeaxanthin might help protect against AMD.

In a multi-center study of 356 subjects aged 55 to 80 years, all diagnosed with advanced stage AMD, a high dietary intake of carotenoids was associated with a 43% lower risk for AMD compared with those consuming low quantities of these carotenoids. Lutein and zeaxanthin were most strongly associated with reduced AMD risk.

Lutein esters, equivalent to 30 milligrams of free lutein per day, given over a period of 140 days, significantly increased macular pigment density in two subjects. A low density of this pigment is believed to be a risk factor for AMD. Controlled clinical trials are needed.

There is also epidemiological evidence that increased lutein and zeaxanthin intake are associated with lower risk of cataract development. In one epidemiological study, those found to have the highest intake of lutein and zeaxanthin had a 22% decreased risk of cataract extraction compared with those who consumed the least amounts of these carotenoids. These findings are consistent with those of similar studies. Again, clinical studies are needed.

CONTRAINDICATIONS, PRECAUTIONS, ADVERSE REACTIONS
CONTRAINDICATIONS
Lutein and zeaxanthin are contraindicated in those hypersensitive to any component of lutein and zeaxanthin-containing products.

PRECAUTIONS
Pregnant women and nursing mothers should try to obtain lutein and zeaxanthin from the consumption of five or more servings daily of fruits and vegetables. Chicken egg yolk is also rich in lutein and zeaxanthin, and pregnant women and nursing mothers who do not have problems with elevated cholesterol levels, should try to include this item in their diets, as well.

Lutein and zeaxanthin supplements should not be used for the treatment of vitamin A deficiency, since these carotenoids are not converted to vitamin A.

ADVERSE REACTIONS
Adverse reactions involving lutein and zeaxanthin have not been reported.

INTERACTIONS
DRUGS
Cholestyramine: Concomitant intake of lutein/zeaxanthin and cholestyramine may decrease the absorption of these carotenoids.

Colestipol: Concomitant intake of lutein/zeaxanthin and colestipol may decrease the absorption of these carotenoids.

Mineral oil: Concomitant intake of mineral oil and lutein/zeaxanthin may reduce the absorption of these carotenoids.

Orlistat: Orlistat may decrease the absorption of lutein/zeaxanthin.

NUTRITIONAL SUPPLEMENTS

Beta-carotene: Concomitant intake of beta-carotene and lutein may decrease the absorption of these carotenoids.

Medium-chain triglycerides: Concomitant intake of medium-chain triglycerides and lutein/zeaxanthin may enhance the absorption of these carotenoids.

Pectin: Concomitant intake of pectin and lutein/zeaxanthin may decrease the absorption of these carotenoids.

FOODS

Oils: Some dietary oil, such as corn oil, may increase the absorption of lutein/zeaxanthin, especially the ester forms of these carotenoids.

Olestra: Concomitant intake of olestra and lutein/zeaxanthin may decrease the absorption of these carotenoids.

OVERDOSAGE

Overdosage of lutein and zeaxanthin have not been reported in the literature.

DOSAGE AND ADMINISTRATION

Lutein/zeaxanthin supplements are available in free (non-esterified) and esterified (with fatty acids) forms, and as single ingredient or combination products. The amount of zeaxanthin in these products is considerably lower than that of zeaxanthin. Products that deliver higher amounts of zeaxanthin are being developed. Dosage is variable, and optimal dosage for ophthalmological health is not known. Dietary intake of lutein of 6.9-11.7 milligrams daily has been associated with a decreased risk of age-related macular degeneration. Nutritional supplements containing lutein deliver from 250 micrograms (0.25 milligrams) to 20 milligrams daily.

Green leafy vegetables are good dietary sources of lutein, but poor sources of zeaxanthin. Good dietary sources of zeaxanthin, include yellow corn, orange pepper, orange juice, honeydew, mango and chicken egg yolk.

LITERATURE

Berendschot TT, Goldbohm RA, Klö pping WA, et al. Influence of lutein supplementation on macular pigment, assessed with two objective techniques. *Invest Opthalmol Vis Sci.* 2000; 41:3322-3326.

Bone RA, Landrum JT, Dixon Z, et al. Lutein and zeaxanthin in the eyes, serum and diet of human subjects. *Exp Eye Res.* 2000; 71:239-245.

Bone RA, Landrum JT, Friedes LM, et al. Distribution of lutein and zeaxanthin stereoisomers in the human retinal. *Exp Eye Res.* 1997; 64:211-218.

Bone RA, Landrum JT, Tarsis SL. Preliminary identification of the human macular pigment. *Vision Res.* 1985; 25:1531-1535.

Bowen PE, Clark JP. *Lutein esters having high bioavailability.* International patent publication number: WO 98/45241. International publication date: 15 October 1998.

Brown L, Rimm EB, Seddon JM, et al. A prospective study of carotenoid intake and risk of cataract extraction in U.S. men. *Am J Clin Nutr.* 1999; 70:517-524.

Chasan-Taber L, Willett WC, Seddon JM, et al. A prospective study of carotenoid and vitamin A intakes and risk of cataract extraction in U.S. women. *Am J Clin Nutr.* 1999; 70:509-516.

Dietary Reference Intakes for Vitamin C, Vitamin E, Selenium, and Carotenoids. Washington, DC: National Academy Press; 2000:325-382.

Erdman JW Jr. Variable bioavailability of carotenoids from vegetables (editorial). *Am J Clin Nutr.* 1999; 70:179-180.

Garnett KM, Glerhart DL, Guerra-Santos LH. *Method of making pure 3R-3' R stereoisomer of zeaxanthin for human ingestion.* United States Patent Number: 5,854,015. Date of Patent: Dec. 29, 1998.

Hammond BR Jr, Wooten BR, Snodderly DM. Density of the human crystalline lens is related to the macular pigment carotenoids, lutein and zeaxanthin. *Optom Vis Sci.* 1997; 74:499-504.

Handelman GJ, Nightingale ZD, Lichtenstein AH, et al. Lutein and zeaxanthin concentrations in plasma after dietary supplementation with egg yolk. *Am J Clin Nutr.* 1999; 70:247-251.

Khachik F. *Process for extraction and purification of lutein, zeaxanthin and rare carotenoids from marigold flowers and plants.* International patent publication number: WO 99/20587. International publication date: 29 April 1999.

Koonsvitsky BP, Berry DA, Jones MB, et al. Olestra affects serum concentrations of alpha-tocopherol and carotenoids but not vitamin D or vitamin K status in free-living subjects. *J Nutr.* 1997; 127(8 Suppl):1636S-1645S.

Kostic D, White WS, Olson JA. Intestinal absorption, serum clearance, and interactions between lutein and beta-carotene when administered to human adults in separate or combined oral doses. *Am J Clin Nutr.* 1995; 62:604-610.

Landrum JT, Bone RA, Joa H, et al. A one year study of the macular pigment: the effect of 140 days of a lutein supplement. *Exp Eye Res.* 1997; 65:57-62.

Mares-Perlman JA. Too soon for lutein supplements (editorial). *Am J Clin Nutr.* 1999; 70:431-432.

Nussbaum JJ, Pruett RC, Delori FC. Historic perspectives. Macular yellow pigment. The first 200 years. *Retina.* 1981; 1:296-310.

Olson JA. Carotenoids. In: Shils ME, Olson JA, Shike M, Ross AC. *Modern Nutrition in Health and Disease.* Baltimore, MD: Williams and Wilkins; 1999:525-541.

Roodenburg AJ, Leenen R, van het Hof KH, et al. Amount of fat in the diet affects bioavailability of lutein esters but not of alpha-carotene, beta-carotene, and vitamin E in humans. *Am J Clin Nutr.* 2000; 71:1187-1193.

Siems WG, Sommerburg O, van Kuijk FJ. Lycopene and beta-carotene decompose more rapidly than lutein and zeaxanthin upon exposure to various pro-oxidants in vitro. *Biofactors.* 1999; 10:105-113.

Sommerburg O, Keunen JE, Bird AC, et al. Fruits and vegetables that are sources for lutein and zeaxanthin: the macular pigment in human eyes. *B J Opthalmol.* 1998; 82:907-910.

Sommerburg OG, Siems WG, Hurst JS, et al. Lutein and zeaxanthin are associated with photoreceptors in the human retina. *Curr Eye Res.* 1999; 19:491-495.

van den Berg H. Effect of lutein on beta-carotene absorption and cleavage. *Int J Vitam Nutr Res.* 1998; 68:360-365.

van het Hof KH, Brouwer IA, West CE, et al. Bioavailability of lutein from vegetables is 5 times higher than that of beta-carotene. *Am J Clin Nutr.* 1999; 70:261-268.

Luteolin

DESCRIPTION

Luteolin is a polyphenolic substance and a member of the flavone subclass of flavonoids.

Conjugated forms of luteolin, including luteolin-7-glucoside, luteolin 7-O-beta-glucuronide and luteolin 7 O-[beta-glucuronosyl-(1>2)-beta-glucuronide] are found naturally in many plants, including celery (*Apium graveolens*), green peppers (*Capsicum annuum*), perilla leaf and seed (*Perilla frutescens*), dandelion (*Taraxacum officinale*), balsamic sage (*Salvia tomentosa*), thyme (*Thymus vulgaris*), chamomile tea (*Matricaria recutita*) and Japanese honeysuckle (*Lonicera japonica*).

Luteolin is chemically described as 2-(3,4-dihydroxyphenyl)-5,7-dihydroxy-4*H*-chromen-4-one. It is also known as 3',4',5,7-tetrahydroxyflavone, 2-(3,4-dihydroxyphenyl)-5,7-dihydroxy-4*H*-1-benzopyran-4-one, digitoflavone, daphneflavonol and flacitran. Its CAS registry number is 491-70-3, its empirical formula is $C_{15}H_{10}O_6$ and its molecular weight is 286.24.

Luteololin is of interest for its possible anti-inflammatory, anticancer and antiatherogenic activities. Recently, it has been found that luteolin may even help to ameliorate the niacin-induced flush.

All flavonoids possess a basic 15-carbon skeleton that can be represented as C_6-C_3-C_6. The common structure is that of a diphenylpropane molecule, consisting of two aromatic rings linked through the three carbons. Flavones possess a carbonyl group on position 4 of the C ring. Luteolin (tetrahydroxyflavone) possesses hydroxyl groups on positions 3' and 4' of the B ring and 5 and 7 of the A ring. The chemical structures below are described within this monograph.

Luteolin

Flavonol Skeleton

Flavonoid Skeleton

ACTIONS AND PHARMACOLOGY

ACTIONS

Luteolin has antioxidant activity and possible activity against the niacin (nicotinic acid)-induced flush. Luteolin may also have antiatherogenic, anticancer, anti-inflammatory, anti-leishmanial and otoprotective activities.

MECHANISM OF ACTION

Activity against the niacin (nicotinic acid)-induced flush: Niacin or nicotinic acid is one of the two forms of vitamin B_3 (See Niacin). At high doses, niacin is an effective lipid-modifying agent, lowering LDL cholesterol, raising HDL cholesterol and lowering triglyceride levels. The problem is that most people cannot tolerate the major adverse event of niacin, the so-called niacin flush, leading to its discontinuation. The niacin-induced flush is thought to involve the release of prostaglandin D_2 (PGD_2) from the skin. Pharmaceutical companies are researching possible PGD_2 and

PGD$_2$-receptor antagonists, but, to date, none are available, and it is not clear that such an antagonist would significantly decrease the symptoms of the niacin flush.

Luteolin was reported to inhibit the niacin-induced flush in a rat model. High-dose niacin was found to increase the ear temperature in rats and also to increase levels of PGD$_2$. When luteolin was administered to the rats 45 minutes prior to the niacin, it inhibited the niacin effect in the animals by 88% and also inhibited the level of PGD$_2$ by 100%. Aspirin, the most famous prostaglandin inhibitor, inhibited the niacin effect by only 30% and reduced PGD$_2$ by 86%. The hunt for a nontoxic substance that would abrogate the niacin-induced flush has been going on for some time. More research with luteolin is awaited to see if the results with this agent are any better than past attempts with other promising molecules.

Antiatherogenic activity: It is now widely accepted that atherosclerosis is an inflammatory disorder that is actually initiated very early in life. The earliest visible lesion of atherosclerosis is the fatty streak, which is due to an accumulation of lipid-laden foam cells in the intimal layer of the artery. The mature atherosclerotic lesion is comprised of three major components. The first is the cellular component composed predominately of smooth muscle cells and macrophages. The second component is the connective tissue matrix and extracellular lipid. The third component is intracellular lipid that accumulates within macrophages, converting them into the so-called foam cells. Inflammatory stimuli and release of various cytokines catalyze the formation of atherosclerotic lesions. The oxidation of LDL (low-density lipoprotein) to oxidized LDL plays a major role in the atherogenic process. Macrophages bind intraluminal LDL via receptors known as scavenger receptors, which recognize LDL only after it has been oxidized. Uptake of oxidized LDL renders the macrophages less mobile and promotes the accumulation of lipid-laden foam cells in the intima of the blood vessel.

Using THP-1 cells, a human monocyte cell line, and human umbilical vein endothelial cells (HUVEC), it was shown that luteolin inhibited THP-1 cell adhesion onto oxidized LDL-activated HUVECs. In addition, luteolin decreased the uptake of oxidized LDL by oxidized LDL-treated HUVACs. This study showed that luteolin might affect early steps in the atherogenic process by its inhibition of oxidized LDL-induced endothelial monocyte adhesion and oxidized LDL uptake.

The mechanism of luteolin's possible antiatherogenic activity is unclear. The antioxidant and anti-inflammatory activities of luteolin may play some roles in this. Further study is necessary and warranted, including animal studies and clinical trials.

Anticancer activity: Luteolin was found to reverse tumor resistance to doxorubicin in human and murine breast cancer cells under hypoxic conditions, but not under conditions of normoxia. These results suggested that luteolin's mechanism of action was via inhibition of glycolysis.

One of the oldest hypotheses of carcinogenesis is that of the German biochemist Otto Warburg, known as the Warburg hypothesis. The hypothesis states that there is a fundamental difference in the way that cancer cells, as opposed to non-cancer cells, produce energy (both in the form of ATP, or adenosine triphosphate). Warburg postulated that cancer cells are good survivors under hypoxic conditions and derive most of their energy from glycolysis, while non-cancer cells derive most of their energy via mitochondrial oxidative phosphorylation. Indeed, a high rate of glycolysis has been observed in a wide range of human cancers. And the metabolic adaptation to cancer cells in response to hypoxia is associated with reduced sensitivity to common anticancer agents. Thus, selectively inhibiting the glycolytic pathway might preferentially sensitize cancer cells to chemotherapeutic agents without significant toxicity to normal cells. And this is what luteolin appeared to do in human and murine breast cancer cells *in vitro*.

Luteolin was also shown to sensitize the anticancer effect of the widely used cancer chemotherapeutic agent, cisplatin (*cis*-diamminediachloroplatinum), but in this case by a different mechanism than that described above. Cisplatin's action as an anticancer agent is through crosslinking DNA, thus interfering with cell division. The damaged DNA elicits DNA repair mechanisms, which in turn activate apoptosis (programmed cell death). p53 is the key regulator for cisplatin-mediated apoptosis in cancer cells. The term p53 is used for both the tumor suppressor gene and its gene product, the transcription factor p53. p53 is arguably one of the most important cancer suppressor genes. The regulation of p53 protein stability is crucial to its anticancer function, and phosphorylation of p53 by c-Jun NH$_2$-terminal kinase (JNK) is central to its stability. If the p53 transcription factor becomes unstable, it winds up in the ubiquitin-proteasome degradation pathway, and if this occurs, cisplatin loses its efficacy as a cancer chemotherapeutic agent. Luteolin was found in cancer cells *in vitro* to activate JNK, resulting in the stabilization of p53 via its phosphorylation and decreased ubiquitination and proteasomal degradation, thus enhancing the anticancer activity of cisplatin. The enhanced cancer therapeutic efficacy of cisplatin via p53 stabilization was confirmed in an *in vivo* nude mouse xenograft model.

There appear to be still other mechanisms by which luteolin may inhibit cancer growth. Luteolin was shown to inhibit the proliferation of the prostate cancer cell lines, PC-3 and DU145. Luteolin also significantly inhibited PC-3 xenograft growth in nude mice. The insulin-like growth factor-1 receptor (IGF-1R), activated by insulin growth factor-1 (IGF-1), is required for prostate cell proliferation. IGF-1 binds to IGF-1R and induces receptor tyrosine phosphorylation, followed by activation of the intracellular PI3K (phosphatidylinositol-3 kinase)/Akt (protein kinase B) signaling pathway. Akt is the major signal for cell survival and proliferation. Luteolin was shown to inhibit tyrosine phosphorylation of IGF-1R and activation of Akt induced by IGF-1, which resulted in apoptosis and in the inhibition of prostate cancer cell proliferation *in vitro*.

Luteolin was found to inhibit the proliferation of HT-29 human colon cancer cells *in vitro*. In this case, it inhibited cyclin-dependent kinase (CDK)2 and CDK4 activity, resulting in arrest of the cell cycle in G1. Luteolin also promoted G2M arrest at 24 hours post-treatment by downregulating cyclin B1 expression and inhibiting cell division cycle (CDC)2 activity. Luteolin also induced apoptosis.

Luteolin was shown to inhibit tumor growth and angiogenesis in a murine xenograft model. The flavonoid inhibited vascular endothelial growth factor (VEGF)–induced angiogenesis in the rabbit cornea assay model. Further, luteolin inhibited VEGF-induced survival and proliferation of human vein endothelial cells (HUVECs). Specifically, luteolin inhibited phosphatidylinositol-3 kinase (PI3K) and Akt activity in the HUVECs. The flavonoid appeared mainly to target the survival signals of the PI3K/Akt signaling pathway, which was responsible for the inhibitory effects of luteolin on VEGF-induced survival of the HUVECs. With regard to the antimitotic effects of luteolin, that appeared to be mediated via inhibition of the PI3K/p 70 S6 kinase signaling pathway. Luteolin inhibited VEGF-induced phosphorylation of the 70 S6 kinase, a downstream effector of PI3K responsible for progression of the G1 phase of the cell cycle.

Anti-inflammatory activity: Luteolin has demonstrated a number of anti-inflammatory activities.

Luteolin has been shown to inhibit lipopolysaccharide (LPS)-induced proinflammatory cytokine signaling pathways in murine macrophages. Exposure of the macrophages to LPS was found to increase phosphorylation of the mitogen-activated protein kinase (MAPK) family members—extracellular signal-regulated kinases (ERKs)1/2, p38 and c-JUN N-terminal kinases (JNK)1/2. Pretreatment of the macrophages with luteolin inhibited the phosphorylation of the LPS-induced proinflammatory signaling molecules ERK 1/2 and p38, but not JNK1/2. It also blocked release of the inflammatory cytokine tumor necrosis factor (TNF)-alpha.

Saibokuto is an herbal medicine used in Kampo medicine (traditional Japanese medicine) as an adjunct in the treatment of a number of inflammatory conditions, such as asthma. Saibokuto is comprised of 10 herbs, including perilla leaf (*Perilla frutescens*), soyo in Japanese. Oral administration of an extract of perilla leaf to mice was shown to inhibit TNF-alpha and to possess anti-inflammatory and antiallergy activities. Of all the constituents isolated from perilla leaf, luteolin appeared to be the only one that showed significant anti-inflammatory and antiallergy activities *in vivo*. Luteolin was found to inhibit serum TNF-alpha production, arachidonic acid-induced ear edema, 12-O-tetradecanoylphorbol-13-acetate (TPA)-induced ear edema and oxazolone-induced allergic edema. The mechanism of the anti-inflammatory and antiallergy activities of luteolin is not completely known.

Luteolin was reported to have modulatory effects on osteoblastic function and inflammatory mediators in the mouse osteoblastic MC3T3-E1 cell line. Bone is remodeled continuously during adulthood via the resorption of old bone by osteoclasts and the subsequent formation of new bone by osteoblasts. A number of inflammatory cytokines are involved in the development of osteoclasts, including interleukin (IL)-1, interleukin (IL)-6 and interleukin (IL)-11. The production of IL-6 is regulated by sex hormones. The loss of gonadal function that occurs with aging leads to an increase in the formation of osteoclasts. Excessive osteoclastogenesis, which is associated with increased production of inflammatory mediators, can lead to osteopenia and osteoporosis. Luteolin was found to inhibit the production of a number of inflammatory mediators in osteoclasts, including IL-6. Further research is necessary and warranted to elucidate the mechanism of this anti-inflammatory activity, as well as the possible role of luteolin in the prevention of osteopenia and osteoporosis.

Luteolin also appears to have possible activity against neuroinflammation. It was recently reported that luteolin reduces production of the cytokine interleukin (IL)-6 in microglia via its inhibition of the JUN N-terminal kinase (JNK) signaling pathway and activation of activator protein (AP)-1. Microglia are specialized macrophages that act as the first and main form of active immune defense in the central nervous system (CNS). A major part of the innate immune system of the body, microglia use proinflammatory cytokines, including IL-6, as their defense molecules. However, excess production of these proinflammatory cytokines by activated microglia can lead to neurodegeneration and behavioral pathology.

A primary murine microglial cell line and BV-2 microglial cells (BV-2 is an immortalized murine microglial cell line) were pretreated with luteolin and then activated by lipopolysaccharide (LPS), which stimulates the production of IL-6 by the microglial cells. Luteolin inhibited the production of IL-6 at both the mRNA transcription and protein translation levels. Luteolin was found to inhibit the phosphorylation of JNK, thereby inhibiting the JNK signaling pathway. *In vivo* studies were also performed on mice that received intraperitoneal injections of LPS. Luteolin consumption by the mice reduced LPS-induced IL-6 levels in plasma and decreased the induction of IL-6 mRNA by LPS in the hippocampus, but not in the cortex or cerebellum.

Antileishmanial activity: Leishmaniasis is a parasitic disease caused by protozoan parasites of the genus *Leishmania* and transmitted by the bite of certain species of the sand fly. A tropical and subtropical disease, leishmaniasis presents with a range of signs and symptoms, from benign cutaneous lesions, through disfiguring mucocutaneous forms, to the often fatal visceral form. Some parasite strains have become resistant to the classic drugs, and some of the newer drugs used for treatment can be quite toxic. Therefore, there is great interest in researching and discovering new effective treatments. *Leishmania* parasites contain a unique DNA structure, the kinetoplast DNA, within their mitochondria. Luteolin has been demonstrated to be a fairly potent antileishmanial agent. It appears to have this effect by inducing topoisomerase II-mediated kinetoplast DNA cleavage leading to apoptosis.

Antioxidant activity: Luteolin, like other polyphenols, has a number of antioxidant activities. Luteolin has been demonstrated to scavenge hydroxyl radicals, superoxide anions and hydrogen peroxide. In addition, luteolin was shown to inhibit lipid peroxidation and the formation of 8-hydroxy-deoxyguanosine (8-OhdG), a product of nucleic acid oxidation.

Luteolin 7-glucoside was reported to protect against hepatic oxidative damage caused by carbon tetrachloride. Carbon tetrachloride increased the levels of 8-OhdG in liver tissue and decreased the levels of reduced glutathione. 8-OhdG is one of the most sensitive markers for oxidative stress. Reduced glutathione is the major intracellular antioxidant. Pretreatment of liver cells with luteolin suppressed the increase in 8OhdG and prevented the reduction in reduced glutathione and also reduced the carbon tetrachloride damage to the liver cells.

Otoprotective activity: Cisplatin is one of the most effective cancer chemotherapeutic agents. However, it has some very serious adverse events, including ototoxicity, nephrotoxicity, bone marrow toxicity and peripheral neuropathy. The loss of hearing appears to be caused by destruction of outer hair cells in the organ of Corti via induction of apoptosis. An active research area in cancer chemotherapy is the discovery of agents that can ameliorate the adverse events of chemotherapeutic agents. Luteolin was reported to suppress cisplatin-induced apoptosis in HEI-OC1 (House Ear Institute-Organ of Corti 1) cells. Luteolin was found to activate the extracellular signal-regulated kinase (ERK)/mitogen-activated protein kinase (MAPK) pathway and also induce heme oxygenase-1 expression. The mechanism of luteolin's otoprotective effect is not completely understood; more research is necessary to clarify it and also to ascertain if luteolin has other otoprotective activities.

PHARMACOKINETICS

Pharmacokinetic studies of luteolin and its conjugates have been performed mainly in experimental animals and are incomplete. An absorption analysis using rat everted small intestine showed that luteolin was converted to its glucuronide during passage through the intestinal mucosa. Luteolin 7 0-beta-glucoside was absorbed following hydrolysis to luteolin via bacteria in the intestinal wall. Free luteolin and its conjugates, including methylated conjugates, were present in rat plasma after dosing, suggesting that some luteolin can escape intestinal conjugation and first pass hepatic sulfation and methylation. The main conjugate circulating in the blood was found to be luteolin 7-glucuronide. Luteolin and its mono-glucuronide were demonstrated in human plasma following ingestion of luteolin. Further study on the absorption, distribution, metabolism and excretion of luteolin and its conjugates following oral intake is needed and warranted.

INDICATIONS AND USAGE

Mostly *in vitro* data suggest that the flavonoid luteolin may have some potentially significant anticancer, anti-inflammatory, cardioprotective and neuroprotective effects. There is very preliminary experimental evidence that luteolin might have some favorable impact on bone health and that it might be an effective antiparasitic, at least with respect to leishmaniasis. Its reported ability to inhibit the niacin-induced flush could be of benefit by increasing compliance in using niacin in the prevention of hyperlipidemia. Luteolin is found in green pepper, celery and perilla leaf among other sources. The Japanese have reportedly used a garnish made with the leaves of *Perilla frutescens* on raw fish and as an antidote to food poisoning. Dried red perilla leaves are also used in Chinese herbal medicine for the treatment of bronchial asthma.

RESEARCH SUMMARY

Building on prior research that had shown that various flavonoids inhibit some cancers, a group of researchers tested luteolin *in vitro*, demonstrating that it can inhibit tumor growth and angiogenesis in a murine xenograft model. They also demonstrated that the flavonoid can inhibit vascular endothelial growth factor-induced angiogenesis *in vivo* in a rabbit corneal assay. In another *in vitro* study, luteolin inhibited insulin-like growth factor 1 receptor signaling in prostate cancer cells. Since activation of this receptor is necessary in order for prostate cells to proliferate, the finding suggests that luteolin might have preventive and/

or therapeutic value in this cancer. Still other research has shown that luteolin may be able to inhibit proliferation of human myeloid leukemia cells, human gastric cancer cells, lung cancer cells, breast cancer cells, colon cancer cells and other cancer cells. Favorable chemosensitizing effects have also been observed when luteolin is combined with the anticancer drug cisplatin, making the latter more effective in *in vitro* tests. It has also been shown to sensitize breast cancer cells to doxorubicin in mice. Luteolin seems to work to inhibit these cancers by several modes of action, including one in which it significantly increases several proapoptotic proteins and decreases some others that are antiapoptotic. Follow-up of these promising studies is needed.

There are other studies indicating that luteolin most likely has significant anti-inflammatory properties. In a number of experiments, it has demonstrated an ability to reduce production of proinflammatory mediators in several cell types, including intestinal epithelial cells, fibroblasts, some macrophages, brain microglia and others. In one *in vivo* study, oral administration of 10 and 50 mg/kg of luteolin significantly suppressed paw edema chemically induced in mice. In a study of mouse alveolar macrophages, luteolin significantly inhibited inflammatory genes and mediators in a dose-dependent fashion, suggesting a possible role for this substance in inflammatory disorders of the lung. Some other experimental data suggest that luteolin might have efficacy in some allergic reactions, though whether it can be effective in allergic asthma has not been established. Its ability to favorably modulate inflammatory mediators in osteoblasts *in vitro* provides an early hint that the flavonoid might be bone-friendly.

Neuroinflammation may also be ameliorated by luteolin, according to preliminary findings. There are *in vivo* mouse data suggesting that luteolin reduces production of the proinflammatory cytokine IL-6 in brain microglia. There is a study indicating that luteolin, through activity in the central cholinergic system, may be able to help learning acquisition and memory. In this rat study, luteolin seemed to achieve its favorable result by blocking the negative effects on learning and memory of various central cholinergic neurotoxins. Luteolin has also exhibited antianxiety effects in an animal model, despite having no or low affinity for the benzodiazepine receptor binding site. More research is indicated in order to further elucidate the effects of this flavonoid in the central nervous system in general.

A possible role in cardiovascular health for luteolin is suggested by some recent data. In a study of human endothelial cells, luteolin was shown to help protect against some of the atherogenic effects of LDL oxidation. In a study of porcine endothelial cells, luteolin inhibited the secretion and gene expression of endothelin-1, a vasoconstrictor

important in blood pressure regulation; over-production of this vasoconstrictor is implicated in vascular disease and atherosclerosis. In addition, another recent study has found that luteolin can inhibit the so-called "niacin flush" that keeps many from using niacin to help regulate blood lipids. Prior research in humans has demonstrated that sustained release niacin is very effective at lowering serum cholesterol, LDL and triglycerides, while concomitantly raising HDL. Unfortunately, some 75 percent of those taking niacin experience unpleasant warmth and itching ("the niacin flush"), leading, in many cases, to discontinuation of the niacin therapy. In a rat study, injected luteolin produced effects consistent with blocking the flush. The researchers concluded that it might be a better inhibitor of the flush than some other substances. More research is needed to determine if luteolin can be effective in blocking the flush in humans and if it can be helpful in preventing/treating cardiovascular disease in general.

Finally, luteolin has been reported to have a potent antileishmanial effect in animal models. It attacks the parasite, a major health problem in developing countries, reportedly by inhibiting DNA synthesis, arresting cell cycle progression and thus inducing apoptosis. Again, more research is needed and warranted.

CONTRAINDICATIONS, PRECAUTIONS, ADVERSE REACTIONS

CONTRAINDICATIONS

Luteolin is contraindicated in those who are hypersensitive to any component of a luteolin- or conjugated luteolin-containing dietary supplement.

PRECAUTIONS

Those who wish to try luteolin supplements for the support of any health condition should first discuss its use with his or her physician.

Pregnant women and nursing mothers should avoid the use of luteolin-containing dietary supplements.

See drug interactions below.

ADVERSE REACTIONS

None known.

INTERACTIONS

DRUGS

Luteolin was found to reverse tumor resistance to doxorubicin in human and murine breast cancer cells under hypoxic conditions.

Luteolin was shown to sensitize the anticancer effect of cisplatin (*cis*-diamminedichloroplatinum).

Luteolin has been found to inhibit the metabolism of the sedative drug, midazolam, by human liver microsomes and cytochrome P450 3A4 (CYP 3A4) and CYP3A5. Midazolam is a probe substrate for CYP 3A4 and CYP3A5 enzymes. CYP 3A4 is located in the intestine and liver, and its inhibition leads to delayed absorption and reduced first pass metabolism in the liver, resulting in higher plasma levels of the drug. It is unclear how clinically relevant this finding might be, and this issue should be further studied. However, given this finding, those using midazolam or other drugs metabolized by CYP 3A4, including the statins—atorvastatin, lovastatin and simvastatin—as well as amiodarone, buspirone, cisapride, etopiside, quinidine, sidenafil, tadalafil, vardenafil and others, should exercise caution in the use of luteolin-containing dietary supplements.

NUTRITIONAL SUPPLEMENTS
None known.

OVERDOSAGE
There are no reports of overdosage.

DOSAGE AND ADMINISTRATION
The optimal doses of luteolin or its conjugates for health benefits are not known.

Dietary supplements containing luteolin or its conjugates in various amounts are available.

Luteolin in the form of its conjugates are found in celery and green peppers in variable amounts.

LITERATURE

Bagli E, Stefaniotou M, Morbidelli L, et al. Luteolin inhibits vascular endothelial growth factor-induced angiogenesis; inhibition of endothelial cell survival and proliferation by targeting phosphatidylinositol 3'-kinase activity. *Cancer Res.* 2004;64(21):7936-7946.

Cai Q, Rahn RO, Zhang R. Dietary flavonoids, quercetin, luteolin and genistein, reduce oxidative DNA damage and lipid peroxidation and quench free radicals. *Cancer Lett.* 1997;119(1):99-107.

Chen CY, Peng WH, Tsai KD, et al. Luteolin suppresses inflammation-associated gene expression by blocking NF-kappaB and AP-1 activation pathway in mouse alveolar macrophages. *Life Sci.* 2007;81(23-24):1602-1614.

Chen T, Li LP, Lu XY, et al. Absorption and excretion of luteolin and apigenin in rats after oral administration of Chrysanthemum morifolium extract. *J Agric Food Chem.* 2007;55(2):273-277.

Choi B-M, Lim D-W, Lee, J-A, et al. Luteolin suppresses cisplatin-induced apoptosis in auditory: possible mediation through induction of heme oxygenase-1 expression. *J Med Food.* 2008; 11(2):230-236.

Choi EM. Modulatory effects of luteolin on osteoblastic function and inflammatory mediators in osteoblastic MC3T3-E1 cells. *Cell Biol Int.* 2007;31(9):870-877.

Chowdhury AR, Sharma S, Mandal S, et al. Luteolin, an emerging anti-cancer flavonoid, poisons eukaryotic DNA topoisomerase I. *Biochem J.* 2002;366(Pt 2):653-661.

Chung JG, Hsia TC, Kuo HM, et al. Inhibitory actions of luteolin on the growth and arylamine N-acetyltransferase activity in strains of Helicobacter pylori from ulcer patients. *Toxicol In Vitro.* 2001;15(3):191-198.

Coleta M, Campos MG, Cotrim MD, et al. Assessment of luteolin (3',4',5,7-tetrahydroxyflavone) neuropharmacological activity. *Behav Brain Res.* 2008;189(1):75-82.

Du GJ, Song ZH, Lin HH, et al. Luteolin as a glycolysis inhibitor offers superior efficacy and lesser toxicity of doxorubicin in breast cancer cells. *Biochem Biophys Res Commun.* 2008;372(3):497-502.

Fang J, Zhou Q, Shi XL, et al. Luteolin inhibits insulin-like growth factor 1 receptor signaling in prostate cancer cells. *Carcinogenesis.* 2007;28(3):713-723.

Harris GK, Qian Y, Leonard SS, et al. Luteolin and chrysin differentially inhibit cyclooxygenase-2 expression and scavenge reactive oxygen species but similarly inhibit prostaglandin-E2 formation in RAW 264.7 cells. *J Nutr.* 2006;136(6):1517-1521.

Hirano T, Arimitsu J, Higa S, et al. Luteolin, a flavonoid, inhibits CD40 ligand expression by activated human basophils. *Int Arch Allergy Immunol.* 2006;140(2):150-156.

Horinaka M, Yoshida T, Shiraishi T, et al. Luteolin induces apoptosis via death receptor 5 upregulation in human malignant tumor cells. *Oncogene.* 2005;24(48):7180-7189.

Hu C, Kitts DD. Luteolin and luteolin-7-O-glucoside from dandelion flower suppress iNOS and COX-2 in RAW264.7 cells. *Mol Cell Biochem.* 2004;265(1-2):107-113.

Jang S, Kelley KW, Johnson RW. Luteolin reduces IL-6 production in microglia by inhibiting JNK phosphorylation and activation of AP-1. *Proc Natl Acad Sci U S A.* 2008;105(21):7534-7539.

Jeong YJ, Choi YJ, Choi JS, et al. Attenuation of monocyte adhesion and oxidised LDL uptake in luteolin-treated human endothelial cells exposed to oxidised LDL. *Br J Nutr.* 2007;97(3):447-457.

Jiang H, Xia Q, Wang X, et al. Luteolin induces vasorelaxion in rat thoracic aorta via calcium and potassium channels. *Pharmazie.* 2005;60(6):444-447.

Ju W, Wang X, Shi H, et al. A critical role of luteolin-induced reactive oxygen species in blockage of tumor necrosis factor-activated nuclear factor-kappaB pathway and sensitization of apoptosis in lung cancer cells. *Mol Pharmacol.* 2007;71(5):1381-1388.

Karrasch T, Kim JS, Jang BI, et al. The flavonoid luteolin worsens chemical-induced colitis in NF-kappaB(EGFP) transgenic mice through blockade of NF-kappaB-dependent protective molecules. *PLoS ONE.* July 2007;2(7):e596.

Kim JA, Kim DK, Kang OH, et al. Inhibitory effect of luteolin on TNF-alpha-induced IL-8 production in human colon epithelial cells. *Int Immunopharmacol.* 2005;5(1):209-217.

Kim JH, Lee EO, Lee HJ, et al. Caspase activation and extracellular signal-regulated kinase/Akt inhibition were involved in luteolin-induced apoptosis in Lewis lung carcinoma cells. *Ann NY Acad Sci.* December 2006;1090:147-60. Erratum in: *Ann NY Acad Sci.* 2007;1095:597. Corrected and republished in: *Ann NY Acad Sci.* 2007;1095:598-611.

Kim JS, Jobin C. The flavonoid luteolin prevents lipopolysaccharide-induced NF-kappaB signaling and gene expression by blocking IkappaB kinase activity in intestinal epithelial cells and bone-marrow derived dendritic cells. *Immunology.* 2005;115(3):375-387.

Kim JS, Lee HJ, Lee MH, et al. Luteolin inhibits LPS-stimulated inducible nitric oxide synthase expression in BV-2 microglial cells. *Planta Med.* 2006;72(1):65-68.

Kim TJ, Kim JH, Jin YR, et al. The inhibitory effect and mechanism of luteolin 7-glucoside on rat aortic vascular smooth muscle cell proliferation. *Arch Pharm Res.* 2006;29(1):67-72.

Kotanidou A, Xagorari A, Bagli E, et al. Luteolin reduces lipopolysaccharide-induced lethal toxicity and expression of proinflammatory molecules in mice. *Am J Respir Crit Care Med.* 2002;165(6):818-823.

Kozakai T, Yamanaka A, Ichiba T, et al. Luteolin inhibits endothelin-1 secretion in cultured endothelial cells. *Biosci Biotechnol Biochem.* 2005;69(8):1613-1615.

Leung HW, Wu CH, Lin CH, et al. Luteolin induced DNA damage leading to human lung squamous carcinoma CH27 cell apoptosis. *Eur J Pharmacol.* 2005;508(1-3):77-83.

Li YC, Hung CF, Yeh FT, et al. Luteolin-inhibited arylamine N-acetyltransferase activity and DNA-2-aminofluorene adduct in human and mouse leukemia cells. *Food Chem Toxicol.* 2001;39(7):641-647.

Manju V, Balasubramaniyan V, Nalini N. Rat colonic lipid peroxidation and antioxidant status: the effects of dietary luteolin on 1,2-dimethylhydrazine challenge. *Cell Mol Biol Lett.* 2005;10(3):535-551.

Manju V, Nalini N. Protective role of luteolin in 1,2-dimethylhydrazine induced experimental colon carcinogenesis. *Cell Biochem Funct.* 2007;25(2):189-194.

Manju V, Nalini N. Chemopreventive potential of luteolin during colon carcinogenesis induced by 1,2-dimethylhydrazine. *Ital J Biochem.* 2005;54(3-4):268-275.

Michels G, Wätjen W, Niering P, et al. Pro-apoptotic effects of the flavonoid luteolin in rat H4IIE cells. *Toxicology.* 2005;206(3):337-348.

Min YS, Bai KL, Yim SH, et al. The effect of luteolin-7-O-beta-D-glucuronopyranoside on gastritis and esophagitis in rats. *Arch Pharm Res.* 2006;29(6):484-489.

Mittra B, Saha A, Chowdhury AR, et al. Luteolin, an abundant dietary component is a potent anti-leishmanial agent that acts by inducing topoisomerase II-mediated kinetoplast DNA cleavage leading to apoptosis. *Mol Med.* 2000;6(6):527-541.

Papaliodis D, Boucher W, Kempuraj D, et al. The flavonoid luteolin inhibits niacin-induced flush. *Br J Pharmacol.* 2008;153(7):1382-1387.

Qiusheng Z, Xiling S, Xubo, et al. Protective effects of luteolin-7-glucoside against liver injury caused by carbon tetrachloride in rats. *Pharmazie.* 2004;59(4):286-289.

Quintieri L, Palatini P, Nassi A, et al. Flavonoids diosmetin and luteolin inhibit midazolam metabolism by human liver microsomes and recombinant CYP 3A4 and CYP3A5 enzymes. *Biochem Pharmacol.* 2008;75(6):1426-1437.

Samy RP, Gopalakrishnakone P, Ignacimuthu S. Anti-tumor promoting potential of luteolin against 7,12-dimethylbenz(a)anthracene-induced mammary tumors in rats. *Chem Biol Interact.* 2006;164(1-2):1-14.

Schlupper D, Giesa S, Gebhardt R. Influence of biotransformation of luteolin, luteolin 7-O-glucoside, 3′,4′-dihydroxyflavone and apigenin by cultured rat hepatocytes on antioxidative capacity and inhibition of EGF receptor tyrosine kinase activity. *Planta Med.* 2006;72(7):596-603.

Shi R, Huang Q, Zhu X, et al. Luteolin sensitizes the anticancer effect of cisplatin via c-Jun NH2-terminal kinase-mediated p53 phosphorylation and stabilization. *Mol Cancer Ther.* 2007;6(4):1338-1347.

Su CC, Chen GW, Yeh CC, et al. Luteolin induces N-acetylation and DNA adduct of 2-aminofluorene accompanying N-acetyltransferase activity and gene expression in human bladder cancer T24 cell line. *Anticancer Res.* 2003;23(1A):355-362.

Theoharides TC, Kempuraj D, Iliopoulou BP. Mast cells, T cells, and inhibition by luteolin: implications for the pathogenesis and treatment of multiple sclerosis. *Adv Exp Med Biol.* 2007;601:423-430.

Tsai FS, Peng WH, Wang WH, et al. Effects of luteolin on learning acquisition in rats: involvement of the central cholinergic system. *Life Sci.* 2007;80(18):1692-1698.

Tsou MF, Chen GW, Hung CF, et al. Luteolin inhibits the growth and arylamine N-acetyl-transferase activity in Neisseria gonorrhoeae. *Microbios.* 2001;104(408):87-97.

Ueda H, Yamazaki C, Yamazaki M. Luteolin as an anti-inflammatory and anti-allergic constituent of Perilla frutescens. *Biol Pharm Bull.* 2002;25(9):1197-1202.

Wang X, Wang Q, Morris ME. Pharmacokinetic interaction between the flavonoid luteolin and gamma-hydroxybutyrate in rats: potential involvement of monocarboxylate transporters. *AAPS J.* 2008;10(1):47-55.

Wang XG, Chen GY, Chen MP. [Effect of luteolin on COX-2 and mPGES-1 expression in LPS-induced RAW264.7 cells] [Article in Chinese.] *Zhong Yao Cai.* 2007;30(10):1263-1266.

Wruck CJ, Claussen M, Fuhrmann G, et al. Luteolin protects rat PC12 and C6 cells against MPP+ induced toxicity via an ERK dependent Keap1-Nrf2-ARE pathway. *J Neural Transm Suppl.* 2007;(72):57-67.

Wu B, Zhang Q, Shen W, et al. Anti-proliferative and chemosensitizing effects of luteolin on human gastric cancer AGS cell line. Mol Cell Biochem. 2008;313(1-2):125-132.

Yang SF, Yang WE, Chang HR, et al. Luteolin induces apoptosis in oral squamous cancer cells. *J Dent Res.* 2008;87(4):401-406.

Zhang FF, Shen HM, Zhu XQ. [Research progress on anti-tumor effects of luteolin] [Article in Chinese.] *Zhejiang Da Xue Xue Bao Yi Xue Ban.* 2006;35(5):573-578.

Zhao W, Liang C, Chen Z, et al. [Luteolin inhibits proliferation and collagen synthesis of hepatic stellate cells] [Article in Chinese.] *Zhonghua Gan Zang Bing Za Zhi.* 2002;10(3):204-206.

Zhou P, Li LP, Luo SQ, et al. Intestinal absorption of luteolin from peanut hull extract is more efficient than that from individual pure luteolin. *J Agric Food Chem.* 2008;56(1):296-300.

Lycopene

DESCRIPTION

Lycopene is a member of the carotenoid family of chemical substances. Lycopene, similar to other carotenoids, is a natural fat-soluble pigment (red, in the case of lycopene) found in certain plants and microorganisms, where it serves as an accessory light-gathering pigment and to protect these organisms against the toxic effects of oxygen and light. Lycopene may also protect humans against certain disorders, such as prostate cancer and perhaps some other cancers, and coronary heart disease.

Carotenoids are the principal pigments responsible for the colors of vegetables and fruits (see Beta-Carotene and Lutein and Zeaxanthin). Lycopene is responsible for the red color of red tomatoes. In addition to tomatoes (*Lycopersicon esculentum*) and tomato-based products, such as ketchup, pizza sauce, tomato juice and tomato paste, lycopene is also found in watermelon, papaya, pink grapefruit and pink guava. Processed tomato products are more available dietary sources of lycopene than fresh tomatoes. The average daily intake of lycopene is approximately 25 milligrams, with 50% of this in the form of processed tomato products.

Lycopene is an acyclic isomer of beta-carotene. Beta-carotene, which contains beta-ionone rings at each end of the molecule, is formed in plants, including tomatoes, via the action of the enzyme lycopene beta-cyclase. Lycopene is a 40 carbon atom, open chain polyisoprenoid with 11 conjugated double bonds. The structural formula of lycopene is represented as follows:

Lycopene

All-trans lycopene is the predominant geometric isomer found in plants. *Cis* isomers of lycopene are also found in nature, including 5-*cis*, 9-*cis*, 13-*cis* and 15-*cis* isomers. Lycopene found in human plasma is a mixture of approximately 50% *cis* lycopene and 50% all-*trans* lycopene. Lycopene in processed foods, is mainly in the form of the *cis*-isomer.

Lycopene is a lipophilic compound and is insoluble in water. Lycopene is also known as psi-carotene. Its molecular formula is $C_{40}H_{56}$ and its molecular weight is 536.88 daltons. In contrast to beta-carotene, lycopene has no vitamin A activity and thus is a nonprovitamin A carotenoid.

ACTIONS AND PHARMACOLOGY

ACTIONS

Lycopene may have anticarcinogenic and antiatherogenic activities.

The intake of tomato-based foods, especially processed tomato products, is associated with a significantly lower risk for prostate cancer, and also appears to be associated with a lower risk for lung cancer. The mechanism of the possible anticarcinogenic activity of lycopene is not well understood, but there are a few hypotheses. Cancer, as well as several other chronic diseases, is linked to oxidative stress. *In vitro* studies have demonstrated that lycopene has the highest antioxidant activity of all the carotenoids. It has the ability to quench singlet oxygen (more so than beta-carotene), to trap peroxyl radicals, to inhibit the oxidation of DNA, to inhibit lipid peroxidation, and in some studies, to inhibit the oxidation of low-density lipoprotein (LDL).

MECHANISM OF ACTION

Non-antioxidant mechanisms have also been proposed. Failure of cell signaling may be a cause of cell overgrowth and eventually cancer. Lycopene may stimulate gap junction communication between cells. It is speculated that lycopene may suppress carcinogen-induced phosphorylation of regulatory proteins such as p53 and Rb antioncogenes and stop cell division at the G_0-G_1 cell cycle phase. One researcher has hypothesized that lycopene-induced modulation of the liver metabolizing enzyme cytochrome P450 2E1 may be the underlying mechanism of protection against carcinogen-induced preneoplastic lesions in the rat liver. Lycopene may also reduce cellular proliferation induced by insulin-like growth factors. There is some preliminary *in vitro* evidence for the latter proposal.

The mechanism of the possible antiatherogenic activity of lycopene is likewise unclear. Lycopene's antioxidant activity is a possibility. Lycopene has also been found to inhibit cholesterol synthesis, to inhibit HMG-CoA (hydroxymethyl-glutaryl coenzyme A) reductase activity and to upregulate LDL receptor activity in macrophages. A small preliminary study in humans, reported an LDL-cholesterol-lowering effect of lycopene.

PHARMACOKINETICS

Lycopene is available in nutritional supplements in the form of an oleoresin, in phospholipid complexes and in oils. In foods, lycopene exists as part of a matrix (in chloroplasts or chromoplasts) within the vegetables or fruit. The efficiency of absorption of lycopene from supplements and foods is variable. The efficiency of absorption of lycopene from tomatoes, in which lycopene is tightly bound within the matrix, is low. It is much higher in processed tomato products. The improved availability of lycopene from processed foods is due to its release from the ruptured plant cells following the mechanical and thermal processing, as well as heat induced-*trans* to *cis* isomerization. *Cis*-lycopene is reported to be more bioavailable than *trans*-lycopene. Lipids increase the absorption of lycopene. For example, the combination of tomato sauce and olive oil delivers more absorbable lycopene than tomato sauce without oil.

Lycopene from supplements or from the matrices of foods is either solubilized in the lipid core of micelles (formed from bile salts and dietary fat) in the lumen of the small intestine or forms clathrate complexes with conjugated bile salts. Micelles and clathrate complexes deliver lycopene to the enterocytes.

Lycopene is released from the enterocytes into the lymphatics in the form of chylomicrons. Lycopene is transported by the lymphatics to the general circulation via the thoracic duct. In the circulation, lipoprotein lipase hydrolyzes much of the triglycerides in the chylomicrons, resulting in the formation of chylomicron remnants. Chylomicron remnants retain apolipoproteins E and B48 on their surfaces and are mainly taken up by hepatocytes and to lesser degrees by other tissues. Within hepatocytes, lycopene is incorporated into lipoproteins. Lycopene is released into the blood from the hepatocytes in the form of very-low density lipoproteins (VLDL) and low-density lipoproteins (LDL). In the plasma, VLDL is converted by lipoprotein lipase to LDL. Lycopene is transported in the plasma predominantly in the form of LDL.

There is much unknown about the pharmacokinetics of lycopene, in particular its distribution and its metabolism.

INDICATIONS AND USAGE

Lycopene may be helpful in preventing and possibly also managing some cancers, particularly prostate cancer, and may confer some protection against cardiovascular disease. Research, though suggestive of these positive effects, is far from conclusive. And there is far too little evidence of efficacy from very preliminary studies to support any indication for lycopene in the management of HIV disease or other immune dysfunction or in the management of neurodegenerative disorders.

RESEARCH SUMMARY

In a prospective study that followed the eating habits of 47,000 men for six years, a positive correlation was found between tomato-based food consumption and apparent resistance to development of prostate cancer. There was a 35% reduction in risk of developing prostate cancer among those who consumed more than 10 servings of tomato products weekly, compared with those who consumed fewer than 1.5 servings weekly. Most of these servings (82%) were in the form of tomatoes, tomato sauce and pizza. Tomato sauce appeared to be the most protective.

This study reinforced the findings of an earlier prospective study that examined the eating habits of Seventh Day Adventist men over a six-year period. This study found that the relative risk of prostate cancer was 0.60 among Adventist men who ate tomatoes more than five times weekly, compared with those who consumed them less than once weekly.

A recent review of 72 studies found 57 reports of inverse associations between tomato consumption or blood lycopene levels and risk of various types of cancer; 35 of these associations were significant. Evidence of lycopene protective effects were highest for cancers of the prostate, lung and stomach.

While cautioning that these associations do not establish a cause-and-effect relationship, the reviewer observed that "the consistency of the results across numerous studies in diverse populations, for case-control and prospective studies, and for dietary-based and blood-based investigations argues against bias or confounding as the explanation for these findings."

Recently, more direct, though still preliminary, evidence emerged suggestive of lycopene protective and, perhaps, interventive effects in prostate cancer. In this study, 33 men scheduled for surgery to remove cancerous prostate glands, were randomized to receive 30 milligrams of lycopene (in two 15-milligram capsules) daily or nothing. Dosing commenced 30 days prior to surgery.

Examination of the prostate glands post-surgery revealed that cancer had spread to the very edge of the glands in seven of the 21 lycopene-treated subjects compared with the same extent of spread in 9 of the 12 subjects who did not receive lycopene. Pre-cancerous tissue in the lycopene group was judged to be less abnormal than pre-cancerous tissue in the group that did not receive lycopene. Prostate specific antigen (PSA) fell 20% in the lycopene group between initial dosing and surgery. PSA levels were unchanged in the group not receiving lycopene. Research is ongoing.

Recent epidemiological studies have reported an inverse relationship between higher tissue and serum levels of lycopene and the risk of coronary artery disease. And a recent study in which 19 healthy subjects consumed a variety of tomato products for three weeks reported no change in serum cholesterol levels but significant decrease in lipid peroxidation and LDL-cholesterol oxidation. Numerous *in vitro* and animal studies have also reported results suggestive of lycopene effects that might help prevent or ameliorate cardiovascular disease. Research continues.

CONTRAINDICATIONS, PRECAUTIONS, ADVERSE REACTIONS

CONTRAINDICATIONS

Lycopene is contraindicated in those hypersensitive to any component of a lycopene-containing product.

PRECAUTIONS

Pregnant women and nursing mothers should obtain their lycopene intake from food sources rather than supplements.

INTERACTIONS

DRUGS

Cholestyramine: Concomitant intake of cholestyramine and lycopene may decrease the absorption of lycopene.

Colestipol: Concomitant intake of colestipol and lycopene may decrease the absorption of lycopene.

Mineral oil: Concomitant intake of mineral oil and lycopene may reduce the absorption of lycopene.

Orlistat: Orlistat may decrease the absorption of lycopene.

NUTRITIONAL SUPPLEMENTS

Beta-carotene: Concomitant intake of beta-carotene and lycopene may increase the absorption of lycopene.

Medium-chain triglycerides: Concomitant intake of medium-chain triglycerides and lycopene may enhance the absorption of lycopene.

Pectin: Concomitant intake of pectin and lycopene may decrease the absorption of lycopene.

FOODS

Oils: Dietary oils, such as olive oil, may enhance the absorption of lycopene.

Olestra: Olestra may reduce the absorption of lycopene.

DOSAGE AND ADMINISTRATION

Lycopene supplements are available as oleoresin preparations, phospholipid preparations and in oils, such as medium chain triglycerides. Doses range from 5 to 15 milligrams daily.

The optimal dose of lycopene is not known.

The following lists the lycopene contents of some foods:

Food	Lycopene content (micrograms/gram wet weight)
Fresh tomatoes	8.8-42.0
Cooked tomatoes	37
Tomato sauce	62
Tomato paste	54-1,500
Tomato powder	1,126-1,265
Tomato soup (condensed)	80
Tomato juice	50-116
Pizza sauce	127
Ketchup	99-134
Watermelon	23-72
Pink guava	54
Pink grapefruit	34
Papaya	20-53

LITERATURE

Agarwal S, Rao AV. Tomato lycopene and its role in human health and chronic diseases. *CMAJ*. 2000; 163:739-744.

Agarwal S, Rao AV. Tomato lycopene and low density lipiprotein oxidation: a human dietary intervention study. *Lipids*. 1998; 33:981-984.

Arab L, Steck S. Lycopene and cardiovascular disease. *Am J Clin Nutr*. 2000; 71(suppl); 1691S-1695S.

Bohm Y, Bitsch R. Intestinal absorption of lycopene from different matrices and interactions to other carotenoids, the lipid status, and the antioxidant capacity of human plasma. *Eur J Nutr*. 1999; 38:118-125.

Boileau AC, Merchen NR, Wasson K, et al. Cis-lycopene is more bioavailable than trans-lycopene in vitro and in vivo in lymph-cannulated ferrets. *J Nutr*. 1999; 129:1176-1181.

Bramley PM. Is lycopene beneficial to human health? *Phytochem*. 2000; 54:233-236.

Clinton SK. Lycopene: chemistry, biology, and implications for human health and disease. *Nutr Rev*. 1998; 56:35-51.

Clinton SK, Emenhiser C, Schwartz SJ, et al. Cis-trans lycopene isomers, carotenoids, and retinol in the human prostate. *Cancer Epidemiol Biomarkers Prev*. 1996; 5:823-833.

Gann PH, Ma J, Giovannucci E, et al. Lower prostate cancer risk in men with elevated plasma lycopene levels: results of a prospective analysis. *Cancer Res*. 1999; 59:1225-1230.

Gartner C, Stahl W, Sies H. Lycopene is more bioavailable from tomato paste than from fresh tomatoes. *Am J Clin Nutr.* 1997; 66:116-122.

Giovannucci E. Tomatoes, tomato-based products, lycopene, and cancer: Review of the epidemiologic literature. *J Natl Cancer Inst.* 1999; 91:317-331.

Giovannucci E, Ascherio A, Rimm EB, et al. Intake of carotenoids and retinol in relation to risk of prostate cancer. *J Natl Cancer Inst.* 1995; 87:1767-1976.

Johnson EJ. The role of lycopene in health and disease. *Nutr Clin Care.* 2000; 3:35-43.

Johnson EJ, Qin J, Krinsky NI, Russell RM. Ingestion by men of a combined dose of beta-carotene and lycopene does not affect the absorption of beta-carotene but improves that of lycopene. *J Nutr.* 1997; 127:1833-1837.

Leal M, Shimada S, Ruiz F, et al. Effect of lycopene on lipid peroxidation and glutathione-dependent enzymes induced by T-2 toxin in vivo. *Toxicol Lett.* 1999; 109:1-10.

Michaud DS, Feskanich D, Rimm EB, et al. Intake of specific carotenoids and risk of lung cancer in 2 prospective U.S. cohorts. *Am J Clin Nutr.* 2000; 72:990-997.

Paetau I, Rao D, Wiley ER, et al. Carotenoids in human buccal mucosa cells after 4 wk of supplementation with tomato juice or lycopene supplements. *Am J Clin Nutr.* 1999; 70:490-494.

Rao AV, Agarwal S. Bioavailability and in vivo antioxidant properties of lycopene from tomato products and their possible role in the prevention of cancer. *Nutr Cancer.* 1998; 31:199-203.

Rao AV, Agarwal S. Role of lycopene as antioxidant carotenoid in the prevention of chronic diseases: a review. *Nutr Res.* 1999; 19:305-323.

Rao AV, Fleshner N, Agarwal S. Serum and tissue lycopene and biomarkers of oxidation in prostate cancer patients: a case-control study. *Nutr Cancer.* 1999; 33:159-164.

Riso P, Pinder A, Santangelo A, Porrini M. Does tomato consumption effectively increase the resistance of lymphocyte DNA to oxidative damage? *Am J Clin Nutr.* 1999; 69:712-718.

Sengupta A, Das S. The anti-carcinogenic role of lycopene, abundantly present in tomato. *Eur J Cancer Prev.* 1999; 8:325-330.

Sies H, Stahl W. Lycopene: antioxidant and biological effects and its bioavailability in the human. *Proc Soc Exp Biol Med.* 1998; 218:121-124.

Sutherland WH, Walker RJ, De Jong SA, Upritchard JE. Supplementation with tomato juice increases plasma lycopene but does not alter susceptibility to oxidation of low-density lipoproteins from renal transplant patients. *Clin Nephrol.* 1999; 52:30-36.

Magnesium

DESCRIPTION

Magnesium is an essential mineral in human nutrition with a wide range of biological functions. Magnesium is involved in over 300 metabolic reactions. It is necessary for every major biological process, including the production of cellular energy and the synthesis of nucleic acids and proteins. It is also important for the electrical stability of cells, the maintenance of membrane integrity, muscle contraction, nerve conduction and the regulation of vascular tone, among other things.

Magnesium is an alkaline earth metal with atomic number 12 and an atomic weight of 24.31 daltons. Its chemical symbol is Mg. Magnesium exists under physiological conditions in its divalent (+2 or II) state. The total body magnesium content of an adult is about 25 grams. About 50%-60% exists in bone. Magnesium is the second most abundant intracellular cation; potassium is the most abundant. Approximately 1% of the body's magnesium is found extracellularly.

Magnesium is intimately interlocked, biologically with calcium. In some reactions, such as the synthesis of nucleic acids and protein, calcium and magnesium are antagonistic. Magnesium is necessary for these processes, while calcium can inhibit them. Magnesium and calcium cooperate, however, in the production of adenosine triphosphate or ATP. Magnesium has been called "nature's physiological calcium channel blocker" since it appears to regulate the intracellular flow of calcium ions.

Symptoms and signs of magnesium deficiency include anorexia, nausea and vomiting, diarrhea, generalized muscle spasticity, paresthesias, confusion, tremor, focal and generalized seizures, confusion, loss of coordination, cardiac arrhythmias, laboratory abnormalities, such as hypokalemia and hypocalcemia, muscle cramps, hypertension and coronary and cerebral vasospasms. Magnesium deficiency may be found in diabetes mellitus, malabsorption syndromes, alcoholism and hyperthyroidism, among other disorders. Use of certain drugs may also lead to magnesium deficiency. These drugs include thiazide diuretics (when used for long periods of time), loop diuretics, cisplatin, amphotericin, pentamidine (when used intravenously), aminoglycosides and cyclosporine. Magnesium deficiency itself is an important cause of hypokalemia.

In addition to its use for the treatment of hypomagnesemia, magnesium is used for the treatment of certain cardiac arrhythmias, in particular torsade de pointes, and eclampsia. It is also used as a laxative and antacid. Magnesium may also have value for the prevention of osteoporosis and for the management of migraine headaches in some. There is preliminary evidence that magnesium may help some with premenstrual syndrome, type 2 diabetes mellitus and hypertension. The role of magnesium, if any, in the management of acute myocardial infarction remains controversial.

Foods rich in magnesium include unpolished grains, nuts and green vegetables. Green leafy vegetables are particularly good sources of magnesium because of their chlorophyll content. Chlorophyll is the magnesium chelate of porphyrin. Meats, starches and milk are less rich sources of magnesium. Refined and processed foods are generally magnesium-poor. The mean daily magnesium intake in the U.S. in males nine years and older is estimated to be about 323 milligrams; for females nine years and older, it is estimated to be 228 milligrams. Some surveys report lower intakes, and some believe that the dietary intake for many may be sub-optimal.

ACTIONS AND PHARMACOLOGY

ACTIONS

Magnesium may have anti-osteoporotic activity. Magnesium has anti-arrhythmic activity. Magnesium has activity in the management of preeclampsia. Magnesium may have antihypertensive, glucose-regulatory and bronchodilatory activities. Magnesium has putative myocardial protective activity during an acute myocardial infarction and putative antimigraine activity.

MECHANISM OF ACTION

Significant reductions in bone mineral content and serum magnesium have been reported in women with postmenopausal osteoporosis compared to age-matched controls. Bone mineral content and bone mineral density have been positively correlated with dietary magnesium in a few, but not all, studies of postmenopausal women. A couple of studies have demonstrated increased bone mineral density in postmenopausal women which was associated with intake of supplemental magnesium. Magnesium influences both matrix and mineral metabolism in bone. Magnesium depletion can cause cessation of bone growth, decreased osteoblastic and osteoclastic activity, osteopenia and increased bone fragility. Bone mineral with decreased magnesium content results in larger and more perfect bone mineral crystals, which may be more brittle than amorphous crystals.

Magnesium depletion is associated with a number of cardiac arrhythmias, including atrial fibrillation, premature atrial and ventricular beats, ventricular tachycardia and ventricular fibrillation. Magnesium is effective in treating these arrhythmias in those who are magnesium deficient. Magnesium may also be effective in treating cardiac arrhythmias in those who are not magnesium deficient. This is especially true for the treatment, by magnesium, of torsade de pointes. The mechanism of the anti-arrhythmic action of magnesium is not fully understood. The anti-arrhythmic effect of magne-sium may be related to its role in maintaining intracellular potassium. It may also be related to its role as a natural calcium channel blocker.

Magnesium sulfate is widely used to prevent eclamptic seizures in pregnant women with hypertension. Vasospasm in preeclampsia is thought to be a consequence of endothelial dysfunction. Magnesium has been found, both *in vitro* and *in vivo*, to increase production of the vasodilator prostacyclin. Magnesium may also protect against damage to the endothelium by reactive oxygen species. The action of magnesium sulfate in the treatment of eclampsia can be accounted for by the release of endothelial prostaglandin by magnesium, its protection against reactive oxygen species damage to the endothelium and by its possible inhibition of platelet aggregation. It may act as an anticonvulsant via neuronal calcium-channel blockade and antagonism of the glutamate N-methyl-D-aspartate (NMDA) receptor.

Some studies have reported that some populations with low dietary intake of magnesium have increased incidence of hypertension. Another study reported dietary intake of magnesium in normotensives to be significantly greater than intake in untreated hypertensive subjects. Intervention studies with magnesium therapy for hypertensives have led to conflicting results. The mechanism of the possible antihypertensive activity of magnesium is unclear. A possibility is that magnesium, acting in a calcium channel blocking capacity, may have a vasodilatory action.

A few studies have reported that magnesium depletion results in insulin resistance as well as impaired secretion of insulin. Insulin resistance and abnormal glucose tolerance may be accounted for, in part, by inadequate magnesium. Some studies have reported improved insulin response in elderly type 2 diabetics who received magnesium. The mechanism of the possible role of magnesium in improving glycemic control is unclear. Magnesium is a cofactor for phosphorylation reactions. Magnesium may affect insulin signal transduction. Magnesium may also alter insulin receptor binding. These are some speculative possibilities.

Intravenous magnesium has been demonstrated to have bronchodilatory activity in some with asthma. The mechanism of this activity is unclear.

The mechanism of the putative myocardial protective activity of magnesium during an acute myocardial infarction is also unclear. Speculative possibilities include magnesium's anti-arrhythmic activity, as well as its possible activity in inhibiting platelet aggregation. Magnesium's possible vasodilatory activity—via its acting as a calcium channel blocker—and possible reduction of reperfusion dysfunction are two additional speculative mechanisms for this putative activity. The mechanism of the possible anti-migraine activity is unknown.

PHARMACOKINETICS

The efficiency of absorption of magnesium is inversely proportional to the amount of magnesium ingested. The fractional absorption of magnesium from 7 to 36 milligrams was found to be 65% to 70% in one study. The same study reported a fractional absorption of 11% to 14% with a magnesium intake of 960 to 1,000 milligrams. One study of magnesium absorption from food sources reported a fractional absorption of 40% to 60% of a daily intake of 380 milligrams of magnesium in healthy older men.

Magnesium appears to be absorbed from both the small intestine and the colon. The sites of maximal magnesium absorption appear to be the distal jejunum and ileum. The efficiency of absorption (fractional absorption) of a magnesium salt appears to principally depend on its solubility in intestinal fluids, as well as on the amount digested. Enteric-coated magnesium salts are less efficiently absorbed than non enteric-coated preparations. Salts with high solubility, e.g., magnesium citrate, appear to be more efficiently absorbed than salts with poor solubility, e.g., magnesium oxide. There are a few reports that suggest that the counter anion of the magnesium salt may influence its absorption. Magnesium aspartate and magnesium orotate are reported by some to be more available forms of magnesium than other magnesium salts. However, there are no compelling data that indicate that the nature of the counter anion makes any significant difference on the availability of magnesium salt, independent of its possible effect on the solubility of the salt.

Magnesium appears to be absorbed by both a saturable active transport mechanism and an unsaturable passive mechanism. The saturable active transport mechanism may account for the higher absorption efficiency at lower magnesium intakes. There is no good evidence that vitamin D and its active metabolite, 1, 25-dihydroxyvitamin D (1, 25(OH)$_2$D) play a significant role in the absorption of magnesium, as some have suggested.

Magnesium is transported to the liver via the portal circulation and to the rest of the body via the systemic circulation. A large fraction of ingested magnesium is taken up by bone. Magnesium transport into cells appears to require the presence of carrier-mediated transport systems. Magnesium is excreted by the kidneys, and the kidney is the principal organ involved in magnesium homeostasis. There is no tubular secretion of magnesium. Magnesium is filtered and reabsorbed. About 65% of filtered magnesium is reabsorbed in the loop of Henle and 20% to 30% in the proximal convoluted tubule.

About 3% to 5% of filtered magnesium is excreted in the urine. The regulatory mechanisms of the kidney in maintaining magnesium homeostasis are unclear.

There is much about the pharmacokinetics of magnesium that is not known. Research is ongoing.

INDICATIONS AND USAGE

Magnesium deficiency is associated with the pathogenesis of numerous serious disorders, notably ischemic heart disease, congestive heart failure, sudden cardiac death, cardiac arrhythmias, diabetes mellitus, pre-eclampsia/eclampsia and hypertension, among others. Treatment with supplemental magnesium is often helpful in these conditions. There is also evidence that it can be of benefit in some with osteoporosis, alcoholism, migraine, asthma, pre-menstrual syndromes, kidney stones and strokes. It may help prevent or reduce the incidence of cerebral palsy and mental retardation in early pre-term infants. There is little or no evidence to support claims that magnesium enhances athletic/exercise performance, that it is an effective antidepressant or that it is helpful in bipolar disorder.

RESEARCH SUMMARY

There is considerable epidemiological data associating low magnesium intake with an increased incidence of cardiovascular disease. Some recent data have suggested the presence of serum magnesium abnormality in sick inpatient and outpatient populations ranging from 12% to 40%. Hypomagnesemia has frequently been associated with those suffering from various forms of cardiovascular disease.

Magnesium's role as a cofactor in various crucial intracellular enzymatic reactions related to myocardial metabolism and contractility is well established. It is not surprising, then, that magnesium deficiencies, perhaps even borderline deficiencies, can negatively impact cardiovascular health. At the same time, due to lack of an accurate assay of intracellular magnesium, it has been difficult to assess the efficacy of supplemental magnesium in some of these conditions. "Also uncertain," two reviewers of the data have stated in an editorial, "is whether magnesium administration merely corrects an underlying deficiency state or exerts specific beneficial pharmacologic effects." That caveat can be applied equally not only to the possible cardiologic indications for the use of supplemental magnesium but to all other possible indications, as well.

In addition to the epidemiological data, there are also some experimental and clinical data supporting the use of magnesium in some with cardiovascular disease. Frank magnesium deficiency has clearly been shown to induce vascular damage in the heart and kidneys and to promote atherosclerosis. In pharmacological concentrations, infusion of magnesium inhibits platelet aggregation, exerts anti-arrhythmic effects and induces vasodilatation of blood vessels. In animals it has protected against ischemia-reperfusion injury.

In some randomized, double-blind, placebo-controlled studies, intravenous magnesium has significantly improved outcome in subjects with acute myocardial infarction. However, in a recent prospective study assessing the effects of early captopril, oral mononitrate and intravenous magnesium in 58,050 patients with suspected acute myocardial infarction, no beneficial effects were observed with magnesium. Some have argued that because the magnesium was administered after iatrogenic or spontaneous reperfusion this difference in timing might explain, at least in part, its poor performance. Reviewers of these data have concluded that there is, as yet, insufficient evidence of magnesium efficacy to recommend it for routine use in patients with suspected myocardial infarction. They have recommended further study. It should also be pointed out that, as of yet, there are no randomized studies showing a magnesium mortality benefit in congestive heart failure.

Epidemiological data indicate that low dietary magnesium intake is associated with a higher incidence of hypertension. Magnesium supplementation has significantly reduced blood pressure in some, but not all, studies. Some of these positive studies have been criticized as being methodologically flawed. Larger, better designed studies are needed. A meta-analysis of 12 randomized, controlled trials showed that magnesium supplementation did not significantly reduce systolic blood pressure but did favorably affect diastolic values. The authors, however, said that the poor quality of the included studies did not support a causal association.

Intravenous administration of magnesium has been effective in suppressing some, but not all, cardiac arrhythmias. It is the treatment of choice for controlling torsade de pointes and is an option for treating refractory or recurrent ventricular fibrillation or tachycardia.

There is also an inverse association between dietary magnesium intake and risk of total stroke in men. In some animal experiments, magnesium has demonstrated significant neuroprotective effects. A large multicenter trial of intravenous magnesium's possible efficacy post-acute stroke is now underway.

Magnesium's possible usefulness in protecting against atherosclerosis was suggested by findings in experimental animals that magnesium deficiency promotes vascular damage and other atherosclerotic processes. In addition, supplemental magnesium has lowered serum cholesterol and triglyceride levels and has inhibited atherosclerotic lesions in other animal studies. More research is needed.

An association has been reported between lower magnesium intake and increased incidence of metabolic syndrome (concurrent hyperglycemia, dyslipidemia, hypertension and visceral obesity). In several studies, however, the association was largely or completely abolished after adjusting for other intakes, particularly fiber. Another recent study examined the relationship between dietary magnesium, calcium, potassium and sodium intake with risk of stroke in a cohort of 26,556 Finnish male smokers, aged 50 to 69 years, all free from stroke at baseline. Over a follow-up period of almost 14 years, they found that a high-magnesium intake was significantly associated with a lower risk of cerebral infarction but not with intracerebral or subarachnoid hemorrhages. Calcium, potassium and sodium intake was not significantly associated with risk of any subtype of stroke.

Magnesium was first used in 1906 to help prevent eclamptic seizures. It is now routinely used for this purpose in hypertensive pregnant women. It showed marked benefit in this condition and significant superiority over diazepam and phenytoin in the Collaborative Eclampsia Trial. There is also good evidence that treating pregnant women with magnesium pre-delivery may reduce the incidence of mental retardation and cerebral palsy in early preterm infants. Intravenous magnesium has also been used to inhibit premature labor with some success in one study.

Recently, the results were released from a multicenter, placebo-controlled, randomized trial involving 2,241 women at risk of imminent preterm birth between 24 and 31 weeks of gestation. No benefit was seen in the offspring of women given intravenous magnesium sulfate, compared with those given placebo, in terms of risk of death or moderate or severe cerebral palsy. Benefit was seen, however, in terms of reduced rate of cerebral palsy overall. More research is needed, a recent editorial in *The New England Journal of Medicine* declared, before magnesium treatment can be widely and routinely recommended in this context, although it acknowledged that the findings to date show promise.

Magnesium deficiency has been implicated in increased insulin resistance and a higher incidence of cardiovascular disease among those with diabetes mellitus. Hypomagnesemia has been reported in 25% to 38% of diabetic patients; its incidence is highest in those with the poorest metabolic control. In a small early study of eight elderly subjects with NIDDM, supplementation with two grams of magnesium daily significantly improved insulin response and action, compared with placebo. Some other small studies have suggested benefits with daily doses as low as 100 milligrams of magnesium daily. Recently, however, the large, well-designed prospective Atherosclerosis Risk in Communities (ARIC) study found no relationship between low dietary magnesium intake and increased risk of type 2 diabetes in a middle-aged population. On the other hand, there was a significant inverse correlation between serum total magnesium levels and incidence in the caucasian subset of this study. The same correlation was not seen in the black subset. More study is needed.

Magnesium has been used with some success in a few studies to promote bronchodilation and improve lung function in some asthmatic patients. In one recent meta-analysis, intravenous magnesium was found to significantly reduce the rate of hospital admissions and to improve pulmonary function in patients treated in emergency departments for severe acute asthma. The same benefit was not reported for those with mild to moderate asthma. Epidemiological data have also shown that higher dietary intakes of magnesium are associated with a lower incidence of airway reactivity and respiratory symptoms. More research is needed to further determine the relative value of supplemental magnesium in the prevention and treatment of asthma and related conditions.

Alcoholics have a high incidence of magnesium deficiency. This deficiency contributes, some research indicates, to an increased incidence of osteoporosis and cardiovascular disease among chronic alcoholics. Alcohol is known to be a potent magnesium diuretic. Supplemental magnesium has shown benefit in some alcoholics. In one randomized study, supplemental magnesium improved a number of metabolic variables and muscle strength, compared with placebo, in chronic alcoholics. Alcohol consumption was the same before and during the trial. The favorable metabolic changes suggested that supplemental magnesium might improve liver cell function and electrolyte status, as well as muscle strength, in chronic alcoholics.

Magnesium and phenobarbital have been reported to be effective in easing the symptoms of alcohol withdrawal. A double-blind, placebo-controlled trial of magnesium in the ethanol withdrawal syndrome, however, found no benefit from intramuscular injections of magnesium, compared with saline control. The researchers concluded that magnesium is not indicated for alcohol withdrawal unless withdrawal is characterized by cardiac arrhythmias.

Other researchers, reviewing the literature on the use of magnesium in delirium tremens between 1954 and 1987, have similarly concluded that there is most likely no causal relationship between hypomagnesemia and delirium tremens. They cite more recent research findings showing that hypomagnesemia is not universal among chronic alcoholics and that magnesium concentrations return to normal in some alcoholics without use of magnesium supplements. They have recommended against the routine use of parenteral magnesium in patients with delirium tremens.

Magnesium supplements may significantly protect post menopausal women from osteoporosis according to researchers who tested the supplement in a group of these women for two years. Magnesium's role in regulating active calcium transport has made its importance in bone metabolism manifest. Women in the two-year study received varying doses of magnesium, from 250 milligrams to 750 milligrams, and were compared with unsupplemented age-matched controls. The magnesium-treated women also had significantly increased bone density by the end of the study while the controls did not. Follow-up is needed.

Magnesium levels have been found to be diminished in some with premenstrual syndrome (PMS). In one double-blind, randomized study, women with PMS received placebo or 360 milligrams of magnesium three times a day from day 15 of the menstrual cycle to the onset of menstrual flow. Magnesium performed better than placebo in some measures related to premenstrual mood changes. Both placebo and magnesium seemed to reduce pain associated with PMS. More rigorous studies are needed before any conclusion can be drawn with respect to magnesium's possible efficacy in alleviating symptoms of PMS. Finally, two double-blind, studies have suggested that chronic oral magnesium supplementation may reduce the frequency of migraine headaches. Refractory patients have, reportedly, been helped with intravenous magnesium. Magnesium concentrations have been shown to affect serotonin receptors, nitric oxide synthesis and release and NMDA receptors, all believed to play some role in migraine. In a multi-center, placebo-controlled, double-blind, randomized study, 81 patients, aged 18-65 years, with a mean migraine frequency attack of 3-6 per month, were given 600 milligrams of magnesium or placebo orally each day for 12 weeks. In weeks 9-12, attack frequency was reduced by 41.6% in the magnesium group and by 15.8% in the placebo group, compared with baseline. More research is warranted.

One recent review of the roles of dietary magnesium in human health has observed that ingestion of this micronutrient worldwide has diminished over the years, owing to "westernization" and attendant dietary changes. These reviewers assert that most US and European populations are getting less than the recommended dietary allowances of magnesium. Climate changes, they add, may also be further depleting populations of this crucial nutrient through increased sweat losses. They hypothesize that this may help account for an association between higher temperatures and higher incidence of heart deaths and diabetes. An increasingly elderly population is another factor that may call for higher magnesium intake. "Higher magnesium intake and, in general, a greater intake of whole grains might be a marker of an overall healthier diet and life-style," they concluded.

Some other authors have recently concluded that magnesium inadequacy is likely associated with the aging process generally. Cellular senescence has been induced in various cell lines through magnesium deprivation, and magnesium-deficient diets have been widely reported to promote disease processes closely associated with aging. They suggest that "broadly correcting the nutritional intake of magnesium might be a simple and inexpensive solution that contributes to healthier aging and the prevention of age-related diseases."

CONTRAINDICATIONS, PRECAUTIONS, ADVERSE REACTIONS

CONTRAINDICATIONS

Magnesium is contraindicated in those with renal failure. It is also contraindicated in those with high-grade atrioventricular (AV) blocks unless those with high-grade AV blocks have artificial pacemakers.

Magnesium is contraindicated in those who are hypersensitive to any component of a magnesium-containing supplement.

PRECAUTIONS

Pregnant women and nursing mothers should avoid magnesium doses greater than 350 milligrams daily (in supplementary form) unless higher doses are prescribed by their physicians.

Those with myasthenia gravis should avoid the use of magnesium supplements. Magnesium supplements may exacerbate weakness and trigger a myasthenic crisis.

ADVERSE REACTIONS

The most common adverse reaction from the use of magnesium supplements is diarrhea. Other gastrointestinal symptoms that may occur with the use of magnesium supplements are nausea and abdominal cramping. If magnesium supplements are taken with food, diarrhea and other gastrointestinal symptoms are less likely to occur. Diarrhea and other gastrointestinal symptoms typically occur with magnesium doses greater than 350 milligrams daily. Doses of 350 milligrams or lower are generally well tolerated.

Those with renal failure may develop hypermagnesemia with use of magnesium supplements (see Contraindications). Serious adverse reactions with the use of oral magnesium supplements in those with normal renal function are rare but they have been reported. An eight week-old infant developed metabolic alkalosis, diarrhea and dehydration after receiving large amounts of magnesium oxide powder on each of two successive days. An adult woman developed metabolic alkalosis and hypokalemia from the repeated daily ingestion of 30 grams of magnesium oxide. Paralytic ileus has been reported in adults taking large, cathartic doses of magnesium. One suicide patient given 465 grams of magnesium sulfate as a cathartic to counteract an intentional drug overdose had a cardiopulmonary arrest. A few deaths have been reported in patients with renal failure who took very large doses of magnesium as magnesium sulfate or magnesium oxide.

INTERACTIONS

DRUGS

Bisphosphonates (alendronate, etidronate, risedronate): Concomitant intake of a bisphosphonate and magnesium may decrease the absorption of the bisphosphonate.

Quinolones (ciprofloxacin, gatifloxacin, levofloxacin, lomefloxacin, moxifloxacin, norfloxacin, ofloxacin, sparfloxacin, trovafloxacin): Concomitant use of a quinolone and magnesium may decrease the absorption of the quinolone.

Tetracyclines (doxycyline, monocycline, tetracycline): Concomitant intake of a tetracycline and magnesium may decrease the absorption of the tetracycline.

NUTRITIONAL SUPPLEMENTS

Boron: Boron may increase magnesium levels.

Calcium: Concomitant intake of high doses of calcium—greater than 2 grams—may decrease the absorption of magnesium. Most studies have shown that concomitant intakes of typical doses of calcium and magnesium do not decrease the absorption of magnesium.

Inositol Hexaphosphate: Concomitant intake of inositol hexaphosphate and magnesium may depress the absorption of magnesium.

Iron: Concomitant intake of magnesium and iron may decrease the absorption of iron.

Manganese: Concomitant intake of magnesium and manganese may decrease the absorption of manganese.

Non-digestible oligosaccharides (fructo-oligosaccharides, inulin): Concomitant use of non-digestible oligosaccharides and magnesium may increase the colonic absorption of magnesium.

Phosphate: Concomitant intake of phosphate and magnesium may decrease the absorption of both phosphate and magnesium.

Sodium Alginate: Concomitant intake of sodium alginate and magnesium may decrease the absorption of magnesium.

FOODS

Concomitant intake of a magnesium supplement with foods rich in oxalic acid (spinach, sweet potatoes, rhubarb and beans) or phytic acid (unleavened bread, raw beans, seeds, nuts and grains and soy isolates) may decrease the absorption of magnesium.

OVERDOSAGE

See Adverse Reactions.

There is a report of a patient having a cardiopulmonary arrest after ingesting 465 grams of magnesium sulfate, and there are a few reports of deaths in those with renal failure who took very large doses of magnesium.

DOSAGE AND ADMINISTRATION

There are several forms of magnesium used for nutritional supplementation. These include: magnesium oxide, magnesium gluconate, magnesium chloride, magnesium citrate, magnesium hydroxide, magnesium aspartate, magnesium orotate, magnesium arginate, magnesium pidolate and other amino acid and oligopeptide chelates of magnesium. Magnesium supplements are available as stand-alone supplements or in combination products. Some products contain mixtures of a few magnesium forms, e.g., magnesium oxide, magnesium chloride and magnesium gluconate. Many combination products are available.

Typical doses of magnesium (expressed as elemental magnesium) range from 100 to 350 milligrams daily.

Taking magnesium supplements with food is less likely to cause diarrhea.

The Food and Nutrition Board of the Institute of Medicine of the United States National Academy of Sciences has recommended the following Adequate Intake (AI) and Recommended Dietary Allowance (RDA) values for magnesium:

Infants	(AI)
0 through 6 months	30 mg/day
7 through 12 months	75 mg/day

Children	(RDA)
1 through 3 years	80 mg/day
4 through 8 years	130 mg/day

Boys	
9 through 13 years	240 mg/day
4 through 18 years	410 mg/day

Girls	
9 through 13 years	240 mg/day
4 through 18 years	360 mg/day

Men	
19 through 30 years	400 mg/day
31 through 50 years	420 mg/day
51 through 70 years	420 mg/day
Older than 70 years	420 mg/day

Women	
19 through 30 years	310 mg/day
31 through 50 years	320 mg/day
51 through 70 years	320 mg/day
Older than 70 years	320 mg/day

Pregnancy	
14 through 18 years	400 mg/day
19 through 30 years	350 mg/day
31 through 50 years	380 mg/day

Lactation	
14 through 18 years	360 mg/day
19 through 30 years	310 mg/day
31 through 50 years	320 mg/day

The Food and Nutrition Board has recommended the following upper limits (UL) for supplementary magnesium (i.e., nonfood source magnesium).

Infants	(UL)
0 through 12 months	Not determinable

Children	
1 through 3 years	65 mg
4 through 8 years	110 mg

Pregnancy	
14 through 50 years	350 mg

Lactation	
14 through 50 years	350 mg

Adolescents and Adults	350 mg

The DV (Daily Value) for magnesium, which is used for determining percentage of nutrient daily values on nutritional supplement and food labels, is 400 mg. The basis for the DV for magnesium is the 1973 U.S. RDA.

The Food and Nutrition Board recognizes that those with certain clinical conditions, such as neonatal tetany, hyperuricemia, hyperlipidemia, lithium toxicity, hyperthyroidism, cardiac arrhythmias and digitalis intoxication, may benefit from the prescribed use of magnesium supplements exceeding the above ULs.

LITERATURE

Abbott L, Nadler J, Rude RK. Magnesium deficiency in alcoholism: possible contribution to osteoporosis and cardiovascular disease in alcoholics. *Alcohol Clin Exp Res.* 1994;18:1076-1082.

Altura BM, Altura BT. Role of magnesium and calcium in alcohol-induced hypertension and strokes as probed by in vivo television microscopy, digital image microscopy, optical spectroscopy, 31P-NMR, spectroscopy and a unique magnesium ion-selective electrode. *Alcohol Clin Exp Res.* 1994;18:1057-1068.

Baxter GF, Sumeray MS, Walker JM. Infant size and magnesium: insights into LIMIT-2 and ISIS-4 from experimental studies. *Lancet*. 1996;348:1424-1426.

Bo S, Pisu E. Role of dietary magnesium in cardiovascular disease prevention, insulin sensitivity and diabetes. *Curr Opin Lipidol*. 2008;19(1):50-56.

Britton J, Pavord I, Richards K, et al. Dietary magnesium, lung function, wheezing, and airway hyper-reactivity in a random adult population sample. *Lancet*. 1994;344:357-362.

Casscells W. Magnesium and myocardial infarction. *Lancet*. 1994;343:807-809.

Christiansen CW, Rieder MA, Silverstein EL, Gencheff NE. Magnesium sulfate reduces myocardial infarct size when administered before but not after coronary reperfusion in a canine model. *Circulation*. 1995;92:2617-2621.

de Lourdes Lima M, Cruz T, Carreiro Pousada J, et al. The effect of magnesium supplementation in increasing doses on the control of type 2 diabetes. *Diabetes Care*. 1998;21:682-686.

Durlach J, Durlach V, Bac P, et al. Magnesium and therapeutics. *Magnes Res*. 1994;7:313-328.

Elisaf M, Merkouropoulos M, Tsianos EV, et al. Pathogenetic mechanisms of hypomagnesemia in alcoholic patients. *J Trace Elem Med Biol*. 1995;9:210-214.

Facchinetti F, Borella P, Sances G, et al. Oral magnesium successfully relieves premenstrual mood changes. *Obstet Gynecol*. 1991;78:177-181.

Gullestad L, Dolva LO, Soyland E, et al. Oral magnesium supplementation improves metabolic variables and muscle strength in alcoholics. *Alcohol Clin Exp Res*. 1992;16:986-990.

Herzog WR, Schlossberg ML, MacMurdy KS, et al. Timing of magnesium therapy affects experimental infarct size. *Circulation*. 1995;92:2622-2626.

Institute of Medicine, Food and Nutrition Board. Dietary Reference Intakes for calcium, phosphorous, magnesium, vitamin D, and fluoride. Washington, DC: National Academy Press, 1997.

Iseri LT, French JH. Magnesium: nature's physiologic calcium blocker. *Am Heart J*. 1984;108:188-193.

ISIS-4 (Fourth International Study of Infarct Survival) Collaborative Group. ISIS-4: a randomised factorial trial assessing early oral captopril, oral mononitrate, and intravenous magnesium sulfate in 58,050 patients with suspected acute myocardial infarction. *Lancet*. 1995;345:669-685.

Jermain DM, Crisman ML, Nisbet RB. Controversies over the use of magnesium sulfate in delirium tremens. *Ann Pharmacother*. 1992;26:650-652.

Kao WHL, Folsom AR, Nieto J, et al. Serum and dietary magnesium and the risk for type 2 diabetes mellitus (editorial). *Arch. Int Med*. 1999;159:2151-2159.

Killilea DW, Ames BN. Magnesium deficiency accelerates cellular senescence in cultured human fibroblasts. *Proc Natl Acad Sci USA*. 2008;105(15):5768-5773.

Killilea DW, Maier JA. A connection between magnesium deficiency and aging: new insights from cellular studies. *Magnes Res*. 2008;21(2):77-82.

Larsson SC, Virtanen MJ, Mars M, et al. Magnesium, calcium, potassium, and sodium intakes and risk of stroke in male smokers. *Arch Intern Med*. 2008;168(5):459-465.

Lim R, Herzog WR. Magnesium for cardiac patients: is it a valuable treatment supplement? *Contemp Int Med*. 1998;10:6-9.

Lucas MJ, Leveno KJ, Cunningham FG. A comparison of magnesium sulfate with phenytoin for the prevention of eclampsia. *N Engl J Med*. 1995;333:201-205.

Marret S, Doyle LW, Crowther CA, et al. Antenatal magnesium sulphate neuroprotection in the preterm infant. *Semin Fetal Neonatal Med*. 2007;12(4):311-317.

Marret S, Marpeau L, Zupan-Simunek V, et al. PREMAG trial group. Magnesium sulphate given before very-preterm birth to protect infant brain: the randomised controlled PREMAG trial. *BJOG*. 2007;114(3):310-318.

Martini LA. Magnesium supplementation and bone turnover. *Nutr Rev*. 1999;57:227-229.

Mauskop A, Altura BM. Role of magnesium in the pathogenesis and treatment of migraines. *Clin Neurosci*. 1998;5:24-27.

Orchard TJ. Magnesium and type 2 diabetes mellitus (editorial). *Arch Int Med*. 1999;159:2119-2120.

Paolisso G, Sgamabato S, Pizza G, et al. Improved insulin response and action by chronic magnesium administration in aged NIDDM. *Diabetes Care*. 1989;12:265-269.

Peikert A, Wilimzig C, Kohne-Volland R. Prophylaxis of migraine with oral magnesium: results from a prospective, multi-center, placebo-controlled and double-blind randomized study. *Cephalalgia*. 1996;16:257-263.

Rivlin RS. Magnesium deficiency and alcohol intake: mechanisms, clinical significance and possible relation to cancer development (a review). *J Am Coll Nutr*. 1994;13:416-423.

Roberts JM. Magnesium for preeclampsia and eclampsia. *N Engl J Med*. 1995;333:250-251.

Roffe C, Fletcher S, Woods KL. Investigation of the effects of intravenous magnesium sulphate on cardiac rhythm in acute myocardial infarction. *Br Heart J*. 1994;71:141-145.

Rouse DJ, Hirtz DG, Thom E, et al. Eunice Kennedy Shriver NICHD Maternal-Fetal Medicine Units Network. A randomized, controlled trial of magnesium sulfate for the prevention of cerebral palsy. *N Engl J Med*. 2008;359(9):895-905.

Saris N-EL, Mervaala E, Karppanen H, et al. Magnesium. An update on physiological, clinical and analytical aspects (review). *Clinica Chimica Acta*. 2000;294:1-26.

Schendel DE, Berg CJ, Yeargin-Allsopp M, et al. Prenatal magnesium sulfate exposure and the risk for cerebral palsy or mental retardation among very low-birth-weight children aged 3 to 5 years. *JAMA*. 1996;276:1805-1810.

Shils ME. Magnesium. In: Shils M, Olson JA, Shike M, Ross AC, eds. *Modern Nutrition in Health and Disease.* 9th ed. Baltimore, MD: Williams and Wilkins; 1999:169-192.

Sojka JE. Magnesium supplementation and osteoporosis. *Nutr Rev.* 1995;53:71-80.

Stanley FJ, Crowther C. Antenatal magnesium sulfate for neuroprotection before preterm birth? *N Engl J Med.* 2008;359(9):962-964.

Terblanche S, Noakes TD, Dennis SC, et al. Failure of magnesium supplementation to influence marathon running performance or recovery in magnesium-replete subjects. *Int J Sports Nutr.* 1992;2:154-164.

Toba Y, Kajita Y, Masuyama R, et al. Dietary magnesium supplementation affects bone metabolism and dynamic strength of bone in ovariectomized rats. *J Nutr.* 2000;130:216-220.

Tosiello L. Hypomagnesemia and diabetes mellitus. A review of clinical implications. *Arch Intern Med.* 1998;156:1143-1148.

Volpe SL. Magnesium, the metabolic syndrome, insulin resistance, and type 2 diabetes mellitus. *Crit Rev Food Sci Nutr.* 2008;48(3):293-300.

Woods KL, Fletcher S. Long-term outcome after intravenous magnesium sulphate in suspected acute myocardial infarction: the second Leicester Intravenous Magnesium Intervention Trial (LIMIT-2). *Lancet.* 1994;343:816-819.

Malic Acid

DESCRIPTION

Malic acid, an alpha-hydroxy organic acid, is sometimes referred to as a fruit acid. This is because malic acid is found in apples and other fruits. It is also found in plants and animals, including humans. In fact, malic acid, in the form of its anion malate, is a key intermediate in the major biochemical energy-producing cycle in cells known as the citric acid or Krebs cycle located in the cells' mitochondria.

Malic acid, also known as apple acid, hydroxybutanedioic acid and hydroxysuccinic acid, is a chiral molecule. The naturally occurring stereoisomer is the L-form. The L-form is also the biologically active one. There is some preliminary evidence that malic acid, in combination with magnesium, may be helpful for some with fibromyalgia. Malic acid sold as a supplement is mainly derived from apples and, therefore, is the L-form. L-malic acid has the following chemical structure:

L-malic Acid

ACTIONS AND PHARMACOLOGY

ACTIONS

Malic acid, in combination with magnesium, has putative antifibromyalgic activity.

MECHANISM OF ACTION

The mechanism of malic acid's putative antifibromyalgic activity is unknown.

PHARMACOKINETICS

Malic acid is absorbed from the gastrointestinal tract from whence it is transported via the portal circulation to the liver. There are a few enzymes that metabolize malic acid. Malic enzyme catalyzes the oxidative decarboxylation of L-malate to pyruvate with concomitant reduction of the cofactor NAD+ (oxidized form of nicotinamide adenine dinucleotide) or NADP+ (oxidized form of nicotinamide adenine dinucleotide phosphate). These reactions require the divalent cations magnesium or manganese. Three isoforms of malic enzyme have been identified in mammals: a cytosolic NADP+-dependent malic enzyme, a mitochondrial NADP+-dependent malic enzyme and a mitochondrial NAD(P)+-dependent malic enzyme. The latter can use either NAD+ or NADP+ as the cofactor but prefers NAD+. Pyruvate formed from malate can itself be metabolized in a number of ways, including metabolism via a number of metabolic steps to glucose. Malate can also be metabolized to oxaloacetate via the citric acid cycle. The mitochondrial malic enzyme, particularly in brain cells, may play a key role in the pyruvate recycling pathway, which utilizes dicarboxylic acids and substrates, such as glutamine, to provide pyruvate to maintain the citric acid cycle activity when glucose and lactate are low.

Clearly, the metabolism of malic acid is complex and what any of the above has to do, if anything, with malic acids' putative activity in those with fibromyalgia is entirely unclear.

INDICATIONS AND USAGE

Malic acid may help some with fibromyalgia.

RESEARCH SUMMARY

Results have been mixed in studies of malic acid's possible effects in those with fibromyalgia. In a double-blind, placebo-controlled crossover study, subjects with primary fibromyalgia syndrome were randomized to receive a combination of 200 milligrams of malic acid and 50 milligrams of magnesium per tablet (three tablets twice a day) or placebo for four weeks. This was followed by a six-month, open-label trial with dose escalating up to six tablets twice a day. Outcome variables were measures of pain and tenderness, as well as functional and psychological measures.

No clear benefit was observed for the malic acid/magnesium combination in the lower-dose blinded trial. But in the open-label trial, at higher doses, there were significant reductions in the severity of all three primary pain/tenderness measures. Follow-up is needed.

CONTRAINDICATIONS, PRECAUTIONS, ADVERSE REACTIONS

CONTRAINDICATIONS
Known hypersensitivity to a malic acid-containing product.

PRECAUTIONS
Because of lack of long-term safety studies, supplementary malic acid should be avoided by pregnant women and lactating mothers. See Magnesium.

INTERACTIONS
None reported for malic acid. See Magnesium.

DOSAGE AND ADMINISTRATION
The doses used in the fibromyalgia studies were L-malic acid, 1200 to 2400 milligrams daily, and magnesium, 300 to 600 milligrams daily.

LITERATURE
Russell IJ, Michalek JE, Flechas JD, Abraham GE. Treatment of fibromyalgia syndrome with Super Malic: a randomized, double-blind, placebo-controlled pilot study. *J Rheumatol.* 1995; 22:953-958.

Young Z, Floyd DL, Loeber G, Tong L. Structure of a closed form of human malic enzyme and implications for catalytic mechanism. *Nature Struct Biol.* 2000; 7:251-257.

Manganese

DESCRIPTION
Manganese is an essential trace mineral in animal nutrition and is believed to be an essential trace mineral in human nutrition, as well. Manganese is a metallic element with atomic number 25 and an atomic weight of 54.94 daltons. Its chemical symbol is Mn. Manganese exists in the oxidation states Mn^{2+} or Mn(II) and Mn^{3+} or Mn(III) under physiological conditions.

Dietary manganese-deficiency in animals results in a wide variety of structural and physiological defects, including growth retardation, skeletal and cartilage malformations, impaired reproductive function, congenital ataxia due to abnormal inner ear development, optic nerve abnormalities, impaired insulin metabolism and abnormal glucose tolerance, alterations in lipoprotein metabolism and an impaired oxidant defense system.

Manganese deficiency states have not been well documented in humans. There is one report of a man maintained for four months on a manganese-deficient diet and also given magnesium-containing antacids. The symptoms which occurred included a decrease in serum cholesterol, depressed growth of hair and nails, scaly dermatitis, weight loss, reddening of his black hair and beard and impaired blood clotting. He responded to a diet containing manganese. In another report, men fed a low-manganese diet manifested low serum cholesterol levels and dermatitis. Short-term manganese supplementation did not reverse these symptoms.

In still another report, young women fed a manganese-poor diet were found to have mildly abnormal glucose tolerance and increased menstrual losses of manganese, calcium, iron and total hemoglobin. Finally a child on long-term total parenteral nutrition (TPN) lacking manganese manifested bone demineralization and impaired growth that were corrected by supplementation with manganese.

Manganese is the preferred metal cofactor for glycosyltransferases. Glycosyltransferases are important in the synthesis of glycoproteins and glycosaminoglycans (GAGs or mucopolysaccharides). Glycoproteins are involved in the synthesis of myelin and the clotting factors, among other things. Manganese-containing metalloenzymes include manganese superoxide dismutase, the principal antioxidant enzyme of mitochondria, arginase, pyruvate carboxylase and glutamine synthetase.

The richest dietary sources of manganese include whole grains, nuts, leafy vegetables and teas. Manganese is concentrated in the bran of grains which is removed during processing. Mean intakes of manganese worldwide range from 0.52 to 10.8 milligrams daily.

ACTIONS AND PHARMACOLOGY

ACTIONS
Manganese may have antioxidant activity. Manganese has putative anti-osteoporotic and anti-arthritic activities.

MECHANISM OF ACTION
Manganese ions have been found to scavenge hydroxyl and superoxide radicals. The mechanism of binding of manganese ions to these reactive oxygen species is not known. Manganese is a crucial component of the metalloenzyme manganese superoxide dismutase (MnSOD). MnSOD is found in mitochondria and is the principal constituent of the mitochondrial oxidant defense system. Rats and mice fed manganese-deficient diets are found to have reduced MnSOD activity in heart muscle and nervous tissue. They also have mitochondrial abnormalities and pathological changes in these tissues. The pathological changes are thought to result from oxidative damage due to the decreased activity of MnSOD which normally would protect against this damage.

Dietary manganese deficiency results in skeletal and cartilage malformations in animals and in one human report. It is thought that this is due to decreased activity of the manganese-dependent glycosyltransferases which, among other things, are involved in the synthesis of glycosaminoglycans or GAGs. GAGs are crucial for healthy cartilage and bone. However, there is as yet only very preliminary evidence that supplemental manganese has any effect on the promotion of bone or cartilage formation in humans who are not manganese-deficient. One study reported that manganese when taken in combination with calcium, copper and zinc may improve bone mineral density in postmenopausal women with osteoporosis.

PHARMACOKINETICS

There is scant information on the pharmacokinetics of manganese in humans. The efficiency of absorption (fractional absorption) of ingested manganese appears to be low, about 5%. Absorption efficiency appears to decrease as dietary intake of manganese increases. It increases with low dietary intake of manganese. Absorption appears to occur throughout the small intestine and appears to occur by both active-transport and passive diffusion mechanisms. Manganese ions are transported via the portal circulation to the liver. In what forms manganese is transported to the liver—bound to albumin, alpha$_2$-macroglobulin, hydrated manganese complexes, etc.—is also unclear. A fraction of manganese is taken up by hepatocytes and a fraction is transported by the systemic circulation to the various tissues of the body. Some manganese is bound to the plasma protein transferrin, but there also appear to be other carriers that transport manganese in the systemic circulation. Manganese is found principally in the mitochondria of cells. Absorbed manganese is excreted primarily via the biliary route. Very little manganese is excreted in the urine.

INDICATIONS AND USAGE

Apart from its uses in rare overt deficiency disorders, manganese might have some efficacy in osteoporosis and osteoarthritis as well as in some with premenstrual syndrome (PMS). Evidence for these benefits is preliminary.

RESEARCH SUMMARY

Manganese supplementation, in combination with calcium, zinc and copper, showed some efficacy in postmenopausal osteoporosis. Manganese ascorbate, in combination with glucosamine hydrochloride and chondroitin sulfate, was helpful in treating knee osteoarthritis pain in a recent randomized, double-blind, placebo-controlled pilot study. Follow-up on these studies is needed. Similarly, there is an isolated study needing follow-up that suggested some possible benefit from manganese in alleviating some PMS symptoms, including anxiety, depression, irritability and mood swings.

CONTRAINDICATIONS, PRECAUTIONS, ADVERSE REACTIONS

CONTRAINDICATIONS

Manganese supplements are contraindicated in those with liver failure. Some patients with end-stage liver disease have been found to accumulate manganese in their basal ganglia. It is thought that manganese may play a role in the hepatic encephalopathy in those with liver failure. Manganese is eliminated primarily through the bile, and hepatic dysfunction leads to depressed manganese excretion.

Manganese supplements are contraindicated in those hypersensitive to any component of a manganese-containing supplement.

PRECAUTIONS

Pregnant women and nursing mothers should avoid intakes of manganese above the upper limit of the estimated safe and adequate daily dietary intake (ESSADI). The ESSADI for those 11 years and older is 2.0 to 5.0 milligrams daily.

ADVERSE REACTIONS

Oral manganese supplements are generally well tolerated. Oral manganese, however, may be neurotoxic in those with liver failure. Manganese is primarily eliminated via the biliary route, and hepatic dysfunction leads to depressed manganese excretion. Manganese may accumulate in the basal ganglia of those with liver failure and may exacerbate hepatic encephalopathy and/or cause Parkinson's disease-like symptoms.

Manganese is toxic under certain conditions. Hepatic failure was discussed above. Mine workers exposed to high concentrations of manganese dust develop what is known in the mining villages of northern Chile, where this disorder has been found, as "locura manganica" or manganese madness. In later stages of this disease, symptoms similar to those of Parkinson's disease are observed. Levodopa is the treatment of the later stages of manganese madness.

There are a few reports of manganese intoxication occurring in those on long-term total parenteral nutrition (TPN) who developed parkinsonism which was treated with levodopa.

INTERACTIONS

DRUGS

Antacids: Magnesium-containing antacids, such as aluminum hydroxide/magnesium hydroxide, aluminum hydroxide/magnesium carbonate and aluminum hydroxide/magnesium trisilicate, may decrease the absorption of manganese if taken concomitantly.

Laxatives: Magnesium-containing laxatives may decrease the absorption of manganese if taken concomitantly.

Tetracycline: Tetracycline may reduce the absorption of manganese if taken concomitantly.

NUTRITIONAL SUPPLEMENTS

Calcium: Calcium supplements may decrease the absorption of manganese if taken concomitantly.

Iron: Non-heme iron supplements may reduce the absorption of manganese if taken concomitantly.

Magnesium: Magnesium supplements may decrease the absorption of manganese if taken concomitantly.

FOODS

Concomitant intake of manganese with foods rich in phytic acid (unleavened bread, raw beans, seeds, nuts and grains and soy isolates) or oxalic acid (spinach, sweet potatoes, rhubarb and beans) may depress the absorption of manganese.

DOSAGE AND ADMINISTRATION

There are several forms of supplementary manganese, including manganese gluconate, manganese sulfate, manganese ascorbate and manganese amino acid chelates. Manganese is available as a stand-alone supplement and also in combination products. One combination product used for bone/joint health contains chondroitin sulfate, glucosamine hydrochloride and manganese ascorbate.

Typical supplemental intake of manganese ranges from 2 to 5 milligrams daily.

A summary of DRIs for various age groups is as follows:

DRI values (milligrams/day)

Infants	Adequate Intake (AI)
0-6 months	0.003
7-12 months	0.6
Children	
1-3 years	1.2
4-8 years	1.5
Boys	
9-13 years	1.9
14-18 years	2.2
Girls	
9-13 years	1.6
14-18 years	1.6
Men	
19-30 years	2.3
31-50 years	2.3
51-70 years	2.3
Older than 70 years	2.3

Women	
19-30 years	1.8
31-50 years	1.8
51-70 years	1.8
Older than 70 years	1.8
Pregnancy	
14-18 years	2.0
19-30 years	2.0
31-50 years	2.0
Lactation	
14-18 years	2.6
19-30 years	2.6
31-50 years	2.6

The following summarizes the Tolerable Upper Intake Level (UL) for various age groups and conditions:

Infants	
0-6 months	ND
7-12 months	ND
Children	
1-3 years	2
4-8 years	3
9-13 years	6
Adolescents	
14-18 years	9
Adults	
19 years and older	11
Pregnancy	
14-18 years	9
19 years and older	11
Lactation	
14-18 years	9
19 years and older	11

ND = Not Determinable

The DV (Daily Value) for manganese, which is used for determining percentage of nutrient daily values on nutritional supplement and food labels, is 2 mg. The basis for the DV for manganese is the1989 Estimated Safe and Adequate Daily Dietary Intake (ESADDI).

LITERATURE

Baly DL, Schneiderman JS, Garcia-Welsh AL. Effect of manganese deficiency on insulin binding, glucose transport and metabolism in rat adipocytes. *J Nutr.* 1990;120:1075-1079.

Fell JME, Reynolds AP, Meadows N, et al. Manganese toxicity in children receiving long-term parenteral nutrition. *Lancet.* 1996;347:1218-1221.

Gong H, Amemiya T. Optic nerve changes in manganese-deficient rats. *Exp Eye Res.* 1999;68:313-320.

Hussain S, Ali SF. Manganese scavenges superoxide and hydroxyl radicals: an in vitro study in rats. *Neuroscience Letters.* 1999;261:21-24.

Institute of Medicine, Food and Nutrition Board. Dietary Reference Intakes for vitamin A, vitamin K, arsenic, boron, chromium, copper, iodine, iron, manganese, molybdenum, nickel, silicon, vanadium, and zinc. Washington, DC: National Academy Press, 2001.

Keen CL, Ensunsa JL, Watson MH, et al. Nutritional aspects of manganese from experimental studies. *Neurotoxicol.* 1999;20:213-223.

Krieger D, Krieger S, Jansen O, et al. Manganese and chronic hepatic encephalopathy. *Lancet.* 1995;346:270-274.

Nagatomo S, Umehara F, Hanada K, et al. Manganese intoxication during total parenteral nutrition: report of two cases and review of the literature. *J Neurol Sci.* 1999;162:102-105.

Nielsen FH. Ultratrace minerals. In: Shils ME, Olson JA, Shike M, Ross AC, eds. *Modern Nutrition in Health and Disease,* 9th ed. Baltimore, MD: Williams and Wilkins;1999:283-303.

Strause L, Saltman P, Glowacki J. The effect of deficiencies of manganese and copper on osteo-induction and on resorption of bone particles in rats. *Calcif Tissue Int.* 1987;41:145-150.

Strause L, Saltman P, Smith KT, et al. Spinal bone loss in postmenopausal women supplemented with calcium and trace minerals. *J Nutr.* 1994;124:1060-1064.

Strause LG, Hegenauer J, Saltman P, et al. Effects of long-term dietary manganese and copper deficiency on rat skeleton. *J Nutr.* 1986;116:135-141.

Medium-Chain Triglycerides

DESCRIPTION

Medium-chain triglycerides, commonly abbreviated MCT or MCTs, are medium-chain fatty acid esters of glycerol. Medium-chain fatty acids are fatty acids containing from six to 12 carbon atoms. These fatty acids are constituents of coconut and palm kernel oils and are also found in camphor tree drupes. Coconut and palm kernel oils are also called lauric oils because of their high content of the 12 carbon fatty acid, lauric or dodecanoic acid.

Medium-chain triglycerides used for nutritional and other commercial purposes are derived from lauric oils. In the process of producing MCTs, lauric oils are hydrolyzed to medium-chain fatty acids and glycerol. The glycerol is drawn off from the resultant mixture, and the medium-chain fatty acids are fractionally distilled. The medium-chain fatty acid fraction used commercially is mainly comprised of the eight carbon caprylic or octanoic acid and the 10 carbon

capric or decanoic acid. There are much smaller amounts of the six carbon caproic or hexanoic acid and the 12 carbon lauric acid in the commercial products. The caprylic- and capric-rich mixture is finally re-esterified to glycerol to produce medium-chain triglycerides that are mainly glyceral esters of caproic (C_6) caprylic (C_8), capric (C_{10}) and lauric acid (C_{12}) in a ratio of approximately 2:55:42:1. MCTs are represented by the following chemical structures:

Medium-chain triglycerides

R represents the alkyl moieties primarily of C_8, caprylic (octanoic) and C_{10}, capric (decanoic) acids.

$$CH_3(CH_2)_5CH_2-C(=O)-OH$$

Caprylic Acid

$$CH_3(CH_2)_7CH_2-C(=O)-OH$$

Capric acid

MCT is also known as fractionated coconut oil. In a process called interesterification, long-chain fatty acids, such as oleic and linoleic acid, are introduced into the final product. MCT derivatives produced by the interesterification process are referred to as structural lipids or structural triglycerides. Unlike most natural oils of animal or vegetable origin, MCT is stable and resistant to oxidation owing mainly to the saturation of the medium-chain fatty acids.

ACTIONS AND PHARMACOLOGY

ACTIONS

MCT's major action is as an energy-yielding substrate, particularly beneficial for those with malabsorption syndromes. MCT is also ketogenic.

MECHANISM OF ACTION

The physiology and biochemistry of medium-chain triglycerides are very different from those of long-chain triglycerides. MCT is rapidly absorbed from the small intestine, intact or following hydrolysis, into the portal circulation. From there, it is transported to the liver. Long-chain triglycerides are first hydrolyzed in the small intestine to long-chain fatty acids. They are in turn re-esterified in the mucosal cells of the small intestine to long-chain triglyerides, which are then carried by chylomicrons and transported via the lymphatic system to the systemic circulation. The systemic circulation in turn distributes the long-chain triglycerides to various tissues of the body, including adipose tissue and the liver.

Since MCT, in contrast with long-chain fatty acids, does not require pancreatic enzymes or bile salts for digestion and absorption, MCT is better handled in those with malabsorption syndromes than are the long-chain fatty acids. These syndromes include pancreatic disorders, hepatic disorders, gastrointestinal disorders and disorders of the lymph system.

Medium-chain fatty acids are taken up by hepatocytes and converted to medium-chain fatty acyl CoA which enters mitochondria without requiring the aid of carnitine. On the other hand, long-chain fatty acids, which are also converted to their coenzyme A esters in cells, including hepatocytes, require that they be converted from coenzyme A esters to carnitine esters in order to be transported across the mitochondrial membrane. Within the hepatocyte mitochondria, medium-chain fatty acyl CoA is converted to acetoacetate and beta-hydroxybutyrate and subsequently to carbon dioxide, water and energy. The oxidation of MCT produces 8.3 kilocalories of energy per gram ingested.

MCTs are therefore easier to metabolize, which could be advantageous to those who are critically ill and those with carnitine deficiencies.

MCT is ketogenic. The metabolism of MCT in hepatocytes produces two so-called ketone bodies, acetoacetate and beta-hydroxybutyrate. These ketone bodies are carried by the bloodstream to other tissues of the body, where they are used for energy production, as well as for other biochemical processes. It is believed that ketosis may raise the seizure threshold and reduce seizure severity. This is still hypothetical but is the rationale for the use of ketogenic diets in the treatment of seizure disorders.

PHARMACOKINETICS

MCT is rapidly absorbed from the small intestine, intact or hydrolyzed, after ingestion and is transported to the liver via the portal circulation. Medium-chain fatty acids are transported into hepatocytes and converted to medium-chain fatty acyl CoA esters. Medium-chain fatty acyl CoAs (mainly of caprylic and capric acids) are transported into mitochondria, where they are metabolized to acetoacetate and beta-hydroxybutyrate. The first mitochondrial enzyme in this process is medium-chain acyl CoA dehydrogenase. Acetoacetate and beta-hydroxybutyrate may be further metabolized in the liver to carbon dioxide, water and energy, and may enter some other metabolic pathways in the liver or be transported by the systemic circulation to other tissues, where they undergo metabolism mainly to CO_2, H_2O and energy. Very little ingested MCT is deposited in the body as fat.

INDICATIONS AND USAGE

Though MCTs are being promoted in the supplement marketplace for weight loss and to increase athletic performance, numerous studies have shown that MCT's are ineffective for achieving these goals. On the other hand, MCT does appear to be helpful for nutritional support in a number of conditions, including enteral and total parenteral nutrition in some infants and surgical patients, as well as in some of those who are critically ill with immunosuppression, pulmonary disease, liver disease, neurologic injury and various malabsorption syndromes. MCT may also be useful in some with epilepsy and other disorders characterized by seizures. There is preliminary evidence that MCT may be helpful in some cancers and may have some positive effects on immunity.

RESEARCH SUMMARY

A large number of studies have sought to determine whether MCT can promote long-chain fatty acid oxidation, inhibit the rate of muscle glycogen depletion, and enhance exercise and athletic performance. Many of these studies have tested subjects, some of them elite athletes, on bicycle ergometers. Some of these trials have been randomized, double-blind, placebo-controlled. Almost all have found no effect of MCT on rates of long-chain fatty acid oxidation, muscle glycogen utilization or performance. "At present," one research group concluded, "there is insufficient scientific evidence to recommend that athletes either ingest fat, in the form of MCT, during exercise, or 'fat adapt' in the weeks prior to a major endurance event to improve athletic performance."

It should be noted that some have reported that exercise performance is actually impaired in some taking high doses of MCT. This diminished performance was associated with increased gastrointestinal complaints, primarily intestinal cramping.

Research on weight loss associated with MCT intake is not as abundant but presents a mixed and mostly negative conclusion. MCT diets have been compared with LCT (long-chain triglyceride) diets and show no superiority. There are no convincing data that diets high in MCT are effective for weight loss.

MCT shows considerable promise, on the other hand, for the nutritional support of some premature infants, surgical patients and the critically ill, particularly those needing total parenteral nutrition (TPN). Lipid emulsions containing significant quantities of MCT as part of TPN have demonstrated significant benefits in some with pulmonary diseases, AIDS, liver disease, neurologic injury and several other illnesses.

AIDS patients, for example, who were suffering from fat malabsorption and chronic diarrhea with weight loss, were significantly benefited by a 12-week regimen of MCT. There was a significant decrease in stool number, stool fat and stool weight compared with baseline, regardless of the etiology of the diarrhea.

Surgical patients have shown more improvement in some studies, using MCT, compared with LCT. The same is true in some patients with some forms of liver disease. MCT is more readily utilized than LCT and is not deposited in the liver. MCT combined with LCT was found to be superior to LCT alone in septic patients with ARDS. Nutritional support with MCT has also helped prevent gestational hyperlipid-emic pancreatitis, with resulting successful childbirth.

MCT's usefulness in drug-resistant epilepsy was demonstrated in a trial with 50 children, eight of whom achieved complete control of seizures (four without further use of anticonvulsant drugs). In another trial, five of 17 MCT-treated subjects with previously intractable drug-resistant seizures achieved complete control of seizures with diminished or discontinued use of drugs. Five others had some improvement. Other types of intractable seizures have also yielded to MCT supplementation. Seven girls with Rett syndrome who suffered from drug-resistant seizures were given MCT therapy; five showed clinical benefit.

There is very preliminary evidence that MCT may have some positive effects on immunity and may exert some anti-cancer effects. Compared with LCT, MCT enhanced macrophage response in an animal model and suppressed *Malassezia* infection *in vitro*. This is significant, in particular, since lipophilic *Malassezia* species frequently grow on standard lipid infusions and can induce catheter-associated sepsis in newborns and immunocompromised patients receiving parenteral lipids.

In an animal model of cachexia-inducing colon adenocarcinoma, an MCT regimen reduced weight loss and was associated with a marked reduction in tumor size. LCT, on the other hand, did not have these effects. *In vitro* studies have indicated that MCT is significantly cytotoxic against some human tumor cells. More research is underway.

CONTRAINDICATIONS, PRECAUTIONS, ADVERSE REACTIONS

CONTRAINDICATIONS

MCT is contraindicated in those with hepatic encephalopathy. Known hypersensitivity to an MCT-containing product.

PRECAUTIONS

Great caution should be exercised in the use of MCT in those with diabetes, acidosis, ketosis, cirrhosis and the inborn error of metabolism, medium-chain acyl CoA dehydrogenase deficiency. Those with cirrhosis may accumulate free fatty acids and glycerol if given MCT.

ADVERSE REACTIONS

Adverse effects reported include diarrhea, nausea, vomiting, irritability and, with high doses (over 80 grams taken at one time), intestinal cramping.

INTERACTIONS

DRUGS

Theoretically, MCT may facilitate the uptake of some lipophilic drugs.

NUTRITIONAL SUPPLEMENTS

MCT may facilitate the absorption of vitamin E, magnesium and calcium. Theoretically, MCT may facilitate the absorption of the fat-soluble vitamins A, D and K, carotenoids, lipophilic polyphenols and supplemental long-chain fatty acids (ALA, EPA, DHA, GLA).

FOODS

MCT may facilitate the absorption of magnesium, calcium, fat-soluble vitamins and other lipophilic nutrients (carotenoids, flavonoids) and long-chain fatty acids in foods.

HERBS

Theoretically, MCT may facilitate the absorption of lipophilic substances in herbs.

OVERDOSAGE

There are no reports of overdosage with MCT.

DOSAGE AND ADMINISTRATION

Medium-chain triglycerides are available in several medical food products, many for use in a hospital setting. Doses of these medical food products are as prescribed by a physician.

MCT (100 percent) is available as a nutritional supplement. Those with malabsorption syndromes typically use one tablespoon up to three times a day with food or as directed by a physician. One tablespoon is equivalent to approximately 15 grams of MCT.

Those who use MCT as a supplement for any other reason typically use one tablespoon once to three times daily taken with food.

Doses greater than 80 grams (over five tablespoons) taken at one time may cause intense intestinal cramping.

LITERATURE

Babayan VK. Medium chain length fatty acid esters and their medical and nutritional applications. *J Am Oil Chem Soc.* 1981; 58:49A-51A.

Bach AC, Ingenbleek Y, Frey A. The usefulness of dietary medium-chain triglycerides in body weight control: fact or fancy? *J Lipid Res*. 1996; 37:708-726.

Bach AC, Babayan VK. Medium-chain triglycerides: an update. *Am J Clin Nutr*. 1982; 36:950-962.

Craig GB, Darnell BE, Weinsier RL, et al. Decreased fat and nitrogen losses in patients with AIDS receiving medium-chain-triglyceride-enriched formula vs. those receiving long-chain-triglyceride-containing formula. *J Am Diet Assoc*. 1997; 97:605-611.

Fan, ST. Review: nutritional support for patients with cirrhosis. *Gastroenterol Hepatol*. 1997; 12:282-286.

Greenberger NJ, Skillman TG. Medium-chain triglycerides. Physiologic consideration and clinical implications. *N Engl J Med*. 1969; 280:1045-1058.

Haas RH, Rice MA, Trauner DA, Merritt TA. Therapeutic effects of a ketogenic diet in Rett syndrome. *Am J Med Genet Suppl*. 1986; 1:225-246.

Hawley JA, Brouns F, Jeukendrup A. Strategies to enhance fat utilization during exercise. *Sports Med*. 1998; 25:241-257.

Hinton PS, Peterson CA, McCarthy DO, Ney DM. Medium-chain compared with long-chain triacylglycerol emulsions enhance macrophage response and increase mucosal mass in parenterally fed rats. *Am J Clin Nutr*. 1998; 67:1265-1272.

Jeukendrup AE, Thielen JJ, Wagenmakers AJ, et al. Effect of medium-chain triacylglycerol and carbohydrate ingestion during exercise on substrate utilization and subsequent cycling performance. *Am J Clin Nutr*. 1998; 67:397-404.

Jiang ZM, Zhang SY, Wang XR, et al. A comparison of medium-chain and long-chain triglycerides in surgical patients. *Ann Surg*. 1993; 217:175-184.

Kimoto Y, Tanji Y, Taguchi T, et al. Antitumor effect of medium-chain triglyceride and its influence on the self-defense system of the body. *Cancer Detect Prev*. 1998; 22:219-224.

Kimura T, Fukui E, Kageyu A, et al. Enhancement of oral bioavailability of d-alpha-tocopherol acetate by lecithin-dispersed aqueous preparation containing medium-chain triglycerides in rats. *Chem Pharm Sci*. 1989; 37:439-441.

Mizushima T, Ochi K, Matsumura N, et al. Prevention of hyperlipidemic acute pancreatitis during pregnancy with medium-chain triglyceride nutritional support. *Int J Pancreatol*. 1998; 23:187-192.

Papamandjaris AA, MacDougall DE, Jones PJ. Medium chain fatty and metabolism and energy expenditure: obesity treatment implications. *Life Sci*. 1998; 62:1203-1215.

Papavassilis C, Mach KK, Mayser PA. Medium-chain triglycerides inhibit growth of Malassezia: implications for prevention of systemic infection. *Crit Care Med*. 1999; 27:1781-1786.

Ruppin DC, Middleton WRJ. Clinical use of medium chain triglycerides. *Drugs*. 1980; 20:216-224.

Sanchez R, Hendler S. Delivery formulation for probucol. 1996; U.S. Patent No. 5, 494, 936

Sills MA, Forsythe WI, Haidukewych D, et al. The medium chain triglyceride diet and intractable epilepsy. *Arch Dis Child*. 1986; 61:1168-1172.

Smirniotis V, Kostopanagiotou G, Vassiliou J, et al. Long chain versus medium chain lipids in patients with ARDS: effects on pulmonary haemodynamics and gas exchange. *Intensive Care Med*. 1998; 24:1029-1033.

Tisdale MJ, Brennan RA. A comparison of long-chain triglycerides and medium-chain triglycerides on weight loss and tumour size in a cachexia model. *Br J Cancer*. 1988; 58:580-583.

Trauner DA. Medium-chain triglyceride (MCT) diet in intractable seizure disorder. *Neurology*. 1985; 35:237-238.

Wanke CA, Pleskow D, Degirolami PC, et al. A medium chain triglyceride-based diet in patients with HIV and chronic diarrhea reduces diarrhea and malabsorption: a prospective, controlled trial. *Nutrition*. 1996; 12:766-771.

Melatonin

DESCRIPTION

Melatonin is the principal hormone of the vertebrate pineal gland, and it is also produced by extra-pineal tissues in amphibians. It is found in plants as well, but at much lower concentrations than in animals. This hormone is involved in setting the timing (entrainment) of mammalian circadian rhythms, as well as regulating seasonal responses to changes in day length in seasonally breeding mammals—so called photoperiodic responses. Photoperiodic responses include changes in reproductive status, behavior and body weight. Seasonal effects on reproduction in humans are subtle, and the role of melatonin here, if any, is unclear. Recently, melatonin supplementation has become popular as a possible aid for sleep disorders among other things.

Melatonin is synthesized endogenously by the pinealocytes of the pineal gland. The essential amino acid L-tryptophan is a precursor in the synthesis of melatonin. In this synthesis, L-tryptophan first gets metabolized to 5-hydroxytryptophan from which 5-hydroxytryptamine, also known as serotonin, is made. 5-hydroxytryptamine is converted to melatonin in a two-step process, occurring mainly in the pineal gland.

Melatonin is also known as N-acetyl-5-methoxytryptamine and N-[2-(5-Methoxy-1H-indol-3-yl) ethyl] acetamide. The structural formula is:

Melatonin

Melatonin is a solid, lipophilic, hydrophobic substance, which is available as a supplement in synthetic form. Melatonin derived from the pineal glands of beef cattle is also marketed.

ACTIONS AND PHARMACOLOGY

ACTIONS

Supplemental melatonin may have a hypnotic action. It may also have antioxidant and anti-apoptotic activity.

MECHANISM OF ACTION

Melatonin is derived in pinealocytes from L-tryptophan. 5-hydroxytryptamine or serotonin is an intermediate in the biosynthetic process. The rate limiting step in the synthesis of melatonin is the n-acetylation of the 5-hydroxytryptamine by the enzyme arylalkylamine N-acetyltransferase (AA-NAT). Melatonin synthesis displays a circadian rhythm that is reflected in serum melatonin levels. The rhythm is generated by a circadian clock located in the suprachiasmatic nucleus (SCN) of the hypothalamus. The SCN clock is set to the 24 hour day by the natural light-dark cycle. Light signals through a direct retinal pathway to the SCN. The SCN clock sends circadian signals over a neural pathway to the pineal gland. This drives rhythmic melatonin synthesis. The neural input to the gland is norepinephrine, and the output is melatonin. Specifically, the rhythm of the enzyme AA-NAT is under SCN control, with the resulting melatonin rhythm characterized by high levels at night. Thus, the synthesis and release of melatonin are stimulated by darkness and inhibited by light.

The effects of hormones are typically mediated through receptors. Two forms of high-affinity melatonin receptors and one form of a low-affinity receptor have been identified. The high-affinity ML1 receptors are designated Mel1a and Mel1b. The low-affinity receptor is designated ML2.

The Mel1a receptor is expressed in the SCN and in the hypophyseal pars tuberalis. The SCN is the putative site of circadian action of melatonin, and the hypophyseal pars tuberalis is the putative site of its reproductive effects. The Mel1b receptor is expressed mainly in the retina. The ML1 melatonin receptors belong to the family of guanadine triphosphate-binding proteins or G protein-coupled receptors. Activation of the ML1 receptors results in inhibition of adenylate cyclase activity in target cells.

The distribution of the ML2 receptors has not yet been determined. These receptors are coupled to the stimulation of phosphoinositide hydrolysis.

In summary, melatonin is a hormone that has biological effects and that signals through a family of G protein-coupled receptors.

Melatonin has antioxidant activity. However, this activity is found only with very high pharmaceutical doses of this substance. The most significant antioxidant activity of melatonin appears to be its ability to inhibit metal ion-catalyzed oxidation processes, specifically the Fenton reaction.

Melatonin has been found to have anti-apoptotic activity in the thymus. Melatonin inhibits apoptosis in the thymus as well as in cultured dexamethasone-treated thymocytes (a standard model for the study of apoptosis). It is thought to do so by down-regulating the glucocorticoid receptor.

The mechanism of action of supplemental melatonin is speculative. The putative effect of melatonin as a hypnotic may be accounted for by receptor-mediated action on the limbic system. Pharmacologic doses of melatonin may produce a hypothermic effect, which may also play a role in its hypnotic effect.

PHARMACOKINETICS

The absorption and bioavailability of melatonin varies widely. Melatonin is absorbed from the small intestine and is transported by the portal circulation to the liver. Variable amounts of ingested melatonin are metabolized in the liver to 6-hydroxymelatonin. After conjugation with sulfuric or glucuronic acid, it is excreted by the kidneys. Nonmetabolized melatonin is transported via the systemic circulation to various tissues in the body. Serum half-life of ingested melatonin is approximately 35 to 50 minutes.

If melatonin causes drowsiness, this effect occurs about 30 minutes after ingestion and lasts for at least an hour. Melatonin given in the early evening appears to advance the nighttime peak of melatonin secretion by about three hours. Ingested melatonin that did not undergo first-pass metabolism in the liver is eventually metabolized, mainly in the liver, by hydroxylation to 6-hydroxymelatonin. After conjugation with sulfuric or glucuronic acid, it is excreted by the kidneys. A single nighttime dose is cleared by the following morning. With chronic dosing, however, some lipid storage occurs.

INDICATIONS AND USAGE

Melatonin may be indicated for some forms of insomnia and other sleep disturbances. Research results are mixed with respect to claims that melatonin can abolish some of the symptoms of jet lag. Use of the supplement in cancer and immune disorders is unsupported by current research; there are some promising findings, but they are very preliminary. There is no evidence to substantiate claims that melatonin can delay aging, be useful in cardiovascular disease, depression, seasonal affective disorder or sexual dysfunction.

RESEARCH SUMMARY

Numerous studies, many of them well-designed, suggest that supplemental melatonin can be effective in some sleep disorders, principally insomnia. These studies show that, in doses that raise serum melatonin levels to those that approximate normal nocturnal levels, sleep can be induced and sustained in some. Through its effects on circadian rhythms and possibly through an induced hypothermic effect, melatonin, in doses administered at carefully timed intervals, may be able to normalize various sleep disorders, such as those sometimes experienced by shift workers, and thus diminish fatigue.

The complexity of appropriate timing and dosage, however, has prompted some researchers to caution against melatonin use for sleep disturbance outside of laboratory settings or without medical supervision—at least until more research sheds further light on these issues. Even marginal drowsiness or lack of mental alertness could prove hazardous for some shift workers, for example.

In addition, a cautionary note has recently been issued with respect to the use of melatonin to treat sleep disturbances in children with neurologic disorders. Six such children, aged nine months to 18 years, were given 5 milligrams of melatonin at bedtime in as effort to treat their sleep disorder. Quality and quantity of sleep quickly increased in five of the six children. But in four of the subjects, all of whom had a prior history of seizures, incidence of seizures increased while taking melatonin. Discontinuance of the supplements led to seizure-incidence returning to pre-supplementation levels. But resumption of melatonin supplementation, this time at a reduced level of 1 milligram doses, again caused an increase in seizures, and the study was halted.

Some criticized these researchers for using inappropriately high doses, but the typical dose range in studies of melatonin's effects on sleep disturbance has been 0.3 milligrams to 5 milligrams, with 2 to 3 milligrams commonly being used. Clearly, more research is needed before melatonin can safely be recommended for use in individuals, whether children or adults, with seizure history. In addition, safety data, in general, is lacking for use of this supplement, particularly for long-term use. Certainly, if more research better defines the proper use of melatonin in sleep disturbances, the supplement might make a significant contribution considering that many sleep-deprived individuals become dependent upon benzodiazepine and other sedating drugs with potentially serious adverse effects in search of insomnia relief.

This point was made in a recent well-designed study that tested the effects of melatonin (2 milligrams daily) in a controlled release formula against placebo. During the course of the study, 34 long-term users of benzodiazepine were encouraged to reduce their benzodiazepine dosage incrementally. The goal was complete discontinuance during weeks five and six. The study proceeded double-blind through the six weeks of period one and then single-blind through the six weeks of period two, during which all subjects received melatonin and efforts to discontinue benzodiazepine resumed.

At the end of the study, 14 of 18 subjects who received melatonin in period one had completely discontinued benzodiazepine use; only four of 16 in the placebo group achieved this goal. An additional six subjects in the placebo group achieved complete discontinuance of benzodiazepine in period two. Sleep quality scores were significantly higher for the melatonin group than for the placebo group. A six-month post-study followup showed that 19 of the 24 subjects who discontinued benzodiazepine therapy continued to maintain good sleep quality. These subjects continued to use melatonin after the study ended and they did not resume use of benzodiazepine.

The use of melatonin to help alleviate some of the symptoms of jet lag has produced mixed results in trials to date. Often some benefit has been noted, but many studies have been criticized for being small and poorly designed. In the largest controlled trial to date, researchers recently reported that melatonin exerts no beneficial physiological effect on jet lag. Melatonin was tested against placebo in two doses and with different administration times. No melatonin regimen was superior to placebo.

Claims that melatonin can be used to prevent or treat cancer or immune dysfunction are unsupported by current research. There is some very preliminary data suggesting some beneficial effects in animal models and in *in vitro* studies. A small amount of clinical work has been done, and more seems warranted.

Claims that melatonin can favorably influence lipids, lower blood pressure and help prevent heart attacks are entirely baseless, as are claims that it can correct sexual dysfunction or otherwise enhance sexual performance. It has demonstrated no effect in seasonal affective disorder and, rather than help dispel depression it has been reported to cause or worsen it in some cases.

The sensational claim that melatonin dramatically delays aging is similarly without foundation. The claim was based, generally, on the long-held belief that endogenous melatonin secretion diminishes with age and, specifically, upon a single mouse study that has been criticized as seriously flawed by several researchers.

The idea that levels of serotonin fall with age was refuted in a recent study of 34 healthy subjects aged 65 to 81 in whom plasma melatonin concentrations were compared with those of a younger subject group (98 healthy individuals aged 18 to 30). No significant difference was noted between the two groups. The researchers have cautioned against the use of melatonin by the elderly, particularly since many of them may be using a variety of prescription drugs for which interactions with melatonin are unknown and could be potentially hazardous.

CONTRAINDICATIONS, PRECAUTIONS, ADVERSE REACTIONS

CONTRAINDICATIONS
Known hypersensitivity to a melatonin-containing product.

PRECAUTIONS
Use of melatonin in children, pregnant women and nursing mothers is not advised.

Adverse reactions of supplemental melatonin include depression. Those who suffer from depression are advised against taking melatonin.

Because melatonin may cause both nighttime and daytime drowsiness, those who operate hazardous machinery are advised against taking melatonin.

Large doses of melatonin (not recommended) have been shown to inhibit ovulation. Women who are trying to conceive should avoid melatonin.

Melatonin use in some children with seizure disorders leads to increased seizure activity. Those with seizure disorders, both children and adults, should avoid melatonin supplements.

Those over 65 years old who take any sedating medications or herbs, or who use alcohol, should exercise caution in the use of melatonin.

ADVERSE REACTIONS
Adverse reactions associated with melatonin include stomach discomfort, morning grogginess, daytime "hangover," feeling of a "heavy head," depression, psychotic episodes (in combination with fluoxetine), headache, lethargy, fragmented disorientation, amnesia, inhibition of fertility, increased seizure activity, suppression of male sexual drive, hypothermia, retinal damage, gynecomastia and low sperm count. Typically, these reports are related to high doses. However, adverse effects have been reported and can occur with low doses as well.

INTERACTIONS

DRUGS
Aspirin and other NSAIDs: Concomitant use may lead to decreased melatonin levels.

Benzodiazepines, sedating antihistamines, sedating antidepressants and other sedating drugs: Concomitant use may cause additive sedation and increase incidence of adverse effects.

Beta blockers: Concomitant use may lead to decreased melatonin levels.

Corticosteroids: Concomitant use may interfere with the efficacy of the corticosteroids.

Fluoxetine: A psychotic episode associated with the use of melatonin in a subject taking the antidepressant fluoxetine has been reported.

Fluvoxamine: The bioavailability of oral melatonin is increased by coadministration of fluvoxamine. This is believed due to inhibition of the elimination of melatonin.

Interleukin-2: There is a report of melatonin augmenting the antitumor effect of this drug.

Isoniazid: There is a report of melatonin enhancing the activity of this antitubercular drug.

Progestin combinations: Melatonin can be additive in inhibiting ovarian function in women.

HERBS
Valerian or kava kava: Concomitant use may lead to additive sedation.

NUTRITIONAL SUPPLEMENTS
5-hydroxytryptophan: Concomitant use may lead to additive sedation.

ALCOHOL
Use of melatonin with alcohol may lead to additive sedation.

FOOD
No interactions are known.

OVERDOSAGE
None known. No apparent serious consequences have been reported in those taking up to 24 grams daily of melatonin for one month, though such doses are not recommended.

DOSAGE AND ADMINISTRATION
Those who use melatonin supplements for sleep disturbance or jet lag usually take no more than 0.3 milligrams to 3 milligrams at bedtime for short periods of time (no longer than two weeks). Higher doses and dosing for longer periods of time requires medical supervision. As with all nutritional supplements, the physician must know if his or her patient is

taking melatonin. Melatonin supplements derived from animals should be avoided.

LITERATURE

Antunes F, Barclay LRC, Ingold KU. On the antioxidant activity of melatonin. *Free Rad Bio Med.* 1999; 26:117-128.

Barni S, Lissoni P, Cazzaniga M, et al. A randomized study of low-dose subcutaneous interleukin-2 plus melatonin versus supportive care alone in metastatic colorectal cancer patients progressing under 5-fluorouracil and folates. *Oncology.* 1995; 52:243-245.

Brzezinski A. Melatonin in humans. *N Engl J Med.* 1997; 336:186-195.

Bursztajn HJ. Melatonin therapy: from benzodiazepine-dependent insomnia to authenticity and autonomy. *Arch Intern Med.* 1999; 159:2393-2395.

Cupp MJ. Melatonin. *Am Fam Physician.* 1997; 56:1421-1425.

Dolberg OT, Hirschmann S, Grunhaus L. Melatonin for the treatment of sleep disturbances in major depressive disorder. *Am J Psychiat.* 1998; 155:1119-1121.

Force RW, Hansen L, Bedell M. Psychotic episode after melatonin [letter]. *Ann Pharmacother.* 1997; 31:1408.

Garfinkel D, Zisapel N, Wainstein J, Laudon M. Facilitation of benzodiazepine discontinuation by melatonin. *Arch Intern Med.* 1999; 159:2456-2460.

Hartter S, Grozinger M, Weigmann H, et al. Increased bioavailability of oral melatonin after fluvoxamine administration. *Clin Pharmacol Therap.* 2000; 67:1-6.

Middleton BA, Stone BM, Arendt J. Melatonin and fragmented sleep patterns. *Lancet.* 1996; 348:551-552.

Murphy PJ, Myers BL, Badia P. Nonsteroidal anti-inflammatory drugs alter body temperature and suppress melatonin in humans. *Physiol Behav.* 1996; 59:133-139.

Reiter RJ. Melatonin, active oxygen species and neurological damage. *Drug News Perspect.* 1998; 11:291-296.

Reppert SM, Weaver DR. Melatonin madness. Cell. 1995; 83:1059-1062.

Sainz RM, Mayo JC, Reiter RJ, et al. Melatonin regulates glucocorticoid receptor: an answer to its antiapoptotic action in thymus. *FASEB J.* 1999; 13:1547-1556.

Turjanski AG, Rosenstein RE, Estrin DA. Reactions of melatonin and related indoles with free radicals: a computational study. *J Med Chem.* 1998; 44:3684-3689.

Voorduow BC, Euser R, Verdonk RE, et al. Melatonin and melatonin-progestin combinations alter pituitary-ovarian function in women and can inhibit ovulation. *J Clin Encocrinol Metab.* 1992; 74:108-117.

Wiid I, Hoal-van Helden E, Hon D. et al. Potentiation of isoniazid activity against *Myobacterium tuberculosis* by melatonin. *Antimicrob Agents Chemother.* 1999; 43:975-977.

Methylsulfonylmethane (MSM)

DESCRIPTION

Methylsulfonylmethane, abbreviated MSM, is an organic sulfur-containing compound that occurs naturally in a variety of fruits, vegetables, grains and in animals, including humans in at least trace amounts. MSM has also been found in such plants as *Equisetem arvense,* also known as horsetail. The biological role of MSM, if any, is not known. MSM is a metabolite of dimethyl sulfoxide or DMSO (see Dimethyl Sulfoxide). It is believed that some of the possible effects of DMSO could be attributed to MSM.

MSM is a water-soluble, solid compound. It is also known as dimethyl sulfone, DMSO2, sulfonylbismethane and methyl sulfone.

ACTIONS AND PHARMACOLOGY

ACTIONS

Known hypersensitivity to an MSM-containing product.

PHARMACOKINETICS

Little is known about the pharmacokinetics of MSM in humans. Sulfur from MSM was found to be incorporated into protein methionine and cysteine when fed to guinea pigs. MSM was also detected in the brain of a normal 62-year old male, following its ingestion, using *in vivo* proton magnetic resonance spectroscopy. Thus, it appears that MSM gets absorbed and can cross the blood-brain barrier.

INDICATIONS AND USAGE

Claims for MSM include pain relief, particularly in arthritis, immune modulation in autoimmune disorders, muscle repair, sleep aid and diabetes therapy. There is no credible evidence to support any of these claims. There is very preliminary research suggesting some possible MSM anti-cancer effects.

RESEARCH SUMMARY

Two animal studies showed that MSM and other bipolar solvents can prolong latency period to time of tumor appearance in chemically induced animal model cancers. In one of these studies, there was no effect on tumor incidence; in the other, MSM seemed to reduce the incidence of poorly differentiated tumors. More research is indicated.

There is no research to support other claims made for MSM.

CONTRAINDICATIONS, PRECAUTIONS, ADVERSE REACTIONS

CONTRAINDICATIONS

Known hypersensivity to an MSM-containing product.

PRECAUTIONS

MSM should be avoided by pregnant women and nursing mothers.

ADVERSE REACTIONS

Reported adverse reactions include nausea, diarrhea and headache.

OVERDOSAGE

There are no reports of overdosage.

DOSAGE AND ADMINISTRATION

Doses used are typically 1 to 3 grams daily.

LITERATURE

Childs SJ. Dimethyl sulfone (DMSO2) in the treatment of interstitial cystitis. *Urol Clin North Am.* 1994; 21:85-98.

Kandorf H, Chirra AR, De Gruccio A, Girman DJ. Dimethyl sulfoxide modulation of diabetes onset in NOD mice. *Diabetes.* 1989; 38:194-197.

Kocsis JJ, Harkaway S, Snyder R. Biological effects of the metabolites of dimethyl sulfoxide. *Ann NY Acad Sci.* 1975; 243:104-109.

Layman DL. Growth inhibitory effects of dimethyl sulfoxide and dimethyl sulfone on vascular smooth muscle and endothelial cells in vitro. *In Vitro Cell Dev Biol.* 1987; 23:422-428.

Morton JI, Siegel BV. Effects of oral dimethyl sulfoxide and dimethyl sulfone on murine autoimmune lymphoproliferative disease. *Proc Soc Exp Biol Med.* 1986; 183; 227-230.

O'Dwyer PJ, McCabe DP, Sickle-Santanello BJ, et al. Use of polar solvents in chemoprevention of 1, 2-dimethylhydrazine-induced colon cancer. *Cancer.* 1988; 62:944-948.

Pearson TW, Dawson HJ, Lackey HB. Natural occurring levels of dimethyl sulfoxide in selected fruits, vegetables, grains and beverages. *J Agric Food Chem.* 1989; 29:1089-1091.

Richmond VL, Incorporation of methylsulfonylmethane sulfur into guinea pig serum proteins. *Life Sci.* 1986; 39:263-268.

Rose SE, Chalk JB, Galloway GJ, Doddrell DM. Detection of dimethyl sulfone in the human brain by in vivo proton magnetic resonance spectroscopy. *Magn Reson Imaging.* 2000; 18:95-98.

Modified Citrus Pectin

DESCRIPTION

Modified citrus pectin refers to citrus pectin which has been hydrolyzed to yield smaller molecular weight molecules which appears to render it more absorbable. Unmodified citrus pectin is not absorbable. Pectin (see Pectin) is a soluble fiber that is found in citrus fruits (oranges, lemons, grapefruits) and apples. Pectin obtained from orange or lemon rinds, both rich sources of pectin, is referred to as citrus pectin. Citrus pectin is a linear polysaccharide containing from about 300 to 1,000 monosaccharide units. D-galacturonic acid, an acid form of the sugar D-galactose, is the principal monosaccharide unit of citrus pectin. The D-galacturonic acid residues are bonded together by alpha-1,4 glycosidic linkages in linear chains. Neutral sugars, present in side chains on the pectin molecule, include D-galactose, L-arabinose, D-xylose and L-frucose. L-Rhamnose is also found in pectin. Some of the galacturonic acid residues in pectin are in the form of methyl esters. The molecular weight of citrus pectin ranges from 20,000 to 400,000 daltons, with the majority of the molecules having molecular weights ranging from 50,000 to 150,000 daltons.

Modified citrus pectin is formed from citrus pectin via a depolymerization process in which citrus pectin is first treated with sodium hydroxide at a pH of 10 for a short time, and then hydrochloric acid at a pH of 3 for a much longer period of time. The pectin fragments that are formed are principally comprised of D-polygalacturonates, absent the methoxyl groups. The molecular weight of modified citrus pectin ranges from 1,000 to 15,000 daltons, with an average weight of about 10,000 daltons. Modified citrus pectin is comprised of linear polygalacturonate chains containing from 5 to 90 galacturonic acid residues, with an average of approximately 55 residues. Also present, are D-galactose residues in side chains. Modified citrus pectin is also known as modified pectin, depolymerized pectin and pH-modified pectin. It is abbreviated as MCP. It is water soluble.

ACTIONS AND PHARMACOLOGY

ACTIONS

Modified citrus pectin has putative anticarcinogenic activity.

MECHANISM OF ACTION

Modified citrus pectin, when administered orally to rats, was found to inhibit spontaneous prostate carcinoma metastasis. It had no effect on the growth of the primary tumor. Injected modified citrus pectin was found to inhibit metastasis of melanoma cells in mice. The mechanism of these anticarcinogenic effects is not clear.

Galectins comprise a family of galactoside-binding mammalian lectins. Lectins themselves comprise a group of hemagglutinating proteins found in plant seeds, which bind the branching carbohydrate molecules of glycoproteins and glycolipids on cell surfaces, resulting in agglutination or proliferation, among other things. Galectins are proteins that can bind to carbohydrates via carbohydrate recognition domains (CRDs). At present, the galactin family includes 10 members. Apparently, galectins are secreted from cells via nonclassical secretory pathways. Galectin-3, one of the members of the family, is thought to be involved in mitosis and proliferation. On the cell surface, galectin-3 mediates cell-cell adhesion and cell-matrix interaction via binding to its complementary glycoconjugates, such as laminin and fibronectin, and thereby is thought to play an important role in the pathogenesis of cancer metastasis.

Some metastic events may involve cellular interactions that are mediated by cell surface components, including galectins. The galactose-containing carbohydrate side chains of modified citrus pectin may interfere with these cellular interactions by competing with the natural ligands of the galectins and by doing so, inhibit the metastatic process. It is thought that galectins may play a role in human prostate cancer, and in particular, human prostate cancer metastasis.

PHARMACOKINETICS

There is little on the pharmacokinetics of modified citrus pectin in humans. Based on rat studies, modified citrus pectin is probably absorbed to some degree following ingestion. However, research is necessary to determine its absorption efficiency, as well as its distribution, metabolism and excretion.

INDICATIONS AND USAGE

Modified citrus pectin has shown some ability to inhibit metastasis of prostate cancer in a rat study. It has also shown some activity against melanoma cells in culture and in mice. More research is needed before there can be any indication for the use of modified citrus pectin in cancer.

RESEARCH SUMMARY

There was the suggestion in one *in vitro* study of modified citrus pectin that it might have some ability to inhibit melanoma metastasis. Stronger, but still preliminary evidence emerged from a rat study that modified citrus pectin might similarly inhibit the spread of prostate cancer. The lungs of rats treated with this substance had significantly fewer metastatic colonies than controls. There was no effect on the primary tumor. Follow-up is needed.

CONTRAINDICATIONS, PRECAUTIONS, ADVERSE REACTIONS

CONTRAINDICATIONS

Modified citrus pectin is contraindicated in those hypersensitive to any component of a modified citrus pectin-containing product.

PRECAUTIONS

The use of modified citrus pectin for the management of prostate cancer or any type of cancer is considered experimental. Those who wish to use modified citrus pectin for the management of prostate cancer or any type of cancer must be under medical supervision.

Modified citrus pectin should be avoided by pregnant women and nursing mothers.

DOSAGE AND ADMINISTRATION

Modified citrus pectin is available as a dietary supplement both as a powder and in capsule form. Dosage is variable. See precautions regarding its use.

LITERATURE

Gopalkrishnan RV, Roberts T, Tuli S, et al. Molecular characterization of prostate carcinoma tumor antigen-1, PCTA-1, a human galectin-8 related gene. *Oncogene.* 2000; 19:4405-4416.

Hsieh TC, Wu JM. Changes in cell growth, cyclin/kinase, endogenous phosphoproteins and nm23 gene expression in human prostatic JCA-1 cells treated with modified citrus pectin. *Biochem Mol Biol Int.* 1995; 37:833-841.

Inohara H, Raz A. Effects of natural complex carbohydrate (citrus pectin) on murine melanoma cell properties related to galectin-3 functions. *Glycoconj J.* 1994; 11:527-532.

Pienta KJ, Naik H, Akhtar A, et al. Inhibition of spontaneous metastasis in a rat prostate cancer model by oral administration of modified citrus pectin. *J Natl Cancer Inst.* 1995; 87:348-353.

Platt D, Raz A. Modulation of the lung colonization of B16-F1 melanoma cells by citrus pectin. *J Natl Cancer Inst.* 1992; 84:438-442.

Rabinovich GA, Riera CM, Landa CA, Sotomayor CE. Galectins: a key intersection between glycobiology and immunology. *Braz J Med Biol Res.* 1999; 32:383-393.

Raz A, Pienta KJ. Method for treatment of cancer by oral administration of modified citrus pectin. United States Patent Number 5,895,784. Date of Patent: Apr. 20, 1999.

Molybdenum

DESCRIPTION

Molybdenum is an essential trace mineral in animal and human nutrition. It is found in several tissues of the human body and is required for the activity of some enzymes that are involved in catabolism, including the catabolism of purines and the sulfur amino acids. Molybdenum is a transition metal with atomic number 42 and an atomic weight of 95.94 daltons. Its symbol is Mo. Compounds of molybdenum are among the scarcer constituents of the earth's crust. In fact, molybdenum is only about three times more abundant than gold. The principal ore of molybdenum is molybdenite (molybdenum disulfide). Organic forms of molybdenum are found in living matter, from bacteria to animals, including humans.

In spite of its low abundance, molybdenum deficiency in humans is rare but it has been described. A patient on long-term total parenteral nutrition (TPN) developed a syndrome characterized by hypouricemia, hypermethioninemia, low urinary sulfate excretion, tachycardia, tachypnea and mental and visual disturbances. The syndrome worsened with the administration of L-methionine and the patient eventually became comatose. The patient improved when molybdenum, in the form of ammonium molybdate, was added to the TPN. The deleterious effects of molybdenum deficiency were primarily due to the accumulation of sulfite coming from the catabolism of L-cysteine. Sulfite is toxic to the nervous system and molybdenum is necessary for its metabolism to a nontoxic form.

Animals can be made molybdenum deficient by feeding them diets containing high amounts of tungsten or copper. Both tungsten and copper are molybdenum antagonists. Molybdenum deficiency has also been produced experimentally in goats by feeding them purified diets, very low in molybdenum. Molybdenum deficiency in animals results in retarded weight gain, decreased food consumption, impaired reproduction and a shortened life expectancy.

High intake of molybdenum is antagonistic to copper and can produce a condition in animals known as molybdenosis. Molybdenum-containing compounds, such as tetrathiomolybdate are currently in clinical trials for the treatment of metastatic cancer and Wilson disease. The use of copper antagonistic substances in these disorders is known as copper depletion therapy.

ACTIONS AND PHARMACOLOGY

ACTIONS

Molybdenum prevents and treats molybdenum deficiency. Molybdenum has putative anticarcinogenic activity.

MECHANISM OF ACTION

The active biological form of molybdenum is known as the molybdenum cofactor or Moco. Moco is comprised of a molybdenum atom coordinated by the dithiolene moiety of a family of tricyclic pyranopterin structures, the simplest of which is known as molybdopterin. Moco is the cofactor for four human enzymes: xanthine dehydrogenase (xanthine: NAD+ oxidoreductase), xanthine oxidase (a form of xanthine dehydrogenase), sulfite oxidase (sulfite dehydrogenase; sulfite: ferricytochrome c oxidoreductase), and aldehyde oxidase (aldehyde: oxygen oxidoreductase). Xanthine dehydrogenase catalyzes the conversion of hypoxanthine to xanthine, and xanthine to uric acid. In addition to uric acid, the end product of purine catabolism, NADH is formed from NAD+ in the reaction. Xanthine oxidase also catalyzes the reactions of purine end metabolism. However, in the case of xanthine oxidase, which is formed from xanthine dehydrogenase, NAD+ is not a participant in the reaction, and a reactive oxygen species, the superoxide anion, is a product of the reaction.

Sulfite oxidase is involved in the degradative metabolism of the sulfur amino acids methionine and cysteine. Sulfite oxidase, which is located in mitochondria, converts sulfite to sulfate. Sulfite is derived from the metabolism of cysteine. It also enters the body in the form of free sulfites which are used as food additives. Aldehyde oxidase is involved in a number of reactions, including the catabolism of pyrimidines and the biotransformation of xenobiotics.

Deficiency of the molybdenum cofactor (Moco) causes a severe disease in humans that usually results in premature death in early childhood and is inherited as an autosomal recessive trait. All of the Moco-dependent enzymes—xanthine dehydrogenase, sulfite oxidase and aldehyde oxidase—are affected. Moco deficiency is rare. Additional signs of this combined enzyme deficiency, are severe neurological abnormalities, dislocated ocular lenses, mental retardation, increased urinary excretion of sulfite, thiosulfate, S-sulfocysteine, taurine, hypoxanthine and xanthine, and reduced serum and urine levels of sulfate and urate. Isolated sulfite oxidase deficiency is also known. This is a rare autosomal-recessive disorder presenting at birth with seizures, severe neurologic disease and lens subluxation.

Lin Xian is a small region in Honan Province in north China which has had one of the highest incidences of esophageal cancer in the world. It was determined that the soil in this area was markedly low in molybdenum. In order for nitrates in the soil to be reduced to nitrogenous substances necessary for plant nutrition, a molybdenum-dependent enzyme, nitrate reductase (found in nitrogen-fixing bacteria), is required. When the molybdenum level in the soil is low, instead of being converted to amines, the nitrates get converted to nitrosamines, known carcinogenic substances. By enriching the soil with molybdenum, as ammonium molybdate, those living in this region are exposed to lower amounts of nitrosamines in their diets, and the incidence of esophageal cancer may be declining.

The possible anticarcinogenic activity in the above example is due to feeding the soil to produce lower amounts of carcinogens. When the inhabitants in the region were administered molybdenum as a supplement, this action did not appear to affect the incidence of esophageal or any other type of cancer. However, molybdenum may have anticarcinogenic activity for a few hypothetical reasons. Aldehyde oxidase may play a role in the detoxification of some carcinogenic xenobiotics. This needs to be studied. Molybdenum is involved in cofactors that are required for enzyme activity by some of the inhabitants of the microflora of the large intestine. Some of these molybdenum-dependent enzymes may also be involved in detoxifying carcinogenic xenobiotics. This, too, needs study. Finally, it has been shown that copper depletion suppresses tumor growth in an animal model. There is some evidence that copper is an important cofactor for angiogenesis, and therefore, copper deficiency may suppress angiogenesis. Tetrathiomolybdate, a molybdenum compound which antagonizes copper, is now in clinical trial to determine if copper depletion therapy via molybdenum is a viable approach for the treatment of cancer.

PHARMACOKINETICS

Molybdenum in nutritional supplements is in the form of either sodium molybdate or ammonium molybdate. Molybdenum in food is principally in the form of the organic molybdenum cofactors. The efficiency of absorption of nutritional supplement forms of molybdenum ranges from 88% to 93%, and the efficiency of absorption of molybdenum from foods ranges from about 57% to 88%. Absorption of molybdenum occurs rapidly from the stomach as well as the small intestine. The mechanism of absorption—passive, active or both—is unclear. Following absorption, molybdenum is transported via the portal circulation to the liver and via the systemic circulation to the other tissues of the body. Molybdate is carried in the blood bound to alpha-macroglobulin and by adsorption to erythrocytes. The liver and kidney retain the highest amounts of molybdenum. Within cells, molybdenum participates in the formation of the molybdenum cofactor. Molybdenum is excreted in the urine as molybdate. Some molybdenum is excreted in the bile. Excretion, rather than absorption, is the principal homeostatic mechanism for molybdenum.

INDICATIONS AND USAGE

Molybdenum is indicated in cases of molybdenum deficiency due to prolonged use of total parenteral nutrition. Despite some epidemiological evidence showing a higher incidence of esophageal carcinoma in those who live in areas where the soil is low in molybdenum, there is as yet no indication for the use of supplemental molybdenum in the prevention of cancer. Claims that molybdenum may help prevent anemia, that it protects against dental caries and helps in cases of sexual impotence have no credible support.

RESEARCH SUMMARY

Except for evidence of supplemental molybdenum's usefulness in some individuals made deficient due to prolonged total parenteral nutrition, research to date has revealed no further indications for the supplemental use of molybdenum.

An epidemiologic association has been made between the high incidence of esophageal cancer and the low intake of molybdenum in an area of China. In one study, supplementing some of those who live in this area with molybdenum for prolonged periods did not lower the incidence of cancer, although supplementation with beta carotene, vitamin E and selenium did reduce the incidence of some cancers in this study group.

Non-dietary forms of molybdenum, however, are being developed as experimental drugs for the treatment of cancer via their ability to deplete copper.

CONTRAINDICATIONS, PRECAUTIONS, ADVERSE REACTIONS

CONTRAINDICATIONS

Molybdenum is contraindicated in those who are hypersensitive to any component of a molybdenum-containing product.

PRECAUTIONS

Pregnant women and nursing mothers should avoid the use of supplemental molybdenum greater than U.S. RDA amounts (75 micrograms daily). Dietary intake of molybdenum in the United States ranges from about 120 to 240 micrograms daily, with an average intake of 180 micrograms daily. A supplementary intake of molybdenum of 75 micrograms daily brings the intake up to the upper limits of the estimated safe and adequate daily dietary intake for molybdenum.

Those with hyperuricemia and/or gout should exercise caution in the use of supplementation with doses of molybdenum greater than U.S. RDA amounts.

The use of molybdenum, specifically tetrathiomolybdate, for the treatment of cancer or Wilson disease is experimental.

ADVERSE REACTIONS

Doses of molybdenum of 10 to 15 milligrams daily have been associated with a gout-like syndrome and hyperuricemia. Supplementary doses of molybdenum of up to 500 micrograms are generally well tolerated. However, there is one report of a male who suffered acute toxicity with a molybdenum dose ranging from 300-800 micrograms daily for 18 days (see Overdosage).

INTERACTIONS

DRUGS

Acetaminophen: High doses of molybdate may inhibit the metabolism of acetaminophen.

NUTRITIONAL SUPPLEMENTS

Copper: High doses of molybdate may antagonize the absorption of copper. Likewise, high doses of copper may antagonize the absorption of molybdenum and overall decrease molybdenum status.

FOODS

High doses of molybdenum may antagonize absorption of copper from foods.

OVERDOSAGE

There is one report of acute clinical poisoning with molybdenum from a dietary molybdenum supplement. The subject, a male in his late thirties, consumed a cumulative dose of 13.5 milligrams of molybdenum over a period of 18 days, at an intake rate of 300-800 micrograms daily. This was followed by the development of acute psychosis (visual and auditory hallucinations), several petit mal seizures and one grand mal seizure. The subject was treated with chelation therapy and his symptoms and signs remitted after several hours. Neuropsychological tests and Spectral Emission Computer Tomography revealed frontal lobe damage of the brain. Major depression and learning disability persisted one year following the molybdenum incident. There are no other reports of overdosage. Further, other reports of those taking doses of molybdenum up to 500 micrograms daily or greater for extended periods of time, have not shown any adverse reactions.

DOSAGE AND ADMINISTRATION

Molybdenum supplements are usually available in the form of sodium molybdate and sometimes in the form of ammonium molybdate. Molybdenum is found in combination products, including multivitamin/multimineral formulas. A typical supplementary dose is 75 micrograms daily. The amounts of molybdenum on nutritional supplement labels are expressed as elemental molybdenum.

The Food and Nutrition Board of the U.S. National Academy of Sciences has recommended the following Dietary Reference Intakes (DRI) for molybdenum. A summary of DRIs for various age groups is as follows:

DRI values (micrograms/day)

Infants	Adequate Intake (AI)
0-6 months	2
7-12 months	3

Children	Recommended Daily Allowance (RDA)
1-3 years	17
4-8 years	22

Boys	
9-13 years	34
14-18 years	43

Girls	
9-13 years	34
14-18 years	43

Men	
19-30 years	45
31-50 years	45
51-70 years	45
Older than 70 years	45

Women	
19-30 years	45
31-50 years	45
51-70 years	45
Older than 70 years	45

Pregnancy	
14-18 years	50
19-30 years	50
31-50 years	50

Lactation	
14-18 years	50
19-30 years	50
31-50 years	50

The following summarizes the Tolerable Upper Intake Level (UL) for various age groups and conditions:

Infants	
0-6 months	ND
7-12 months	ND

Children	
1-3 years	300
4-8 years	600
9-13 years	1,100

Adolescents	
14-18 years	1,700

Adults	
19 years and older	2,000

Pregnancy	
14-18 years	1,700
19 years and older	2,000

Lactation	
14-18 years	1,700
19 years and older	2,000

ND = Not Determinable

The DV (Daily Value) for molybdenum, which is used for determining percentage of nutrient daily values on nutritional supplement and food labels, is 75 micrograms. The basis for the DV for molybdenum is the 1989 Estimated Safe and Adequate Daily Dietary Intake (ESADDI).

The richest dietary sources of molybdenum include legumes, cereal grains, leafy vegetables, milk, beans, liver and kidney.

LITERATURE

Anon. Molybdenum deficiency in TPN. *Nutr Rev.* 1987;45:337-341.

Barceloux DG. Molybdenum. *J Toxicol Clin Toxicol.* 1999;37:231-237.

Barch DH. Esophageal cancer and microelements. *J Am Coll Nutr.* 1989;8:99-107.

Beedham C. Molybdenum hydroxylases as drug-metabolizing enzymes. *Drug Metab Rev.* 1985;16:119-156.

Blot WJ, Li JY, Taylor PR, et al. Nutrition intervention trials in Linxian, China: supplementation with specific vitamin/mineral combinations, cancer incidence, and disease-specific mortality in the general population. *J Natl Cancer Inst.* 1993;85:1483-1492.

Boles JW, Klaassen CD. Effects of molybdate and pentachlorophenol on the sulfation of acetaminophen. *Toxicology.* 2000;146:23-35.

Brewer GJ, Dick RD, Grover DK, et al. Treatment of metastatic cancer with tetrathiomolybdate, an anticopper, antiangiogenic agent: Phase I study. *Clin Cancer Res.* 2000;6:1-10.

Brewer GJ, Johnson V, Dick RD, et al. Treatment of Wilson disease with ammonium tetrathiomolybdate. II. Initial therapy in 33 neurologically affected patients and follow-up with zinc therapy. *Arch Neurol.* 1996;53:1017-1025.

Edwards MC, Johnson JL, Marriage B, et al. Isolated sulfite oxidase deficiency: review of two cases in one family. *Ophthalmology.* 1999;106:1957-1961.

Hille R. Molybdenum enzymes. *Essays Biochem.* 1999;34:125-137.

Institute of Medicine, Food and Nutrition Board. Dietary Reference Intakes for vitamin A, vitamin K, arsenic, boron, chromium, copper, iodine, iron, manganese, molybdenum, nickel, silicon, vanadium, and zinc. Washington, DC: National Academy Press, 2001.

Johnson JL, Cohen HJ, Rajagopalan KV. Molecular basis of the biological function of molybdenum. *J Biol Chem.* 1974;249:5046-5055.

Johnson JL, Waud WR, Rajagopalan KV, et al. Inborn errors of molybdenum metabolism: Combined deficiencies of sulfite oxidase and xanthine dehydrogenase in a patient lacking the molybdenum cofactor. *Proc Natl Acad Sci USA.* 1980;77:3715-3719.

Luo XM, Wei HJ, Hu GG, et al. Molybdenum and esophageal cancer in China. *Federation Proceedings.* 1981;46:928 (Abstract #3962).

Mendel RR. The role of the molybdenum cofactor in humans. *Biofactors.* 2000;11:147-148.

Momcilovic B. A case of acute human molybdenum toxicity from a dietary molybdenum supplement—a new member of the "Lucor metallicum" family. *Arh Hig Rada Toksikol.* 1999;50:289-297.

Nielsen FH. Ultratrace minerals. In: Shils ME, Olson JA, Shike M, Ross AC, eds. *Modern Nutrition in Health and Disease.* 9th ed. Baltimore, MD: Williams and Wilkins;1999:283-303.

Rajagopalan KV. Molybdenum—an essential trace element. *Nutr Rev.* 1987;45:321-328.

Thompson KH, Scott KC, Turnlund JR. Molybdenum metabolism in men with increasing molybdenum intakes: changes in kinetic parameters. *J Appl Physiol.* 1996;81:1404-1409.

Turnland JR, Keyes WR, Peiffer GL. Molybdenum absorption, excretion, and retention studied with stable isotopes in young men at five intakes of dietary molybdenum. *Am J Clin Nutr.* 1995;62:790-796.

Vyskocil A, Viau C. Assessment of molybdenum toxicity in humans. *J Appl Toxicol.* 1999;19:185-192.

Wuebbens MW, Liu MTW, Rajagopalan KV, et al. Insights into molybdenum cofactor deficiency provided by the crystal structure of the molybdenum cofactor biosynthesis protein MoaC. *Structure.* 2000;8:709-718.

Myco-Polysaccharides

DESCRIPTION

Some mushrooms and other fungal entities have possible immunomodulatory activities and possible other health benefits. It is thought these health benefits are mainly due to polysaccharides and polysaccharide-protein complexes, which comprise the cell walls of these organisms. The principal bioactive substances are believed to be the beta-D-glucans. Beta-D-glucans, usually called beta-glucans, are nondigestible polysaccharides found in nature in such sources as cereal grains, including oats and barley, as well as in yeast, bacteria, algae and mushrooms.

It is likely that the activities of the various myco-beta-D-glucans depend on such chemical characteristics as their molecular weight, their branching patterns, their solubility in water and their tertiary structure. The most studied mushroom beta-glucans, all of which are available in Japan for use as biological response modifiers, are lentinan from *Lentinus edodes*; grifolan (also called GRN and grifolan LE) from *Grifola frondosa*; schizophyllan (also called SPG, sonifilan, sizofiran and sizofilan) from *Schizophyllum commune*; SSG from *Sclerotinia sclerotiorum*; PSK (also called krestin) from *Coriolus versicolor*; and PSP (polysaccharide peptide), also from *Coriolus versicolor*.

The beta-glucan lentinan is comprised of a beta-$(1{\rightarrow}3)$-D-glucan backbone with beta-$(1{\rightarrow}6)$-glucan side chains. The molecular weight of lentinan is approximately 5×10^5 daltons, the degree of branching is 2/5, and the tertiary structure of lentinan is a triple helix. Grifolan is also comprised of a beta-$(1{\rightarrow}3)$-D-glucan backbone with beta-$(1{\rightarrow}6)$-glucan side chains. The molecular weight of grifolan is approximately 5×10^5 daltons, the degree of branching is 1/3, and its tertiary structure is a triple helix. Both schizophyllan and SSG also contain beta-$(1{\rightarrow}3)$-D-glucan backbones and beta-$(1{\rightarrow}6)$-glucan side chains; they have triple helix tertiary structures. The degree of branching in schizophyllan is 1/3; in SSG, it is 1/3. PSK and PSP are glycoproteins containing beta-glucans.

ACTIONS AND PHARMACOLOGY

ACTIONS

Myco-polysaccharides may have immunomodulatory, antitumor, antimicrobial, lipid-lowering and glucose-regulating activities.

MECHANISM OF ACTION

The best studied of the mushroom beta-glucans is lentinan. Lentinan is typically used parenterally and appears to have little antitumor activity when administered orally. Parenterally administered lentinan has been demonstrated to have immunomodulatory activity. Lentinan appears to stimulate such cells as macrophages, monocytes, neutrophils, NK (natural killer) cells and LAK (lymphokine-activated killer) cells. Stimulation of these cells by lentinan may release a number of different cytokines, including TNF (tumor necrosis factor)-alpha, IL (interleukin)-1, IL-2 and IL-6; lentinan may also stimulate the production of nitric oxide (NO) in macrophages. These effects may result in antimicrobial and tumoricidal activities. Grifolan, schizophyllan and SSG have been shown to have similar effects when used parenterally.

The possible immunomodulatory effects of oral mushroom beta-glucans remain unclear. They may have immunological activity by virtue of their interaction with gut-associated lymphoid tissue (GALT). Immune cells associated with GALT, activated by contact with mushroom or other myco-beta-glucans in the gut, may migrate to other tissues where they might exert immunomodulatory effects. Further, there may be some digestion of myco-beta-glucans in the large intestine, via bacterial beta-glucosidases, to produce some oligosaccharides, which may be absorbed and may have immunomodulatory activity. However, this is unclear. There also may be substances in mushrooms other than beta-glucans that have immunomodulatory activity.

The possible antitumor and antimicrobial activities of the myco-beta-glucans are thought to be accounted for, in large part, by their possible immunomodulatory activities.

The mechanism of the possible cholesterol-lowering activity of the myco-beta-glucans is unclear. The myco-beta-glucans are somewhat similar in structure to oat beta-glucan. It is thought that the cholesterol-lowering effect of oat beta-glucan may be accounted for, in large part, by promoting the excretion of bile acids. Myco-beta-glucans may also promote the excretion of bile acids.

The mechanism of the possible glucose-regulatory activity of myco-beta-glucans is poorly understood.

PHARMACOKINETICS

Following ingestion, there is virtually no digestion of myco-beta-glucans in the small intestine. There are no beta-glucosidases among the digestive enzymes. Some digestion of myco-beta-glucans does take place in the large intestine via the action of bacterial beta-glucosidases. Some oligosaccharides (up to molecular weights of 20,000 daltons) that are produced via the bacterial beta-glucosidases may get absorbed. A large percentage of the ingested myco-beta-glucans is excreted in the feces.

INDICATIONS AND USAGE

The myco-polysaccharides may have anticarcinogenic, immune-modulating, antimicrobial, anti-inflammatory, cardioprotective, hepatoprotective, nephroprotective, hypoglycemic and anticaries effects.

RESEARCH SUMMARY

Many myco-polysaccharides, particularly those derived from *Lentinus edodes* (the shiitake mushroom), *Grifold frondosa* (the maitake mushroom), *Sclerotinia sclerotiorum* and *Schizophyllum commune*, have demonstrated anticarcinogenic effects in both animals and humans. The beta-glucan constituents of these polysaccharides are believed to be their most active anticancer components. These beta-glucans are lentinan from *Lentinus edodes*, GRN from *Grifola frondosa*, SPG from *Schizophyllum commune* and SSG from *Sclerotinia sclerotiorum*.

In *in vitro* studies, lentinan demonstrated anticancer effects by significantly boosting the cytotoxic capabilities of macrophages, enhancing production of macrophage tumor necrosis factor-alpha. It also increased production of interleukin (IL)-1. GRN also produced macrophage-stimulating activity in mouse macrophages, as did (though to lesser extents) SPG and SSG.

In animal experiments, these beta-glucans have shown varying activity against sarcomas, mammary cancer, some chemically induced cancers, adenocarcinoma, colon cancer and some leukemias, among others.

In humans, lentinan and SPG are approved for clinical use in Japan. Injected lentinan has reportedly increased survival time in patients with gastric and colorectal cancers, while SPG has shown clinical activity against cervical cancer, prolonging survival time and time to recurrence in stage II, but not stage III, cervical cancer patients. Its efficacy against gastric cancer is low.

Lentinan, combined with some other anticancer agents, prolonged survival times in some patients with advanced cancers of different types, including gastric cancer. SPG similarly enhanced the efficacy of several cancer treatments, including surgery and radiotherapy. Combining these treatments with SPG resulted in significantly longer survival times. In one recently concluded multi-center prospective study of lentinan's use in advanced gastric cancer patients, the combination of lentinan, tegafur and cisplatin resulted in median survival of 297 days versus 199 days for those controls receiving the two cancer drugs without lentinan.

Some substances, other than the beta-glucans identified above, have been isolated from these mushrooms, which also show anticancer activity in *in vitro* and animal experiments. Research continues.

The non-specific (macrophage-activating) immune-enhancing effects of the myco-polysaccharides most likely account for much of their reported anti-inflammatory and antimicrobial activities. Preliminary trials of intravenous lentinan have not produced significant results in HIV-positive subjects. One recent study found that lentinan significantly stimulated expression of IL-2 receptors on peripheral blood mononuclear cells in patients with chronic hepatitis B.

Another recent study identified three antibacterial substances in shiitake mushrooms. They showed efficient activity against *Streptococcus spp.* and *Actinomyces spp.*, among others. They were far less effective against *Enterococcus spp.*, *Staphylococcus spp.* and some others.

Cordyceps sinensis has enhanced cellular immune function in subjects with chronic renal failure and has boosted natural killer activity in cells from both healthy individuals and some with leukemia. NK activities were also boosted by an extract of *Cordyceps sinensis* in mice with lung melanoma.

Ganoderma lucidum has immunologically active polysaccharides. Some of these have shown some activity against HIV-1 *in vitro* but not *in vivo*. Various extracts of the mushroom have exhibited some antibacterial activity *in vitro*, especially against *Micrococcus luteus*, and have been shown to have microbial additive effects with some antibiotics and antagonistic effects with others. Clearly, more research is needed before ganoderma preparations can be recommended for use with antibiotic drugs.

Recently, two patients with postherpetic neuralgia that had not yielded to other therapies and two patients with severe pain due to herpes zoster infection were said to receive dramatic pain relief upon administration of hot water soluble extracts of *Ganoderma lucidum* (36 to 72 grams dry weight per day). More recently still, various ganoderma polysaccharides have been isolated that show significant antiherpetic activity *in vitro* against both HSV-1 and HSV-2. Research is ongoing.

Various constituents of shiitake have shown effects that could be cardioprotective. Inhibition of platelet aggregation and some hypocholesterolemic effects have been noted *in vitro*. Dietary shiitake significantly lowered plasma-free cholesterol, triglycerides and phospholipids in spontaneously hypertensive rats, compared with controls. Shiitake, however, did not reduce blood pressure in these animals.

Maitake, on the other hand, significantly lowered blood pressure but had no significant effect on lipids in this study. In some other animal studies, however, maitake did have favorable lipid effects.

A constituent of *Cordyceps sinensis* has been shown to have hypotensive and vasorelaxant effects in animal studies. Another extract has reportedly counteracted chemically induced arrhythmias in rats.

Ganoderma lucidum was said to significantly inhibit platelet aggregation in 15 healthy volunteers and 33 subjects with atherosclerotic disease.

Cordyceps sinensis protected animals from the nephrotoxic effects of cyclosporin A in one experiment. *Ganoderma lucidum* was hepatoprotective in another animal model.

Maitake and some of its constituents have shown some anti-diabetic activity in animals. Blood glucose reductions were observed in genetically diabetic mice given these substances, compared with controls in which blood glucose levels rose with age. In an animal model of NIDDM, maitake again produced significant reductions in blood glucose levels, compared with controls. Researchers in this study concluded that maitake does not inhibit glucose absorption at the enteron but, rather, inhibits the metabolism of absorbed glucose.

Cordyceps sinensis extracts have also shown some ability to lower plasma glucose levels in animal models of diabetes. A *cordyceps sinensis* polysaccharide was said to have potent hypoglycemic effects, via intraperitoneal administration, in genetic diabetic mice.

Finally, a polysaccharide constituent of shiitake has been reported to have an anticaries effect. A significantly lower caries score was seen in shiitake-supplemented rats fed a cariogenic diet, compared with controls on the same diet but without shiitake extract.

CONTRAINDICATIONS, PRECAUTIONS, ADVERSE REACTIONS

CONTRAINDICATIONS

Myco-beta-glucans and myco-polysaccharides are contraindicated in those who are hypersensitive to mushrooms, to mushroom extracts and to any component in a mushroom-containing supplement, a mushroom extract-containing supplement, a mushroom polysaccharide-containing supplement or a mushroom beta-glucan-containing supplements.

PRECAUTIONS

Pregnant women and nursing mothers should avoid supplementation with mushroom extracts and should avoid mushroom polysaccharide-containing supplements and mushroom beta-glucan-containing supplements.

Those with cancer, immune deficiencies and other medical problems should only use mushroom supplementation, mushroom polysaccharide or mushroom beta-glucan supplements under medical supervision.

ADVERSE REACTIONS

The most commonly reported adverse reactions from the use of the various beta-glucan-containing fungal products are gastrointestinal, including nausea and epigastric distress. Eosinophilia has been reported in subjects taking 4 grams daily of shiitake mushroom powder. Contact dermatitis has also been reported in some cases, from the handling of shiitake mushrooms.

INTERACTIONS

DRUGS

Antibiotics and chemotherapeutic agents: In vitro studies, animal studies and parenteral use of the mushroom beta-glucans suggest that they may enhance the efficacy of various chemotherapeutic agents, as well as antibiotics. However, it is unclear if oral use of these substances, either in concentrated forms or in the form of mushrooms, would produce similar interactions.

Antiplatelet drugs: Ganoderma may enhance the effect of antiplatelet drugs.

OVERDOSAGE

There are no reports of overdosage of any of the products mentioned in this monograph.

DOSAGE AND ADMINISTRATION

The beta-glucans lentinan, grifolan, schizophyllan and SSG are available in Japan. Lentinan and schizophyllan are approved in Japan as drugs for the treatment of cancer. Edible mushrooms rich in beta-glucans include the shiitake mushroom (*Lentinus edodes*), the maitake mushroom (*Grifola frondosa*), the himematsutake mushroom (*Agaricus blazei*), the button mushrooms (*Schizophyllum commune* and *Sclerotina sclerotiorium*), the wood ear mushroom (*Auricularia auricula*), the tremella mushroom (*Tremella fuciformis*), the poria mushroom (*Wolfporia cocos*) and the enoki mushroom (*Flammulina velutipes*). Huitlacoche (*Ustilago maydis*) is not a true mushroom, but it is an edible fungus and also rich in beta-glucans. Non-edible mushrooms that are rich in beta-glucans include the reishi mushroom (*Ganoderma lucidum*) and the coriolus mushroom (*Coriolus versicolor*). *Cordyceps sinensis* is a fungus, not a mushroom.

Nutritional supplements containing extracts of the above edible and non-edible mushrooms are available and are typically marketed with emphasis on their beta-glucan content.

One supplement contains a mixture of reishi, maitake, shiitake, hericium, cordyceps, coriolus, wood ear, tremella, poria and umbellatus/polyporus (*Grifola umbellatus*). There is no typical dose of this supplement.

A beta-glucan-enriched maitake supplement, called the maitake D fraction, is available. The maitake D fraction comprises a mixed beta-D-glucan fraction prepared from the maitake mushroom. The supplement is available in solid and liquid form. Maitake in the form of a crude dried mushroom is also available. Crude dried reishi mushrooms, reishi powders and reishi tinctures are available, as are crude dried shiitake mushrooms and shiitake powders. *Cordyceps sinensis* is available in powdered form. No specific doses of these products can be recommended at this time.

LITERATURE

Borchers AT, Stern JS, Hackman RM, Keen CL, Gershwin ME. Mushrooms, tumors, and immunity. *Proc Soc Exp Biol Med.* 1999; 221:281-293.

Chang R. Functional properties of edible mushrooms. *Nutr Rev.* 1996; 54:S91-S93.

Chang RY. Potential application of *Ganoderma* polysaccharides in the immune surveillance and chemoprevention of cancer. In: Royse DJ, ed. *Mushroom Biology and Mushroom Products.* 1996; Penn State Univ:153-159.

Chen AW, Miles PG. Biomedical research and the application of mushroom nutriceuticals from *Ganoderma lucidum.* In: Royse DJ, ed. *Mushroom Biology and Mushroom Products.* 1996; Penn State Univ:161-175.

Eo SK, Kim YS, Lee CK, Han SS. Antiherpetic activities of various protein bound polysaccharides isolated from Ganoderma lucidum. *J Ethnopharmacol.* 1999; 68:175-181.

Fujimiya Y, Suzuki Y, Oshiman K, et al. Selective tumoricidal effect of soluble proteoglucan extracted from the basidiomycete, *Agaricus blazei* Murill, mediated via natural killer cell activation and apoptosis. *Canc Immunol Immunotherapy.* 1998; 46:147-159.

Gordon M, Bihari B, Goosby E, et al. A placebo-controlled trial of the immune modulator, lentinan in HIV-positive patients: a phase I/II trial. *J Med.* 1998; 29:305-330.

He Y, Li R, Chen Q, et al. [Chemical studies on immunologically active polysaccharides of Ganoderma lucidum (Leyss ex Fr.) Karst.] [Article in Chinese.] *Chung Kuo Chung Yao Tsa Chih.* 1992; 17:226-228,256.

Kidd P. The use of mushroom glucans and proteoglycans in cancer treatment. *Altern Med Rev.* 2000; 5:4-27.

Kiho T, Yamane A, Hui J, et al. Polysaccharides in fungi. XXXVI. Hypoglycemic activity of a polysaccharide (CS-F30) from the cultural mycelium of Cordyceps sinensis and its effect on glucose metabolism in mouse liver. *Biol Pharm Bull.* 1996; 19:294-296.

Kubo K, Nanba H. Anti-diabetic mechanism of maitake (*Grifola frondosa*). In: Royse DJ, ed. *Mushroom Biology and Mushroom Products.* 1996; Penn State Univ:215-222.

Kuo YC, Tsai WJ, Shiao MS, et al. Cordyceps sinensis as an immunomodulatory agent. *Am J Chin Med*. 1996; 24:111-125.

Ladanyi A, Timar J, Lapis K. Effect of lentinan on macrophage cytotoxicity against metastatic tumor cells. *Cancer Immunol Immunother*. 1993; 36:123-126.

Levy AM, Kita H, Phillips SF, et al. Eosinophilia and gastrointestinal symptoms after ingestion of shiitake mushrooms. *J Allergy Clin Immunol*. 1998; 101:613-620.

Manzi P, Pizzoferrato L. Beta-glucans in edible mushrooms. *Food Chemistry*. 2000; 68:315-318.

Matsuoka H, Seo Y, Wakasugi H, et al. Lentinan potentiates immunity and prolongs the survival time of some patients. *Anticancer Res*. 1997; 17:2751-2755.

Mitamura T, Sakamoto S, Suzuki S, et al. Effects of lentinan on colorectal carcinogenesis in mice with ulceractive colitis. *Oncol Rep*. 2000; 7:559-601.

Mizuno M, Minato K, Ito H, et al. Anti-tumor polysaccharide from the mycelium of liquid-cultured Agaricus blazei mill. *Biochem Mol Biol Int*. 1999; 47:707-714.

Murata T, Hatayama I, Kakizaki I, et al. Lentinan enhances sensitivity of mouse colon 26 tumor to cis-diamminedichloroplatinum (II) and decreases glutathionine transferase expression. *Jpn J Cancer Res*. 1996; 87:1171-1178.

Nakano H, Namatame K, Nemoto H, et al. A multi-institutional prospective study of lentinan in advanced gastric cancer patients with unresectable and recurrent diseases: effect on prolongation of survival and improvement of quality of life. Kanagawa Lentinin Research Group. *Hepatogastroenterology*. 1999; 46:2662-2668.

Nakumara T. Shiitake (Lentinus edodes) dermatitis. *Contact Dermatitis*. 1992; 27:65-70.

Shouji N, Takada K, Fukushima K, Hirasawa M. Anticaries effect of a component from shiitake (an edible mushroom). *Caries Res*. 2000; 34:94-98.

Tari K, Satake I, Nakagomi K, et al. [Effect of lentinan for advanced prostate carcinoma.] [Article in Japanese.] *Hinyokika Kiyo*. 1994; 40:119-123.

Wan K. [Effects of lentinan of peripheral blood mononuclear cell expression of interleukin-2 receptor in patients with chronic hepatitis B *in vivo* and *in vitro*.] [Article in Chinese.] *Hunan I Ko Ta Hsueh Hsueh*. 1998; 23:90-92.

Wasser SP, Weis AL. Therapeutic effects of substances occurring in higher Basidiomycetes mushrooms: a modern prospective. *Crit Rev Immunol*. 1999; 19:65-96.

Yoon SY, Eo SK, Kim YS, et al. Antimicrobial activity of Ganoderma lucidum extract alone and in combination with some antibiotics. *Arch Pharm Res*. 1994; 17:438-442.

Myo-Inositol

DESCRIPTION

Myo-inositol, the major nutritionally active form of inositol, is vital to many biological processes of the body, participating in a diverse range of activities. *Myo*-inositol is one of nine distinct isomers of inositol. It is essential for the growth of rodents, but not for most animals, including humans. Humans can make *myo*-inositol endogenously, which they do from glucose, and, even though *myo*-inositol is sometimes referred to as a vitamin, it is not a vitamin for humans or most animals. However, the dietary intake of *myo*-inositol can influence the levels of circulating and bound *myo*-inositol in the body and may influence certain biological activities. Nutritional supplementation of this cyclitol may affect behavior and may have anti-depressant and anti-anxiety activities. For more information on Inositol supplementation, see Inositol Hexanicotinate.

Myo-inositol intake from the average diet is approximately one gram daily. The major dietary forms of *myo*-inositol are inositol hexaphosphate or phytic acid, which is widely found in cereals and legumes and associated with dietary fiber, and *myo*-inositol-containing phospholipids from animal and plant sources.

Myo-inositol is also known as inositol, hexahydroxycyclohexane, cyclohexanehexol, mouse antialopecia factor and, chemically, as cis-1,2,3,5-trans-4,6-cyclohexanehexol. *Myo*-inositol is abbreviated as Ins and sometimes as just I. It is represented by the following chemical structure:

myo-Inositol

Another naturally occurring isomer of inositol, D-*chiro*-inositol, has been found to have activity against insulin resistance. However, at present, D-*chiro*-inositol is neither available as a nutritional supplement nor as a drug. A hexanicotinate conjugate of *myo*-inositol, inositol niacinate or inositol nicotinate, is available in Europe as a drug for the treatment of circulatory problems.

ACTIONS AND PHARMACOLOGY

ACTIONS

Myo-inositol may have antidepressant and antianxiety activity.

MECHANISM OF ACTION

The mechanism of action of *myo*-inositol has yet to be fully elucidated. However, much is known about the biological roles of *myo*-inositol and some speculation can be made. *Myo*-inositol is metabolized to phosphatidylinositol, which makes up a small, but very significant, component of cell membranes. Phosphatidylinositol can be converted to phosphatidylinositol-4,5-bisphosphate, a key intermediate in biological signaling. Phosphatidylinositol-4,5-bisphosphate is the precursor of at least three second-messenger molecules. These are inositol-1,4,5-triphosphate, which modifies intracellular calcium levels, diacylglycerol, which regulates some members of the protein kinase C family, and phosphatidylinositol-3,4,5-triphosphate, which is involved in signal transduction.

Some of the second-messenger activity is related to activation of serotonin receptors. It is hypothesized that the mechanism of action of *myo*-inositol's possible benefit in the management of depression, panic attacks and obsessive-compulsive behavior may be explained by *myo*-inositol's role as a second-messenger precursor.

PHARMACOKINETICS

Myo-inositol is absorbed from the small intestine following ingestion and is transported by the portal circulation to the liver and then by the systemic circulation to various tissues in the body, including the brain. *Myo*-inositol crosses the blood-brain barrier.

Within the liver and the various tissues of the body, *myo*-inositol enters into a wide range of diverse biochemical pathways. *Myo*-inositol reacts with CDP-diacylglycerol to form the phospholipid phosphatidylinositol, which can be incorporated into membrane structure. Phosphatidylinositol, via kinase reactions, forms phosphatidyl-4,5-bisphosphate, which is the precursor to inositol-1,4,5-triphosphate, diacylglycerol, phosphatidylinositol-3,4,5-triphosphate, *myo*-inositol 1,3,4-triphosphate and *myo*-inositol 1,3,4,5-tetrakisphosphate, among others. The *myo*-inositol phosphates can be dephosphorylated via phosphatases.

It is believed that the mechanism of action of lithium is due, in part, to its inhibition of the phosphatase that converts *myo*-inositol-monophosphate back to *myo*-inositol.

INDICATIONS AND USAGE

Myo-inositol has exhibited positive effects in a number of studies related to depression, panic attacks and obsessive-compulsive disorder. On the other hand, it generally has not been effective in treating Alzheimer's disease, autism, schizophrenia and electroconvulsive therapy-induced memory impairment. The suggestion, from animal studies, that *myo*-inositol might be helpful in preventing neural tube defects has not been tested in humans.

RESEARCH SUMMARY

Inositol levels in cerebrospinal fluid are decreased, compared with general populations, in many suffering from depression. In one double-blind study, 28 depressed patients received placebo or high-dose (12 grams daily) *myo*-inositol for four weeks. Overall, significant improvement was achieved in the treatment group but not in the placebo group. There was improvement in both monopolar and bipolar depression in this pilot study. *Myo*-inositol, however, was not shown, in another study, to enhance or speed the response of depressed subjects to SSRIs (selective serotonin reuptake inhibitors). More research is needed in this area.

In another double-blind study, 21 patients with panic disorder, with or without agoraphobia, received 12 grams daily of *myo*-inositol or placebo for four weeks. Again, the treated group, overall, achieved improvement (frequency and severity of both panic attacks and agoraphobia declined significantly), compared with no significant improvement in the placebo group.

And in a third double-blind study, this one with a crossover component, 13 patients with obsessive-compulsive disorder (OCD) received 18 grams of inositol or placebo for six weeks each. Subjects improved significantly more, as reflected by significantly lower scores on the Yale-Brown Obsessive Compulsive Scale, when taking *myo*-inositol than when taking placebo. *Myo*-inositol, in a subsequent study, did not enhance the effects of SSRIs in subjects with treatment-refractory OCD. Again, more research is needed to confirm and further elucidate *myo*-inositol's role in treating OCD. Its effectiveness, to the extent demonstrated to date, combined with its general lack of serious side effects, make it an attractive potential therapy in these psychiatric disorders.

Myo-inositol has not demonstrated the same promise in Alzheimer's disease, autism, schizophrenia and electroconvulsive therapy-induced memory impairment. Studies related to these conditions have produced negative results. And in children with attention deficit disorder, *myo*-inositol aggravated rather than ameliorated symptoms in one small study.

In general, it appears that *myo*-inositol may be effective in many of the same disorders in which the SSRIs have shown some usefulness. This may not be surprising since *myo*-inositol has been shown to help reverse desensitization of serotonin receptors.

Myo-inositol is also being investigated for possible use in pediatric respiratory depression syndrome and for prevention of neural tube defects. Its usefulness with respect to the latter has been demonstrated in embryonic mice, but its use in humans may be curtailed or limited due to the fact that it has also been shown to induce uterine contractions.

CONTRAINDICATIONS, PRECAUTIONS, ADVERSE REACTIONS

CONTRAINDICATIONS

Known hypersensitivity to a *myo*-inositol-containing product.

PRECAUTIONS

Because of lack of long-term safety data, *myo*-inositol should be avoided by pregnant women and nursing mothers. Also, high-dose *myo*-inositol may induce uterine contractions.

Because of the hypothetical possibility that *myo*-inositol may exacerbate hypomanic or manic symptoms in those with bipolar disorder, those with this condition should use supplemental *myo*-inositol with caution and under medical supervision.

ADVERSE REACTIONS

Myo-inositol supplementation is generally well tolerated. Gastrointestinal effects such as nausea and diarrhea are occasionally reported.

INTERACTIONS

DRUGS

Theoretically, high-dose *myo*-inositol may have additive effects with selective serotonin reuptake inhibitors (SSRIs) such as fluoxetine, sertraline, paroxetine, fluvoxamine and citalopram, and with 5-hydroxytrytamine receptor agonists, such as sumatriptan.

NUTRITIONAL SUPPLEMENTS

No interactions known.

FOODS

Very small amounts of the inositol isomer, *scyllo*-inositol, are present in some foods. *Scyllo*-inositol has been reported to inhibit uptake of *myo*-inositol into the brain. Since the amount of *scyllo*-inositol intake is likely to be very little, this potential interaction is insignificant.

HERBS

Theoretically, high-dose *myo*-inositol may have additive effects with St. John's Wort.

OVERDOSAGE

Not reported.

DOSAGE AND ADMINISTRATION

For the management of depression and panic attacks, 12 grams of *myo*-inositol daily, in divided doses, were used in clinical studies. In the clinical studies performed with *myo*-inositol, effects, if any, were seen in about one month. Compliance with such doses may be a problem.

LITERATURE

Barak Y, Levine J, Glassman A, et al. Inositol treatment of Alzheimer's disease: a double blind, cross-over placebo controlled trial. *Prog Neuropsychopharmacol Biol Psychiatry*. 1996; 20:729-735.

Benjamin J, Levine J, Fox M, et al. Double-blind, placebo-controlled, crossover trial of inositol treatment for panic disorder. *Am J Psyvhiatry*. 1995; 152:1084-1086.

Cohen RA, MacGregory LC, Spokes KC, et al. Effect of *myo*-inositol on renal Na-K-ATPase in experimental diabetes. *Metabol*. 1990; 39:1026-1032.

Colodny L, Hoffman RL. Inositol-clinical applications for exogenous use. *Altern Med Rev*. 1998; 3:432-447.

Downes CP. The cellular functions of *myo*-inositol. *Biochem Soc Trans*. 1989; 17:259-268.

Einat H, Belmaker RH, Kopilov M, et al. Rat brain monomines after acute and chronic *myo*-inositol treatment. *Eur Neuropsychopharmacol*. 1999; 10:27-30.

Einat H, Karbovski H, Korik J, et al. Inositol reduces depressive-like behaviors in two different models of depression. *Psychopharmacology*. 1999; 144:158-162.

Fox M, Levine J, Aviv A, Belmaker RH. Inositol treatment of obsessive-compulsive disorder. *Am J Psychiat*. 1996; 153:1219-1221.

Holub BJ. Metabolism and function of *myo*-inositol and inositol phospholipids. *Annu Rev Nutr*. 1986; 6:563-597.

Holub BJ. The cellular forms and functions of the inositol phospholipids and their metabolic derivates. *Nutr Rev*. 1987; 45:65-71.

Khandelwal M, Reece EA, Wu YK, Borenstein M. Dietary *myo*-inositol therapy in hyperglycemic-induced embryopathy. *Teratology*. 1998; 57:79-84.

Larner J, Allan G, Kessler C, et al. Phosphoinositol glycan derived mediators and insulin resistance. Prospects for diagnosis and therapy. *J Basic Clin Physiol Pharmacol*. 1998; 9:127-137.

Levine J. Controlled trials of inositol in psychiatry. *Eur Neuropsychopharmacol*. 1997; 7:147-155.

Levine J, Aviram A, Holan A, et al. Inositol treatment of action, *J Neural Transm*. 1997; 104:307-310.

Levine J, Barak Y, Gonzalues M, et al. Double-blind, controlled-trial of inositol treatment of depression. *Am J Psychiatry*. 1995; 152:792-794.

Levine J, Goldberger I, Rapaport A, et al. CSF inositol in schizophrenia and high-dose inositol treatment of schizophrenic. *Eur Neuropsychopharmacol*. 1994; 4:487-490.

Levine J, Kurtzman L, Rapoport A, et al. CSF inositol does not predict antidepressant response to inositol. *J Neural Transm*. 1996; 103:1457-1462.

Nestler JE, Jakabowicz DJ, Reamer P, et al. Ovulatory and metabolic effects of D-*chiro*-inositol in the polycystic ovary syndrome. *N Engl J Med*. 1999; 340:1314-1320.

Seedat S, Stein DJ. Inositol augmentation of serotonin reuptake inhibitors in treatment-refractory obsessive-compulsive disorder: an open trial. *Int Clin Psychopharmacol*. 1999; 14:353-356.

NADH

DESCRIPTION

NADH is a natural substance found in most life forms and is necessary for energy production. NADH is located both in the mitochondria and cytosol of cells. It is a dinucleotide comprised of the nucleotide adenylic acid and a second nucleotide in which nicotinamide, a B vitamin, is the nitrogenous base. NADH is a key member of the electron transfer chain in mitochondria. The nicotinamide moiety is the portion of the dinucleotide that undergoes reversible reduction. NADH is the reduced form of the dinucleotide. The passage of electrons along the electron transport chain is coupled to the formation of ATP by the process known as oxidative phosphorylation.

NADH is synthesized by the body and thus is not an essential nutrient. It does require the essential nutrient nicotinamide for its synthesis, and its role in energy production is certainly an essential one. In addition to its role in the mitochondrial electron transport chain, NADH is produced in the cytosol. The mitochondrial membrane is impermeable to NADH, and this permeability barrier effectively separates the cytoplasmic from the mitochondrial NADH pools. However, cytoplasmic NADH can be used for biologic energy production. This occurs when the malate-aspartate shuttle introduces reducing equivalents from NADH in the cytosol to the electron transport chain of the mitochondria. This shuttle mainly occurs in the liver and heart.

NADH is the abbreviation for the reduced form of nicotinamide adenine dinucleotide. It is also known as coenzyme I. An older name was diphosphopyridine nucleotide reduced or DPNH. NADH has the following chemical structure:

NADH

ACTIONS AND PHARMACOLOGY

ACTIONS

The action of supplemental NADH is unclear.

MECHANISM OF ACTION

Any comments on the mechanism of action are speculative. NADH is a redox active substance and participates in biologic energy production. However, how the known roles of endogenous NADH relate to any possible action of supplemental NADH is not known. There is some evidence that a mitochondrial DNA mutation appears to cause a defective complex I in the mitochondria of Parkinson's disease patients. Complex I is comprised of NADH: ubiquinone oxidoreductase. Exogenous NADH may improve symptoms in some with ideopathic Parkinson's disease, and it is speculated that this is due to stimulation of levodopa biosynthesis.

PHARMACOKINETICS

There is scant pharmacokinetic data on supplemental NADH. It is unclear how much of an administered dose is absorbed and what the metabolic course is of any absorbed NADH. If NADH were to be transported into cells, it is highly unlikely that any would enter mitochondria.

INDICATIONS AND USAGE

There is very preliminary evidence suggesting that NADH might be useful in Parkinson's disease, chronic fatigue syndrome, Alzheimer's disease and cardiovascular disease.

RESEARCH SUMMARY

Reports that NADH may stimulate endogenous dopamine biosynthesis have led to its experimental use in Parkinson's disease. Some favorable results have been reported in case studies and open-label trials using both intravenous and oral NADH. In one open-label study of 885 subjects with Parkinson's disease, half received oral NADH and half received parenteral NADH with similar results. Some 80% of patients were said to have benefited clinically, with 19.3% showing good improvement, 58.8% moderate improvement and 21.8% non-responding. Younger patients and those with the shortest duration of disease showed the most improvement.

Only one very small double-blind study (with five Parkinson's patients) has been conducted to date. This was a short-term study. It found no benefit from NADH. More research is needed to determine the therapeutic role, if any, of NADH in Parkinson's disease.

Hope that NADH might be helpful in treating chronic fatigue syndrome was raised recently by a double-blind, placebo-controlled cross-over study of 26 patients. In the first phase of the study, subjects were randomly assigned to receive either 10 milligrams of NADH or a placebo for four weeks.

After a four-week washout period, subjects were assigned to the alternate regimen for the final four-week trial period. Among the NADH-treated patients, 31% were judged to have notable improvement, while 8% of controls were similarly improved. Larger trials are indicated.

In another pilot study, 17 patients with dementia associated with Alzheimer's disease were treated with NADH for eight to 12 weeks. Researchers reported improvement in cognitive function in all 17 patients in this open-label trial, but they cautioned that "a double-blind, placebo-controlled study is necessary to demonstrate the clinical efficacy of NADH."

Yet another recent study sought to see whether oral NADH might lower blood pressure and affect lipids in a hypertensive animal model. This was a blinded, placebo-controlled, 10-week study. Systolic blood pressure was the same in the treated and placebo groups over the first month but thereafter was significantly reduced in the NADH group. Total cholesterol and LDL cholesterol were significantly reduced in the NADH group. No significant differences were noted in blood levels of glucose, insulin, triglyceride or HDL cholesterol. More research is warranted to see whether NADH might be useful in cardiovascular disease.

CONTRAINDICATIONS, PRECAUTIONS, ADVERSE REACTIONS

CONTRAINDICATIONS
Known hypersensitivity to an-NADH-containing product.

PRECAUTIONS
Because of lack of long-term safety studies, NADH should be avoided by children, pregnant women and nursing mothers.

ADVERSE REACTIONS
There are a few reports of gastrointestinal side effects, including nausea and loss of appetite.

INTERACTIONS
There are no reported drug, nutritional supplement, food or herb interactions.

OVERDOSAGE
None reported.

DOSAGE AND ADMINISTRATION
Those who use NADH typically take either 5 milligrams once daily or 5 milligrams twice a day. Enteric-coated preparations are claimed to have better stability.

LITERATURE
Birkmayer JG. Coenzyme nicotinamide adenine dinucleotide: new therapeutic approach for improving dementia of the Alzheimer type. *Ann Clin Lab Sci.* 1996; 26:1-9.

Birkmayer JG, Vrecko C, Volc D, Birkmayer W. Nicotinamide adenine dinucleotide (NADH)—a new therapeutic approach to Parkinson's disease. Comparison of oral and parenteral application. *Acta Neurol Scand Suppl.* 1993; 146:32-35.

Bushehri N, Jarrell ST, Lieberman S, et al. Oral reduced B-nicotinamide adenine dinucleotide (NADH) affects blood pressure, lipid peroxidation, and lipid profile in hypertensive rats (SHR). *Geriatr Nephrol Urol.* 1998; 8:95-100.

Dizdar N, Kagedal B, Lindvall B. Treatment of Parkinson's disease with NADH. *Acta Neurol Scand.* 1994; 90:345-347.

Forsyth LM, Preuss HG, MacDowell AL, et al. Therapeutic effects of oral NADH on the symptoms of patients with chronic fatigue syndrome. *Ann Allergy Asthma Immunol.* 1999; 82:185-191.

Kuhn W, Muller T, Winkel R, et al. Parenteral application of NADH in Parkinson's disease: clinical improvement partially due to stimulation of endogenous levodopa biosynthesis. *J Neural Transm.* 1996; 103:1187-1193.

Swerdlow RH. Is NADH effective in the treatment of Parkinson's disease? *Drugs Aging.* 1998; 13:263-268.

Swerdlow RH, Parks JK, Miller SW, et al. Origin and functional consequences of the complex I defect in Parkinson's disease. *Ann Neurol.* 1996; 40:663-671.

Nattokinase (Subtilisin NAT)

DESCRIPTION
Nattokinase, also called subtilisin NAT, is a serine protease enzyme that possesses fibrinolytic activity. Fibrinolysis is the biochemical process that degrades blood clots or thrombi. Recently, it has been found that some proteases contained in indigenous fermented foods have the ability to prevent blood clots. The most studied of these proteases is nattokinase, which is derived from natto. Natto is a soybean-fermented food that has been a traditional Japanese staple for over 1,000 years. Natto is made by steaming or boiling soybeans and then fermenting them with the bacterium *Bacillus subtilis* natto. Nattokinase is isolated and purified from the fermented product.

Nattokinase is comprised of 275 amino acid residues and has a molecular weight of 27.728 kDa (kilo Daltons). It has four times the fibrinolytic activity of the natural fibrinolytic substance plasmin, both *in vitro* and *in vivo*. Discovered in 1987, nattokinase was named after the fibrinolytic enzyme urokinase. In addition to its ability to potentiate fibrinolysis, nattokinase has also been demonstrated to induce posterior vitreous detachment by intravitreal injection, an action that may have usefulness for pharmacologic vitreolysis.

ACTIONS AND PHARMACOLOGY

ACTIONS

Nattokinase has antithrombotic and fibrinolytic activity.

MECHANISM OF ACTION

The coagulation of blood is the body's major response to the threat of fatal hemorrhage. The interaction between platelets and clotting factors, especially fibrin, results in the generation of the protective hemostatic plug, the function of which is to stop the flow of blood at the site of the vascular injury. Obviously, this mechanism was of utmost importance to primitive man and woman, who constantly faced threats that could lead to fatal hemorrhaging. Modern humans are exposed to different types of threats that can activate the coagulation cascade/waterfall. Hypertension and elevated cholesterol and LDL-cholesterol levels are associated to a large degree with modern dietary and physical activity habits and can lead to injury of vascular endothelium via oxidative and inflammatory mechanisms, setting the stage for the subsequent aggregation of platelets, the activation of the coagulation cascade/waterfall and the formation of a fibrin clot, which adheres to the unbroken wall of blood vessels. Fibrin is the main protein of the fibrin blood clot, or thrombus, and is formed from fibrinogen by the action of thrombin in the final steps of the coagulation cascade/ waterfall. Accumulation of fibrin in the blood vessels usually increases thrombosis, leading to myocardial infarction and stroke. In this case, the blood clot is anything but protective.

Fortunately, there is another system to balance the coagulation cascade/waterfall system. This is the fibrinolytic cascade system. The fibrinolytic system has evolved to recanalize the occluded blood vessels as healing occurs to restore perfusion through an injured blood vessel in which the clot has formed. The fibrinolytic system is another type of cascade. Plasmin, the major fibrinolytic factor, is produced from fibrinogen via its activation by tissue plasminogen activator (tPA). The fibrinolytic system works very well for the fibrin plugs formed secondary to hemorrhaging but, unfortunately, not nearly as well for thrombi in coronary and cerebral arteries, the cause of myocardial infarctions and strokes. Pharmaceutical fibrinolytics, also known as clot busters, used in an intensive care setting are streptokinase alteplase (recombinant plasminogen activator), reteplase and tenecteplase. Streptokinase works by combining with plasminogen to form an active complex which degrades fibrin, breaking up the thrombus. The others are modified forms of plasminogen activator.

Nattokinase was the first protease fibrinolytic isolated from fermented foods, and in contrast to the parenteral fibrinolytics mentioned above, is an oral fibrinolytic agent. The exact mechanism of action of nattokinase is still not fully understood, but there is much that we do know. Nattokinase does not have plasminogen activator activity, unlike streptokinase, alteplase, reteplase and tenecteplase, but does digest fibrin to some degree by limited proteolysis. It also activates the production of (tPA), which results in the conversion of plasminogen to plasmin. Nattokinase has been demonstrated to cleave and inactivate the plasminogen activator inhibitor type-1 (PAI-1). PAI-1 is the primary inhibitor of fibrinolysis and regulates total fibrinolytic activity by its relative ratio with tPA.

PHARMACOKINETICS

The pharmacokinetics of nattokinase is incomplete. It is known that nattokinase can be absorbed across the rat intestine after intraduodenal administration. Following absorption, it does induce fibrinolysis. Nattokinase is a fairly stable protein, but the exact mechanism of its absorption across the intestine is not known. Possibly it is via the enteropancreatic circulation. Nattokinase has been demonstrated to dissolve thrombi in experimental animals following oral administration. Also, a human trial showed that oral administration of nattokinase enhanced the ability of the subjects to dissolve blood clots.

In both the animal and human cases, it can be inferred that nattokinase was absorbed from the intestines.

Research is needed and warranted to understand the absorption, distribution, metabolism and excretion of nattokinase in humans.

INDICATIONS AND USAGE

Nattokinase, an extract of the traditional Japanese fermented soybean preparation known as natto, has antithrombotic and fibrinolytic activities and may thus be useful in reducing risk of thrombosis, including venous thrombosis that some suffer during or after long-haul airline flights. It is contraindicated in those with bleeding disorders and should be avoided in those receiving antiplatelet or anticoagulation agents.

RESEARCH SUMMARY

Natto is a cheese-like fermented soybean product that has been a traditional food in Japan for about 1,000 years. Nattokinase is an enzyme derived from this product which has been found to have significant thrombolytic properties superior to several other agents used for this purpose. In one animal thrombosis model, carotid blockage was induced with acetic acid. After administration of nattokinase, blood flow was restored in a dose-dependent fashion, reaching 62 per cent recovery at the highest dose. Other agents tested in this study were significantly inferior to nattokinase. Only 15.8 per cent of the blood flow was regained using plasmin, and no recovery at all was noted when using elastase.

In another study, blood clots were induced in a major leg vein of male dogs. The clots reportedly dissolved within five hours of administering nattokinase, and normal circulation was restored.

In a study involving 12 healthy Japanese adults given 200 grams of natto before breakfast daily, fibrinolytic activity was evaluated in a series of blood plasma tests.

The results indicated that the natto had anticlotting effects in these subjects. The measured fibrinolytic effects persisted for two to eight hours after administration of the natto.

In another human study, a proprietary blend containing nattokinase (in an undisclosed dosage) and pycnogenol (see Pycnogenol) was given to subjects at high risk for developing deep vein thrombosis (DVT) two hours before a long-haul airline flight (seven to eight hours in duration) and six hours later. Potentially dangerous DVT has long been associated with prolonged sitting, such as occurs on prolonged airline flights, in susceptible individuals. The subjects' venous systems were scanned with ultrasound within 90 minutes of departure and again within 90 minutes of landing. There was a significant reduction in thrombotic events in those receiving the proprietary blend (called Pinokinase). None of the experimentals suffered any adverse events, whereas seven subjects (7.6% of the controls) who did not receive the blend did suffer such events. It was not possible to ascertain whether one ingredient or the other or the two in combination exerted the observed positive effects.

A recent review of the natto and nattokinase literature concluded that while human data are very limited, there exists the possibility that nattokinase may improve circulation and overall cardiovascular health, reducing, in particular, the risk of blood clots. Clearly more research is needed and indicated.

Nattokinase should not be used by anyone with a bleeding problem or any kind of coagulation disorder or by anyone taking any type of anti-coagulant or anti-platelet agent, as excessive bleeding could result from the combination. There is one report of a patient using aspirin as an agent for secondary stroke prevention who suffered acute cerebral hemorrhage after additionally taking 400 mg of nattokinase for seven consecutive days. Magnetic resonance imagery revealed multiple microbleeds in addition to the hemorrhage.

CONTRAINDICATIONS, PRECAUTIONS, ADVERSE REACTIONS

CONTRAINDICATIONS

Nattokinase is contraindicated in anyone who is allergic to any component of a nattokinase-containing product. Nattokinase is contraindicated in anyone who has a bleeding problem, including hemophilia and von Willebrand disease. It is also contraindicated in those taking the anticoagulant warfarin (Coumadin).

PRECAUTIONS

The use of nattokinase should be discussed with ones physician before starting its use.

Pregnant women and nursing mothers should avoid the use of nattokinase.

Pending long-term safety studies, nattokinase should be avoided by those on antiplatelet drugs or on anticoagulant therapy (see following list).

Antiplatelet drugs, Oral
    Aspirin
    Dipyridamole (Persantine)
    Clopidogrel (Plavix)
    Ticlopidine (Ticlid)

Antiplatelet Drugs, Parenteral
    GPIIB/IIA Inhibitors
    Abciximab (Reopro)
    Eptifibatide (Integrilin)
    Tirofiban (Aggrastat)

Anticoagulants, Oral
    Warfarin (Coumadin)

Anticoagulants, Parenteral
    Unfractionated heparin
    Low-molecular weight heparin
    Enoxaparin (Lovenox)
    Dalteparin (Fragmin)
    Tinzaparin (Innohep)

Direct Thrombin Inhibitors
    Argatroban
    Lepirudin (Refludan)
    Bivalirudin (Angiomax)

Nattokinase supplementation should be stopped at least one week before surgical procedures, including dental surgical procedures.

ADVERSE REACTIONS

The fermented food natto has been consumed for many years by the Japanese and it appears to be quite safe. However, long-term safety studies are necessary for the natto-derived enzyme, nattokinase.

Recently, a case of a cerebral hemorrhage provoked by combined use of nattokinase and aspirin in a 52-year old woman with cerebral bleeds has been reported. The authors of the report concluded that they "suggest that nattokinase may increase risk of intracerebral hemorrhage in patients who have bleeding-prone cerebral microangiopathy and are receiving other antithrombotic agents at the same time." (See Precautions above.)

INTERACTIONS

DRUGS

The use of nattokinase along with any of the antiplatelet drugs or anticoagulants listed below may cause serious adverse events, especially excessive bleeding.

Antiplatelet drugs, Oral
> Aspirin
> Dipyridamole (Persantine)
> Clopidogrel (Plavix)
> Ticlopidine (Ticlid)

Antiplatelet Drugs, Parenteral
> GPIIB/IIA Inhibitors
> Abciximab (Reopro)
> Eptifibatide (Integrilin)
> Tirofiban (Aggrastat)

Anticoagulants, Oral
> Warfarin (Coumadin)

Anticoagulants, Parenteral
> Unfractionated heparin
> Low-molecular-weight-heparin
> Enoxaparin (Lovenox)
> Dalteparin (Fragmin)
> Tinzaparin (Innohep)

Direct Thrombin Inhibitors
> Argatroban
> Lepirudin (Refludan)
> Bivalirudin (Angiomax)

FOODS

No known interactions.

NUTRITIONAL SUPPLEMENTS

Although never reported, the theoretical possibility exists that coadministration of nattokinase with fish oil, garlic (*Allium sativa*), ginkgo (*Ginkgo biloba*), ginseng or curcuminoid supplements may result in increased bleeding tendencies, manifested by increased susceptibility to bruising, nosebleeds, hemoptysis, hematemesis, hematuria and blood in the stool. All of the above dietary supplements may affect platelets to some degree.

OVERDOSAGE

No reports.

DOSAGE AND ADMINISTRATION

Nattokinase is available in 25 mg, 50 mg and 100 mg dose forms. These preparations contain 20 fibrinolytic units (FU) per mg. Optimal dose is not known. Many users of nattokinase take 100 mg of the substance three times daily, which comes to 6,000 FU daily. Review Contraindications and Precautions above.

LITERATURE

Cesarone MR, Belcaro G, Nicolaides AN, et al. Prevention of venous thrombosis in long-haul flights with Flite Tabs: the LONFLIT-FLITE randomized, controlled trial. *Angiology*. 2003;54(5):531-539.

Chang CT, Fan MH, Kuo FC, et al. Potent fibrinolytic enzyme from a mutant of Bacillus subtilis IMR-NK1. *J Agric Food Chem*. 2000;48(8):3210-3216.

Chang YY, Liu JS, Lai SL, et al. Cerebellar hemorrhage provoked by combined use of nattokinase and aspirin in a patient with cerebral microbleeds. *Intern Med*. 2008;47(5):467-469.

Chen PT, Chiang CJ, Chao YP. Medium optimization for the production of recombinant nattokinase by Bacillus subtilis using response surface methodology. *Biotechnol Prog*. 2007;23(6):1327-1332.

Fujita M, Hong K, Ito Y, et al. Thrombolytic effect of nattokinase on a chemically induced thrombosis model in rat. *Biol Pharm Bull*. 1995;18(10):1387-1391.

Fujita M, Hong K, Ito Y, et al. Transport of nattokinase across the rat intestinal tract. *Biol Pharm Bull*. 1995;18(9):1194-1196.

Fujita M, Nomura K, Hong K, et al. Purification and characterization of a strong fibrinolytic enzyme (nattokinase) in the vegetable cheese natto, a popular soybean fermented food in Japan. *Biochem Biophys Res Commun*. 1993;197(3):1340-1347.

Guo J, Sun Y, Su Y. [Preparation of natto and its function in health care] [Article in Chinese.] *Zhong Yao Cai*. 2002;25(1):61-64.

Pais E, Alexy T, Holsworth RE Jr, et al. Effects of nattokinase, a pro-fibrinolytic enzyme, on red blood cell aggregation and whole blood viscosity. *Clin Hemorheol Microcirc*. 2006;35(1-2):139-142.

Peng Y, Yang X, Zhang Y. Microbial fibrinolytic enzymes: an overview of source, production, properties, and thrombolytic activity in vivo. *Appl Microbiol Biotechnol*. 2005;69(2):126-132.

Sugimoto S, Fujii T, Morimiya T, et al. The fibrinolytic activity of a novel protease derived from a tempeh producing fungus, Fusarium sp. BLB. *Biosci Biotechnol Biochem*. 2007;71(9):2184-2189.

Sumi H, Hamada H, Nakanishi K, et al. Enhancement of the fibrinolytic activity in plasma by oral administration of nattokinase. *Acta Haematol*. 1990;84(3):139-143.

Sumi H, Hamada H, Tsushima H, et al. A novel fibrinolytic enzyme (nattokinase) in the vegetable cheese Natto; a typical and popular soybean food in the Japanese diet. *Experientia*. 1987;43(10):1110-1111.

Suzuki Y, Kondo K, Matsumoto Y, et al. Dietary supplementation of fermented soybean, natto, suppresses intimal thickening and modulates the lysis of mural thrombi after endothelial injury in rat femoral artery. *Life Sci*. 2003;73(10):1289-1298.

Takano A, Hirata A, Ogasawara K, et al. Posterior vitreous detachment induced by nattokinase (subtilisin NAT): a novel enzyme for pharmacologic vitreolysis. *Invest Ophthalmol Vis Sci.* 2006;47(5):2075-2079.

Urano T, Ihara H, Umemura K, et al. The profibrinolytic enzyme subtilisin NAT purified from Bacillus subtilis Cleaves and inactivates plasminogen activator inhibitor type 1. *J Biol Chem.* 2001;276(27):24690-24696.

Wu S, Feng C, Zhong J, et al. Roles of s3 site residues of nattokinase on its activity and substrate specificity. *J Biochem.* 2007;142(3):357-364.

Zheng ZL, Zuo ZY, Liu ZG, et al. Construction of a 3D model of nattokinase, a novel fibrinolytic enzyme from Bacillus natto. A novel nucleophilic catalytic mechanism for nattokinase. *J Mol Graph Model.* 2005;23(4):373-380.

Niacin (Nicotinic Acid)

DESCRIPTION

The term niacin is used in two different ways. As a collective term, it refers to both nicotinic acid and nicotinamide. It is also used synonymously with nicotinic acid. In this monograph, the biochemistry and pharmacology of niacin—nicotinic acid and nicotinamide—will be discussed, as well as the actions of and indications for nicotinic acid. The actions of and indications for nicotinamide will be discussed in a separate monograph (see Nicotinamide). Nicotinic acid and nicotinamide have identical vitamin activities, but have very different pharmacological activities.

Niacin is a member of the B-vitamin family. It is sometimes referred to as vitamin B_3. Nicotinic acid was first discovered as an oxidation product of nicotine and thus, the origin of its name. In fact, much of the confusion caused by the use of the term niacin for both nicotinic acid and nicotinamide, as well as for nicotinic acid alone, was created by the attempt to dissociate nicotinic acid from its nicotine origins. Niacin, via its metabolites, is involved in a wide range of biological processes, including the production of energy, the synthesis of fatty acids, cholesterol and steroids, signal transduction, the regulation of gene expression and the maintenance of genomic integrity. Nicotinic acid, in pharmacological doses, is used as an antihyperlipidemic agent.

Niacin and substances that are convertible to niacin are found naturally in meat (especially red meat), poultry, fish, legumes and yeast. In addition to preformed niacin, some L-tryptophan found in the proteins of these foods is metabolized to niacin. Niacin is also present in cereal grains, such as corn and wheat. However, consumption of corn-rich diets has resulted in niacin deficiency in certain populations. The reason for this is that niacin exists in cereal grains in bound forms, such as the glycoside niacytin, which exhibit little or no nutritional availability. Interestingly, niacin deficiency is not common in Mexico and Central America even though the diets of those in these countries are based on corn. Alkaline treatment, such as soaking corn in a lime solution, the process used by the populations of Mexico and Central America in the production of corn tortillas, yields release of bound niacin and increased availability of the vitamin.

The well-known disorder of niacin deficiency is pellagra. The term pellagra is derived from the Italian words pelle agra meaning rough or smarting skin. Pellagra is characterized by the triad of dermatitis, diarrhea and dementia. A fourth d, death, is the final outcome of the disease, if not treated. The skin lesions are primarily located on sun-exposed areas of the face, hands, arms and feet. The dermatitis progresses from an erythematous, often pruritic rash, to vesicles and blisters with scales and fissures, and finally, to thickened, lichenified, hyperpigmented skin. Casal's necklace refers to characteristic advanced skin lesions of pellagra. Casal's necklace is named for Gaspar Casal, the physician to King Ferdinand of Spain, who first reported on the symptoms and signs of pellagra in modern times. He called the disease mal de la rosa (disease of the rose), because of the red and glossy color of the skin lesions. Casal attributed the disorder to the diets of the poor laborers; diets which were mainly comprised of corn. Although pellagra was commonly found in the United States through the 1930s, the disorder is rare today in industrialized countries. This is due, in large part, to the enrichment of refined flours with niacin.

Niacin deficiency, however, can and does occur under certain conditions. These conditions include alcoholism, malabsorption syndromes, cirrhosis and in those receiving total parenteral nutrition (TPN) with inadequate niacin. It may also occur in Hartnup's syndrome, an autosomal recessive disorder in which there is defective conversion of tryptophan to niacin; carcinoid syndrome, in which tryptophan metabolism is diverted to form 5-hydroxytryptamine, also known as serotonin; and in those receiving isoniazid for the treatment of tuberculosis.

The biochemical effects of niacin are principally mediated by its metabolite nicotinamide adenine dinucleotide or NAD^+. NAD^+ serves both coenzyme and substrate functions. NAD^+ was originally called cozymase and was also known as coenzyme I and DPN or diphosphopyridine nucleotide. The positive sign in NAD^+ refers to the fact that the nitrogen in the pyridine ring of niacin is positively charged in the NAD^+ structure. NAD^+ and its reduced form NADH (reduced nicotinamide dinucleotide) are the major hydrogen acceptor and donor, respectively, in many biological redox reactions. NAD^+ is used in metabolic reactions to transfer the potential free energy stored in carbohydrates, lipids and proteins to NADH, which is used to form ATP (adenosine triphosphate).

NADP+ or nicotinamide adenine dinucleotide phosphate is formed from NAD+ via a kinase-catalyzed phosphorylation. NADP+ participates as a coenzyme in the oxidation of glucose 6-phosphate via the enzyme glucose 6-phosphate dehydrogenase. This is the oxidative reaction in the pentose phosphate pathway which produces, among other things, ribose 5-phosphate. During the oxidation of glucose 6-phosphate, NADP+ is reduced to NADPH or reduced nicotinamide adenine dinucleotide phosphate. NADPH serves as the reducing agent in fatty acid and steroid biosyntheses and serves to maintain glutathione in its reduced form.

In addition to its coenzyme role in many metabolic reactions, NAD+ also serves as a substrate in a number of biochemical reactions. The beta-N-glycosylic bond of NAD+ can be cleaved by three types of enzymes. In the process, nicotinamide and ADP (adenosine diphosphate)-ribose are formed. One type of enzyme catalyzes mono(ADP-ribosyl)ation of proteins—a posttranslational modification—by transferring ADP-ribose from NAD+ to target proteins. The enzymes are known as mono(ADP-ribosyl)transferases (mADPRTs). Mono(ADP-ribosyl)ation of endogenous proteins by bacterial toxins, such as diphtheria toxin and cholera toxin, accounts, in large part, for the pathogenic effects of these toxins. The physiological functions of endogenous mono(ADP-ribosyl)transferases are not clear. Another type of enzyme catalyzes poly(ADP-ribosyl)ation of target proteins. This enzyme is known as poly(ADP-ribose)polymerase or PARP. PARP is also known as poly(ADP-ribose) synthetase (PARS), poly(ADP-ribose)transferase (pADPRT) and PARP1. PARP is believed to be involved in DNA repair, among other things.

NAD+ is also involved in the biosynthesis of signaling molecules. A third type of beta-N-glycosylic bond-cleaving enzymes catalyzes the formation of cyclic ADP-ribose (cADPR). Cyclic ADP-ribose is an intracellular calcium mobilizing agent. The enzyme that catalyzes the synthesis of cyclic ADP-ribose is called ADP-ribosyl cyclase. NADP+ is also involved in the biosynthesis of signaling molecules. NADP+ leads to the formation of NAADP+ (nicotinic acid adenine dinucleotide phosphate) and cADPRP (2'-phospho cyclic ADP-ribose). NAADP+ and cADPRP are also intracellular calcium mobilizing agents.

The enzyme poly(ADP-ribose) polymerase(PARP) is a highly abundant nuclear protein, the physiological role of which is not yet clear. PARP poly(ADP-ribosyl)ates various nuclear proteins as well as itself. PARP is thought to be involved in a number of biological processes, including DNA repair and replication, cell differentiation and cellular apoptosis. DNA damage appears to enhance the activity of PARP. In damaged cells, PARP binds to DNA and becomes enzymatically activated. Once activated, PARP automodifies itself through poly(ADP-ribosyl)ation. This results in its inactivation and its dissociation from DNA breaks. This dissociation is necessary for DNA repair.

Recently, it has been found that NAD+ plays a key role in life-span extension by calorie restriction in the yeast *Saccharomyces cerevisiae*. It does so by serving as the cofactor for an NAD+-dependent histone deacetylase, an enzyme that removes acetyl groups from the lysine residues of histone proteins, thus promoting genomic silencing. Maintenance of genomic silencing may be critical to longevity either by repressing genomic instability or by preventing inappropriate gene expression. A similar mechanism may operate in metazoans, including humans.

As mentioned above, niacin is used either to refer to both nicotinic acid and nicotinamide or to nicotinic acid itself. Nicotinic acid, in addition to being known as niacin, is also known as pyridine-3-carboxylic acid, vitamin B_3, 3-pyridine-carboxylic acid, pyridine-beta-carboxylic acid, antipellagra vitamin and pellagra preventive factor. The molecular formula of nicotinic acid is $C_6H_5NO_2$. The molecular weight of nicotinic acid is 123.11 daltons and the structural formula is:

Nicotinic Acid

Nicotinamide is also known as pyridine-3-carboxamide, niacinamide and nicotinic acid amide. Its molecular formula is $C_6H_6N_2O$ and its molecular weight is 122.13 daltons.

ACTIONS AND PHARMACOLOGY
ACTIONS
Nicotinic acid has antihyperlipidemic activity and may have anti-atherogenic activity.

MECHANISM OF ACTION
Nicotinic acid in gram doses, but not nicotinamide, lowers serum levels of total cholesterol, low-density lipoprotein cholesterol (LDL-C), very low-density lipoprotein (VLDL) and triglycerides. High-dose nicotinic acid also increases serum levels of high-density lipoprotein cholesterol (HDL-C) and decreases serum levels of lipoprotein (a) [Lp(a)] and apolipoprotein B-100 (Apo B). The mechanism of the antihyperlipidemic action of nicotinic acid is not well understood. It is thought that this effect is mediated, in part,

via decreases in the release of free fatty acids from adipose tissue, thereby decreasing the influx of free fatty acids into the liver, the hepatic reesterification of free fatty acids and the rate of production of hepatic very low-density lipoprotein (VLDL). A decrease in the hepatic production of VLDL reduces the level of circulating VLDL available for conversion to LDL. Another hypothesis holds that nicotinic acid directly inhibits hepatic synthesis or secretion of apolipoprotein B-containing lipoproteins. Still another hypothesis holds that nicotinic acid has the potential to cause a generalized inhibition of synthetic function in the liver. This mechanism may be considered a manifestation of nicotinic acid hepatotoxicity resulting in decreased LDL-cholesterol. However, this liver-damaging hypothesis would not explain the HDL-elevating effect of nicotinic acid. The mechanism by which nicotinic acid elevates HDL is unclear. A recent study suggested that the mechanism may have something to do with nicotinic acid's inhibition of the cell surface expression of the ATP synthase beta chain, leading to a reduced hepatic removal of HDL proteins, and thus implicating a potential cellular target for nicotinic action to raise HDL. This possibility is certainly worthwhile to pursue.

High dose nicotinic acid has been found to significantly decrease cardiovascular and cerebrovascular events in those with coronary heart disease. It is thought that this effect is due, in part, to nicotinic acid's antihyperlipidemic activity.

PHARMACOKINETICS
Both nicotinic acid and nicotinamide are efficiently absorbed from the stomach and small intestine. At low amounts, absorption is mediated by sodium-dependent facilitated diffusion. Passive diffusion is the principal mechanism of absorption at higher doses. Doses of up to three to four grams of nicotinic acid and niacinamide are almost completely absorbed. Nicotinic acid and nicotinamide are transported via the portal circulation to the liver and via the systemic circulation to the various tissues of the body. Nicotinic acid and nicotinamide enter most cells by passive diffusion and enter erythrocytes by facilitated transport.

Nicotinic acid and nicotinamide are metabolized through different pathways. Nicotinic acid is not directly metabolized to nicotinamide. It undergoes a number of metabolic steps to yield NAD^+ which in turn can be converted to nicotinamide. Nicotinamide can be directly converted to nicotinic acid. Nicotinic acid is metabolized to nicotinic acid mononucleotide (NicMN, nicotinic acid ribonucleotide). NicMN is also the first niacin metabolite to which dietary L-tryptophan is converted. NicMN is converted to nicotinic acid adenine dinucleotide (NicAD, desamido-NAD^+). NicAD is converted in turn to NAD^+. NAD^+ has a number of metabolic opportunities. These include, the formation of nicotinamide, $NADP^+$, nicotinamide 5'-mononucleotide (NMN), cyclic

ADP-ribose and nicotinic acid dinucleotide phosphate (NAADP). NAD^+ also serves as the substrate for mono-(ADP-ribosyl)ation and poly(ADP-ribosyl)ation reactions. Nicotinamide is converted to nicotinic acid via the enzyme nicotinamidase. Nicotinamide is also metabolized to NMN which in turn is converted to NAD^+.

In the liver, the principal catabolic product of high doses of nicotinic acid is the glycine conjugate of nicotinic acid called nicotinuric acid. The principal catabolic products of nicotinamide are N'-methylnicotinamide, N'-methyl-5-carboxamide-2-pyridone, N'-methyl-5-carboxamide-4-pyridone and nicotinamide-N-oxide.

High doses of nicotinic acid are excreted in the urine as unchanged nicotinic acid and the glycine conjugate of nicotinic acid nicotinuric acid. High doses of nicotinamide are excreted in the urine as unchanged nicotinamide, N'-methylnicotinamide, N'-methyl-5-carboxamide-2-pyridone, N'-methyl-5-carboxamide-4-pyridone and nicotinamide-N-oxide.

The pharmacokinetics of the various forms of nicotinic acid (immediate-release, intermediate-release, extended-release) differs in certain particulars. The time to reach peak serum concentrations of the immediate-release or crystalline form of nicotinic acid is approximately 45 minutes following ingestion. The time to reach peak serum concentrations of the extended-release form of nicotinic acid is from 4-5 hours following ingestion. Administration of nicotinic acid with food maximizes its availability. Nicotinic acid-induced flushing, which is due to vasodilation, occurs within 20 minutes following ingestion of immediate-release nicotinic acid and may last for up to one hour.

INDICATIONS AND USAGE
Nicotinic acid has demonstrated an ability to lower LDL-cholesterol and triglycerides and to protect against atherosclerosis. Recently, researchers have begun focusing on its abilities to boost the "good" HDL-cholesterol and on ways to diminish the so-called "niacin flush" that has prevented some from using this helpful agent.

RESEARCH SUMMARY
Nicotinic acid has been tested for its effects on cardiovascular-disease risk factors in a number of major trials. In the largest of these, the effect of nicotinic acid monotherapy on cardiovascular endpoints was investigated. The study included 8,341 men who had suffered myocardial infarction. In this randomized, six-year study, nicotinic acid, given in 1 gram doses three times a day, decreased cholesterol levels by 10% and triglyceride levels by 26%. There was a decrease of 27% in recurrent non-fatal heart attacks among the nicotinic-acid treated subjects. They also experienced 26% fewer cerebrovascular events.

In a five-year randomized, placebo-controlled study of 555 survivors of myocardial infarction, nicotinic acid, in combination with clofibrate, was found to significantly decrease total and cardiac mortality. Total mortality declined by 26%. Nicotinic acid was given in 1 gram doses three times daily. Clofibrate was given in 1 gram doses twice daily.

In another well-controlled study of men aged 40 to 59 who had undergone coronary artery bypass, nicotinic acid used in combination with colestipol significantly decreased disease progression in some and significantly increased disease regression in some others, compared with placebo.

Various studies have shown that nicotinic acid can significantly lower total cholesterol, LDL-cholesterol, triglycerides and lipoprotein (a) levels. It can also increase HDL-cholesterol levels.

Nicotinic acid may be an effective and safe lipid-modifying agent even among those with diabetes. A recent report of the analysis of data from the Arterial Disease Multiple Intervention Trial (ADMIT), showed that those with and without diabetes who received crystalline nicotinic acid (3,000 milligrams/day) had significantly increased levels of HDL-cholesterol and decreased levels of LDL-cholesterol and triglycerides after 18 weeks of treatment. Glucose levels were only modestly increased among subjects with and without diabetes. Among those with diabetes, HbA_{1c} levels were unchanged in the nicotinic acid group, but decreased in the placebo group. No significant differences in nicotinic acid discontinuation or hypoglycemic therapy were noted in those with diabetes assigned to nicotinic acid vs. placebo.

A newer extended-release nicotinic acid, used once daily, either as monotherapy or in combination with lipid-lowering drugs, has demonstrated the same favorable effects on lipids in clinical trials. This form may be less hepatotoxic than slow-release nicotinic acid.

More-recent studies continue to produce positive results for nicotinic acid. In one of these, it was shown to inhibit vascular oxidative stress, redox-sensitive genes and monocyte adhesion to human aortic endothelial cells. All of this provides evidence that niacin inhibits vascular inflammation and has antiatherosclerotic properties independent of, and in addition to, its lipid-modulating effects. In a recent double-blind, placebo-controlled study, niacin, either alone or in combination with statins, was found to reduce coronary heart disease morbidity and mortality in patients with confirmed coronary heart disease and low levels of HDL-cholesterol.

Studies have shown that the cutaneous vasodilation niacin induces—resulting in the so-called "niacin flush" that is harmless but causes some people discomfort and prevents them from continuing to use niacin—can be blocked to some extent by pretreatment with aspirin. Some further research has identified prostaglandin receptors involved in this flushing process and has raised hopes that even more effective and safe antagonists of these receptors may be found. Other strategies for minimizing the flush have lately been proposed, including regular consistent dosing; the use of extended-release formulations as discussed above; patient education; dosing with meals or at bedtime; and avoidance of alcohol, hot beverages, spicy foods and hot baths or showers near the time of dosing or soon after.

A number of other new discoveries have further revived interest in niacin as a unique agent for the promotion of heart health. Findings related to its influence on HDL-cholesterol, in particular, have excited much recent interest. Niacin is now recognized, as one group of researchers recently stated, as "the most potent available lipid-regulating agent to increase HDL levels." HDL particles have antiatherogenic properties owing to their ability to take up cholesterol and remove it from blood vessels; additionally, it has been shown to have antiinflammatory and anticoagulatory properties. And as important as reducing plasma concentrations of harmful LDL-cholesterol is (through use of statins, for example), researchers note that this is insufficient in itself for purposes of substantially reducing cardiovascular disease. Low HDL is an established independent risk factor; thus increasing attention is being focused on strategies to increase HDL. One reviewer recently observed that "though there are several novel strategies being pursued, the oldest lipid-modifying drug, nicotinic acid, has recently enjoyed a renaissance owing to its strong HDL-cholesterol elevating effect, which is unique among the drugs currently approved for clinical use." Another reviewer, similarly hailing the re-emergence of niacin as an important therapy in cardiovascular disease, added that concerns about niacin's safety have been largely assuaged by results seen over the long course of its use: "Evidence is also accumulating that hyperglycemic responses are minor and manageable, that liver toxicity is very infrequent when appropriately dosed, and that myopathic potential is absent or minimal in combination with statins."

CONTRAINDICATIONS, PRECAUTIONS, ADVERSE REACTIONS
CONTRAINDICATIONS

Niacin is contraindicated in those who are hypersensitive to any component of a niacin-containing product. High-dose nicotinic acid is contraindicated in those with hepatic dysfunction, unexplained elevations of serum aminotransferases (transaminases), active peptic ulcer disease and arterial bleeding.

PRECAUTIONS

Pregnant women and nursing mothers should avoid supplement doses of niacin greater than U.S. RDA amounts (20 milligrams daily) unless higher doses are prescribed by their physicians.

The use of nicotinic acid as an antihyperlipidemic agent should only be undertaken under medical supervision.

Those with a past history of hepatobiliary disease, jaundice, peptic ulcer disease or gastritis should exercise caution in the use of high-dose nicotinic acid. Those with a history of diabetes, renal dysfunction, cardiovascular disease (especially acute myocardial infarction and unstable angina) and gout should exercise caution in the use of high-dose nicotinic acid. Those who consume substantial amounts of alcohol should also exercise caution in the use of high-dose nicotinic acid.

Those who take high-dose nicotinic acid should have their serum aminotransferase levels monitored. Aspartate aminotransferase (AST, also known as SGOT or serum glutamate oxaloacetate transaminase) and alanine aminotransferase (ALT, also known as SGPT or serum glutamate pyruvate transaminase) levels should be determined prior to starting high-dose nicotinic acid therapy, then every 6-12 weeks for one year and after one year, periodically. High-dose nicotinic acid should be discontinued if the aminotransferase levels are equal to greater than three times the upper limit of normal.

Intermediate-release (extended-release) and slow-release forms of nicotinic acid should not be substituted for equivalent doses of immediate-release (crystalline) nicotinic acid. Cases of severe hepatic toxicity, including fulminant hepatic necrosis, have occurred in subjects who have substituted sustained-release nicotinic acid products for immediate-release nicotinic acid at equivalent doses. Those who switch from immediate-release nicotinic acid to sustained-release forms of nicotinic acid, should start off with low doses of sustained-release nicotinic acid and the dose should then be slowly increased in order to obtain the desired therapeutic response.

High-dose nicotinic acid may negatively affect glucose tolerance. Diabetics who take nicotinic acid for lipid-lowering, should have their serum glucose levels carefully monitored and the dose of their antidiabetic medications adjusted as necessary.

ADVERSE REACTIONS

Nicotinic acid can cause vasodilation of cutaneous blood vessels, resulting in increased blood flow, principally in the face, neck and chest. This produces the niacin- or nicotinic acid-flush. The niacin-flush is thought to be mediated via the vasodilatory eicosanoids, particularly prostaglandin D_2 (PGD_2). It is thought that an antagonist to the PGD_2 receptor subtype might significantly reduce the flush, and at least one pharmaceutical company is developing such a drug. Histamine may also play some role in the niacin-flush. Flushing is the adverse reaction first observed after intake of a large dose of nicotinic acid, and the most bothersome one. It is the principal reason for compliance issues with the use of high-dose nicotinic acid for the treatment of hyperlipidemia. Nicotinamide does not appear to be associated with flushing. However, high-dose nicotinamide does not possess antihyperlipidemic activity. The symptoms of flushing include a burning, tingling and itching sensation. A reddened flush occurs primarily on the face, arms and chest. Flushing is often accompanied by pruritus and headaches. In one study, 5% of subjects ingesting 50 milligrams of nicotinic acid experienced flushing, 50% experienced flushing after ingesting 100 milligrams of nicotinic acid and 100% of subjects ingesting 500 milligrams of nicotinic acid experienced flushing. In another study, 66% of subjects experienced a flushing sensation after ingestion of 50 milligrams of nicotinic acid. Based on these studies, the Food and Nutrition Board of the Institute of Medicine has established a LOAEL (lowest-observed-adverse-effect level) for niacin of 50 mg/day. Based on this LOAEL, the Tolerable Upper Intake Level (UL) for niacin, for adults, is set at 35 mg/day. To obtain this UL, the LOAEL of 50 mg/day was divided by an uncertainty factor (UF) of 1.5 and rounded off.

The flushing effect of nicotinic acid is transient and tolerance to this effect occurs with continued administration of the vitamin. The flushing effect, as mentioned above, is prostaglandin mediated, and tolerance results from reduction in prostaglandin levels with continued administration.

Other adverse reactions of nicotinic acid include dizziness, palpitations, tachycardia, shortness of breath, sweating, chills, skin rashes, insomnia, nausea, vomiting, abdominal pain and myalgia. Nicotinic acid can cause hepatotoxicity. In the most severe cases, subjects develop liver dysfunction and fulminant hepatitis and may progress to stage 3 and 4 encephalopathy requiring liver transplantation. The most frequently observed manifestations of nicotinic acid-induced hepatitis are increased levels of serum aminotransferases (transaminases) and jaundice. Many, if not most of the subjects who developed hepatoxicity from nicotinic acid appeared to be taking the slow-release form. A recent double-blind comparison suggested that the slow-release form is more hepatotoxic than the immediate-release form. However, not all studies find this to be the case. Another recent study reported that both the slow release and immediate-release forms of nicotinic acid are hepatotoxic.

High-dose nicotinic acid (approximately 3 grams daily) has caused impaired glucose tolerance in otherwise healthy individuals. Further, glucose tolerance in some diabetics may be worsened by nicotinic acid therapy. High doses of nicotinic acid (1.5 to 5 grams/day) have also caused ocular effects, including blurred vision, macular edema, toxic amblyopia and cystic maculopathy. Nicotinic acid-induced ocular effects do not appear to be common and appear to be reversible. Elevated uric acid levels have also occurred with nicotinic acid therapy.

INTERACTIONS

DRUGS

Alpha$_1$-blockers (doxazosin, prazosin, tamsulosin, terazosin): Concomitant use of high-dose nicotinic acid and an alpha$_1$-blocker may potentiate the hypotensive effect of the alpha$_1$-blocker and may cause postural hypotension.

Alpha-glucosidase inhibitors (acarbose, miglitol): High-dose nicotinic acid may antagonize the antidiabetic action of alpha-glucosidase inhibitors, requiring adjustment of their dosage.

Biguanides (metformin): High-dose nicotinic acid may antagonize the antidiabetic activity of metformin, requiring adjustment of its dosage,

Calcium channel blockers: Concomitant use of high-dose nicotinic acid and a calcium channel blocker may potentiate the hypotensive effect of the calcium channel blocker.

Cholestyramine: Concomitant use of high-dose nicotinic acid and cholestyramine may reduce the absorption of nicotinic acid. It is recommended that a 4 to 6 hour interval elapse between the ingestion of cholestyramine and the administration of nicotinic acid. Administration of high-dose nicotinic acid and cholestyramine may produce complementary antihyperlipidemic effects.

Colestipol: Concomitant use of high-dose nicotinic acid and colestipol may reduce the absorption of nicotinic acid. It is recommended that a 4 to 6 hour interval elapse between the ingestion of colestipol and the administration of nicotinic acid. Administration of high-dose nicotinic acid and colestipol may produce complementary antihyperlipidemic effects.

Ganglionic blocking agents (mecamylamine HCL, trimethaphan): Nicotinic acid may potentiate the effects of ganglionic blocking agents resulting in postural hypotension.

Gemfibrozil: Administration of high-dose nicotinic acid and gemfibrozil may produce complementary antihyperlipidemic effects.

HMG-CoA reductase inhibitors or "statins" (atorvastatin, cerivastatin, fluvastatin, lovastatin, pravastatin, simvastatin): Concomitant administration of high-dose nicotinic acid and HMG-CoA reductase inhibitors have resulted in rare cases of rhabdomyolysis. Those receiving concomitant high-dose nicotinic acid and an HMG-CoA reductase inhibitor should be carefully monitored for any signs or symptoms of muscle pain, tenderness or weakness. Administration of high-dose nicotinic acid and a statin may produce complementary antihyperlipidemic effects.

Meglitinides (repaglinide): High-dose nicotinic acid may antagonize the antidiabetic action of repaglinide, a meglitinide analogue, requiring adjustment of its dosage.

Nicotine patch: Concomitant use of a transdermal nicotine patch and nicotinic acid may enhance the flushing reaction.

Nitrates: Concomitant use of high-dose nicotinic acid and a nitrate may potentiate the hypotensive effect of the nitrate.

NSAIDs (ibuprofen, etc.) and aspirin: The use of aspirin (80 to 325 milligrams), ibuprofen (200 to 400 milligrams) or other NSAIDs, taken 30 minutes to one hour before a dose of nicotinic acid, may blunt the flushing effect of high-dose nicotinic acid. Nicotinic acid induces the release of vasodilatory eicosanoids, particularly prostaglandin D_2 (PGD$_2$). Prostaglandin D_2 (PGD$_2$) is thought to account for, in large part, nicotinic- acid-induced flushing. Aspirin may help to antagonize the effect of PGD$_2$ and also may decrease the metabolic clearance of nicotinic acid.

Sulfonylureas (chlorpropamide, glimepiride, glipizide, glyburide): High-dose nicotinic acid may antagonize the antidiabetic action of sulfonylureas, requiring adjustment of their dosage.

Thiazolidinediones (pioglitazone, rosiglitazone): High-dose nicotinic acid may antagonize the antidiabetic action of thiazolidinediones, requiring adjustment of their dosage.

Warfarin: Extended-release (intermediate-release) forms of nicotinic acid have been associated with small but statistically significant increases in prothrombin time. Concomitant use of extended-release forms of nicotinic acid, as well as other forms of nicotinic acid, may enhance the anticoagulant activity of warfarin. INRs should be closely monitored in those taking high-dose nicotinic acid concomitantly with warfarin.

NUTRITIONAL SUPPLEMENTS

Red yeast rice: The nutritional supplement red yeast rice contains HMG-CoA reductase inhibitors, including lovastatin. Concomitant administration of high-dose nicotinic acid and HMG-CoA reductase inhibitors, including lovastatin, has resulted in rare cases of rhabdomyolysis. Otherwise, high-dose nicotinic acid and red yeast rice may produce complementary antihyperlipidemic effects.

Luteolin: Animal studies suggest that the flavonoid luteolin may help to ameliorate the niacin-induced flush.

FOODS

Ethanol-containing beverages: Concomitant intake of nicotinic acid and ethanol-containing beverages may cause an increase in nicotinic acid-induced flushing.

Hot beverages and hot foods: Concomitant intake of hot beverages or hot foods and nicotinic acid may cause an increase in nicotinic acid-induced flushing.

OVERDOSAGE

There are no reports of niacin overdosage in the literature.

DOSAGE AND ADMINISTRATION

Niacin, as nicotinamide (niacinamide) is the principal form used for nutritional supplementation. It is available as a single ingredient product (see Nicotinamide) and in multivitamin and multivitamin/multimineral products. Typical supplemental dosage, ranges from 20 to 100 milligrams daily. Nicotinamide is also the form of niacin used in food fortification.

The Food and Nutrition Board of the Institute of Medicine of the National Academy of Sciences has recommended the following dietary reference intakes (DRIs) for niacin: (Preformed niacin refers to nicotinic acid and nicotinamide; niacin equivalents refer to nicotinic acid, to nicotinamide and the contribution to niacin obtained by conversion from dietary L-Tryptophan. The relative contribution of tryptophan is estimated as follows: 60 mg of L-tryptophan = one mg of niacin = 1 mg of niacin equivalents.)

The most recent Dietary Reference Intakes (DRI) and the Tolerable Upper Intake Level (UL) for niacin are as follows:

Infants	Adequate Intake (AI)	Tolerable Upper Intake Level (UL)
0-6 months	2 mg/day of preformed niacin ~ 0.2 mg/Kg	ND
7-12 months	4 mg/day of niacin equivalents ~ 0.4 mg/Kg	ND

Children	Recommended Dietary Allowances (RDA)	Tolerable Upper Intake Level (UL)
1-3 years	6 mg/day of niacin equivalents	10 mg/day
4-8 years	8 mg/day of niacin equivalents	15 mg/day
Boys		
9-13 years	12 mg/day of niacin equivalents	20 mg/day
14-18 years	16 mg/day of niacin equivalents	30 mg/day
Girls		
9-13 years	12 mg/day of niacin equivalents	20 mg/day
14-18 years	14 mg/day of niacin equivalents	30 mg/day
Men		
≥19 years	16 mg/day of niacin equivalents	35 mg/day
Women		
≥19 years	14 mg/day of niacin equivalents	35 mg/day
Pregnancy		
14-18 years	18 mg/day of niacin equivalents	30 mg/day
19-50 years	18 mg/day of niacin equivalents	35 mg/day
Lactation		
14-18 years	17 mg/day of niacin equivalents	30 mg/day
19-50 years	17 mg/day of niacin equivalents	35 mg/day

ND = Not determinable

The DV (Daily Value) for niacin (nicotinamide and nicotinic acid), which is used for determining percentage of nutrient daily values on nutritional supplement and food labels, is 20 milligrams. This is based on the U.S. RDA for niacin.

Nicotinic acid is available as a single ingredient product. It is available both as an OTC product and as a prescription product. The use of nicotinic acid as an antihyperlipidemic agent should only be undertaken under medical supervision. Three different formulations are available for antihyperlipidemic use: immediate-release (crystalline) nicotinic acid, extended-release (intermediate-release) nicotinic acid and slow-release nicotinic acid. Recommended adult doses are up to 3 grams daily of the immediate-release form or 1 to 2 grams of the extended-release forms. It is recommended that nicotinic acid be started at low doses and slowly titrated to the desired therapeutic dose. Administration on an empty stomach is *not* recommended. The use of an NSAID taken $1/2$ hour before nicotinic acid may blunt the flushing reaction. The flushing is less severe with extended-release and slow-release forms than it is with immediate-release forms. However, the slow-release form may lead to an increased incidence of gastrointestinal problems and hepatotoxicity. The intermediate-release form may be less hepatotoxic than the slow-release form.

LITERATURE

Alsheikh-Ali AA, Karas RH. The safety of niacin in the US Food and Drug Administration adverse event reporting database. *Am J Cardiol.* 2008;101(8A):9B-13B.

Bays H. Safety of niacin and simvastatin combination therapy. *Am J Cardiol.* 2008;101(8A):3B-8B.

Bodor ET, Offermanns S. Nicotinic acid: an old drug with a promising future. *Br J Pharmacol.* 2008;153 Suppl 1:S68-75.

Canner PL, Berge KG, Wenger NK, et al. Fifteen year mortality in Coronary Drug Project patients: long-term benefit with niacin. *J Am Coll Cardiol.* 1986;8:1245-1255.

Capuzzi DM, Guyton JR, Morgan JM, et al. Efficacy and safety of an extended-release niacin (Niaspan): a long-term study. *Am J Cardiol.* 1998;82(12A):74U-81U.

Carlson LA, Rosenhamer G. Reduction of mortality in the Stockholm ischemic Heart Disease Secondary Prevention Study by combined treatment with clofibrate and nicotinic acid. *Acta Med Scand.* 1988;223:405-418.

Cervantes-Laurean D, McElvaney NG, Moss J. Niacin. In: Shils ME, Olson JA, Shike M, Ross AC, eds. *Modern Nutrition in Health and Disease.* 9th ed. Baltimore, MD: Williams and Wilkins; 1999:401-411.

Cheng K, Wu TJ, Wu KK, et al. Antagonism of the prostaglandin D2 receptor 1 suppresses nicotinic acid-induced vasodilation in mice and humans. *Proc Natl Acad Sci USA.* 2006;103(17):6682-6687.

Chojnowska-Jezierska J, Adamska-Dyniewska H. [Prolonged treatment with slow release nicotinic acid in patients with type II hyperlipidemia]. [Article in Polish]. *Pol Arch Med Wewn.* 1997;98:391-399.

Colletti RB, Neufeld EJ, Roff NK, et al. Niacin treatment of hypercholesterolemia in children. *Pediatrics.* 1993;92:78-82.

Davidson MH. Niacin use and cutaneous flushing: mechanisms and strategies for prevention. *Am J Cardiol.* 2008;101(8A):14B-19B.

Elam MB, Hunninghake DB, Davis KB, et al. Effect of niacin on lipid and lipoprotein levels and glycemic control in patients with diabetes and peripheral arterial disease: The ADMIT Study: A randomized trial. *JAMA.* 2000;284:1263-1270.

Ganji SH, Qin S, Zhang L, et al. Niacin inhibits vascular oxidative stress, redox-sensitive genes, and monocyte adhesion to human aortic endothelial cells. *Atherosclerosis.* Epub: 2008 May 9.

Gille A, Bodor ET, Ahmed K, et al. Nicotinic acid: pharmacological effects and mechanisms of action. *Annu Rev Pharmacol Toxicol.* 2008;48:79-106.

Goldberg A, Alagona P Jr, Capuzzi DM, et al. Multiple-dose efficacy and safety of an extended-release form of niacin in the management of hyperlipidemia. *Am J Cardiol.* 2000;85:1100-1105.

Gray DR, Morgan T, Chretian SD, et al. Efficacy and safety of controlled-release niacin in dyslipoproteinemic veterans. *Ann Intern Med.* 1994;121:252-258.

Guyton JR. Effect of niacin on atherosclerotic cardiovascular disease. *Am J Cardiol.* 1998;82:18U-23U.

Guyton JR. Niacin in cardiovascular prevention: mechanisms, efficacy, and safety. *Curr Opin Lipidol.* 2007;18(4):415-420.

Guyton JR, Blazing MA, Hagar J, et al. Extended-release niacin vs gemfibrozil for the treatment of low levels of high-density lipoprotein cholesterol. Niaspan-Gemfibrozil Study Group. *Arch Int Med.* 2000;160:1177-1184.

Henkin Y, Oberman A, Hurst DC. Niacin revisited: clinical observations on an important but underutilized drug. *Am J Med.* 1991;91:239-246.

Illingworth DR, Stein EA, Mitchel YB, et al. Comparative effects of lovastatin and niacin in primary hypercholesterolemia. *Arch Intern Med.* 1994;154:1586-1595.

Institute of Medicine. Food and Nutrition Board. Dietary Reference Intakes for thiamin, riboflavin, niacin, vitamin B_6, folate, vitamin B_{12}, pantothenic acid, biotin, and choline. Washington, DC: National Academy Press, 1998.

Johansson JO, Egberg N, Asplund-Carlson A, et al. Nicotinic acid treatment shifts the fibrinolytic balance favorably and decreases plasma fibrinogen in hypertriglyceridaemic men. *J Cardiovasc Risk.* 1997;4:165-171.

Kamanna VS, Kashyap ML. Mechanism of action of niacin. *Am J Cardiol.* 2008;101(8A):20B-26B.

Kamanna VS, Kashyap ML. Nicotinic acid (niacin) receptor agonists: will they be useful therapeutic agents? *Am J Cardiol.* 2007;100(11 A):S53-61.

Kamanna VS, Vo A, Kashyap ML. Nicotinic acid: recent developments. *Curr Opin Cardiol.* 2008;23(4):393-398.

King JM, Crouse JR, Terry JG, et al. Evaluation of effects of unmodified niacin on fasting and postprandial plasma lipids in normolipidemic men with hypoalphalipoproteinemia. *Am J Med.* 1994;97:323-331.

Lai E, De Lepeleire I, Crumley TM, et al. Suppression of niacin-induced vasodilation with an antagonist to prostaglandin D2 receptor subtype 1. *Clin Pharmacol Ther.* 2007;81(6):849-857.

Lin S-J, Defossez P-A, Guarente L. Requirement of NAD and SIR2 for life-span extension by calorie restriction in *Saccharomyces cerevisiae. Science.* 2000;289:2126-2128.

McKenney JM, Proctor JD, Harris S, et al. A comparison of the efficacy and toxic effects of sustained-vs immediate-release niacin in hypercholesterolemic patients. *JAMA.* 1994;271:672-677.

Rader JI, Calvert RJ, Hathcock JN. Hepatic toxicity of unmodified and time-release preparations of niacin. *Am J Med.* 1992;92:77-81.

Saareks V, Mucha I, Sievi E, et al. Nicotinic acid and pyridoxine modulate arachidonic acid metabolism in vitro and ex vivo in man. *Pharmacol Toxicol.* 1999;84:274-280.

Tato F, Vega GL, Grundy SM. Effects of crystalline nicotinic acid-induced hepatic dysfunction on serum low-density lipoprotein cholesterol and lecithin cholesteryl acyl transferase. *Am J Cardiology.* 1998;81:805-807.

Taylor AJ, Sullenberger LE, Lee HJ, et al. Arterial Biology for the Investigation of the Treatment Effects of Reducing Cholesterol (ARBITER) 2: a double-blind, placebo-controlled study of extended-release niacin on atherosclerosis progression in secondary prevention patients treated with statins. *Circulation.* 2004;110(23):3512-3517.

Trueblood NA, Ramasamy R, Wang LF, et al. Niacin protects the isolated heart from ischemia-reperfusion injury. *Am J Physiol Heart Circ Physiol.* 2000;279:H764-H771.

Tsalamandris C, Panagiotopoulos S, Sinha A, et al. Complementary effects of pravastatin and nicotinic acid in the treatment of combined hyperlipidaemia in diabetic and non-diabetic patients. *J Cardiovasc Risk.* 1994;1:231-239.

Vispé S, Yung TMC, Ritchot J, et al. A cellular defense pathway regulating transcription through poly(ADP-ribosyl)ation in response to DNA damage. *Proc Natl Acad Sci USA.* 2000;97:9886-9891.

Wang W, Basinger A, Neese RA, et al. Effects of nicotinic acid on fatty acid kinetics, fuel selection, and pathways of glucose production in women. *Am J Physiol Endocrinol Metab.* 2000;279:E50-E59.

Zhang LH, Kamanna VS, Zhang MC, et al. Niacin inhibits surface expression of ATP synthase beta chain in HepG2 cells: implications for raising HDL. *J Lipid Res.* 2008;49(6):1195-1201.

Ziegler M. New Functions of a long-known molecule. Emerging roles of NAD in cellular signaling. *Eur J Biochem.* 2000;267:1550-1564.

Nickel

DESCRIPTION

Nickel is a hard, malleable and ductile metal with atomic number 28 and symbol Ni. It occurs in igneous rock and as a free metal and, together with iron, it is a component of the earth's core. Nickel also occurs in living organisms, mainly in plants.

Nickel is not currently considered an essential nutrient for humans. Nickel deficiency states have been reported in some animals. Rats and goats fed nickel-deficient diets have depressed growth, reproductive performance and plasma glucose, as well as abnormalities in mineral status. Nickel is conjectured to play a role in processes related to the vitamin B$_{12}$-and folic acid-dependent pathway in methione metabolism.

The major dietary source of nickel is plant foods. Nickel-rich food items include nuts, beans, peas, grains and chocolate. Animal foods are low in nickel. Total daily dietary intakes of nickel vary depending on the amount of plant and animal foods consumed. Diets high in plant foods, such as the ones listed above, supply about 900 micrograms daily of nickel. Nickel intake in the United States ranges from 69 to 162 micrograms daily. A daily dietary requirement of 25 to 35 micrograms has been suggested.

Nickel allergies are not uncommon and usually manifested as hand eczema. The results of one open, prospective trial suggested that low-nickel diets may benefit some nickel-sensitive individuals.

ACTIONS AND PHARMACOLOGY

ACTIONS

The actions of dietary nickel are not known.

PHARMACOKINETICS

Little is known about the pharmacokinetics of dietary nickel in humans. Apparently nickel is poorly absorbed when ingested in typical diets. The mechanism of absorption is unclear. Following absorption, nickel is transported in blood bound to serum albumin. Nickel is not significantly accumulated by any tissue in the body, although the thyroid and adrenal glands have relatively high nickel concentrations compared with other tissues. Most of the absorbed nickel is excreted by the kidney as low-molecular weight complexes. Nickel is also lost in sweat and bile.

INDICATIONS AND USAGE

There is no indication for the use of supplemental nickel.

RESEARCH SUMMARY

Though decreased levels of nickel have been reported in some conditions, there is no evidence that supplemental nickel is of any benefit in any of these conditions.

CONTRAINDICATIONS, PRECAUTIONS, ADVERSE REACTIONS

CONTRAINDICATIONS

Known hypersensitivity to a nickel-containing product.

PRECAUTIONS

Those with nickel-sensitivity should avoid nickel supplementation.

ADVERSE REACTIONS

None known.

DOSAGE AND ADMINISTRATION

No recommendation.

Nickel is available in some multivitamin preparations, typically at a dose of about 5 micrograms. Nickel may also be present in colloidal or liquid mineral supplements.

In NHANES III, the adult median intake of nickel from supplements was approximately 5 micrograms/day.

Except for tolerable upper intake levels (UL—see table below), no DRI (dietary reference intake) has yet been established for nickel.

The Food and Nutrition Board of the U.S. National Academy of Sciences has published the following Dietary Reference Intakes (DRI) for nickel. A summary of DRIs for various age groups is as follows:

DRI values (milligrams/day)

	UL
Infants	
0-6 months	ND
7-12 months	ND
Children	
1-3 years	0.2
4-8 years	0.3
Boys	
9-13 years	0.6
14-18 years	1.0
Girls	
9-13 years	0.6
14-18 years	1.0
Men	
19-30 years	1.0
31-50 years	1.0
51-70 years	1.0
Older than 70 years	1.0
Women	
19-30 years	1.0
31-50 years	1.0
51-70 years	1.0
Older than 70 years	1.0
Pregnancy	
14-18 years	1.0
19-30 years	1.0
31-50 years	1.0
Lactation	
14-18 years	1.0
19-30 years	1.0
31-50 years	1.0

ND = Not Determinable. The value is not determinable because of the lack of data on adverse effects in this age group and concern regarding the lack of ability to handle excess amounts. To prevent high levels of intake, the only source of nickel for infants should be from food and formula.

There are no Recommended Dietary Allowances (RDA), Estimated Average Requirements (EAR) or Adequate Intake levels established for nickel.

The UL is the Tolerable Upper Intake Level and usually represents the total intake from food, water and supplements.

LITERATURE

Institute of Medicine, Food and Nutrition Board. Dietary Reference Intakes for vitamin A, vitamin K, arsenic, boron, chromium, copper, iodine, iron, manganese, molybdenum, nickel, silicon, vanadium, and zinc. Washington, DC: National Academy Press, 2001.

Nielsen FH. Ultratrace minerals. In: Shils ME, Olson JA, Shike M, Ross AC, eds. *Modern Nutrition in Health and Disease*. 9th ed. Baltimore MD: Williams and Wilkins; 1999;283-303.

Uthus EO, Poellot RA. Dietary nickel and folic acid interact to affect folate and methionine metabolism in the rat. *Biol Trace Elem Res.* 1997;58:25-33.

Veien NK, Hattel T, Laurberg G. Low nickel diet: an open prospective trial. *J Am Acad Dermatol.* 1993;29:1001-1007.

Nicotinamide

DESCRIPTION

Nicotinamide (niacinamide) is one of the two principal forms of the B-complex vitamin niacin (see Niacin). The term niacin is used as a collective term to refer to both nicotinamide and nicotinic acid, the other principal form of niacin, or the term is used synonymously with nicotinic acid. Nicotinamide and nicotinic acid have identical vitamin activities, but they have very different pharmacological activities.

Nicotinamide, via its major metabolite NAD^+ (nicotinamide adenine dinucleotide), is involved in a wide range of biological processes, including the production of energy, the synthesis of fatty acids, cholesterol and steroids, signal transduction and the maintenance of the integrity of the genome. Nicotinic acid, in pharmacological doses, is used as an antihyperlipidemic agent. It also causes vasodilation of cutaneous blood vessels resulting in the so-called niacin flush. Nicotinamide in pharmacological doses does not have antihyperlipidemic activity, nor does it cause a niacin-flush. There is evidence, however, that pharmacological doses of nicotinamide may prevent type 1 diabetes mellitus. And, interestingly, pyrazinamide, an important drug in the treatment of tuberculosis, is an analogue of and shares the same biochemical mechanism with nicotinamide.

Nicotinamide, in addition to being known as niacinamide, is also known as 3-pyridinecarboxamide, pyridine-3-carboxamide, nicotinic acid amide, vitamin B_3 and vitamin PP. Its molecular formula is $C_6H_6N_2O$ and its molecular weight is 122.13 daltons and the structural formula is:

Nicotinamide

Nicotinamide is the principal form of niacin used in nutritional supplements and in food fortification. See also Niacin (Nicotinic Acid).

ACTIONS AND PHARMACOLOGY

ACTIONS

Nicotinamide may have anti-diabetogenic activity in some. It may also have antioxidant, anti-inflammatory and anticarcinogenic activities. Nicotinamide has putative activity against osteoarthritis and granuloma annulare.

MECHANISM OF ACTION

Nicotinamide is being investigated as an agent for the possible prevention or delaying of the onset of type 1 diabetes mellitus (insulin-dependent diabetes mellitus or IDDM). The rationale for using nicotinamide to prevent type 1 diabetes mellitus is derived from human and animal studies as well as *in vitro* investigations. Nicotinamide has been found to prevent diabetes in alloxan- and streptozotocin-treated mice and rats and in non-obese diabetic (NOD) mice. *In vitro* studies have shown that nicotinamide can prevent macrophage- or interleukin-1beta-induced beta-cell damage. An intervention study in New Zealand using nicotinamide treatment showed a 50% reduction in the development of IDDM over a five-year period.

The mechanism of the possible anti-diabetogenic activity of nicotinamide is not well understood. The pathogenesis of IDDM involves the autoimmune destruction of beta-cells, which is accompanied by the appearance of beta-cell specific antibodies, such as islet cell antibodies (ICA) and antibodies to glutamic acid decarboxylase (GAD), many years before the onset of the disease. Macrophages and T lymphocytes are the first cells to appear in the islets of the pancreas during the development of autoimmune diabetes. It is thought that cytokines released by macrophages/monocytes, such as interleukin (IL)-12 and tumor necrosis factor (TNF)-alpha, might play a role in early beta-cell damage. IL-12 may play a role in the initiation of the autoimmune process by enhancing T helper 1 lymphocyte (Th1) responses. Nicotinamide has been shown to decrease the production of IL-12 and TNF-alpha in cultures of whole blood from prediabetic and diabetic subjects and also in healthy controls. Inhibition of IL-12 production by nicotinamide could play an important role in the modulation of the immune response leading to IDDM. Further, since the cytokine-inhibitory activity was observed in healthy controls, as well as in prediabetic and diabetic subjects, nicotinamide may have application in other autoimmune disorders.

Nicotinamide has been demonstrated, in one study, to affect glucose tolerance and insulitis in NOD mice, slowing down diabetes progression. In this study, nicotinamide decreased MHC class II expression (but not MHC class I), enhanced intercellular adhesion molecule-1 (ICAM-1) expression, counteracted the fall of superoxide dismutase (observed in untreated NOD mice) and increased the levels of interleukin (IL)-4, a T helper 2 lymphocyte (Th2) protective cytokine.

The anti-diabetogenic effect of nicotinamide may be due, in part, to an increase in the pool size of NAD+ in beta-cells. NAD+ is the principal metabolite of nicotinamide. It appears that the pool size of NAD+ in beta-cells in pre-diabetics and diabetics is significantly reduced. Damage and destruction of beta-cells may occur via oxidative stress. Increased levels of reactive oxygen species in beta-cells may result in, among other things, oxidative damage to DNA resulting in DNA strand breaks. The enzyme poly(ADP-ribose)polymerase or PARP is believed to play a role in DNA repair. PARP uses NAD+ as its substrate. In the context of a reduced level of NAD+, PARP activity may essentially use most of the cellular NAD+. This could result in cellular apoptosis. Nicotinamide is an inhibitor of PARP. It also has antioxidant activity and, of course, is metabolized to NAD+. All of these effects may play some role in the possible anti-diabetogenic action of nicotinamide.

Nicotinamide has been shown to have antioxidant activity. *In vitro*, it has been found to inhibit protein oxidation and lipid peroxidation. It has also been found to inhibit reactive oxygen species-induced apoptosis, to inhibit phagocytic generation of reactive oxygen species, to scavenge reactive oxygen species and to inhibit the oxidative activity of nitric oxide.

Nicotinamide has demonstrated a number of anti-inflammatory activities. Nicotinamide has been shown to inhibit lipopolysaccharide-induced TNF-alpha in the mouse, in a dose-dependent manner. It is thought that this inhibition of

TNF-alpha is mediated via inhibition, at the gene transcription level, of NF-Kappa B, which in turn inhibits TNF-alpha. Nicotinamide has also been shown to decrease the production of IL-12 and TNF-alpha in cultures of whole blood from prediabetic and diabetic subjects and also in healthy subjects.

Niacin deficiency has been found to inhibit DNA repair in cell culture models. NAD+ is the substrate for PARP, an enzyme thought to be involved in DNA repair. Extensive damage to DNA may result in depletion of NAD+ secondary to its use by PARP. Depletion of NAD+ may trigger cellular apoptosis. DNA repair by PARP, as well as its possible role in apoptosis, may contribute to protection against carcinogenesis. These mechanisms may account, in part, for the possible anticarcinogenic activity of nicotinamide. Nicotinamide, via NAD+, modulates the expression of the p53 tumor suppressor protein in human breast, lung, skin and lung cells. This is another mechanism for nicotinamide's possible anticarcinogenic activity.

A pilot study suggests that nicotinamide may be beneficial in some with osteoarthritis. The mechanism of this putative activity is unknown. The mechanism of the putative activity of nicotinamide in granuloma annulare is also unknown.

PHARMACOKINETICS

Nicotinamide is efficiently absorbed from the gastrointestinal tract. At low doses, absorption is mediated via sodium-dependent facilitated diffusion. Passive diffusion is the principal mechanism of absorption at higher doses. Doses of up to three to four grams of nicotinamide are almost completely absorbed. Nicotinamide is transported via the portal circulation to the liver and via the systemic circulation to the various tissues of the body. Nicotinamide enters most cells by passive diffusion and enters erythrocytes by facilitated transport.

Nicotinamide is metabolized to NAD+ which in turn has a number of metabolic opportunities, including the formation of nicotinamide, NADP+ (nicotinamide adenine dinucleotide phosphate), NMN (nicotinamide 5'-mononucleotide), cyclic ADP-ribose and NAADP (nicotinic acid dinucleotide phosphate). NAD+ also serves as the substrate for mono(ADP-ribosyl)ation and poly(ADP-ribosyl)ation. Poly(ADP-ribosyl)ation is catalyzed by PARP. Nicotinamide may be converted to nicotinic acid via the enzyme nicotinamidase.

In the liver, the principal catabolic products of high-dose nicotinamide are N'-methylnicotinamide, N'-methyl-5-carboxamide-2-pyridone, N'-methyl-5-carboxamide-4-pyridone and nicotinamide-N-oxide. High-dose nicotinamide is excreted in the urine as unchanged nicotinamide, N'-methylnicotinamide, N'-methyl-5-carboxamide-2-pyridone, N'-methyl-5-carboxamide-4-pyridone and nicotinamide-N-oxide.

INDICATIONS AND USAGE

Nicotinamide, unlike nicotinic acid (niacin), does not have significant effects on lipids, and its efficacy in diabetes is unclear. It demonstrates antiinflammatory properties, and it is emerging as a possible potent neuroprotective agent. It may also be an effective depigmenter in some with skin hyperpigmentation. It was recently shown to suppress hyperphosphatemia in hemodialysis patients. There is preliminary evidence it might help some with generalized granuloma annulare and osteoarthritis, but little evidence that it is helpful in rheumatoid arthritis or schizophrenia. There is a suggestion that it might aid in some cancer therapies. There is little evidence that it is useful in tinnitus.

RESEARCH SUMMARY

Nicotinamide was shown to protect the non-obese diabetic (NOD) mouse from type 1 (IDDM) diabetes if given early enough and at high enough doses. It was hoped that nicotinamide might similarly intervene in human type 1 diabetes as evidenced, among other things, by its observed ability to protect isolated islets of Langerhans *in vitro* from various toxic agents. *In vitro* experiments also showed that nicotinamide could reduce beta cell impairment and death caused by macrophages and exposure to various cytokines involved in this autoimmune disease.

Since nicotinamide has not been shown to have significant, prolonged effects when introduced after the onset of type 1 diabetes, its efficacy has been researched as an interventive therapy. It shows some ability to extend the remission phase when administered to subjects newly diagnosed with the disease. During the remission phase, the need for exogenous insulin is decreased or obliterated, but insulin-dependence reasserts itself, usually within one year despite nicotinamide supplementation. On the other hand, nicotinamide appears to be far more effective as a preventive.

In one 5-year intervention study, nicotinamide was administered prior to the clinical onset of IDDM. Using antibody markers that predict the onset of IDDM within 5 years, 150 young subjects were selected to receive nicotinamide at a dose of 1.2 grams per square meter of body surface area daily. It was concluded that nicotinamide supplementation reduced the expected incidence of IDDM 50% over a 5-year period. After all this positive news, it was hoped that nicotinamide might continue to show benefit in a larger, better-controlled study of type 1 (insulin-dependent) diabetes. However, high-dose nicotinamide has now failed to provide protection in a double-blind, placebo-controlled, randomized trial in individuals with a first-degree family history of type-1 diabetes. This five-year study involved 552 individuals. Of 159 participants who developed diabetes during the study period, 82 were taking nicotinamide and 77 were receiving placebo. With this result, nicotinamide's future as a significant therapy in type 1 diabetes is in doubt.

There is one recent single-blind, placebo-controlled study indicating that nicotinamide improves insulin secretion and metabolic control in lean type 2 diabetic patients with secondary failure to sulfonylureas. Follow-up is needed.

Recently nicotinamide reversed neurological and neurovascular deficits in streptozotocin diabetic rats, leading the researchers to conclude that nicotinamide "deserves consideration as an attractive, nontoxic therapy for the treatment of diabetic peripheral neuropathy." Other research adds further evidence that nicotinamide may be a significant neuroprotectant in a number of contexts. High-dose nicotinamide prevented oxidative mitochondrial dysfunction in a cellular model and improved motor deficit in a *Drosphilia* model of Parkinson's disease. It has also shown to have a broad range of neuroprotective effects in some mouse models of chemically induced Parkinsonism. In still other tests, nicotinamide has exerted protective effects in animal models of traumatic brain injury and ischemia, including reduced infarct size and improved functional recovery. Acute neuroprotection and edema reductions were achieved in one such recent study. A number of acute pathophysiological processes were said to be favorably modulated by nicotinamide in this study, indicating, among other things, that the agent can inhibit cortical neuronal death.

In another recent study, nicotinamide demonstrated potent antiinflammatory activity, inhibiting various proinflammatory cytokines. These *in vitro* results encouraged the researchers to speculate that nicotinamide might have some future role in the treatment of human inflammatory diseases.

Nicotinamide suppressed hyperphosphatemia in hemodialysis patients. Hyperphosphatemia is a considerable problem in hemodialysis, and the available remedies are often toxic in the long term. Thus, the observation that nicotinamide inhibits sodium-dependent phosphate transport in rat renal tubule and small intestine encouraged researchers to recently examine whether nicotinamide could reduce serum levels of phosphorous and intact parathyroid hormone in patients undergoing hemodialysis. Mean dose of nicotinamide in this study was 1,080 milligrams per day for 12 weeks. Beneficial effects were sufficient for the researchers to conclude: "Nicotinamide may provide an alternative for controlling hyperphosphatemia and hyperparathyroidism without inducing hypercalcemia in hemodialysis patients."

Also recently, researchers reported that a niacinamide (nicotinamide) moisturizing cream reduced facial hyperpigmentation compared with a control vehicle, in Asian women. A significant lightening of skin was noted after four weeks of treatment and was attributed to an inhibition of melano-

some transfer from melanocytes to keratinocytes. More research is needed to further explore this finding. There is a case study showing pronounced improvement in a patient with generalized granuloma annulare treated with high-dose (1,500 milligrams daily) niacinamide for six months. This patient's disease had previously resisted treatment with topical adrenal steroids, oral erythromycin and oral zinc.

A recent double-blind, placebo-controlled, pilot study examined the effect of nicotinamide in subjects with osteoarthritis. In the study, 72 subjects with osteoarthritis were randomly assigned to receive nicotinamide (500 milligrams six times per day) or placebo. The study lasted 12 weeks. Subjects who received nicotinamide reduced their non-steroidal anti-inflammatory (NSAID) medication by 13% compared with those in the placebo group. Pain levels were no different in the two groups. Nicotinamide reduced the sedimentation rate by 22% and increased joint mobility by 22% over controls. Follow-up is needed.

Some preliminary evidence suggests that nicotinamide may increase the irradiation response of experimental tumors. More research is needed in this area.

Nicotinamide produced effects no better than placebo when used in a double-blind trial involving 48 subjects with tinnitus.

CONTRAINDICATIONS, PRECAUTIONS, ADVERSE REACTIONS

CONTRAINDICATIONS

Nicotinamide is contraindicated in those hypersensitive to any component of a nicotinamide-containing preparation.

High-dose nicotinamide (doses greater than 500 milligrams/day) is contraindicated in those with liver disease and in those with active peptic ulcer disease.

PRECAUTIONS

Pregnant women and nursing mothers should avoid supplemental doses of nicotinamide greater than the U.S. RDA (20 milligrams/day), unless higher doses are prescribed by their physicians.

The use of nicotinamide for any medical indication requires medical supervision.

Those with a history of peptic ulcer disease, gastritis, liver disease, gallbladder disease, diabetes and gout, should exercise caution in the use of high-dose nicotinamide.

ADVERSE REACTIONS

In contrast to nicotinic acid, nicotinamide does not cause flushing and has only very rarely been associated with diabetogenic effects. There are rare reports of elevations in liver tests and liver damage, including jaundice and parenchymal liver cell injury. These reports were in those using very high doses of nicotinamide (10 grams or greater, daily).

Adverse reactions in those using high-dose nicotinamide, include nausea, vomiting, diarrhea, headache and dizziness.

INTERACTIONS

DRUGS

Carbamazepine: Concomitant use of nicotinamide and carbamazepine may decrease carbamazepine clearance.

OVERDOSAGE

Nicotinamide overdosage is not reported in the literature.

DOSAGE AND ADMINISTRATION

Nicotinamide is the form of niacin which is typically used for nutritional supplementation. It is also the form of niacin used in food fortification. It is available as a single ingredient product (immediate-release and sustained-release) and in multivitamin and multivitamin/multimineral products. Typical supplemental dosage ranges from 20 to 100 milligrams daily. Pre- and postnatal vitamin/mineral supplements typically deliver a dose of 20 milligrams daily.

LITERATURE

Akabane A, Kato I, Takasawa S, et al. Nicotinamide inhibits IRF-1mRNA induction and prevents IL-1 beta-induced nitric oxide synthase expression in pancreatic beta cells. *Biochem Biophys Res Commun.* 1995;215:524-530.

Anderson DW, Bradbury KA, Schneider JS. Broad neuroprotective profile of nicotinamide in different mouse models of MPTP-induced parkinsonism. *Eur J Neurosci.* 2008;28(3):610-617.

Behme MT. Nicotinamide and diabetes prevention. *Nutr Rev.* 1995;53:137-139.

Boyonoski AC, Gallacher LM, ApSimon MM, et al. Niacin deficiency increases the sensitivity of rats to the short and long term effects of ethylnitrosourea treatment. *Mol Cellular Biochem.* 1999;193:83-87.

Chaplin DJ, Horsman MR, Trotter MJ. Effect of nicotinamide on the microregional hetereogeneity of oxygen delivery within a murine tumor. *J Natl Cancer Inst.* 1990;82:672-676.

Crowley CL, Payne CM, Bernstein H, et al. The NAD+ precursors, nicotinic acid and nicotinamide protect cells against apoptosis induced by a multiple stress inducer, deoxycholate. *Cell Death Differ.* 2000;7:314-326.

Elliott RB, Pilcher CC, Stewart A, et al. The use of nicotinamide in the prevention of type 1 diabetes. *Ann NY Acad Sci.* 1993;696:333-341.

Gale EA. Molecular mechanisms of beta-cell destruction in IDDM: the role of nicotinamide. *Horm Res.* 1996;45 Suppl:39-43.

Gale EA, Bingley PJ, Emmett CL, et al. European Nicotinamide Diabetes Intervention Trial (ENDIT) Group. European Nicotinamide Diabetes Intervention Trial (ENDIT): a randomized controlled trial of intervention before the onset of type 1 diabetes. *Lancet.* 2004;363(9413):925-931.

Greenbaum CJ, Kahn SE, Palmer JP. Nicotinamide's effect on glucose metabolism in subjects at risk for IDDM. *Diabetes.* 1996;45:1631-1634.

Hakozaki T, Minwalla L, Zhuang J, et al. The effect of niacinamide on reducing cutaneous pigmentation and suppression of melanosome transfer. *Br J Dermatol.* 2002;147(1):20-31.

Hiromatsu Y, Yang D, Miyake I, et al. Nicotinamide decreases cytokine-induced activation of orbital fibroblasts from patients with thyroid-associated ophthalmopathy. *J Clin Endocrinol Metab.* 1998;83:121-124.

Hoane MR, Kaplan SA, Ellis AL. The effects of nicotinamide on apoptosis and blood-brain barrier breakdown following traumatic brain injury. Brain Res. 2006;1125(1):185-193.

Hoane MR, Pierce JL, Holland MA, et al. Nicotinamide treatment induces behavioral recovery when administered up to 4 hours following cortical contusion injury in the rat. *Neuroscience.* 2008;154(3):861-868.

Hoane MR, Tan AA, Pierce JL, et al. Nicotinamide treatment reduces behavioral impairments and provides cortical protection after fluid percussion injury in the rat. *J Neurotrauma.* 2006;23(10):1535-1548.

Holland MA, Tan AA, Smith DC, et al. Nicotinamide treatment provides acute neuroprotection and GFAP regulation following fluid percussion injury. *J Neurotrauma.* 2008;25(2):140-152.

Hoorens A, Pipeleers D. Nicotinamide protects human beta cells against chemically-induced necrosis, but not against cytokine-induced apoptosis. *Diabetologia.* 1999;42:55-59.

Jacobson EL, Shieh WM, Huang AC. Mapping the role of NAD metabolism in prevention and treatment of carcinogenesis. *Mol Cellular Biochem.* 1999;193:69-74.

Jia H, Li X, Gao H, et al. High doses of nicotinamide prevent oxidative mitochondrial dysfunction in a cellular model and improve motor deficit in a Drosophila model of Parkinson's disease. *J Neurosci Res.* 2008;86(9):2083-2090.

Jonas WB, Rapoza CP, Blair WF. The effect of niacinamide on osteoarthritis: a pilot study. *Inflamm Res.* 1996;45:330-334.

Kamat JP, Devasagayam TP. Nicotinamide (vitamin B3) as an effective antioxidant against oxidative damage in rat brain mitochondria. *Redox Rep.* 1999;4:179-184.

Klaidman LK, Mukherjee SK, Hutchin TP, Adams JD. Nicotinamide as a precursor for NAD+ prevents apoptosis in the mouse brain induced by tertiary-butylhydroperoxide. *Neurosci Lett.* 1996;206:5-8.

Kolb H, Burkart V. Nicotinamide in type 1 diabetes. Mechanism of action revisited. *Diabetes Care.* 1999;22 Supp 2:B16-B20.

Kretowski A, Myliwiec J, Szelachowaska M, et al. Nicotinamide inhibits enhanced *in vitro* production of interleukin-12 and tumor necrosis factor-alpha in peripheral whole blood of people at high risk of developing Type 1 diabetes and people with newly diagnosed Type 1 diabetes. *Diabetes Res Clin Pract.* 2000;47:81-86.

Kroger H, Hauschild A, Ohde M, et al. Nicotinamide and methionine reduce the liver toxic effect of methotrexate. *Gen Pharmacol.* 1999;33:203-206.

Lewis CM, Canafax DM, Sprafka JM, Barbosa JJ. Double-blind randomized trial of nicotinamide on early-onset diabetes. *Diabetes Care.* 1992;15:121-123.

Ma A, Medenica M. Response of generalized granuloma annulare to high-dose niacinamide. *Arch Dermatol.* 1983;119:836-839.

McCarty MF, Russell AL. Niacinamide therapy for osteoarthritis—does it inhibit nitric oxide synthase induction by interleukin 1 in chondrocytes? *Med Hypotheses.* 1999;53:350-360.

Melo SS, Arantes MR, Meirelles MS, et al. Lipid peroxidation in nicotinamide-deficient and nicotinamide-supplemented rats with streptozotocin-induced diabetes. *Acta Diabetol.* 2000;37:33-39.

Miesel R, Kurpisz M, Kroger H. Modulation of inflammatory arthritis by inhibition of poly(ADPribose)polymerase. *Inflammation.* 1995;19:379-387.

Olsson AR, Sheng Y, Pero RW, et al. DNA damage and repair in tumour and non-tumour tissues. *Br J Cancer.* 1996;74:368-373.

Papaccio G, Ammendola E, Pisanti FA. Nicotinamide decreases MHC class II but not MHC class I expression and increases intercellular adhesion molecule-1 structures in non-obese diabetic mouse pancreas. *J Endocrinol.* 1999;160:389-400.

Pero RW, Axelsson B, Siemann D, et al. Newly discovered anti-inflammatory properties of the benzamides and nicotinamides. *Mol Cellular Biochem.* 1999;193:119-125.

Petley A, Macklin B, Renwick AG, Wilkin TJ. The pharmacokinetics of nicotinamide in humans and rodents. *Diabetes.* 1995;44:152-155.

Polo V, Saibene A, Portiroli AE. Nicotinamide improves insulin secretion and metabolic control in lean type 2 diabetic patients with secondary failure to sulphonylureas. *Acta Diabetol.* 1998;35:61-64.

Pozzilli P, Browne PD, Kolb H. Meta-analysis of nicotinamide treatment in patients with recent-onset IDDM. The Nicotinamide Trialists. *Diabetes Care.* 1996;19:1357-1363.

Stevens MJ, Li F, Drel VR, et al. Nicotinamide reverses neurological and neurovascular deficits in streptozotocin diabetic rats. *J Pharmacol Exp Ther.* 2007;320(1):458-464.

Takahashi Y, Tanaka A, Nakamura T, et al. Nicotinamide suppresses hyperphosphatemia in hemodialysis patients. *Kidney Int.* 2004;65(3):1099-1104.

Ungerstedt JS, Blömback M, Söderström T. Nicotinamide is a potent inhibitor of proinflammatory cytokines. *Clin Exp Immunol.* 2003;131(1):48-52.

Vidal J, Fernandez-Balsells M, Sesmilo G, et al. Effects of nicotinamide and intravenous insulin therapy in newly diagnosed type 1 diabetes. *Diabetes Care.* 2000;23:360-364.

Wan FJ, Lin HC, Kang BH, et al. D-amphetamine-induced depletion of energy and dopamine in the rat striatum is attenuated by nicotinamide pretreatment. *Brain Res Bull.* 1999;50:167-191.

Zimhony O, Cox JS, Welch JT, et al. Pyrazinamide inhibits the eukaryotic-like fatty acid synthetase I (FASI) of *Mycobacterium tuberculosis. Nature Med.* 2000;6:1043-1047.

Nobiletin

DESCRIPTION

Nobiletin is a member of the polymethoxyflavone family of flavones. Flavones themselves comprise a subclass of the large class of plant substances, the flavonoids. Polymethoxylated flavones (PMFs) exist almost exclusively in the *Citrus* genus, particularly in the peels and tissues of sweet oranges (*Citrus sinensis*), the peels and tissues of bitter oranges (*Citrus aurantium* L.) and, especially, the peels and tissues of tangerines (*Citrus reticulata* Blanco), including Dancy and Cleopatra tangerines and clementines. The two most common PMFs found in citrus peels are nobiletin and tangeretin (see Tangeretin). Sinensetin is the third most common PMF found in the peels and tissues of citrus fruits.

Nobiletin, like other flavonoids, is a plant secondary metabolite. Plant secondary metabolites comprise the defense system of plants against fungi, predators and pests, among other things. Mal seco is a fungal disease of citrus varieties, mainly lemons, caused by the pathogenic fungus *Deuterophoma tracheiphila* (or *Phoma tracheiphila)* and is widespread throughout the Mediterranean region. There is almost no nobiletin in lemons. Nobiletin, when inoculated in lemon seedlings infected with the mal seco fungus, was demonstrated to have strong fungistatic activity. Tangeretin was found to be weakly active. Nobiletin-containing citrus fruits are quite resistant to mal seco. Lemons (*Citrus limon*) and grapefruits (*Citrus paradisi*) are virtually devoid of nobiletin and other PMFs.

Recently, there has been great interest in studying nobiletin for its possible anti-inflammatory, anticarcinogenic, antiatherogenic and neuroprotective activities. It turns out that nobiletin and other PMFs appear to have greater oral bioavailability than their polyphenolic cousins.

Nobiletin is chemically described as 5,6,7,8-tetramethoxy-2-(3,4-dimethoxyphenyl)-4H-1-benzopyran-4-one. Nobiletin is also known as 3′,4′,5,6,7,8-hexamethoxyflavone, and 5,6,7,8,3′,4′-hexamethoxyflavone. Its empirical formula is $C_{21}H_{22}O_8$ and its molecular weight is 402,39. The chemical structures below are described within this monograph.

Nobiletin

Flavone Skeleton

Flavonoid Skeleton

All flavonoids possess a basic 15-carbon skeleton that can be represented as C_6-C_3-C_6 (see figure). The common structure is that of a diphenylpropane molecule, consisting of two aromatic rings linked through the three carbons. Flavonoids differ in the saturation of the heteroatomic ring C, in the placement of the aromatic ring B at positions C-2 or C-3 of ring C and in the overall hydroxylation or methoxylation patterns. The polymethoxylated flavones have a benzo-gamma-pyrone skeleton with a carbonyl group at the C-3 position and methoxy groups in different positions on the benzo-gamma-pyrone skeleton. Polymethoxylated flavones (PMFs) typically do not possess free phenolic hydroxyl groups in their native structures (plants). And, in contrast to polyphenolic flavonoids that exist in their native states (in plants) as glycones, PMFs are typically aglycones in their native states.

ACTIONS AND PHARMACOLOGY

ACTIONS

Nobiletin has antifungal activity, particularly against the citrus pathogenic fungus *Deuterophoma tracheiphilia,* or *Phoma tracheiphila*. Nobiletin may have antiarthritic, antiatherogenic, anticarcinogenic, anti-inflammatory/immuno-modulatory, neuroprotective, and cognitive-enhancing activities.

MECHANISM OF ACTION

Antiarthritic activity: In addition to the inflammatory processes that take place in the various arthritic disorders, there are other degenerative changes that lead to articular cartilage destruction.

The extracellular matrix in cartilage is mainly composed of type II cartilage, hyaluronic acid and aggrecan, a large aggregating proteoglycan. The loss of aggrecan in the matrix occurs early in the destruction of articular cartilage. This results in the disruption of the structural and functional integrity of cartilage. The enzymes aggrecanase-1 and aggrecanase-2 appear to play major roles in cartilage destruction in arthritic disorders. Nobiletin was shown to interfere with the IL(interleukin)-1beta-mediated aggrecanase-1 and aggrecanase-2 expression in cultured human synovial fibroblasts. And, in collagen-induced arthritic mice, nobiletin was found to suppress aggrecanase-1 and aggrecanase-2 mRNA expression in joint tissue, and to effectively inhibit aggrecanase-mediated degradation of aggrecan in cartilage, preventing cartilage destruction.

Antiatherogenic: Citrus polymethoxylated flavones, especially tangeretin, were found to significantly lower total cholesterol and LDL-cholesterol in hamsters. The mechanism of this putative lipid-lowering effect is unclear.

Unregulated uptake of oxidized low-density lipoproteins (ox-LDL), as well as modified LDL by macrophage scavenger receptors, are thought to be key events in the pathogenesis of atherosclerosis. The uptake of ox-LDL into the macrophage leads to their conversion to foam cells, a precursor to atheromas. Also, LDL modified by acetylation (acetyl-LDL) can be taken up by macrophage scavenger receptors into macrophages, where it undergoes oxidation, inducing foam cell formation. Nobiletin was found to inhibit the metabolism of acetylated LDL, suggesting a possible antiatherogenic role for this citrus flavone.

Anticarcinogenic activity: Nobiletin has been reported to induce differentiation of mouse myeloid leukemia cells, to show antiproliferative activity toward a human squamous cell line and to exert antimutagenic activity.

TPA (12,0-tetradecanoylphorbol-13-acetate) is a carcinogen that is known to cause malignant tumors in mouse skin. Nitric oxide (NO) appears to be closely associated with the pathogenesis of epithelial carcinogenesis. NO and superoxide (O_2^-) anions are generated when TPA is applied to human-differentiated promyelocyte HL-60 cells. When topical TPA is applied to ICR mouse skin, inflammatory and premalignant changes occur almost immediately, accompanied by the production of reactive oxygen and reactive nitrogen species. When nobiletin was applied to the mouse skin prior to the application of TPA, it was found to inhibit skin inflammation, oxidative stress and tumor promotion in the skin. The specific mechanism of this anticarcinogenic effect is not completely understood.

Nobiletin might have chemopreventive effects against colon carcinogenesis, partly via regulation of leptin levels.

Adipocytokines, including leptin, adiponectin and tumor necrosis factor–alpha (TNF-alpha), represent a group of adipocyte-secreted proteins that affect the metabolism of lipids and carbohydrates. It is thought that adipocytokines may be involved in the metabolic syndrome, the growing obesity epidemic, and other disorders. Recent studies suggest that some adipocytokines may even significantly influence the proliferation of malignant cells *in vitro*, and, possibly, *in vivo*, as well. When mice were injected with the carcinogen azomethane, the serum leptin levels in these mice were six times higher than in untreated mice. There were no significant differences in the levels of adiponectin, IL-6 or triglycerides. Colon tumors were also found in the mice. However, in mice that received azomethane and then given nobiletin orally, nobiletin was found to abolish colonic malignancy and significantly decreased leptin levels. In an HT-29 colon cancer cell line, nobiletin suppressed the leptin-dependent, but not the leptin-independent proliferation of cancer cells. Further, nobiletin decreased leptin secretion, but not that of adiponectin in differentiated 3T3-L1 mouse adipocytes, thought to be via inactivation of mitogen activated protein/extracellular signaling-regulated kinase (MEK). Thus, it appears that high levels of serum leptin may help promote colon carcinogenesis in mice, while nobiletin may have chemopreventive action against colon carcinogenesis, partly through regulation of leptin levels.

The activation of MEK is well known to be associated with tumor invasion and metastasis. Nobiletin has been shown to inhibit the phosphorylation of MEK, thereby suppressing MMP (matrix metalloproteinase) expression in a tumor-metastasis stimulator, TPA (12,0-tetradecanoylphorbol-13-acetate)-stimulated human fibrosarcoma HT-1080 cells. TPA was found to augment MEK activity in HT-1080 cells. However, the augmented MEK activity was diminished by nobiletin. This decrease was also found to inhibit the phosphorylation of extracellular regulated kinase, or ERK. Nobiletin appears to inhibit MEK activity and decrease the sequential phosphorylation of ERK, thus exhibiting antitumor metastatic activity by suppressing matrix metalloproteinase activity in HT-1080 cells.

Antifungal activity: The antifungal mechanism of action of nobiletin (see Description above) is not entirely clear.

Anti-inflammatory/immunodulatory: Articular cartilage destruction is a common feature in osteoarthritis, rheumatoid arthritis and other arthritic conditions. Matrix metalloproteinases (MMPs) appear to play important roles in the destruction of matrix components in the connective tissue of those with rheumatoid arthritis and osteoarthritis. Proinflammatory

cytokines such as interleukin 1 (IL-1), TNF-alpha and interleukin-6 (IL-6) enhance the synthesis of precursors of MMPs, or proMMPs, and prostaglandin E2 (PGE2) from mesenchymal cells at inflammatory sites.

Nobiletin has been shown to effectively interfere with the production of proMMP-9/progelatinase B in rabbit synovial fibroblasts, to suppress the (IL-1)-induced production of PGE2 in human synovial fibroblasts, to selectively down-regulate COX (cyclooxygenase)-2 but not COX-1 mRNA expression, to interfere with the lipopolysaccharide-induced production of PGE2 and the gene expression of proinflammatory cytokines, including IL-1alpha, IL-2beta, TNF-alpha and IL-6 in a mouse macrophage cell line, to downregulate the IL-2-induced gene expression and production of proMMP-1/procollagenase-1 and pro-MMP-3, or prostromelysin-1, in human synovial fibroblasts, and to upregulate the production of TIMP (tissue inhibitor of metalloproteinases)-1, the endogenous MMP inhibitor. These anti-inflammatory and immunomodulatory actions of nobiletin are similar in several particulars to that of the anti-inflammatory and immunomodulatory corticosteroids. The mechanism of action by which nobiletin suppresses the production of proMMPs while upregulating TIMP-1 production is unclear and further studies are needed and warranted to clarify the mechanism of the anti-inflammatory and immunomodulatory actions of this polymethoxylated flavone.

Asthma is a chronic airway inflammatory disease. The pathophysiology of airway inflammation may involve eosinophilic infiltration (especially if there is an allergic component to the asthma), mucous hypersecretion, epithelial denudation and airway remodeling. This may all be accounted for by the sustained activation of inflammatory cells (eosinophils, lymphocytes, macrophages, basophils and mast cells) and synthesis of proinflammatory mediators and cytokines. Nobiletin was demonstrated to inhibit eosinophilic airway inflammation in asthmatic rats. The mechanism of action of this effect is not clear but may have something to do with the lowering of levels of the chemokine eotaxin, relieving airway inflammation of eosinophils and promoting apoptosis of eosinophils via enhancing expression of fas-RNA. Clearly, more research is needed to understand the anti-inflammatory/antiasthma effect of nobiletin.

The synthesis of proinflammatory mediators is mainly regulated at the level of DNA to RNA transcription via the activity of transcription factors. Arguably, the most important of these is the transcription factor NF-kappaB (nuclear factor-kappaB). NF-kappaB is activated by a number of signals, including oxidative stress, cytokines and bacterial lipopolysaccharides (LPS). Inhibition of the expression of NF-kappaB is a major target in the development of anti-inflammatory substances. Nobiletin has been shown to inhibit LPS-induced NF-kappaB transcriptional activation in mouse macrophages, as well as to inhibit NO and PGE2 production, iNOS (inducible nitric oxide synthase) and CPX-2 protein expression. Significantly, nobiletin was found to inhibit the DNA-binding activity of NF-kappaB and also to inhibit intracellular reactive oxygen species (ROS) production in the cells. ROS are known to regulate the activation of NF-kappaB. The mechanism of this anti-inflammatory action is not entirely clear.

The worst complication of pathogenic bacterial or fungal infection, short of death, is septic shock. In gram-negative bacterial sepsis, lipopolysaccharide (LPS) endotoxin is released from the bacteria and activates monocytes, endothelial cells, and epithelial cells, triggering a massive inflammatory response that is orchestrated by monocytes. In addition, the gram-negative, sepsis procoagulant molecule tissue factor (TF) is inducibly expressed via LPS stimulation by vascular endothelial cells, circulating monocytes, and renal and pulmonary epithelial cells. TF is a membrane glycoprotein that triggers the coagulation cascade/waterfall into motion, leading to a dangerous thrombotic situation.

The human-derived monocytic cell line THP-1, when stimulated with LPS, shows increased expression of both TF protein and mRNA levels. Also, binding of nuclear proteins from LPS-stimulated THP-1 cells to NF-kappaB and the AP (activator protein)-1 transcription factor is increased. Pretreatment with nobiletin leads to inhibition of LPS-induced expression of both TF protein and mRNA levels, as well as reduced binding of NF-kappaB and AP-1 to nuclear proteins. Sp1 (sequence-specific activator protein) is an essential transcription factor for LPS-induced TF expression in THP-1 cells. Nobiletin was demonstrated to prevent LPS-induced TF expression via the inhibition of Sp1, as well as by NF-kappaB and AP-1 activation.

Recently, it was found that some metabolites of nobiletin—3′,4′-didemethylnobiletin and 4′-demethylnobiletin—may have even greater anti-inflammatory activity than nobiletin itself. These metabolites may exert their anti-inflammatory activity by suppressing iNOS and COX-2 gene expression. (See PHARMACOKINETICS below).

Neuroprotective and Cognitive-Enhancing Activities: Alzheimer's disease (AD) is the most dramatic and most serious example of cognitive impairment. It is characterized by progressive decline in cognitive function and is associated with elevated levels of beta-amyloid (Abeta), cleaved from amyloid precursor protein (APP) and amyloid plaques in the brain. In addition, neuroinflammatory activity produced mainly by activation of microglia in the brain also appears to play a major role in the pathogenesis of AD.

Long-term potentiation (LTP) is the long-lasting enhancement in communication between two neurons that results from stimulating them simultaneously. An enormous effort has been made to understand the mechanism by which strengthening of synaptic connections can be achieved, and in this effort, the importance of LTP cannot be overestimated. Since neurons communicate by chemical synapses, LTP and its opposite process, long-term depression, are arguably the major cellular mechanisms that underlie learning and memory. LTP is dependent on a cascade of cellular signaling events that are stimulated by an increase in cAMP (cyclic adenosine monophosphate) concentrations. These events include activation of PKA (protein kinase A), which leads to the activation of ERK (extracellular signal-regulated kinase) and, ultimately, to the activation of transcription factors such as CREB (cAMP response element-binding protein) and translation into proteins. cAMP and PKA activation is enhanced after induction of LTP.

Nobiletin has been found to enhance PKA/ERK/CREB signaling in cell cultures, including cultured rat hippocampal neurons. It has also been shown to induce LTP via the activation of PKA-dependent phosphorylation of the AMPA (alpha-amino-3-hydroxy-5-methyl-4-isoxazolepropionic acid) receptor subunit GluR1 (human glutamate receptor type1), in the hippocampus. Nobiletin has also been demonstrated to rescue Abeta-induced memory deterioration in AD model rats and to exert a preventive action on the Abeta-induced inhibition of phosphorylation of PKA and CREB in hippocampal neurons in cultures. Nobiletin also has been demonstrated to reverse learning impairment associated with NMDA (N-methyl-D-aspartate) receptor antagonism by activation of ERK signaling in the mouse hippocampus and to improve impaired memory in olfactory-bulbectomized mice.

Recently, it has been demonstrated that nobiletin improves cognitive deficits in amyloid precursor protein (APP) transgenic mice that overexpress human AP695 and markedly reduces the quantity of guanidine-soluble Abeta1-40 and Abeta1-42 in the brain. These studies should be continued.

PHARMACOKINETICS

The pharmacokinetics (PK) of nobiletin is interesting, but incomplete. Most of the PK of nobiletin has been studied in animals. Nobiletin is absorbed across the small intestine to some degree. Nobiletin has very low solubility in water, but its permeability is quite high, which ultimately contributes to a fair bioavailability for this citrus flavone. Nobiletin, following absorption, most likely enters first into the lymphatics and is transported to the systemic circulation, which transports it to various tissues and organs of the body, including the liver. In contrast to polyphenolic flavonoids, nobiletin is not glucuronidated by UDP-glucuronosyltransferase to a glucuronide. Nor does it get sulfated by sulfotransferases to a sulfate. This is because the hydroxyl groups are methylated.

Metabolites found in mouse urine following administration of nobiletin were 3'-demethylnobiletin, 4'-demethylnobiletin and 3',4'-didemethylnobiletin. Some nobiletin was also found in the urine. Both 3'4'-didemethylnobiletin and 4'-demethylnobiletin were found to have anti-inflammatory activity, thought to be accounted for by the suppression of inducible NOS and COX-2 gene expression. Much more study is needed in order to understand the PK of nobiletin.

INDICATIONS AND USAGE

Though clinical data are lacking, experimental data suggest a number of possible uses for nobiletin, pending confirmatory studies: anticancer, anti-inflammatory (including antiarthritic), anti-hyperlipidemic, anti-neurodegenerative (including help in memory disorders and possibly Alzheimer's disease), skin depigmenter and possible acne treatment.

RESEARCH SUMMARY

Nobiletin, a dietary phytochemical derived from citrus peel and other sources, has demonstrated some anticancer effects *in vitro*. It inhibits various human cancer cell lines quite effectively *in vitro*, but, like a related substance, tangeretin (see Tangeretin), it seems to lack efficacy in some *in vivo* trials. It was inactive in a chemically induced hamster cheek pouch cancer model and failed to have significant effect on early rat hepatocarcinogenesis *in vivo*. Nonetheless, the researchers concluded that more study was warranted as there were indications that nobiletin might be more effective in late stages of hepatocarcinoma. Far more research will be needed, extending into the clinical arena, before it can be concluded that this substance shows any promise as a human anticancer agent.

Various *in vitro* and preliminary animal experiments indicate that nobiletin may have some significant anti-inflammatory effects. Nobiletin has exhibited anti-inflammatory actions similar to those achieved with such anti-inflammatory steroids as dexamethasone. Among other actions, nobiletin has demonstrated an ability to suppress interleukin-1-induced production of prostaglandin in human synovial cells in a dose-dependent manner and to favorably modulate a wide array of other proinflammatory processes. In one study, nobiletin effectively inhibited cartilage destruction in collagen-induced arthritic mice. Acne vulgaris, an inflammatory disease in sebaceous glands, might also be helped by nobiletin according to other researchers who showed that the flavonoid can inhibit sebum production and sebocyte proliferation, while also enhancing sebum excretion, in hamsters. Clearly more research in this area is warranted.

An *in vitro* study of mouse macrophages demonstrated an antiatherogenic effect separate from previously reported nobiletin-associated cholesterol-lowering effects. In this study, a favorable modulation of macrophage metabolism attributed to the flavonoid was observed. Three other flavonoids failed to show the same beneficial effects. Another study suggested that nobiletin might help inhibit oxidation of low-density lipoprotein, an important contributor to atherosclerosis. Yet another study suggests that nobiletin might be able to regulate fat cells in ways that could help prevent arteriosclerosis and diabetes. Again, far more study will be needed before any conclusions can be drawn with respect to the efficacy of this substance in human disease, but such study is again clearly warranted.

Researchers have reported that nobiletin can improve memory impairment and protect against neurodegeneration in mice. These findings are thought to have implications for Alzheimer's disease. In another study, this one using a rat model of Alzheimer's disease, memory deterioration was said to be inhibited by the use of nobiletin. It is hoped that this research may eventually lead to the development of a new drug for the treatment of memory impairment and Alzheimer's disease.

Finally, it has been reported that nobiletin is a tyrosinase inhibitor and, as such, may be an effective skin lightener for use in pigmentation problems. The search for inhibitors of tyrosinase, which catalyzes the oxidation of tyrosine and other substances in a process that gives rise to melanin, has been intense for some years, owing to the cosmetic potential of such products. Noting that citrus peel has been used in traditional Japanese medicine for some time as a skin lightener, one group of researchers tested nobiletin for its potential effectiveness, using a known skin lightener called Kojic acid as a positive control. In this *in vitro* test, nobiletin was shown to have significant tyrosinase inhibiting potency, double that of Kojic acid. More study is needed to determine whether nobiletin can be used as an effective topical treatment for human pigmentation problems.

CONTRAINDICATIONS, PRECAUTIONS, ADVERSE REACTIONS

CONTRAINDICATIONS

Nobiletin is contraindicated in those who are hypersensitive to any component of a nobiletin-containing product.

PRECAUTIONS

Those who wish to try nobiletin for the support of any health condition should discuss its use with his or her physician.

ADVERSE REACTIONS

None known.

INTERACTIONS

DRUGS, DIETARY SUPPLEMENTS, FOODS, HERBS

None reported.

OVERDOSAGE

There are no reports of overdosage.

DOSAGE AND ADMINISTRATION

The optimal dose of nobiletin is not known.

At present, only one dietary supplement containing a mixture of polymethoxylated flavones (PMF), tocotrienols and ascorbyl palmitate is being marketed in the U.S. The PMF-tocotrienol mixture contains a total of 150 mg per capsule; those using this supplement take about two per day.

The amount of nobiletin in citrus peel and juice is variable. One of the highest concentrations of nobiletin is found in the tangerine and a lime cross, *Citrus depressa* or shiikuwasha, which contains approximately 26.7 mg per gram of dry weight.

It is expected that other nobiletin dietary supplements will enter the dietary supplement marketplace.

LITERATURE

Ben-Aziz A. Nobiletin Is Main Fungistat in Tangerines Resistant to Mal Secco. *Science.* 1967;155(3765):1026-1027.

Choi SY, Hwang JH, Ko HC, et al. Nobiletin from citrus fruit peel inhibits the DNA-binding activity of NF-kappaB and ROS production in LPS-activated RAW 264.7 cells. *J Ethnopharmacol.* 2007;113(1):149-155.

Eguchi A, Murakami A, Ohigashi H. Nobiletin, a citrus flavonoid, suppresses phorbol ester-induced expression of multiple scavenger receptor genes in THP-1 human monocytic cells. *FEBS Lett.* 2006;580(13):3321-3328.

Hirata Y, Masuda Y, Kakutani H, et al. Sp1 is an essential transcription factor for LPS-induced tissue factor expression in THP-1 monocytic cells, and nobiletin represses the expression through inhibition of NF-kappaB, AP-1, and Sp1 activation. *Biochem Pharmacol.* 2008;75(7):1504-1514.

Ishiwa J, Sato T, Mimaki Y, et al. A citrus flavonoid, nobiletin, suppresses production and gene expression of matrix metalloproteinase 9/gelatinase B in rabbit synovial fibroblasts. *J Rheumatol.* 2000;27(1):20-25.

Ito A, Ishiwa J, Sato T, et al. The citrus flavonoid nobiletin suppresses the production and gene expression of matrix metalloproteinases-9/gelatinase B in rabbit synovial cells. *Ann N Y Acad Sci.* 1999;878:632-634.

Li S, Sang S, Pan MH, et al. Anti-inflammatory property of the urinary metabolites of nobiletin in mouse. *Bioorg Med Chem Lett.* 2007;17(18):5177-5181.

Li S, Wang Z, Sang S, et al. Identification of nobiletin metabolites in mouse urine. *Mol Nutr Food Res.* 2006;50(3):291-299.

Li S, Yu H, Ho CT. Nobiletin: efficient and large quantity isolation from orange peel extract. *Biomed Chromatogr.* 2006;20(1):133-138.

Lin N, Sato T, Takayama Y, et al. Novel anti-inflammatory actions of nobiletin, a citrus polymethoxy flavonoid, on human synovial fibroblasts and mouse macrophages. *Biochem Pharmacol.* 2003;65(12):2065-2071.

Luo G, Guan X, Zhou L. Apoptotic effect of citrus fruit extract Nobiletin on Lung Cancer cell line A549 in vitro and in vivo. *Cancer Biol Ther.* 2008;7(6):966-973.

Matsuzaki K, Miyazaki K, Sakai S, et al. Nobiletin, a citrus flavonoid with neurotrophic action, augments protein kinase A-mediated phosphorylation of the AMPA receptor subunit, GluR1, and the postsynaptic receptor response to glutamate in murine hippocampus. *Eur J Pharmacol.* 2008;578(2-3):194-200.

Matsuzaki K, Yamakuni T, Hashimoto M, et al. Nobiletin restoring beta-amyloid-impaired CREB phosphorylation rescues memory deterioration in Alzheimer's disease model rats. *Neurosci Lett.* 2006;400(3):230-234.

Minagawa A, Otani Y, Kubota T, et al. The citrus flavonoid, nobiletin, inhibits peritoneal dissemination of human gastric carcinoma in SCID mice. *Jpn J Cancer Res.* 2001;92(12):1322-1328.

Miyamoto S, Yasui Y, Tanaka T, et al. Suppressive effects of nobiletin on hyperleptinemia and colitis-related colon carcinogenesis in male ICR mice. *Carcinogenesis.* 2008;29(5):1057-1063.

Miyata Y, Sato T, Imada K, et al. A citrus polymethoxyflavonoid, nobiletin, is a novel MEK inhibitor that exhibits antitumor metastasis in human fibrosarcoma HT-1080 cells. *Biochem Biophys Res Commun.* 2008;366(1):168-173.

Miyata Y, Sato T, Yano M, et al. Activation of protein kinase C betaII/epsilon-c-Jun NH2-terminal kinase pathway and inhibition of mitogen-activated protein/extracellular signal-regulated kinase 1/2 phosphorylation in antitumor invasive activity induced by the polymethoxy flavonoid, nobiletin. *Mol Cancer Ther.* 2004;3(7):839-847.

Murakami A, Koshimizu K, Ohigashi H, et al. Characteristic rat tissue accumulation of nobiletin, a chemopreventive polymethoxyflavonoid, in comparison with luteolin. *Biofactors.* 2002;16(3-4):73-82.

Murakami A, Kuwahara S, Takahashi Y, et al. In vitro absorption and metabolism of nobiletin, a chemopreventive polymethoxyflavonoid in citrus fruits. *Biosci Biotechnol Biochem.* 2001;65(1):194-197.

Murakami A, Nakamura Y, Torikai K, et al. Inhibitory effect of citrus nobiletin on phorbol ester-induced skin inflammation, oxidative stress, and tumor promotion in mice. *Cancer Res.* 2000;60(18):5059-5066.

Murakami A, Song M, Katsumata S, et al. Citrus nobiletin suppresses bone loss in ovariectomized ddY mice and collagen-induced arthritis in DBA/1J mice: Possible involvement of receptor activator of NF-kappaB ligand (RANKL)-induced osteoclastogenesis regulation. *Biofactors*. 2007;30(3):179-192.

Nagase H, Omae N, Omori A, et al. Nobiletin and its related flavonoids with CRE-dependent transcription-stimulating and neuritegenic activities. *Biochem Biophys Res Commun*. 2005;337(4):1330-1336.

Nagase H, Yamakuni T, Matsuzaki K, et al. Mechanism of neurotrophic action of nobiletin in PC12D cells. *Biochemistry*. 2005;44(42):13683-13691.

Nakajima A, Yamakuni T, Haraguchi M, et al. Nobiletin, a citrus flavonoid that improves memory impairment, rescues bulbectomy-induced cholinergic neurodegeneration in mice. *J Pharmacol Sci*. 2007;105(1):122-126.

Nakajima A, Yamakuni T, Matsuzaki K, et al. Nobiletin, a citrus flavonoid, reverses learning impairment associated with N-methyl-D-aspartate receptor antagonism by activation of extracellular signal-regulated kinase signaling. *J Pharmacol Exp Ther*. 2007;321(2):784-790.

Nogata Y, Sakamoto K, Shiratsuchi H, et al. Flavonoid composition of fruit tissues of citrus species. *Biosci Biotechnol Biochem*. 2006;70(1):178-192.

Okuno Y, Miyazawa M. Biotransformation of nobiletin by Aspergillus niger and the antimutagenic activity of a metabolite, 4′-hydroxy-5,6,7,8,3′-pentamethoxyflavone. *J Nat Prod*. 2004;67(11):1876-1878.

Onozuka H, Nakajima A, Matsuzaki K, et al. Nobiletin, a citrus flavonoid, improves memory impairment and Aβ pathology in a transgenic mouse model of Alzheimer's disease. *J Pharmacol Exp Ther*. 2008;326(3):739-744.

Saito T, Abe D, Sekiya K. Nobiletin enhances differentiation and lipolysis of 3T3-L1 adipocytes. *Biochem Biophys Res Commun*. 2007;357(2):371-376.

Sasaki K, Yoshizaki F. Nobiletin as a tyrosinase inhibitor from the peel of Citrus fruit. *Biol Pharm Bull*. 2002;25(6):806-808.

Sato T, Koike L, Miyata Y, et al. Inhibition of activator protein-1 binding activity and phosphatidylinositol 3-kinase pathway by nobiletin, a polymethoxy flavonoid, results in augmentation of tissue inhibitor of metalloproteinases-1 production and suppression of production of matrix metalloproteinases-1 and -9 in human fibrosarcoma HT-1080 cells. *Cancer Res*. 2002;62(4):1025-1029.

Sato T, Takahashi A, Kojima M, et al. A citrus polymethoxy flavonoid, nobiletin inhibits sebum production and sebocyte proliferation, and augments sebum excretion in hamsters. *J Invest Dermatol*. 2007;127(12):2740-2748.

Suzuki R, Kohno H, Murakami A, et al. Citrus nobiletin inhibits azoxymethane-induced large bowel carcinogenesis in rats. *Biofactors*. 2004;22(1-4):111-114.

Tanaka S, Sato T, Akimoto N, et al. Prevention of UVB-induced photoinflammation and photoaging by a polymethoxy flavonoid, nobiletin, in human keratinocytes in vivo and in vitro. *Biochem Pharmacol*. 2004;68(3):433-439.

Wu YQ, Zhou CH, Tao J, et al. Antagonistic effects of nobiletin, a polymethoxyflavonoid, on eosinophilic airway inflammation of asthmatic rats and relevant mechanisms. *Life Sci*. 2006;78(23):2689-2696.

Yasuda T, Yoshimura Y, Yabuki H, et al. Urinary metabolites of nobiletin orally administered to rats. *Chem Pharm Bull* (Tokyo). 2003;51(12):1426-1428.

Yoshimizu N, Otani Y, Saikawa Y, et al. Anti-tumour effects of nobiletin, a citrus flavonoid, on gastric cancer include: antiproliferative effects, induction of apoptosis and cell cycle deregulation. *Aliment Pharmacol Ther*. 2004;20(Suppl 1):95-101.

Zhang HQ, Ge H, Cheng MY. [Antitumor effects of nobiletin on Heps and its mechanism] [Article in Chinese.] *Yao Xue Xue Bao*. 2006;41(8):797-800.

Nucleic Acids/Nucleotides

DESCRIPTION

DNA (deoxyribonucleic acid), the molecule that comprises the genome, and RNA (ribonucleic acid) are marketed as nutritional supplements. DNA, which makes up the genetic material, is comprised of units called nucleotides. A nucleotide consists of a base, a sugar and a phosphate group. The major bases in DNA are the purines adenine and guanine and the pyrimidines cytosine and thymine. The sugar moiety of the nucleotide is 2′-deoxyribose. RNA, which is more abundant in tissues than DNA by about an order of magnitude, is also comprised of nucleotide units. In the case of RNA, the major bases are again the purines adenine and guanine, and the pyrimidines are cytosine and uracil. One of the major differences between DNA and RNA is the presence of uracil in RNA and of thymine in DNA. The other major difference is in the sugar moiety. In RNA, the sugar moiety of the nucleotide is ribose, whereas in DNA it is deoxyribose.

For years, nucleic acids and nucleotides were not considered essential nutrients. It was thought that the body can synthesize sufficient nucleotides to meet its physiological demands via *de novo* nucleotide synthetic pathways. Some research during the last several years indicates that this may not be completely correct. There are certain conditions in which the body requires dietary nucleic acids/nucleotides to meet its physiological requirements. These conditions include rapid growth, limited food supply and metabolic stress. Under these conditions, metabolic demand exceeds the capacity of *de novo* synthesis. Under these conditions, dietary nucleosides, nucleotides and nucleic acids become conditionally essential nutrients. Dietary nucleotides may spare the energetic cost of *de novo* synthesis of nucleotides.

Dietary nucleic acids are found in plant and animal foods. The dietary intake of RNA is typically about an order of magnitude greater than DNA. The nucleotide salts disodium inosinate and disodium guanylate are present in many food products as seasoning substances, contributing to the dietary nucleotide intake. Interestingly, mother's milk is a rich source of nucleic acids, especially RNA, and nucleotides. There are a few medical foods and enteral supplements containing RNA and nucleotides, which are used for immune-enhancement under conditions of metabolic stress. RNA and nucleotides are sometimes referred to as immuno-nutrients. Nutritional supplements of RNA, DNA, nucleo-tides, nucleosides and bases are also being marketed.

ACTIONS AND PHARMACOLOGY

ACTIONS
Nucleic acids and nucleotides may have immune-enhancing and tissue-regenerating activities.

MECHANISM OF ACTION
Nucleotides have been demonstrated to affect a number of immune functions, including reversing malnutrition and starvation-induced immunosuppression, enhancing T-cell maturation and function, enhancing natural killer cell activi-ty, improving delayed cutaneous hypersensitivity, aiding in resistance to such infectious agents as *Staphylococcus aureus* and *Candida albicans,* and modulating T-cell responses toward type 1 CD4 helper lymphocytes or Th1 cells. Mice fed a nucleotide-free diet have both impaired cellular and humoral immune responses. Addition of dietary nucleotides restores both types of responses. Both RNA, which can be considered a delivery form of nucleotides, and ribonucleo-tides were used in these studies. The mechanism of the immune-enhancing activity of nucleic acids/nucleotides is unclear.

RNA and nucleotides have been shown to have stimulatory effects on recovery from hepatectomy in animals. They have also been shown to stimulate intestinal repair, in animals. The mechanism of the tissue-regenerating effects of RNA and nucleotides is unclear. Possibly the regenerating activity may be explained, in part, by the nucleotides serving as precursors of nucleic acid synthesis via the salvage pathways of nucleotide synthesis. Utilization of the salvage pathways may spare the energetic cost of *de novo* nucleotide synthesis.

PHARMACOKINETICS
RNA is digested in the small intestine via the action of the pancreatic enzyme ribonuclease to the nucleotides adeno-sine-5′ -monophosphate (AMP), guanosine-5′-monophos-phate (GMP), cytidine-5′ -monophosphate (CMP) and uridine-5′-monophosphate (UMP). These nucleotides are then hydrolyzed to the nucleosides adenosine, guanosine, cytidine and uridine, respectively, via the action of the

enzymes alkaline phosphatase and nucleotidase. The nucleo-sides may be further hydrolyzed to the purine bases adenine and guanine and the pyrimidine bases cytosine and uracil.

The nucleosides are transported in the enterocytes by both facilitated diffusion and sodium-dependent carrier mediated processes. Under normal conditions, that is, under conditions where the body is not under metabolic stress, the nucleosides undergo extensive catabolism in the enterocytes. The end product of purine catabolism is uric acid. An end product of pyrimidine metabolism is beta-alanine. Nucleosides and bases that are not catabolized in the enterocytes are transported via the portal circulation to the liver, where they are also catabolized. A small percentage of ingested RNA and nucleotides reach the systemic circulation and is transported to various tissues of the body.

Even under normal conditions, a small percentage (from 2% to 5%) of dietary RNA and dietary nucleotides is incorporat-ed into nucleic acids, especially in the small intestine, liver and skeletal muscle. This occurs via the salvage pathways of purine nucleotide and pyrimidine nucleotide synthesis. During conditions of metabolic stress, including trauma, rapid growth and limited food supply, there is apparently greater conversion of dietary RNA and nucleotides into tissue nucleotides and nucleic acids.

DNA is digested in the small intestine via the action of the pancreatic enzyme deoxyribonuclease to deoxynucleotides; these, in turn, are hydrolyzed to deoxynucleosides and finally to the pyrimidine bases cytosine and thymine and the purine bases adenine and guanine. The deoxynucleosides and bases are absorbed by the enterocytes and processed as described above for the nucleosides.

INDICATIONS AND USAGE
The nucleotides appear to be effective in boosting immune response in some circumstances. They may also promote tissue repair in some conditions. Claims that they are an effective treatment for Alzheimer's disease, depression, skin disorders, sexual dysfunction, fatigue and aging are unsubstantiated.

RESEARCH SUMMARY
Numerous studies have shown that nucleotides can help restore immune function in malnourished animals, can enhance the activity of T-cells and natural killer cells, and can increase resistance to some pathogenic agents. Infants fed formulas supplemented with nucleotides had a lower incidence of diarrhea, higher natural killer cell activity and higher antibody titers following *Haemophilus influenzae* type b vaccination, compared with unsupplemented controls. In another study, post-operative immune response, evidenced by several measures, was enhanced in patients with upper-

gastrointestinal cancer who were given supplements of RNA, arginine and omega-3 fatty acids.

Nucleosides have promoted tissue repair in a number of animal studies. They have shortened recovery time in animals with liver injury and have enhanced healing of experimental intestinal ulcers. They have shortened recovery time following small and large bowel injuries.

CONTRAINDICATIONS, PRECAUTIONS, ADVERSE REACTIONS

CONTRAINDICATIONS

Supplemental RNA, DNA, nucleotides and nucleosides are contraindicated in those hypersensitive to any component of products containing these substances.

PRECAUTIONS

Pregnant women and nursing mothers should avoid nucleic acid and nucleotide supplements unless recommended by their physicians.

Those with a history of hyperuricemia should be extremely cautious about use of nucleic acid and nucleotide supplements.

ADVERSE REACTIONS

No reports of adverse reactions.

DOSAGE AND ADMINISTRATION

Medical foods are available containing RNA as a delivery form of nucleotides/nucleosides, sometimes along with L-arginine and fish oils. These medical foods are used to support the immune system under conditions of metabolic stress.

RNA and DNA nutritional supplements are available, with RNA supplements being more popular. Typical doses range from 0.5 to 1.5 grams daily.

Brewer's yeast is a rich source of RNA (see Brewer's Yeast). Inosine is a nucleoside (see Inosine).

LITERATURE

Adjei AA, Yamamoto S. A dietary nucleoside-nucleotide mixture ihibits endotoxin-induced bacterial translocation in mice fed protein-free diet. *J Nutr.* 1995; 125:42-48.

Carver JD. Dietary nucleotides: effects on the immune and gastrointestinal systems. *Acta Paediatr Suppl.* 1999; 88:83-88.

Carver JD, Cox WI, Barness LA. Dietary nucleotide effects upon murine natural killer cell activity and macrophage activation. *J Parenter Enteral Nutr.* 1990; 14:18-22.

Carver JD, Walker A. The role of nucleotides in human nutrition. *Nutr Biochem.* 1995; 6:58-72.

De Jong JW, Vander Meer P, Owen P, Opie LH. Prevention and treatment of ischemic injury with nucleosides. *Bratisl Lek Listy.* 1991; 92(3-4):165-173.

Fanslow WC, Kulkarni AD, Van Buren CT, Rudolph FB. Effect of nucleotide restriction and supplementation of resistance to experimental murine candidiasis. *J Parenter Enteral Nutr.* 1988; 12:49-52.

Frank BS. *Nucleic Acid and Antioxidant Therapy of Aging and Degeneration.* New York, NT: Rainstone Publishing; 1977.

Grimble GK. Dietary nucleotides and gut mucosal defense. *Gut.* 1994; 35(Suppl 1):S46-S51.

Jackson CD, Weis C, Miller BJ, et al. Comparison of cell proliferation following partial hepatectomy in rats fed NIH-31 or semipurified AIN-76A diets: effects of nucleic acid supplementation. *Nutr Res.* 1995; 15:1487-1495.

Jyonouchi H, Sun S, Abiru T, et al. Dietary nucleotides modulate antigen-specific type 1 and type 2 T-cell responses in young C57BL/6 mice. *Nutrition.* 2000; 16:442-446.

Leach JL, Baxter JH, Molitor BE, et al. Total potentially available nucleosides of human milk by stage of lactation. *Am J Clin Nutr.* 1995; 61:1224-1230.

Pickering LK, Granoff DM, Erickson JR, et al. Modulation of the immune system by human milk and infant formula containing nucleotides. *Pediatrics.* 1998; 101:242-249.

Rudoph FB, Kulkarni AD, Fanslow WC, et al. Role of RNA as a dietary source of pyrimidines and purines in immune function. *Nutr.* 1990; 6:45-52.

Torres-Lopé z MI, Fernandez I, Fontana L, et al. Influence of dietary nucleotides on liver structural recovery and hepatocyte binuclearity in cirrhosis induced by thioacetamide. *Gut.* 1996; 38:260-264.

Tsujinaka T, Kishibuchi M, Iijima S, et al. Nucleotides and intestine. *J Parenter Enteral Nutr.* 1999; 23:S74-S77.

Yu VY. The role of dietary nucleotides in neonatal and infant nutrition. *Singapore Med J.* 1998; 39:145-150.

Oat Beta-D-Glucan

DESCRIPTION

In 1998, the Food and Drug Administration (FDA) issued its final rule allowing health claims to be made on the labels of foods containing soluble fiber from whole oats (oat bran, oat flour and rolled oats), noting that these foods, in conjunction with a diet low in saturated fat and cholesterol, may reduce the risk of heart disease. In order to qualify for the health claim, the whole oat-containing food must provide at least 0.75 grams of soluble fiber per serving. The soluble fiber in whole oats comprises a class of polysaccharides known as beta-D-glucans.

Beta-D-glucans, usually referred to as beta-glucans, comprise a class of non-digestible polysaccharides widely found in nature in such sources as oats, barley, yeast, bacteria, algae and mushrooms.

Beta-glucans are located primarily in the cell walls. In oats, barley and other cereal grains, they are located primarily in the endosperm cell wall.

Oat beta-glucan is a soluble fiber. It is a viscous polysaccharide made up of units of the sugar D-glucose. Oat beta-glucan is comprised of mixed-linkage polysaccharides. This means that the bonds between the D-glucose or D-glucopyranosyl units are either beta-1, 3 linkages or beta-1, 4 linkages. This type of beta-glucan is also referred to as a mixed-linkage $(1\rightarrow3)$, $(1\rightarrow4)$-beta-D-glucan. Most of the oat bran beta-glucan molecules consist of cellotriose and cellotetraose blocks separated by $(1\rightarrow3)$-linkages. There is, however, a smaller amount of sequences of $(1\rightarrow4)$-linkages longer than the tetraose type. The $(1\rightarrow3)$-linkages break up the uniform structure of the beta-D-glucan molecule and make it soluble and flexible. In comparison, the nondigestible polysaccharide cellulose is also a beta-glucan but is non-soluble. The reason that it is non-soluble is that cellulose consists only of $(1\rightarrow4)$-beta-D-linkages. The percentages of beta-glucan in the various whole oat products are: oat bran, greater than 5.5%; rolled oats, about 4%; whole oat flour about 4%.

ACTIONS AND PHARMACOLOGY

ACTIONS

Oat beta-glucan may have hypocholesterolemic and glucose-regulating activity. It also has putative immunomodulatory activity.

MECHANISM OF ACTION

The exact mechanism of oat beta-glucan's possible hypocholesterolemic effect is not clear. Oat beta-glucan does not appear to have any effect on the biosynthesis of cholesterol. It appears to promote increased excretion of bile acids, which could explain, in large part, its possible cholesterol-lowering activity. Oat beta-glucan may also promote cholesterol clearance from the plasma via reverse cholesterol transport.

The mechanism of the possible glucose-regulatory activity of oat beta-glucan is also not well understood. Oat beta-glucan may delay gastric emptying time and consequently affect the rate of uptake of D-glucose from the small intestine. This may be one possible mechanism; the high viscosity of oat beta-glucan may delay absorption of glucose, which may be another possible mechanism. Oat beta-glucan has been found to have immunomodulatory activity in tissue culture and in mice. It appears to activate macrophages to release certain cytokines. Such activity, in mice, has been found to be protective against bacterial infection. It is unclear whether oat beta-glucan has immunomodulatory activity in humans.

PHARMACOKINETICS

Following ingestion, there is virtually no digestion of oat beta-glucan in the small intestine. Some digestion of oat beta-glucan does take place in the large intestine via bacterial beta-glucosidases. Some smaller oligosaccharides produced by the bacterial transformation of oat beta-glucan may get absorbed, but this is unclear. A large percentage of the ingested beta-glucan is excreted in the feces.

INDICATIONS AND USAGE

Oat beta-glucan has hypocholesterolemic effects and may also favorably affect some other lipids. It has demonstrated some immune-enhancing effects and may be helpful in some with diabetes.

RESEARCH SUMMARY

Evidence that oat beta-glucan can reduce cholesterol levels was sufficient to induce the FDA to allow health claims on whole oat products that provide at least 0.75 grams of soluble fiber per serving. The allowed health claim is that these products reduce the risk of heart disease by reducing levels of cholesterol.

In one study, mildly hypercholesterolemic subjects on a "typical" diet, in which 35% of calories was derived from fat, were given an oat beta-glucan extract containing 1% or 10% oat beta-glucan. There was a significant reduction in total cholesterol levels in those receiving the 10% oat beta-glucan preparation after three weeks. Cholesterol levels declined significantly in the 1% group, as well, but not as quickly. There was also a significant decline in LDL-cholesterol levels in both groups. Triglyceride and HDL-cholesterol levels were not significantly changed. Some other studies have reported similar results.

Improved glucose and insulin responses have been reported in a study of moderately hypercholesterolemic healthy subjects. Oat extracts containing 1% and 10% beta-glucan both demonstrated these beneficial effects on glucose tolerance factors.

NIDDM patients given varying concentrations of oat beta-glucan also had significantly improved glucose and insulin responses. Higher doses of the oat beta-glucan correlated with greater improvement.

There are *in vitro* and animal studies demonstrating that oat beta-glucan, like those extracted from yeast and other fungi, has favorable immunomodulatory activities. These include the ability to activate macrophages and stimulate their release of interleukin (IL)-1 and tumor necrosis factor (TNF)-alpha, among other activities

Intraperitoneal administration of oat beta-glucan has enhanced a non-specific resistance to bacterial challenge in mice. Survival times have been improved in mice pre-treated with oat beta-glucan and then challenged with *Staphylococcus aureus*. Similarly, resistance to *Eimeria vermiformis* has been significantly increased in immunosuppressed mice given oat beta-glucan intragastrically or parenterally.

CONTRAINDICATIONS, PRECAUTIONS, ADVERSE REACTIONS

CONTRAINDICATIONS

Known hypersensitivity to an oat beta-D-glucan-containing product.

PRECAUTIONS

None known.

ADVERSE REACTIONS

Oat beta-glucans are generally well tolerated. Occasional flatulence is reported.

OVERDOSAGE

There are no reports of overdosage.

DOSAGE AND ADMINISTRATION

Dosage of oat beta-glucan required for a possible hypocholesterolemic effect ranges from 3 to 6 grams daily. This can be obtained from a whole oat product. There is some marketed oat beta-glucan nutritional supplements.

LITERATURE

Anderson JW, Gustafson NJ. Hypocholesterolemic effects of oat and bean products. *Am J Clin Nutr.* 1988; 48:749-753.

Anderson JW, Story L, Sieling B, et al. Hypocholesterolemic effects of oat-bran or bean intake for hypercholesterolemic men. *Am J Clin Nutr.* 1984; 40:1146-1155.

Behall KM, Scholfield DJ, Hallfrisch J. Effect of beta-glucan level in oat fiber extracts on blood lipids in men and women. *J Am Coll Nutr.* 1997; 16:46-51.

Bell S, Goldman VM, Bistrian BR, et al. Effect of beta-glucan from oats and yeast on serum lipids. *Crit Rev Food Sci Nutr.* 1999; 39:189-202.

Braaten JT, Wood PJ, Scott FW, et al. Oat beta-glucan reduces blood cholesterol concentration in hypercholesterolemic subjects. *Eur J Clin Nutr.* 1994; 48:465-474.

Davidson MH, Dugan LD, Burns JH, et al. The hypocholesterolemic effects of beta-glucan in oatmeal and oat bran. A dose-controlled study. *JAMA.* 1991; 265:1833-1839.

Estrada A, Yun CH, Van Kessel A, et al. Immunomodulatory activities of oat beta-glucan in vitro and in vivo. *Microbiol Immunol.* 1997; 41:991-998.

Food and Drug Administration. Food labeling: health claims; soluble fiber from certain foods and coronary heart disease: final rule 21 CFR Part 101. *Federal Reg.* Feb 18,1998; 63(32): 8103.

Hallfrisch J, Scholfield DJ, Behall KM. Diets containing soluble oat extracts improve glucose and insulin responses of moderately hypercholesterolemic men and women. *Am J Clin Nutr.* 1995; 61:379-384.

Johansson L, Virkki L, Maunu S, et al. Structural characterization of water soluble beta-glucan of oat bran. *Carbohydrate Polymers.* 2000; 42:143-148.

Lia A, Andersson H, Mekki N, et al. Postprandial lipemia in relation to sterol and fat excretion in ileostomy subjects given oat-bran and wheat test meals. *Am J Clin Nutr.* 1997; 66:357-365.

Lia A, Hallmans G, Sandberg AS, et al. Oat beta-glucan increases bile acid excretion and a fiber-rich barley fraction increases cholesterol excretion in ileostomy subjects. *Am Clin Nutr J.* 1995; 62:1245-1251.

Wood PJ, Braaten JT, Scott FW, et al. Effect of dose and modifications of viscous properties of oat gum on plasma glucose and insulin following an oral glucose load. *Br J Nutr.* 1994; 72:731-743.

Octacosanol

DESCRIPTION

Octacosanol is a 28 carbon long-chain saturated primary alcohol. It is a constituent of vegetable waxes. Octacosanol is isolated from the wax found on green blades of wheat. It is the major long-chain alcohol isolated from the waxes of sugar cane and yams. It is also found in wheat germ oil.

Octacosanol is also known as l-octacosanol, n-octacosanol and octacosyl alcohol. It has the following chemical formula:

$$CH_3(CH_2)_{26}CH_2OH$$

Octacosanol (1-Octacosanol)

Octacosanol is a solid waxy substance that is insoluble in water. Octacosanol belongs to the family of fatty alcohols.

ACTIONS AND PHARMACOLOGY

ACTIONS

The action of octacosanol is unknown. It is the major long-chain alcohol in policosanol (see Policosanol), and policosanol appears to lower cholesterol and LDL-cholesterol levels. However, the role of octacosanol in the putative cholesterol-lowering activity of policosanol is unclear.

PHARMACOKINETICS

The absorption of octacosanol is variable and low. Octacosanol absorption, following ingestion, ranges from about 11% in rats and humans to about 28% in rabbits. Less octacosanol is absorbed on an empty stomach and more with food. The higher the lipid content of food, the greater the absorption. Octacosanol is absorbed from the small intestine into the lymph and from there enters the bloodstream. Distribution is mainly to the liver, digestive tract, skeletal muscle and adipose tissue. Octacosanol may be partly oxidized to the long-chain fatty acid, octacosanoic acid, which then undergoes beta-oxidation.

Following a single dose of octacosanol in experimental animals, peak plasma levels are observed between 30 minutes to two hours. Following a single dose of octacosanol in human volunteers, peak plasma levels are observed at one hour and four hours later. Bile is the main route of excretion. Renal excretion is negligible.

INDICATIONS AND USAGE

Octacosanol, like policosanol (see Policosanol), may have cholesterol-lowering effects but research will have to be done to confirm this. Similarly, there is preliminary evidence suggesting that octacosanol may increase physical endurance and that it may benefit some with Parkinson's disease. Octacosanol is not indicated for use in amyotrophic lateral sclerosis despite some claims of efficacy in this disorder.

RESEARCH SUMMARY

There is limited evidence that octacosanol itself may lower cholesterol levels. This needs to be researched. (See Policosanol.) There are claims that octacosanol is useful in building strength and endurance, and these claims have made the supplement popular with some body builders and athletes. There is preliminary evidence, limited to animal experiments, that octacosanol may increase voluntary exercise in the animals.

Evidence that octacosanol may help in the treatment of Parkinson's disease is very preliminary, and the use of this substance in a well-designed study of those suffering from amyotrophic lateral sclerosis showed no benefit. Neither neurologic nor pulmonary functions were improved.

CONTRAINDICATIONS, PRECAUTIONS, ADVERSE REACTIONS

CONTRAINDICATIONS

Known hypersensitivity to an octacosanol-containing product.

PRECAUTIONS

Octacosanol is not recommended for children, pregnant women and nursing mothers. Parkinson's disease patients taking carbidopa-levodopa may experience side effects (see Adverse Reactions).

ADVERSE REACTIONS

Side effects of octacosanol taken up to 20 milligrams daily are infrequent. Mild position-related nonrotational dizziness, increased nervous tension and worsening of carbidopa-levodopa-related dyskinesias have been reported in a few Parkinson's disease patients taking octacosanol.

INTERACTIONS

Carbidopa-levodopa: Octacosanol has been reported to worsen dyskinesias in a few Parkinson's disease patients taking carbidopa-levodopa.

No other nutritional supplement, herb or food interactions are known.

OVERDOSAGE

There are no reports of overdosage.

DOSAGE AND ADMINISTRATION

Typical doses used are 1 to 8 milligrams (1,000 to 8,000 micrograms) daily taken with food. A dose of 20 milligrams daily should not be exceeded. Octacosanol frequently comes in mixtures with other long-chain alcohols.

LITERATURE

Kabir Y, Kimura S. Distribution of radioactive octacosanol in response to exercise in rats. *Nahrung.* 1994; 38:373-377.

Kato S, Hasegawa S, Nagasawa J, et al. Octacosanol affects lipid metabolism in rats fed on a high-fat diet. *Br J Nutr.* 1995; 73:433-441.

Norris FH, Denys EH, Fallat RJ. Trial of octacosanol in amyotrophic lateral sclerosis. *Neurol.* 1986; 36:1263-1264.

Snider SR. Octacosanol in Parkinsonism. *Ann Neurol.* 1984; 16:723.

Oleocanthal

DESCRIPTION

A number of observational studies have shown that those who follow the Mediterranean diet have a lower incidence of cardiovascular disease, including heart attacks, and also a lower incidence of cancer, including breast, prostate and colorectal cancer, and other chronic degenerative diseases. The principal components of this diet are fruits, vegetables, fish, wine and olive oil. The consumption of red meat is relatively low, and olive oil is the major source of lipids in the diet. The health benefits are mainly attributed to the consumption of olive oil.

The specific substances in olive oil that appear to confer the health benefits include the monounsaturated fatty acid oleic acid and especially the polyphenolic lignans (+)-1-acetoxypinoresinol and (+)-pinoresinol and the polyphenolics hydroxytyrosol and oleuropein aglycone.

In September 2005, a short communication appeared in the international science journal *Nature* describing the anti-inflammatory effects of a recently discovered (1993) olive oil polyphenol, which the authors named oleocanthal. The press immediately picked up on the article, not only because it made for an interesting story, but also because of the possibility that the substance may be the key to understanding the health benefits of olive oil.

The study reported in *Nature* was directed by Paul Breslin, Ph.D. and Gary Beauchamp, Ph.D., both of the Monell Chemical Senses Center in Philadelphia. The researchers were led to the discovery by the serendipitous observation that fresh extra-virgin olive oil irritates the back of the throat in a unique and unusual manner. To quote Dr. Beauchamp, "I had considerable experience swallowing and being stung in the throat by ibuprofen from previous studies on its sensory properties. So when I tasted newly-pressed olive oil while attending a meeting on molecular gastronomy in Sicily, I was startled to notice that the throat sensations were virtually identical."

The researchers systematically evaluated the sensory properties of a number of compounds and found one that was thought to be responsible for the irritating property of premium extra-virgin olive oil. Chemically, the molecule that conferred the throaty bite was found to be the dialdehydic form of (-) decetoxy-ligstroside aglycone, which had been isolated by another group in 1993. The Monell researchers named this compound oleocanthal, oleo for olive, canth for sting and al for aldehyde. They also proceeded to synthesize the molecule and found that the synthetic molecule produced the same throat irritant effect as did premium extra-virgin olive oil and that the effect was dependent on the dose.

The nonsteroidal anti-inflammatory drug (NSAID) ibuprofen is widely used as an analgesic and anti-inflammatory for such disorders as osteoarthritis and many more. It inhibits both cyclooxygenase-1 (COX-1) and cyclooxygenase-2 (COX-2), as does aspirin, but does not inhibit the lipoxygenases. The chemical structures of ibuprofen and oleocanthal are quite different. However, oleocanthal, like ibuprofen, was found to inhibit COX-1 and COX-2, but not 15-lipoxygenase (15-LOX).

Oleocanthal is chemically described as 2-(4-hydroxyphenyl)ethyl (3S,4E)-4-formyl-3-(2-oxorthyl)hex-4-enoate. Oleocanthal is also known as deacetoxy ligstroside aglycone. There are two enantiomers of oleocanthal. (Enantiomers are one of two stereoisomers that are nonsuperimposable, complete mirror images of each other.) (-)-Oleocanthal is the naturally occurring enantiomer. Oleocanthal's CAS Registration number is 289030-99-5, its empirical formula is $C_{17}H_{20}O_5$, and its molecular weight is 304.34. Oleocanthal is a member of the secoiridoid family. It was first isolated and described in 1993 by Gianfrancesco Montedoro and his co-workers. The secoiridoid family also includes the olive polyphenols oleuropein (see Oleuropein), the bitter principle of olives, and hydroxytyrosol (see Hydroxytyrosol), which is responsible for the high stability of olive oil. Chemically, the secoiridoids are monoterpinoid lactones. Oleocanthal is represented by the following chemical structure.

Oleocanthal

The types of phenols in extra-virgin olive oil are different from those of the olive fruit. The olives mainly contain the polar glycosides, oleuropein and ligstroside. Oleuropein is the ester of elenoic acid with 3,4'-dihydroxyphenylethanol (hydroxytyrosol), and ligstroside is the ester of of elenolic acid with 4-hydoxyphenylethanol (tyrosol). Oleuropein and ligstroside are the parent compounds of the less polar oleuropein- and ligstroside-aglycones (eg, oleocanthal). Oleuropein- and ligstroside-aglycones are formed by removal of the glucose moiety from the oleuropein- and ligstroside-glycosides via beta-glucosidase during ripening. Those aglycones and their various derivatives are the most abundant phenols in olive oil.

ACTIONS AND PHARMACOLOGY

ACTIONS

Oleocanthal may have antioxidant and anti-inflammatory activities.

MECHANISM OF ACTION

Few studies have been performed on the possible antioxidant activity of oleocanthal. However, given that oleocanthal is a polyphenolic substance, it is likely to possess scavenging activity against a wide range of radicals, including hydroxyl, peroxyl, and superoxide anion radicals. It might also inhibit the oxidation of LDL. Oxidized LDL is thought to be a crucial event in the pathogenesis of atherosclerosis. *In vitro* and *in vivo* studies determining if oleocanthal does indeed inhibit the oxidation of LDL should be performed.

Oleocanthal has been shown to inhibit COX-1 and COX-2, but not 15-lipoxygenase (15-LOX). Thus, it does possess ibuprofen-like anti-inflammatory activity. However, a large range of high-quality clinical studies are needed and warranted to determine if this anti-inflammatory effect has any significance regarding prevention of cardiovascular disease, cancer and cognitive disorders, such as Alzheimer's disease.

PHARMACOKINETICS

Little is known about the pharmacokinetics (PK) of oleocanthal in either experimental animals or in humans. PK studies on oleocanthal in humans are needed to fill in all the details of its ADME (absorption, distribution, metabolism and excretion).

INDICATIONS AND USAGE

Oleocanthal, an olive polyphenol, has reported antioxidative and antiinflammatory activity. One report stirred wide interest in the substance by claiming it has ibuprofen-like activity. In common with what has been claimed for other olive polyphenols (see Hydroxytyrosol and Oleuropein), it may have some cardioprotective and anticancer activity, as well, although clinical evidence for this is lacking.

RESEARCH SUMMARY

A brief communication in the journal *Nature* excited interest in oleocanthal when researchers reported that this substance, derived from newly pressed extra-virgin olive oil, has some characteristics in common with the anti-inflammatory drug ibuprofen. They noted that both induce very similar stinging sensations in the throat and thereafter determined that the two substances have structural and pharmacological similarities. They found that oleocanthal, like ibuprofen, is an inhibitor of the COX-1 and COX-2 enzymes in a dose-dependent manner. Thus they hypothesized that, through consistent long-term consumption of extra-virgin olive oil, some ibuprofen-like relief from inflammation and pain might be realized in some individuals. Others, however, have questioned whether plasma levels of the polyphenol could thus ever be high enough to have a meaningful effect. Research is needed to see whether supplements of this substance could safely and effectively be used in the same way that ibuprofen is used. If so, it might have application in a number of situations since there are data suggesting that ibuprofen, apart from providing pain relief, may, when used long-term, have some inhibiting effect on various inflammatory processes, including Alzheimer's disease.

CONTRAINDICATIONS, PRECAUTIONS, ADVERSE REACTIONS

CONTRAINDICATIONS

Oleocanthal is contraindicated in those hypersensitive to any component of an oleocanthal-containing product. Hypersensitivity to oleocanthal is probably very rare.

PRECAUTIONS

Those who wish to use oleocanthal for health reasons should first discuss this with his or her physician.

ADVERSE REACTIONS

No reports.

INTERACTIONS

No reports.

OVERDOSAGE

There are no reports of overdosage.

DOSAGE AND ADMINISTRATION

The concentration of oleocanthal in extra-virgin olive oil is variable. Premium extra-virgin olive oil contains up to 200 micrograms of oleocanthal per milliliter. Fifty grams of premium extra-virgin olive oil contains about nine milligrams of oleocanthal. The potency of oleocanthal and ibuprofen is approximately the same. Therefore, nine milligrams of oleocanthal is approximately equal to nine milligrams of ibuprofen, which is about 10% percent of a low dose (100 milligrams) of ibuprofen.

Dietary supplements of oleocanthal are currently unavailable.

LITERATURE

Andrewes P, Busch JL, de Joode T, et al. Sensory properties of virgin olive oil polyphenols: identification of deacetoxy-ligstroside aglycon as a key contributor to pungency. *Agric Food Chem.* 2003;51(5):1415-1420.

Beauchamp GK, Keast RS, Morel D, et al. Phytochemistry: ibuprofen-like activity in extra-virgin olive oil. *Nature.* 2005;437(7055):45-46.

Fini L, Hotchkiss E, Fogliano V, et al. Chemopreventive properties of pinoresinol-rich olive oil involve a selective activation of the ATM-p53 cascade in colon cancer cell lines. *Carcinogenesis.* 2008;29(1):139-46.

Fogliano V, Sacchi R. Oleocanthal in olive oil: between myth and reality. *Mol Nutr Food Res.* 2006;50(1):5-6.

Impellizzeri J, Lin J. A simple high-performance liquid chromatography method for the determination of throat-burning oleocanthal with probated antiinflammatory activity in extra virgin olive oils. *J Agric Food Chem.* 2006;54(9):3204-3208.

Joshi K, Hankey A, Patwardhan B. Traditional phytochemistry: identification of drug by 'taste'. *Evid Based Complement Alternat Med.* 2007;4(2):145-148.

Smith AB 3rd, Sperry JB, Han Q. Syntheses of (-)-oleocanthal, a natural NSAID found in extra virgin olive oil, the (-)-deacetoxy-oleuropein aglycone, and related analogues. *J Org Chem.* 2007;72(18):6891-6900.

Smith AB 3rd, Han Q, Breslin PA, et al. Synthesis and assignment of absolute configuration of (-)-oleocanthal: a potent, naturally occurring non-steroidal anti-inflammatory and anti-oxidant agent derived from extra virgin olive oils. *Org Lett.* 2005;7(22):5075-5078.

Oleuropein and Oleuropein Aglycone

DESCRIPTION

Olive oil is the principal fat component in the Mediterranean diet, and the consumption of olive oil by those who live in the Mediterranean basin has been associated with a lower incidence of coronary heart disease (CHD), some cancers, including prostate, breast and colorectal cancer, and other chronic degenerative diseases. A large number of phenolic compounds are found in olive oil, and it is thought that some of these compounds might help to confer those health benefits.

The phenolic compounds found in olive oil can be broken down into simple phenols (eg, tyrosol, hydroxytyrosol and elenolic acid), lignans (eg, pinoresinol and acetoxypinoresinol) and secoiridoids (eg, oleuropein aglycone, deacetoxy oleuropein aglycone, and ligstroside aglycone).

Oleuropein aglycone is the most abundant polyphenol in olive oil and is responsible for the characteristic bitter, pungent taste of the oil. Oleuropein (oleuropein glycoside) is found in olive fruit, in the leaves and bark of the olive tree (*Olea europaea* L.), and in olive mill wastewater. Oleuropein is also found in the fruits and leaves of the Japanese privet tree (*Ligustrum japonicum*) and the Chinese privet tree (*Ligustrum lucidum*). Oleuropein, known as the bitter principle of the olive tree, is present in high amounts in the leaves. It is a secondary metabolite of the olive tree and confers resistance to disease and to insect infestation. Olive leaf extracts, mainly oleuropein, were used by the ancient Egyptians to mummify their pharaohs and, in the 1800s, by the British to treat tropical diseases, including malaria.

The types of phenols in extra-virgin olive oil are different from those of the olive fruit. The olives mainly contain the polar glycosides oleuropein and ligstroside. Oleuropein is the ester of elenoic acid with 3,4'-dihydroxyphenylethanol (hydroxytyrosol), and ligstroside is the ester of elenolic acid with 4-hydroxyphenylethanol (tyrosol). Oleuropein and ligstroside are the parent compounds of the less polar oleuropein aglycone and ligstroside aglycone. Oleuropein aglycone and ligstroside aglycone are formed during ripening by removal of the glucose moiety from the oleuropein- and ligstroside-glycosides via the enzyme beta-glucosidase. Those aglycones and their various derivatives are the most abundant phenols in olive oil. Hydroxytyrosol is mainly formed from the hydrolysis of the secoiridoid oleuropein aglycone (see Hydroxytyrosol).

The name "oleuropein" refers to the glycoside form and is sometimes called oleuropein glycoside; the aglycone form is always called, or should always be called, oleuropein aglycone. These names are not always used correctly.

Oleuropein is chemically described as methyl (4*S*,5*E*,6*S*)-4-[2-[2-(3,4-dihydroxyphenyl)ethoxy]-2-oxoethyl]-5-ethylidene-6-[(2*S*,3*R*,4*S*,5*S*,6*R*)-3,4,5-trihydroxy-6-(hydroxymethyl)oxan-2-yl]oxy-4*H*-pyran-3-carboxylate. It is also known as [2*S*-(2alpha,3*E*,4beta)]-3-ethylidene-2-(beta-D-glucopyranosyloxy)-3,4-dihydro-5-(methoxycarbonyl)-2*H*-pyran-4-acetic acid 2-(3,4-dihydroxyphenyl)ethyl ester.

Oleuropein's empirical formula is $C_{25}H_{32}O_{13}$, its molecular weight is 540.51 and its CAS Registry Number is 32619-42-

4. Oleuropein is represented by the following chemical structure.

Oleuropein

Oleuropein is moderately soluble in water; oleuropein aglycone is much less so.

ACTIONS AND PHARMACOLOGY

ACTIONS

Oleuropein has antioxidant activity. It may also have anticancer, anti-inflammatory, antimicrobial, antithrombotic, cardioprotective and rejuvenating/antiaging activities.

MECHANISM OF ACTION

Anticancer activity: Oleuropein was shown to inhibit the proliferation and migration of advanced-grade human tumor cell lines dose-dependently. The tumor cell lines included LN-18, poorly differentiated glioblastoma, TF-1a, erythroleukemia, 786-0, renal cell adenocarcinoma, T-47D, infiltrating ductal carcinoma of the breast-pleural effusion, MCF-7, mammary gland adenocarcinoma, pleural effusion, RPMI-7952, malignant melanoma of the skin, node metastasis, and L_0V_0, colorectal adenocarcinoma and suprascapular region metastasis.

Oleuropein was shown to induce the production of irreversibly rounded cells, preventing their replication, motility and invasiveness. No viable cells could be recovered from those tumors. Oleuropein directly disrupted actin filaments in cells and in a cell-free system. Only very high doses of the olive polyphenol caused growth inhibition in normal fibroblasts. In order to see if the glucose moiety in oleuropein affected its biological activity, it was removed with beta-glucosidase to produce oleuropein aglycone. Beta-glucosidase treated oleuropein was less effective in inhibiting cell proliferation than the nontreated phenol. Possibly, the glucose transporters (GLUTs) were necessary to facilitate the diffusion of oleuropein into the cells, and they didn't work as well for oleuropein aglycone. The mechanism of this interesting anticancer activity of oleuropein is unclear. Continued research in this promising area is needed and warranted.

Human epidermal growth factor receptor 2 (HER2) is an important prognostic and predictive marker of treatment response in women with breast cancer in the adjuvant setting and advanced disease. An oncogene is a protein encoding gene, which when deregulated, participates in the onset and development of cancer. The HER2 gene, also known as HER2/neu or c-erbB2, an oncogene, is amplified and the HER2 protein is overexpressed in about 20% to 35% of breast cancers, with resulting poor prognosis and shortened overall survival. The gene encodes a transmembrane tyrosine kinase growth factor receptor, which mediates signaling for cell proliferation and survival. HER2 gene amplification and resultant protein overexpression are associated with a more aggressive clinical course. Trastuzumab (Herceptin) is a humanized monoclonal antibody that binds to the HER2 receptor. The combination of trastuzumab with chemotherapy has significantly improved the outlook of women with HER2-positive tumors. However, many women who achieve an initial response to trastuzumab-based therapy acquire resistance to the drug within one year.

Oleuropein aglycone was reported to reverse acquired autoresistance to trastuzumab in HER2-overexpressing - breast cancer. Among extra-virgin olive oil polyphenols, oleuropein aglycone was the most potent one in decreasing breast cancer viability. An up to 50-fold increase in the efficacy of trastuzumab occurred in the presence of oleuropein aglycone. A preclinical model of acquired autoresistance to trastuzumab completely recovered trastuzumab sensitivity when co-cultured in the presence of oleuropein aglycone. Oleuropein aglycone significantly reduced HER2 ECD (extracellular domain) cleavage and subsequent HER2 autophosphorylation, while it dramatically enhanced trastuzumab-induced downregulation of HER2 expression. Hydroxytyrosol slightly, but significantly, reduced cell viability at the highest concentrations tested. Oleuropein glycoside was ineffective at inducing any significant cytostatic or cytotoxic effect, regardless of the HER2 status of breast cancer cells.

In the first study mentioned above, oleuropein had more effective anticancer activity against a number of advanced-grade human cancer cell lines than did oleuropein aglycone. This is very different than the present study under consideration. In the present study, a significantly higher cytotoxic activity of the aglyconic form compared with the glycosidic form of oleuropein was observed in all the breast cancer cell lines employed in the study. The authors speculated that the difference possibly derived from the greater lipophilicity of the aglyconic form, a property that, they suggest, should allow better cell membrane incorporation and/or interaction with other lipids.

The above study suggests that oleuropein aglycone, through the specific inhibition of the HER2 oncogene, may exert protective effects not only in the promotion (risk) but also in the progression (invasion and metastasis) of human breast cancer.

However, there are many questions to answer regarding this important work. Oleuropein aglycone, following ingestion, is mainly converted to hydroxytyrosol. The anticancer activity of hydroxytyrosol was lower than that of oleuropein in the study. The mechanism of action of the anticancer effect of oleuropein aglycone is far from being understood. The authors themselves state "caution must be applied when extrapolating *in vitro* results into clinical practice." This research is potentially very important and, before it can be put into clinical practice, much work needs to be done, including human pharmacokinetic studies (via oral and parenteral routes), safety studies and large, prospective, placebo-controlled and randomized clinical trials to investigate the possible anticancer effects of oleuropein aglycone and to determine the optimal dosage of the olive oil phenol for these possible effects.

Anti-inflammatory activity: Oleuropein is discussed in this section. However, oleuropein aglycone has similar properties.

Oleuropein was assessed in experimental sepsis in rabbits caused by the bacteria *Pseudomonas aeruginosa*. Oleuropein was found to significantly prolong the survival of the animals. Rabbits administered oleuropein intravenously had lower levels of the inflammatory cytokine, tumor necrosis factor-alpha (TNF-alpha). It was thought that the positive result with the olive phenol could be explained, at least in part, by an anti-inflammatory mechanism. Promotion of phagocytosis by oleuropein was another possibility.

Oleuropein was demonstrated to have protective effects on bone mass in an ovariectomy/inflammation experimental rat model of bone loss induced by talc granulomatosis. Castration in the animals was associated with decreased mineral density. Inflammation, as characterized by an increase in spleen weight and plasma fibrinogen levels, exacerbated the bone loss. Oleuropein was found to reduce bone loss and to improve the biomarkers of inflammation, such as fibrinogen and spleen weight. The mechanism of action of the possible anti-inflammatory effect of oleuropein is not clear. An antioxidant mechanism was ruled out. This research should continue, since these preliminary results suggest that oleuropein might play a role in the treatment and prevention of osteoporosis.

There are a couple of reports of oleuropein inhibiting the proinflammatory 5-lipoxygenase (5-LOX) enzyme. The inhibition of 5-LOX interferes with eicosanoid metabolism, thereby reducing leukotriene B4 production in leukocytes. The exact mechanism of action of the possible anti-inflammatory effects of oleuropein is unclear.

Antimicrobial: Phenols have long been known to have antimicrobial activity, including antibacterial, antiviral and antifungal activities. The antimicrobial action of phenols is related to their ability to denature proteins, and they are generally classified as surface-acting agents. They act by causing leakage of cytoplasmic constituents. High concentrations precipitate proteins, while lower concentrations inactivate enzymes.

Oleuropein and its aglycone (oleuropein aglycone) have been found to possess antibacterial activity against both gram-negative and gram-positive strains of bacteria, including *Pseudomonas* sp., *Enterococcus* sp. *Salmonella* sp., *Bacillus* sp., *Vibrio* sp. and *Staphylococcus* sp. They have also been shown to inhibit various mycoplasma strains, including *Mycoplasma hominis* and *Mycoplasma fermentans*. The antimicrobial effect of plant secondary metabolites, such as the olive phenolics, represents the plant's defense against microbes, insects and an occasional omnivore that might injure it. Continued research in this area is necessary in order to determine the role oleuropein and oleuropein aglycone might have in the treatment and prevention of bacterial and other microbial infections in humans. It is not clear whether either oleuropein or its aglycone retains its antimicrobial properties in *vivo*.

Antioxidant activity: Oleuropein is discussed in this section. However, oleuropein aglycone has similar properties.

It is known that compounds that share an orthodiphenolic (catecholic) structure possess antioxidant activity. Oleuropein and oleuropein aglycone, like hydroxytyrosol, possess this type of structure. Several studies, for the most part *in vitro* studies, have evaluated the antioxidant properties of oleuropein. The polyphenol has scavenging activity against a wide range of radicals, including hydroxyl, peroxyl, peroxynitrite and superoxide anion radicals. Oleuropein has been found to inhibit the respiratory burst of neutrophils caused by the enzyme NADPH oxidase and the production of hypochlorous acid-derived radicals.

Prevention of free radical formation by oleuropein may occur through its ability to chelate metal ions, such as copper and ferric ions, which catalyze free radical generation reactions.

Oleuropein has also been found to inhibit the oxidation of LDL (low-density lipoprotein). Oxidized LDL is thought to be a crucial factor in the pathogenesis of atherosclerosis. When comparing the radical scavenging ability of oleuropein with that of hydroxytyrosol, hydroxytyrosol was found to generally have more potent antioxidant activity.

In one study, diabetes was induced in rabbits by alloxan. After induction of diabetes, there is a significant rise in malondialdehyde (MDA, a marker of oxidative stress) and blood glucose as well as alteration in enzymatic and non-enzymatic antioxidants in the diabetic animals. Essentially, all of this was attributed to oxidative stress. When the animals were treated with the antioxidant oleuropein, the levels of MDA and blood glucose, as well as the levels of both the non-enzymatic and enzymatic antioxidants, were restored to near normal levels.

Antithrombotic activity: Oleuropein is discussed in this section. However, oleuropein aglycone has similar properties.

Inhibition of platelet aggregation by oleuropein was found in a recent study that examined a few olive oil phenols, their effect on platelet aggregation, and the role cyclic adenosine monophosphate phosphodiesterase (cAMP-PDE) inhibition may play in the effect. Oleuropein was found to inhibit platelet aggregation, but in contrast to hydroxytyrosol, which turned out to be a less potent inhibitor of platelet aggregation, oleuropein inhibited (cAMP-PDE), while hydroxytyrosol did not.

Phosphodiesterase inhibitors possess anti-aggregatory activity.

Cardioprotective activity: Rat hearts were made ischemic and then reperfused. At different times, the coronary effluent was collected and assayed for creatine kinase activity and for reduced and oxidized glutathione. Lipid peroxidation was also assayed by measuring thiobarbituric acid reactive substances (TBARS) concentration in cardiac muscle. (TBARS is used as an assay for lipid peroxidation, a major indicator of oxidative stress.) Pretreatment of the rat hearts with oleuropein prior to ischemia resulted in a decrease of creatine kinase and reduced glutathione release in the perfusate. The protective effect of oleuropein against the post-ischemic oxidative burst was assayed by measuring the release in the coronary effluent of oxidized glutathione, a sensitive marker of the heart's exposure to oxidative stress. Reflow in ischemic hearts was accompanied by prompt release of oxidized glutathione. In ischemic hearts treated with oleuropein, the release of oxidized glutathione was significantly reduced. Membrane lipid peroxidation was also prevented by oleuropein. The mechanism by which oleuropein prevents oxidative myocardial injury induced by ischemia and reperfusion can be explained, in part, by the antioxidant activity of oleuropein.

In another study, oleuropein was demonstrated to exhibit anti-ischemic, antioxidative and hypolipidemic effects in anesthetized rabbits. Oleuropein reduced the infarct size, conferred strong antioxidant protection and reduced the circulating lipids. Again, the mechanism of these effects can be explained, in part, by the antioxidant activity of oleuropein.

Rejuvenation/anti-aging activity: Aging can be characterized as increasing damage to the various tissues of the body and increasing inability to repair the damage, thus leading to chronic degenerative diseases and disorders.

Some of the deleterious changes that occur are the accumulation of damaged proteins. Proteasomes are large protein complexes within most of our cells, whose major function is to degrade unneeded or damaged proteins via proteolysis. The proteins are tagged for degradation by a small protein called ubiquitin. In time, this repair mechanism becomes less efficient and damaged proteins accumulate in the cells. The accumulation of damaged proteins accelerates cell senescence. Human fibroblasts undergo a limited number of divisions in cell culture and progressively reach a state of irreversible growth arrest, a process termed replicative senescence. The fibroblasts remain viable and functional, but they exhibit several biochemical and morphological changes.

Oxidative distress is a major factor in the aging process. Oxidative distress can be defined as the accumulation of reactive oxygen and nitrogen species to the point where the antioxidative mechanisms of the cell are overwhelmed. In the process, DNA, lipids and proteins are damaged. If the proteasome has difficulty handling the damaged proteins, a vicious cycle develops, which hastens the aging process and all the degenerative disorders associated with it. So, what does all of this have to do with olives?

Oleuropein was demonstrated to enhance the proteasome activities *in vitro*. At the same time, continuous treatment of early passage human embryonic fibroblasts with oleuropein was found to decrease the intracellular levels of reactive oxygen species, to reduce the amount of oxidized proteins through increased proteasome-mediated degradation rates and to retain proteasome function during replicative senescence. Further, oleuropein-treated cultures exhibited a delay in the appearance of senescence morphology and their life spans were extended by about 15%. Basically, the antioxidant oleuropein slowed down the oxidative damage of the proteasome and the fibroblasts, leading to an increase in the life span of the fibroblasts, *in vitro*.

There has been great interest in attempting to increase life span in experimental animals by manipulating antioxidant mechanisms. The results to date have been mixed.

PHARMACOKINETICS
The pharmacokinetics (PK) of oleuropein aglycone in humans, as well as that of oleuropein, is incomplete, but some studies are available. The following PK picture of oleuropein represents a composite of those studies.

Oleuropein aglycone, the form found in olive oil, is poorly absorbed in the small intestine. Virtually no oleuropein aglycone is transferred across human Caco-2 cell monolayers or rat segments of jejunum and ileum in *in vitro* models of absorption. In comparison, hydroxytyrosol is efficiently transferred across the monolayers and the intestinal segments. It appears that a certain amount of oleuropein aglycone is hydrolyzed in the stomach to produce hydroxytyrosol. A much greater amount is rapidly degraded by the colonic microflora, resulting in the formation of hydroxytyrosol. A small amount of oleuropein aglycone may get absorbed in the small intestine. Most of an ingested dose of oleuropein aglycone, however, will wind up as hydroxytyrosol. Oleuropein, the form found in olive leaves, has its glucose removed via a glucosidase prior to its being converted to hydroxytyrosol in the stomach and colon.

Hydroxytyrosol is efficiently absorbed from the lumen of the small intestine into the enterocytes via passive diffusion. From the enterocytes, hydroxytyrosol enters the portal circulation, which takes it to the liver from whence it enters the systemic circulation. Hydroxytyrosol produced in the colon is absorbed and also enters the portal circulation and then the systemic circulation. The systemic circulation transports hydroxytyrosol to the various tissues of the body. Hydroxytyrosol appears to cross the blood-brain barrier, entering the brain where it can mix with hydroxytyrosol that is produced from the catabolism of dopamine. The major metabolites of hydroxytyrosol in humans are 4-hydroxy-3-methoxyphenylethanol, also called homovanillyl alcohol, produced from hydroxytyrosol via the enzyme catechol-O-methyltransferase (COMT), 4-hydroxy-3-methoxyphenylacetic acid (homovanillic acid) and the glucuronide conjugates of hydroxytyrosol, as well as of homovanillyl alcohol and homovanillic acid. Most of the ingested hydroxytyrosol is ultimately excreted in the urine as its glucuronide conjugate. Homovanillyl alcohol and homovanillic acid and their glucuronide conjugates and some unconjugated hydroxytyrosol are also found in the urine. Glucuronidation of hydroxytyrosol appears to occur in both the small intestine and in the liver.

Further PK studies on oleuropein and oleuropein aglycone in humans are needed in order to fill in all the details on their ADME (absorption, distribution, metabolism and excretion). PK studies on parenterally administered oleuropein and oleuropein aglycone would also be valuable.

INDICATIONS AND USAGE
Oleuropein, a polyphenol component of olive leaves, and oleuropein aglycone derived from olive oil, have antioxidative and anti-inflammatory activity that may confer upon them cardioprotective and anticancer effects. There is also preliminary evidence these substances might be helpful in

treating and preventing some of the complications of diabetes, protecting against UVB irradiation and preventing inflammation-induced bone loss. They may have also some antimicrobial effects. Clinical studies are lacking.

RESEARCH SUMMARY

Oleuropein has been more extensively studied than some of the other olive polyphenols (see Hydroxytyrosol and Oleocanthal). It is said to have potent antioxidative effects (though, according to one review of the literature, not as potent as hydroxytyrosol). *In vitro* and animal studies suggest that oleurpein's antioxidative and anti-inflammatory activities may have effects that could be cardioprotective. In one study, oleuropein enhanced nitric oxide production in mouse macrophages. In a study of isolated rat heart, it prevented oxidative myocardial injury induced by ischemia and reperfusion. Membrane lipid peroxidation was prevented by the polyphenol in this study, and reperfusion-related release of oxidized glutathione was significantly inhibited. In other research, oleuropein has demonstrated antithrombotic activity. In a study utilizing rabbits, oleuropein exhibited anti-ischemic, antioxidative and hypolipidemic effects. Treatment for six weeks with varying doses of the polyphenol resulted in decreases in both total cholesterol and triglyceride levels in these animals. Both hypoglycemic and antioxidant effects were observed in alloxan-induced diabetic rabbits administered oleuropein. During 16 weeks of treatment with the polyphenol, oxidative stress markers and glucose levels were largely restored to normal. Further research is needed and warranted.

Like hydroxytyrosol, oleuropein has shown some antimicrobial activity against both gram-positive and gram-negative bacterial species of several types. In a study of acute pyelonephritis induced in 70 rabbits, oleuropein prolonged survival through immunomodulating effects which, the researchers concluded, might include promotion of phagocytosis and/or inhibition of biosynthesis of proinflammatory cytokines. In other research, oleuropein has demonstrated antimycoplasma effects. More research is needed before any conclusions can be drawn about a possible role for this substance as a useful clinical antimicrobial agent.

There is some evidence of an oleuropein anticancer effect. In one study, oleuropein inhibited the proliferation and migration of advanced-grade human tumor cell lines in a dose-dependent manner. In a mouse model of spontaneous tumor, the substance was said to achieve complete tumor regression in 9-12 days. One group of researchers has concluded that oleuropein may be a potent antitumor agent. These promising results need follow-up.

Oleuropein reduced bone loss and several inflammatory biomarkers in an ovariectomy/inflammation experimental model of bone loss in the rat. The level of response was dose-dependent. Further research is warranted.

A gel containing oleuropein has shown some efficacy against UVB irradiation.

CONTRAINDICATIONS, PRECAUTIONS, ADVERSE REACTIONS

CONTRAINDICATIONS

Oleuropein- and oleuropein aglycone-containing dietary supplements are contraindicated in those hypersensitive to any component of an oleuropein- or oleuropein aglycone-containing dietary supplement. Hypersensitivity to oleuropein or oleuropein aglycone is probably very rare.

PRECAUTIONS

Those who wish to use oleuropein- or oleuropein aglycone-containing dietary supplements for a health condition should first discuss this with his or her physician.

Because of the possible antithrombotic effect of oleuropein or oleuropein aglycone, hemophiliacs and those taking warfarin (Coumadin) should exercise caution in its use. Oleuropein- or oleuropein aglycone-containing dietary supplements should be stopped a few days before any surgery and can be resumed following the surgery.

Because of the lack of long-term studies on the safety of oleuropein- and oleuropein aglycone-containing dietary supplements, pregnant women and nursing mothers should be cautious in their use.

ADVERSE REACTIONS

No reports.

INTERACTIONS

DRUGS

Oleuropein aglycone was reported to reverse acquired autoresistance to trastuzumab in HER2-overexpressing breast cancer. (See Anticancer activity above.)

NUTRITIONAL SUPPLEMENTS

None known.

HERBS

None known.

FOODS

None known.

OVERDOSAGE

There are no reports of overdosage.

DOSAGE AND ADMINISTRATION

Oleuropein-containing dietary supplements, mainly in the form of olive leaf extracts, are available in capsules. Doses higher than those recommended on the label should generally not be exceeded.

Oleuropein aglycone is present in extra-virgin olive oil from about 23.3% to 37.7%.

LITERATURE

Al-Azzawie HF, Alhamdani MS. Hypoglycemic and antioxidant effect of oleuropein in alloxan-diabetic rabbits. *Life Sci.* 2006;78(12):1371-1377.

Andreadou I, Sigala F, Iliodromitis EK, et al. Acute doxorubicin cardiotoxicity is successfully treated with the phytochemical oleuropein through suppression of oxidative and nitrosative stress. *J Mol Cell Cardiol.* 2007;42(3):549-558.

Bianco AD, Muzzalupo I, Piperno A, et al. Bioactive derivatives of oleuropein from olive fruits. *J Agric Food Chem.* 1999;47(9):3531-3534.

Bitler CM, Viale TM, Damaj B, et al Hydrolyzed olive vegetation water in mice has anti-inflammatory activity. *J Nutr.* 2005;135(6):1475-1479.

Briante R, La Cara F, Febbraio F, et al. Bioactive derivatives from oleuropein by a biotransformation on Olea europaea leaf extracts. *J Biotechnol.* 2002;93(2):109-119.

Christian MS, Sharper VA, Hoberman AM, et al. The toxicity profile of hydrolyzed aqueous olive pulp extract. *Drug Chem Toxicol.* 2004;27(4):309-330.

Ciafardini G, Marsilio V, Lanza B, et al. Hydrolysis of Oleuropein by Lactobacillus plantarum Strains Associated with Olive Fermentation. *Appl Environ Microbiol.* 1994;60(11):4142-4147.

Coni E, Di Benedetto R, Di Pasquale M, et al. Protective effect of oleuropein, an olive oil biophenol, on low density lipoprotein oxidizability in rabbits. *Lipids.* 2000;35(1):45-54.

Edgecombe SC, Stretch GL, Hayball PJ. Oleuropein, an antioxidant polyphenol from olive oil, is poorly absorbed from isolated perfused rat intestine. *J Nutr.* 2000;130(12):2996-3002.

Fleming HP, Walter WM Jr, Etchells JL. Antimicrobial properties of oleuropein and products of its hydrolysis from green olives. *Appl Microbiol.* 1973 Nov;26(5):777-782.

Furneri PM, Marino A, Saija A, et al. In vitro antimycoplasmal activity of oleuropein. *Int J Antimicrob Agents.* 2002;20(4):293-296.

Giamarellos-Bourboulis EJ, Geladopoulos T, Chrisofos M, et al. Oleuropein: a novel immunomodulator conferring prolonged survival in experimental sepsis by Pseudomonas aeruginosa. *Shock.* 2006;26(4):410-416.

Hamdi HK, Castellon R. Oleuropein, a non-toxic olive iridoid, is an anti-tumor agent and cytoskeleton disruptor. *Biochem Biophys Res Commun.* 2005;334(3):769-778.

Juven B, Henis Y, Jacoby B. Studies on the mechanism of the antimicrobial action of oleuropein. *J Appl Bacteriol.* 1972;35(4):559-567.

Katsiki M, Chondrogianni N, Chinou I, et al. The olive constituent oleuropein exhibits proteasome stimulatory properties in vitro and confers life span extension of human embryonic fibroblasts. *Rejuvenation Res.* 2007;10(2):157-172.

Manna C, Migliardi V, Golino P, et al. Oleuropein prevents oxidative myocardial injury induced by ischemia and reperfusion. *J Nutr Biochem.* 2004;15(8):461-466.

Menendez JA, Vazquez-Martin A, Colomer R, et al. Olive oil's bitter principle reverses acquired autoresistance to trastuzumab (Herceptin) in HER2-overexpressing breast cancer cells. *BMC Cancer.* 2007;7:80.

Perugini P, Vettor M, Rona C, et al. Efficacy of oleuropein against UVB irradiation: preliminary evaluation. *Int J Cosmet Sci.* 2008;30(2):1131-1120.

Puel C, Mathey J, Agalias A, et al. Dose-response study of effect of oleuropein, an olive oil polyphenol, in an ovariectomy/inflammation experimental model of bone loss in the rat. *Clin Nutr.* 2006 Oct;25(5):859-868.

Puel C, Quintin A, Agalias A, et al. Olive oil and its main phenolic micronutrient (oleuropein) prevent inflammation-induced bone loss in the ovariectomised rat. *Br J Nutr.* 2004 Jul;92(1):119-127.

Sivakumar G, Briccoli Bati C, et al. Demethyloleuropein and beta-glucosidase activity in olive fruits. *Biotechnol J.* 2007 Mar;2(3):381-385.

Soni MG, Burdock GA, Christian MS, et al. Safety assessment of aqueous olive pulp extract as an antioxidant or antimicrobial agent in foods. *Food Chem Toxicol.* 2006;44(7):903-915.

Tsarbopoulos A, Gikas E, Papadopoulos N, et al. Simultaneous determination of oleuropein and its metabolites in plasma by high-performance liquid chromatography. *J Chromatogr B Analyt Technol Biomed Life Sci.* 2003;785(1):157-164.

Tuck KL, Hayball PJ. Major phenolic compounds in olive oil: metabolism and health effects. *J Nutr Biochem.* 2002;13(11):636-644.

Visioli F, Bellosta S, Galli C. Oleuropein, the bitter principle of olives, enhances nitric oxide production by mouse macrophages. *Life Sci.* 1998;62(6):541-546.

Visioli F, Galli C. Oleuropein protects low density lipoprotein from oxidation. *Life Sci.* 1994;55(24):1965-1971.

Vissers MN, Zock PL, Roodenburg AJ, et al. Olive oil phenols are absorbed in humans. *J Nutr.* 2002;132(3):409-417.

Zanichelli D, Baker TA, Clifford MN, et al. Inhibition of Staphylococcus aureus by oleuropein is mediated by hydrogen peroxide. *J Food Prot.* 2005;68(7):1492-1496.

Ornithine Alpha-Ketoglutarate

DESCRIPTION

Ornithine alpha-ketoglutarate, abbreviated OKG, also known as ornithine 2-oxoglutarate or ornithine oxoglutarate (OGO), is a salt formed of two molecules of the non-protein amino acid, L-ornithine, and one molecule of the Krebs cycle dicarboxylic acid, alpha-ketoglutarate. OKG has been used both enterally and parenterally in burn, trauma, surgical and chronically malnourished patients. It appears to decrease protein catabolism and/or increase protein synthesis under these conditions. OKG is a popular nutritional supplement for athletes, among others.

ACTIONS AND PHARMACOLOGY

ACTIONS

OKG, under certain conditions, may have immunomodulatory and anticatabolic and/or anabolic actions. OKG is a delivery form of L-glutamine and L-arginine precursors.

MECHANISM OF ACTION

The actions of OKG can be attributed to the metabolites that the OKG components, L-ornithine and alpha-ketoglutarate, give rise to. These metabolites are L-arginine, L-glutamine, L-proline and polyamines. The metabolism of L-glutamine and L-arginine is altered in trauma, and this alteration is linked to immune dysfunction.

One of the major biochemical events that occurs following a burn injury is a fall in intramuscular L-glutamine. This amino acid is released from muscle tissue to meet the increased needs of other cells, in particular immune cells and intestinal cells. L-glutamine is now known to be essential for sustaining the proliferation and activation of immune cells. In the intestine it is essential for maintaining the integrity of the mucosal barrier and its metabolic and immune function. Immune and gastrointestinal dysfunctions occur when *de novo* L-glutamine synthesis is insufficient to maintain normal function of immune cells and enterocytes. Under these conditions, for example a burn injury, the normally non-essential (meaning the body can make it) L-glutamine becomes a conditionally essential amino acid (meaning the body can't make enough of it). OKG is a delivery form of L-glutamine.

L-arginine is also essential for immune cells. It is thought that the role of L-arginine in immunity is mediated by its metabolite nitric oxide. Burn injury and some other traumas affect the status of both L-glutamine and L-arginine in the various tissues of the body, especially muscle, the immune system and the gastrointestinal tract. As in the case of L-glutamine, *de novo* synthesis of L-arginine during these conditions is probably not sufficient for normal immune and gastrointestinal function, nor for normal protein synthesis. OKG, in addition to being a delivery form of L-glutamine, is also a delivery form of L-arginine or more precisely L-ornithine, which is converted to L-arginine.

It is unclear if OKG has immunomodulatory or anticatabolic/anabolic actions under normal conditions.

See L-Glutamine and L-Arginine.

PHARMACOKINETICS

Following ingestion, OKG is absorbed from the small intestine from whence it is transported to the liver. In the liver, OKG enters various metabolic pathways. L-ornithine is a precursor in the synthesis of L-arginine and polyamines, among others. Alpha-ketoglutarate is metabolized to L-glutamine, among other molecules. OKG not metabolized by the liver is transported via the systemic circulation and distributed to various tissues of the body, including the brain, where it undergoes metabolic reactions similar to those above. Under conditions of trauma or burn injury, OKG may be metabolized in immune cells, enterocytes and muscle tissue to produce L-arginine and L-glutamine.

INDICATIONS AND USAGE

OKG has demonstrated significant usefulness in the nutritional support of burn and other trauma patients, as well as in chronically malnourished subjects and post-surgery in the elderly. It has been shown to speed wound healing. It has exhibited some immunomodulating effects. Claims that it enhances athletic performance have not been confirmed.

RESEARCH SUMMARY

OKG has shown significant effects related to nutritional support in burn, trauma, surgical, elderly and chronically malnourished subjects. These effects have been achieved with both enteral and parenteral administration. OKG has been shown, in varying conditions, to decrease muscle protein catabolism and/or increase muscle protein synthesis. It has also been shown to enhance wound healing. Its ability to increase synthesis of L-glutamine and L-arginine may account for these positive effects. In a recent double-blind, placebo-controlled study, 60 severely burned subjects were randomized to receive 20 grams of OKG daily or placebo for 21 days beginning mean four days post-injury. Significant improvement was achieved in the OKG-treated group, compared with controls, as measured by both biological and clinical end points. Previous studies of OKG-treated burn patients have reported shorter hospitalizations and fewer fatalities.

No conclusions can yet be drawn from scant, preliminary evidence that OKG may exert some positive effects on immunity. And there is no credible research to support claims that OKG can build muscle in healthy individuals or that it can enhance exercise/athletic performance.

CONTRAINDICATIONS, PRECAUTIONS, ADVERSE REACTIONS

CONTRAINDICATIONS

OKG is contraindicated in those with deficiency of ornithine-delta-aminotransferase (OAT). This is a genetic disease resulting in gyrate atrophy of the choroid and retina and progressive blinding chorioretinal degeneration. It is rare.

PRECAUTIONS

Pregnant women and nursing mothers should avoid supplemental OKG. OKG supplementation may potentially cause hypoglycemia in starved individuals. Those with eating disorders or those who are on very-low-calorie diets should exercise caution in using OKG.

ADVERSE REACTIONS

None reported for those using supplemental OKG.

DOSAGE AND ADMINISTRATION

There are no typical doses for OKG supplementation. Some athletes use about 2.5 grams before and after exercise, as well as before breakfast and at bedtime.

Doses of 20 to 30 grams daily, given enterally, have been used in burn and trauma patients.

LITERATURE

Czernichow B, Nsi-Emvo E, Galluser M, et al. Enteral supplementation with ornithine alpha ketoglutarate improves the early adaptive response to resection. *Gut*. 1997; 40:67-72.

De Bandt JP, Coudray-Lucas C, Lioret N, et al. A randomized controlled trial of the influence of the mode of enteral ornithine alpha-ketoglutarate administration in burn patients. *J Nutr*. 1998; 128:563-569.

Dumas F, De Bandt JP, Colomb V, et al. Enteral ornithine alpha-ketoglutarate enhances intestinal adaptation to massive resection in rats. *Metabolism*. 1998; 47:1366-1371.

Donati L, Ziegler F, Pongelli G, Signorini MS. Nutritional and clinical efficacy of ornithine alpha-ketoglutarate in severe burn patients. *Clin Nutr*. 1999; 18:307-311.

Duranton B, Schleiffer R, Gosse F, Raul F. Preventive administration of ornithine alpha-ketoglutarate improves intestinal mucosal repair after transient ischemia in rats. *Crit Care Med*. 1998; 26:120-125.

Jeevanandam M, Holaday NJ, Petersen SR. Ornithine-alpha-ketoglutarate(OKG) supplementation is more effective than its component salts in traumatized rats. *J Nutr*. 1996; 126:2141-2150.

Jeevanandam M, Petersen SR. Substrate fuel kinetics in enterally fed trauma patients supplemented with ornithine alpha-ketoglutarate. *Clin Nutr*. 1999; 18; 209-217.

Le Boucher J, Eurengbiol, Farges MC, et al. Modulation of immune response with ornithine A-ketoglutarate in burn injury: an arginine or glutamine dependency? *Nutrition*. 1999; 15; 773-777.

Le Bricon T, Cynober L, Baracos VE. Ornithine alpha-ketoglutarate limits muscle protein breakdown without stimulating tumor growth in rats bearing Yoshida ascites hepatoma. *Metabolism*. 1994; 43; 899-905.

Le Bricon T, Cynober L. Field CJ, Baracos VE. Supplemental nutrition with ornithine alpha-ketoglutarate in rats with cancer-associated cachexia: surgical treatment of the tumor improves efficacy of nutritional support. *Nutr. J* 1995; 125:2999-3010.

Robinson LE, Bussiere FI, Le Boucher J, et al. Amino acid nutrition and immune function in tumour-bearing rats: a comparison of glutamine-, arginine- and ornithine 2-oxoglutarate-supplemented diets. Clin Sci (Colch). 1999; 97:657-669.

Roch-Arveiller M, Fontagne J, Coudray-Lucas C, et al. Ornithine alpha-ketoglutarate counteracts the decrease of liver cytochrome p-450 content in burned rats. *Nutrition*.1999; 15:379-383.

Roch-Arveiller M, Tissat M, Coudray-Lucas C, et al. Immunomodulatory effects of ornithine alpha-ketoglutarate in rats with burn injuries. *Arch Surg*. 1996; 131:718-723.

Varanasi RV, Saltzman JR. Ornithine oxoglutarate therapy improves nutrition status. *Nutr Rev*. 1996; 53:96-97.

Pantethine

DESCRIPTION

Pantethine is the disulfide dimer of pantetheine, the 4'-phosphate derivative of which is an intermediate in the conversion of the B vitamin pantothenic acid to coenzyme A (see Pantothenic Acid). Pantethine is found naturally in small quantities in most forms of life, and therefore, in food sources. Very large doses of pantethine have been found to have lipid-lowering effects, and pantethine is used in Europe and Japan as a lipid-lowering agent. Pantethine is marketed in the United States as a nutritional supplement.

Pantethine is also known as D-bis(N-pantothenyl-beta-aminoethyl)disulfide and (R)-N,N'-[dithiobis(ethyleneiminocarbonylethylene]bis(2,4-dihydroxy-3,3-dimethylbutyramide). Its molecular formula is $C_{22}H_{42}N_4O_8S_2$ and its molecular weight is 554.73 daltons. Pantetine is represented by the following chemical structure:

Pantethine

ACTIONS AND PHARMACOLOGY

ACTIONS

Pantethine may have lipid-modulating activity. It has putative antiatherogenic, ophthalmoprotective and detoxification activities.

MECHANISM OF ACTION

Pantethine has been found to decrease serum levels of total cholesterol, low-density lipoprotein cholesterol (LDL-C), apolipoprotein B and triglycerides. It has also been found to increase high-density lipoprotein cholesterol (HDL-C) and apolipoprotein A1 levels. The mechanism of the possible lipid-modulating activity of pantethine is not understood. In isolated hepatocytes, pantethine has been shown to inhibit both cholesterol and fatty acid synthesis. It is speculated that pantethine, by acting as a precursor of coenzyme A, may enhance the beta-oxidation of fatty acids. However, this has not been confirmed. Another hypothesis is that the lipid-modulating effect of pantethine may be mediated via its metabolite cysteamine. It is argued that there is little pantethine found in the serum following its ingestion and that most of a dose is metabolized to pantothenic acid and cysteamine. Since pantothenic acid does not possess lipid-modulatory activity, cysteamine might. This lipid-modulatory activity could occur via the inhibition of acetyl coenzyme A carboxylase activity and the stimulation of hepatic fatty acid oxidation, resulting in lowered triglyceride levels, and via the inhibition of HMG-CoA reductase activity, resulting in lowered cholesterol levels. Again, this has not been confirmed. Further, cysteamine, a treatment for cystinosis, has not been found to have lipid-lowering activity in those with this rare genetic disorder. Nor, does pantethine appear to be efficacious in the treatment of cystinosis.

The putative antiatherogenic activity may be accounted for, in large part, by pantethine's possible lipid-modulatory activity. In addition, pantethine may have antioxidant activity and also may decrease platelet aggregability. A few studies suggest that pantethine may have antioxidant activity. One *in vitro* study found inhibition of peroxidation of LDL, but only under certain concentrations.

The mechanism of pantethine's possible antioxidant activity is unclear. Other studies have reported that pantethine may decrease platelet aggregability. Possible mechanisms, include decreased thromboxane production and modulation of platelet membrane fluidity. Treatment with pantethine has been found to decrease the cholesterol content of platelet membranes. This could result in increased platelet membrane fluidity and decreased platelet aggregability.

Parenterally administered pantethine has been demonstrated to inhibit lens opacification, in some animal studies. The mechanism of this possible ophthalmoprotective effect is not understood. One possibility is that pantethine may inhibit the formation of protein aggregates in the lens of the eye by forming mixed disulfides with cysteine residues of certain lens proteins. There is no evidence that orally administered pantethine has any activity in inhibiting lens opacification.

Other animal experiments have demonstrated that pantethine protects the liver against certain hepatotoxins, such as carbon tetrachloride. Again, pantethine was administered parenterally in these studies. This hepatoprotective activity may be accounted for, in part, by the possible antioxidant activity of pantethine.

Pantethine has been shown to lower serum acetaldehyde in a small human study, following ethanol ingestion. Acetaldehyde is thought to mediate some of the hepatotoxic effects of ethanol. It is speculated that pantethine-induced lowering of blood acetaldehyde levels following alcohol ingestion is due, in part, to accelerated acetaldehyde oxidation by an interaction between hepatic aldehyde dehydrogenase and pantethine-related intermediates formed in the liver.

PHARMACOKINETICS

The pharmacokinetics of pantethine in humans are incomplete. Following ingestion, pantethine is absorbed from the small intestine into the enterocytes where some is reduced, via glutathione reductase, to pantetheine. Some pantetheine is metabolized in the enterocytes to coenzyme A and the rest, along with pantethine, is released by the enterocytes into the portal circulation. It appears that pantethine undergoes significant metabolism in the blood to pantothenic acid and cysteamine. These metabolites, along with pantethine and pantetheine, are transported to the liver where they are extracted by the hepatocytes and undergo various metabolic reactions. In the liver, some pantethine is reduced to pantetheine and the pantetheine pool in that organ is metabolized to coenzyme A. There appears to be significant first-pass extraction, as well as first-pass metabolism, of pantethine by the liver. There does not appear to be much pantethine circulating in the blood, following ingestion. Coenzyme A itself is catabolized by a number of hydrolytic steps resulting in the production of pantothenate and cysteamine. There is some evidence that pantethine is more efficiently converted to coenzyme A than is pantothenic acid.

INDICATIONS AND USAGE

Pantethine may favorably affect lipids and protect against cardiovascular disease. There is evidence, in animal research, that it can inhibit cataract formation. It also exhibits some hepatoprotective effects in animal models. Additionally, it has been shown to protect against a number of toxins, including alcohol. Preliminary research suggests that pantethine may influence various central nervous system and adrenal junctions, but no useful conclusions can yet be drawn from these early investigations. There is no credible evidence that pantethine enhances exercise performance or that it inhibits hair loss and graying of hair.

RESEARCH SUMMARY

Several studies have shown that pantethine can significantly lower levels of both cholesterol and triglycerides. Doses used in these studies have ranged from 600 to 1,200 milligrams daily. In one of these studies, seven children and 65 adults suffering from hypercholesterolemia alone or combined with hypertriglyceridemia achieved significant reductions in total cholesterol, LDL-cholesterol, triglycerides and apo-B, as well as significant increases in HDL-cholesterol and apo-A1.

They received 900-1,200 milligrams of pantethine daily for three to six months.

Pantethine has also proved helpful in treating diabetics with dyslipidemia, reducing triglyceride levels by 37% in one study (utilizing 600 milligram daily doses). In general, looking at all studies to date, pantethine typically reduces total cholesterol by 15-25% and triglycerides by 25-40%.

Additionally, there is *in vitro* and clinical evidence that pantethine can help maintain normal platelet functions, favorably affecting platelet lipid composition and cell membrane fluidity. These effects may provide further protection against atherosclerosis.

Animal research indicates that pantethine can inhibit cataract formation. This has been demonstrated in several animal models. Reversal of existing opacities has not been demonstrated. More research is needed to see whether these findings extend to humans.

There is also considerable animal data suggesting that pantethine may have significant hepatoprotective effects. It has demonstrated protection against carbon tetrachloride, halocarbon, autoxidized linoleate, acetaldehyde, ethanol and other hepatotoxins.

There is no evidence that pantethine can prevent hair loss or graying of hair. Similarly there is no evidence that pantethine can enhance athletic performance. A recent study showed that a combination of pantethine, pantothenic acid and allithiamin had no effect on exercise performance.

CONTRAINDICATIONS, PRECAUTIONS, ADVERSE REACTIONS

CONTRAINDICATIONS

Pantethine is contraindicated in those hypersensitive to any component of a pantethine-containing product.

PRECAUTIONS

Pregnant women and nursing mothers should avoid the use of pantethine.

The use of pantethine for its possible lipid-lowering effects should only be undertaken under medical supervision.

ADVERSE REACTIONS

Doses up to 1,200 milligrams daily have been well tolerated. There are a few reports of gastrointestinal effects, including nausea and heartburn.

INTERACTIONS

DRUGS

HMG-CoA reductase inhibitors (atorvastatin, cerivastatin, fluvastatin, lovastatin, pravastatin, simvastatin): Concomitant use of pantethine and a HMG-CoA reductase inhibitor may produce additive lipid-modulatory effects.

NUTRITIONAL SUPPLEMENTS

Nicotinic acid: Concomitant use of pantethine and high-dose nicotinic acid may produce additive lipid-modulatory effects.

OVERDOSAGE

There are no reports of pantethine overdosage in the literature.

DOSAGE AND ADMINISTRATION

Single component and combination products (e.g., with pantothenic acid) are available. Possible lipid-lowering dosage typically ranges from 600 to 1,200 milligrams daily, taken in divided doses. See Precautions.

LITERATURE

Arsenio L, Bodria P, Magnati G, et al. Effectiveness of long-term treatment with pantethine inpatients with dyslipidemia. *Clin Ther.* 1986; 8:537-545.

Bertolini S, Donati C, Elicio N, et al. Lipoprotein changes induced by pantethine in hyperlipoproteinemic patients: adults and children. *Int J Clin Pharmacol Ther Toxicol.* 1986; 24:630-637.

Bon GB, Cazzolato G, Zago S, Avogaro P. Effects of pantothine on in vitro peroxidation of low density lipoproteins. *Atherosclerosis.* 1985; 57:99-106.

Branca D, Scutari G, Siliprandi N. Pantethine and pantothenate effect on the CoA content of rat liver. *Internat J Vit Nutr Res.* 1984; 54:211-216.

Carrara P, Matturri L, Galbussera M, et al. Pantethine reduces plasma cholesterol and the severity of arterial lesions in experimental hypercholesterolemic rabbits. *Atherosclerosis.* 1984; 53:255-264.

Cighetti G, Del Puppo M, Paroni R, et al. Pantethine inhibits cholesterol and fatty acid syntheses and stimulates carbon dioxide formation in isolated rat hepatocytes. *J Lipid Res.* 1987; 28:152-161.

Clark JI, Livesey JC, Steele JE. Delay or inhibition of rat lens opacification using pantethine and WR-77913. *Exp Eye Res.* 1996; 62:75-84.

Congdon NT, West ST, Duncan DT, et al. The effect of pantethine and ultraviolet-B radiation on the development of lenticular opacity in the emory mouse. *Curr Eye Res.* 2000; 20:17-24.

Donati C, Barbi G, Cairo G, et al. Pantethine improves the lipid abnormalities of chronic hemodialysis patients: results of a multicenter clinical trial. *Clin Nephrol.* 1986; 25:70-74.

Donati C, Bertieri RS, Barbi G. [Pantethine, diabetes mellitus and atherosclerosis. Clinical study of 1045 patients]. [Article in Italian]. *Clin Ter.* 1989; 128:411-422.

Friberg G, Pande J, Ogun O, Benedek GB. Pantethine inhibits the formation of high-Tc protein aggregates in gamma B crystallin solutions. *Curr Eye Res.* 1996; 15:1182-1190.

Gaddi A, Descovich GC, Noseda G, et al. Controlled evaluation of pantethine, a natural hypolipidemic compound, in patients with different forms of hyperlipoproteinemia. *Atherosclerosis.* 1984; 50:73-83.

Galeone F, Scalabrino A, Giuntoli F, et al. The lipid-lowering effect of pantethine in hyperlipidemic patients: a clinical investigation. *Curr Ther Res.* 1983; 34:383-390.

Gensini GF, Prisco D, Rogasi PG, et al. Changes in fatty acid composition of the single platelet phospholipids induced by pantethine treatment. *Int J Clin Pharm Res.* 1985; 5:309-318.

Hayashi H, Kobayashi A, Terada H, et al. Effect of pantethine on action potential of canine papillary muscle during hypoxic perfusion. *Jap Heart J.* 1985; 26:289-296.

Hiramatsu N, Kishida T, Hamano T, Natake M. Effects of dietary pantethine levels on contents of fatty acids and thiobarbituric acid reactive substances in the liver of rats orally administered varying amounts of autoxidized linoleate. *J Nutr Sci Vitaminol (Tokyo).* 1991; 37:73-87.

Hoffman B, Lang A, Ostermann G, et al. Effect of pantethine on platelet functions *in vitro. Curr Ther Res.* 1987; 41:791-801.

Iida J, Nishimura K, Ukei S, Azuma I. Macrophage activation with pantethine and pantetheine-4'-phosphate. *Int J Vitam Nutr Res.* 1985; 55:405-411.

Kumerova AO, Silova AA, Utno Lia. [Effect of pantethine on post-heparin lipolytic activity and lipid peroxidation in the myocardium]. [Article in Russian]. *Biull Eksp Biol Med.* 1991; 111:33-35.

Maggi GC, Donati C, Criscuoli G. Pantethine: a physiological lipomodulating agent in the treatment of hyperlipidemias. *Curr Ther Res.* 1982; 32:380-386.

Nagiel-Ostaszewski I, Lau-Cam CA. Protection by pantethine, pantothenic acid and cystamine against carbon tetrachloride-induced hepatotoxicity in the rat. *Res Commun Chem Pathol Pharmacol.* 1990; 67:289-292.

Prisco D, Rogasi PG, Matucci M, et al. Effect of pantethine treatment on platelet aggregation and thromboxane A_2 production. *Curr Ther Res.* 1984; 35:700-706.

Vecsei L, Alling C, Widerlov E. Comparative studies of intracerebroventricularly administered cysteamine and pantethine in different behavioral tests and on brain catechols in rats. *Arch Int Pharmacodyn Ther.* 1990; 305:140-151.

Watanabe A, Hobara BS, Kobayashi M, et al. Lowering of blood acetaldehyde but not ethanol concentrations by pantethine following alcohol ingestion: different effects in flushing and nonflushing subjects. *Alcoholism: Clin Exper Res.* 1985; 9:272-276.

Webster MJ. Physiological and performance responses to supplementation with thiamin and pantothenic acid derivatives. *Eur J Appl Physiol.* 1998; 77:486-491.

Wittwer CT, Graves CP, Peterson MA, et al. Pantethine lipomodulation: evidence for cysteamine mediation *in vitro* and *in vivo. Atherosclerosis.* 1987; 68:41-49.

Yoon SB, Kajiyama K, Ogura R. [Effect of pantethine on adriamycin-induced cardiotoxicity]. [Article in Japanese]. *Kurume Igakkai Zasshi.* 1982; 45:598-606.

Pantothenic Acid

DESCRIPTION

Pantothenic acid, a member of the B-vitamin family, is an essential nutrient in human nutrition. It is sometimes referred to as vitamin B_5. Pantothenic acid is involved in a number of biological reactions, including the production of energy, the catabolism of fatty acids and amino acids, the synthesis of fatty acids, phospholipids, sphingolipids, cholesterol and steroid hormones, and the synthesis of heme and the neurotransmitter acetylcholine. It also appears to be involved in the regulation of gene expression and in signal transduction. Roger J. Williams, the discoverer of pantothenic acid and a scientist who pioneered the use of nutrients for the prevention and treatment of disease, thought that pantothenic acid might be helpful in the management of certain medical disorders, such as rheumatoid arthritis.

The term pantothenic acid is derived from the Greek word pantos, meaning everywhere. Pantothenic acid is widely distributed in plant and animal food sources, where it occurs in both bound and free forms. Rich sources of the vitamin, include organ meats (liver, kidney), egg yolk, avocados, cashew nuts and peanuts, brown rice, soya, lentils, broccoli and milk. Royal jelly and brewer's yeast, both of which are used as nutritional supplements, are two of the richest sources of pantothenic acid. The richest sources of the vitamin are the ovaries of cod and tuna. Pantothenic acid is synthesized by intestinal microflora and this may also contribute to the body's pantothenic acid requirements.

Pantothenic acid deficiency in humans is rare. Symptoms of pantothenic acid deficiency, which has occurred under conditions of severe malnutrition, include numbness in the toes and painful burning in the feet (melalgia). Experimentally-induced pantothenic acid deficiency in humans, produced headache, fatigue, insomnia, intestinal disturbances, paresthesias of the hands and feet, impaired antibody production, an elevated sedimentation rate and an impaired eosinopenic response to ACTH. Most of these symptoms and signs resolved with administration of pantothenic acid.

The principal biologically active forms of pantothenic acid are coenzyme A (CoA) and acyl carrier protein (ACP). In both CoA and ACP, the business center of the molecule is the pantothenic acid metabolite 4'-phosphopantetheine. Coenzyme A is comprised of 4'-phosphopantetheine linked by an anhydride bond to the nucleotide adenosine 5'-monophosphate. 4'-Phosphopantetheine itself is comprised of pantothenic acid linked at one end, via an amide bond, to beta-mercaptoethylamine, derived from L-cysteine, and at the other end to a phosphate group. The sulfhydryl group of 4'-phosphopantetheine, which is the business end of the coenzyme, forms thioesters with acyl groups producing acyl-CoA derivatives, including acetyl-CoA.

Acetyl-CoA is produced via beta-oxidation of fatty acids, via the metabolism of carbohydrates—glucose 6-phosphate to pyruvate to acetyl-CoA—and via the catabolism of amino acids. Acetyl-CoA has a number of metabolic opportunities. It is metabolized in the tricarboxylic acid cycle to produce carbon dioxide, water and energy. It can also be metabolized to fatty acids, cholesterol and steroid hormones. Acetyl-CoA also participates in a number of acetylation reactions, including the formation of acetylcholine, melatonin, N-acetylglucosamine, N-acetylgalactosamine and N-acetylneuraminic acid. Finally, acetyl-CoA is involved in the acetylation of proteins and peptides. Histone acetylation is an epigenetic mechanism of gene regulation. In general, chromatin fractions enriched in actively transcribed genes are also enriched in highly acetylated core histones, whereas silent genes are associated with nucleosomes with a low level of acetylation. Nucleosomes are the fundamental units of chromosomes.

The other major form of pantothenic acid is acyl carrier protein or ACP. Acyl carrier protein (ACP) functions as a coenzyme in the fatty acid synthetase complex which is central to the *de novo* synthesis of fatty acids. The prosthetic group of acyl carrier protein is again, 4'-phosphopantetheine. 4'-Phosphopantetheine binds to acyl carrier protein via a phosphodiester linkage to a serine residue of acyl carrier protein. The function of ACP in fatty acid synthesis is analogous to that of coenzyme A in the beta-oxidation of fatty acids. ACP serves as an anchor to which the acyl intermediates are esterified. The acyl intermediates are esterified to the sulfhydryl group of 4'-phosphopantetheine. 4'-Phosphopantetheine is added to ACP in a posttranslational modification reaction which is catalyzed by a transferase enzyme acting on CoA. In the case of coenzyme A, the sulfhydryl groups are also esterified to acyl groups, such as the acetyl group. However, the 4'-phosphopantetheine part of the structure is not esterified to a serine residue in a protein (ACP), but is bound to the nucleotide adenosine 5'-monophosphate.

In addition to acetyl-CoA, other forms of CoA also play important biological roles. Malonyl-CoA supplies two-carbon units for the synthesis of fatty acids up until palmitic acid, and succinyl-CoA reacts with delta-aminolevulinic acid in the first reaction of heme biosynthesis. Myristoyl-CoA, derived from the 14-carbon saturated fatty acid myristic acid, is involved in the myristoylation of proteins; palmitoyl-CoA is involved in the palmitoylation of proteins, and farnesyl-CoA and geranylgeranyl-CoA are involved in protein isoprenylation. Protein isoprenylation, myristoylation and palmitoylation appear to play roles in signal transduction, among other biological activities.

The principal supplemental form of pantothenic acid is calcium D-pantothenate (D-calcium pantothenate). This marketed supplement is usually made synthetically. Dexpanthenol, the corresponding alcohol of pantothenic acid is also available. Dexpanthenol is a synthetic form which is not found naturally. Dexpanthenol is converted to pantothenic acid in the body, and therefore can be considered a provitamin form of pantothenic acid. Dexpanthenol is used topically to promote wound healing. It is also used in various cosmetic products.

In addition to being known as vitamin B_5, pantothenic acid is also known as D(+)-pantothenic acid, D-pantothenic acid, D(+)-*N*-(2,4-dihydroxy-3,3-dimethylbutyryl)-beta-alanine and (*R*)-*N*-(2,4-dihydroxy-3,3-dimethyl-1-oxobutyl)-beta-alanine. D-pantothenic acid is the biologically active enantiomer of the vitamin and is comprised of beta-alanine and a dihydroxy acid called pantoic acid. Its molecular formula is $C_9H_{17}NO_5$, its molecular weight is 219.24 daltons and its structural formula is as follows:

Pantothenic Acid

Dexpanthenol, the corresponding alcohol of pantothenic acid, is also known as pantothenol, provitamin B_5 and (*R*)-2,4-dihydroxy-*N*-(3-hydroxypropyl)-3,3-dimethylbutyramide. Its molecular formula is $C_9H_{19}NO_4$ and its molecular weight is 205.3 daltons.

ACTIONS AND PHARMACOLOGY

ACTIONS

Pantothenic acid may have antioxidant and radioprotective activities. It has putative anti-inflammatory, wound healing and antiviral activities. It also has putative activity in the management of rheumatoid arthritis.

MECHANISM OF ACTION

Pantothenic acid and its derivatives, 4'-phosphopantothenic acid, pantothenol and pantethine, have been shown, *in vitro*, to protect cells against lipid peroxidation. This protective effect does not appear to be due to the scavenging of the reactive oxygen species by pantothenic acid. It is thought that the antioxidant effect of pantothenic acid is due to its stimulation of increased cellular levels of coenzyme A. Coenzyme A may facilitate removal of lipid peroxides by increasing mobilization of fatty acids, and promote repair of plasma membranes by activating phospholipid synthesis. Pantothenic acid has also been shown to increase levels of cellular reduced glutathione. The mechanism by which pantothenic acid increases glutathione levels is unknown. However, increased levels of glutathione may play a large role in the protective effect of pantothenic acid against peroxidative damage of cell membranes.

Pantothenol has been demonstrated to protect rats against some of the deleterious effects of gamma radiation. The deleterious effects of gamma radiation occur via the generation of reactive oxygen species resulting in the peroxidation of lipid membranes. It is thought that the protective effects of pantothenol, which is a precursor of pantothenic acid, is due, in part, to its promotion of coenzyme A biosynthesis and to its increasing cellular levels of reduced glutathione (see above).

There is some evidence that pantothenic acid may be helpful in the management of some with rheumatoid arthritis. The mechanism of this putative effect is unclear. Activated granulocytes play a role in the inflammatory response by production of reactive oxygen species. Pantothenic acid, in the form of calcium D-pantothenate, was found to significantly inhibit the release of myeloperoxidase from granulocytes *in vitro*, as well as to inhibit the production of reactive oxygen species by these cells. This effect of pantothenic acid as well as the antioxidant effect of the vitamin discussed above, may account, in part, for the putative action of pantothenic acid in rheumatoid arthritis.

Pantothenic acid has been shown to accelerate wound healing in experimental animals. The mechanism of the putative wound healing effect of pantothenic acid is unclear. In human dermal fibroblasts in culture, calcium D-pantothenate was demonstrated to accelerate the wound healing process by increasing the number of cells migrating into a wounded area, as well as their mean migration speed. Dexpanthenol (pantothenol), the corresponding alcohol of pantothenic acid, is used topically for the treatment of various minor skin disorders and to promote wound healing. Topical dexpanthenol has been found to improve stratum corneum hydration, reduce tranepidermal water loss and to stabilize the epidermal barrier function. The putative wound healing activity of pantothenic acid, may also be accounted for, in part, by its possible antiinflammatory activity.

PHARMACOKINETICS

Dietary sources of pantothenic acid include bound and unbound forms. The principal bound form of the vitamin is coenzyme A. The principal supplementary form of the vitamin is calcium D-pantothenate, Dietary coenzyme A is hydrolyzed in the intestine to dephospho-CoA, phosphopantetheine and pantetheine. Pantetheine, in turn, is hydrolyzed to pantothenic acid. Pantothenic acid is efficiently absorbed from the small intestine. Absorption at low intakes occurs via a sodium-dependent carrier-mediated active transport process, and at higher intakes, by passive diffusion. Pantothenic acid is transported via the portal circulation to the liver and via the systemic circulation to other tissues of the body. Uptake of pantothenic acid by most cells of the body is by a sodium-dependent process.

Pantothenic acid is metabolized to coenzyme A via a sequence of steps. Coenzyme A is a precursor of acyl carrier protein. Approximately 95% of CoA is found in the mitochondria. Coenzyme A is catabolized by a number of hydrolytic steps resulting in pantothenate and cysteamine. Unchanged pantothenate is the major urinary excretion product of pantothenic acid. In dogs, a glycosylated catabolite of the vitamin, pantothenyl-4'-beta-glucoside, has been identified in the urine. Glycosylated catabolites of pantothenic acid have not, to date, been reported in humans.

INDICATIONS AND USAGE

There is some dated evidence that pantothenic acid may be of some benefit in some with rheumatoid arthritis. Research results are mixed, but overall not encouraging, with respect to claims that pantothenic acid enhances exercise performance. There is some animal and *in vitro* evidence that pantothenic acid may aid in wound healing. However, one human clinical study did not show a wound healing effect for oral pantothenic acid. A topical form of the provitamin, dexpanthenol (pantothenol) is used for the treatment of minor skin disorders, including for the promotion of wound healing. There is preliminary evidence that pantothenic acid may be helpful in treating those with hepatitis A and a suggestion from animal studies that it may be helpful in some with Duchenne muscular dystrophy. There is no evidence that it prevents loss of hair and graying of hair.

RESEARCH SUMMARY

Decades ago there were reports that supplemental pantothenic acid could ameliorate some bone and cartilage disorders in acutely pantothenic acid-deficient young rats. Years later, it was noted that blood levels of pantothenic acid are significantly reduced in rheumatoid arthritis (RA) patients. A clinical trial tested 50 milligrams daily of injected calcium pantothenate. Blood levels rose to normal, and significant symptomatic relief was achieved in many of the test subjects. When the pantothenate was withdrawn, symptoms returned. The best results were achieved in a subgroup of vegetarians, and still better results were reported in vegetarians who were given a combination of pantothenic acid and royal jelly. (See Royal Jelly). This study was conducted in 1963.

In 1980, a double-blind, placebo-controlled study followed-up on the initial report. Subjects with various forms of arthritis were randomized to receive oral calcium pantothenate or placebo. Dosage was as follows: one tablet (500 milligrams) daily for two days, then one twice a day for three days, then one three times a day for four days and, finally, one four times a day thereafter.

Calcium pantothenate was no better than placebo in treating all forms of arthritis—except RA. In the subset of subjects with RA, pantothenic acid produced significant results. The researchers noted, in particular, that "highly significant effects were recorded for calcium pantothenate in reducing the duration of morning stiffness, degree of disability and severity of pain, whereas placebo produced no effects on these symptoms." As these researchers noted, further investigation is warranted.

There have been reports that pantothenic acid speeds wound healing in animal models. However, recent, double-blind, prospective, randomized trial found "no major improvement" of the human skin wound healing process. This 21-day study tested a combination of 1 gram of ascorbic acid and 0.2 grams of pantothenic acid daily on 49 subjects. Further investigation is needed to determine if oral pantothenic acid has any role in wound healing. A topical forms of the provitamin, pantothenol, appears to play some role in the management of minor skin disorders.

Claims that pantothenic acid enhances exercise performance rest, primarily, in the results of one study in which experienced distance runners received 2 grams of pantothenic acid daily for 14 days. Their performance was significantly better than that of equally well-trained distance runners who received placebo.

In another study, however, 1 gram of pantothenic acid daily for two weeks did not enhance the performance of distance runners compared with distance runners given placebo.

More recently, highly trained cyclists performed no better with a combination of 1 gram of allithiamin and 1.8 grams of a 55%/45% pantethine/pantothenic acid mixture than they did with placebo. The substances were administered for seven days prior to each exercise performance test. The researchers concluded: "we found the oral administration of these compounds to have no effect on any physiological or performance parameters during steady-state or high-intensity exercise."

There is preliminary evidence that pantothenic acid, in combination with pantetheine, may be helpful in the treatment of hepatitis A. Pantetheine is thought to be more active in this respect than pantothenic acid.

Administration of pantothenic acid increased skeletal muscle energy metabolism in the murine model of Duchenne muscular dystrophy, the mdx mouse. Reduced energy metabolism in slow-and fast-twitch skeletal muscle fibers has been reported in the mdx mouse. It is thought that this is due to a decreased oxidative utilization of glucose and free fatty acids. It is speculated that inefficiency of coenzyme A transport in the mitochondria might account for the reduced energy metabolism. Administration of pantothenic acid to mdx mice increased the cytoplasmic synthesis of CoA, and increased the thermogenic response to glucose, more in the muscles of mdx mice than in control muscles. Human studies are warranted.

CONTRAINDICATIONS, PRECAUTIONS, ADVERSE REACTIONS

CONTRAINDICATIONS

Pantothenic acid is contraindicated in those hypersensitive to any component of a pantothenic acid-containing product.

Dexpanthenol (pantothenol), the alcohol analog of pantothenic acid, is contraindicated in those hypersensitive to any component of a dexpanthenol-containing product. Oral and parenteral dexpanthenol are also contraindicated in those with ileus due to mechanical obstruction and those with hemophilia.

PRECAUTIONS

Pregnant women and nursing mothers should avoid doses of pantothenic acid greater than the U.S. RDA (10 milligrams/day) unless a higher dosage is prescribed by their physicians.

Those who have developed contact dermatitis from use of dexpanthenol may develop eczema from the use of oral pantothenic acid. Dexpanthenol, also known as pantothenol and provitamin B_5, in addition to being used for the treatment of various minor skin disorders, is an ingredient in many cosmetic products.

The use of pantothenic acid for any medical condition must be medically supervised.

ADVERSE REACTIONS

Contact dermatitis has been reported with topical use of dexpanthenol.

INTERACTIONS

NUTRITIONAL SUPPLEMENTS

Biotin: High doses of pantothenic acid may inhibit the absorption of biotin produced by the microflora in the large intestine. Pantothenic acid and biotin appear to use the same uptake carrier in colonocytes.

OVERDOSAGE

There are no reports of pantothenic acid overdosage in the literature.

DOSAGE AND ADMINISTRATION

The principal form of supplementary pantothenic acid is calcium D-pantothenate. Calcium D-pantothenate is available in multivitamin, multivitamin/multimineral and B-complex products, as well as single ingredient products. Typical doses of pantothenic acid range from 10-50 milligrams/day. Single ingredient tablets and capsules of pantothenic acid are available in doses ranging from 100 to 500 milligrams.

The Food and Nutrition Board of the Institute of Medicine of the U.S. National Academy of Sciences has recommended the following Dietary Reference Intakes (RDI) for pantothenic acid:

Infants	Adequate Intakes (AI)
0 through 6 months	1.7 milligrams/day ≈ 0.2 mg/Kg
7 through 12 months	1.8 milligrams/day ≈ 0.2 mg/Kg
Children	
1 through 3 years	2 milligrams/day
4 through 8 years	3 milligrams/day
Boys	
9 through 13 years	4 milligrams/day
14 through 18 years	5 milligrams/day
Girls	
9 through 13 years	4 milligrams/day
14 through 18 years	5 milligrams/day
Men	
19 years and older	5 milligrams/day
Women	
19 years and older	5 milligrams/day
Pregnancy	
14 through 50 years	6 milligrams/day
Lactation	
14 through 50 years	7 milligrams/day

There is no evidence of toxicity associated with the ingestion of pantothenic acid. Therefore, a lowest-observed-adverse-effect level (LOAEL) and an associated no-observed-adverse-effect level (NOAEL) cannot be determined.

The optimal intakes of pantothenic acid are not known.

The DV (Daily Value) for pantothenic acid, which is used for determining percentage of nutrient daily values on nutritional supplement and food labels, is 10 mg. This is based on the U.S. RDA for pantothenic acid.

LITERATURE

Anon. Calcium pantothenate in arthritic conditions. A report from the General Practitioner Research Group. *Practitioner*. 1980; 224:208-211.

Aprahamian M, Dentinger A, Stock-Damge C, et al. Effects of supplemental pantothenic acid on wound healing: experimental study in rabbit. *Am J Clin Nutr*. 1985; 41:578-589.

Barton-Wright EC, Elliot WA. The pantothenic acid metabolism of rheumatoid arthritis. *Lancet*. 1963; 2:862-863.

Dietary Reference Intakes for Thiamin, Riboflavin, Niacin, Vitamin B₆, Folate, Vitamin B₁₂, Pantothenic Acid, Biotin, and Choline. Washington, DC: National Academy Press; 1998.

Even PC, Decrouy A, Chinet A. Defective regulation of energy metabolism in mdx-mouse skeletal muscles. *Biochem J*. 1994; 304:649-654.

Gehring W, Gloor M. Effect of topically applied dexpanthenol on epidermal barrier function and stratum corneum hydration. Results of a human *in vivo* study. *Arzneimittelforschung*. 2000; 50:659-663.

Hahn C, Roseler S, Fritzsche R, et al. Allergic contact reaction to dexpanthenol: lymphocyte transformation test and evidence for microsomal-dependent metabolism of the allergen. *Contact Dermatitis*. 1993; 28:81-83.

Kapp A, Zeak-Kapp G. Effect of Ca-pantothenate on human granulocyte oxidative metabolism. *Allerg Immunol (Leipz)*. 1991; 37:145-150.

Kehrl W, Sonnemann U. [Dexpanthenol nasal spray as an effective therapeutic principle for treatment of rhinitis sicca anterior]. [Article in German]. *Laryngorhinootologie*. 1998; 77:506-512.

Komar VI. [The use of pantothenic acid preparations in treating patients with viral hepatitis A]. [Article in Russian]. *Ter Arkh*. 1991; 63:58-60.

Kumerova AO, Utno LIa, Lipsberga ZE, Shkestere IIa. [Study of pantothenic acid derivatives as cardiac protectors in a model of experimental ischemia and reperfusion of the isolated heart]. [Article in Russian]. *Biull Eksp Biol Med*. 1992; 113:373-375.

Litoff D, Scherzer H, Harrison J. Effects of pantothenic acid supplementation on human exercise. *Med Sci Sports Exercise*. 1985; 17:287(Abstract 17).

Loftus EV Jr, Tremaine WJ, Nelson RA, et al. Dexpanthenol enemas in ulcerative colitis: a pilot study. *Mayo Clin Proc*. 1997; 72:616-620.

Moiseenok AG, Dorofeev BF, Omel'ianchik SN. [The protective effect of pantothenic acid derivatives and changes in the system of acetyl CoA metabolism in acute ethanol poisoning]. [Article in Russian]. *Farmakol Toksikol*. 1988; 51:82-86.

Nice C, Reeves AG, Brinck-Johnsen T, Noll W. The effects of pantothenic acid on human exercise capacity. *J Sports Med*. 1984; 24:26-29.

Plesofsky-Vig N. Pantothenic acid. In: Shils, ME, Olson JA, Shike M, Ross AC, eds. *Modern Nutrition in Health and*

Disease. 9th ed. Baltimore MD: Williams and Wilkins; 1999:423-432.

Rychlik M. Quantification of free and bound pantothenic acid in foods and blood plasma by a stable isotope dilution assay. *J Agric Food Chem.* 2000; 48:1175-1181.

Sachs M, Asskali F, Lanaros C, et al. [The metabolism of panthenol in patients with postoperative intestinal atony]. [Article in German]. *Z Ernahrungswiss.* 1990; 29:270-283.

Slyshenkov VS, Moiseenok AG, Wojtczak L. Noxious effects of oxygen reactive species on energy-coupling processes in Ehrlich ascites tumor mitochondria and the protection by pantothenic acid. *Free Rad Biol Med.* 1996; 20:793-800.

Slyshenkov VS, Omelyanchik SN, Moiseenok AG, et al. Panthenol protects rats against some deleterious effects of gamma radiation. *Free Rad Biol Med.* 1998; 24:894-899.

Slyshenkov VS, Rakowska M, Moiseenok AG, Wojtczak L. Pantothenic acid and its derivatives protect Ehrlich ascites tumor cells against lipid peroxidation. *Free Rad Biol Med.* 1995; 19:767-772.

Slyshenkov VS, Rakowska M, Wojtczak L. Protective effect of pantothenic acid and related compounds against permeabilization of Ehrlich ascites tumor cells by digitonin. *Acta Biochim Pol.* 1996; 43:407-410.

Vaxman F, Olender S, Lambert A, et al. Effect of pantothenic acid and ascorbic acid supplementation on human skin wound healing process. A double-blind, prospective and randomized trial. *Eur Surg Res.* 1995; 27:158-166.

Webster MJ. Physiological and performance responses to supplementation with thiamin and pantothenic acid derivatives. *Eur J Appl Physiol.* 1998; 77:486-491.

Weimann BI, Hermann D. Studies on wound healing: effects of calcium-D-pantothenate on the migration, proliferation and protein synthesis of human dermal fibroblasts in culture. *Int J Vitam Nutr Res.* 1999; 69:113-119.

Williams RJ. *Biochemical Individuality.* New York, NY: John Wiley and Sons, Inc; 1963.

Para-Aminobenzoic Acid (PABA)

DESCRIPTION

Para-aminobenzoic acid or PABA is a non-protein amino acid that is widely distributed in nature. It is sometimes referred to as vitamin Bx, but it is neither a vitamin nor an essential nutrient for humans. PABA is an intermediate in the synthesis of folic acid in bacteria. The sulfonamide antibiotics are structurally similar to PABA and interfere with the synthesis of nucleic acids in sensitive micro-organisms by blocking the conversion of PABA to the co-enzyme dihydrofolic acid, a reduced form of folic acid. In humans, dihydrofolic acid is obtained from dietary folic acid; thus sulfonamides do not affect human cells. PABA is also known as 4-aminobenzoic acid. It is a solid substance with slight solubility in water. Its chemical structure is:

PABA (p-Aminobenzoic acid)

ACTIONS AND PHARMACOLOGY

ACTIONS

PABA may have antifibrosis activity.

MECHANISM OF ACTION

The mechanism of action of PABA's reputed antifibrosis effect in not known. It has been speculated that PABA mediates increased oxygen uptake at the tissue level, but this has never been established.

PHARMACOKINETICS

Following ingestion, PABA is passively absorbed mainly from the small intestine. From there, it enters the portal circulation. Some metabolism of PABA occurs in the liver. A major metabolite is N-acetyl PABA. PABA and its metabolites are mainly excreted in the urine. Small amounts are eliminated in the feces and in bile, milk and other secretions.

INDICATIONS AND USAGE

Pharmaceutical doses of PABA are indicated for Peyronie's disease, scleroderma, morphea and linear scleroderma. There is less evidence to indicate it for pemphigus and dermato-myositis. Claims that it can halt hair loss and restore color to graying hair are entirely anecdotal.

RESEARCH SUMMARY

A retrospective review reported on 32 Peyronie's disease patients treated for at least three months with 12 grams daily of a potassium PABA preparation (POTABA) and followed for 8 to 24 months. Improvement in penile discomfort was demonstrated in 8 of 18 patients, decreased plaque size was reported in 18 of 32 patients, improvement in penile angulation in 18 of 31 patients. No significant adverse effects were noted. Additional research is needed to confirm these findings.

Another retrospective review analyzed skin responses of scleroderma patients to potassium para-aminobenzoate thera-py. Ninety percent of 224 patients treated with about 12 grams daily of potassium para-benzoate (POTABA) experienced mild, moderate or marked skin softening. Among a parallel group of 96 evaluable scleroderma patients who did not receive potassium para-benzoate, less than 20% had mild or moderate improvement at the end of follow-up. The difference in skin softening in the treated group, compared to the untreated group, was statistically significant, and no significant adverse events were reported. Again, these findings require confirmation. Clinical improvement was noted in two dermatomyositis patients treated with 15 to 20 grams of potassium para-benzoate daily. Adequate clinical trials are necessary before any conclusion can be drawn regarding the possible effectiveness of PABA for dermatomyositis.

There are anecdotal reports that PABA can halt hair loss and restore color to graying hair; there are at least as many reports that contradict these claims.

CONTRAINDICATIONS, PRECAUTIONS, ADVERSE REACTIONS

CONTRAINDICATIONS

PABA should not be administered to anyone taking sulfonamides or to anyone who is hypersensitive to it.

PRECAUTIONS

PABA should be avoided by children, pregnant women and nursing mothers. PABA should be used with caution in those with renal disease. If anorexia or nausea occurs, PABA should be stopped until the person is eating normally again. PABA should be stopped if hypersensitivity develops. Those taking pharmaceutical doses of PABA must be under medical supervision.

ADVERSE REACTIONS

Anorexia, nausea, vomiting, fever and rash have been reported in those taking PABA, particularly with larger doses. These symptoms resolve when PABA is stopped.

INTERACTIONS

Sulfonamides: PABA can decrease the effectiveness of sulfonamides and is contraindicated in anyone taking sulfonamides.

No other drug, nutritional supplement, herb or food interaction is known.

OVERDOSAGE

There are no known reports of overdosage.

DOSAGE AND ADMINISTRATION

In addition to PABA, the potassium salt of PABA called POTABA is available on prescription. POTABA is indicated for Peyronie's Disease and scleroderma. (See *Physicians' Desk Reference* for complete prescribing information.)

The dose for Peyronie's disease and scleroderma is high and must only be used under medical supervision. The dose used for these disorders is 12 grams daily taken in four to six divided doses with meals. The tablets must be dissolved in plenty of liquid to prevent gastrointestinal upset. Because of the high doses needed to achieve clinical efficacy, patient compliance is typically poor.

LITERATURE

Carson CC. Potassium para-aminobenzoate for treatment of Peyronie's disease: is it effective? *Tech Urol.* 1997; 3:135-139.

Hasche-Klunder R. Treatment of Peyronie's disease with para-aminobenzoacidic potassium. *Urologe[A].* 1978; 17:224-227.

Kierkegaard E, Nielsen B. Peyronie's diseases treated with K-para-aminobenzoate and vitamin E. *Ugeskr Laeger.* 1979; 141:2052-2053.

Physicians' Desk Reference. 54th edition. Montvale, NJ: Medical Economics Company; 2000.

Zarafonetis CJ, Dabich L, Skovronski JJ, et al. Retrospective studies in scleroderma: skin responses to potassium para-aminobenzoate therapy. *Clin Exp Rheumatol.* 1998; 6:261-268.

Zuckerman JE, Hollinger MA, Giri SN. Evaluation of antifibrotic drugs in bleomycin-induced pulmonary fibrosis in hamsters. *J Pharmacol Exp Ther.* 1980; 213:425-431.

Pectin

DESCRIPTION

Pectin is classified as a soluble fiber. It is found in most plants, but is most concentrated in citrus fruits (oranges, lemons, grapefruits) and apples. Pectin is obtained by the aqueous extraction of citrus peels and apple pulp under mildly acidic conditions. Pectin obtained from citrus peels is referred to as citrus pectin.

Pectin is widely used in the food industry as a gelling agent to impart a gelled texture to foods, mainly fruit-based foods such as jams and jellies. It also has pharmaceutical applications. Pectin is used in combination with the clay kaolin (hydrated aluminum silicate) for the management of diarrhea. It is used as a component in the adhesive part of ostomy rings. Pectin is also marketed as a nutritional supplement for the management of elevated cholesterol.

Chemically, pectin is a linear polysaccharide containing from about 300 to 1,000 monosaccharide units. D-Galacturonic acid is the principal monosaccharide unit of pectin. Some neutral sugars are also present in the substance. The D-galacturonic acid residues are linked together by alpha-1, 4 glycosidic linkages. The molecular weight of pectin ranges from 50,000 to 150,000 daltons. The galacturonic acid residues in pectin may be esterified with methyl groups. There are different types of pectin. Pectin in which more than 50% of the galacturonic acid residues are esterified is called high methoxyl or HM pectin. Pectin in which less than

50% of the galacturonic acid residues are esterified is called low methoxy or LM pectin. Pectin is a nondigestible polysaccharide. So-called modified citrus pectin is pectin that has been hydrolyzed and otherwise modified to make it more digestible and absorbable.

ACTIONS AND PHARMACOLOGY

ACTIONS

Pectin may have hypocholesterolemic and antithrombotic activities. It has a putative protective action against colorectal cancer.

MECHANISM OF ACTION

The mechanism of the possible hypocholesterolemic activity of pectin is not well understood. It appears that the viscosity of pectin is related to its possible hypocholesterolemic activity. Pectin preparations with high viscosity appear to be more effective in lowering cholesterol than are pectin preparations with lower viscosity. High-viscosity pectin is thought to lower cholesterol levels by raising the excretion of fecal bile acids and neutral sterols. High-viscosity pectin may interfere with the formation of micelles and/or lower the diffusion rate of bile acid and cholesterol-containing micelles through the bolus, consequently diminishing the uptake of cholesterol and bile acids.

Pectin has been found to alter the characteristics of the fibrin-network architecture, suggesting that it may have some antithrombotic activity. Fibrin networks, following pectin supplementation, were found to have lower tensile strength, and to be more lysable and permeable. Acetate supplementation was found to have similar activity on fibrin networks. It is thought that the acetate resulting from bacterial fermentation of pectin in the large intestine may account for pectin's possible effect on fibrin networks.

The putative protective activity of pectin against colorectal cancer may be accounted for by its fermentation in the large intestine to butyric acid. Butyric acid may upregulate apoptosis.

PHARMACOKINETICS

Following ingestion of pectin, very little of it gets digested in the small intestine. Some fermentation of pectin takes place in the large intestine via the action of bacteria. The final products of fermentation of pectin are the short-chain fatty acids, acetate, propionate and butyrate, as well as hydrogen and carbon dioxide. The short-chain fatty acids that escape colonic metabolism are transported via the portal circulation to the liver where they undergo metabolism. The short-chain fatty acids that are not metabolized in the liver enter the systemic circulation and are distributed to the various tissues of the body. Acetate appears to be the principal short-chain fatty acid to reach the systemic circulation from the liver.

INDICATIONS AND USAGE

Pectin appears to have hypocholesterolemic effects and may be antiatherogenic in some. It is used in some multi-ingredient preparations for the treatment of constipation and diarrhea. Claims that it is an effective antiobesity agent are unsubstantiated. There is a recent preliminary animal study suggesting that pectin could have some anticancer activity. (See also Modified Citrus Pectin.)

RESEARCH SUMMARY

Numerous studies have demonstrated that pectin has favorable effects on lipids. In a small early study, administration of 15 grams of pectin daily for three weeks resulted in a mean 13% reduction in plasma cholesterol levels. There was no effect on plasma triglyceride concentrations. Subsequently, giving 40 to 50 grams of pectin daily significantly lowered cholesterol levels in both normolipidemic and hyperlipidemic subjects. In another study, a pectin-supplemented diet (without other dietary or lifestyle changes), significantly reduced plasma cholesterol in volunteers evaluated to be at medium to high risk for coronary heart disease due to hypercholesterolemia. This was a double-blind, placebo-controlled trial. Treatment continued for 16 weeks. The pectin was credited with decreasing plasma cholesterol 7.6% and LDL-cholesterol 10.8%.

Pectin's adsorbent and bulk-forming properties have promoted its use in some multi-ingredient anticonstipation and antidiarrheal preparations.

Recently, pectin was found to be associated with higher apoptotic index in colonocytes of rats, suggesting that it might be useful in protecting against development of colorectal cancer. Followup is needed. Modified citrus pectin has also demonstrated some anti-carcinogenic activity. (See Modified Citrus Pectin.)

CONTRAINDICATIONS, PRECAUTIONS, ADVERSE REACTIONS

CONTRAINDICATIONS

Pectin is contraindicated in those hypersensitive to any component of a pectin-containing supplement.

PRECAUTIONS

Pregnant women and nursing mothers should avoid pectin supplementation.

ADVERSE REACTIONS

Pectin may cause such gastrointestinal symptoms as flatulence, cramps, gas and diarrhea.

INTERACTIONS

DRUGS

Lovastatin: Pectin when used concomitantly may decrease the absorption of lovastatin. There are no reports of interactions between pectin and other statins.

Clindamycin, Tetracycline, Digoxin: Concomitant use of a kaolin-pectin antidiarrheal suspension with clindamycin, tetracycline and digoxin has been reported to decrease the absorption of those drugs. However, it is unclear as to which component (kaolin or pectin or both) is responsible for this interaction. Kaolin (hydrated aluminum silicate) is known to adsorb a wide variety of drugs and other substances.

NUTRITIONAL SUPPLEMENTS

Carotenoids: Concomitant use of pectin and lycopene, lutein and beta-carotene has been reported to decrease the absorption of these carotenoids.

Minerals: Pectin may decrease the absorption of such minerals as zinc, copper, iron, calcium and magnesium if used concomitantly.

FOODS

Pectin may decrease the absorption of such minerals in foods as zinc, copper, iron and calcium.

Pectin, when used concomitantly with lovastatin, caused a paradoxical increase in LDL-cholesterol. It was thought that the pectin reduced the absorption of lovastatin.

DOSAGE AND ADMINISTRATION

There are no typical doses of pectin supplements. Doses of 10 to 15 grams daily have been used in studies showing cholesterol-lowering effects in hypercholesterolemic individuals. Pectin supplements should be used with plenty of fluid.

LITERATURE

Anderson JW, Jones AE, Riddell-Mason S. Ten different dietary fibers have significantly different effects on serum and liver lipids of cholesterol-fed rats. *J Nutr.* 1994; 124:78-83.

Avivi-Green C, Polak-Charcon S, Madar Z, Schwartz B. Dietary regulation and localization of apoptosis cascade proteins in the colonic crypt. *J Cell Biochem.* 2000; 77:18-29.

Cerda JJ, Normann SJ, Sullivan MP, et al. Inhibition of atherosclerosis by dietary pectin in microswine with sustained hypercholesterolemia. *Circulation.* 1994; 89:1247-1253.

Cerda JJ, Robbins FL, Burgin CW, et al. The effects of grapefruit pectin on patients at risk for coronary heart disease without altering diet or lifestyle. *Clin Cardiol.* 1988; 11:589-594.

Ebihara K, Kiriyama S, Manabe M. Cholesterol-lowering activity of various natural pectins and synthetic pectin-derivatives with different physico-chemical properties. *Nutr Rep Int.* 1979; 20:519-526.

Hillman LC, Peters SG, Fisher CA, Pomare EW. The effects of the fiber components pectin, cellulose and lignin on serum cholesterol levels. *Am J Clin Nutr.* 1985; 42:207-213.

Judd PA, Truswell AS. The hypocholesterolemic effects of pectins in rats. *Br J Nutr.* 1985; 53:409-425.

Kay RM, Truswell AS. Effects of citrus pectin on blood lipids and fecal steroid excretion in man. *Am J Clin Nutr.* 1977; 30:171-175.

Platt D, Raz A. Modulation of the lung colonization of B16-F1 melanoma cells by citrus pectin. *J Natl Cancer Inst.* 1992; 84:438-442.

Richter WO, Jacob BG, Schwandt P. Interaction between fibre and lovastatin. *Lancet.* 1991; 338:706.

Riedl J, Linseisen J, Hoffman J, Wolfran G. Some dietary fibers reduce the absorption of carotenoids in women. *J Nutr.* 1999; 129:2170-2176.

Rock CL, Swendseid ME. Plasma beta-carotene response in humans after meals supplemented with dietary pectin. *Am J Clin Nutr.* 1992; 55:96-99.

Terpstra AHM, Lapre JA, de Vries HT, Beynen AC. Dietary pectin with high viscosity lowers plasma and liver cholesterol concentration and plasma ester transfer protein activity in hamsters. *J Nutr.* 1998; 128:1944-1949.

Veldman FJ, Nair CH, Vorster HH, et al. Possible mechanism through which dietary pectin influences fibrin network architecture in hypercholesterolaemic subjects. *Thromb Res.* 1999; 93:253-264.

Perilla Oil

DESCRIPTION

Perilla oil is derived from the seed of the plant *Perilla frutescens*. Perilla oil is a very rich source of alpha-linolenic acid. About 50 to 60% of perilla oil is alpha-linolenic acid. Alpha-linolenic acid is an n-3 (omega-3) all-cis polyunsaturated fatty acid containing 18 carbon atoms and three double bonds. It is also known as ALA; ALA, 18:3n-3; 9,12, 15-octadecatrienoic acid and (Z,Z, Z)-9,12,15-octadecatrienoic acid. ALA has the following chemical formula:

Alpha-linolenic acid

Alpha-linolenic acid is found in perilla oil as a triacylglycerol or triglyceride. The Mediterranean diet, high in ALA, appears to lower the risk of coronary artery disease and certain types of cancer.

ACTIONS AND PHARMACOLOGY

ACTIONS

Perilla oil may have anti-inflammatory, antithrombotic and anti-proliferative activities.

MECHANISM OF ACTION

The possible actions of perilla oil are probably dependent on the presence of ALA. ALA is metabolized to eicosapaentenoic acid (EPA) and docosahexaenoic acid (DHA). EPA is a precursor of the series-3 prostaglandins, the series-5 leukotrienes and the series-3 thromboxanes. These eicosanoids have anti-inflammatory and anti-atherogenic properties. The incorporation of metabolites of ALA in cell membranes may play a role in anti-inflammatory activity, inhibition of platelet aggregation and possibly in anti-proliferative actions of ALA.

PHARMACOKINETICS

ALA-laden triacylglycerols (TAGs), following ingestion, undergo hydrolysis via lipases to form monoglycerides and free fatty acids. Once formed, the monoglycerides and the free fatty acids are absorbed by the enterocytes. In the enterocytes, reacylation takes place reforming TAGs, which are then reassembled with phospholipids, cholesterol and apolipoproteins into chylomicrons. The chylomicrons are released into the lymphatics from whence they are transported to the systemic circulation. In the circulation, the chylomicrons are degraded by lipoprotein lipase, and the fatty acids, including ALA, are taken up in part by the endothelial cells where ALA is metabolized to phospholipids. ALA is transported via the circulation to various tissues in the body where it is metabolized to EPA, DHA and series-3 prostaglandins, series-5 leukotrienes and series-3 thromboxanes. Most of this metabolism occurs in cell membrane phospholipids.

An intake of from 3 to 4 grams daily of ALA is estimated to be equivalent to an intake of 0.3 grams daily of EPA, which one would get from a diet rich in fish.

INDICATIONS AND USAGE

Perilla oil may be indicated as a cardioprotective supplement, to help prevent blood clots and to ameliorate some of the symptoms of inflammatory bowel disease. Animal studies suggest that perilla oil might eventually prove useful in the prevention or management of some cancers.

RESEARCH SUMMARY

Perilla oil is a rich source of alpha-linolenic acid (ALA). Perilla oil has cardio-protective effects. It decreases platelet-activating factor, helping to prevent arterial blood clots.

One group of researchers suggests that perilla oil may be superior to either eicosapaentoic acid (EPA) or docahexaenoic acid (DHA) in ameliorating the colitis of experimental Crohn's disease. Perilla oil may be a palatable alternative to those who find fish oils effective in colitis but cannot tolerate taking them for prolonged periods.

In animal experiments, perilla oil proved superior to either soybean or safflower oils in inhibiting mammary, colon and kidney cancers. In one animal study, a relatively small amount of perilla oil, constituting 25% of total dietary fat, significantly protected against colon cancer. In another recent animal study, perilla oil suppressed the development of liver cell carcinoma.

CONTRAINDICATIONS, PRECAUTIONS, ADVERSE REACTIONS

CONTRAINDICATIONS

Known hypersensitivity to a perilla oil-containing product.

PRECAUTIONS

Infants, young children, pregnant women and nursing mothers should only use perilla oil if recommended and monitored by a physician. Because of perilla oil's possible antithrombotic activity, hemophiliacs and those taking warfarin should exercise caution in its use. Perilla oil intake should be stopped in those having surgical procedures.

ADVERSE REACTIONS

Perilla oil may cause some mild gastrointestinal symptoms such as diarrhea.

INTERACTIONS

Interactions may occur between ALA in perilla oil and aspirin, other NSAIDs or herbs, such as *Allium sativum* (garlic) and *Ginkgo biloba* (ginkgo). Such interactions, if they were to occur, might be manifested by nosebleeds and increased susceptibility to bruising. If this does occur, consideration should be given to lowering or stopping intake.

OVERDOSAGE

There are no reports of overdosage.

DOSAGE AND ADMINISTRATION

One-gram capsules of perilla oil containing 55% ALA are available. A usual dose for any of the indications is about 6 grams daily in divided doses with meals. This provides an intake of 3.3 grams of ALA.

LITERATURE

Indu M. Ghafoorunissa n-3 Fatty acids in Indian diets: comparison of the effects of precursor (alpha-linolenic acid) vs product (long-chain n-3 polyunsaturated fatty acids). *Nutr Res.* 1992; 12:569-582.

Narisawa T, Fukaura Y, Yazawa K, et al. Colon cancer prevention with a small amount of dietary perilla oil high in alpha-linolenic acid in an animal model. *Cancer.* 1994; 73:2069-2075.

Oh-hashi K, Takehashi T, Watanabe S. Possible mechanisms for the differential effects high linoleate safflower oil and high alpha-linolenate perilla oil diets on platelet-activating factor production by rat polymorphonuclear leukocytes. *J Lipid Mediat Cell Signal.* 1997; 17:207-220.

Shoda R, Matsuedo K, Yamato S, Umeda N. Therapeutic efficacy of n-3 fatty acid in experimental Crohn's disease. *J Gastroenterol.* 1995; 30 Suppl 8:98-101.

Phosphatidylcholine

DESCRIPTION

Phosphatidylcholine is a phospholipid that is a major constituent of cell membranes. Phosphatidylcholine is also known as 1, 2-diacyl-sn-glycero-3-phosphocholine, PtdCho and lecithin. It is represented by the following chemical structure:

Phosphatidylcholine

The term lecithin itself has different meanings when used in chemistry and biochemistry than when used commercially. Chemically, lecithin is phosphatidylcholine. Commercially, it refers to a natural mixture of neutral and polar lipids. Phosphatidylcholine, which is a polar lipid, is present in commercial lecithin in concentrations of 20 to 90%. Most of the commercial lecithin products contain about 20% phosphatidylcholine.

Lecithins containing phosphatidylcholine are produced from vegetable, animal and microbial sources, but mainly from vegetable sources. Soybean, sunflower and rapeseed are the major plant sources of commercial lecithin. Soybean is the most common source. Plant lecithins are considered to be GRAS (generally regarded as safe). Egg yolk lecithin is not a major source of lecithin in nutritional supplements. Eggs themselves naturally contain from 68 to 72% phosphatidylcholine, while soya contains from 20 to 22% phosphatidylcholine.

The fatty acid makeups of phosphatidylcholine from plant and animal sources differ. Saturated fatty acids, such as palmitic and stearic, make up 19 to 24% of soya lecithin; the monounsaturated oleic acid contributes 9 to 11%; linoleic acid provides 56 to 60%; and alpha-linolenic acid makes up 6 to 9%. In egg yolk lecithin, the saturated fatty acids, palmitic and stearic, make up 41 to 46% of egg lecithin, oleic acid 35 to 38%, linoleic acid 15 to 18% and alpha-linolenic 0 to 1%. Soya lecithin is clearly richer in polyunsaturated fatty acids than egg lecithin. Unsaturated fatty acids are mainly bound to the second or middle carbon of glycerol.

Choline comprises about 15% of the weight of phosphatidylcholine. (See monograph on Choline.)

ACTIONS AND PHARMACOLOGY

ACTIONS

Phosphatidylcholine may have hepatoprotective activity.

Phosphatidylcholine is important for normal cellular membrane composition and repair. Phosphatidylcholine is also the major delivery form of the essential nutrient choline. Choline itself is a precursor in the synthesis of the neurotransmitter acetylcholine, the methyl donor betaine and phospholipids, including phosphatidylcholine and sphingomyelin among others. (See the Choline monograph for further discussion.) Phosphatidylcholine is involved in the hepatic export of very-low-density lipoproteins.

MECHANISM OF ACTION

Phosphatidylcholine's role in the maintenance of cell-membrane integrity is vital to all of the basic biological processes. These are: information flow that occurs within cells from DNA to RNA to proteins; the formation of cellular energy and intracellular communication or signal transduction. Phosphatidylcholine, particularly phosphatidylcholine rich in polyunsaturated fatty acids, has a marked fluidizing effect on cellular membranes. Decreased cell-membrane fluidization and breakdown of cell-membrane integrity, as well as impairment of cell-membrane repair mechanisms, are associated with a number of disorders, including liver disease, neurological diseases, various cancers and cell death.

PHARMACOKINETICS

Phosphatidylcholine is absorbed into the mucosal cells of the small intestine, mainly in the duodenum and upper jejunum, following some digestion by the pancreatic enzyme phospholipase, producing lysophosphatidylcholine (lysolecithin). Re-acylation of lysolecithin takes place in the intestinal mucosal cells, reforming phosphatidylcholine, which is then transported by the lymphatics in the form of chylomicrons to the blood. Phosphatidylcholine is transported in the blood in various lipoprotein particles, including very-low-density lipoproteins (VLDL), low-density lipoproteins (LDL) and high-density lipoproteins (HDL); it is then distributed to the various tissues of the body. Some phosphatidylcholine is incorporated into cell membranes.

Phosphatidylcholine is also metabolized to choline, fatty acids and glycerol. The fatty acids and glycerol either get oxidized to produce energy or become involved in lipogenesis. Choline is a precursor of acetylcholine. Serum choline levels peak between 2 to 6 hours after oral intake.

INDICATIONS AND USAGE

Phosphatidylcholine may be indicated to help restore liver function in a number of disorders, including alcoholic fibrosis, and possibly viral hepatitis. It may also be indicated for the treatment of some manic conditions. There is some evidence that Phosphatidylcholine may be useful in the management of Alzheimer's disease and some other cognitive disorders. A possible future role in cancer therapy is also suggested by recent research. It may also be indicated in some with tardive dyskinesia.

RESEARCH SUMMARY

Clinical studies have demonstrated that choline is essential for normal liver function. Phosphatidylcholine is a better delivery form and is also more tolerable than choline. But, in addition, research has shown that phosphatidylcholine, independent of its choline content, has striking hepatoprotective effects. In two animal studies using baboons fed diets high in alcohol, some supplemented with a soy-derived polyunsaturated lecithin (60% phosphatidylcholine) and some unsupplemented, both fibrosis and cirrhosis were largely prevented in the phosphatidylcholine group. Most of the unsupplemented animals in these studies, which continued for up to eight years, developed fibrosis or cirrhosis.

Because these researchers had previously found that choline, equal in amounts contained in the phosphatidylcholine-rich lecithin they subsequently used, had no comparable protective effects on the liver, they concluded that the polyunsaturated phospholipids themselves may have been responsible for the benefits observed.

In vitro studies have shown that these phospholipids increase hepatic collagenase activity and may thus help prevent fibrosis and cirrhosis by encouraging collagen breakdown. Several other mechanisms under investigation may also contribute.

Others have reported similarly encouraging results in animal models. Clearly, human trials are warranted.

In addition, phosphatidylcholine has demonstrated other protective effects in non-alcoholic liver disorders, including protection against various other toxic substances. Its benefits in viral hepatitis were reported some years ago by several different research groups in Europe and elsewhere. In one of these studies, individuals suffering from hepatitis type A and B were given 1.8 grams of phosphatidylcholine daily. Compared with unsupplemented controls, the phosphatidylcholine group enjoyed quicker recoveries, fewer relapses and quicker normalization of liver function tests.

Researchers in Great Britain treated chronic active hepatitis C patients with 3 grams daily of phosphatidylcholine in double-blind fashion. The phosphatidylcholine patients had significantly reduced symptoms, compared with controls. All histologic evidence of the disease disappeared in some cases. These researchers, like others, have hypothesized that phosphatidylcholine's possible antiviral effects are related to the supplement's apparent ability to increase cellular membrane fluidity and repair the membranes of liver cells.

Phosphatidylcholine may help some with tardive dyskinesia, a neurological disorder characterized by defective cholinergic nerve activity. Both supplemental choline and phosphatidylcholine were found to reduce the muscular hyperactivity of this disorder by about 50% in some studies. However, one significant trial did not see a beneficial effect.

There is some very preliminary evidence that phosphatidylcholine may help control manic symptoms in some.

There has been hope, for some time, that phosphatidylcholine would demonstrate clear-cut benefits in cognitive disorders, such as age-related memory loss and Alzheimer's disease. There are a few reports that supplemental choline can improve short-term memory skills and enhance the memories of those who are initial poor learners.

Those with Alzheimer's disease have a diminished ability to synthesize and/or utilize the neurotransmitter acetylcholine, particularly in those areas of the brain related to memory, thus the hope that supplemental choline/phosphatidylcholine might be of benefit. A few studies have suggested some small benefit in memory restoration, but most have not. Research continues.

Recently it has been suggested that phosphatidylcholine might eventually have some therapeutic role in some cancers. There is no evidence of this to date, but animal studies indicate that deficiencies in choline and phosphatidylcholine may disrupt cell membrane signal transduction in ways that could lead to various cancers. There is ample evidence that liver cancer is promoted in various animals by choline-deficient diets, and it has been shown that excess choline can protect against liver cancer in a mouse model.

Phosphatidylcholine has been used to lower serum cholesterol levels, based on the premise that lecithin cholesterol acyltransferase (LCAT) activity has an important role in the removal of cholesterol from tissues. A few studies have shown reduction in serum cholesterol with phosphatidylcholine intake. The results were quite modest, and most studies have not shown any significant cholesterol-lowering activity.

CONTRAINDICATIONS, PRECAUTIONS, ADVERSE REACTIONS

CONTRAINDICATIONS

Known hypersensitivity to a phosphatidylcholine-containing product.

PRECAUTIONS

Those with malabsorption problems may develop diarrhea or steatorrhea when using phosphatidylcholine supplements. Those with the antiphospholipid-antibody syndrome should exercise caution in the use of phosphatidylcholine supplements.

ADVERSE REACTIONS

No major side effects have been reported. Mild side effects have been noted occasionally such as nausea, diarrhea and increased salivation in some. This holds for all forms of phosphatidylcholine.

INTERACTIONS

There are no known interactions.

OVERDOSAGE

There are no reports of overdosage.

DOSAGE AND ADMINISTRATION

There are several forms of phosphatidylcholine supplements. Typical commercial lecithin supplements contain 20 to 30% phosphatidylcholine. Softgel capsules containing 55% and 90% phosphatidylcholine are available. Liquid concentrates containing 3 grams of phosphatidylcholine per 5 milliliters (one teaspoon) are also available.

Recommended doses range from 3 to 9 grams of phosphatidylcholine daily in divided doses.

LITERATURE

Atoba MA, Ayoola EA, Ogunseyinde O. Effects of essential phospholipid choline on the course of acute hepatitis-B infection. *Trop Gastroenterol*. 1985; 6:96-9.

Buko V, Lukivskaya O, Nikitin V, et al. Hepatic and pancreatic effects of polyenoylphosphatidylcholine in rats with alloxan-induced diabetes. *Cell Biochem Funct*. 1996; 14:131-137.

Canty DJ, Zeisel SH. Lecithin and choline in human health and disease. *Nutr Rev*. 1994; 52:327-339.

Cohen BM, Lipinski JF, Altesman RI. Lecithin in the treatment of mania: double-blind, placebo-controlled trials. *Am J Psychiatry*. 1982; 139:1162-1164.

Gelenberg AJ, Dorer DJ, Wojcik JD, et al. A crossover study of lecithin treatment of tardive dyskinesia. *J Clin Psychiatry*. 1990; 51:149-153.

Growdon JH, Gelenberg AJ, Doller J, et al. Lecithin can suppress tardive dyskinesia. *N Engl J Med*. 1978; 298:1029-1030.

Hanin I, Ansell GB, eds. *Lecithin. Technological, Biological and Therapeutic Aspects*. New York and London: Plenum Press; 1987.

Hirsch MJ, Growdon JH, Wurtman RJ. Relations between dietary choline or lecithin intake, serum choline levels, and various metabolic indices. *Metabolism*. 1978; 27:953-960.

Jackson IV, Nuttall EA, Ibe IO, Perez-Cruet J. Treatment of tardive dyskinesia with lecithin. *Am J Psychiatry*. 1979; 136:1458-1460.

Jenkins PJ, Portmann BP, Eddleston AL, Williams R. Use of polyunsaturated phosphatidylcholine in HBsAg negative chronic active hepatitis: results of prospective double-blind controlled trial. *Liver*. 1982; 2:7-81.

Kosina F, Budka K, Kolouch Z, et al. Essential cholinephospholipids in the treatment of virus hepatitis. *Cas Lek Cesk*. 1981; 120:957-960.

Lieber CS, Leo MA, Aleynik SI, et al. *Alcohol Clin Exp Res*. 1997; 21:375-379.

Lieber CS, De Carl LM, Mak KM, et al. Attenuation of alcohol-induced hepatic fibrosis by polyunsaturated lecithin. *Hepatol*. 1990; 12:1390-1398.

Little A, Levy R, Chuaqui-Kidd P, Hand D. A double-blind, placebo-controlled trial of high-dose lecithin in Alzheimer's disease. *J Neur Neurosurg Psych*. 1985; 48:736-742.

Visco G. Polyunsaturated phosphatidylcholine in association with vitamin B complex in the treatment of acute viral hepatitis B. results of a randomized double-blind clinical study. *Clin Ter*. 1985; 114:183-188.

Wurtman RJ, Hefti F, Melamed E. Precursor control of neurotransmitter synthesis. *Pharmac Rev*. 1981; 32:315-335.

Wurtman RJ, Hirsch MJ, Growdon JH. Lecithin consumption raises serum-free-choline levels. *Lancet*. 1977; 2(8028):68-69.

Phosphatidylserine

DESCRIPTION

Phosphatidylserine is a phospholipid that is a structural component of biological membranes of plants, animals and other life forms. Phosphatidylserine was first isolated from brain lipids called cephalins. The major cephalins are phosphatidylserine and phophatidylethanolamine. Another major phospholipid found in egg yolks and soya is phosphatidylcholine, also known, chemically, as lecithin. Phosphatidylserine is also isolated from soya and egg yolks.

Phosphatidylserine is made up of a glycerophosphate skeleton linked to two fatty acid molecules and the amino acid L-serine. It is an amphiphilic molecule because it is made up of the lipophilic fatty acid tails on one side and the hydrophilic head group containing phosphate and serine on the other side of the molecule. Phosphatidylserine is located in the internal layers of biologic membranes, facing the cytoplasm with its polar head group. In animal tissues, phosphatidylserine is formed from phosphatidylethanolamine by exchange of the ethanolamine head for L-serine. Phosphatidylethanolamine itself is synthesized from diacylglycerol and CDP-ethanolamine.

Phosphatidylserine is known chemically as 1,2-diacyl-sn-glycerol-(3)-L-phosphoserine. It is abbreviated as Ptd Ser, $Acyl_2$ Gro PSer and PS. Most commonly, it is called phosphatidylserine or PS. It has the following chemical structure:

Phosphatidylserine

The fatty acid composition of phosphatidylserine derived from bovine brain and soya lecithin differ. Phosphatidylserine from soya lecithin contains mainly polyunsaturated fatty acids, while phosphatidylserine derived from bovine brain contains mainly saturated and monounsaturated fatty acids, as well as some docosahexaenoic acid.

Phosphatidylserine is involved in signal transduction activity as well as being a basic structural component of biologic membranes.

ACTIONS AND PHARMACOLOGY

ACTIONS

Supplemental phosphatidylserine may have cognition enhancing activity.

MECHANISM OF ACTION

Since the action of phosphatidylserine has not been established, any discussion of the mechanism of action is speculative. However, some findings from animal studies are of interest. Cholinergic hypofunction is thought to account in part for the cognitive deficits found in Alzheimer's disease. The most commonly used drugs for the treatment of Alzheimer's disease are reversible acetylcholinesterase inhibitors. The rationale of these drugs is to increase acetylcholine levels in the brains of Alzheimer's patients, and they may be somewhat effective in some cases. Animal studies indicate that phosphatidylserine restores acetylcholine release in aging rats by maintaining an adequate supply of the molecule and is able to increase the availability of endogenous choline for *de novo* acetylcholine synthesis.

The hippocampus of the brain is believed to be important for cognitive processes and is affected in those with Alzheimer's disease. The dendritic spines of pyramidal cells, the post-synaptic target of the excitatory input to the hippocampus, have been proposed as a substrate for information storage. Age-dependent dendritic spine loss in pyramidal neurons has been reported in the human brain, and the extent of synaptic loss appears to correlate with the degree of cognitive impairment. Rat experiments indicate that phosphatidylserine treatment prevents the age-related reduction in dendritic spine density in rat hippocampus. Protein kinase C facilitation of acetylcholine release has been reported in rats.

Phosphatidylserine was found to restore protein kinase C activity in aging rats. Stimulation of calcium uptake by brain synaptosomes and activation of protein kinase C are yet other speculative mechanisms of phosphatidylserine's putative cognition-enhancing action.

PHARMACOKINETICS

Pharmacokinetic studies of phosphatidylserine have been performed in rats. Little is known of the pharmacokinetics of oral phosphatidylserine in humans. In rats, it appears that there is extensive digestion of phosphatidylserine in the small intestine, producing, among other things, lysophosphatidylserine, a substance that contains only one fatty acid, and phosphatidylethanolamine.

Following absorption, lysophosphatidylserine is metabolized in intestinal mucosa cells, and its metabolites, which include some phosphatidylserine, enter the lymphatics draining the small intestine. It appears that only a small fraction of ingested phosphatidylserine reaches the systemic circulation as part of the phospholipid pool. The amount that reaches the brain, after either intraperitoneal injection or oral administration, is very small. Most of the behavioral and neurochemical effects noted in animal studies have been observed only after repeated intraperitoneal and oral phosphatidylserine dosing.

INDICATIONS AND USAGE

Phosphatidylserine has demonstrated some usefulness in treating cognitive impairment, including Alzheimer's disease, age-associated memory impairment and some non-Alzheimer's dementias. More research is needed before phosphatidylserine can be indicated for immune enhancement or for reduction of exercise stress.

RESEARCH SUMMARY

Several double-blind studies suggest that phosphatidylserine can help maintain cognitive function in older individuals and may be able to improve memory and learning skill in some. These results, while encouraging, are not, to date, dramatic.

Various animal experiments have also demonstrated some benefits including stimulation of brain catechecholaminergic turnover and increased acetylcholine output from the cerebral cortex of adult and old rats, as well as enhanced neurotransmitter and central nervous system signal transduction. There is evidence that phosphatidylserine can help maintain the hippocampal dendritic spine population of aging rats. It has been suggested that these spines serve as a substrate for information storage. There are several studies demonstrating improved cognitive function in several animal models.

In the largest multicenter study to date of phosphatidylserine and Alzheimer's disease, 142 subjects aged 40 to 80 were given 200 milligrams of phosphatidylserine per day or placebo over a three-month period. Those treated with phosphatidylserine exhibited improvement on several items on the scales normally used to assess Alzheimer's status. The differences between placebo and experimental groups were small but statistically significant. Researchers directing a smaller study, also achieving statistical significance with respect to several measures, characterized the therapeutic effects of phosphatidylserine in their Alzheimer's subjects as "mild."

Phosphatidylserine has also shown some efficacy in some non-Alzheimer's dementias, in age-associated memory impairment and general mental deterioration. More clinical trials need to be conducted before anything conclusive can be said about phosphatidylserine in the treatment of cognition impairment. But, given the results to date and the fact that there are so few side effects associated with phosphatidylserine and so few treatment options for Alzheimer's disease, one research group concludes that "the therapeutic possibilities offered by phosphatidylserine should not be dismissed." There are some animal studies demonstrating positive immunomodulatory effects but, as yet, no human studies showing similar effects. There is preliminary research indicating that phosphatidylserine, at doses of 400 to 800 milligrams per day, can inhibit exercise-induced increases in cortisol.

CONTRAINDICATIONS, PRECAUTIONS, ADVERSE REACTIONS

CONTRAINDICATIONS

Phosphatidylserine supplementation is contraindicated in those hypersensitive to any component of the preparation.

PRECAUTIONS

Because of lack of long-term safety studies, phosphatidylserine should be avoided by children, pregnant women and nursing mothers. Those with the antiphospholipid-antibody syndrome should exercise caution in the use of phosphatidylserine and only take it under medical supervision and monitoring.

ADVERSE REACTIONS

Occasional gastrointestinal side effects, such as nausea and indigestion, are reported.

INTERACTIONS

There are no reported drug, nutritional supplement, food or herb interactions with phosphatidylserine.

OVERDOSAGE

There are no reports of overdosage.

LD_{50} in rats is more than 5g/kg, and in rabbits is more than 2g/kg.

DOSAGE AND ADMINISTRATION

Phosphatidylserine supplements derived from both bovine brain and from soya lecithin are available. Phosphatidylserine derived from soya lecithin undergoes an enzymatic process that converts phosphatidylcholine to phosphatidylserine. Because of the hypothetical possibility of bovine spongiform encephalopathy, the soya-derived phosphatidylserine is preferred. Typical doses are 100 milligrams three time daily.

LITERATURE

Amaducc L, SMID Group. Phosphatidylserine in the treatment of Alzheimer's disease. Results of a multicenter study. *Psychopharmacol Bull*. 1988; 24:130-134.

Baer E, Maurukas J. Phosphatidyl serine. *J Biol Chem*. 1955; 212:25-38.

Blokland A, Honig W, Brouns F, Jolles J. Cognition-enhancing properties of subchronic phosphatidylserine (PS) treatment in middle-aged rats: comparison of bovine cortex PS with eggs PS and soybean PS. *Nutr*. 1999; 15: 778-783.

Casamenti F, Scali C, Pepeu G. Phosphatidylserine reverses the age-development decrease in cortical acetylcholine release: a microdialysis study. *Eur J Pharmac*. 1991; 194:11-16.

Crook T, Petrie W, Wells C, et al. Effects of phosphatidylserine in Alzheimer's disease. *Psychopharmacol Bull*. 1992; 28:61-66.

Crook TH, Tinklenberg J, Yesavage J, et al. Effects of phosphatidylserine in age-associated memory impairment. *Neurol*. 1991; 41:644-649.

Folch J. Brain cephalin, a mixture of phosphatides. Separation from it of phosphatidyl serine, phosphatidyl ethanolamine, and a fraction containing an inositol phosphatide. *J Biol Chem*. 1942; 146:35-41.

Monteleleone P, Maj M, Reinat L, et al. Blunting by chronic phosphatidylserine administration of the stress-induced activation of the hypothalamo-pituitary-adrenal axis in healthy men. *Eur J Pharmacol*. 1992; 41:385-388.

Nunzi MG, Milan F, Guidolin D, Toffano G. Dendritic spine loss in hippocampus of aged rats. Effect of brain phosphatidylserine. *Neurobiol Aging*. 1987; 8:501-510.

Pepeu G, Marconcini Pepeu I, Amaducc L. A review of phosphatidylserine pharmacological and clinical effects. Is phosphatidylserine a drug for the ageing brain? *Pharmacol Res*. 1996; 33:73-80.

Phosphatidylserine- a novel pharmacological approach to brain ageing. *Clin Trials J*. 1987; 24:1-130.

Villardita C, Grioli S, Salmeri G, et al. Multicentre clinical trial of brain phophatidylserine in elderly patients with intellectual deterioration. *Clinic Trials J*. 1987; 24:84-93.

Zanott A, Valzelli L, Toffano G. Chronic phosphatidylserine treatment improves spatial memory and passive avoidance in aged rats. *Psychopharmacol*. 1989; 99:316-321.

Phosphorus

DESCRIPTION

Phosphorus is an essential macromineral in human nutrition and plays pivotal roles in the structure and function of the body. Phosphorus, in its pentavalent phosphate form, is essential for the process of bone mineralization and makes up the structure of bone. Approximately 85% of phosphorus in the adult body is in bone. Phosphorus in the form of phospholipids makes up the structure of cellular membranes. Phosphorus also makes up the structure of nucleic acids and nucleotides, including adenosine triphosphate, among other things. Life has been said to be built around phosphorus.

The ability of cells to actively transport phosphate is recognized as a requirement for mineralization in bone. There is some recent evidence that phosphate may regulate the expression of a gene that might be involved in bone mineralization. Phosphate has been found to regulate the expression of the phosphorylated glycoprotein osteopontin. Osteopontin is thought to modulate hydroxyapatite crystal elongation, among other things.

Phosphorus is a non-metallic element with atomic number 15 and an average atomic weight of 30.97 daltons. Its symbol is P. Phosphorus occurs in nature as phosphates in the soil and, in particular, the mineral apatite. The total adult body content of phosphorus is about 700 grams. It accounts for about 2%-4% of the dry weight of most cells.

Phosphorus, mainly in the form of phosphates, is widely distributed in the food supply, and phosphorus intake from the normal diet is usually sufficient to meet the body's phosphorus needs. Milk and milk products are particularly rich sources of phosphorus. One liter of milk contains about 1,000 milligrams of phosphorus. Phosphorus deficiency states, however, do occur but usually they are caused by some disease process. For example, those with malabsorption syndromes and those with diseases causing renal tubular losses of phosphorus can become phosphorus depleted. In addition, those with malnutrition, alcoholics and critically ill patients, such as those being treated for diabetic ketoacidosis, are at risk for phosphorus deficiency, as well as phosphorus imbalance. The so-called refeeding syndrome can cause hypophosphotemia which may be life-threatening.

Phosphorus deficiency can result in anorexia, impaired growth, osteomalacia, skeletal demineralization, proximal muscle atrophy and weakness, cardiac arrhythmias, respiratory insufficiency, increased erythrocyte and lymphocyte dysfunction, susceptibility to infectious rickets, nervous system disorders and even death. Phosphate salts are used in the treatment of phosphorus deficiency. Besides their use for the treatment of phosphorus deficiency, phosphorus supplements are not widely used in the United States. The one exception is calcium phosphate, which is mainly used as a delivery form of calcium.

ACTIONS AND PHARMACOLOGY

ACTIONS

Supplemental phosphorus is used to treat phosphorus deficiency. Calcium phosphate is mainly used as a delivery form of calcium. Phosphorus has putative ergogenic (exercise performance-enhancement) activity.

MECHANISM OF ACTION

Phosphate salts are delivery forms of phosphorus and are used parenterally and orally under conditions of phosphate deficiency.

See Calcium for actions and mechanism of actions of that nutrient.

Short term phosphate-loading, using phosphate salts such as dibasic calcium phosphate ($CaHPO_4$), tribasic sodium phosphate (Na_3PO_4) or dibasic sodium and dibasic potassium phosphates, are used by some athletes who are not phosphorus deficient for performance enhancement.

The effectiveness of phosphate-loading is questionable. The mechanism proposed for this putative effect is attributed to the possible increase of 2, 3-diphosphoglycerate (2,3-DPG) with increased intake of phosphate. 2,3-DPG shifts the oxyhemoglobin dissociation curve to the right, thus allowing a greater unloading of oxygen at the tissue level. Although a few studies suggest that phosphate supplementation in phosphorus-sufficient subjects may increase 2,3-DPG levels in erythrocytes, most studies have reported that it does not have this effect.

PHARMACOKINETICS

Phosphorus supplements are inorganic phosphate salts of sodium, potassium or calcium. Calcium phosphate is a supplement used to supply both calcium and phosphorus. The efficiency of absorption of inorganic forms of phosphorus from the gastrointestinal tract ranges from 55% to 70% in adults. The efficiency of absorption of food phosphorus, which is a mixture of inorganic and organic forms of phosphorus, is similar. Organic forms of phosphorus are hydrolyzed by phosphatases, and therefore most phosphorus absorption occurs as absorption of inorganic phosphate. Absorption of phosphate occurs by both a saturable, active transport process and by passive diffusion. The saturable, active transport process is stimulated by the active form of vitamin D, 1, 25 dihydroxycholecalciferol (1, 25 (OH_2) D_3). The absorption of phosphorus is mainly via the passive, concentration-dependent process.

Phosphorus is transported via the portal circulation to the liver where the hepatocytes extract a fraction of it for their metabolic requirements. Phosphorus is transported via the systemic circulation to the various tissues of the body, where it is used for the metabolic requirements of these tissues. Excretion of phosphorus is mainly via the kidneys. Phosphorus is freely filtered in the glomerulus. Greater than 80% of the filtered phosphorus is reabsorbed in the proximal tubule and a small amount in the distal tubule. Parathyroid hormone adjusts the renal clearance of phosphorus. In the healthy adult, urine phosphorus is essentially equal to absorbed phosphorus.

INDICATIONS AND USAGE

Apart from its use in conditions of phosphorus deficiency, supplemental phosphorus has produced mixed results in tests of its putative ability to enhance exercise performance.

RESEARCH SUMMARY

Oral, enteral and parenteral phosphorus are used as replacement therapy in hypophosphatemia, a condition seen in some with chronic alcoholism or diabetic ketoacidosis, among others.

Claims that supplemental phosphorus enhances athletic performance are supported by some studies and are refuted by others. The majority of studies provide some support. In an early study, phosphate loading in ten trained distance runners attenuated increases in blood lactate after exercise. In another study, 1,000 milligrams of tribasic sodium phosphate four times a day for six days significantly increased maximal oxygen uptake and ventilatory anaerobic threshold. Phosphate loading did not, however, significantly improve five-mile run times compared with placebo, in these subjects.

Tribasic sodium phosphate loading enhanced endurance performance in competitive cyclists and triathletes in a placebo-controlled study. Dosage was 1 gram of phosphate four times a day for three days prior to exercise testing. Another study has suggested that athletes on caloric-restricted diets may benefit from increased dietary phosphorus intake. Researchers have cited limited data indicating that low-phosphorus status may increase incidence of muscle cramps. Again, increased dietary intake of, rather than supplementation with, phosphorus has been suggested. Long-term phosphate supplementation may pose serious health risks.

Not all studies have found benefit from phosphate loading. In a double-blind trial, 1.24 grams of sodium acid phosphate and potassium phosphate, administered one hour before exercise, produced results no better than placebo in male subjects, in terms of leg power and performance on a high-intensity treadmill exercise. Calcium phosphate loading similarly failed to improve work tolerance or aerobic capacity among male runners, compared with placebo, and,

in yet another trial, dibasic calcium phosphate loading was found to be ineffective as an ergogenic aid in subjects of different aerobic fitness levels.

More study will be needed to determine whether phosphate loading has significant benefits in exercise performance.

CONTRAINDICATIONS, PRECAUTIONS, ADVERSE REACTIONS

CONTRAINDICATIONS

Phosphorus supplements are contraindicated in those with hyperphosphatemia and in those with severely impaired renal function (less than 30% of normal). In addition, potassium phosphate is contraindicated in those with hyperkalemia, and calcium phosphate is contraindicated in those with hypercalcemia.

Inorganic phosphates are contraindicated in those with hypersensitivity to any component of an inorganic phosphate-containing supplement.

PRECAUTIONS

The use of supplementary phosphorus in those with phosphorus deficiency requires medical supervision.

Pregnant women and nursing mothers should avoid phosphorus intakes greater than RDA amounts.

Athletes who use supplementary phosphorus should avoid using such supplements for more than four to six days since they may cause hypocalcemia.

ADVERSE REACTIONS

The most common adverse reaction with use of sodium or potassium phosphate is diarrhea. The salts are less likely to cause diarrhea when they are used by phosphorus-deficient individuals than when used by those with normal phosphorus status. Other gastrointestinal symptoms that may occur include nausea, vomiting and stomach pain. Those with renal failure may develop hyperphosphatemia and hypocalcemia with potassium or sodium phosphate supplementation. Hyperphosphatemia can result in ectopic calcification. Prolonged use of high doses of inorganic phosphate salts may result in hypocalcemia even in healthy individuals with normal renal function.

INTERACTIONS

DRUGS

Aluminum-containing antacids: Aluminum-containing antacids are used in the treatment of hyperphosphatemia. Concomitant intake of aluminum-containing antacids and phosphorus will decrease absorption of phosphorus (in the phosphate form).

NUTRITIONAL SUPPLEMENTS

Zinc: Concomitant intake of zinc and phosphate salts (sodium phosphate, potassium phosphate, calcium phosphate) may decrease the absorption of zinc.

OVERDOSAGE

There are no reports of overdosage with oral phosphorus supplements in healthy individuals.

DOSAGE AND ADMINISTRATION

Sodium phosphate is available as monobasic sodium phosphate (NaH_2PO_4), dibasic sodium phosphate (Na_2HPO_4) and tribasic sodium phosphate (Na_3PO_4). Potassium phosphate is available as monobasic potassium phosphate (KH_2PO_4), dibasic potassium phosphate (K_2HPO_4) and tribasic potassium phosphate (K_3PO_4). There are also preparations which are mixtures of the different forms. Monobasic sodium and potassium phosphates are the least basic, and tribasic sodium and potassium phosphate are the most basic of these salts. Use of these salts for the treatment of phosphorus deficiency requires medical supervision.

Calcium phosphate salts used for nutritional supplementation are tribasic calcium phosphate ($Ca_3(PO_4)_2$) and dibasic calcium phosphate ($CaHPO_4$). These are used mainly as calcium supplements (see Calcium for dosage).

Some athletes use calcium phosphate for phosphate-loading.

Several homeopathic remedies are phosphate salts. They include kali phosphoricum (potassium phosphate), ferrum phosphoricum (iron phosphate), magnesia phosphorica (magnesium phosphate), natrum phosphoricum (sodium phosphate) and mixtures of phosphates called biochemic phosphates.

Milk is frequently recommended for phosphorus supplementation in phosphorus-deficient individuuals. One milliliter of milk contains approximately one milligram of phosphorus.

The Food and Nutrition Board of the Institute of Medicine of the National Academy of Sciences has recommended the following adequate intakes (AI) and Recommended Dietary Allowance (RDA) for phosphorus:

Infants	(AI)
0 through 6 months	100 mg/day
7 through 12 months	275 mg/day

Children	(RDA)
1 through 3 years	460 mg/day
4 through 8 years	500 mg/day

Boys	
9 through 18 years	1,250 mg/day

Girls	
9 through 18 years	1,250 mg/day

Men	
19 years and greater	700 mg/day

Women	
19 years and greater	700 mg/day

Pregnancy	
14 through 18 years	1,250 mg/day
19 through 50 years	700 mg/day

Lactation	
14 through 18 years	1,250 mg/day
19 through 50 years	700 mg/day

A NOAEL (No-Observed-Adverse-Effect Level) for phosphorus for adults is 10.2 grams/day.

Tolerable upper Intake Levels (UL) for phosphorus for adults is calculated by the Food and Nutrition Board by dividing the NOAEL for phosphorus by an uncertainty factor (UF) of 2.5.

Adults	(UL)
19 through 70 years	4.0 g/day

Infants	
0 through 12 months	Not possible to establish.

Children	
1 through 8 years	3.0 g/day
9 through 18 years	4.0 g/day

Older Adults	
Greater than 70 years	3.0 g/day

Pregnancy	
14 through 50 years	3.5 g/day

Lactation	
14 through 50 years	4.0 g/day

LITERATURE

Beck GR Jr, Zerler B, Moran E. Phosphate is a specific signal for induction of osteopontin gene expression. *Proc Natl Acad Sci USA.* 2000; 97:8352-8357.

Berner YN, Shike M. Consequences of phosphate imbalance. *Ann Rev Nutr.* 1988; 8:121-148.

Bredle DL, Stager JM, Brechue WF, Farber MO. Phosphate supplementation, cardiovascular function, and exercise performance in humans. *J Appl Physiol.* 1988; 65:1821-1826.

Cade R, Conte M, Zauner C, et al. Effects of phosphate loading on 2, 3-diphosphoglycerate and maximal oxygen uptake. *Med Sci Sports Exerc.* 1984; 16:263-268.

Dietary Reference Intake for Calcium, Phosphorous, Magnesium, Vitamin D and Fluoride. Washington, DC: National Academy Press; 1997.

Duffy DJ, Conlee RK. Effects of phosphate loading on leg power and high intensity treadmill exercise. *Med Sci Sports Exerc.* 1986; 18:674-677.

Galloway SD, Tremblay MS. Sexsmith JR, Roberts CJ. The effects of phosphate supplementation in subjects of different aerobic fitness levels. *Eur J Appl Physiol Occup Physiol.* 1996; 72:224-230.

Knochel JP. Phosphorus. In: Shils ME, Olson JA, Shike M, Ross AC, eds. *Modern Nutrition in Health and Disease.* 9th ed. Baltimore, MD: Williams and Wilkins; 1999:157-167.

Kreider RB, Miller GW, Schenk D, et al. Effects of phosphate loading on metabolic and myocardial responses to maximal and endurance exercise. *Int J Sport Nutr.* 1992; 2:20-47.

Kreider RB, Miller GW, Williams MH, et al. Effects of phosphate loading on oxygen uptake, ventilatory anaerobic threshold, and run performance. *Med Sci Sports Exerc.* 1990; 22:250-256.

Loghman-Adham M. Phosphate binders for control of phosphate retention in chronic renal failure. *Pediatr Nephrol.* 1999; 13:701-708.

Stewart I, McNaughton L, Davies P, Tristram S. Phosphate loading and the effects on VO₂ max in trained cyclists. *Res Q Exerc Sport.* 1990; 61:80-84.

Tremblay MS, Galloway SD, Sexsmith JR. Ergogenic effects of phosphate loading: physiological fact or methodological fiction? *Can J Appl Physiol.* 1994; 19:1-11.

Weisinger JR, Bellorí n-Font E. Magnesium and phosphorus. *Lancet.* 1998; 352:391-396.

Zorbas YG, Federenko YF, Naexu KA. Phosphate-loading test influences on endurance-trained volunteers during restriction of muscular activity and chronic hyperhydration. *Biol Trace Elem Res.* 1995; 48:51-65.

Phytostanols

DESCRIPTION

Phytostanols are saturated phytosterols. (See Phytosterols and Beta-Sitosterol.) That is, they have no double bonds in the sterol ring. Phytosterols, widely found in the plant kingdom, resemble cholesterol. Cholesterol, however, does not occur in plants. The cyclopentanoperhydrophenanthrene ring structure is common to all sterols; the differences among the various sterols are primarily in the structure of the side chains. Beta-sitostanol has the following chemical structure:

Beta-sitostanol

Phytosterols are present in the diet. Typical daily dietary intakes of phytosterols range from 100 to 300 milligrams. It is higher in vegetarians. Saturated phytosterols or phytostanols are also present in the diet in much smaller quantities, usually making up approximately 10 to 20% of the phytosterol intake. There are over 40 phytosterols, but beta-sitosterol is the most abundant one, comprising about 50% of dietary phytosterols. The next most abundant phytosterols are campesterol (about 33%) and stigmasterol (about 2 to 5%).

Phytostanols are potentially atherogenic like cholesterol, but except in the rare genetic disorders, cerebrotendinotic xanthomatosis and sitosterolemia, they are not. This is because so little of the phytosterols, and even less of the phytostanols, is absorbed. On the other hand, phytosterols can lower cholesterol levels. As early as 1951, it was shown that phytosterols lowered cholesterol in chickens, and subsequently they were found to lower cholesterol in other animals and in humans.

Recently, functional foods, containing phytostanols esterified with fatty acids, have entered the marketplace in the form of margarines, spreads and salad dressings. In the case of most of these products, the esterified phytostanols are derived from tall oil from the *Pinaceae* family. Tall oil is a byproduct of the pulp and paper industry. The phytosterols and phytostanols derived from tall oil undergo hydrogenation to produce mainly beta-sitostanol, campestanol and stigmastanol and then, in an esterification step with fatty acids derived from such vegetable oils as rapeseed oil, arrive at the finished product.

Phytostanols are also known as plant stanols and saturated plant sterols. Phytostanols themselves have extremely poor solubility in both aqueous and lipid media. Esterification of phytostanols with long-chain fatty acids increases their lipid solubility.

ACTIONS AND PHARMACOLOGY

ACTIONS

Phytostanols have cholesterol-lowering activity.

MECHANISM OF ACTION

The mechanism of the cholesterol-lowering activity of phytostanols is not fully understood. Phytostanols appear to inhibit the absorption of dietary cholesterol and the reabsorption (via the enterohepatic circulation) of endogenous cholesterol from the gastrointestinal tract. Consequently, the excretion of cholesterol in the feces leads to decreased serum levels of this sterol. Phytostanols do not appear to affect the absorption of bile acids.

It is believed that phytostanols displace cholesterol from bile salt micelles. Another proposed mechanism is the inhibition of the rate of cholesterol esterification in the intestinal mucosa. Much more research is needed on the mechanism of the cholesterol-lowering effect of phytostanols.

PHARMACOKINETICS

Supplemental esterified phytostanols, following ingestion, undergo hydrolysis in the small intestine catalyzed by such enzymes as cholesterol esterase to yield the phytostanols sitostanol, campestanol and stigmastanol. Less than 1% of ingested phytostanols are distributed rapidly and mainly to the liver where some proportion is glucuronidated. The phytostanols are excreted either in the free or glucuronidated form mainly via the biliary route. Virtually all of ingested phytostanols are excreted in the feces.

INDICATIONS AND USAGE

Phytostanols may be indicated for the management of hypercholesterolemia.

RESEARCH SUMMARY

In a double-blind study, 153 subjects with mild hypercholesterolemia were randomized to receive a control margarine or a margarine containing sitostanol ester (1.8 or 2.6 grams of sitostanol daily). The study continued for one year, at the conclusion of which there was a mean reduction in serum cholesterol of 10.2% in the sitostanol groups, compared with a 0.1% increase in the control group. LDL-cholesterol was reduced 14.1% in the sitostanol groups versus 1.1% in the control group. Sitostanol was significantly superior to the control margarine at both dose levels, but the higher dose was significantly more effective than the lower dose. Neither LDL-cholesterol nor triglycerides were affected by sitostanol.

In a more recent study, 318 mildly hypercholesterolemic subjects were randomized to receive margarine containing no phytostanols (placebo control) or margarines with 2 grams or 3 grams of stanol esters daily. Both stanol esters doses were effective, but the 3-gram dose was more effective, lowering total cholesterol by 6.4% and LDL-cholesterol by 10.1%. There was no effect on triglycerides or HDL-cholesterol.

Several other studies have confirmed these results. In a study of post-menopausal women with documented cardiovascular disease, stanol esters decreased total cholesterol by 13% and LDL-cholesterol by 20%, administered in a margarine that delivered 3 grams of sitostanol daily. These women were not taking lipid-lowering medication. In another study, stanol esters augmented the effects of simvastatin in further lowering LDL-cholesterol levels.

Recently, studies have been conducted to compare the relative efficacies of vegetable-oil stanol esters and wood stanol esters. They have found them to be equal in their LDL-cholesterol lowering effects.

Another study has compared a phytostanol ester-supplemented margarine with a soybean margarine that primarily contains sterol esters (see Phytosterols). Both of these, used in similar quantities, were equally significant in reducing LDL-cholesterol by 13%.

The authors of a recent review of the relevant literature continue to find benefit in supplementing diet with phytostanol-enriched foods. They have concluded that "the effective dose is 1 to 3 grams daily, expressed as free stanol, which, in placebo-controlled studies, decreased LDL cholesterol by 6 per cent to 15 per cent." They further observed that this effect is maintained with once-daily or divided dosage and is independent of the fat content of the food vehicle. They concluded, as well, that equivalent amounts of plant sterol esters and plant stanol esters have about equal effectiveness in lowering LDL cholesterol. They noted one unexpected finding—that plasma plant sterol levels increase on plant sterols and decrease on plant stanols. What the clinical significance of this is, if anything, remains to be elucidated. They recommend regular intake of food products enriched with stanol and/or sterol esters, such as some margarines and yogurts.

CONTRAINDICATIONS, PRECAUTIONS, ADVERSE REACTIONS

CONTRAINDICATIONS

Phytostanol supplementation is contraindicated in those with the rare genetic disorders sitosterolemia and cerebrotendinotic xanthomatosis.

PRECAUTIONS

Phytostanol supplementation should be avoided by pregnant women and nursing mothers.

ADVERSE REACTIONS

Adverse reactions reported with phytostanol or phytosterol ingestion are mainly mild gastrointestinal ones, including occasional indigestion, feeling of fullness, gas, diarrhea and constipation. Phytostanol supplementation is generally well tolerated.

INTERACTIONS

DRUGS

None known to date. Phytostanol supplementation may be additive to the cholesterol-lowering effects of such cholesterol-lowering drugs as the statins.

NUTRITIONAL SUPPLEMENTS AND FOOD

Some randomized trials have indicated that phytostanols, as well as phytosterols, may lower serum levels of alpha- and beta-carotene, lycopene and vitamin E, probably by interfering with their absorption. Neither vitamin A nor vitamin D levels appear to be affected by phytostanol ingestion. There are no data yet available on the effect of phytostanols on other carotenoids, flavonoids or polyphenols.

DOSAGE AND ADMINISTRATION

At present, phytostanols, in the form of fatty acid esters, are available in some functional foods, including margarines, spreads and salad dressing. Phytostanols and phytostanol esters are being developed as nutritional supplements in capsule form.

A few studies indicate a dose of 2 grams of phytostanols daily to be optimal. Doses used are 1.5 to 4.5 grams daily. Capsules, when available, should be taken with meals.

LITERATURE

Calpe-Berdiel L, Escolà-Gil JC, Blanco-Vaca F. Are LXR-regulated genes a major molecular target of plant sterols/stanols? *Atherosclerosis.* 2007;195(1):210-211.

Calpe-Berdiel L, Escolà-Gil JC, Blanco-Vaca F. New insights into the molecular actions of plant sterols and stanols in cholesterol metabolism. *Atherosclerosis.* Epub: 2008 Jul 6.

Grundy SM. Stanol esters as a component of maximal dietary therapy in the National Cholesterol Education Program Adult Treatment Panel III report. *Am J Cardiol.* 2005;96(1A):47D-50D.

Gylling H, Miettinen TA. Cholesterol reduction by different plant stand mixtures and with variable fat intake. *Metabolism.* 1999;48:575-580.

Gylling H, Puska P, Vartiainen E, et al. Retinol, vitamin D, carotenes and alpha-tocopherol in serum of a moderately hypercholesterolemic population consuming sitostanol ester margarine. *Atherosclerosis.* 1999;145:279-285.

Gylling H, Puska P, Vartiainen E, et al. Serum sterols during stanol ester feeding in a mildly hypercholesterolemic population. *J Lipid Res.* 1999;4:593-600.

Gylling H, Radhakrishnan R, Miettinen TA. Reduction of serum cholesterol in post menopausal women with previous myocardial infarction and cholesterol malabsorption induced by dietary sitostanol ester margarine: women and dietary sitostanol. *Circulation.* 1997;96:4226-4231.

Hallbrook T, Kristiannsson B, Hildebrand H, et al. [Phytosterolemia is an unknown but serious disease. Xanthomatosis in childhood is a warning signal.] *Lakartidningen.* 1996;93:4275-4277.

Hallikainen MA, Sarkkinen ES, Uusitupa MI. Effects of low-fat stanol ester enriched margarines on concentrations of serum carotenoids in subjects with elevated serum cholesterol concentrations. *Eur J Clin Nutr.* 1999;53:966-969.

Hallikainen MA, Sarkkinen ES, Uusitupa MI. Plant stanol esters affect serum cholesterol concentrations of hypercholesterolemic men and women in a dose-dependent manner. *J Nutr.* 2000;130:767-776.

Hallikainen MA, Uusitupa MI. Effects of 2 low-fat stanol ester-containing margarines on serum cholesterol concentrations as part of a low-fat diet in hypercholesterolemic subjects. *Am J Clin Nutr.* 1999;69:403-410.

Jones PJ, Ntanios FY, Rainini-Sarjaz M, et al. Cholesterol-lowering efficacy of a sitostanol-containing phytosterol mixture with a prudent diet in hyperlipidemic men. *Am J Clin Nutr.* 1999;69:1144-1150.

Jones PJ, Raeini-Sarjaz M, Ntanios FY, et al. Modulation of plasma lipid levels and cholesterol kinetics by phytosterol versus phytostanol esters. *J Lipid Res.* 2000;41(5):697-705.

Law M. Plant sterol and stanol margarines and health. *BMJ.* 2000;320:861-864.

Ling WH, Jones PJ. Enhanced efficacy of sitostanol-containing versus sitostanol-free phytosterol mixtures in altering lipoprotein cholesterol levels and synthesis in rats. *Atherosclerosis.* 1995;118:319-331.

Miettinen TA, Gylling H. Effect of statins on noncholesterol sterol levels: implications for use of plant stanols and sterols. *Am J Cardiol.* 2005;96(1A):40D-46D.

Miettinen TA, Puska P, Gylling H, et al. Reduction of serum cholesterol with sitostanol-ester margarine in a mildly hypercholesterolemic population. *N Engl J Med.* 1995;333:1308-1312.

Moruisi KG, Oosthuizen W, Opperman AM. Phytosterols/stanols lower cholesterol concentrations in familial hypercholesterolemic subjects: a systematic review with meta-analysis. *J Am Coll Nutr.* 2006;25(1):41-48.

Nakamura T, Matsuzawa Y. [Cerebrotendinous xanthomatosis and phytosterolemia.] [Article in Japanese.] *Tanpakushitsu Kakusan Koso.* 1998;33:794-797.

Nguyen TT, Dale LC. Plant stanol esters and vitamin K. Mayo *Clin Proc.* 1999;74:642-643.

Nguyen TT, Dale LC, von Bergmann K, et al. Cholesterol-lowering effect of stanol ester in a US population of mildly hypercholesterolemic men and women: a randomized controlled trial. *Mayo Clin Proc.* 1999;74:1198-1206.

Normén L, Dutta P, Lia A, Andersson H. Soy sterol esters and beta-sitostanol esters as inhibitors of cholesterol absorption in human small bowel. *Am J Clin Nutr.* 2000;71:908-913.

O'Neill FH, Sanders TA, Thompson GR. Comparison of efficacy of plant stanol ester and sterol ester: short-term and longer-term studies. *Am J Cardiol.* 2005;96(1A):29D-36D.

Plat J, Mensink RP. Increased intestinal ABCA1 expression contributes to the decrease in cholesterol absorption after plant stanol consumption. *FASEB J.* 2002;16(10):1248-1253.

Plat J, Mensink RP. Vegetable oil based versus wood based stanol ester mixtures: effects on serum lipids and hemostatic factors in non-hypercholesterolemic subjects. *Atherosclerosis.* 2000;148:101-112.

Plat J, Nichols JA, Mensink RP. Plant sterols and stanols: effects on mixed micellar composition and LXR (target gene) activation. *J Lipid Res.* 2005;46(11):2468-2476.

Thompson GR. Additive effects of plant sterol and stanol esters to statin therapy. *Am J Cardiol.* 2005;96(1A):37D-39D.

Thompson GR, Grundy SM. History and development of plant sterol and stanol esters for cholesterol-lowering purposes. *Am J Cardiol.* 2005;96(1A):3D-9D.

Turnbull D, Frankos VH, Leeman WR, Jonker D. Short-term tests of estrogenic potential of plant stanols and plant stanol esters. *Regul Toxicol Pharmacol.* 1999;29(2 Pt 1):211-215.

Vuorio AF, Gylling H, Turtola H, et al. Stanol ester margarine alone and with simvastatin lowers serum cholesterol in families with familial hypercholesterolemia caused by the FH—North Karelia mutation. *Arterioscler Thromb Vasc Biol.* 2000;20:500-506.

Phytosterols

DESCRIPTION
Phytosterols (also see Phytostanols and Beta-Sitosterol), widely found in the plant kingdom, are chemically similar to cholesterol. Cholesterol, however, only occurs in animals and is not found in plants. The cyclopentanoper-hydrophenanthrene ring structure of the sterol molecule is common to all sterols; the differences are primarily in the structure of the side chains.

Phytosterols are present in the diet. Typical daily dietary intakes of phytosterols range from 100 to 300 milligrams. It is higher in vegetarians. There are over 40 phytosterols, but beta-sitosterol is the most abundant one, comprising about 50% of dietary phytosterols. The next most abundant phytosterols are campesterol (about 33%) and stigmasterol (about 2 to 5%). Other phytosterols found in the diet include brassicasterol, delta-7-stigmasterol and delta-7-avenasterol.

Beta-sitosterol differs from cholesterol by the presence of an ethyl group at the 24th carbon position of the side chain. In the case of campesterol, this position is occupied by a methyl group. Chemically, the phytosterols are classified as 4-desmethylsterols of the cholestane series. Beta-sitosterol has the following chemical structure:

Beta-sitosterol

Phytosterols are potentially atherogenic like cholesterol, but except in the rare genetic disorders, sitosterolemia and cerebrotendinotic xanthomatosis, they are not. This is because so little of the phytosterols are absorbed. On the other hand, phytosterols can lower cholesterol levels. As early as 1951, it was shown that phytosterols lowered cholesterol in chickens, and subsequently they were found to lower cholesterol in humans. Recently, functional foods containing phytosterols have become available. These functional foods are in the form of margarines, spreads and salad dressings. In the case of most of these products, phytosterols are found esterified with long-chain fatty acids. These phytosterols are derived from soybean oil and are mainly beta-sitosterol, campesterol and stigmasterol.

Phytosterols are also known as plant sterols and, owing to their large sitosterol content, are sometimes called sitosterol. Phytosterols are virtually insoluble in aqueous media and are poorly soluble in lipid media. Esterification of phytosterols with long-chain fatty acids increases their lipid solubility.

ACTIONS AND PHARMACOLOGY
ACTIONS
Phytosterols have cholesterol-lowering activity.

MECHANISM OF ACTION
The mechanism of the cholesterol-lowering activity of phytosterols is not fully understood. Phytosterols appear to inhibit the absorption of dietary cholesterol and the reabsorption (via the enterohepatic circulation) of endogenous cholesterol from the gastrointestinal tract. Consequently, the excretion of cholesterol in the feces leads to decreased serum levels of this sterol. Phytosterols do not appear to affect the absorption of bile acids.

It is believed that phytosterols displace cholesterol from bile salt micelles. Another proposed mechanism is the possible inhibition of the rate of cholesterol esterification in the intestinal mucosa.

PHARMACOKINETICS

Supplemental esterified phytosterols, following ingestion, undergo hydrolysis in the small intestine, catalyzed by such enzymes as cholesterol esterase, to yield the phytosterols beta-sitosterol, campesterol and stigmasterol. Of course, unesterified phytosterols do not undergo hydrolysis. About 5% of the ingested beta-sitosterol and about 15% of the campesterol are absorbed and transported via the portal circulation to the liver where some fraction of these phytosterols is glucuronidated. The phytosterols are excreted either in the free or glucuronidated form mainly via the biliary route.

INDICATIONS AND USAGE

Phytosterols may be indicated for the management of hypercholesterolemia.

RESEARCH SUMMARY

Phytosterols have been compared with phytostanols to assess their relative efficacy in lowering total cholesterol and LDL-cholesterol. These studies confirm that both are effective in lowering these lipids. A recent review concluded that plant sterols and stanols, in the studies analyzed, reduce, on average, total cholesterol by 10% and LDL-cholesterol by 13%. They have no significant effect in either HDL-cholesterol or triglycerides. (See Phytostanols.)

Given ongoing positive results in studies of phytosterols, the United States National Cholesterol Education Program recommends dietary phytosterol supplementation of 2 grams daily for cholesterol reduction. It is believed that this will lower LDL-cholesterol by approximately 10%.

CONTRAINDICATIONS, PRECAUTIONS, ADVERSE REACTIONS

CONTRAINDICATIONS

Phytosterol supplementation is contraindicated in those with the rare genetic disorders sitosterolemia and cerebrotendinotic xanthomatosis.

PRECAUTIONS

Phytosterol supplementation should be avoided by pregnant women and nursing mothers.

ADVERSE REACTIONS

Adverse reactions are mainly mild gastrointestinal ones, including occasional indigestion, feeling of fullness, gas, diarrhea and constipation. Phytosterol supplementation is generally well tolerated.

INTERACTIONS

DRUGS

None known to date. Phytosterol supplementation may be additive to the cholesterol-lowering effects of such cholesterol-lowering drugs as the statins.

NUTRITIONAL SUPPLEMENTS AND FOOD

Some randomized trials have indicated that phytosterols may lower serum levels of alpha- and beta-carotene, lycopene and vitamin E, probably by interfering with their absorption. Neither vitamin A nor vitamin D levels appear to be affected by phytosterol ingestion. There are no data yet available on the effect of phytosterols on other carotenoids (lutein, zeaxanthin), flavonoids or polyphenols.

OVERDOSAGE

No reports of overdosage.

DOSAGE AND ADMINISTRATION

Phytosterols are available in the form of fatty acid esters in some functional food products, including margarines, spreads and salad dressing. Unesterified phytosterols are available in capsules. Doses of the phytosterol esters range from 1.12 to 2.24 grams daily. Doses of the unesterified phytosterols are about 1 gram daily. Capsules, if used, should be taken with meals.

LITERATURE

Awad AB, Fink CS. Phytosterols as anticancer dietary components: evidence and mechanism of action. *J Nutr.* 2000;130(9):2127-2130.

Ayesh R, Westrate JA, Drewitt PN, et al. Safety evaluation of phytosterol esters. Part 5. Faecal short-chain fatty acid and microflora content, faecal bacterial enzyme activity and serum female sex hormones in healthy hormolipidaemic volunteers consuming a controlled diet either with or without a phytosterol ester-enriched margarine. *Food Chem Toxicol.* 1999;37:1127-1138.

Baker VA, Hepburn PA, Kennedy SJ, et al. Safety evaluation of phytosterol esters. Part 1. Assessment of oestrogenicity using a combination of in vivo and *in vitro* assays. *Food Chem Toxicol.* 1999;37:13-22.

Bays HE, Neff D, Tomassini JE, et al. Ezetimibe: cholesterol lowering and beyond. *Expert Rev Cardiovasc Ther.* 2008;6(4):447-470.

Bradford PG, Awad AB. Phytosterols as anticancer compounds. *Mol Nutr Food Res.* 2007;51(2):161-170.

Calpe-Berdiel L, Escolà-Gil JC, Benítez S, et al. Dietary phytosterols modulate T-helper immune response but do not induce apparent anti-inflammatory effects in a mouse model of acute, aseptic inflammation. *Life Sci.* 2007;80(21):1951-1956.

Calpe-Berdiel L, Escolà-Gil JC, Blanco-Vaca F. Are LXR-regulated genes a major molecular target of plant sterols/stanols? *Atherosclerosis.* 2007;195(1):210-211.

Calpe-Berdiel L, Escolà-Gil JC, Blanco-Vaca F. New insights into the molecular actions of plant sterols and stanols in cholesterol metabolism. *Atherosclerosis.* Epub: 2008 Jul 6.

Calpe-Berdiel L, Escolà-Gil JC, Blanco-Vaca F. Phytosterol-mediated inhibition of intestinal cholesterol absorption is independent of ATP-binding cassette transporter A1. *Br J Nutr.* 2006;95(3):618-622.

Calpe-Berdiel L, Escolà-Gil JC, Julve J, et al. Differential intestinal mucosal protein expression in hypercholesterolemic mice fed a phytosterol-enriched diet. *Proteomics.* 2007;7(15):2659-2666.

Calpe-Berdiel L, Escolà-Gil JC, Ribas V, et al. Changes in intestinal and liver global gene expression in response to a phytosterol-enriched diet. *Atherosclerosis.* 2005;181(1):75-85.

Ellegård LH, Andersson SW, Normén AL, et al. Dietary plant sterols and cholesterol metabolism. *Nutr Rev.* 2007;65(1):39-45.

Hallbrook T, Kristiannsson B, Hildebrand H, et al. [Phytosterolemia is an unknown but serious disease. Xanthomatosis in childhood is a warning signal.] *Lakartidningen.* 1996;93:4275-4277.

Hendriks HF, Westrate JA, van Vliet T, et al. Spreads enriched with three different levels of vegetable oil sterols and the degree of cholesterol lowering in normocholesterolaemic and mildly hypercholesterolaemic subjects. *Eur J Clin Nutr.* 1999;53:319-327.

Hepburn PA, Horner SA, Smith M. Safety evaluation of phytosterol esters. Part 2. Subchronic 90-day oral toxicity study on phytosterol esters—a novel functional food. *Food Chem Toxicol.* 1999;37:521-532.

Howell TJ, MacDougall DE, Jones PJ. Phytosterols partially explain differences in cholesterol metabolism caused by corn or olive oil feeding. *J Lipid Res.* 1998;39:892-900.

John S, Sorokin AV, Thompson PD. Phytosterols and vascular disease. *Curr Opin Lipidol.* 2007;18(1):35-44.

Jones PJ, Howell T, MacDougall DE, et al. Short-term administration of tall oil phytosterols improves plasma lipid profiles in subjects with different cholesterol levels. *Metabolism.* 1998;47:751-756.

Jones PJ, MacDougall DE, Ntanios F, et al. Dietary phytosterols as cholesterol-lowering agents in human diet. *Can J Physiol Pharmacol.* 1997;75:217-227.

Jones PJ, Raeini-Sarjaz M, Ntanios FY, et al. Modulation of plasma lipid levels and cholesterol kinetics by phytosterol versus phytostanol esters. *J Lipid Res.* 2000;41(5):697-705.

Kidambi S, Patel SB. Cholesterol and non-cholesterol sterol transporters: ABCG5, ABCG8 and NPC1L1: a review. *Xenobiotica.* 2008;38(7):1119-1139.

Kidambi S, Patel SB. Sitosterolaemia: pathophysiology, clinical presentation and laboratory diagnosis. *J Clin Pathol.* 2008;61(5):588-594.

Law M. Plant sterol and stanol margarines and health. *BMJ.* 2000;320:861-864.

Ling WH, Jones PJ. Dietary phytosterols: a review of metabolism, benefits and side effects. *Life Sci.* 1995;57:195-206.

Miettinen TA, Gylling H. Effect of statins on noncholesterol sterol levels: implications for use of plant stanols and sterols. *Am J Cardiol.* 2005;96(1A):40D-46D.

Moghadasian MH, Frohlich JJ. Effects of dietary phytosterols on cholesterol metabolism and atherosclerosis: clinical and experimental evidence. *Am J Med.* 1999;107:588-594.

Moghadasian MH, McManus BM, Pritchard PH, et al. "Tall oil"-derived phytosterols reduce atherosclerosis in ApoE-deficient mice. *Arterioscler Thomb Vasc Biol.* 1997;17:119-126.

Moruisi KG, Oosthuizen W, Opperman AM. Phytosterols/stanols lower cholesterol concentrations in familial hypercholesterolemic subjects: a systematic review with meta-analysis. *J Am Coll Nutr.* 2006;25(1):41-48.

Nakamura T, Matsuzawa Y. [Cerebrotendinous xanthomatosis and phytosterolemia.] [Article in Japanese.] *Tanpakushitsu Kakusan Koso.* 1998;33:794-797.

Normén L, Dutta P, Lia A, et al. Soy sterol esters and beta-sitostanol esters as inhibitors of cholesterol absorption in human small bowel. *Am J Clin Nutr.* 2000;71:908-913.

Ntanios FY, MacDougall DE, Jones PJ. Gender effects of tall oil versus soybean phytosterols as cholesterol-lowering agents in hamsters. *Can J Physiol Pharmacol.* 1988;76:780-787.

O'Neill FH, Sanders TA, Thompson GR. Comparison of efficacy of plant stanol ester and sterol ester: short-term and longer-term studies. *Am J Cardiol.* 2005;96(1A):29D-36D.

Ostlund RE Jr. Phytosterols and cholesterol metabolism. *Curr Opin Lipidol.* 2004;15(1):37-41.

Patch CS, Tapsell LC, Williams PG, et al. Plant sterols as dietary adjuvants in the reduction of cardiovascular risk: theory and evidence. *Vasc Health Risk Manag.* 2006;2(2):157-162.

Patel MD, Thompson PD. Phytosterols and vascular disease. *Atherosclerosis.* 2006;186(1):12-19.

Pinedo S, Vissers MN, von Bergmann K, et al. Plasma levels of plant sterols and the risk of coronary artery disease: the prospective EPIC-Norfolk Population Study. *J Lipid Res.* 2007;48(1):139-144.

Plat J, Nichols JA, Mensink RP. Plant sterols and stanols: effects on mixed micellar composition and LXR (target gene) activation. *J Lipid Res.* 2005;46(11):2468-2476.

Sierksma A, Westrate JA, Meijer GW. Spreads enriched with plant sterols, either esterified 4,4-dimethylsterols or free 4-desmethylsterols, and plasma total-and LDL-cholesterol concentrations. *Br J Nutr* 1999;82:273-282.

Thompson GR. Additive effects of plant sterol and stanol esters to statin therapy. *Am J Cardiol.* 2005;96(1A):37D-39D.

Thompson GR, Grundy SM. History and development of plant sterol and stanol esters for cholesterol-lowering purposes. *Am J Cardiol.* 2005;96(1A):3D-9D.

Von Bergmann K, Sudhop T, Lütjohann D. Cholesterol and plant sterol absorption: recent insights. *Am J Cardiol.* 2005;96(1A):10D-14D.

Waalkens-Beredsen DH, Wolterbeek AP, Wijnands MV, et al. Safety evaluation of phytosterol esters. Part 3. Two generation study in rats with phytosterol ester—a novel functional food. *Food Chem Toxicol.* 1999;37:683-696.

Westrate JA, Ayesh R, Bauer-Plank C, et al. Safety evaluation of phytosterol esters. Part 4. Faecal concentrations of bile acids and neutral sterols in healthy normolipidaemic volunteers consuming a controlled diet either with or without a phytosterol ester-enriched margarine. *Food Chem Toxicol.* 1999;37:1063-1071.

Westrate JA, Ayesh R, Meijer GW. Plant sterl-enriched margarines and reduction of plasma total-and LDL-cholesterol concentrations in normocholesterolaemic subjects. *Eur JClin Nutr.* 1998;52:334-343.

Yu L. The structure and function of Niemann-Pick C1-like 1 protein. *Curr Opin Lipidol.* 2008;19(3):263-269.

Piperine

DESCRIPTION

Piperine is an alkaloid found naturally in plants belonging to the *Piperaceae* family, such as *Piper nigrum* L, commonly known as black pepper, and *Piper longum* L, commonly known as long pepper. Piperine is the major pungent substance in these plants and is isolated from the fruit of the black pepper and long pepper plants. Piperine comprises 1 to 99% of these plants. The term black pepper is used both for the plant *Piper nigrum* and the spice that is mainly in the fruit of the plant.

Piperine is a solid substance essentially insoluble in water. It is a weak base that is tasteless at first, but leaves a burning aftertaste. Piperine belongs to the vanilloid family of compounds, a family that also includes capsaicin, the pungent substance in hot chili peppers. Its molecular formula is $C_{17}H_{19}NO_3$, and its molecular weight is 285.34 daltons. Piperine is the trans-trans stereoisomer of 1-piperoylpiperidine. It is also known as (*E, E*)-1-piperoylpiperidine and (*E, E*)-1-[5-(1, 3-benzodioxol-5-y1)-1-oxo-2, 4-pentdienyl] piperidine. It is represented by the following chemical structure:

Piperine

Black pepper and long pepper have been used in Ayurvedic medicine for the treatment of various diseases. One such preparation is known by the Sanskrit name trikatu and consists of black pepper, long pepper and ginger. Another preparation, known by the Sanskrit name pippali, consists of long pepper. It is thought that piperine is one of the major bioactive substances of these Ayurvedic remedies. Black pepper has also been used in traditional Chinese medicine to treat seizure disorders. A derivative of piperine, antiepilepsirine, has also been used in China to treat seizure disorders. Some recent research suggests that piperine may enhance the bioavailability of some drugs and nutritional substances.

ACTIONS AND PHARMACOLOGY

ACTIONS

Piperine may have bioavailability-enhancing activity for some nutritional substances and for some drugs. It has putative anti-inflammatory activity and may have activity in promoting digestive processes. It has recently been shown to have melanocyte stimulatory activity and antivitiligo activity, when applied topically.

MECHANISM OF ACTION

Piperine has been demonstrated to increase the serum levels and lengthen the serum half lives of some nutritional substances, such as coenzyme Q_{10} and beta-carotene. The mechanism of this action is unknown. It is speculated that piperine may act as a so-called thermonutrient and increase the absorption of certain nutritional substances from the gastrointestinal tract by producing a local thermogenic action. There is no evidence for this.

Piperine has also been found to increase the serum levels and lengthen the serum half lives of some drugs, such as propanolol and theophylline. The mechanism is thought to be by inhibition of certain enzymes involved in the biotransformation of the affected drugs. Piperine has been found to be a nonspecific inhibitor of drug and xenobiotic metabolism. It appears to inhibit many different cytochrome P450 isoforms, as well as UDP-glucuronyltransferase and hepatic arylhydrocarbon hydroxylase and other enzymes involved in drug and xenobiotic metabolism.

The mechanism of piperine's putative anti-inflammatory activity may be accounted for, in part, by piperine's possible antioxidant activity. There are a few studies suggesting that piperine may inhibit lipid peroxidation. Piperine has been shown to stimulate the secretion of the digestive enzymes pancreatic amylase, trypsin, chymotrypsin and lipase in rats. However, piperine appears to have this activity when administered with other spice bioactives, such as capsaicin and curcumin, and not when administered by itself.

The antivitiligo action of piperine is not completely understood.

PHARMACOKINETICS

The pharmacokinetics of piperine in humans remains incompletely understood. In rats, piperine is absorbed following ingestion, and some metabolites have been identified: piperonylic acid, piperonyl alcohol, piperonal and vanillic acid are found in the urine. One metabolite, piperic acid, is found in the bile. Human pharmacokinetic studies are needed.

INDICATIONS AND USAGE

Piperine, in appropriate doses, may be useful in increasing the bioavailability of some drugs and nutrients. There is very preliminary evidence suggesting that piperine may aid in the digestion of food. There is also preliminary evidence that it may have some anticonvulsant, anticarcinogenic and anti-inflammatory properties. On the other hand, there is also preliminary evidence that it might be carcinogenic and cytotoxic in some circumstances and that it might interfere with reproductive processes and have negative effects on sperm. When applied topically, piperine shows antivitiligo activity.

RESEARCH SUMMARY

There are in vitro, animal and human studies demonstrating that piperine can significantly increase the bioavailability of numerous drugs and some nutritional supplements. Reportedly, it has demonstrated this effect with some antimicrobial, antiprotozoal, antihelmintic, antihistaminic, non-steroidal anti-inflammatory, muscle-relaxant and anticancer drugs, among others. It has also increased the bioavailability of coenzyme Q_{10}, curcumin and beta-carotene.

In humans given 2-gram doses of curcumin alone, levels of curcumin in serum were undetectable to very low one hour post-administration. Concomitant administration of 20 mg of piperine was said to significantly increase absorption and bioavailability (by 2000%). Similar results were reported in rats.

In a double-blind crossover study, 5 mg of piperine daily for 14-day periods resulted in significant increases in serum beta-carotene levels. The same dose of piperine produced similar results in another study, this one involving coenzyme Q_{10}.

The claim that piperine may aid in the digestion of food is based on some experimental animal data showing that dietary piperine seems to enhance pancreatic amylase lipase, trypsin and chymotrypsin activity.

The claim that piperine may have some anticonvulsant activity comes, in part, from China, where the substance is used in an effort to treat some forms of epilepsy. In mice, piperine injected intraperitoneally inhibited clonic convulsions induced by kainate. It did not significantly block seizure activity induced by L-glutamate, N-methyl-D-aspartate or guanidinosuccinate.

In a rat intestinal model, piperine was said to provide protection against oxidative changes induced by a number of chemical carcinogens. In another study, this one in vitro, piperine reportedly reduced the cytotoxicity of aflatoxin B1 in rat hepatoma cells.

Piperine exhibited significant anti-inflammatory activity in carageenan-induced rat paw edema and in some other experimental models of inflammation. In one animal study, piperine reduced liver lipid peroxidation, acid phosphatase and edema induced by carageenan.

On the negative side, piperine has shown some evidence of being mutagenic and potentially carcinogenic under some circumstances. It has reportedly given rise to mutagenic products on reaction with nitrites. This causes concern since nitrites and piperine may be consumed simultaneously. Risk might increase with high-dose piperine supplementation. In another study, piperine appeared to enhance the bioavailability of aflatoxin B1 in rat tissues. And in yet another study, piperine was found to be cytotoxic to cultured brain neurons. Piperine was said to be non-mutagenic, however, in a study examining effects of the substance on the germ cells of Swiss albino mice.

In a recent study utilizing albino rats, piperine, given at doses of 5 and 10 mg/kg body weight for 30 days, resulted (at the 10-mg/kg dose level) in significant reduction in the weights of testes and accessory sex organs as well as severe damage to seminiferous tubules. The 5-mg/kg dose resulted in partial degeneration of germ cells.

Decreased mating performance, decreased fertility and anti-implantation activity, along with some other adverse reproductive events, were observed in mice given very high doses of piperine.

CONTRAINDICATIONS, PRECAUTIONS, ADVERSE REACTIONS

CONTRAINDICATIONS

Piperine is contraindicated for those who are hypersensitive to any component of a piperine-containing preparation.

PRECAUTIONS

Pregnant women and nursing mothers should avoid piperine supplementation.

Piperine at doses generally higher than 15 mg daily may affect the metabolism of a wide range of drugs and xenobiotics (see Interactions). In some cases, doses lower than 15 mg daily may affect the metabolism of these substances. Those using the drugs listed in Interactions should exercise caution in the use of piperine supplements.

Piperine may form mutagenic and possibly carcinogenic substances with nitrites. Those who eat processed food containing nitrites and nitrates as food preservatives should exercise caution in the use of piperine supplements.

ADVERSE REACTIONS

The typical dose of piperine in nutritional formulas is 5 milligrams, and doses of 15 milligrams daily are rarely exceeded. No adverse reactions have been reported with these doses. Piperine, if exposed to the tongue, is tasteless at first but leaves a burning aftertaste.

INTERACTIONS

DRUGS

Piperine, usually at a dose of 20 mg or greater, has been shown to inhibit the metabolism of the following drugs: propanolol, theophylline, phenytoin, sulfadiazene, rifampicin, isoniazid, ethambutol, pyrazinamide and dapsone. This list is not inclusive. Piperine is a nonspecific inhibitor of drugs and xenobiotics. Most drugs metabolized via cytochrome P450 enzymes would likely be affected by piperine.

NUTRITIONAL SUPPLEMENTS

Piperine at a dose of 5 mg daily has been found to enhance the absorption of beta-carotene and coenzyme Q_{10}. At a dose of 20 mg daily, it has been found to enhance the absorption of curcumin. Piperine may also enhance the absorption of vitamin B_6, vitamin C and the mineral selenium in the form of L-selenomethionine.

FOOD

Piperine may enhance the absorption of beta-carotene, vitamin B_6, Vitamin C and L-selenomethionine found in certain foods.

DOSAGE AND ADMINISTRATION

The content of piperine in black pepper ranges from 5 to 9%. The daily consumption of piperine in populations that use black pepper regularly is approximately 17 to 31 milligrams daily.

Piperine is available in stand-alone supplements and in combination products. A typical dose is 5 mg daily.

LITERATURE

Atal CK, Dubey RK, Singh J. Biochemical basis of enhanced drug bioavailability by piperine: evidence that piperine is a potent inhibitor of drug metabolism. *J Pharmacol Exp Ther.* 1985;232:258-262.

Badmaev V, Majeed M, Norkus EP. Piperine, an alkaloid derived from black pepper increases serum response of beta-carotene during 14-days of oral beta-carotene supplementation. *Nutr Res.* 1999;19:381-388.

Badmaev V. Majeed M, Prakash L. Piperine derived from black pepper increases the plasma levels of coenzyme Q_{10} following oral supplementation. *J Nutr Biochem.* 2000;11:109-113.

Bano G, Raina RK, Zutshi U, et al. Effect of piperine on bioavailability and pharmacokinetics of propanolol and theophylline in healthy volunteers. *Eur J Clin Pharmacol.* 1991;41:615-617.

D'Hooge R, Pei YQ, Raes A, et al. Anticonvulsant activity of piperine on seizures induced by excitatory amino acid receptor agonists. *Arzneimittelforschung.* 1996;46:557-560.

Dhuley JN, Raman PH, Mujumdar AM, et al. Inhibition of lipid peroxidation by piperine during experimental inflammation in rats. *Indian J Exp Biol.* 1993;31:443-445.

Faas L, Venkatasamy R, Hider RC, et al. In vivo evaluation of piperine and synthetic analogues as potential treatments for vitiligo using a sparsely pigmented mouse model. *Br J Dermatol.* 2008;158(5):941-950.

Karekar VR, Mujumdar AM, Joshi SS, et al. Assessment of genotoxic effect of piperine using Salmonella typhimurium and somatic and somatic and germ cells of Swiss albino mice. *Arzneimittelforschung.* 1996;46:972-975.

Khajuria A, Thusu N, Zutshi U, et al. Piperine modulation of carcinogen induced oxidative stress in intestinal mucosa. *Mol Cell Biochem.* 1998;189:113-118.

Khajuria A, Zutshi U, Bedi KL. Permeability characteristics of piperine on oral absorption—an active alkaloid from peppers and a bioavailability enhancer. *Ind J Exp Biol.* 1998;36:46-50.

Majeed M, Badmaev V, Rajendran R. Use of piperine as a bioavailability enhancer. United States Patent No. 5,972,382. Oct. 26, 1999.

Malini T, Manimaran RR, Arunakaran J, et al. Effects of piperine on testis of albino rats. *J Ethnopharmacol.* 1999;64:219-225.

Mujumdar AM, Dhuley JN, Deshmukh VK, et al. Anti-inflammatory activity of piperine. *Jpn J Med Sci Biol.* 1990;433:95-100.

Pei YQ. A review of pharmacology and clinical use of piperine and its derivatives. *Epilepsia.* 1983; 24:177-182.

Platel K, Srinivasan K. Influence of digestive spices and their active principles on pancreatic digestive enzymes in albino rats. *Nahrung.* 2000;44:42-46.

Shenoy NR, Choughuley AS. Characterization of potentially mutagenic products from the nitrosation of piperine. *Cancer Lett.* 1992;64:235-239.

Shoba G, Joy D, Joseph TM, et al. Influence of piperine on the pharmacokinetics of curcumin in animals and human volunteers. *Planta Med.* 1998;64:353-356.

Srinivasan K. Black pepper and its pungent principle-piperine: a review of diverse physiological effects. *Crit Rev Food Sci Nutr.* 2007;47(8):735-748.

Unchern S, Nagata K, Saito H, et al. Piperine, a pungent alkaloid, is cytotoxic to cultured neutrons from the embryonic rat brain. *Biol Pharm Bull.* 1994;17:403-406.

Policosanol (PPG)

DESCRIPTION

PPG, also known as policosanol, D-001, Ateromixal and Vasoactol, is a Cuban proprietary mixture of long-chain primary aliphatic saturated alcohols. These alcohols are derived from the wax of Cuban sugar cane (*Saccharum officinarium*). The main long-chain alcohol in the Cuban policosanol is the 28 carbon 1-octacosanol, and next most abundant is the 30 carbon 1-triacontanol. Other long-chain alcohols present in much lower concentrations are: 1-docosanol (C22), 1-tetracosanol (C24), 1-hexacosanol (C26), 1-heptacosanol (C27), 1-nonacosanol (C29), 1-dotriacontanol (C32) and 1-tetracontanol (C34). These long-chain alcohols are solid waxy substances and are insoluble in water. They are known collectively as fatty alcohols. In sugar cane, the wax alcohols are found esterified to long-chain fatty acids.

There have been more than 60 well-designed, high-quality PPG clinical trials involving over 3,000 subjects. Most of these studies demonstrated that PPG had significant LDL-cholesterol-lowering activity. The studies mainly took place in Cuba, but some were conducted in Argentina, Russia, Venezuela and Mexico. To date, no trials with PPG have been performed in the United States owing to the U.S. embargo against Cuba. PPG would be an important addition to lipid-lowering therapy if similar results could be obtained in the United States. A couple of recent clinical studies—one in Germany, and one in Italy claiming to have used the Cuban PPG product—did not find significant lipid-lowering effects.

PPG (policosanol) is marketed mainly to Latin-American countries, but, because of the embargo, not to the United States, by Laboratios DALMER S.A., the commercial arm of CNIC (Centro Nacional de Investigaciones Cientificas, or the National Center for Scientific Research in Havana, Cuba).

There are dietary supplements derived from sugar cane, bees wax or other plant sources of fatty alcohols that are marketed in the United States and called policosanol. However, these preparations are different from the Cuban PPG product in several ways. Their wax alcohols occur in different proportions than in the Cuban product, they have a higher content of unidentified components and the finished products have different physico-chemical properties than the PPG product. A Cuban clinical study concluded that these alternative "policosanols" have at best only very modest cholesterol-lowering efficacy, by no means comparable to that seen with statins or PPG; some anecdotal experience in the U.S. appears to corroborate this conclusion.

Hopefully, a clinical study with the Cuban PPG product will one day be allowed in the U.S. The results of such a trial could finally settle the issue of whether or not PPG works.

ACTIONS AND PHARMACOLOGY

ACTIONS

Policosanol may reduce total serum cholesterol and low-density lipoprotein-cholesterol (LDL-C) levels in some.

MECHANISM OF ACTION

The mechanism of action of reported cholesterol-lowering activity is unknown. Some animal studies suggest that policosanol may inhibit cholesterol syntheses in the liver. It is also unclear if the putative cholesterol-lowering activity is due to octacosanol. The long-chain alcohols appear to have different biological activities, and octacosanol by itself may not have the same activities as policosanol. They may work synergistically.

PHARMACOKINETICS

Pharmacokinetic studies have been performed on octacosanol, the major alcohol in policosanol, in experimental animals and human volunteers. The absorption of octacosanol is variable and low. Octacosanol absorption ranges from about 11% in rats and humans to about 28% in rabbits. Octacosanol is absorbed from the small intestine into the lymph and from there enters the blood stream.

Distribution is primarily to the liver digestive tract, skeletal muscle and adipose tissues. Octacosanol may be partly oxidized to the long-chain saturated fatty acid, octacosanoic acid which undergoes beta-oxidation.

Following a single dose of octacosanol in experimental animals, peak plasma levels are seen between 30 minutes to 2 hours. Following a single dose of octacosanol in human volunteers, peak plasma levels are seen at one hour and four hours later. Bile is the main route of excretion. Renal excretion is negligible.

INDICATIONS AND USAGE

Claims that policosanol may be an effective lipid-lowering agent, while having some basis in seemingly sound research, have become controversial. The issue is unresolved. Some recent research, however, suggests that policosanol might be effective, not only as a lipid-lowering agent, but also as a glucose-controlling agent in type 2 diabetes. Reports that policosanol can boost energy and enhance sexual performance are anecdotal.

RESEARCH SUMMARY

A mixture of higher aliphatic primary alcohols derived from sugar cane wax has become popular in such places as Cuba for its reputed cholesterol-lowering benefits, energizing effects and enhancement of sexual function. It is also the source of another increasingly popular supplement—octacosanol (the primary long-chain alcohol in policosanol).

There are a number of animal studies suggesting that policosanol can lower cholesterol, that it can inhibit experimentally induced atherosclerotic lesions of cerebral ischemia, that it can help prevent the peroxidation of lipoprotein and inhibit platelet aggregation.

There are a number of human clinical trials with Cuban policosanol. In one study, patients with LDL-cholesterol greater than 160 mg/dl were randomized in double-blind fashion to receive policosanol (10 milligrams daily), lovastatin (20 milligrams daily) or simvastatin (10 milligrams daily). After eight weeks of therapy, LDL-cholesterol was reduced 24% in the policosanol groups, 22% in the lovastatin group and 15% with simvastatin. HDL-cholesterol increased significantly in the policosanol group but not in the other two groups. Policosanol was judged to be "a safe and effective cholesterol reducing agent.'

In another double-blind study of policosanol's possible effects in hypercholesterolemia, patients received 5 milligrams of policosanol or placebo daily for 12 weeks followed by 10 milligrams of policosanol or placebo for a subsequent 12 weeks. Policosanol (5 and 10 milligrams daily) appeared to significantly reduce LDL-cholesterol (18.2% and 25.6% respectively) and reduce total cholesterol (13% and 17.4%). It appeared to raise HDL-cholesterol (15.5% and 28.4%). Triglycerides were unchanged in the first 12-week period but were significantly reduced (5.2%) by the end of the second 12-week period. Side effects were few and minor. There were 11 serious (7 of these were vascular) adverse events among those in the placebo group, but none in the policosanol group.

In one study, policosanol appeared to significantly reduce platelet aggregation in both healthy and hypercholesterolemic individuals, apparently proving as effective (at 20 milligrams daily doses) as aspirin (100 milligrams per day). The substance also appears to demonstrate beneficial effect in patients with intermittent claudication. Long-term therapy (20 months) using 5 milligrams of policosanol twice a day resulted in significant improvement in treadmill exercise performance and exercise — ECG responses in a group of coronary heart disease patients. The addition of 125 milligrams of aspirin daily further enhanced these results. It is hoped that others will confirm these very promising, largely Cuban studies.

A review of the policosanol literature, originating in Germany, declared a few years ago that "policosanol seems to be a very promising phytochemical alternative to classic lipid-lowering agents such as the statins and deserves further evaluation." These same authors, in collaboration with two other authors in Germany, have more recently arrived at the opposite conclusion following a multicenter, randomized, double-blind, placebo-controlled trial involving patients with hypercholesterolemia or combined hyperlipidemia. Patients were randomized to receive varying doses (10-80 mg daily) of, reportedly, Cuban sugar-cane-derived policosanol or placebo for 12 weeks. The policosanol was said to exert no effect on lipid levels beyond those observed for placebo. Unaccountably, this study was concluded in 2001, prior to publication in 2002 by two of the same authors of the review finding "very promising" lipid-lowering policosanol effects.

A group of Italian researchers have also reported no sugar cane policosanol efficacy in lowering plasma cholesterol in hypercholesterolemic patients who received 10 mg daily of supposed Cuban policosanol for eight weeks.

In contrast, another meta-analysis, published a few years ago and based on 4,596 patients and 52 studies, found policosanol to have lipid-modulating effects "approaching antilipidemic drug efficacy." About the same time, other researchers reported no effect from sugar cane policosanol on plasma cholesterol in golden Syrian hamsters. Still others reported a mild-to-moderate decrease in LDL-cholesterol in patients intolerant of statin therapy and in those receiving adjunctive policosanol with statin therapy. These remarkably divergent results demand further research and explication. A clinical trial in the United States with Cuban policosanol would certainly help.

Other researchers have recently further elucidated how policosanol inhibits cholesterol synthesis, adding support to those who continue to believe that the substance is an effective lipid modulator. In this research, policosanol inhibited cholesterol synthesis in cultured rat hepatoma cells by activation of AMP-kinase, an enzyme involved in cellular energy homeostasis. A three-fold increase in AMP-kinase phosphorylation was detected in policosanol-treated cells. AMP-kinase has been shown to suppress other activity that increases cholesterol synthesis. These researchers have observed that policosanol's activation of AMP-kinase "is reminiscent of the mechanism of metformin, a drug widely used to treat type 2 diabetes. Metformin acts through AMP-kinase to reduce blood glucose levels, enhance glucose uptake into skeletal muscle, decrease circulating lipids and inhibit hepatic gluconeogenesis." These researchers further reported that policosanol is "considerably more potent" than metformin in its ability to stimulate AMP-kinase phosphorylation in the human hepatoma cell line. These findings, they add, "suggest that an evaluation of the ability of policosanol to moderate blood glucose levels in type 2 diabetes may be warranted."

Far from going away, policosanol may thus be further researched in coming years, not only to try to clarify its possible role as a lipid-modulating agent but also as a possible therapy in type 2 diabetes.

Policosanol's reputed efficacy in boosting energy and enhancing sexual function, particularly male sexual function, is entirely anecdotal.

CONTRAINDICATIONS, PRECAUTIONS, ADVERSE REACTIONS

CONTRAINDICATIONS

Hypersensitivity to any component of policosanol.

PRECAUTIONS

Policosanol is not recommended for children, pregnant women and nursing mothers. Because of possible antithrombotic activity, those taking warfarin and hemophiliacs should exercise caution in the use of policosanol. Policosanol supplementation should be stopped before any surgery.

ADVERSE REACTIONS

Mild gastrointestinal side effects, skin rash, headache, insomnia and weight loss have been reported. The incidence of these adverse reactions is low. Policosanol is generally well tolerated.

Except for possible lowering of serum total cholesterol and LDL-cholesterol, policosanol does not appear to affect any other laboratory test results.

INTERACTIONS

Aspirin: Policosanol showed a synergism with the antithrombotic properties of aspirin in different experimental models.

No adverse interactions have been found with policosanol use in combination with beta-blockers, diuretics, calcium-channel blockers, NSAIDs, anxiolytics, oral hypoglycemic agents, digoxin, nitroglycerin, neuroleptics or antidepressants.

No known adverse interactions with nutritional supplements, herbs or foods.

OVERDOSAGE

There are no reports of overdosage. A single dose of 1 gram (50 times the maximum recommended dose) was well tolerated by healthy volunteers. Oral LD_{50} in mice, rats and rabbits is higher than 5 grams per kilogram. Policosanol did not induce genotoxic changes in somatic or germ cells, and it does not act as a mutagenic agent. Teratogenic and carcinogenic testing to date has been negative.

DOSAGE AND ADMINISTRATION

The recommended starting dose of policosanol is 5 milligrams daily taken at dinner time. An effect may take up to 12 weeks to be observed. The dose can be doubled to 5 milligrams twice a day, taken at lunch and dinner. A dose of 20 milligrams daily should not be exceeded. It should be noted that sale and use of Cuban policosanol (PPG) in the United States are not legal. Policosanol products marketed in the United States are not Cuban policosanol, and there is not much support for the effectiveness of the non-Cuban products.

LITERATURE

Arruzazabala, ML, Carbajal D, Mas R, et al. Cholesterol-lowering effects of policosanol in rabbits. *Biol Res.* 1994;27:205-208.

Arruzazabala ML, Mas R, Molina V, et al. Effect of policosanol on platelet aggregation in type II hypercholesterolemic patients. *Int J Tissue React.* 1998;20:119-124.

Arruzazabala ML, Valdes S, Mas R, et al. Comparative study of policosanol, aspirin and the combination therapy policosanol-aspirin on platelet aggregation in healthy volunteers. *Pharmacol Res.* 1997;36:293-297.

Berthold HK, Unverdorben S, Degenhardt R, et al. Effect of policosanol on lipid levels among patients with hypercholesterolemia or combined hyperlipidemia: a randomized controlled trial. *JAMA.* 2006;295(19):2262-2269.

Castano G, Mas R, Roca J, et al. A double-blind, placebo-controlled study of the effects of policosanol in patients with intermittent claudication. *Angiology.* 1999;50:123-130.

Francini-Pesenti F, Beltramolli D, Dall'acqua S, et al. Effect of sugar cane policosanol on lipid profile in primary hypercholesterolemia. *Phytother Res.* 2008;22(3):318-322.

Francini-Pesenti F, Brocadello F, Beltramolli D, et al. Sugar cane policosanol failed to lower plasma cholesterol in primitive, diet-resistant hypercholesterolaemia: a double blind, controlled study. *Complement Ther Med.* 2008;16(2):61-65.

Gouni-Berthold I, Berthold HK. Policosanol: clinical pharmacology and therapeutic significance of a new lipid-lowering agent. *Am Heart J.* 2002;143(2):356-365.

Hernandez F, Illnait J, Mas R, et al. Effect of policosanol on serum lipids and lipoproteins in healthy volunteers. *Current Therap Res.* 1992;52:568-575.

Kassis AN, Marinangeli CP, Jain D, et al. Lack of effect of sugar cane policosanol on plasma cholesterol in Golden Syrian hamsters. *Atherosclerosis.* 2007;194(1):153-158.

Mas R, Castano G, Illnait J, et al. Effects of policosanol in patients with type II hypercholesterolemia and additional coronary risk factors. *Clin Pharmaco Ther.* 1999;64:439-447.

Menéndez R, Frago V, Amor GM, et al. Oral administration of policosanol inhibits in vitro copper ion-induced rat lipoprotein peroxidation. *Physiol Behav.* 1999;67:1-7.

Menéndez R, Marrero D, Más R, et al. In vitro and in vivo study of octacosanol metabolism. *Arch Med Res.* 2005;36(2):113-119.

Prat H, Roman O, Piro E. Comparative effects of policosanol and two HMG-CoA reductase inhibitors on type II hypercholesterolemia. *Rev Med Chil.* 1999;127:286-294.

Stusser R, Batista J, Padron R, et al. Long-term therapy with policosanol improves treadmill exercise-ECG testing performance of coronary heart disease patients. *Int J Clin Pharmacol Ther.* 1998;36:469-473.

Torres O, Agramante AJ, Illnait J, et al. Treatment of hypercholesterolemia in NIDDM with policosanol. *Diabet Care.* 1995;18:393-396.

Potassium

DESCRIPTION

Potassium is an essential macromineral in human nutrition with a wide range of biochemical and physiological roles. Among other things, it is important in the transmission of nerve impulses, the contraction of cardiac, skeletal and smooth muscle, the production of energy, the synthesis of nucleic acids, the maintenance of intracellular tonicity and the maintenance of normal blood pressure. In 1928, it was first suggested that high potassium intake could exert an anti-hypertensive effect. Accumulating evidence suggests that diets high in potassium may be protective not only against hypertension, but also strokes and cardiovascular disease and possibly other degenerative diseases, as well.

Potassium is a metallic element with atomic number 19 and an average atomic weight of 39.09 daltons. Its symbol is K. It is an alkali metal and belongs to the same group as lithium, sodium, rubidium, cesium and francium. The only non-alkali element that it shares some similarities with is thallium. The thallous cation is similar in size to the potassium cation, which is the basis of the use of thallium for myocardial perfusion imaging. The thallous cation is considered a potassium cation analogue. Potassium exists physiologically in its univalent cationic state. It is the principal intracellular cation with an intracellular concentration of about 145 milliequivalents or millimoles per liter. This is 30 to 40 times greater than its extracellular concentration, which is normally 3.5 to 5.0 milliequivalents or millimoles per liter. About 98% of the body's potassium is in intracellular fluid.

The major cause of potassium deficiency is excessive losses of potassium through the alimentary tract or through the kidneys. Potassium depletion typically occurs as a consequence of prolonged use of oral diuretics, from severe diarrhea and from primary or secondary hyperaldosteronism, diabetic ketoacidosis or in those on long-term total parenteral nutrition who have received inadequate potassium. Signs and symptoms of potassium deficiency include hypokalemia, metabolic alkalosis, anorexia, weakness, fatigue, listlessness and cardiac dysrhythmias. Prominent U-waves are seen in the electrocardiograms of those with hypokalemia.

The intake of potassium in the American diet ranges from about 1,560 to 4,680 milligrams (40 to 120 milliequivalents or millimoles) daily. The potassium intake of vegetarians is at the high end. Foods that are rich in potassium are fresh vegetables and fruits. A medium-size banana supplies 630 milligrams of potassium or about 75 milligrams per inch; a medium orange, 365 milligrams; half a cantaloupe, 885 milligrams; half an avocado, 385 milligrams; raw spinach, 780 milligrams per three to four ounces; raw cabbage, 230 milligrams a cup; raw celery, 300 milligrams a cup. Some vegetable juices supply up to 800 milligrams per serving. A dietary intake of about 3.5 grams of potassium is considered to be a desirable intake of potassium for adults.

ACTIONS AND PHARMACOLOGY

ACTIONS

Supplementary potassium is used to treat potassium depletion states, e.g., from prolonged use of diuretics. It is also used to prevent potassium depletion in those on diuretics. Potassium may also have antihypertensive and cerebrovascular- and cardiovascular-protective activities.

MECHANISM OF ACTION

Potassium chloride, in the form of potassium-rich foods or potassium chloride supplements, is used in the management of potassium-deficiency associated with metabolic alkalosis. The fundamental cause of the deficiency is also treated whenever possible. Potassium deficiency may also be associated with metabolic acidosis, e.g., in those with renal tubular acidosis. In those cases, potassium salts other than potassium chloride are used, including potassium citrate, potassium acetate or potassium carbonate.

Potassium supplementation has been demonstrated to bring about small but significant reductions in blood pressure in those with mild to moderate hypertension. The mechanism of this effect is unclear. Possible mechanisms for this antihypertensive effect include a decrease in plasma renin activity, effects on resistance vessels related either to a high potassium concentration or to a decrease in the number of angiotensin II receptors and natriuresis (potassium inhibits sodium reabsorption in the proximal tubules).

The mechanism by which increased potassium intake may prevent stroke is not known. Possible mechanisms include potassium's hypotensive effect, inhibition of free radical formation, prevention of vascular smooth muscle proliferation and prevention of arterial thrombosis. In *in vitro* and in animal studies, elevation of extracellular potassium concentration within the physiological range has been shown to inhibit free radical formation from macrophages and endothelial cells, as well as to inhibit proliferation and thymidine incorporation of vascular smooth muscle cells and to reduce platelet sensitivity to thrombin and other agonists. High potassium diets have also been shown to reduce oxidative stress on the endothelium of high sodium chloride-fed, stroke-prone, spontaneously hypertensive rats independent of blood pressure changes.

PHARMACOKINETICS

The efficiency of absorption of supplementary potassium from the gastrointestinal tract is high. Greater than 90% of an ingested dose of potassium is absorbed. The efficiency of absorption of dietary potassium is similar. Potassium is delivered to the liver via the portal circulation and the rest of the body via the systemic circulation. Insulin and catecholamines promote potassium transport into cells. Potassium is lost from the body in the urine and, to a lesser degree, in gastrointestinal secretions.

INDICATIONS AND USAGE

Potassium may be useful in the prevention and treatment of hypertension in some, notably African Americans. Epidemiological studies have suggested that high dietary intake of potassium may protect many populations against stroke. More recent analyses suggest that this protection may be restricted to black men and hypertensive men. There is experimental data indicating that high potassium intake may have a number of cardioprotective effects. There is no credible evidence that supplemental potassium has anticarcinogenic effects or that it can enhance athletic performance other than, possibly, in those who are potassium deficient.

RESEARCH SUMMARY

Epidemiological studies have shown an inverse relationship between potassium intake and blood pressure. A major meta-analysis designed to assess the effects of potassium supplements on blood pressure examined data from 33 randomized, controlled trials involving 2,609 subjects. The researchers concluded that low potassium intake may be an important contributor to hypertension and that increased potassium intake can both prevent and treat hypertension, particularly in those who cannot or will not reduce their sodium intake.

The study found that potassium supplementation resulted in a significant reduction in mean systolic blood pressure of 3.11 mmHg and a significant reduction in mean diastolic blood pressure of 3.42 mmHg. Greater reductions were also seen in black Americans, compared with Caucasians. Better results were reported in hypertensives than in normotensives, but effects in the latter were sufficient to suggest that supplemental potassium may help significantly prevent hypertension.

Studies have shown that diets high in potassium, magnesium and fiber reduce the risk of strokes. Other studies have reported an inverse relationship between potassium intake and stroke. One of these studies found that, among men with the highest potassium intakes, risk of any type of stroke was

38% lower than among those with the lowest potassium intakes. Potassium supplementation has specifically been inversely associated with the risk of stroke, especially among hypertensive men.

In perhaps the best analysis to date, increased potassium intake was significantly associated with decreased risk of stroke mortality — but only among black men and hypertensive men. Research is ongoing.

There are an abundance of *in vitro* and animal data suggesting that high potassium intake may protect against cardiovascular disease. Various studies have reported that potassium reduces vascular and plasma lipids, macrophage adherence to the vascular wall and endothelial permeability in hypertensive animals. Other animal studies have demonstrated that potassium can reduce atherosclerotic cholesterol ester deposition in the aorta. Research continues.

CONTRAINDICATIONS, PRECAUTIONS, ADVERSE REACTIONS

CONTRAINDICATIONS

Potassium supplements are contraindicated in those with hyperkalemia.

Potassium supplements are also contraindicated in those with hypersensitivity to any component of a potassium-containing supplement.

PRECAUTIONS

The use of potassium supplements in those with potassium deficiency requires medical supervision.

Pregnant women and nursing mothers should avoid potassium supplements unless they are prescribed by their physicians.

ADVERSE REACTIONS

The most common adverse reactions of potassium supplements are gastrointestinal ones and include nausea, vomiting, abdominal discomfort, flatulence and diarrhea. Taking potassium supplements with meals may reduce these adverse reactions. Rashes are occasionally reported. The most serious adverse reaction is hyperkalemia. Hyperkalemia is rare in those with normal renal function.

INTERACTIONS

DRUGS

Angiotensin Converting Enzyme (ACE) inhibitors (benazepril, captopril, enalapril, fosinopril, lisinopril, moexipril, perindopril, quinapril, ramipril, trandolapril): ACE inhibitors will produce some potassium retention by inhibiting aldosterone production. Potassium supplements should be given to those receiving ACE inhibitors only with close monitoring.

Potassium sparing diuretics (amiloride, triamterene, spironolactone): The concomitant administration of a potassium-sparing diuretic and a potassium supplement can produce severe hyperkalemia.

OVERDOSAGE

The use of oral potassium supplements in those with normal renal function very rarely causes serious hyperkalemia. However, overdoses with oral potassium supplements in those with normal renal function have been reported. For example, a 46 year-old woman ingested 31 grams of potassium chloride in a suicide attempt and developed severe hyperkalemia associated with life-threatening arrhythmias. The woman died two weeks later as a result of cerebral anoxia during cardiopulmonary arrest. Oral doses greater than 18 grams of potassium taken at one time may lead to severe hyperkalemia in those with normal renal function.

DOSAGE AND ADMINISTRATION

The use of potassium supplements in those with potassium deficiency requires medical supervision.

There are several potassium supplemental forms available, including potassium chloride, potassium citrate, potassium gluconate, potassium bicarbonate, potassium aspartate and potassium orotate.

Multivitamin, multimineral supplements do not contain more than 99 milligrams of potassium per serving. One milliequivalent or millimole is equal to 39.09 milligrams.

High-potassium (up to 800 milligrams per serving), low-sodium vegetable juices are available. Some soft drinks are rich in potassium. Some soft drinks contain potassium gluconate which has a less bitter taste than some other potassium supplements. Salt substitutes are high in potassium.

Potassium-rich foods and drinks are the best ways to increase potassium intake.

LITERATURE

Addison WLT, The use of sodium chloride, potassium chloride, sodium bromide and potassium bromide in cases of arterial hypertension which are amenable to potassium chloride. *Can Med Assoc J.* 1928; 18:281-285.

Cappuccio FP, MacGregor GA. Does potassium supplementation lower blood pressure? A meta-analysis of published trials. *J Hypertens.* 1991; 9:465-473.

Fang J, Madhavan S, Alderman MH. Dietary potassium intake and stroke mortality. *Stroke.* 2000; 31:1532-1537.

Hermans JJ, Fischer MA, Schiffers PM, Struijker-Boudier HA. High dietary potassium chloride intake augments rat renal mineralocorticoid receptor selectivity via 11beta-hydroxysteroid dehydrogenase. *Biochim Biophys Acta.* 1999; 1472:537-549.

Hermansen K. Diet, blood pressure and hypertension. *Br J Nutr.* 2000; 83 Suppl:S113-S119.

Ishimitsu T, Tobian L. High potassium diets reduce endothelial permeability in stroke-prone spontaneously hypertensive rats. *Clin Exp Pharmacol Physiol.* 1997; 23:241-245.

Ishimitsu T, Tobian L, Sugimoto K, Everson T. High potassium diets reduce vascular and plasma lipid peroxides in stroke-prone spontaneously hypertensive rats. *Clin Exp Hypertens.* 1996; 18:659-673.

Ishimitsu T, Tobian L, Sugimoto K, Lange JM. High potassium diets reduce macrophage adherence to vascular wall in stroke-prone spontaneously hypertensive rats. *J Vasc Res.* 1995; 32:406-412.

Ishimitsu T, Tobian L, Uehara Y, et al. Effect of high potassium diets on the vascular and renal prostaglandin system in stroke-prone spontaneously hypertensive rats. *Prostaglandins Leukot Essent Fatty Acids.* 1995; 53:255-260.

Jin L, ChaoL, Chao J. Potassium supplement upregulates the expression of renal kalikrein and bradykinin B_2 receptor in SHR. *Am J Physiol.* 1999; 276:F476-F484.

Khaw K-T, Barrett-Conner E. Dietary potassium and stroke-associated mortality. *N Engl J Med.* 1987; 316:235-240.

Krishna GG, Miller E, Kapoor S. Increased blood pressure during potassium depletion in normotensive men. *N Engl J Med.* 1989; 320:1177-1182.

Lin H, Young DB. Interactions between plasma potassium and epinephrine in coronary thrombosis in dogs. *Circulation.* 1994; 89:331-338.

Ma G, Young DB, Clower BR. Inverse relationship between potassium intake and coronary artery disease in the cholesterol-fed rabbit. *Am J Hypertens.* 1999; 12:821-825.

McCabe RD, Backarich MA, Srivastava K, Young DB. Potassium inhibits free radical formation. *Hypertension.* 1994; 24:77-82.

McCabe RD, Young DB. Potassium inhibits cultural vascular smooth muscle proliferation. *Am J Hypertens.* 1994; 7:346-350.

Sugimoto T, Tobian L, Ganguli MC. High potassium diets protect against dysfunction of endothelial cells in stroke-prone spontaneously hypertensive rats. *Hypertension.* 1988:11:579-585.

Sugimoto K, Tobian L, Ishimutsu T, Lange JM. High potassium diets greatly increase growth-inhibiting agents in aortas of hypertensive rats. *Hypertension.* 1992; 19:749-752.

Tannen RL. Effects of potassium on blood pressure control. *Ann Intern Med.* 1983; 98(part 2):773-780.

Tobian L. Salt and hypertension. Lessons from animal models that relate to human hypertension. *Hypertension.* 1991; 17:152-158.

West SG, Light KC, Hinderliter AL, et al. Potassium supplementation induces beneficial cardiovascular changes during rest and stress in salt sensitive individuals. *Health Psychol.* 1999; 18:229-240.

Whelton PK, He J, Cutler JA, et al. Effects of oral potassium on blood pressure. Meta-analysis of randomized controlled clinical triglyceride trials. *JAMA.* 1997; 277:1624-1632.

Young DB, Lin H, McCabe RD. Potassium's cardiovascular protective mechanisms. *Am J Physiol.* 1995; 268:R825-R837.

Young DB, Ma G. Vascular protective effects of potassium. *Semin Nephrol.* 1999; 19:477-486.

Zhou MS, Nishida Y, Yoneyama H, et al. Potassium supplementation increases sodium excretion in hypertensive Dahl rats. *Clin Exp Hypertens.* 1999; 21:1397-1411.

Prebiotics

DESCRIPTION

Prebiotics are defined as nondigestible food ingredients that may beneficially affect the host by selectively stimulating the growth and/or the activity of a limited number of bacteria in the colon. Thus, to be effective, prebiotics must escape digestion in the upper gastrointestinal tract and be used by a limited number of the microorganisms comprising the colonic microflora. Prebiotics are principally oligosaccharides. They mainly stimulate the growth of bifidobacteria, for which reason they are referred to as bifidogenic factors.

The following describes the various oligosaccharides which are classified as prebiotics.

FRUCTO-OLIGOSACCHARIDES

Fructo-oligosaccharides or FOS (see Fructo-Oligosaccharides) typically refer to short-chain oligosaccharides comprised of D-fructose and D-glucose, containing from three to five monosaccharide units. FOS, also called neosugar and short-chain FOS (sc FOS), are produced on a commercial scale from sucrose using a fungal fructosyltransferase enzyme. FOS are resistant to digestion in the upper gastrointestinal tract. They act to stimulate the growth of *Bifidobacterium* species in the large intestine. FOS are marketed in the United States in combination with probiotic bacteria and in some functional food products.

INULINS

Inulins (see Inulins) refer to a group of naturally-occurring fructose-containing oligosaccharides. Inulins belong to a class of carbohydrates known as fructans. They are derived from the roots of chicory *(Cichorium intybus)* and Jerusalem artichokes. Inulins are mainly comprised of fructose units and typically have a terminal glucose. The bond between fructose units in inulins is a beta-(2-1) glycosidic linkage. The average degreee of polymerization of inulins marketed as nutritional supplements is 10 to 12. Inulins stimulate the growth of *Bifidobacterium* species in the large intestine.

ISOMALTO-OLIGOSACCHARIDES

Isomalto-oligosaccharides comprise a mixture of alpha-D-(1→6)-linked glucose oligomers, including isomaltose, panose, isomaltotetraose, isomaltopentaose, nigerose, kojibiose, isopanose and higher branched oligo-saccharides. Isomalto-oligosaccharides are produced by various enzymatic processes. They act to stimulate the growth of *Bifidobacterium* species and *Lactobacillus* species in the large intestine. Isomalto-oligosaccharides are marketed in Japan as dietary supplements and in functional foods. They are being developed in the United States for similar uses.

LACTILOL

Lactilol is a disaccharide analogue of lactulose. Its pharmaceutical use is in the treatment of constipation and hepatic encephalopathy. Lactilol is also used in Japan as a prebiotic. It is resistant to digestion in the upper gastrointestinal tract and it is fermented by a limited number of colonic bacteria, resulting in an increase in the biomass of bifidobacteria and lactobacilli in the colon. Lactilol is known chemically as 4-0-(beta-D-galactopyranosyl)-D-glucitol. Lactilol is not approved for the treatment of hepatic encephalopathy or constipation in the U.S., and its use as a prebiotic is considered experimental. Lactilol is used in Europe as a food sweetener.

LACTOSUCROSE

Lactosucrose is a trisaccharide comprised of D-galactose, D-glucose and D-fructose. Lactosucrose is produced enzymatically by the enzymatic transfer of the galactosyl residue in lactose to sucrose. Lactosucrose is resistant to digestion in the stomach and small intestine. It is selectively utilized by intestinal *Bifidobacterium* species resulting in significant induction of growth of these bacteria in the colon. Therefore, under physiological conditions, lactosucrose acts on the intestinal microflora as a growth factor for *Bifidobacterium* species. Lactosucrose is also known as 4G-beta-D-galactosylsucrose. It is widely used in Japan as a dietary supplement and in functional foods, including yogurt. Lactosucrose is being developed in the United States for similar uses.

LACTULOSE

Lactulose (see Lactulose) is a semisynthetic disaccharide comprised of the sugars D-galactose and D-fructose. The sugars are joined by a beta-glycosidic linkage, making it resistant to hydrolysis by human digestive enzymes. Lactulose is, however, fermented by a limited number of colonic bacteria. This can lead to changes in the colonic ecosystem in favor of bacteria, such as lactobacilli and bifidobacteria, which may confer some health benefits. Lactulose is a prescription drug in the United States for the treatment of constipation and hepatic encephalopathy. It is marketed in Japan for use as a dietary supplement and in functional foods. Its use in the United States as a prebiotic substance is still experimental.

PYRODEXTRINS

Pyrodextrins comprise a mixture of glucose-containing oligosaccharides that is derived from the hydrolysis of starch. Pyrodextrins have been found to promote the proliferation of *Bifidobacterium* species in the large intestine. They are resistant to digestion in the upper gastrointestinal tract. Pyrodextrins are being developed for the nutritional supplement market place.

SOY OLIGOSACCHARIDES

Soy oligosaccharides refer to oligosaccharides found in soybeans and also in other beans and peas. The two principal soy oligosaccharides are the trisaccharide raffinose and the tetrasaccharide stachyose. Raffinose is comprised of one molecule each of D-galactose, D-glucose and D-fructose. Stachyose is comprised of two molecules of D-galactose, one molecule of D-glucose and one molecule of D-fructose. Soy oligosaccharides act to stimulate the growth of *Bifidobacterium* species in the large intestine. They are marketed in Japan as dietary supplements and in functional foods. They are being developed in the United States for similar uses.

TRANSGALACTO-OLIGOSACCHARIDES

Transgalacto-oligosaccharides (TOS) are a mixture of oligosaccharides consisting of D-glucose and D-galactose. TOS are produced from D-lactose via the action of the enzyme beta-galactosidase obtained from *Aspergillus oryzae*. TOS are resistant to digestion in the upper gastrointestinal tract and stimulate the growth of bifidobacteria in the large intestine. TOS are marketed in Japan and Europe as dietary supplements and are used in functional foods. They are being developed for similar use in the United States. (See Transgalacto-Oligosaccharides).

XYLO-OLIGOSACCHARIDES

Xylo-oligosaccharides are comprised of oligosaccharides containing beta (1→4) linked xylose residues. The degree of polymerization of xylo-oligosaccharides is from two to four. Xylo-oligosaccharides are obtained by enzymatic hydrolysis of the polysaccharide xylan. They are marketed in Japan as prebiotics and are being developed for similar use in the United States.

ACTIONS AND PHARMACOLOGY

ACTIONS

Prebiotics may have anticarcinogenic, antimicrobial, hypolipidemic and glucose-modulatory activities. They may also have activity in improving mineral absorption and balance and may have anti-osteoporotic activity.

MECHANISM OF ACTION

The possible anticarcinogenic activity of prebiotics is not well understood. It may be accounted for, in part, by the possible anticarcinogenic activity of butyrate. Butyrate, along with other short-chain fatty acids, is produced by bacterial fermentation of the various prebiotic oligosaccharides in the colon. Some studies suggest that butyrate may induce growth arrest and cell differentiation and may also upregulate apoptosis, three activities which could be significant for its possible anticarcinogenic activity. The prebiotic oligosaccharides may also aid in increasing the concentrations of calcium and magnesium in the colon. Elevated concentrations of these cations in the colon may help to control the rate of cell turnover. Elevated concentrations of calcium in the colon may help to control the formation of insoluble bile or salts of fatty acids. This might reduce the potential damaging effects of bile or fatty acids on colonocytes. The prebiotics may stimulate the growth of bifidobacteria and lactobacilli in the large intestine. There are *in vitro* and animal data suggesting that these bacteria can bind to and inactivate some carcinogens, can directly inhibit the growth of some tumors and can inhibit bacteria that may convert precarcinogens into carcinogens.

The possible antimicrobial activity of the prebiotics may be accounted for by their growth-promoting effects on bifidobacteria and lactobacilli. These bacteria can reinforce the barrier function of the intestinal mucosa, helping in the prevention of the attachment of pathogenic bacteria, essentially by crowding them out. These bacteria may also produce antimicrobial substances and stimulate antigen specific and nonspecific immune responses.

The prebiotics may lower triglyceride levels in some. The mechanism of this possible effect is unclear. Decreased hepatocyte *de novo* synthesis of triglycerides is one hypothetical possibility. The prebiotics may also lower total cholesterol and LDL-cholesterol levels in some. Again, the mechanism of this possible effect is unclear. Propionate, a product of oligosaccharide fermentation in the colon, may inhibit HMG-CoA reductase, the rate limiting step in cholesterol synthesis.

The possible effects of the prebiotics on blood glucose may be accounted for in a few ways. The oligosaccharides may delay gastric emptying and/or shorten small intestinal tract transit time. This may be via the short-chain fatty acids produced from the oligosaccharides in the colon. Short-chain fatty acids may be involved in the so-called "ileocolonic brake," which refers to the inhibition of gastric emptying by nutrients reaching the ileo-colonic junction. Short-chain fatty acids may also stimulate contractions of the ileum and shorten ileal emptying. In addition, propionate may inhibit gluconeogenesis by its metabolic conversion to methylmalonyl-CoA and succinyl-CoA. These metabolites could inhibit pyruvate carboxylase. Propionate may also reduce plasma levels of free fatty acids. High levels of free fatty acids lower glucose utilization and induce insulin resistance. Finally, propionate may enhance glycolysis via depletion of citrate in hepatocytes. Citrate is an allosteric inhibitor of phosphofructokinase. In short, the mechanism of the possible effects of prebiotics on glucose tolerance are not well understood.

The oligosaccharides may bind/sequester such minerals as calcium and magnesium in the small intestine. The short-chain fatty acids formed from the bacterial fermentation of the oligosaccharides may facilitate the colonic absorption of calcium and, possibly, also magnesium ions. This could be beneficial in the prevention of osteoporosis and osteopenia.

PHARMACOKINETICS

Following ingestion, the prebiotic oligosaccharides reach the colon with very little of them being digested in the upper gastrointestinal tract. The oligosaccharides are fermented by bifidobacteria, lactobacilli and some other bacteria in the colon to produce the short-chain fatty acids acetate, propionate and butyrate; the gases hydrogen, hydrogen sulfide, carbon dioxide and methane; and lactate, pyruvate, succinate and formate. Acetate, propionate and butyrate that are not metabolized in colonocytes are absorbed from the colon and transported via the portal circulation to the liver. These short-chain fatty acids are extensively metabolized in hepatocytes. Acetate, propionate and butyrate that are not metabolized in hepatocytes are transported by the circulation to various tissues where they undergo further metabolism. Butyrate is an important respiratory fuel for colonocytes.

INDICATIONS AND USAGE

Some prebiotics are used, pharmaceutically, for the treatment of constipation and hepatic encephalopathy. Prebiotics may protect against some intestinal pathogens and may be helpful in some inflammatory bowel disease. They may have some anticarcinogenic effects and may exert favorable lipid effects in some. They may, in some instances, enhance mineral absorption and might help protect against osteoporosis. There is some preliminary research that certain prebiotics might be of some benefit in diabetes mellitus.

RESEARCH SUMMARY

Lactulose is a prescription drug in the United States. It is used to treat constipation and hepatic encephalopathy. Lactilol, similarly, is used pharmaceutically in Europe and elsewhere to treat the same conditions. These prebiotics, as well as several others, including transgalacto-oligosaccharides (TOS), fructo-oligosaccharides (FOS) and various of the experimental prebiotics, have shown benefits in favorably modulating the microbial ecology of the gut, protecting against various intestinal pathogens and, in some instances, boosting gastrointestinal immunity. Lactulose has exhibited some ability to ameliorate symptoms of idiopathic, as well as infectious, inflammatory bowel disease.

Both lactulose and inulins have suppressed experimentally induced colonic aberrant crypt foci in rats, and lactulose helped protect colonic mucosa against a known colon carcinogen in another study. FOS has also shown experimental anticarcinogenic effects, significantly reducing incidence of colon tumors, for example, in one animal study.

In one clinical study, patients who had undergone endoscopic removal of colorectal polyps were administered antioxidant vitamins or lactulose to see if these substances could reduce the recurrence rate of adenomatous polyps. The study continued for five years. During this period polyps recurred in 5.7% of those taking the vitamins (A, C and E) and in 14.7% of those taking lactulose. The recurrence rate in untreated controls was 35.9%.

TOS have exerted hypocholesterolemic effects in animals. They have also shown some preliminary, experimental ability to lower triglycerides. A fermented milk product containing FOS lowered LDL-cholesterol levels in male subjects with borderline elevated serum cholesterol levels in a double-blind, placebo-controlled study. There is a small study in which inulins reportedly lowered plasma total cholesterol and triglyceride levels significantly in healthy male volunteers. Results have been mixed, however, with respect to prebiotic effects on lipids, and more research is needed.

TOS have demonstrated positive effects on calcium absorption and have prevented bone loss in some animal research. Lactulose has significantly stimulated calcium absorption in postmenopausal women in preliminary clinical work.

Lactulose and some of the other prebiotics have also shown some ability to improve glucose tolerance and have other effects on carbohydrate metabolism that could prove helpful in some with diabetes mellitus. This research, too, is very preliminary and ongoing.

CONTRAINDICATIONS, PRECAUTIONS, ADVERSE REACTIONS

CONTRAINDICATIONS

Prebiotics are contraindicated in those who are hypersensitive to any component of a prebiotic-containing supplement.

Some lactulose preparations contain galactose. Therefore, lactulose is contraindicated in those who require a low galactose diet.

PRECAUTIONS

In the United States, lactulose is a prescription drug. Its use requires medical supervision. Its use as a dietary supplement is considered experimental.

Those with lactose intolerance should exercise caution in the use of lactulose, lactilol and transgalacto-oligosaccharides.

Those who develop gastrointestinal symptoms (flatus, bloating, diarrhea) with the use of dietary fiber should exercise some degree of caution in the use of prebiotics. Those receiving whole body radiation or radiation to the gastrointestinal tract should avoid prebiotic supplements.

Pregnant women and nursing mothers should only use prebiotic supplements if prescribed by their physicians.

ADVERSE REACTIONS
Doses of prebiotic oligosaccharides up to 10 grams daily are well tolerated. Higher doses may cause gastrointestinal symptoms, such as flatulence, bloating and diarrhea.

INTERACTIONS
NUTRITIONAL SUPPLEMENTS
Alpha-galactosidase: Concomitant use of alpha-galactosidase (see Supplemental Enzymes) and soy oligosaccharides may decrease the effectiveness of the soy oligosaccharides.

Minerals (calcium, magnesium): Concomitant intake of calcium or magnesium and prebiotics may enhance the colonic absorption of these minerals.

Probiotics: Concomitant intake of probiotics and prebiotics may enhance the possible effectiveness of both the probiotics and the prebiotics.

FOODS
Prebiotic oligosaccharides may enhance the colonic absorption of calcium and magnesium in foods.

DOSAGE AND ADMINISTRATION
Fructo-oligosaccharides, (FOS) and inulins are available in nutritional supplements and in functional foods. Dosage is variable for both FOS and inulins and ranges from 4 to 10 grams. Those who use more than 10 grams daily of FOS or inulins should split the dosage throughout the day. Doses higher than 30 grams daily of FOS or inulins may cause significant gastrointestinal discomfort (flatulence, bloating, cramping, diarrhea).

LITERATURE

Amarowicz R. [Nutritional importance of oligosaccharides]. [Article in Polish]. *Rocz Panstw Zakl Hig.* 1999; 50:89-95.

Flickinger EA, Wolf BW, Garleb KA, et al. Glucose-based oligosaccharides exhibit different in vitro fermentation patterns and affect in vivo apparent nutrient digestibility and microbial populations in dogs. *J Nutr.* 2000; 130:1267-1273.

Gibson GR. Dietary modulation of the human gut microflora using prebiotics. *Br J Nutr.* 1998; 80:S209-S212.

Grizard D, Barthomeuf C. Non-digestible oligosaccharides used as prebiotic agents: mode of production and beneficial effects on animal and human health. *Reprod Nutr Dev.* 1999; 39:563-588.

Macfarlane GT, Cummings JH. Probiotics and prebiotics: can regulating the activities of intestinal bacteria benefit health. *West J Med.* 1999; 171:187-191.

Murosaki S, Muroyama K, Yamamoto Y, et al. Immunopotentiating activity of nigerooligosaccharides for the T helper 1-like immune response in mice. *Biosci Biotechnol Biochem.* 1999; 63:373-378.

Ohkusa T, Ozaki Y, Sato C, et al. Long-term ingestion of lactosucrose increases *Bifidobacterium sp.* in human fecal flora. *Digestion.* 1995; 56:415-420.

Roberfroid MB. Chicory fructooligosaccharides and the gastrointestinal tract. *Nutrition.* 2000; 16:677-679.

Roberfroid MB. Health benefits of non-digestible oligosaccharides. *Adv Exp Med Bull.* 1997; 427:211-219.

Roberfroid MB. Prebiotics and synbiotics: concepts and nutritional properties. *Br J Nutr.* 1998; 80:S197-S202.

Roberfroid MB. Prebiotics and probiotics: are they functional foods. *Am Clin Nutr.* 2000; 71 (6 Suppl):1682S-1687S, discussion 1688S-1690S.

Soontornchai S, Sirichakwal P, Puwastien P, et al. Lactilol tolerance in healthy Thai adults. *Eur J Nutr.* 2000; 38:218-226.

Teramoto F, Rokutan K, Kawakami Y, et al. Effect of 4G-beta-D-galactosylsucrose (lactosucrose) on fecal microflora in patients with chronic inflammatory bowel disease. *J Gastrenterol.* 1996; 31:33-39.

Wang X-D, Rakshit SK. Biosynthesis of nutraceutical iso-oligosaccharides by multiple forms of transferase produced by *Aspergillus foetidus. Nahrung.* 2000; 44:207-210.

For additional Literature, see Fructo-Oligosaccharides, Inulins, Lactulose, Transgalacto-Oligosaccharides.

Pregnenolone

DESCRIPTION
Pregnenolone is a steroid naturally found in animal tissues, especially in the gonads, adrenal gland and brain. Pregnenolone is synthesized from cholesterol and is a precursor for the biosynthesis of steroid hormones. In the adrenal gland, pregnenolone is a precursor to the mineralocorticoid aldosterone, the glucocorticoid cortisol, as well as dehydroepiandrosterone (DHEA) and progesterone. In the ovary, pregnenolone is a precursor to estrogens and progesterone, and, in the testis, pregnenolone is a precursor to testosterone.

Pregnenolone and its metabolite pregnenolone sulfate are now known to be synthesized in the brain either *de novo* from cholesterol or from other metabolites. Pregnenolone and pregnenolone sulfate found in the brain and central nervous system are referred to as neurosteroids.

Pregnenolone is known chemically as 3-Hydroxypregn-5-en-20-one; delta 5-pregnen-3 beta-ol-20-one, and 17 beta-(1-

ketoethyl)-delta 5-androstene-3 beta-ol. Its abbreviation is PREG and the abbreviation of its metabolite, progesterone sulfate, is PREG S. Pregnenolone is a lipophilic solid substance that is sparingly soluble in water. Pregnenolone has the following chemical structure:

Pregnenolone

ACTIONS AND PHARMACOLOGY

ACTIONS

Supplemental pregnenolone has putative memory-enhancing activity.

MECHANISM OF ACTION

Memory enhancement has been observed in aged animals when given pregnenolone or pregnenolone sulfate. Pregnenolone sulfate is both a gamma-aminobutyrate (GABA) antagonist and a positive allosteric modulator at the N-methyl-D-asparatate (NMDA) receptor and may reinforce neurotransmitter systems that may decline with age.

Pregnenolone sulfate was found to stimulate acetylcholine release in the adult rat hippocampus. Acetylcholine release may be due to pregnenolone sulfate's negative modulation of the GABA (A) receptor complex and positive modulation of the NMDA receptor. While a modest increase in acetylcholine release facilities memory processes, elevation of acetylcholine beyond an optimal level is ineffective in doing so.

PHARMACOKINETICS

Little is known about the pharmacokinetics (PK) of pregnenolone in humans. Some PK studies have been done in animals. The absorption of pregnenolone, similar to the absorption of most steroids, is variable. It appears that some pregnenolone is absorbed from the small intestine and distributed throughout the body. How much is taken up by the liver and metabolized is unclear. Likewise, it is unclear how much of an ingested pregnenolone dose is taken up by the brain. Metabolites of injected pregnenolone in the rat brain include pregnenolone sulfate, progesterone, 5 alpha-pregnane-3, 20-dione, 3 alpha-hydroxy-5 alpha-pregnan-20-one or allopregnanolone and DHEA. In other tissues, pregnenolone may be metabolized to DHEA, testosterone, estrogens, cortisol and aldosterone.

INDICATIONS AND USAGE

Pregnenolone may have some efficacy as a memory enhancer; this has so far been demonstrated in various animal models but not yet in humans. There are unsubstantiated claims that pregnenolone is useful in Alzheimer's disease, some forms of cancer and arthritis, in degenerative diseases associated with aging in general and in obesity.

RESEARCH SUMMARY

There are several studies showing a correlation between deficiencies in cognitive performance in aged animals and low pregnenolone levels in the brains of these animals, especially in the hippocampus. Performance or memory tests have been shown to improve in these animals when hippocampal pregnenolone levels were increased via intra-peritoneal or bilateral intrahippocampal injection of pregnenolone sulfate.

There is direct evidence from many of these studies that pregnenolone sulfate stimulates release of acetylcholine in the hippocampus. There is additional evidence that suggests that exogenous pregnenolone can reinforce neurotransmitter systems that normally decline with age. A "global stimulatory effect on central cholinergic neurotransmission" has been suggested by one research group.

Though significant favorable results have been obtained with respect to memory enhancement in aged animals, human studies have yet to commence. These are warranted. Meanwhile, claims that supplemental pregnenolone is helpful in Alzheimer's disease are unsubstantiated. And there is no credible evidence that pregnenolone is useful in the treatment of arthritis, cancer, degenerative diseases or obesity.

CONTRAINDICATIONS, PRECAUTIONS, ADVERSE REACTIONS

CONTRAINDICATIONS

Pregnenolone is contraindicated in those with prostate, breast and uterine cancer. Known hypersensitivity to a pregnenolone-containing product.

PRECAUTIONS

Pregnenolone should be avoided by children, pregnant women and nursing mothers.

Because of the theoretical possibility that pregnenolone may lower seizure threshold—pregnenolone sulfate negatively modulates GABA (A) receptors in animals—those with seizure disorders should avoid pregnenolone.

ADVERSE REACTIONS

To date there are no reported significant adverse effects. Mild gastrointestinal effects, such as nausea, have been noted. However, pregnenolone may be converted to steroids such as DHEA, and DHEA does cause various adverse effects such as acne and hair loss, especially in women.

INTERACTIONS

There are no reported drug, nutritional supplement, food or herb interactions to date.

OVERDOSAGE

No reported overdosage.

DOSAGE AND ADMINISTRATION

Typical pregnenolone doses are 5 to 50 milligrams daily. The safety of taking pregnenolone at any dose, especially long term, is unknown.

LITERATURE

Akawa Y, Baulieu EE. Neurosteroids: behavioral aspects and physiological implications. *J Soc Biol*. 1999; 193:293-298.

Barrot M, Vallee M, Gingras MA, et al. The neurosteroid pregnenolone sulfate increases dopamine release and the dopaminergic response to morphine in the rat nucleus accumbens. *Eur J Neurosci*. 1999; 10:3757-3760.

Darnaudery M, Koehl M, Pallares M, et al. The neurosteroid pregnenolone sulfate increases cortical acetylcholine release: a microdialysis study in freely moving rats. *J Neurochem*. 1998; 71:2018-2022.

Darnaudery M, Koehl M, Piazza PV, et al. Pregnenolone sulfate increases hippocompal acetylcholine release and spatial recognition. *Brain Res*. 2000; 852:173-179.

Kokate TG, Juhng KN, Kirkby RD, et al. Convulsant actions of the neurosteroid pregnenolone sulfate in mice. *Brain Res*. 1999; 831:119-124.

Legrand A, Alfonso G. Pregnenolone reverses the age-dependent accumulation of glial fibrillary acidic protein within astrocytes of specific regions of the rat brain. *Brain Res*. 1998; 802:125-133.

Pallares M, Darnaudery M, Day J, et al. The neurosteroid pregnenolone sulfate infused into the nucleus basalis increases both acetylcholine release in the frontal cortex or amygdala and spatial memory. *Neuroscience*. 1998; 87:551-558.

Vallee M, Mayo W, Darnaudery M, et al. Neurosteroids: deficient cognitive performance in aged rats depends on low pregnenolone sulfate levels in the hippocampus. *Proc Natl Accd Sci*. 1997; 94:14865-14870.

Probiotics

DESCRIPTION

Probiotics are defined as live microorganisms, including *Lactobacillus* species, *Bifidobacterium* species and yeasts, that may beneficially affect the host upon ingestion by improving the balance of the intestinal microflora. The dietary use of live microorganisms has a long history. Mention of cultured dairy products is found in the Bible and the sacred books of Hinduism. Soured milks and cultured dairy products, such as kefir, koumiss, leben and dahi, were often used therapeutically before the existence of microorganisms was recognized. The use of microorganisms in food fermentation is one of the oldest methods for producing and preserving food. Much of the world depends upon various fermented foods that are staples in the diet.

Élie Metchnikoff, the father of modern immunology, spoke highly about the possible health benefits of the lactic acid-bacteria (LAB) *Lactobacillus bulgaricus* and *Streptococcus thermophilus* in his writings at the turn of the last century. He wrote in his book, *The Prolongation of Life*, that consumption of live bacteria, such as *Lactobacillus bulgaricus* and *Streptococcus thermophilus*, in the form of yogurt was beneficial for gastrointestinal health, as well as for health in general, and for longevity. Some recent research suggests that certain live microorganisms may have immuno-modulatory and anticarcinogenic effects, as well as other health benefits. There is presently much active research focusing on the development of target-specific probiotics containing well-characterized bacteria that are selected for their health-enhancing characteristics. These new probiotics are entering the marketplace in the form of nutritional supplements and functional foods, such as yogurt functional food products.

The gastrointestinal tract represents a complex ecosystem in which a delicate balance exists between the intestinal microflora and the host. The microflora are principally comprised of facultative anaerobes and obligate anaerobes. Approximately 95% of the intestinal bacterial population in humans is comprised of obligate anaerobes, including *Bifidobacterium, Clostridium, Eubacterium, Fusobacterium, Peptococcus, Peptostreptococcus* and *Bacteroides*. Approximately 1% to 10% of the intestinal population is comprised of facultative anaerobes, including *Lactobacillus, Escherichia coli, Klebsiella, Streptococcus, Staphylococcus* and *Bacillus*. Aerobic organisms are not present in the intestinal tract of healthy individuals with the exception of *Pseudomonas*, which is present in very small amounts. Most of the bacteria are present in the colon where the bacterial concentration ranges between 10^{11} to 10^{12} colony-forming units (CPU) per milliliter.

The intestinal microflora are important for maturation of the immune system, the development of normal intestinal morphology and in order to maintain a chronic and immunologically balanced inflammatory response. The microflora reinforce the barrier function of the intestinal mucosa, helping in the prevention of the attachment of pathogenic microorganisms and the entry of allergens. Some members of the microflora may contribute to the body's requirements for certain vitamins, including biotin, pantothenic acid and vitamin B_{12}. Alteration of the microbial flora of the intestine, such as may occur with antibiotic use, disease and aging, can negatively affect its beneficial role.

The probiotics that are marketed as nutritional supplements and in functional foods, such as yogurts, are principally the *Bifidobacterium* species and the *Lactobacillus* species. Probiotics are sometimes called colonic foods. Most of the presently available probiotics are bacteria. *Saccharomyces boulardii* is an example of a probiotic yeast.

The following describe the various bacteria and yeasts used as probiotics:

BIFIDOBACTERIUM

Bifidobacteria are normal inhabitants of the human and animal colon. Newborns, especially those that are breast-fed, are colonized with bifidobacteria within days after birth. Bifidobacteria were first isolated from the feces of breast-fed infants. The population of these bacteria in the colon appears to be relatively stable until advanced age when it appears to decline. The bifidobacteria population is influenced by a number of factors, including diet, antibiotics and stress. Bifidobacteria are gram-positive anaerobes. They are non-motile, non-spore forming and catalase-negative. They have various shapes, including short, curved rods, club-shaped rods and bifurcated Y-shaped rods. Their name is derived from the observation that they often exist in a Y-shaped or bifid form. The guanine and cytosine content of their DNA is between 54 mol% and 67 mol%. They are saccharolytic organisms that produce acetic and lactic acids without generation of CO_2, except during degradation of gluconate. They are also classified as lactic acid bacteria (LAB). To date, 30 species of bifidobacteria have been isolated. Bifidobacteria used as probiotics include *Bifidobacterium adolescentis, Bifidobacterium bifidum, Bifidobacterium animalis, Bifidobacterium thermophilum, Bifidobacterium breve, Bifidobacterium longum, Bifidobacterium infantis* and *Bifidobacterium lactis*. Specific strains of bifidobacteria used as probiotics include *Bifidobacterium breve* strain Yakult, *Bifidobacterium breve* RO7O, *Bifidobacterium lactis* Bb12, *Bifidobacterium longum* RO23, *Bifidobacterium bifidum* RO71, *Bifidobacterium infantis* RO33, *Bifidobacterium longum* BB536 and *Bifidobacterium longum* SBT-2928.

LACTOBACILLUS

Lactobacilli are normal inhabitants of the human intestine and vagina. Lactobacilli are gram-positive facultative anaerobes. They are non-spore forming and non-flagellated rod or coccobacilli. The guanine and cytosine content of their DNA is between 32 mol% and 51 mol%. They are either aerotolerant or anaerobic and strictly fermentative. In the homofermentative case, glucose is fermented predominantly to lactic acid. Lactobacilli are also classified as lactic acid bacteria (LAB). To date, 56 species of the genus *Lactobacil-*

lus have been identified. Lactobacilli used as probiotics include *Lactobacillus acidophilus, Lactobacillus brevis, Lactobacillus bulgaricus, Lactobacillus casei, Lactobacillus cellobiosus, Lactobacillus crispatus, Lactobacillus curvatus, Lactobacillus fermentum, Lactobacillus* GG *(Lactobacillus rhamnosus* or *Lactobacillus casei* subspecies *rhamnosus), Lactobacillus gasseri, Lactobacillus johnsonii, Lactobacillus plantarum* and *Lactobacillus salivarus. Lactobacillus plantarum* 299v strain originates from sour dough. *Lactobacillus plantarum* itself is of human origin. Other probiotic strains of *Lactobacillus* are *Lactobacillus acidophilus* BG2FO4, *Lactobacillus acidophilus* INT-9, *Lactobacillus plantarum* ST31, *Lactobacillus reuteri, Lactobacillus johnsonii* LA1, *Lactobacillus acidophilus* NCFB 1748, *Lactobacillus casei* Shirota, *Lactobacillus acidophilus* NCFM, *Lactobacillus acidophilus* DDS-1, *Lactobacillus delbrueckii* subspecies *delbrueckii, Lactobacillus delbrueckii* subspecies *bulgaricus* type 2038, *Lactobacillus acidophilus* SBT-2062, *Lactobacillus brevis, Lactobacillus salivarius* UCC 118 and *Lactobacillus paracasei* subsp *paracasei* F19.

LACTOCOCCUS

Lactococci are gram-positive facultative anaerobes. They are also classified as lactic acid bacteria (LAB). *Lactococcus lactis* (formerly known as *Streptococcus lactis*) is found in dairy products and is commonly responsible for the souring of milk. Lactococci that are used or are being developed as probiotics include *Lactococcus lactis, Lactococcus lactis* subspecies *cremoris (Streptococcus cremoris), Lactococcus lactis* subspecies *lactis* NCDO 712, *Lactococcus lactis* subspecies *lactis* NIAI 527, *Lactococcus lactis* subspecies *lactis* NIAI 1061, *Lactococcus lactis* subspecies *lactis* biovar diacetylactis NIAI 8 W and *Lactococcus lactis* subspecies *lactis* biovar diacetylactis ATCC 13675.

SACCHAROMYCES

Saccharomyces belongs to the yeast family. The principal probiotic yeast is *Saccharomyces boulardii. Saccharomyces boulardii* is also known as *Saccharomyces cerevisiae* Hansen CBS 5296 and *S. boulardii. S. boulardii* is normally a nonpathogenic yeast. *S. boulardii* has been used to treat diarrhea associated with antibiotic use.

STREPTOCOCCUS THERMOPHILUS

Streptococcus thermophilus is a gram-positive facultative anaerobe. It is a cytochrome-, oxidase- and catalase-negative organism that is nonmotile, non-spore forming and homofermentative. *Streptococcus thermophilus* is an alpha-hemolytic species of the *viridans* group. It is also classified as a lactic acid bacteria (LAB). *Steptococcus thermophilus* is found in milk and milk products. It is a probiotic and used in the production of yogurt. *Streptococcus salivarus* subspecies *thermophilus* type 1131 is another probiotic strain.

ENTEROCOCCUS

Enterococci are gram-positive, facultative anaerobic cocci of the Streptococcaceae family. They are spherical to ovoid and occur in pairs or short chains. Enterococci are catalase-negative, non-spore forming and usually nonmotile. Entero-cocci are part of the intestinal microflora of humans and animals. *Enterococcus faecium* SF68 is a probiotic strain that has been used in the management of diarrheal illnesses.

ACTIONS AND PHARMACOLOGY

ACTIONS

Probiotics may have antimicrobial, immunomodulatory, anticarcinogenic, antidiarrheal, antiallergenic and antioxidant activities.

MECHANISM OF ACTION

Lactobacillus plantarum 299v, which is derived from sour dough and which is used to ferment sauerkraut and salami, has been demonstrated to improve the recovery of patients with enteric bacterial infections. This bacterium adheres to reinforce the barrier function of the intestinal mucosa, thus preventing the attachment of the pathogenic bacteria to the intestinal wall. *Bifidobacterium breve* was found to eradicate *Campylobacter jejuni* from the stools of children with enteritis, although less rapidly than in those treated with erythromycin. *Lactobacillus* GG was found to eradicate *Clostridium difficile* in patients with relapsing colitis, and supplementation of infant formula milk with *Bifidobacterium bifidum* and *Streptococcus thermophilus* reduced rotavirus shedding and episodes of diarrhea in hospitalized children.

The antimicrobial activity of probiotics is thought to be accounted for, in large part, by their ability to colonize the colon and reinforce the barrier function of the intestinal mucosa. Probiotics, such as *Lactobacillus bulgaricus,* which do not adhere as well to the intestinal mucosa, are much less effective against enteric pathogens. In addition, some probi-otics have been found to secrete antimicrobial substances. These substances are known as bacteriocins. Such a bacter-iocin has been isolated from *Lactobacillus plantarum* ST31, a probiotic derived from sour dough. The substance was found to be a 20 amino acid peptide. A different bacteriocin was isolated from another strain of *Lactobacillus plantarum*. The bacteriocin has 27 amino acids and contains lanthionine residues. This type of bacteriocin is classified as a lantibiotic.

Lactobacillus casei has been demonstrated to increase levels of circulating immunoglobulin A (IgA) in infants infected with rotavirus. This has been found to be correlated with shortened duration of rotavirus-induced diarrhea. *Lactobacil-lus* GG has also been shown to potentiate intestinal immune response to rotavirus infection in children. *Lactobacillus acidophilus* and *Bifidobacterium bifidum* appear to enhance the nonspecific immune phagocytic activity of circulating blood granulocytes. This effect may account, in part, for the stimulation of IgA responses in infants infected with rotavirus. In healthy individuals, *Lactobacillus salivarius* UCC118 and *Lactobacillus johnsonii* LA1 were demon-strated to produce an increase in the phagocytic activity of peripheral blood monocytes and granulocytes. Also, *Lacto-bacillus johnsonii* LA1, but not *Lactobacillus salivarius* UCC118, was found to increase the frequency of interferon-gamma-producing peripheral blood monocytes.

Lactobacillus GG has been shown to inhibit chemically induced intestinal tumors in rats. The probiotic appears to alter the initiation and/or promotional events of the chemi-cally-induced tumors. *Lactobacillus* GG also binds to some chemical carcinogens.

Saccharomyces boulardii has been shown to prevent antibi-otic-associated diarrhea and also to prevent diarrhea in critically ill tube-fed patients. The mechanism of this antidiarrheal effect is not well understood. *S. boulardii* has been found to secrete a protease which digests two protein exotoxins, toxin A and toxin B, which appear to mediate diarrhea and colitis caused by *Clostridium difficile*. The protective effects of *S. boulardii* on *C. difficile*-induced inflammatory diarrhea may, in part, be due to proteolytic digestion of toxin A and toxin B by a secreted protease.

Dietary antigens may induce an immunoinflammatory re-sponse that impairs the barrier function of the intestine, resulting in aberrant absorption of intralumenal antigens. This may account, in part, for food allergies. Probiotics that colonize the colon may be helpful in the management of some with food allergies by reinforcing the barrier function of the intestinal mucosa. *Lactobacillus rhamnosus* GG and *Bifidobacterium lactis* Bb12 were found to produce signifi-cant improvement of atopic eczema in children with food allergies. The decrease in the signs and symptoms of atopic eczema occurred in parallel with a reduction in the concen-tration of circulating CD4+ T lymphocytes and an increase in transforming growth factor beta1 (TGF-beta1), indicating suppressive effects on T cell functions in this disorder. These probiotics may help restore the Th1/Th2 balance in atopic eczema.

Lactobacillus GG was found to scavenge superoxide anion radicals, inhibit lipid peroxidation and chelate iron *in vitro*. The iron chelating active of *Lactobacillus* GG may account, in part, for its antioxidant activity. Other lactic acid bacteria, including strains of *Lactobacillus acidophilus, Lactobacillus bulgaricus, Bifidobaterium longum* and *Streptococcus ther-mophilus*, have also demonstrated antioxidative ability. Mechanisms include chelation of metal ions (iron, copper), scavenging of reactive oxygen species and reducing activity.

PHARMACOKINETICS

The effectiveness of probiotics is related to their ability to survive in the acidic stomach environment and the alkaline conditions in the duodenum, as well as their ability to adhere to the intestinal mucosa of the colon and to colonize the colon. Some probiotics, such as *Lactobacillus* GG and *Lactobacillus plantarum* 299v, are better able to colonize the colon than others. After passage through the stomach and the small intestine, those probiotics that do survive become established transiently in the colon.

INDICATIONS AND USAGE

Probiotics have been used with some benefit in the prevention and treatment of some gastrointestinal disorders, including antibiotic-associated diarrhea and some infectious and viral diarrheas, most notably rotavirus-induced diarrhea in infants and children, lactose intolerance, sucrase and maltase deficiencies and inflammatory bowel disease. Probiotics may be of benefit in some with food allergies, but supporting evidence is preliminary. They may favorably modulate immunity in some circumstances and may have anticarcinogenic effects. There is the suggestion in some preliminary research that they may have some hypocholesterolemic activity. There is some evidence to support the use of probiotics to re-colonize the vaginas of women with recurrent vaginosis.

RESEARCH SUMMARY

Among the probiotics, only *S. boulardii, E. faecium* and *Lactobacillus sp.* have been useful in preventing antibiotic-related diarrhea. In one double-blind study, 180 hospitalized patients on antibiotic therapy were randomized to receive placebo or *S. boulardii* supplementation. Incidence of diarrhea was significantly lower among those receiving the probiotic, compared with controls (9% and 22%, respectively). These results have been confirmed in other controlled studies.

Lactobacillus GG significantly reduced the severity and duration of rotavirus diarrhea in infants in a double-blind, placebo-controlled study. Other researchers have demonstrated that the incidence of acute diarrhea and rotavirus shedding can be significantly reduced among infants admitted to the hospital by adding *Bifidobacterium bifidum* and *Streptococcus thermophilus* to infant formula. *Lactobacillus* GG has been shown helpful in the treatment of diarrhea associated with relapsing colitis due to *Clostridium difficile*. These studies, however, were small and uncontrolled. In a double-blind, placebo-controlled trial, *Saccharomyces boulardii* was significantly superior to placebo in treating diarrhea despite having no apparent effect on *Clostridium difficile* toxin. The use of probiotics in the attempted prevention and treatment of traveler's diarrhea, most commonly caused by enterotoxigenic *E. coli*, has produced inconclusive results. More study is needed.

Reduced fecal concentrations of various probiotics have been noted, although without conclusive power, in some with active ulcerative colitis, Crohn's disease, active pouchitis and some other inflammatory gastrointestinal conditions. *Lactobacillus* species prevented development of spontaneous colitis in interleukin 10-deficient mice. *Lactobacillus plantarum* ameliorated colitis that was already established in the same animal model.

In a clinical trial, subjects with chronic relapsing pouchitis given a probiotic preparation for nine months, consisting of *L. casei, L. plantarum, L. acidophilus* and *L. delbruekii* subspecies *bulgaricus*, had significantly fewer relapses than did unsupplemented subjects receiving placebo. No side effects were seen. Some researchers believe that *Lactobacillus* GG may also be useful in treating pouchitis.

Some lactic acid bacteria, including *L. plantarum, L. rhamnosus, L. casei* and *Lactobacillus bulgaricus,* have demonstrated immuno-regulatory effects that might help protect against some allergic disorders. There is some evidence that some of these probiotic strains can reduce the intestinal inflammation associated with some food allergies, including cow's milk allergy among neonates. Breast-fed infants of nursing mothers given *Lactobacillus* GG had significantly improved atopic dermatitis, compared with infants not exposed to this probiotic.

There are *in vitro*, animal and some preliminary human data suggesting that some probiotics can bind and inactivate some carcinogens, can directly inhibit the growth of some tumors and can inhibit bacteria that may convert precarcinogens into carcinogens. *L. acidophilus* and *L. casei* have exhibited the latter activity in human volunteers. There is some preliminary evidence that *L. casei* may have reduced the recurrence of bladder tumors in humans. Confirmatory trials are needed. Animal work has suggested that some lactic-acid bacteria might help protect against colon cancer. Again, more research is needed.

Dairy products containing *L. acidophilus* have been credited with lowering cholesterol levels in some animal experiments. It has been hypothesized that bacterial assimilation of cholesterol in the intestine might reduce cholesterol stores available for absorption into the blood. To date, there is no credible evidence showing that any of the probiotics can lower cholesterol levels in humans. More study may be warranted. Yogurt has been used for some time as an "alternative" treatment for vaginitis. In an early test of this hypothesis, women with recurrent candidal vaginitis were treated with yogurt for six months. This was a crossover trial with subjects serving as their own controls. Daily ingestion of 8 ounces of yogurt significantly decreased both candidal colonization and infection.

Recently *L. acidophilus, L. crispatus* and *L. delbrueckii* subspecies *delbrueckii* all inhibited bacterial vaginosis-associated bacterial species *in vitro*. The researchers concluded that these probiotics might be useful for vaginal recolonization in women with recurrent vaginosis.

Owing to the fact that yogurt and some other probiotic-containing products are foods, rather than regulated pharmaceuticals, and owing to the fact that the probiotic content and potential of these food products may be highly variable, some researchers and clinicians have questioned the use of these products to treat vaginitis. In any event, larger better controlled studies are needed to further evaluate their reliability and efficacy in this context.

CONTRAINDICATIONS, PRECAUTIONS, ADVERSE REACTIONS

CONTRAINDICATIONS

Probiotics are contraindicated in those hypersensitive to any component of a probiotic-containing product.

PRECAUTIONS

Pregnant women and nursing mothers should only use probiotic nutritional supplements if recommended by their physicians.

The use of probiotics for the treatment of any disorder must be medically supervised.

ADVERSE REACTIONS

The most common adverse reactions with use of probiotics are gastrointestinal and include flatulence and constipation. Probiotics are generally well tolerated.

Four cases of *Saccharomyces boulardii* fungemia have been reported. All of the patients had indwelling catheters, and the fungemia was thought to be due to catheter contamination.

There are a few reports of *Lactobacillus* bacteremia and endocarditis. In all cases, there were underlying conditions, including cancer, diabetes mellitus and recent surgery. There is one death reported secondary to *Lactobacillus* bacteremia.

There is one report of meningitis caused by *Bifidobacterium* in an infant.

INTERACTIONS

NUTRITIONAL SUPPLEMENTS

Prebiotics: Concomitant use of prebiotics and probiotics may enhance the effectiveness of the probiotics. See Prebiotics. See Symbiotics.

DOSAGE AND ADMINISTRATION

There are many probiotic products available. These products contain various *Lactobacillus* strains, various *Bifidobacterium* strains, combinations of lactobacilli and bifidobacteria and combinations of probiotics and prebiotics. Typical doses of probiotics range from one to ten billion colony-forming units (CFU) a few times a week. Probiotics need to be consumed at least a few times a week to maintain their effect on the intestinal microecology.

The development of probiotic-containing yogurt products is actively being pursued by major food companies. These yogurt products are functional yogurt food products.

LITERATURE

Arunachalam K, Gill HS, Chandra RK. Enhancement of natural immune function by dietary consumption of bifidobacterium lactis. *Eur J Clin Nutr.* 2000; 54:263-267.

Arunachalam KD. Role of bifidobacteria in nutrition, medicine and technology. *Nutr Res.* 1999; 19:1559-1597.

Bielecka M, Biedrzycka E, Biedrzycka E, et al. Interaction of Bifidobacterium and Salmonella during associated growth. *Int J Food Microbiol.* 1998; 45:151-155.

Bleichner G, Blehaut H, Mentec H, Moyse D. *Saccharomyces boulardii* prevents diarrhea in critically ill tube-fed patients. A multicenter, randomized, double-blind, placebo-controlled trial. *Intensive Care Med.* 1997; 23:517-523.

Blum S, Reniero R, Schiffrin EJ, et al. Adhesion studies for probiotics: need for validation and refinement. *Trends Food Sci Technol.* 1999; 10:405-410.

Castagliuolo I, Riegler MF, Valenick L, et al. *Saccharomyces boulardii* protease inhibits the effects of *Clostridium difficile* toxins A and B in human colonic mucosa. *Infect Immun.* 1999; 67:302-307.

Czerucka D, Rampal P. Effect of *Saccharomyces boulardii* on cAMP- and Ca^{2+}-dependent Cl^- secretion in T84 cells. *Dig Dis Sci.* 1999; 44:2359-2368.

Dugas B, Mercenier A, Lenoir-Wijnkoop I, et al. Immunity and probiotics. *Immunol Today.* 1999; 20:387-390.

Elmer GW, McFarland LV, Surawicz CM, et al. Behavior of *Saccharomyces boulardii* in recurrent *Clostridium difficile* disease patients. *Aliment Pharmacol Ther.* 1999; 13:1663-1668.

Fredenucci I, Chomarat M, Boucaud C, Flandrois JP. *Saccharomyces boulardii fungemia* in a patient receiving Ultra-levure therapy. *Clin Infect Dis.* 1998; 27:222-223.

Gionchetti P, Rizzello F, Venturi A, Campieri M. Probiotics in infective diarrhoea and inflammatory bowel diseases. *J Gastroenterol Hepatol.* 2000; 15:489-493.

Gomes AMP, Malcata FX. *Bifidobacterium* spp. and *Lactobacillus acidophilus*: biological, biochemical, technological and therapeutical properties relevant for use as probiotics. *Trends Food Sci Technol.* 1999; 10:139-157.

Herias MV, Hessle C, Telemo E, et al. Immunomodulatory effects of *Lactobacillus plantarum* colonizing the intestine of gnotobiotic rats. *Clin Exp Immunol.* 1999; 116:283-290.

Hilton E, Isenberg HD, Alperstein P, et al. Ingestion of yogurt containing *Lactobacillus acidophilus. Ann Int Med.* 1992; 116:353-357.

Jahn HU, Ullrich R, Schneider T, et al. Immunological and trophical effects of *Saccharomyces boulardii* on the small intestine in healthy human volunteers. *Digestion.* 1996; 57:95-104.

Kimoto H, Kurisaki MN, Tsuji, et al. Lactococci as probiotic strains: adhesion to human enterocyte-like Caco-2 cells and tolerance to low pH and bile. *Lett Applied Microbiol.* 1999; 29:313-316.

Kirjavainen PV, Ouwehand AC, Isolauri E, Salminen SJ. The ability of probiotic bacteria to bind to human intestinal mucus. *FEMS Microbiol Lett.* 1998; 167:185-189.

Lactobacillus GG. *Nutrition Today.* 1996; 31:1S-52S.

Lin M-Y, Yen C-L. Antioxidative ability of lactic acid bacteria. *J Agric Food Chem.* 1999; 47:1460-1466.

Mack DR, Michail S, Wei S, et al. Probiotics inhibit enteropathogenic *E. coli* adherence in vitro by inducing intestinal mucin gene expression. *Am J. Physiol.* 1999; 276(4 Pt 1):G941-G950.

Majamaa H, Isolauri E. Probiotics: a novel approach in the management of food allergy. *J Allergy Clin Immunol.* 1997; 99:179-185.

Matilla-Sandholm T, Blum S, Collins JK, et al. Probiotics: towards demonstrating efficacy. *Trends Food Sci Technol.* 1999; 10:393-399.

Mattila-Sandholm T. The PROBDEMO project: demonstration of the nutritional functionality of probiotic foods. *Trends Food Sci Technol.* 1999; 10:385-386.

McFarland LV, Surawicz CM, Greenberg RN, et al. A randomized placebo-controlled trial of *Saccharomyces boulardii* in combination with standard antibiotics for *Clostridium difficile* disease. *JAMA.* 1994; 271:1913-1918.

Metchnikoff E. *The Prolongation of Life: Optimistic Studies.* The English translation. Mitchell PC, ed. 1908; New York:GP6

O'Brien J, Crittenden R, Ouwehand AC, Salminen S. Safety evaluation of probiotics. *Trends Food Sci Technol.* 1999; 10:418-424.

Ouwehand AC, Tölkkö S, Kulmala J, et al. Adhesion of inactivated probiotic strains to intestinal mucus. *Lett Applied Microbiol.* 2000; 31:82-86.

Pletinex M, Legein J, Vandenplas Y. Fungemia with *Saccharomyces boulardii* in a 1-year old girl with protracted diarrhea. *J Pediatr Gastroenterol Nutr.* 1995; 21:113-115.

Saavedra J. Probiotics and infectious diarrhea. *Am J Gastroenterol.* 2000; 95 (1 Suppl):S16-S18.

Saxelin M, Grenov B, Svensson U, et al. The technology of probiotics. *Trends Food Sci Technol.* 1999; 10:387-392.

Shortt C. The probiotic century: historical and current perspectives. *Trends Food Sci Technol.* 1999; 10:411-417.

Symposium: Probiotic Bacteria: Implications for Human Health. *J Nutr.* 2000; 130:382S-409S.

Todorov S, Onno B, Sorokine O, et al. Detection and characterization of a novel antibacterial substance produced by *Lactobacillus plantarum* ST31 isolated from sourdough. *Int J Food Microbiol.* 1999; 48:167-177.

Turner DL, Brennan L, Meyer HE, et al. Solution structure of *plantaricin C*, a novel lantibiotic. *Eur J Biochem.* 1999; 264: 833-839.

Vaughan EE, Heilig HGHJ, Zoetendal EG, et al. Molecular approaches to study probiotic bacteria. *Trends Food Sci Technology.* 1999; 10:400-404.

Wollowski I, Ji S-T. Bakalinsky AT, et al. Bacteria used for the production of yogurt inactivate carcinogens and prevent DNA damage in the colon of rats. *J Nutr.* 1999; 129:77-82.

Propolis

DESCRIPTION

Propolis, also known as bee glue and bee propolis, is a brownish resinous substance collected by bees, mainly from poplar and conifer buds, and used to seal their hives. Because of antimicrobial properties of propolis, it helps keep hives free of germs. Propolis has a long history of use in folk medicine and was even used as an official drug in London in the 1600s. Over time, propolis has been used for many purposes and marketed as lozenges, cough syrups, tooth-pastes, mouth rinses, lipsticks, cosmetics and even for the varnishing of Stradivarius violins. It appears to have antimicrobial and anti-inflammatory activities.

The composition of propolis is variable, depending on the locale and variety of trees and other plant species used for the collection. For example, unique constituents have been identified in propolis collected in Cuba and Brazil. The main chemical classes found in propolis are flavonoids, phenolics and terpenes. The flavonoids include quercetin, apegenin, galangin, kaempferol, luteolin, pinocembrin, pinostrobin and pinobanksin. The phenolic ester (caffeic acid phenethyl ester or CAPE) present in propolis is receiving much attention in the medical research community because of its potential for the treatment of a number of disorders, including spinal cord injury. Most of the substances in propolis are poorly soluble in water.

ACTIONS AND PHARMACOLOGY

ACTIONS

A list of possible actions of propolis includes: antibacterial, antifungal, antiviral (including anti HIV-1 activity), antioxidant, anticarcinogenic, antithrombotic and immunomodulatory.

MECHANISM OF ACTION

The mechanism of the possible actions of propolis may be understood by reviewing research findings on some of the individual compounds found in it. It is difficult to study the mechanism of actions of more than one compound at a time. Therefore, the following descriptions apply only to single compounds. The contribution of any single compound to the possible action of such a complex substance as propolis is difficult to know.

Caffeic acid phenethyl ester (CAPE) inhibits the lipoxygenase pathway of arachidonic acid, resulting in anti-inflammatory activity. CAPE is also known to have anticarcinogenic, antimitogenic and immunomodulatory properties. CAPE has been found to completely inhibit the activation of the nuclear transcription factor NF-Kappa B by tumor necrosis factor (TNF), as well as by other pro-inflammatory agents. The inhibition of NF-Kappa B activation may provide the molecular basis for its immunomodulatory, anticarcinogenic, anti-inflammatory and antiviral activities. It is possible that CAPE exerts its effects by inhibiting reactive oxygen species (ROS) production. ROS are known to play a major role in the activation of NF-Kappa B.

Compounds in propolis found to have antibacterial activity include a polyisoprenylated benzophenone, galangin, pinobanksin and pinocembrin. The exact mechanism of antimicrobial action of these compounds is not known.

INDICATIONS AND USAGE

There is evidence that propolis has some broad antimicrobial activity and that it may have anti-inflammatory effects that could make it useful in the treatment of some forms of arthritis, among other disorders. There is also some evidence of anti-cancer activity.

RESEARCH SUMMARY

In vitro and animal studies of propolis and derivative constituents have shown anti-bacterial, anti-viral and anti-fungal effects. It shows activity in culture against a broad spectrum of pathogens, including influenza and herpes viruses, as well as HIV and various fungal and bacterial organisms.

In a study of school children, an aqueous propolis extract was judged effective in reducing the incidence and intensity of acute and chronic rhinopharyngitis. In another study involving 10 volunteers, it exerted activity against oral bacteria. A Cuban study concluded that propolis is more effective than tinidazole against giardia.

Propolis has a high concentration of caffeic acid esters that some believe may give it some antitumor properties. In two studies, extracts of propolis fed to rats have inhibited azoxymethane-induced colonic tumors.

In vitro studies have shown propolis-related anti-inflammatory effects. Various extracts of propolis have also shown anti-inflammatory activity in animal models, particularly against adjuvant-induced arthritis.

More research is needed to further explore these preliminary findings.

CONTRAINDICATIONS, PRECAUTIONS, ADVERSE REACTIONS

CONTRAINDICATIONS

Propolis is contraindicated in those who are allergic or hypersensitive to any of its components.

PRECAUTIONS

Pregnant women and nursing mothers should avoid using propolis supplements.

ADVERSE REACTIONS

There are reported adverse reactions in those using topical preparations of propolis. These reactions are manifested as a dermatitis. There are reports of hypersensitivity reactions to ingested propolis, including rhinitis, conjunctivitis, skin rashes and bronchospasm.

OVERDOSAGE

No reported overdosage of propolis.

DOSAGE AND ADMINISTRATION

No typical dose. Propolis is available in several different preparations, including lozenges, tablets, creams, gels, mouth rinses, toothpastes and cough syrups.

LITERATURE

Burdock GA. Review of the biological properties and toxicity of bee propolis (propolis). *Food Chem Toxicol.* 1998; 36:347-363.

Chopra S, Pillai KK, Husain SZ, Giri DK. Propolis protects against doxorubicin-induced myocardiopathy in rats. *Exp Mol Pathol.* 1995; 62:190-198.

El-Ghazaly MA, Khayyal MT. The use of aqueous propolis extract against radiation-induced damage. *Drugs Exp Clin Res.* 1995; 21:229-236.

Grange JM, Davey RW. Antibacterial properties of propolis (bee glue). *J.R Soc Med.* 1990; 83:159-160.

Harish Z, Rubinstein A, Golodner M, et al. Suppression of HIV-1 replication by propolis and its immunoregulatory effect. *Drugs Exp Clin Res.* 1997; 23:89-96.

Khayyal MT, el-Ghazaly MA, el-Khatib AS. Mechanism involved in the anti-inflammatory effect of propolis extract. *Drugs Exp Clin Res.* 1993; 19:197-203.

Kujumgiev A, Tsverkova I, Serkedjieva Y, et al. Antibacterial, antifungal and antiviral activity of propolis of different geographic origins. *J Ethnopharmacol.* 1999; 64:235-240.

Ledon N, Casaco A, Gonzales R, et al. Antipsoriatic, anti-inflammatory and analgesic effects of an extract of red propolis. *Chung Kuo Yao Li Hsueh Pao.* 1997; 18:274-276.

Lin SC, Lin YH, Chen CF, et al. The hepatoprotective and therapeutic effects of propolis ethanol extract on chronic alcohol-induced liver injuries. *Am J Chin Med* 1997; 25:325-332.

Matsuno T, Jung SK, Matsumoto Y, et al. Preferential cytotoxicity to tumor cells of 3, 5-diprenyl-4-hydroxycinnamic acid (artipillin C) isolated from propolis. *Anticancer Res.* 1997; 17(5A):3565-3568.

Mirzoeva OK, Calder PC. The effect of propolis and its components on eicosanoid production during the inflammatory response. *Prostaglandins Leukot Essent Fatty Acids.* 1996; 55:441-449.

Mirzoeva OK, Grishanin RN, Calder PC. Antimicrobial actin of propolis and some of its components: the effects on growth, membrane potential and motility of bacteria. *Microbiol Res.* 1997; 152:239-246.

Natarajan K, Singh S, Burke TR Jr, et al. Caffeic acid phenethyl ester is a potent and specific inhibitor of activation of nuclear transcription factor NF-Kappa B. *Proc Natl Acad Sci.* 1996; 93:9090-9095.

Ozturk F, Kurt E, Cerci M, et al. The effect of propolis extract in experimental chemical corneal injury. *Ophthalmic Res.* 2000; 32:13-18.

Park EH, Kahng JH. Suppressive effects of propolis in rat adjuvant arthritis. *Arch Pharm Res.* 1999; 22:554-558.

Rao CV, Desai D, Simi B, et al. Inhibitory effect of caffeic acid esters on azoxymethane-induced biochemical change and aberrant crypt foci formation in rat colon. *Cancer Res.* 1993; 53:4182-4188.

Psyllium

DESCRIPTION

In 1998, the Food and Drug Administration (FDA) issued its final rule allowing health claims to be made on the labels of foods containing soluble fiber from whole oats (see Oat Beta-D-Glucan), noting that these foods, in conjunction with a diet low in saturated fat and cholesterol, may reduce the risk of heart disease. Shortly afterward, the FDA amended this to include the soluble fiber psyllium in the health claim. The FDA requires that there be at least 1.7 grams of soluble fiber from psyllium seed husk per serving in any food for which this health claim is made. To achieve heart-health benefits, the consumption of 7 grams of soluble fiber from psyllium are required.

Psyllium or *Plantago ovata* Forsk is an annual plant grown primarily in India, southern Europe and the United States. Psyllium is cultivated primarily for its use as a laxative or as a dietary fiber ingredient in foods, such as ready-to-eat cereals. It is also known as blond psyllium, Indian psyllium and plantain. Although the seed alone contains the bioactive mucilage polysaccharide, the refined psyllium seed husk, known as the Ispaghula husk, is the psyllium component principally used as the soluble fiber source for laxatives, ready-to-eat cereals and nutritional supplements.

The term psyllium is used interchangeably for the seed husk, the seed and the plant. Psyllium seed husk is comprised primarily of xylans. Xylans are polysaccharides built from the five-carbon sugar D-xylose. Xylans in psyllium seed husk occur in association with cellulose. The soluble fiber derived from psyllium seed husk is also known as psyllium hydrophilic mucilloid, psyllium hydrocolloid and psyllium seed gum. It is a white to cream-colored, slightly granular powder with a slight acid taste.

ACTIONS AND PHARMACOLOGY

ACTIONS

Psyllium may have hypocholesterolemic, glucose-regulatory and bowel-regulatory actions.

MECHANISM OF ACTION

The mechanism of psyllium's possible hypocholesterolemic activity is not fully understood. The bioactive agent of psyllium is a soluble, viscous xylan fiber. It is thought that this polysaccharide stimulates the conversion of cholesterol to bile acids and that it stimulates fecal excretion of bile acids. Psyllium may also decrease the intestinal absorption of cholesterol.

Some studies indicate that psyllium may improve glycemic control in type 2 diabetics. The mechanism of the effect is unclear. Psyllium may delay the absorption of carbohydrates by increasing gastric-emptying time and/or decreasing small intestinal transit time.

The laxative effect of psyllium is thought to be due to the swelling of psyllium from absorption of water with consequent increase in stool bulk and stimulation of peristalsis.

PHARMACOKINETICS

Following ingestion of psyllium, very little is digested in the small intestine. The psyllium polysaccharides are resistant to hydrolysis by the digestive enzymes. Some fermentation of the psyllium polysaccharides takes place in the large intestine via the action of colonic bacteria. The products of fermentation include the short-chain fatty acids acetate, propionate and butyrate, as well as hydrogen and carbon dioxide. The short-chain fatty acids that escape colonic metabolism are transported via the portal circulation to the liver, where they undergo metabolism.

INDICATIONS AND USAGE

The FDA allows a health claim for psyllium to the effect that, in conjunction with a low-fat diet, it may reduce risk of heart disease if used in adequate amounts. Numerous studies have shown that psyllium is effective in lowering total cholesterol and LDL-cholesterol levels in some with hypercholesterolemia. It is also helpful in some with constipation and may have benefit in some with diabetes. Claims that it is useful in preventing and treating anal fissures and hemorrhoids appear related to psyllium's efficacy in preventing and treating constipation. There is no credible evidence to support claims that psyllium is helpful in those with psoriasis or that it is effective in treating obesity.

RESEARCH SUMMARY

A recent meta-analysis of eight controlled trials investigating the effects of psyllium on lipids concluded that this supplement significantly lowered serum total and LDL-cholesterol concentrations in both male and female subjects who consumed a low-fat diet. Consumption of 10.2 grams of psyllium per day lowered serum total cholesterol 4% and LDL-cholesterol by 7%, compared with controls also consuming a low-fat diet but not supplementing with psyllium. No significant effects were seen in this meta-analysis on either serum HDL-cholesterol or triacylglycerol concentrations.

In one recent animal model of hypertension induced by salt ingestion, psyllium supplementation significantly attenuated salt-accelerated hypertension. The proposed possible mechanism of action was increased fecal excretion of sodium taken up by the psyllium.

In a recent study, psyllium was used adjunctively with a traditional diabetes diet to treat men with mild-to-moderate hypercholesterolemia and type 2 diabetes. Subjects were randomized to receive 5.1 grams of psyllium or cellulose placebo twice daily for eight weeks. Those receiving psyllium had significant improvement in glucose and lipid values compared with controls. Concentrations of serum total and LDL-cholesterol were 8.9% and 13% lower, respectively, in the psyllium group than in the control group.

Psyllium has been used for some time as a major ingredient in bulk laxatives. The FDA has approved this use, and the German Commission E has indicated that psyllium may be helpful in those with chronic constipation and some of the possible complications of constipation, including anal fissures and hemorrhoids. It may also be useful in some forms of diarrhea and in those who have had anal/rectal surgery. Some pregnant women are said to benefit from it as well.

CONTRAINDICATIONS, PRECAUTIONS, ADVERSE REACTIONS

CONTRAINDICATIONS

Psyllium is contraindicated in those hypersensitive to psyllium or to any component of a psyllium-containing product. It is also contraindicated in those with intestinal obstruction, fecal impaction, difficulty in swallowing and esophageal narrowing.

PRECAUTIONS

Pregnant women and nursing mothers should only use psyllium supplements if recommended by their physicians.

Supplemental psyllium must be taken with adequate amounts of fluids. Inadequate fluid intake may cause psyllium to swell and block the throat, esophagus or intestines.

Supplemental psyllium should not be taken right before going to bed.

ADVERSE REACTIONS

The most common adverse reactions are flatulence and abdominal distention. Potentially severe allergic reactions, including anaphylaxis, have been reported. These are not common.

INTERACTIONS

DRUGS

Concomitant use of psyllium and lithium may reduce the absorption of lithium. Concomitant use of psyllium and carbamazepine, digoxin and warfarin may reduce the absorption of those drugs.

Psyllium may enhance the cholesterol-lowering action of cholestyramine.

NUTRITIONAL SUPPLEMENTS

Psyllium may decrease the absorption of such minerals as zinc, copper, iron, calcium and magnesium if used concomitantly.

OVERDOSAGE

No reports.

DOSAGE AND ADMINISTRATION

Psyllium supplements are typically used in powder form, along with adequate amounts of fluids.

A dose of at least 7 grams daily taken with adequate amounts of fluid (water, juice) is used by some for management of elevated cholesterol.

There are a number of psyllium products used for constipation. The usual dose is about 3.5 grams twice a day. Again, the psyllium should be taken with adequate amounts of fluid.

Psyllium is a component of several ready-to-eat cereals.

LITERATURE

Anderson JW, Allgood LD, Lawrence A, et al. Cholesterol-lowering effects of psyllium intake adjunctive to diet therapy in men and women with hypercholesterolemia: meta-analysis of 8 controlled studies. *Am J Clin Nutr.* 2000; 71:472-479.

Anderson JW, Allgood LD, Turner J, et al. Effects of psyllium on glucose and serum lipid responses in men with type 2 diabetes and hypercholesterolemia. *Am J Clin Nutr.* 1999; 70:466-473.

Anderson JW, Davidson MH, Blonde L, et al. Long-term cholesterol-lowering effects of psyllium as an adjunct in the treatment of hypercholesterolemia. *Am J Clin Nutr*. 2000; 71:1433-1438.

Lantner RR, Espiritu BR, Zumerchik P, Tobin MC. Anaphylaxis following ingestion of a psyllium-containing cereal. *JAMA*. 1990; 264:2534-2536.

Levin EG, Miller VT, Muesing RA, et al. Comparison of psyllium hydrophilic mucilloid and cellulose in the treatment of mild to moderate hypercholesterolemia. *Arch Intern Med*. 1990; 150:1822-1827.

Turley SD, Daggy BP, Dietschy JM. Effect of feeding psyllium and cholestyramine in combination on low density lipoprotein metabolism and fecal bile acid excretion in hamsters with dietary-induced hypercholesterolemia. *J Cardiovasc Pharmacol*. 1996; 27:71-79.

Pycnogenol

DESCRIPTION

The term pycnogenol refers to a specific mixture of procyanidins extracted from the bark of the French maritime pine, *Pinus maritima*. The French maritime pine grows in Bay of Biscay in the Landes de Gascogne in France. Although the term pycnogenol is now confined to procyanidins from the French maritime pine, the term was originally intended to serve as scientific name for this class of flavonoids.

Procyanidins are derivatives of the flavan-3-ol class of flavonoids. This class includes epicatechin and catechin. Procyanidins consisting of dimers of catechin and oligomers of epicatechin and catechin are found in pycnogenol. Pycnogenol has a high amount of oligomers containing 5 to 7 units. Procyanidin oligomers are also known as oligomeric procyanidins (OPC), oligomeric proanthocyanidins (also OPCs) and procyanidolic oligomers (PCOs). In addition to OPCs, pycnogenol contains catechin, epicatechin and taxifolin, and such phenolic acids as caffeic, ferulic and para-hydroxybenzoic acids as minor constituents. It also contains glycosylation products of flavonols and phenolic acids as minute constituents. Pycnogenol is abbreviated PYC.

Procyanidins, including oligomeric procyanidins, are also found in such foods as cocoa and chocolate, grape seeds, apples, peanuts, almonds, cranberries and blueberries. They are also found in such medicinal herbs as "Sangre de drago" (*Croton lechleri*).

Procyanidins are also known as leucocyanidins. Procyanidins and prodelphinidins comprise a class of polyphenolic compounds called proanthocyanidins. Whereas procyanidins are oligomers of catechin and epicatechin and their gallic acid esters, prodelphinidins are oligomers of gallocatechin and epigallocatechin and their galloylated derivatives. Proanthocyanidins are also known as condensed tannins.

ACTIONS AND PHARMACOLOGY

ACTIONS

Pycnogenol has antioxidant activity. It may also have anti-inflammatory activity and has putative cardiovascular-protective activity.

MECHANISM OF ACTION

Pycnogenol has demonstrated a number of antioxidant activities in the laboratory. These include scavenging of the superoxide radical anion, the hydroxyl radical, the lipid peroxyl radical, the peroxynitrite radical and singlet oxygen. It has also been shown to protect low-density lipoprotein (LDL) from oxidation. The oligomeric procyanidins appear to have especially potent antioxidant activity when compared with smaller molecules, such as catechin and epicatechin. The extent of the antioxidant potential of pycnogenol in *vivo* is unclear. Some studies suggest that the antioxidant potential is at least partially available *in vivo*. Pycnogenol has been shown to have anti-inflammatory activity, again in the laboratory. This activity is thought to be due, in large part, to pycnogenol's capacity as a scavenger of reactive oxygen and reactive nitrogen species.

Pycnogenol appears to inhibit the activation of the transcription factors NF-kappa B and AP-1. NF-kappa B and AP-1 upregulate the expression of several inflammatory mediators such as intercellular adhesion molecule-1 (ICAM-1). NF-kappa B is itself activated by reactive oxygen species. Pycnogenol has been found to inhibit the inducible expression of ICAM-1. Inhibition of ICAM-1 may be accounted for by inhibition, by pycnogenol, of the activation of NF-Kappa B and AP-1. Further, the inflammatory cytokine interferon-gamma (IFN-gamma) may upregulate ICAM-1 expression in keratinocytes. This has been noted in some inflammatory skin conditions, such as lupus erythematous, atopic dermatitis and psoriasis. Pycnogenol appears to inhibit IFN-gamma activation of STAT (signal transducer and activator of transcription) 1. Inhibition of ICAM-1 expression by pycnogenol could account for possible anti-inflammatory and anti-atherogenic activities of pycnogenol.

PHARMACOKINETICS

Little is known about the pharmacokinetics of pycnogenol in humans. It appears that at least some of it is absorbed. However, the extent of absorption appears to vary widely, not only among the various components of pycnogenol, but also among subjects.

Some of the components of pycnogenol (e.g., catechin) appear to undergo extensive glucuronidation and sulfation following and/or during absorption. The glucuronides and sulfates are excreted in the urine.

INDICATIONS AND USAGE

Claims made for pycnogenol are sweeping. It has been demonstrated to have free-radical-scavenging properties, but far from established are claims that it is useful in immune and neuro-degenerative disorders, that it is an effective anti-allergen, anticancer agent, antidiabetic agent and that it speeds healing of injuries, fights arthritis and is useful in cirrhosis of the liver and aging. Clinical trials are in short supply. Current research suggests that pycnogenol might have some cardioprotective effects and might be helpful in some vascular disorders. It is possible that some immune-modulating, anti-inflammatory and anticancer effects will emerge.

RESEARCH SUMMARY

In vitro studies have demonstrated that pycnogenol can protect some cells from lipid peroxidation and damage induced by various oxidative toxins.

In vivo, pycnogenol has shown some ability to minimize ischemic reperfusion injury in an animal model. There is some preliminary suggestion that pycnogenol may exhibit vasorelaxation activity, inhibit angiotensin-converting enzyme and enhance microcirculation by promoting increased capillary resistance. It may inhibit platelet aggregation and LDL-cholesterol oxidation. It may help maintain levels of some other antioxidants, principally vitamins C and E. Many of these effects have only been demonstrated *in vitro*.

In one of the few clinical trials of pycnogenol, the substance significantly inhibited smoking-induced platelet aggregation, more significantly with doses of 200 mg than with doses of 100 or 150 mg of pycnogenol. A single 200 mg dose of pycnogenol was reported to significantly inhibit platelet aggregation for longer than three days in smokers.

Pycnogenol has reportedly met with some success in treating certain vascular disorders, including varicose veins and chronic venous insufficiency. Pycnogenol has also inhibited some localized inflammation experimentally induced in animals.

Using doses of pycnogenol higher than could likely be administered to humans, researchers have restored some immune functions in an animal model of HIV-infection. In other animals, oral feeding of pycnogenol has resulted in significant improvement in T- and B-cell function. Natural killer cell cytotoxicity has been enhanced in animals given pycnogenol. Clinical trials are needed.

Pycnogenol has shown preliminary chemoprotective effects against NKK, a tobacco-specific nitrosamine, in rats exposed to this substance.

CONTRAINDICATIONS, PRECAUTIONS, ADVERSE REACTIONS

CONTRAINDICATIONS

Pycnogenol is contraindicated in those with known hypersensitivity to any of the ingredients of a pycnogenol-containing product.

PRECAUTIONS

Pycnogenol supplementation should be avoided by pregnant women and nursing mothers.

ADVERSE REACTIONS

None reported.

INTERACTIONS

DRUGS

The use of pycnogenol and dextroamphetamine appeared superior to dextroamphetamine alone in the management of attention deficit-hyperactivity disorder, in one case report.

OVERDOSAGE

There are no reports of overdosage.

DOSAGE AND ADMINISTRATION

Dosage ranges from 25 to 200 mg daily.

LITERATURE

Bito T, Roy S, Sen CK, Packer L. Pine bark extract pycnogenol downregulates IFN-gamma-induced adhesion of T cells to human keratinocytes by inhibiting inducible ICAM-1 expression. *Free Rad Biol Med.* 2000; 28:219-227.

Heimann SW. Pycnogenol for ADHD. *J Am Acad Child Adolesc Psychiatry.* 1999; 38:357-358.

Huynh HT, Teel RW. Effects of pycnogenol on the microsomal metabolism of the tobacco-specific nitrosamine NNK as a function of age. *Cancer Lett.* 1998; 132:135-139.

Liu FJ, Zhang YX, Lau BH. Pycnogenol enhances immune and haemopoietic functions in senescence-accelerated mice. *Cell Mol Life Sci.* 1998; 54:1168-1172.

Packer LK, Rimbach G, Virgili F. Antioxidant activity and biological propertes of a procyanidin-rich extract from pine (*Pinus maritima*) bark, pycnogenol. *Free Rad Biol Med.* 1999; 27:704-724.

Putter M, Grotemeyer KH, Wurthwein G, et al. Inhibition of smoking-induced platelet aggregation by aspirin and pycnogenol. *Thromb Res.* 1999; 95:155-161.

Pyruvate

DESCRIPTION

Pyruvate is the anionic form of the three-carbon organic acid, pyruvic acid. Pyruvate is a key intermediate in the glycolytic and pyruvate dehydrogenase pathways, which are involved in biological energy production. Pyruvate is widely found in living organisms. It is not an essential nutrient since it can be synthesized in the cells of the body. Pyruvate, however, is consumed in the diet. The average daily intake of this substance ranges between about 100 milligrams and 1 to 2 grams. Certain fruits and vegetables are rich in pyruvate. For example, an average-size red apple contains approximately 450 milligrams. Dark beer and red wine are also rich sources of pyruvate.

Recent research suggests that pyruvate in supraphysiological concentrations may have a role in cardiovascular therapy, as an inotropic agent. Supraphysiological amounts of this dietary substance may also have bariatric and ergogenic applications.

Pyruvate is also known as 2-oxopropanoate, alpha-ketopropionate, acetylformate and pyroracemate. Pyruvate and pyruvic acid are frequently use interchangeably, even though pyruvate is the anion of pyruvic acid and the form that occurs in living organisms. Pyruvic acid is represented by the following chemical structure:

Pyruvic Acid

ACTIONS AND PHARMACOLOGY

ACTIONS

Pyruvate is a biological fuel source. It may also have cardiac and skeletal muscle inotropic activity as well as bariatric activity. Pyruvate also has antioxidant activity.

MECHANISM OF ACTION

Pyruvate serves as a biological fuel by being converted to acetyl coenzyme A, which enters the tricarboxylic acid or Krebs cycle where it is metabolized to produce ATP aerobically. Energy can also be obtained anaerobically from pyruvate via its conversion to lactate.

At supraphysiological levels, pyruvate increases contractile function of hearts when metabolizing glucose or fatty acids. This inotropic effect is striking in hearts stunned by ischemia/reperfusion. The inotropic effect of pyruvate requires intracoronary infusion.

Among possible mechanisms for this effect are increased generation of ATP and an increase in ATP phosphorylation potential. Another is activation of pyruvate dehydrogenase, promoting its own oxidation by inhibiting pyruvate dehydrogenase kinase. Pyruvate dehydrogenase is inactivated in ischemia myocardium. Yet another is reduction of cytosolic inorganic phosphate concentration. There are other possible mechanisms, such as enhanced sarcoplasmic reticular ion uptake and release, and reactive oxygen species scavenging.

Supraphysiological levels of pyruvate are reported to enhance aerobic endurance capacity. Again, the mechanism of this action is far from being well understood. Some studies indicate that pyruvate at supraphysiological levels increases the transport of glucose into muscle cells in a process known as blood glucose extraction. This could spare skeletal muscle glycogen stores.

The mechanism by which supraphysiological levels of pyruvate may lead to fat loss is unclear. Rats that consumed a diet supplemented with pyruvate and dihydroxyacetone reportedly had a lower respiratory quotient (RQ), indicating an increased utilization of fat as an energy source, as well as elevated resting metabolic rate. In addition, the rats that received pyruvate and dihydroxyacetone had elevated levels of thyroxine, lower levels of plasma insulin and lower rates of lipid synthesis in adipose tissue. Fat oxidation may be enhanced in some obese individuals administered pyruvate.

Regarding pyruvate's antioxidant action, pyruvate is known to scavenge such reactive oxygen species as hydrogen peroxide and lipid peroxides. This is a direct antioxidant effect. Indirectly, supraphysiological levels of pyruvate may increase cellular reduced glutathione.

PHARMACOKINETICS

Pyruvate is absorbed from the gastrointestinal tract from whence it is transported to the liver via the portal circulation. In the liver, pyruvate is metabolized via several pathways. Pyruvate may be converted to acetyl coenzyme A, which can enter the tricarboxylic acid or Krebs cycle for aerobic production of ATP. Energy can also be obtained from pyruvate anaerobically via its reduction to lactate. Via an aminotransferase reaction, pyruvate may be converted to L-alanine. And via its conversion to oxaloacetate by pyruvate carboxylase, it can become a precursor in the synthesis of glucose and glycogen by the process known as gluconeogenesis. Pyruvate not metabolized in the liver can be transported via the systemic circulation to other tissues in the body and undergo similar metabolic processes as described above.

INDICATIONS AND USAGE

Pyruvate may help some obese individuals lose weight. There is also the suggestion in current research that it might help some overweight individuals lower their blood pressure, and it may favorably modify lipid profiles. It also appears to enhance exercise endurance in some and may be protective in others with cardiac ischemia. There is a suggestion in animal work that it might have an ability to reduce insulin resistance.

RESEARCH SUMMARY

Obese women were given a 1000-calorie liquid diet that included 30 grams of pyruvate daily or placebo in the form of matching liquid diet without pyruvate for 21 days. The pyruvate-supplemented women lost significantly more weight, including weight in the form of fat, than did the controls.

In a subsequent trial, hyperlipidemic subjects were randomized to receive 36 to 53 grams of pyruvate daily or 21 to 37 grams of polyglucose as placebo. There was a significant reduction in plasma cholesterol and LDL concentrations in the pyruvate-treated subjects but not in the controls. Plasma HDL cholesterol and triglyceride concentrations did not show significant change. Resting heart rate, diastolic blood pressure and rate-pressure product decreased 9%, 6% and 12% respectively in the treated group, but were unchanged in the untreated group.

In a recent double-blind study, a much lower dose of pyruvate was tested in overweight men and women. Twenty-six subjects were randomized to receive 6 grams of pyruvate daily or placebo. All subjects participated in 45 to 60 minutes of aerobics three times a week. At the conclusion of the six-week trial, there were significant decreases in body weight, body fat and percent body fat in the pyruvate group, compared with controls.

Pyruvate has also shown some ability to enhance exercise endurance capacity. Used in combination with dihydroxyacetone (DHA), pyruvate (100 grams for seven days) significantly enhanced submaximal arm endurance capacity in untrained males (20 to 26 years old). This placebo-controlled study demonstrated pyruvate's ability to significantly increase arm muscle glucose extraction before and during exercise.

A follow-up study demonstrated similar positive effects in enhancing leg exercise endurance. On the other hand, a recent study showed no pyruvate effect on anaerobic performance and body composition in football players except when it was combined with creatine. More research in needed.

There is evidence from *in vitro*, animal and preliminary human research that pyruvate, in doses and modes of administration not relevant to supplementation, may be effective in some with cardiac ischemia through its inhibition of free-radical generation, among other things.

A study in female Zucker obese rats showed that pyruvate can favorably alter metabolism in these animals; it appeared to reduce the insulin resistance that spontaneously develops in this animal model.

CONTRAINDICATIONS, PRECAUTIONS, ADVERSE REACTIONS

CONTRAINDICATIONS
Known hypersensitivity to a pyruvate-containing product.

PRECAUTIONS
Pregnant women and nursing mothers should avoid pyruvate supplementation.

ADVERSE REACTIONS
Those taking large doses of supplemental pyruvate—usually greater than 5 grams daily—have reported gastrointestinal symptoms, including abdominal discomfort and bloating, gas and diarrhea. One child receiving pyruvate intravenously for restrictive cardiomyopathy died.

INTERACTIONS
Acetyl-L-carnitine has been reported to reverse the age-related decrease in mitochondrial pyruvate metabolism in rats.

OVERDOSAGE
There are no reports of overdosage with supplemental pyruvate.

DOSAGE AND ADMINISTRATION
Dosage has been variable. The most current research suggests a dose of 5 to 6 grams daily for a possible bariatric action or for athletic use.

LITERATURE
Hermann H-P, Pieske B, Schwarzmü ller E, et al. Haemodynamic effects of intracoronary pyruvate in patients with congestive heart failure: an open study. *Lancet.* 1999; 353:1321-1323.

Ivy JL. Effect of pyruvate and dihydroxyacetone on metabolism and aerobic endurance capacity. *Med Sci Sports Exer.* 1998; 30:837-843.

Ivy JL, Cortez MY, Chandler RM, et al. Effects of pyruvate on the metabolism and insulin resistance of obese Zucker rats. *Am J Clin Nutr.* 1994; 59:331-337.

Kalman D, Colker CM, Wilets I, et al. The effects of pyruvate supplementation on body composition in overweight individuals. *Nutrition.* 1999; 15:337-340.

Mallet RT. Pyruvate: metabolic protector of cardiac performance. *Proc Soc Exp Biol Med.* 2000; 223:136-148

Mallet RT, Sun J. Mitochondrial metabolism of pyruvate is required for its enhancement of cardiac function and energetics. *Cardiovasc Res.* 1999; 42:149-161.

Matthys D, Van Coster R, Verhaaren H. Fatal outcome of pyruvate loading test in child with restrictive cardiomyopathy. *Lancet.* 1991; 338:1020-1021.

Robertson RJ, Stanko RT, Goss FL. Blood glucose extraction as a mediator of perceived exertion during prolonged exercise. *Eur J Appl Physiol.* 1990; 61:100-105.

Stanko RT, Arch JE. Inhibition of regain in body weight and fat with addition of 3-carbon compounds to the diet with hyperenergetic refeeding after weight reduction. *Int J Obes Relat Metab Disord.* 1996; 20:925-930.

Stanko RT, Mullick P, Clarke MR, et al. Pyruvate inhibits growth of mammary adenocarcinoma 13762 in rats. *Cancer Res.* 1994; 54:1004-1007.

Stanko RT Reynolds HR, Hoyson R, et al. Pyruvate supplementation of a low-cholesterol, low-fat diet: effects on plasma lipid concentrations and body composition in hyperlipidemic patients. *Am J Clin Nutr.* 1994; 59:423-427.

Stanko RT, Reynolds HR, Lonchar KD, Arch JE. Plasma lipid concentrations in hyperlipidemic patients consuming a high-fat diet supplemented with pyruvate for 6 weeks. *Am J Clin Nutr.* 1992; 56:950-954.

Stanko RT, Tietze DL, Arch JE. Body composition, energy utilization, and nitrogen metabolism with a 4.25 MJ/d low-energy diet supplemented with pyruvate. *Am J Clin Nutr.* 1992; 56:630-635.

Quercetin

DESCRIPTION

Quercetin belongs to a group of polyphenolic substances known as flavonoids. Quercetin is a member of the class of flavonoids called flavonols. It is widely distributed in the plant kingdom in rinds and barks. Especially rich sources of quercetin include onions, red wine, green tea and St. John's wort.

Quercetin is typically found in plants as glycone or carbohydrate conjugates. Quercetin itself is an aglycone or aglucon. That is, quercetin does not possess a carbohydrate moiety in its structure. Quercetin glycone conjugates include rutin and thujin. Rutin is also known as quercetin-3-rutinoside. Thujin is also known as quercitrin, quercetin-3-alpha-L-rhamnoside, and 3-rhamnosylquercetin. Onions contain conjugates of quercetin and the carbohydrate isorhamnetin, including quercetin-3,4'-di-O-beta glucoside, isorhamnetin-4'-0-beta-glucoside and quercetin-4'-0-beta-glucoside. Quercetin itself is practically insoluble in water. The quercetin carbohydrate conjugates have much greater water solubility then quercetin.

Quercetin is known chemically as 2-(3, 4-dihydroxyphenyl)-3,5,7-trihydroxy-4H-1-benzopyran-4-one and 3,3',4'5,7-pentahydroxy flavone. It is also known as meletin and sophretin and is represented by the following structural formula:

Quercetin

ACTIONS AND PHARMACOLOGY

ACTIONS

Quercetin may have antioxidant, anti-inflammatory, antivral, immunomodulatory, anticancer and gastroprotective activities. It may also have anti-allergy activity and activity in preventing secondary complications of diabetes.

MECHANISM OF ACTION

Quercetin is a phenolic antioxidant and has been shown to inhibit lipid peroxidation. The putative anti-ulcer and gastro-protective effects of quercetin may, in part, be accounted for by this activity. *In vitro* and animal studies have shown that quercetin inhibits degranulation of mast cells, basophils and neutrophils. Such activity could account, in part, for quercetin's putative anti-inflammatory, anti-allergy and immunomodulating activities. Other *in vitro* and animal studies suggest that quercetin inhibits tyrosine kinase and nitric oxide synthase and that it modulates the activity of the inflammatory mediator, NF-kappaB. The mechanisms of anti-viral (in some cases enhanced with vitamin C) and anti-cancer activity that have been observed, again in *in vitro* and in animal studies, are unknown.

Aldose reductase, also known as alditol: NADP+ oxidoreductase, is the first enzyme of the polyol pathway. Hyperglycemia enhances the flow rate of the polyol pathway and this has been linked to such diabetic complications as cataracts, retinopathy, neuropathy and nephropathy. Quercetin is known to inhibit aldose reductase.

PHARMACOKINETICS

About 25% of an ingested dose of quercetin is absorbed from the small intestine and is transported to the liver via the portal circulation, where it undergoes significant first pass metabolism. Quercetin and its metabolites are distributed from the liver to various tissues in the body. Quercetin is strongly bound to albumin in the plasma. Peak levels of plasma quercetin occur from 0.7 to 7 hours following ingestion, and the elimination half-life of quercetin is approximately 25 hours.

Regarding pharmacokinetics of the quercetin glycoside conjugates, it appears that the main determinant of absorption of these conjugates is the nature of the sugar moiety. For example, quercetin glucoside is absorbed from the small intestine, whereas quercetin rutinoside is absorbed from the colon after removal of the carbohydrate moiety by bacterial enzymes.

INDICATIONS AND USAGE

It has been claimed that quercetin protects against heart attacks and stroke, but recent research found no support for this claim. Quercetin may, however, have benefit in some allergies, in conditions characterized by capillary fragility, in chronic prostatis and in some cancers. It may have beneficial effects on immunity and may have gastro-protective effects. It may also protect against the development of such diabetic complications as cataracts, retinopathy, neuropathy and nephropathy.

RESEARCH SUMMARY

Epidemiological evidence has suggested for some time that dietary intake of flavonols and flavones is inversely associated with coronary heart disease. It has been hypothesized that the ability of flavonoids to inhibit lipid peroxidation, demonstrated both *in vitro* and in various animal models, might, at least partially, account for this association.

More recently, however, a double-blind, placebo-controlled study compared one-gram daily of oral quercetin with placebo in 27 healthy subjects. This dose was said to be about 50-fold greater than dietary intakes associated, epidemiologically, with reduced risk of coronary heart disease mortality. The study continued for 28 days, during which period subjects receiving quercetin achieved plasma quercetin levels 23-fold higher than levels in those on placebo.

The results showed no quercetin effect on serum total cholesterol, LDL-cholesterol, HDL-cholesterol or triglyceride levels. Nor was there any effect on other factors considered to be indicators of risk for cardiovascular/thrombogenic disease, including platelet aggregation, platelet thromboxane B_2 production, blood pressure and resting heart rate. There was no effect on levels of (n-6) or (n-3) polyunsaturated fatty acids in serum or platelet phospholipids.

The researchers noted that the previous studies indicating that flavonoids, including quercetin, might be beneficial in heart disease were all performed *in vitro* or in animal models. They further observed that prior studies showing a quercetin platelet aggregation-inhibiting effect, for example, used doses far higher than those used in this study and thus amounts greatly in excess of those present in normal diet.

The researchers concluded: "Our results suggest that any protective effect of foods containing quercetin may be mediated via effects on risk factors other than those we have measured... Alternatively, the protective effect of quercetin-containing foods may be due to factors other than quercetin in those foods."

Another recent study increased plasma quercetin concentrations in 18 healthy subjects, via increased intake of quercetin-rich foods, such as onions. But, again, there was no effect on platelet aggregation, thromboxane B_2 production, factor VII or other hemostatic variables.

Quercetin is one of several flavonoids that have effects on mast cells and basophils; thus, some research suggests, it might be useful in some allergies, such as hay fever. Quercetin can help prevent the release of histamine and other mediators of allergic reactions, possibly by stabilizing cell membranes so that they are less reactive to allergens. Quercetin also exhibits anti-inflammatory properties, inhibiting formation of inflammatory prostaglandins and leukotrienes.

It was suggested in an open-label study that quercetin might be helpful in category III chronic prostatitis syndromes (nonbacterial chronic prostatitis and prostatodynia). Recently, this was confirmed in a prospective, randomized, double-blind, placebo-controlled trial.

Thirty men with these disorders received either placebo or 500 milligrams of quercetin twice daily for one month. Significant improvement was achieved in the treated group, as measured by the National Institutes of Health chronic prostatitis score. Some 67% of the treated subjects had at least 25% improvement in symptoms, compared with 20% of the placebo group achieving this same level of improvement.

In a follow-up, unblind, open-label study, 17 additional men received the same amount of quercetin for one month, but this time the quercetin was combined with bromelain and papain, which may enhance its absorption. In this study, 82% achieved a minimum 25% improvement score.

Several of quercetin's activities, including anti-inflammatory, antioxidant and immune-modulating actions, are believed to play roles in achieving these effects. There was evidence that quercetin prevented oxidative-mediated cellular injury, which the researchers suggested would apply whether the injury was due to infective, inflammatory or auto-immune mechanisms.

The researchers concluded: "Few therapies have shown durable efficacy with these disorders. Quercetin is efficacious, inexpensive, well tolerated and safe."

Fears that quercetin might be carcinogenic have not been supported by recent research. On the contrary, quercetin appears to have some anticancer effects, as demonstrated *in vitro* and in some animal models. Several processes that contribute to some cancers have been inhibited by quercetin. Some experiments have suggested a chemopreventive role for quercetin in colorectal carcinogenesis. Quercetin is reported to be one of very few substances that inhibit an animal model of basophil leukemia.

These preliminary results, as well as tentative findings that quercetin can have favorable immune-modulating and (in combination with vitamin C) some antiviral activity (against picomaviruses) need more vigorous follow up studies.

There are reports that quercetin may have some gastroprotective effects in animal models. High-dose quercetin promoted mucus production and helped diminish the severity of gastric lesions in animals injured with absolute thanol. Thiobarbituric acid reactive substances in gastric mucosa, a measure of lipid peroxidation, was significantly decreased by quercetin in ethanol-injured animals. Whether these findings will have relevance in humans remains to be seen.

Finally, quercetin has been shown to inhibit aldose reductase, the first enzyme in the polyol pathway. Experimental data link glucose metabolism via this pathway to long-term diabetic complications, such as cataract, nephropathy, retinopathy and neuropathy. Again, whether inhibition of aldose reductase will have any relevance in humans remains to be proven by well-controlled clinical trials.

CONTRAINDICATIONS, PRECAUTIONS, ADVERSE REACTIONS

CONTRAINDICATIONS

Known hypersensitivity to a quercetin-containing product.

WARNINGS AND PRECAUTIONS

Because of lack of long-term safety data, quercetin should be avoided by pregnant women and nursing mothers.

ADVERSE REACTIONS

Adverse effects reported with oral quercetin include gastrointestinal effects such as nausea, and rare reports of headache and mild tingling of the extremities. Oral quercetin is generally well tolerated. Intravenous administration of quercetin has been associated with nausea, vomiting, diaphoresis, flushing and dyspnea.

INTERACTIONS

DRUGS

Quinolone Antibiotics: Quercetin binds, *in vitro*, to the DNA gyrase site in bacteria. Therefore, theoretically, it can serve as a competitive inhibitor to the quinolone antibiotics which also bind to this site.

Cisplatin: Because of the theoretical risk of genotoxicity in normal tissues in those using cisplatin along with quercetin, those taking cisplatin should avoid quercetin supplements.

NUTRITIONAL SUPPLEMENTS

Bromelain and papain are reported to increase absorption of quercetin.

OVERDOSAGE

There are no reports of overdosage with oral quercetin. Intravenous administration of doses greater than 945 milligram per square meter has been associated with nephrotoxicity.

DOSAGE AND ADMINISTRATION

Doses of quercetin used range from 200 to 1,200 milligrams daily.

In the study showing possible benefit of quercetin for chronic prostatitis (see Research Summary), a quercetin dose of 500 milligrams was used, administered twice a day for one month.

LITERATURE

Alarcon de la Lastra C. Martin MJ, Motilve V. Antiulcer and gastroprotective effects of quercetin: a gross and histologic study. *Pharmacol.* 1994; 48:56-62.

Boulton DW, Walle UK, Walle T. Extensive binding of the bioflavonoid quercetin to human plasma proteins. *J Pharm Pharmacol.* 1998; 50:243-249.

Conquer JA, Maiani G, Azzini E, et al. Supplementation with quercetin markedly increases plasma quercetin concentration without effect on selected risk factors for heart disease in healthy subjects. *J Nutr.* 1998; 128:593-597.

Costantino L, Rastelli G, Gamberini MC, et al. 1-Benzopyran-4-one antioxidants as aldose reductase inhibitors. *J Med Chem.* 1999; 42:1881-1893.

de Vries JH, Jenssen PL, Hollman PC, et al. Consumption of quercetin and kaempferol in free-living subjects eating a variety of diets. *Cancer Lett.* 1997. 114:141-144.

Ferry DR, Smith A, Malkhandi J, et al. Phase I clinical trial of the flavonoid quercetine: phonmacokinetics and evidence for tyrosine kinase inhibition. *Clin Cancer Res.* 1996; 2:659-668.

Hilliard JJ, Krause HM, Bernstein JI, et al. A comparison of active site binding of 4-quinolones and novel flavone gyrase inhibitors to DNA gyrase. *Adv Exp Med Biol.* 1995; 390:59-69.

Hollman PC, Bijsman MN, van Gameren Y, et al. The sugar moiety is a major determinant of the absorption of dietary flavonoid glycosides in man. *Free Rad Res.* 1999; 31:569-573.

Hollman PC, de Vries JH, van Leeuwen SD, et al. Absorption of dietary quercetin glycosides and quercetin in healthy ileostomy volunteers. *Am J Clin Nutr.* 1995; 62:1276-1282.

Hollman PCH, van Trijp JMP, Mengelers MJB, et al. Bioavailability of the dietary antioxidant flavonol quercetin in man. *Cancer Lett.* 1997; 114:139-140.

Hollman PCH, Gaag MVD, Mengelers MJB, et al. Absorpotion and disposition kinetics of the dietary antioxidant quercetin in man. *Free Red Biol Med*. 1996; 21:703-707.

Ito N, Hagiwara A, Tamano S, et al. Lack of carcinogencity of quercetin in F344/DuCrj rats. *Jpn J Cancer Res*. 1989; 80:317-325.

Martin MJ, La-Casa C, Alarcon-de-la-Lastra C, et al. Antioxidant mechanisms involved in gastroprotective effects of quercetin. *Z Naturforsch[C]*. 1998; 53:82-88.

Middleton Jr E, Anne S. Quercetin inhibits lipopolysaccharide-induced expression of endothelial cell intracellular adhesion molecule-1. *Int Arch Allergy Immunol*. 1995; 107:435-436.

Sato M, Miyazaki T, Kambe F, et al. Quercetin, a bioflavonoid, inhibits the induction of interlenkin 8 and monocyte chemoattractant protein-1 expression by tumor necrosis factor-alpha in cultured human synovial cells. *J Rheumatol*. 1997; 24:1680-1684.

Shoskes DA. Effect of the bioflavonoids quercetin and curcumin on ischemic renal injury: a new class of renoprotective agents. *Transplantation*. 1998; 66:147-152.

Shoskes DA, Zeitlin SI, Shahed A, Rajfer J. Quercetin in men with category III chronic prostatitis: a preliminary prospective double-blind, placebo-controlled trial. *Urology*. 1999; 54:960-963.

Stavric B. Quercetin in our diet: from potent mutagen to probable anticarcinogen. *Clin Biochem*. 1994; 27:245-248.

Varma SD, Kinoshita JH. Inhibition of lens aldose reductase by flavonoids. Their possible role in the prevention of diabetic cataracts. *Biochem Pharmacol*. 1976; 25:2505-2513.

Red Yeast Rice

DESCRIPTION

Red yeast rice refers to the product of fermentation of rice with various strains of the yeast *Monascus purpureus* (Went). Red yeast rice has been used for centuries in China in foods and in medicines. It was introduced in the U.S. during the latter half of the 1990s as a dietary supplement for the promotion of healthy serum lipid levels. However, because it contains the HMG-CoA reductase inhibitor lovastatin, among other things, the U.S. FDA has contended that it is not a dietary supplement, but an unapproved drug. Presently, it is unclear what the final determination of this product will be; dietary supplement or unapproved drug.

The use of red yeast rice was apparently first noted in the Tang dynasty and was introduced to Taiwan by wine makers of Fukien about a century ago. It is used by the Chinese as a coloring agent in the preparation of foods, including fish, fish sauce, fish paste, rice wine (fu chiu), red soybean curd (hung-lu chiu, a cheese-like product used as a spice), pickled vegetables and salted meats. In addition to adding color, it adds flavor to foods. It has also been used in Chinese folk medicine for treating indigestion, diarrhea, and for improving blood circulation, among other things.

In addition to natural pigments such as monascorubin and monascin (azaphilone derivatives), red yeast rice contains starch, fatty acids (oleic, linoleic, linolenic, palmitic, stearic), phytosterols (beta-sitosterol, stigmasterol), isoflavones and monacolins. Monacolins possess hydroxymethyglutaryl coenzyme A (HMG-CoA) reductase-inhibitory activity. HMG-CoA reductase inhibitors are commonly known as statins. The first statin introduced in the U.S., for use as a cholesterol lowering agent, was lovastatin. Lovastatin was originally derived from *Monascus ruber*, and was first called monacolin K. Monacolin K is a lactone which is converted in the body to the active form of the statin, the corresponding beta-hydroxy acid of monacolin K (lovastastin, mevinolin).

The proprietary red yeast rice product that was first introduced in the U.S. was processed to yield 0.4% HMG-CoA reductase inhibitors in the final product. In addition to monacolin K or lovastatin, which comprises 0.2% of this product, it contains the corresponding beta-hydroxy acid of monacolin K at a concentration of 0.1%, and much smaller amounts of dihydromonacolin, monacolin I, monacolin II (hydroxy acid form), monacolin III, monacolin IV, monacolin V and monacolin VI, to give a total of 9 HMG-CoA reductase inhibitors. Traditional red yeast rice does not contain as high an amount of these substances. The yeast in red yeast rice is inactive.

The legal status surrounding red yeast rice as a dietary supplement has become an ongoing battle. In May, 1998, the FDA determined that the proprietary red yeast rice was an unapproved drug and not a dietary supplement. The FDA argued that although red yeast rice had been used as a food product for many years, neither it nor lovastatin were marketed as dietary supplements prior to the drug approval of the lovastatin drug product in 1987. They further argued that because of that situation, the product would not be covered under the Dietary Supplement Health and Education Act (DSHEA) which was passed in 1994. This meant that the product would be regulated by the FDA.

The manufacturer of the proprietary product argued that the FDA approved the lovastatin drug product and not the drug active (lovastatin) and also, that the product is a food product that had been used for centuries in China and thus, would fall under DSHEA. In February, 1999, the Federal District Court in Utah ruled against the FDA, stating that the proprietary red yeast rice product was not a drug but a dietary supplement. This decision came about as a result of a law suit brought by the manufacturer against the FDA. In the most recent legal turn of events, the 10th U.S. Circuit Court of Appeals ruled on July 24, 2000 that the proprietary red yeast product *is* subject to regulation by the U.S. FDA. The future of red yeast rice as a dietary supplement is unclear. Lovastatin has the following structural formula:

Lovastatin

Red yeast rice is known by various names, including Chinese red yeast rice, red rice, *Monascus purpureus*-fermented rice, red yeast, anka, ang-kak, ankak, angquac, beni-koji, beni-Jiuqu, aga-Jiuqu, aka-koji, xuezhikang, hung-chu and hongqu.

ACTIONS AND PHARMACOLOGY

ACTIONS

Red yeast rice may have hypocholesterolemic and hypotriglyceridemic activities in some.

MECHANISM OF ACTION

The mechanism of the hypolipidemic activity of red yeast rice is not entirely clear. The possible hypocholesterolemic activity of red yeast rice can be accounted for, in part, by the presence of HMG-CoA reductase inhibitors, especially monacolin I (lovastatin, mevinolin) and its corresponding beta-hydroxy acid, monacolin II. Lovastatin is converted in the body to its corresponding beta-hydroxy acid, which is the form that inhibits HMG-CoA reductase. HMG-CoA reductase catalyzes the conversion of HMG-CoA to mevalonate, which is an early and rate limiting step in cholesterol biosynthesis. Lovastatin is known to lower plasma total cholesterol, low-density lipoprotein cholesterol (LDL-C), the total cholesterol/HDL-C ratio and the LDL-C/HDL-C ratio. Lovastatin may also produce a modest increase in HDL-cholesterol and modest decreases in VLDL-C and triglyceride levels in some.

LDL is formed from VLDL and is principally catabolized via the high affinity LDL receptor. Lovastatin's mechanism in lowering LDL appears also to involve reduction of VLDL-C levels and upregulation of the LDL receptor, resulting in reduced production of LDL-C, as well as increased catabolism of LDL-C.

The hypolipidemic effects of red yeast rice have been found to be greater than those obtained from equivalent doses of the pharmaceutical form of lovastatin. To be clear about this, the amount of lovastatin delivered by red yeast rice is typically 7.2 milligrams. The amount of lovastatin in the pharmaceutical form of lovastatin ranges from 10 to 40 milligrams. It is unclear why a lovastatin dose of 7.2 milligrams in red yeast rice appears to have more potent lipid-lowering activity than higher doses of pharmaceutical lovastatin. It is speculated that other substances in red yeast rice besides the HMG-CoA reductase inhibitors may have lipid-lowering activity themselves or may work synergistically with the HMG-CoA reductase inhibitors. What these substances are and how they may work synergistically with the HMG-CoA reductase inhibitors is entirely unclear. Beta-sitosterol (see Beta-Sitosterol) is found in red yeast and it is known to have hypocholesterolemic activity. However, the amount of this substance found in red yeast rice is too small to make much of a cholesterol-lowering contribution.

PHARMACOKINETICS

There is little on the pharmacokinetics of red yeast rice in humans. However, the pharmacokinetics of lovastatin, which appears to be the principal bioactive substance in red yeast rice, are known. The efficiency of absorption of lovastatin is approximately 30%. The efficiency of absorption is greater when it is given with food. Following absorption, lovastatin is transported to the liver via the portal circulation where it undergoes extensive first-pass extraction. The liver is the principal site of action of lovastatin. Less than 5% of an oral dose of lovastatin reaches the systemic circulation. Lovastatin is metabolized in the liver to its corresponding beta-hydroxy acid, which is the active HMG-CoA reductase inhibitor. In addition to the beta-hydroxy acid of lovastatin, lovastatin is metabolized to a few other metabolites, including its 6'-hydroxy derivative. Lovastatin is metabolized by the cytochrome P450 3A4 system. Excretion is mainly via the biliary route. Approximately 83% of an oral dose of lovastatin is excreted in the feces (biliary excretion and unabsorbed lovastatin), and approximately 10% is excreted in the urine.

INDICATIONS AND USAGE

Red yeast rice may have favorable effects on lipids, lowering cholesterol and triglycerides in some. However, there is an ongoing legal issue regarding the status of red yeast rice, particularly those preparations that contain statins, as a dietary supplement.

RESEARCH SUMMARY

Recent clinical studies have demonstrated that red yeast rice can significantly lower triglyceride and cholesterol levels in some individuals. In one multi-center, randomized, single-blind trial of the substance in 502 patients with hyperlipidemia, there was a 17% reduction of total cholesterol in the treated group. LDL-cholesterol was reduced an average of 24.6%, and serum triglyceride levels fell an average of 19.8%. HDL-cholesterol rose by 12.8% in the treatment group.

These results were measured after four weeks of treatment. Dosage was 600 milligrams of red yeast rice twice daily for a total of 1,200 milligrams daily. At the end of eight weeks of red yeast rice supplementation, still better results were reported for the treatment group: total cholesterol reduced by 22.7%, LDL-cholesterol reduced by 30.9%, triglycerides reduced by 34.1%, HDL-cholesterol increased by 19.9%.

In another recent study, this one conducted in a double-blind, placebo-controlled fashion, 83 hyperlipidemic subjects who were not being treated with lipid-lowering drugs were randomized to receive red yeast rice, 2.4 grams daily, or placebo. Subjects were instructed to consume a diet deriving 30% of energy from fat (with no more than 10% of this from saturated fat and no more than 300 milligrams of cholesterol daily).

The study continued for 12 weeks. Red yeast rice was found to significantly reduce total cholesterol, LDL-cholesterol and total triacylglycerol concentrations, compared with placebo. HDL-cholesterol was not affected in this study. Research is ongoing. Also ongoing is the legal issue regarding the status of lipid-lowering red yeast rice as a dietary supplement.

CONTRAINDICATIONS, PRECAUTIONS, ADVERSE REACTIONS

CONTRAINDICATIONS

Red yeast rice is contraindicated in those who are hypersensitive to any component of a red yeast rice-containing product. Red yeast rice is also contraindicated in pregnant women, nursing mothers, women of childbearing age who are likely to conceive, those with active liver disease and those with unexplained aminotransferase (transaminase) elevations.

PRECAUTIONS

Since the principal bioactive substance in red yeast rice is lovastatin, all of the warnings, precautions and interactions of pharmaceutical lovastatin apply to red yeast rice, as well.

The use of red yeast rice for the management of hyperlipidemia must be medically supervised.

Those with a past history of liver disease and those who routinely use alcoholic beverages should exercise caution in the use of red yeast rice.

Lovastatin and other HMG-CoA reductase inhibitors occasionally cause myopathy. This is manifested as muscle pain or weakness associated with elevated levels of creatine kinase. Rhabdomyolysis with or without acute renal failure secondary to myoglobinuria, has been reported rarely and can occur at any time. Those using red yeast rice should report promptly to their physicians unexplained muscle pain, tenderness or weakness.

Bleeding and/or increased INR values have been reported in a few patients taking warfarin concomitantly with lovastatin.

Persistent increases (to more than 3 times the upper limit of normal) in serum aminotransferases (transaminases) occurred in 1.9% of adults who received lovastatin for at least one year in some early clinical trials. It is recommended that liver tests be performed before starting red yeast rice, at 6 and 12 weeks after starting its use, and periodically thereafter.

Lovastatin has been reported to lower coenzyme Q (CoQ$_{10}$) levels.

ADVERSE REACTIONS

In clinical studies of red yeast rice, few adverse reactions were reported. Adverse reactions reported, included flatulence and heartburn. There is one report of anaphylaxis resulting from inhalation of red yeast rice. Adverse reactions from the pharmaceutical form of lovastatin, include elevated liver tests, elevated creatine kinase levels (noncardiac), myopathy and liver dysfunction. Overall, lovastatin is generally well tolerated; adverse reactions usually have been mild and transient.

INTERACTIONS

DRUGS

Azole antifungals (fluconazole, ketoconazole, itraconazole): Concomitant use of red yeast rice and an azole antifungal may increase the risk of myopathy.

Cyclosporine: Concomitant use of red yeast rice and cyclosporine may increase the risk of myopathy.

Fibrates (clofibrate, fenofibrate): Concomitant use of red yeast rice and a fibrate may increase the risk of myopathy.

Gemfibrozil: Concomitant use of red yeast rice and gemfibrozil may increase the risk of myopathy.

Macrolide antibiotics (clarithromycin, erythromycin): Concomitant use of red yeast rice and certain macrolide antibiotics may increase the risk of myopathy.

Nefazodone: Concomitant use of red yeast rice and nefazodone may increase the risk of myopathy.

Protease inhibitors (amprenavir, indinavir, nelfinavir, ritonavir, saquinavir): Concomitant use of red yeast rice and a protease inhibitor may increase the risk of myopathy.

Statins (atorvastatin, cerivastatin, fluvastatin, lovastatin, pravastatin, simvastatin): Concomitant use of red yeast rice with a pharmaceutical statin may increase the risk of adverse reactions.

Warfarin: Concomitant use of red yeast rice and warfarin may result in an increase in the INR as well as bleeding.

NUTRITIONAL SUPPLEMENTS
Nicotinic acid: Concomitant use of red yeast rice and high doses of nicotinic acid may increase the risk of myopathy.

FOODS
Grapefruit juice: Grapefruit juice contains some substances, such as the furanocoumarin bergamottin, which inhibit cytochrome P450 3A4, the enzyme that metabolizes lovastatin, among other substances. Therefore, concomitant use of red yeast rice and grapefruit juice may increase the risk of myopathy.

Meals: When lovastatin was given under fasting conditions, plasma concentrations of lovastatin and its active metabolite were on the average two-thirds those found when lovastatin was administered immediately following a meal.

OVERDOSAGE

There are no reports of overdosage with red yeast rice. A few cases of accidental overdosage have been reported with the pharmaceutical form of lovastatin. The maximum dose taken was 5-6 grams. No patients had any specific symptoms and they completely recovered.

DOSAGE AND ADMINISTRATION

Red yeast rice is currently available in single ingredient and combination products. The red yeast rice dietary supplements are standardized to 0.4% HMG-CoA reductase inhibitors, with 0.3% coming from lovastatin equivalents. A dose of 2,400 milligrams daily delivers 9.6 milligrams of HMG-CoA reductase inhibitors, including 7.2 milligrams of lovastatin equivalents. Red yeast rice typically comes in 600 milligram capsules. The usual dose has been 2,400 milligrams daily. See Precautions.

LITERATURE

Baens-Arcega L, Ardisher AG, Beddows CG, et al. Indigenous amino acid/peptide sauces and pastes with meat-like flavors. Chinese soy sauce, Japanese shoyu, Japanese miso, Southeast Asian fish sauces and pastes, and related fermented foods. In: Steinkraus KH, ed. *Handbook of Indigenous Fermented Foods.* 2nd ed. New York, NY: Marcel Dekker, Inc; 1996:625-633.

Endo A. Monacolin K. A new hypocholesterolemic agent produced by a *Monascus* species. *J Antibiot (Tokyo).* 1979; 32:852-854.

Havel RJ. Dietary supplement or drug? The case of Cholestin (editorial). *Am J Clin Nutr.* 1999; 69:175-176.

Heber D, Yip I, Ashley JM, et al. Cholesterol-lowering effects of a proprietary Chinese red-yeast-rice dietary supplement. *Am J Clin Nutr.* 1999; 69:231-236.

Kou W, Lu Z, Guo J. [Effect of xuezhikang on the treatment of primary hyperlipidemia]. [Article in Chinese]. *Chung Hua Nei Ko Tsa Chih.* 1997; 36:529-531.

Li C, Wang Y, et al. *Monascus purpureus*-fermented rice (red yeast rice): a natural food product that lowers blood cholesterol in animal models of hypercholesterolemia. *Nutr Res.* 1998; 18:71-81.

SoRelle R. Appeals Court says Food and Drug Administration can regulate Cholestin. *Circulation.* 2000; 102:E9012-E9013.

Wigger-Alberti W, Bauer A, Hipler UC, Elsner P. Anaphylaxis due to *Monascus purpureus*-fermented rice (red yeast rice). *Allergy* 1999; 54:1330-1331.

Zhang ML, Pong CX, Chang MN. *Methods and Compositions Employing Red Yeast Fermentation Products.* International patent publication number: WO 98/14177. International publication date: 9 April 1998.

Resistant Starch

DESCRIPTION

Resistant starch is defined as the starch and starch degradation products that, on average, resist digestion in the small intestine. And, since resistant starch has similar physiological and metabolic features, like those of soluble and insoluble dietary fibers, resistant starch is now considered one of the three types of dietary fibers, along with soluble fiber and insoluble fiber. (See Pectin, Psyllium and Oat Beta-Glucan).

Starch represents the primary energy source for many animals, including humans. The rate of starch digestion and glucose release and absorption play major roles in human health by helping maintain normal plasma glucose and insulin levels. There are various ways of classifying native starches, including based on the structure as determined by X-ray diffraction, based on the rate of digestion and based on nutritional characteristics. Based on the rate of digestion, starch is classified as rapidly digestible starch (RDS), slowly digestible starch (SDS) and resistant starch (RS). RDS typically leads to rapid increases in plasma glucose and insulin levels. SDS leads to a moderate glycemic and insulinemic response and decreased excursions of plasma glucose when compared with RDS. Chronic consumption of foods with high levels of RDS can cause substantial fluctuations in glucose homeostasis, which is associated with a number of health conditions, including diabetes, obesity and cardiovascular disease. The development of foods and nutritional supplements with higher amounts of SDS and RS could very well make a big impact on these growing health conditions.

Chemically, starches are polysaccharides composed of a number of glucose molecules linked together via alpha-D-(1>4) and/or alpha-D-(1>6) linkages. Starches are packed in granules, and following disruption and dissociation of the granules, starches can be fractionated into the two polysaccharide forms, amylose and amylopectin, which are contained in the granules. Amylose consists of approximately 20% to 30% of the starch in the granules, and amylopectin about 70%-80%.

Amylose is a generally linear polymer of D-glucose units connected by alpha-(1>4) glycosidic linkages. Amylose possesses infrequent alpha-(1>6) glycosidic linkages. Its molecular weight ranges from 200,000 to 700,000. Amylopectin is a large, highly branched polymer, again made up of D-glucose units. The backbone glycosidic linkages in amylopectin are alpha (1>4), similar to those in amylose, but the frequent branch points have alpha (1>6) glycosidic linkages. The molecular weight of amylopectin ranges from 50 to 200 million. The degree of polymerization of amylose is <2,000, while the degree of polymerization of amylopectin is >5,000. (Degree of polymerization refers to the number of monomer units in a polymer.)

The enzyme pancreatic alpha-amylase plays a major role in the digestion of starch. Pancreatic alpha-amylase hydrolyzes alpha (1>4) linkages randomly to produce maltodextrins, maltotriose, other glucose oligosaccharides, maltose and some D-glucose. Although alpha-amylase hydrolyzes the alpha (1>4) linkages in amylopectin, it cannot hydrolyze the alpha (1>6) linkages, which occur at the branch points of amylopectin, consequently forming a highly branched core called limit dextrin. A debranching enzyme, alpha (1>6) glycosidase, hydrolyzes the alpha (1>6) linkages at the branch points, producing D-glucose. The brush border of the cells lining the lumen of the small intestine contains enzymes called glucosidases that convert glucose oligosaccharides and disaccharides to D-glucose. Alpha-glucosidases convert maltose and maltotriose to D-glucose. Thus, D-glucose is the major endproduct of the complete digestion of starch. Importantly, D-glucose is the only carbohydrate derived from the breakdown of starch that can be absorbed in the small intestine.

Starch itself, or any of the products of starch digestion, including maltose, maltotriose and maltodextrin, which have escaped digestion in the small intestine are not absorbed in the small intestine and pass into the large intestine where they are fermented by the colonic microflora. These carbohydrates are collectively called "resistant starch."

The recognition of incomplete digestion and absorption of starch (actually of glucose) in the intestine as a normal phenomenon is relatively recent and has raised great interest in nondigestible starch fractions. Excessive consumption of starch plays a large role in the growing obesity pandemic. The production of starch that resists digestion decreases the effective caloric content of the starch (from four kilocalories per gram to about two to three kilocalories per gram) and at the same time increases its dietary fiber content, which could translate into better glucose control, among other things. There is much ongoing research in this area, and products are being designed with RS starch that retain all of the desirable organoleptic (mouthfeel) qualities of starch.

There are four types of RS: RS1, RS2, RS3 and RS4.

RS1 results from the starch being physically inaccessible to alpha-amylase. For example, starch embedded in a protein or a fiber matrix, such as found in whole grains, partially milled grains, seeds and legumes. The starch resistance can be minimized by milling and chewing.

RS2 is intact, ungelatinized native starch granules that, like uncooked starch, have a physical structure that is digestive-resistant. It can be slowly hydrolyzed by alpha-amylase. Examples of **RS2** include raw potatoes, green (unripe) bananas, high amylose corn and some legumes. The starch resistance can be minimized by food processing and cooking.

RS3, also known as retrograded starch, is a starch that has been cooked and gelatinized (gelatinization is the swelling of starch granules when heated in a water medium) and cooled and crystallized post-gelatinization. In this way, the native structure has been destroyed and the starch molecules have reassociated themselves during the process so that the starch is alpha-amylase resistant after cooking. This type of starch is also referred to as retrograded starch. Retrogradation is the process in which additional bonds form in gels and increase their rigidity after cooking. Storage and cooling of starch pastes increase the retrogradation, and water is pushed out of the cells, causing watery areas in the starch paste. A cornstarch paste will retrograde with storage. Examples of RS3 include cooked and cooled potatoes, bread, cornflakes and food products with repeated moist heat treatments. Starch resistance is minimized by processing conditions.

Recently, a maltodextrin has been reported that is physiologically and metabolically similar to type 3 resistant starch and has been classified as a type 3 retrograded resistant starch.

RS4 is chemically modified starch produced by cross-linking with chemical reagents. RS4 is constructed to resist digestion. RS4 does not occur naturally in foods. Foods in which

RS4 starches have been used include breads and cakes. RS4 is less susceptible to digestion *in vivo*.

In cooked foods, amylose molecules reassociate rapidly on cooling, forming complexes that resist digestion, whereas amylopectin molecules reassociate slowly and are more readily digested.

ACTIONS AND PHARMACOLOGY

ACTIONS

Resistant starch has prebiotic activity. Resistant starch may also have anticarcinogenic activity in the colon, colon-protective activity and glucose-modulating activity.

MECHANISM OF ACTION

Prebiotic activity: Substances such as resistant starch may promote the growth of beneficial bacteria in the colon. In this capacity, resistant starch can be said to demonstrate prebiotic activity. Prebiotics are typically nondigestible oligosaccharides. The beneficial bacteria contained in the colon microbiota are called probiotics. (Probiotics are considered "good" microorganisms.) Type 3 resistant starch has been demonstrated to induce the growth of *Bifidobacterium* spp. in human subjects.

Anticarcinogenic activity in the colon: Resistant starch in the form of raw potato starch (type 2 resistant starch) was found to suppress azomethane (AOM)-induced colonic preneoplastic aberrant crypt foci at the promotion stage of carcinogenesis in Wistar rats, but not at the preinitiation stage.

In another animal study (with male Sprague-Dawley rats), retrograded amylose corn starch (type 3 resistant starch) was shown to prevent 1,2-dimethylhydrazine-induced colon carcinogenesis. This was mediated by enhanced apoptosis of damaged cells and accompanied by changes in parameters of dedifferentiation in the colonic mucosa.

The above anticarcinogenic activities of resistant starch might be accounted for, in part, by the possible anticarcinogenic action of butyrate. Butyrate, a short-chain fatty acid, is the main endproduct of intestinal microbial fermentation of resistant starch. Of all the short-chain fatty acids produced via intestinal fermentation of resistant starch, butyrate appears to play the major role, particularly with regard to the colon. It is considered to be the major nutrient of the colonocytes and has been shown to trigger differentiation and apoptosis of colon-derived cells in culture. It has also been shown to cause growth arrest, induce apoptosis and regulate the expression of proteins involved in cellular dedifferentiation in various tumor cell lines in culture. Butyrate has also been found to reduce aberrant crypt foci formation (preneoplastic lesions used as a marker of early carcinogenesis) in rats (see above).

The exact mechanism of the anticancer effect of resistant starch is unclear. Also unclear is the exact role of butyrate in this effect. Butyrate has been demonstrated to inhibit histone deacetylase (HDAC), and it is conceivable that this activity of butyrate plays a major role in the possible anticancer effect of resistant starch. Histone acetylation plays an important role in the regulation of gene expression. Hyperacetylated chromatin is transcriptionally active, and hypoacetylated chromatin is silent. HDAC inhibition by butyrate unsilences the chromatin and may activate its transcription.

Recently, there has been much interest in HDAC inhibitors for cancer chemotherapy. For example, suberoylanilide hydroxamic acid (SAHA) is a potent inhibitor of HDAC that causes growth arrest, differentiation, and/or apoptosis of many tumor types *in vitro* and *in vivo*. Butyrate and SAHA might have additive/synergistic activities against certain cancers. This should be explored.

Colonic protective activity: Resistant starch may also have general effects on colonic health.

Raw potato starch (type 2 resistant starch) was administered to growing pigs for a period of 14 weeks and its effects on colonic mucosal integrity and immunity were studied. It was reported that long-term administration of the resistant starch reduced damage to the colonocytes, improved colonic mucosal integrity and demonstrated anti-inflammatory activity. The mechanism of these effects was not clear, but it was thought that the butyrate derived from fermentation of the resistant starch by the colonic microflora probably played an important role.

Dose-dependent reduction by high amylose maize starch (type 2 resistant starch) of dietary-induced colonocyte DNA damage was reported in a rat study. The reduction in DNA damage by the resistant starch was found to correlate more highly with caecal butyrate than with the other short-chain fatty acids produced via colonic fermentation of the starch, including acetate and propionate.

High amylose corn starch (type 2 resistant starch) was also found to protect rats against trinitrobenzene sulfonic acid-induced colitis.

Raw potato starch (type 2 resistant starch) was shown to lead to a reduction of colonocyte apoptosis and shifted apoptosis to the stem cell department in order to counteract excessive proliferation of crypts in the pig colon. Again, increased butyrate formation in the pig colon was thought to account for these actions.

Recently, it has been reported that short-chain fatty acids, produced via colonic fermentation of resistant starch, enhance the barrier function of the colonic epithelium via their interaction with cholesterol-rich microdomains in the plasma membranes. This study was performed in rats and in cell culture.

Glucose-modulating activity: The "second meal effect" refers to a meal's ability to diminish the glucose response to carbohydrates eaten during the following meal. Basically, it is the first meal's ability to blunt plasma glucose and insulin excursions during the next meal.

The glycemic index, or GI, is a measure of the effect of carbohydrates on blood glucose levels. The GI of a food is defined by the area under a two-hour blood glucose response curve following the ingestion of a fixed portion of carbohydrates, usually 50 grams. The current validated methods use glucose as the reference food, giving it a glycemic index value of 100 by definition.

Carbohydrates that break down rapidly during digestion (rapidly digestible starch), releasing glucose rapidly into the blood, have a high GI. Carbohydrates that break down slowly (slowly digestible starch), releasing glucose gradually into the blood, have a low GI.

It had been thought that the reduced glycemia elicited by low GI foods consumed during the first meal is the main mechanism for the second meal effect. However, that is now not thought to be the whole story. Low GI foods may increase colonic fermentation secondary to the presence of dietary fibers, such as resistant starch. The products of the fermentation may account, in part, for the second meal effect.

In a study with human volunteers, it was found that fermentable carbohydrates, like RS, independent of their effect on GI, have the potential to regulate postprandial responses to a second meal by reducing nonesterified fatty acid competition for glucose disposal and, to a lesser extent, by affecting intestinal motility. The exact mechanism of this effect is unknown.

Better glucose management and consequent insulin sensitivity might also have a hunger suppressing effect. Thus, the effect of RS discussed above may not only have value for controlling plasma glucose and insulin excursions, but might also have a weight-controlling effect. Further investigation is needed and warranted.

Dietary supplementation with resistant starch has been shown to have the potential to improve insulin sensitivity. The mechanism of this effect is unknown.

In a study with healthy human volunteers, it was reported that a cereal-based evening meal containing RS was capable of improving glucose excursion and increased satiety after a subsequent standardized high GI breakfast. This is another demonstration of the "second meal effect." Among other things, the researchers concluded that it may be possible to tailor novel high-grain foods capable of facilitating glycemic regulation not only at the acute meal, but also at a meal ingested several hours afterwards. It was thought that the overall benefits to glucose control and satiety were probably mediated by mechanisms emanating from colonic fermentation of the resistant starch, and the researchers suggested that specific combinations of indigestible carbohydrates may prove to have even more potent prebiotic effects. Significantly, the benefits were associated with decreased levels of free fatty acids (FFA) and interleukin (IL)-6 and increased levels of GLP (glucagon-like peptide)-1 and adiponectin at the time of breakfast, suggesting a link between the gut microbial metabolism and key factors associated with insulin resistance.

In still another study, chronic feeding of rats with resistant starch compared to diets high in digestible starch, was reported to decrease postprandial lipogenesis in white adipose tissue (WAT) and to lead to reduced fat cell size. The mechanism of action of this effect is unclear.

PHARMACOKINETICS

Little digestion of resistant starch occurs in the stomach and small intestine following ingestion of RS, which is fermented in the colon by the colonic microflora to produce the short-chain fatty acids (SCFA) acetate, propionate and butyrate; the gases hydrogen, hydrogen sulfide, carbon dioxide and methane; and lactate, pyruvate and succinate. The major short-chain fatty acid produced is butyrate. Some acetate, propionate and butyrate is absorbed from the colon and transported by the circulation to various tissues where these SCFA undergo further metabolism. Much of these SCFA, especially butyrate, are metabolized by the colonocytes. Butyrate is an important respiratory fuel for the colonocytes.

Those with ileostomies may have a microbial population colonizing their ileums. In those cases, RS could be fermented by some of the bacteria much as they are in the colon.

INDICATIONS AND USAGE

A number of studies, mostly conducted *in vitro* and in animals, suggest that RS may be helpful in maintaining good colonic health. There is very preliminary evidence that RS might be helpful in preventing diabetes and obesity and that it might favorably modulate some lipids.

RESEARCH SUMMARY

That portion of dietary starch that eludes digestion in the small intestine and passes into the large bowel is called RS. A number of researchers have concluded that this is one of the most important components of dietary fiber in terms of health benefit. Fermentation of RS by microflora in the bowel gives rise to, among other things, SCFA, including butyrate, which has been shown in various *in vitro* and animal studies to protect against colon cancer by multiple mechanisms. It has demonstrated growth arrest, apoptosis and an ability to regulate proteins involved in cellular dedifferentiation in tumor cell lines. It inhibited preneoplastic lesions (aberrant crypt foci) in rats and pigs.

In one of these many animal experiments, pigs were fed a diet for 14 weeks high in either RS or digestible starch. The butyrate content of the proximal colon digesta was twofold higher in the RS-fed animals than in the digestible starch group. Indices of colonic health were generally significantly higher in the RS group, including reduced damage to colonocytes, improved mucosal integrity, and reduced colonic and systemic immune reactivity. The researchers concluded that RS might thus have significant health benefits in inflammatory conditions of the gut.

In another study, dietary RS supplementation exerted a protective effect against trinitrobenzene sulfonic acid-induced colitis in rats. Rats fed RS both before and after the induced colitis enjoyed reduced colonic permeability among other benefits. In a clinical study, 12 healthy men and 12 healthy women were given fiber supplements for two weeks. Those receiving the RS supplements exhibited significantly increased fecal butyrate levels and fecal bulk. The RS, however, did not produce better results than wheat bran or fiber supplements in terms of glycemic index and serum lipids.

However, in addition to increasing production of short-chain fatty acids, as discussed above, RS has also been observed, in some studies, to reduce plasma cholesterol levels, to increase caecal and large intestinal contents, to favorably alter microbial populations in the gut, to improve glucose tolerance, to lower inflammatory markers and to increase satiety, suggesting possible benefits (beyond promotion of colon health), including antiobesity, antiatherosclerotic and antidiabetic effects.

A number of *in vitro* and animal studies suggest that RS reduces fat cell size. In one of these studies, feeding RS to rats decreased postprandial lipogenesis in white adipose tissue at a level that encouraged the researchers to conclude that RS might have significant potential as an antiobesity agent. In a mouse study, dietary RS demonstrated effects on adipocyte and glucose metabolism, as well as on neuronal activity in hypothalamic regions associated with satiety, suggesting to the researchers, once again, that the substance might have potential as a weight control agent.

In a study of 10 healthy subjects supplemented with 30 grams of RS daily for one month, an effect consistent with improved insulin sensitivity was observed. Adding RS to the evening meals of another group of healthy human subjects resulted in improved glucose tolerance, reduced inflammatory markers and evidence of increased satiety.

All of these positive results need further investigation. One group of reviewers, while finding much that is promising in the RS research, have cautioned that some of the animal data may not "translate" at all well to humans. They point out, for example, that the rat may be particularly unsuitable as a model for testing the effects of RS in the bowel since the rat is a fecal refector. They also caution that there is far from sufficient data to conclude that RS can effectively substitute for dietary fiber derived from many cereal products; at most, currently, it should be regarded as a component of dietary fiber, not a substitute. They also conclude that it is very unlikely that RS has a significant effect on plasma cholesterol.

Nonetheless, some others have concluded that the evidence that has accumulated to date with respect to RS's probable impact on colonic health make it a good candidate to be added to wheat and other products as a functional food.

CONTRAINDICATIONS, PRECAUTIONS, ADVERSE REACTIONS

CONTRAINDICATIONS

Resistant-starch is contraindicated in those who are hypersensitive to these substances.

PRECAUTIONS

Those who develop gastrointestinal symptoms with the use of RS should exercise some caution in its use. Gastrointestinal side effects are unlikely with RS except at high doses. Those with irritable bowel syndrome should exercise caution in the use of RS and start with low doses and gradually work their way up to higher doses, as tolerated. Those receiving whole-body radiation or radiation to the gastrointestinal tract should avoid RS-containing products until the course of radiation treatments has been completed.

Those with gluten sensitivities should avoid wheat-based RS products.

ADVERSE REACTIONS

RS doses up to 25 grams daily or higher are usually well tolerated. Higher doses may cause gastrointestinal symptoms, including flatus, abdominal cramping and diarrhea. Some people are more sensitive to RS and may develop gastrointestinal symptoms at lower doses.

INTERACTIONS

No known interactions with drugs, nutritional supplements, foods or herbs.

OVERDOSAGE

No reports.

DOSAGE AND ADMINISTRATION

The typical daily consumption of dietary fiber by adult Americans is 14 grams a day. The typical consumption of RS by adult Americans ranges from 3 to 7 grams daily. This is much lower than doses recommended by the World Health Organization (WHO), the British Nutrition Foundation, the American Diabetes Association (ADA) and the Food and Nutrition Board (FNB) of the National Academy of Sciences (NAS) Research Council. In 2002, the FNB issued dietary reference intakes (DRIs) for dietary fiber. The recommendation for adult men was 38 grams daily and for adult women, 25 grams daily.

Including RS in ones' dietary fiber intake is an excellent way of reaching the desired goals, since RS can be incorporated into foods without significantly altering or compromising the neuroleptic quality of the foods. Adding RS to a smoothie is a good way to start.

RS is contained in certain foods (see list below), including green (unripe) bananas and navy beans, and in some functional foods. High amylose cornstarch flour is available (RS2) and can be added to soups, sauces, dietary supplements and smoothies. Digestion-resistant maltodextrins are also available and can be used to increase the dietary fiber content of practically any food, beverage or dietary supplement. Dosing is variable and ranges from 5 to 25 grams daily and sometimes higher. Those who use more than 25 grams daily should split the dosage throughout the day.

Foods with High Natural Resistant Starch Content

Food	Serving size	Amount of Resistant Starch (grams)**
Green (unripe) banana	one medium, peeled	4.7
Pearl barley	one-half cup, cooked	1.6
Cold pasta	one cup	1.9
Cold potato	one, 2' diameter, cooked	3.2
Lentils	one-half cup, cooked	2.5
Navy beans	one-half cup, cooked	9.8
Oatmeal	one cup, cooked	0.7
Wholegrain bread	two slices	0.5

** The amount of RS in various foods is variable. The amounts listed represent averages.

LITERATURE

Annison G, Topping DL. Nutritional role of resistant starch: chemical structure vs physiological function. *Annu Rev Nutr.* 1994;14:297-320.

Bauer-Marinovic M, Florian S, Müller-Schmehl K, et al. Dietary resistant starch type 3 prevents tumor induction by 1,2-dimethylhydrazine and alters proliferation, apoptosis and dedifferentiation in rat colon. *Carcinogenesis.* 2006;27(9):1849-1859.

Bird AR, Brown IL, Topping DL. Starches, resistant starches, the gut microflora and human health. *Curr Issues Intest Microbiol.* 2000;1(1):25-37.

Bird AR, Vuaran M, Brown I, et al. Two high-amylose maize starches with different amounts of resistant starch vary in their effects on fermentation, tissue and digesta mass accretion, and bacterial populations in the large bowel of pigs. *Br J Nutr.* 2007;97(1):134-144.

Brighenti F, Benini L, Del Rio D, et al. Colonic fermentation of indigestible carbohydrates contributes to the second-meal effect. *Am J Clin Nutr.* 2006;83(4):817-822.

Brouns F, Arrigoni E, Langkilde AM, et al. Physiological and metabolic properties of a digestion-resistant maltodextrin, classified as type 3 retrograded resistant starch. *J Agric Food Chem.* 2007;55(4):1574-1581.

Champ MM. Physiological aspects of resistant starch and in vivo measurements. *J AOAC Int.* 2004;87(3):749-755.

Chen L, Li X, Pang Y, Li L, et al. Resistant starch as a carrier for oral colon-targeting drug matrix system. *J Mater Sci Mater Med.* 2007;18(11):2199-2203.

de Deckere EA, Kloots WJ, van Amelsvoort JM. Resistant starch decreases serum total cholesterol and triacylglycerol concentrations in rats. *J Nutr.* 1993;123(12):2142-2151.

Englyst HN, Cummings JH. Digestion of the carbohydrates of banana (Musa paradisiaca sapientum) in the human small intestine. *Am J Clin Nutr.* 1986;44(1):42-50.

Englyst HN, Cummings JH. Digestion of the polysaccharides of some cereal foods in the human small intestine. *Am J Clin Nutr.* 1985;42(5):778-787.

Englyst HN, Trowell H, Southgate DA, et al. Dietary fiber and resistant starch. *Am J Clin Nutr.* 1987;46(6):873-874.

Grubben MJ, van den Braak CC, Essenberg M, et al. Effect of resistant starch on potential biomarkers for colonic cancer risk in patients with colonic adenomas: a controlled trial. *Dig Dis Sci.* 2001;46(4):750-756.

Han KH, Fukushima M, Shimizu K, et al. Resistant starches of beans reduce the serum cholesterol concentration in rats. *J Nutr Sci Vitaminol* (Tokyo). 2003;49(4):281-286.

Higgins JA, Brown MA, Storlien LH. Consumption of resistant starch decreases postprandial lipogenesis in white adipose tissue of the rat. *Nutr J.* 2006;5:25.

Iur'ev VP, Gapparov MM, Genkina NK, et al. [Resistant starches. Part 1. General description and physiologic aspects] [Article in Russian.] *Vopr Pitan.* 2005;74(6):11-16.

Iur'ev VP, Gapparov MM, Vasserman LA, et al. [Resistant starches. Part II. Physico-chemical and technological aspects solution medico-biological problems] [Article in Russian.] *Vopr Pitan.* 2006;75(1):3-9.

Jenkins DJ, Kendall CW. Resistant starches. *Curr Opin Gastroenterol.* 2000;16(2):178-183.

Jenkins DJ, Vuksan V, Kendall CW, et al. Physiological effects of resistant starches on fecal bulk, short chain fatty acids, blood lipids and glycemic index. *J Am Coll Nutr*. 1998;17(6):609-616.

Keenan MJ, Zhou J, McCutcheon KL, et al. Effects of resistant starch, a non-digestible fermentable fiber, on reducing body fat. *Obesity* (Silver Spring). 2006;14(9):1523-1534.

Kendall CW, Emam A, Augustin LS, et al. Resistant starches and health. *J AOAC Int*. 2004;87(3):769-774.

Kestell P, Zhu S, Ferguson LR. Mechanisms by which resistant starches and non-starch polysaccharide sources affect the metabolism and disposition of the food carcinogen, 2-amino-3-methylimidazo[4,5-f]quinoline. *J Chromatogr B Analyt Technol Biomed Life Sci*. 2004;802(1):201-210.

Le Leu RK, Brown IL, Hu Y, et al. A synbiotic combination of resistant starch and Bifidobacterium lactis facilitates apoptotic deletion of carcinogen-damaged cells in rat colon. *J Nutr*. 2005;135(5):996-1001.

Le Leu RK, Brown IL, Hu Y, et al. Effect of resistant starch on genotoxin-induced apoptosis, colonic epithelium, and lumenal contents in rats. *Carcinogenesis*. 2003;24(8):1347-1352.

Lesmes U, Beards EJ, Gibson GR, et al. Effects of Resistant Starch Type III Polymorphs on Human Colon Microbiota and Short Chain Fatty Acids in Human Gut Models. *J Agric Food Chem*. 2008;56(13):5415-5421

Liu R, Xu G. Effects of resistant starch on colonic preneoplastic aberrant crypt foci in rats. Food Chem Toxicol. *Food Chem Toxicol*. 2008;46(8):2672-2679.

Liu X, Ogawa H, Kishida T, et al. Hypolipidaemic effect of maize starch with different amylose content in ovariectomized rats depends on intake amount of resistant starch. *Br J Nutr*. June 2008:1-12. [Epub ahead of print]

Lopez-Rubio A, Flanagan BM, Shrestha AK, et al. Molecular Rearrangement Of Starch During In Vitro Digestion: Toward A Better Understanding Of Enzyme Resistant Starch Formation In Processed Starches. *Biomacromolecules*. 2008;9(7):1951-1958.

Mathers JC, Mickleburgh I, Chapman PC, et al. Concerted Action Polyp Prevention (CAPP) 1 Study. Can resistant starch and/or aspirin prevent the development of colonic neoplasia? The Concerted Action Polyp Prevention (CAPP) 1 Study. *Proc Nutr Soc*. 2003;62(1):51-57.

Suzuki T, Yoshida S, Hara H. Physiological concentrations of short-chain fatty acids immediately suppress colonic epithelial permeability. *Br J Nutr*. 2008;100(2):297-305.

Resveratrol

DESCRIPTION

Resveratrol is a naturally occurring phytoalexin produced by some higher plants in response to injury or fungal infection. Phytoalexins are chemical substances produced by plants as a defense against infection by pathogenic microorganisms, such as fungi. Alexin is from the Greek, meaning to ward off or to protect. Resveratrol may also have alexin-like activity for humans. Epidemiological, *in vitro* and animal studies suggest that a high resveratrol intake is associated with a reduced incidence of cardiovascular disease, and a reduced risk for cancer.

Resveratrol is found in grapevines (*Vitis vinifera* L). It occurs in the vines, roots, seeds and stalks, but its highest concentration is in grape skins. Wine also contains resveratrol. The concentration of resveratrol in red wine is much higher than that of white wine. The main difference between red and white wine production, besides the grapes used, is that for red wine the skins and seeds are involved in the process, while white wine is mainly prepared from the juice, essentially avoiding the use of grape skins and seeds. During the wine making process, resveratrol, as well as other polyphenols, including quercetin, catechins, gallocatechins, procyanidins and prodelphidins (condensed tannins), are extracted from the grape skins via a process called maceration.

Resveratrol, as well as the other polyphenols in wine, is thought to account in large part for the so-called French Paradox. The French Paradox—the finding that the rate of coronary heart disease mortality in France is lower than observed in other industrialized countries with a similar risk factor profile—has been attributed to frequent consumption of red wine.

In addition to grapes and wine, dietary sources of resveratrol include peanuts and mulberries. Resveratrol is also found in significant amounts in the dried roots and stems of the plant *Polygonium cuspidatum* Sieb. Et Zucc., also known as the Japanese knotweed. The dried root and stem of this plant is used in traditional Chinese and Japanese medicine as a circulatory tonic, among other things. This traditional Chinese and Japanese remedy is also known as Hu Zhang, Hu Chang, tiger cane, kojo-kon and hadori-kon. Most of the resveratrol-containing supplements which are marketed in the U.S. contain extracts of the root of *Polygonium cuspidatum*. Darakchasava, an ayurvedic herbal remedy, has as its principal ingredient *Vitis vinifera* L, and therefore, contains resveratrol. It is mainly used in ayurvedic medicine as a cardiotonic.

Resveratrol, which is also known as 3,4',5 trihydroxystilbene and 3,4',5-stilbenetriol, exists in *cis-* and *trans*-stereoisomeric forms. Resveratrol is the parent molecule of a family of polymers called viniferins. *Cis-* and *trans*-resveratrol occur naturally as do their glucosides. Resveratrol-3-O-beta-D-glucoside is also known as piceid, and the respective *cis-* and *trans*-glucosides are called *cis*-piceid and *trans*-piceid. The molecular formula of resveratrol is $C_{14}H_{12}O_3$ and its molecular weight is 228.25 daltons. It is represented by the following structural formula:

Resveratrol

The stereoisomer of resveratrol found in grapes and peanuts is the *trans*-form. Both *cis*- and *trans*-resveratrol are found in *Polygonium cuspidatum*. Therefore, dietary supplements containing resveratrol, which are principally derived from this plant, contain both stereoisomers. The amount of resveratrol (*trans*-resveratrol) in peanuts ranges from 0.02 to 1.79 micrograms per gram. Red wine contains from 0.6 to 0.8 micrograms per milliliter, and fresh grape skin, approximately 50 to 100 micrograms per gram. A glass of red wine delivers on the average, between 600 to 700 micrograms of resveratrol.

ACTIONS AND PHARMACOLOGY

ACTIONS

Resveratrol may have cardioprotective and antiproliferative actions.

MECHANISM OF ACTION

Resveratrol has several activities that may account for its possible cardioprotective action. These include inhibition of the oxidation of low-density lipoprotein (LDL), inhibition of smooth muscle cell proliferation and inhibition of platelet aggregation. Resveratrol has also been found to reduce the synthesis of lipids in rat liver and to inhibit the production of proatherogenic eicosanoids by human platelets and neutrophils.

Resveratrol's antioxidant activity may play an important role in its possible cardioprotective action. Above, was mentioned its ability to inhibit the oxidation of LDL. Resveratrol also has been found to exert a strong inhibitory effect on superoxide anion and hydrogen peroxide production by macrophages stimulated by lipopolysaccharides or phorbol esters. It also has been demonstrated to decrease arachidonic acid release induced by lipopolysaccharides or phorbol esters, or by exposure to superoxide or hydrogen peroxide. It has hydroxyl-radical scavenging activity and has recently been found to possess glutathione-sparing activity.

In a rat study of the effect of resveratrol on ischemia-reperfusion, it was found that the substance had a dramatic effect against ischemia-reperfusion-induced arrhythmias and mortality. Resveratrol pretreatment both reduced the incidence and duration of ventricular dysrhythmias, including ventricular tachycardia and ventricular fibrillation. Resveratrol pretreatment also increased nitric oxide and decreased lactate dehydrogenase levels in the carotid blood. In this example, the cardioprotective effect of resveratrol may be correlated with its antioxidant activity, upregulation of nitric oxide synthesis and protection against endothelial dysfunction.

Resveratrol's possible phytoestrogenic activity may also contribute to its possible cardioprotective action. Resveratrol appears to act as a mixed agonist/antagonist for estrogen receptors alpha and beta. It has been found to bind estrogen receptor beta and estrogen receptor alpha with comparable affinity but with 7,000-fold lower affinity than estradiol. Resveratrol differs from other phytoestrogens, which bind estrogen receptor beta with higher affinity than they bind estrogen receptor alpha. Resveratrol also shows estradiol antagonistic behavior for estrogen receptor alpha with some estrogen receptors. It does not show estradiol antagonistic activity with estrogen receptor beta.

Resveratrol's possible antiproliferative activity also may be accounted for in several different ways. Resveratrol's antioxidant activity was discussed above. It also has antimutagenic activity, as illustrated by its dose-dependent inhibition of the mutagenic response induced by treatment of *Salmonella typhimurium* strain TM677 with 7,12-dimethyl-benz(*a*)anthracene (DMBA). Resveratrol has been found to inhibit cellular events associated with tumor initiation, promotion and progression. It has been found to inhibit cyclooxygenase (COX) activities in different cancer models, suggesting an effect at the level of tumor promotion. It has also been found to reverse tumor-promoter-induced inhibition of gap-junctional intracellular communication in rat epithelial cells. Inhibition of gap-junctional intracellular communication is an important mechanism of tumor promotion.

Resveratrol has demonstrated inhibition of growth of several cancer cell lines and tumors, suggesting that it has an inhibitory effect on cancer promotion/progression. It has been found to inhibit ribonucleotide reductase, DNA polymerase, the transcription of COX-2 in human mammary epithelial cells and the activity of ornithine decarboxylase. Ornithine decarboxylase is a key enzyme of polyamine biosynthesis, which is enhanced in tumor growth.

Resveratrol has also been found to induce phase II metabolizing enzymes which are involved in the detoxification of carcinogens, to upregulate apoptosis, to inhibit the progression of cancer by inducing cell differentiation and to inhibit protein kinase D and possibly protein kinase C. Recently, resveratrol has been shown to inhibit both NF-kappaB activation and NF-kappaB-dependent gene expression via its ability to inhibit IkappaB kinase activity, the key regulator of NF-kappaB activation. This appears to upregulate apoptosis.

It is clear that resveratrol has a wide range of activities that may account for its possible antiproliferative action. It is also clear that the mechanism of this possible action is far from being understood.

PHARMACOKINETICS
From animal studies and from limited human studies, it appears that resveratrol is absorbed from the gastrointestinal tract following its ingestion. However, the efficiency of its absorption, as well as its distribution, metabolism and excretion, are not well understood. Much research needs to be done in order to elucidate the pharmacokinetics of resveratrol in its various forms.

INDICATIONS AND USAGE
Resveratrol, a naturally occurring phytoalexin found in grape skins and wine, as well as some other sources, made a splash in the media when some researchers suggested that it might be a genuine antiaging substance. While some animal data are suggestive of an antiaging effect, there is no evidence for the safe or effective use of resveratrol in humans for this purpose.

Epidemiological, *in vitro* and animal studies suggest that resveratrol has anti-atherosclerotic activity and that it might have some immune-stimulating and anti-cancer effects. Human studies are few in number and inconclusive due to short duration and poor design.

RESEARCH SUMMARY
A few years ago, researchers reported that resveratrol significantly extended the lifespan of a yeast. One of the same research groups subsequently reported that it also prolonged the lifespan of a worm (*Caenorhabditis elegans*) and the fruit fly (*Drosophilia melanogaster*). More recently, another group failed to consistently reproduce these results in either the fruit fly or the worm. An Italian group reported extended lifespan in a short-lived fish (*Northobranchius furzeri*), which it attributed to resveratrol. Also, more recently, one of the same groups that made the original reports stated that mice fed 22 mg/kg resveratrol daily had lower death rates whether fed a standard diet or a high-fat diet. Another group using an even higher dose of resveratrol reported that the supplementation helped the animals control weight and increase physical endurance. Suddenly the media were broadcasting stories of a "miracle" substance that might allow the sedentary to eat whatever they wanted and still lose weight and extend lifespan. Some hoped that drinking copious amounts of wine alone might help confer these putative benefits.

Scientists quickly pointed out that one would have to imbibe hundreds of glasses of wine per day to approach the doses used in these preliminary animal studies—or take fistfuls of resveratrol pills daily at a cost of many thousands of dollars per year and at considerable risk of significant toxicity. Far more research will be required in order for these findings to be validated, even in animals. At present there is no evidence whatsoever that resveratrol can replicate any of the reported benefits in humans or that it is safe to take in equivalent doses. Nonetheless, the research is worthy of follow-up and extension. There is some indication that resveratrol may at least partially mimic some of the effects of caloric restriction, which has been shown to retard aging in some animals. There are reports that it activates a gene (known as SIRT1 in humans) that some say controls factors capable of prolonging cell life through favorable effects on metabolism, increased mitochondrial biogenesis and other modes of action that make for a more efficient and "cleaner burning" organism. Others dispute that resveratrol has meaningful, consistent effects on SIRT1 in humans or on the equivalent gene in other animals—or even that the functions of SIRT1 are well understood in humans.

In one of the most recent positive reports, researchers stated that resveratrol induced gene expression patterns in multiple tissues in mice that they say parallel some of those induced by caloric restriction. They reported reduced albuminuria, decreased inflammation, decreased apoptosis in vascular endothelium, increased aortic elasticity, greater motor coordination, reduced cataract formation and preserved bone mineral density in mice supplemented with resveratrol. Despite all this, however, mice fed a standard diet did not live longer when treated with resveratrol beginning at 12 months of age (midlife). Even some of those most involved in the current resveratrol research acknowledge that it may not be possible to find a caloric restriction mimetic, whether resveratrol or some other agent, that is efficacious and safe for long-term consumption. In the animal work to date, many of the benefits seen in caloric restriction work are not mimicked by the use of resveratrol, and the dosages that have generally been used in the animal resveratrol work may far exceed what humans could safely tolerate. Possible estrogenic effects of resveratrol, among other things, could pose peril. Mortality has been very high in rats and mice administered very high dosages of resveratrol. Even if resveratrol itself does not turn out to be a useful antiaging substance, it is possible that new drugs will be developed that utilize the SIRT1 pathway. Research is ongoing.

There has been a suggestion from epidemiological data for some time that moderate consumption of red wine is associated with a reduced incidence of mortality and morbidity from coronary heart disease. *In vitro* and animal work has strongly suggested that resveratrol and other polyphenols found in grapes and wines are at least partially responsible for often-observed anti-platelet aggregating anti-inflammatory and anti-oxidant effects.

Red wine has been shown, in some experiments, to be more effective than other alcoholic beverages in decreasing some of the risk factors of coronary heart disease. Compared, in one study, with ethanol, resveratrol had superior anti-platelet-aggregation effects; it was superior in this respect, as well, to catechin, epicatechin, alpha-tocopherol, hydroquinone and butylated hydroxytoluene. Resveratrol also inhibited the synthesis of thromboxane B2 and hydroxyheptadecatrienoate from arachidonate in a dose-dependent manner.

Other studies, in animals and *in vitro*, have shown that resveratrol can inhibit the oxidation of LDL-cholesterol and, more recently, that it can reduce smooth-muscle-cell proliferation, believed to be one of the requisites of atherogenesis, by 70-90%, in a dose-dependent pattern. Red wine extract and resveratrol have shown equally significant cardioprotective effects in animal models of myocardial ischemic reperfusion injury.

Additional evidence suggests that resveratrol also has estrogenic effects that may also provide cardiovascular protection. Bearing a structural resemblance to diethylstilbestrol, *trans*-resveratrol is a phytoestrogen found to have variable degrees of estrogen-receptor agonisms in different test systems.

The clinical data that would confirm or refute the relevance of these findings are largely lacking. In one small, short-term study, 24 healthy human subjects aged 26-45 consumed red wine, white wine, commercial grape juice and the same grape juice fortified with resveratrol over periods of 4 weeks. Results were mixed and conflicting, suggesting some positive benefit from resveratrol while also suggesting lack of activity in other measures related to coronary heart disease. The researchers themselves acknowledged multiple weaknesses in their study design. Further, better-controlled, longer-term studies are needed to determine whether red wine, high-resveratrol grape juice, or resveratrol supplements are efficacious in preventing atherosclerosis or in ameliorating it once it is present.

More preliminary yet are findings of some resveratrol-related anti-cancer and immune-stimulating effects. In a number of mostly *in vitro* studies, resveratrol has demonstrated an ability to inhibit tumor initiation, promotion and progression. Some of its antiproliferative activity is attributed to its observed ability to inhibit ribonucleotide reductase and DNA synthesis in mammalian cells. It has been shown to induce apoptotic cell death in human leukemia cell lines, as well as in some breast carcinoma cells.

Its antiestrogenic activity is also believed to play a role in its inhibition of human breast cancer cells *in vitro*. A partial estrogen-receptor agonist itself, resveratrol is believed by some researchers to be an estrogen-receptor antagonist in the presence of estrogen, resulting in breast cancer inhibition.

Resveratrol has shown activity against herpes simplex virus types 1 and 2 in a dose-dependent manner. It appears to disrupt a critical early event in the viral reproduction cycle. More research is needed.

Claims that resveratrol can help control weight are unproved, but some recent research is suggestive of possible favorable resveratrol effects on adipocytes. In an *in vitro* study both curcumin and resveratrol significantly reduced cytokine expression in adipocytes, suggesting that they might be of benefit in reducing some of the chronic inflammatory processes that originate in adipocytes.

CONTRAINDICATIONS, PRECAUTIONS, ADVERSE REACTIONS

CONTRAINDICATIONS

Resveratrol is contraindicated in those hypersensitive to any component of a resveratrol-containing product.

PRECAUTIONS

Pregnant women and nursing mothers should avoid the use of resveratrol-containing supplements. They should also avoid the use of wine as a resveratrol source. Purple grape juice is a good and safe source of resveratrol, as well as other polyphenolic antioxidants.

DOSAGE AND ADMINISTRATION

Resveratrol, marketed as a nutritional supplement, is typically an extract of *Polygonum cuspidatum* (see Description). Such an extract contains both *cis*- and *trans*-resveratrol. The extracts are usually standardized to deliver about 8% resveratrol in its various forms. Many of the products currently marketed have resveratrol in combination with other phytonutrients and vitamins. Some supplements deliver 16 milligrams per serving or higher. There is no typical dosage. Functional food products containing resveratrol are being developed.

LITERATURE

Aubin MC, Lajoie C, Clément R, et al. Female rats fed a high-fat diet were associated with vascular dysfunction and cardiac fibrosis in the absence of overt obesity and hyperlipidemia: therapeutic potential of resveratrol. *J Pharmacol Exp Ther.* 2008;325(3):961-968.

Barger JL, Kayo T, Vann JM, et al. A low dose of dietary resveratrol partially mimics caloric restriction and retards aging parameters in mice. *PLoS ONE.* 2008;3(6):e2264.

Baur JA, Pearson KJ, Price NL, et al. Resveratrol improves health and survival of mice on a high-calorie diet. *Nature*. 2006;444(7117):337-342.

Baur JA, Sinclair DA. Therapeutic potential of resveratrol: the in vivo evidence. *Nat Rev Drug Discov*. 2006;5(6):493-506.

Bowers JL, Tyulmenkov VV, Jernigan SC, Klinge CM. Resveratrol acts as a mixed agonist/antagonist for estrogen receptors alpha and beta. *Endocrinology*. 2000;141:3657-3667.

Burkitt MJ, Duncan J. Effects of *trans*-resveratrol on copper-dependent hydroxyl-radical formation and DNA damage: Evidence for hydroxyl-radical scavenging and a novel. Glutathione-sparing mechanism of action. *Arch Biochem Biophys*. 2000;381:253-263.

Cao G, Prior RL. Red wine in moderation: Potential health benefits independent of alcohol. *Nutr Clin Care*. 2000;3:76-82.

Chun YJ, Kim MY, Guengerich FP. Resveratrol is a selective human cytochrome P450 1A1 inhibitor. *Biochem Biophys Res Commun*. 1999;262:20-24.

Cichewicz RH, Kouzi SA, Hamann MT. Dimerization of resveratrol by the grapevine pathogen. *Botrytis cinerea. J Natl Prod*. 2000;63:29-33.

Ciolino HP, Yeh GC. Inhibition of aryl hydrocarbon-induced cytochrome P450 1A1 enzyme activity and CYP1A1 expression by resveratrol. *Mol Pharmacol*. 1999;56:760-767.

Dasgupta B, Milbrandt J. Resveratrol stimulates AMP kinase activity in neurons. *Proc Natl Acad Sci USA*. 2007;104(17):7217-7222.

Doherty JJ, Fu MM, Stiffer BS, et al. Resveratrol inhibition of herpes simplex virus replication. *Antiviral Res*. 1999;43:145-155.

Donnelly LE, Newton R, Kennedy GE, et al. Anti-inflammatory effects of resveratrol in lung epithelial cells: molecular mechanisms. *Am J Physiol Lung Cell Mol Physiol*. 2004;287(4):L774-783.

dos Santos AQ, Nardin P, Funchal C, et al. Resveratrol increases glutamate uptake and glutamine synthetase activity in C6 glioma cells. *Arch Biochem Biophys*. 2006;453(2):161-167.

Dubash BD, Zheng BL, Kim CH, et al. Inhibitory effect of resveratrol and related compounds on the macromolecular synthesis in HL-60 cells and the metabolism of 7,12-dimethylbenz[a]anthracene by mouse liver microsomes. In: Shahidi F, Ho C-T, eds. *Phytochemicals and Phytopharmaceuticals*. Champaign, IL: AOCS Press; 2000;314-320.

Fontecave M, Lepoivre M, Elleingand E, et al. Resveratrol, a remarkable inhibitor of ribonucleotide reductase. *FEBS Lett*. 1998;421:277-279.

Frémont L. Biological effects of resveratrol. *Life Sci*. 2000;66:663-673.

Frémont L, Belguendouz L, Delpal S. Antioxidant activity of resveratrol and alcohol-free wine polyphenols related to LDL oxidation and polyunsaturated fatty acids. *Life Sci*. 1999;64:2511-2521.

Gehm BD, McAndrews JM, Chien P-Y, Jameson JL. Resveratrol, a polyphenolic compound found in grapes and wine, is an agonist for the estrogen receptor. *Proc Natl Acad Sci USA*. 1997;94:14138-14143.

Gonzales AM, Orlando RA. Curcumin and resveratrol inhibit nuclear factor-kappaB-mediated cytokine expression in adipocytes. *Nutr Metab* (Lond). 2008;5:17.

Holme AL, Pervaiz S. Resveratrol in cell fate decisions. *J Bioenerg Biomembr*. 2007;39(1):59-63.

Holmes-McNary M, Baldwin AS Jr. Chemopreventive properties of trans-resveratrol are associated with inhibition of activation of the IkappaB kinase. *Cancer Res*. 2000;60:3477-3483.

Hsieh TC, Juan G, Darzynkiewicz Z, Wu JM. Resveratrol increases nitric oxide synthase, induces accumulation of p53 and p21 (WAF1/CIP1), and suppresses cultured bovine pulmonary artery endothelial cell proliferation by perturbing progression through S and G2. *Cancer Res*. 1999;59:2596-2601.

Hung L-M, Chen J-K, Huang S-S, et al. Cardioprotective effect of resveratrol, a natural antioxidant derived from grapes. *Cardiovascular Res*. 2000;47:549-555.

Jang M, Cai L, Udeani GO, et al. Cancer chemopreventive activity of resveratrol, a natural product derived from grapes. *Science*. 1997;275:218-220.

Jang M, Pezzuto JM. Cancer chemopreventive activity of resveratrol. *Drugs Exp Clin Res*. 1999;25:65-77.

Kirk RI, Deitch JA, Wu JM, Lerea KM. Resveratrol decreases early signaling events in washed platelets but has little effect on platelet aggregation in whole blood. *Blood Cells Mol Dis*. 2000;26:144-150.

Koo SH, Montminy M. In vino veritas: a tale of two sirt1s? *Cell*. 2006;127(6):1091-1093.

Lagouge M, Argmann C, Gerhart-Hines Z, et al. Resveratrol improves mitochondrial function and protects against metabolic disease by activating SIRT1 and PGC-1alpha. *Cell*. 2006;127(6):1109-1122.

Lin HY, Sun M, Tang HY, et al. Resveratrol causes COX-2- and p53-dependent apoptosis in head and neck squamous cell cancer cells. *J Cell Biochem*. 2008;104(6):2131-2142.

Lu KT, Chiou RY, Chen LG, et al. Neuroprotective effects of resveratrol on cerebral ischemia-induced neuron loss mediated by free radical scavenging and cerebral blood flow elevation. *J Agric Food Chem*. 2006;54(8):3126-3131.

Marambaud P, Zhao H, Davies P. Resveratrol promotes clearance of Alzheimer's disease amyloid-beta peptides. *J Biol Chem*. 2005;280(45):37377-37382.

Martinez J, Moreno JJ. Effect of resveratrol, a natural polyphenolic compound, on reactive oxygen species and prostaglandin production. *Biochem Pharmacol*. 2000;59:865-870.

Nielsen M, Ruch RJ, Vang O. Resveratrol reverses tumor-promoter-induced inhibition of gap-junctional intercellular communication. *Biochem Biophys Res Commun*. 2000;275:804-809.

Orallo F. Comparative studies of the antioxidant effects of cis- and trans-resveratrol. *Curr Med Chem.* 2006;13(1):87-98.

Pace-Asciak CR, Hahn S, Diamandis EP, et al. The red wine phenolics trans-resveratrol and quercetin block human platelet aggregation and eicosanoid synthesis: implications for protection against coronary heart disease. *Clin Chim Acta.* 1995;235:207-219.

Palamara AT, Nencioni L, Aquilano K, et al. Inhibition of influenza A virus replication by resveratrol. *J Infect Dis.* 2005;191(10):1719-1729.

Paul B, Masih I, Deopujari J, Charpentier C. Occurrence of resveratrol and pterostilbene in age-old darakchasava, an ayurvedic medicine from India. *J Ethnopharmacol.* 1999;68:71-76.

Pearson KJ, Baur JA, Lewis KN, et al. Resveratrol delays age-related deterioration and mimics transcriptional aspects of dietary restriction without extending life span. *Cell Metab.* 2008;8(2):157-168.

Pinto MC, García-Barrado JA, Macías P. Resveratrol is a potent inhibitor of the dioxygenase activity of lipoxygenase. *J Agric Food Chem.* 1999;47:4842-4846.

Prokop J, Abrman P, Seligson AL, et al. Resveratrol and its glycon piceid are stable polyphenols. *J Med Food.* 2006;9(1):11-14.

Raval AP, Lin HW, Dave KR, Defazio RA, Della Morte D, Kim EJ, Perez-Pinzon MA. Resveratrol and ischemic preconditioning in the brain. *Curr Med Chem.* 2008;15(15):1545-1551.

Ray PS, Maulik G, Cordis GA, et al. The red wine antioxidant resveratrol protects isolated rat hearts from ischemia reperfusion injury. *Free Rad Biol Med.* 1999;27:160-169.

Sanders TH, McMichael RW Jr, Hendrix KW. Occurrence of resveratrol in edible peanuts. *J Agric Food Chem.* 2000;48:1243-1246.

Schneider Y, Vincent F, Duranton B, et al. Anti-proliferative effect of resveratrol, a natural component of grapes and wine, on human colonic cancer cells. *Cancer Lett.* 2000;158:85-91.

Seeni A, Takahashi S, Takeshita K, et al. Suppression of Prostate Cancer Growth by Resveratrol in The Transgenic Rat for Adenocarcinoma of Prostate (TRAP) Model. *Asian Pac J Cancer Prev.* 2008;9(1):7-14.

Soleas GJ, Diamandis EP, Goldberg DM. Resveratrol: A molecule whose time has come? And gone? *Clin Biochem.* 1997;30:91-113.

Sovak M. Grape Extract, Resveratrol, and Its Analogs: A Review. *J Med Food.* 2001;4(2):93-105.

Stewart JR, Christman KL, O'Brian CA. Effects of resveratrol on the autophosphorylation of phorbol ester-responsive protein kinases. *Biochem Pharmacol.* 2000;60:1355-1359.

Subbaramaiah K, Chung WJ, Michaluart P, et al. Resveratrol inhibits cyclooxygenase-2 transcription and activity in phorbol ester-treated human mammary epithelial cells. *J Biol Chem.* 1998;273:21875-21882.

Subbaramaiah K, Michaluart P, Chung WJ, et al. Resveratrol inhibits cyclooxygenase-2 transcription in human mammary epithelial cells. *Ann NY Acad Sci.* 2000;889:214-223.

Tang FY, Chiang EP, Sun YC. Resveratrol inhibits heregulin-beta1-mediated matrix metalloproteinase-9 expression and cell invasion in human breast cancer cells. *J Nutr Biochem.* 2008;19(5):287-294.

Tang FY, Su YC, Chen NC, et al. Resveratrol inhibits migration and invasion of human breast-cancer cells. *Mol Nutr Food Res.* 2008;52(6):683-691.

Tang W, Eisenbrand G. *Chinese Drugs of Plant Origin.* Berlin: Springer-Verlag: 1992;787-791.

Tessitore L, Davit A, Sarotto I, Caderni G. Resveratrol depresses the growth of colorectal aberrant crypt foci by affecting *bax* and *p21*$_{CIP}$ expression. *Carcinogenesis.* 2000;21:1619-1622.

Tomera JF. Current knowledge of the health benefits and disadvantages of wine consumption. *Trends Food Sci Technol.* 1999;10:129-138.

Tsai SH, Lin-Shiau SY, Lin JK. Suppression of nitric oxide synthase and the down-regulation of the activation of NFkappaB in macrophages by resveratrol. *Br J Pharmacol.* 1999;126:673-680.

Zou J, Huang Y, Chen Q, et al. Suppression of mitogenesis and regulation of cell cycle traverse by resveratrol in cultured smooth muscle cells. *Int J Oncol.* 1999;15:647-651.

Riboflavin (Vitamin B2)

DESCRIPTION

Riboflavin or vitamin B$_2$ is an essential nutrient in human nutrition and plays a key role in the production of energy. It is the precursor of flavin mononucleotide (FMN, riboflavin monophosphate) and flavin adenine dinucleotide (FAD). FMN and FAD serve as cofactors for a family of proteins called flavoenzymes. Flavoenzymes catalyze a wide range of biochemical reactions, typically of the redox type. They are key elements in cellular respiration, among other things. In cellular respiration, FAD and FMN act as intermediate hydrogen acceptors in the mitochondrial electron transport chain, accepting hydrogens derived from foodstuffs, and passing on electrons to the cytochrome system. During this process, cellular energy is produced. Recent research suggests that riboflavin may be effective in the prophylaxis of migraine headaches in some with altered cerebral bioenergetics.

Riboflavin deficiency or ariboflavinosis was originally known as *pellagra sin pellagra*. The most common cause of riboflavin deficiency is dietary inadequacy, which occurs in those who do not consume rich dietary sources of the vitamin, such as organ meats, eggs, milk, cheese, yogurt, leafy green vegetables and whole grains. Deficiency of the vitamin can occur in the elderly subsisting on tea or coffee, toast and cookies. Riboflavin deficiency also occurs in those with chronic liver disease, chronic alcoholics and those who receive total parenteral nutrition (TPN) with inadequate riboflavin. Marginal riboflavin deficiency, in the context of nucleoside analog antiretroviral therapy, has been known to cause severe lactic acidosis.

The signs and symptoms of riboflavin deficiency include, cheilosis (fissuring of the vermilion surfaces of the lips), angular stomatitis, glossitis (magenta tongue), seborrheic dermatitis (particularly affecting the scrotum or labia majora and the nasolabial folds), sore throat, hyperemia and edema of the pharyngeal and oral mucous membranes and a normochromic, normocytic anemia associated with pure erythrocyte cytoplasia of the bone marrow. Isolated riboflavin deficiency is rare. Typically, riboflavin deficiency is accompanied by deficiency of other vitamins and other nutrients. Futher, the skin and mucosal signs of riboflavin deficiency may be difficult to interpret in the elderly. Esophageal lesions in the Turkoman people of Iran have been related to chronic riboflavin deficiency, and the greater incidence of esophageal cancer in this group has created interest in the relationship between esophageal cancer and riboflavin deficiency.

Riboflavin, in addition to being known as vitamin B$_2$, is also known as riboflavine, 7, 8-dimethyl-10- (1^1-D-ribityl)isoalloxazine, 7, 8-dimethyl-10- (D-ribo-2, 3, 4, 5-tetrahydroxypentyl)isoalloxazine and 7, 8-dimethyl-10-ribitylisoalloxazine. Its molecular formula is C$_{17}$H$_{20}$N$_4$O$_6$ and its molecular weight is 376.4 daltons. It has the following structure:

Riboflavin

Riboflavin is an orange powder, and water solutions have intense greenish yellow fluorescence. The 5^1-hydroxymethyl group of the ribityl side chain of riboflavin is metabolized in the body to form the coenzyme flavin mononucleotide or FMN. FMN is also known as riboflavin monophosphate, riboflavin-5^1-phosphate and riboflavin-5^1-(dihydrogen phosphate). FMN is metabolized in the body to form flavin adenine dinucleotide (FAD).

ACTIONS AND PHARMACOLOGY

ACTIONS

Riboflavin has antioxidant activity. It may have activity in the prophylaxis of migraine headaches and may have activity against esophageal cancer. It has putative anti-atherosclerotic activity and putative antimalarial activity.

MECHANISM OF ACTION

The antioxidant activity of riboflavin is principally derived from its role as a precursor of FAD and the role of this cofactor in the production of the antioxidant reduced glutathione. Reduced glutathione is the cofactor of the selenium-containing glutathione peroxidases (see Selenium), among other things. The glutathione peroxidases are major antioxidant enzymes. Reduced glutathione is generated by the FAD-containing enzyme glutathione reductase. Riboflavin deficiency is reported to be associated with compromised oxidant defense resulting in increased lipid peroxidation. Increased lipid peroxidation under conditions of riboflavin deficiency may be accounted for, in large part, by decreased regeneration of reduced glutathione which is necessary for the function of the antioxidant glutathione peroxidases. Riboflavin deficiency may also affect the mitochondrial pool of reduced glutathione which in turn may affect the activities of the flavoenzymes NADPH-cytochrome P450 reductase and NADPH-cytochrome b reductase. Elevated riboflavin levels have been reported to provide protection against oxidative forms of hemeproteins. Oxidative forms of hemeproteins have been implicated in reperfusion injury. Riboflavin has also been shown to protect against reperfusion injury in isolated rabbit hearts. The protection by riboflavin against oxidative damage caused by oxidized forms of hemeproteins may be mediated by an NADPH-dependent methemoglobin reductase which is also known as flavin reductase. In this case, riboflavin itself appears to act as an antioxidant via its conversion to dihydroriboflavin. Riboflavin has been found to protect the lungs, brain and heart from cellular oxidative injury, The protection has been proposed to be mediated through flavin reductase. It has been demonstrated that higher oxidation states of hemeproteins are rapidly reduced by dihydroriboflavin.

High-dose riboflavin has recently been demonstrated to be effective in the prophylaxis of migraine headaches in some. The rationale for studying riboflavin for migraine prophylaxis came from the findings, in migraine sufferers, of a decreased mitochondrial phosphorylation potential between migraine attacks. This indicates that those with a history of migraines have decreased brain mitochondrial energy reserve between attacks. The studies were conducted using ^{31}P-NMR spectroscopy. Riboflavin is the precursor of flavin adenine mononucleotide (FMN) and flavin adenine dinucleotide (FAD), which are required for the activity of flavoenzymes involved in the electron transport chain and in the production of cellular energy. Riboflavin's effect on cerebral bioenergetics is a possible mechanism of riboflavin's antimigraine activity. There are most likely other mechanisms at work, as well.

Riboflavin deficiency has been associated with an increased incidence of esophageal cancer in certain parts of the world. Riboflavin supplementation has been found to reduce the prevalence of micronuclei in esophageal cells in a study performed in Huixan, People's Republic of China. Micronuclei are considered precancerous lesions. People living in this region have a high risk of esophageal cancer and poor riboflavin status. It remains unclear, however, whether riboflavin supplementation can decrease the incidence of esophageal cancer. The mechanism of the possible anticarcinogenic activity of riboflavin is also unclear. Riboflavin deficiency has been found to enhance the carcinogenicity of certain xenobiotics, such as azo dyes. The azo dyes are inactivated by a microsomal hydroxylase enzyme system that uses FAD. Riboflavin, as FAD, plays a key role in glutathione metabolism (see above). Glutathione is involved in the detoxification of xenobiotic substances. Riboflavin is also important for the maintenance of epithelial integrity.

The putative anti-atherosclerotic activity of riboflavin may be accounted for, in part, by its role in the metabolism of homocysteine. Elevated serum homocysteine is considered to be an independent risk factor for coronary heart disease. Vitamin B_6, folate and vitamin B_{12} are involved in the metabolism of homocysteine. The riboflavin metabolites FMN and FAD serve as cofactors for enzymes involved in the metabolism of vitamin B_6, folate and vitamin B_{12}. FMN serves as a cofactor for pyridoxine-5^1-phosphate oxidase, which is important for the formation of the active form of vitamin B_6, pyridoxal-5^1 - phosphate. FAD is a cofactor for methylenetetrahydrofolate reductase, which is important for the formation of 5-methyltetrahydrofolate. FMN and FAD are involved in vitamin B_{12} metabolism and serve as cofactors for methionine synthase reductase. Studies on riboflavin deficient subjects are needed to evaluate the usefulness of riboflavin supplementation in hyperhomocysteinemia. Riboflavin may also have anti-atherosclerotic activity secondary to its antioxidant action. Riboflavin, in the form of FAD, is necessary for the formation of reduced glutathione via the FAD-containing enzyme glutathione reductase. Glutathione is the cofactor of the glutathione peroxidases, antioxidant enzymes which protect against lipid peroxidation and oxidation of low-density lipoprotein (LDL).

Oxidized-LDL is thought to be a key etiological factor in the pathophysiology of atherosclerosis.

Recently, riboflavin has been demonstrated to have antimalarial activity. The malarial parasite ingests a significant proportion of host cell hemoglobin in an acidic organelle called the food vacuole. The acidic pH of the food vacuole is favorable to the oxidation of hemoglobin to methemoglobin. The malarial parasite also digests hemoglobin and polymerizes the released free heme into hemozoin, also in the food vacuole. It has recently been shown that treatment of erythrocytes infected with *Plasmodium falciparum* with riboflavin decreased the production of methemoglobin and hemozoin, decreased the size of the food vacuole and inhibited asexual parasite growth in cultures. It is thought that the mechanism of the possible antimalarial action of riboflavin is via its acting as a substrate for the enzyme NADPH-methemoglobin reductase. During this reaction, methemoglobin is reduced while riboflavin is oxided to dihydroriboflavin. Thus, riboflavin acts as a reducing agent. Reduction of methemoglobin is correlated with inhibition of hemazoin formation and food vacuole development and arrest of asexual development to schizogony. It is thought that the reduction of methemoglobin plays a role in limiting the amount of hemoglobin which is available to the malarial parasite for further processing. The effects of riboflavin in this recent research differ from earlier studies showing that riboflavin deficiency has an antimalarial effect. The mechanism of antimalarial activity of riboflavin deficiency may be accounted for by a decrease in the activity of reductive enzymes, such as riboflavin reductase, which require riboflavin as a cofactor. This decreased activity lowers glutathione levels. This results in increased oxidative stress and lipid peroxidation, conditions detrimental to the malarial parasite. The use of high-dose riboflavin as an antimalarial strategy appears more attractive than that of causing riboflavin deficiency to treat malaria. Riboflavin deficiency may not only be detrimental to the malarial parasite, but can be detrimental to the host, as well. Continued research in this most important area is warranted and needed to determine, among other things, which approach—riboflavin treatment or riboflavin deficiency—should be the one to pursue regarding a possible new treatment of malaria.

PHARMACOKINETICS

In food, riboflavin is found mainly in the form of flavin mononucleotide (FMN, riboflavin-5^1-phosphate) and flavin adenine dinucleotide (FAD). Riboflavin is used for food fortification. Riboflavin and riboflavin-5^1 -phosphate are the principal nutritional supplement forms of riboflavin, with riboflavin being the major form. Coenzyme forms of riboflavin (FAD, FMN) that are not covalently bound to proteins are released from proteins in the acid environment of the stomach. Covalently bound forms or riboflavin (e.g., in mitochondrial succinate dehydrogenase) are released from the proteins they are bound to following proteolysis. FAD and FMN are converted to riboflavin in the small intestine via the action of pyrophosphatase and phosphatase, respectively. Riboflavin is mainly absorbed in the proximal small intestine by a saturable transport system. The rate of absorption increases when riboflavin is ingested with food. The presence of bile salts appears to facilitate absorption of riboflavin. The maximal amount of riboflavin that is absorbed from a single oral dose appears to be about 27 milligrams. The amount of absorption of riboflavin-5^1-phosphate and FAD appears to be very low. During the process of absorption, riboflavin, in part, appears to be converted to FMN which is either used by the enterocytes for their metabolic requirements, or converted back to riboflavin for further processing. Riboflavin is transported via the portal circulation to the liver and by the systemic circulation to the various tissues of the body.

A large percentage of serum riboflavin is carried by immunoglobulins. Some serum riboflavin is carried by albumin. Riboflavin is transported into cells via facilitated diffusion at physiological concentrations, and by passive diffusion at higher concentrations. Within cells, riboflavin is converted to FMN via flavokinase. FMN is converted to FAD via FAD synthetase. FAD is the predominant form of riboflavin in tissues.

Very little riboflavin is stored in tissues. Riboflavin in excess of body requirements is excreted mainly by the kidneys. A number of riboflavin metabolites are also found in the urine, including 7-hydromethylriboflavin, 8-hydroxymethylribofla-vin, 8 alpha-sulfonylriboflavin, 5^1-riboflavinyl peptide, 10-hydroxyethylflavin, lumiflavin, 10-formylmethylflavin and carboxymethylflavins. A significant percentage of large intakes of riboflavin—greater than 30 milligrams in a single dose—is excreted in the feces.

INDICATIONS AND USAGE

Riboflavin has been found to be an effective migraine prophylaxis in some. Riboflavin supplementation has resulted in full recovery of several patients who developed a sometimes fatal syndrome characterized by lactic acidosis and hepatic steatosis caused by treatment with nucleoside reverse-transcriptase inhibitors. Riboflavin has significant antioxidant-promoting activity which, experimentally, has protected against cardiac injury produced by reperfusion following ischemia. It has also exhibited notable ability to inhibit lipid oxidation and has protected against a number of oxidative injuries in the laboratory. It has demonstrated some activity against esophageal cancer. Intriguingly, riboflavin deficiency has been shown to be protective against malaria in both animals and humans. On the other hand, high doses of riboflavin may have antimalarial activity.

RESEARCH SUMMARY

Riboflavin has been called "a significant breakthrough" in migraine prophylaxis with "an outstanding efficacy-side effect profile" by one recent reviewer of migraine research developments.

In an open study, high-dose riboflavin showed significant effectiveness as a migraine prophylaxis. In a subsequent randomized trial, 400 milligrams of riboflavin and placebo were tested for three months in 55 migraine patients. In the riboflavin group, 59% improved by at least 50%, compared with 15% of the placebo group showing at least 50% improvement.

In a more recent clinical trial (open label), the efficacy of high-dose riboflavin—400 mg daily—for the prevention of migraine headaches was studied in 23 patients in a specialized headache outpatient clinic. Headache frequency, duration, intensity and the use of abortive drugs were recorded at baseline and 3 and 6 months after start of treatment. Headache frequency was significantly reduced from 4 days per month at baseline to 2 days per month after 3 and 6 months. The use of abortive drugs also significantly decreased after 3 and 6 months of treatment. The number of headache hours and headache intensity did not significantly change. The researchers concluded that "riboflavin is a safe and well-tolerated alternative in migraine prophylaxis." Further research on the effect of riboflavin on migraine headaches is needed and warranted.

Both riboflavin and beta-blockers were tested for their effects on the intensity dependence of auditory evoked cortical potentials. Intensity dependence is usually increased during migraines. In this study, the beta-blockers significantly decreased the intensity dependence, and this decrease correlated with significant clinical improvement. Riboflavin treatment did not affect intensity dependence but was, nonetheless, also associated with significant improvement. Thus, given that the two agents apparently act via two distinct pathophysiological mechanisms, the researchers concluded that a combination of the two treatments might enhance their efficacy without increasing central nervous system side effects. This hypothesis warrants investigation.

A 46-year-old woman who had been treated for AIDS with triple anti-retroviral therapy for four months developed lactic acidosis and marked hepatic steatosis. Suspecting that a riboflavin deficiency induced by amitriptyline, which she was also taking (see Interactions), might be contributing to these potentially life-threatening metabolic abnormalities, the physicians treated her with 50 milligrams of riboflavin daily. This was followed by rapid recovery.

Subsequently, these researchers similarly identified two other HIV-infected patients with less severe lactic acidosis. These patients had also been on triple drug therapy. Riboflavin again rapidly resolved the acidosis. This condition, they believed, results, in part, from impaired mitochondrial DNA replication caused by the HIV drug therapies.

Another researcher has also reported that 50 milligrams of riboflavin daily resolved the severe lactic acidosis of a 35-year-old pregnant HIV-infected patient. Blood lactate levels returned to normal within four days of beginning treatment. This syndrome is a rare complication of treatment with nucleoside reverse-transcriptase inhibitors, but, since it can be fatal, it is a significant one, as is riboflavin's apparent role in resolving it.

Riboflavin's antioxidant-promoting activity has been shown to provide protection against oxidative damage caused by oxidized forms of hemeproteins. In an animal model of ischemic reperfusion injury, riboflavin was significantly cardioprotective. In an *in vivo* animal experiment, it protected rat lungs from the oxidative injury initiated by injection of cobra venom factor. It also significantly protected rat brains from swelling after four hours of ischemia. Riboflavin is the precursor of co-enzymes that are required in potent antioxidant processes. Some researchers have concluded that riboflavin nutriture plays a crucial role in inactivation of lipid peroxides. Riboflavin supplementation has been shown to prevent hepatic lipid peroxidation both in *in vitro* and in animal studies.

Some studies have shown a synergy between Vitamin E and riboflavin as antioxidants. Riboflavin, for example, diminished lipid peroxidation and prevented the oxidation of Vitamin E in the livers of experimental animals. It has been suggested that riboflavin has a sparing effect on vitamin E or may help regenerate Vitamin E via production of reduced glutathione.

There is an epidemiological association between riboflavin and esophageal cancer. The incidence of this cancer is particularly high in parts of the world (some areas of China, Iran and Africa) where riboflavin deficiency is high. One study suggested that riboflavin supplementation might reduce the number of precancerous cells in the esophagus. This needs followup.

There is a finding, in both animals and humans, that a deficiency in riboflavin has significant antimalarial effects. Dietary riboflavin deficiency dramatically decreases malarial parasitemia with concomitant diminution of symptoms. Further, specific riboflavin antagonists have demonstrated antimalarial activity. Whether these findings can become the basis for a new pharmacological approach to the treatment of this challenging disease remains to be seen. On the other hand, a recent study reported that high doses of riboflavin may have antimalarial activity. Further research is necessary and warranted in order to resolve these seemingly contradictory findings.

CONTRAINDICATIONS, PRECAUTIONS, ADVERSE REACTIONS

CONTRAINDICATIONS

Riboflavin is contraindicated in those hypersensitive to any component of a riboflavin-containing product.

PRECAUTIONS

The use of riboflavin for the treatment of riboflavin deficiency or for any medical indication must be medically supervised.

Most pre- and postnatal vitamin/mineral supplements deliver 3.4 milligrams daily of riboflavin. Pregnant women and nursing mothers should avoid intakes of riboflavin greater than this amount unless higher amounts are prescribed by their physicians.

High dose intake of riboflavin may interfere with the Abbott TDX drugs-of-abuse assay.

Riboflavin absorption is increased in hypothyroidism and decreased in hyperthyroidism.

Those who use nucleoside reverse-transcriptase inhibitors (see Interactions) should be aware that even mild riboflavin deficiency may increase the risk of lactic acidosis.

ADVERSE REACTIONS

Riboflavin is well tolerated. Doses of 400 milligrams daily for four months were found to cause diarrhea and polyuria in two out of 28 subjects who participated in a migraine prophylaxis study. Riboflavin supplements impart a yellow-orange discoloration to urine. This color has no pathological implication.

INTERACTIONS

DRUGS

Cholestyramine: Concomitant intake of cholestyramine and riboflavin may decrease the absorption of riboflavin.

Chlorpromazine: Chlorpromazine may inhibit the conversion of riboflavin to FMN and FAD.

Colestipol: Concomitant intake of colestipol and riboflavin may decrease the absorption of riboflavin.

Doxorubicin: Doxorubicin may inhibit the conversion of riboflavin to FMN and FAD.

Metoclopramide: Metoclopramide may decrease the absorption of riboflavin.

Nucleoside reverse-transcriptase inhibitors (didanosine, lamivudine, stavudine, zidovudine): Riboflavin has been found to reverse nucleoside analogue-induced lactic acidosis in patients with mild riboflavin deficiencies. These mild riboflavin deficiencies may result from the use of drugs, such as amitriptyline, which may adversely affect riboflavin status.

Oral Contraceptive Agents: Use of oral contraceptive agents may result in decreased serum levels of riboflavin.

Probenecid: Probenecid may inhibit the absorption of riboflavin. It may also inhibit renal tubular secretion of riboflavin.

Propantheline bromide: Propantheline bromide may enhance the absorption of riboflavin by allowing the vitamin to remain at intestinal absorption sites for longer periods of time.

Quinacrine: Quinacrine may inhibit the conversion of riboflavin to FMN and FAD.

Tricyclic Antidepressants (amitriptyline, imipramine): Tricyclic antidepressant drugs may inhibit the conversion of riboflavin to FMN and FAD.

NUTRITIONAL SUPPLEMENTS
Boron: Boric acid may induce riboflavin deficiency, since it displaces riboflavin from plasma-binding sites and results in increased urinary excretion of the vitamin. Most forms of boron (see Boron) used for nutritional supplementation are readily converted to boric acid. High intakes of these boron supplements may result in riboflavin deficiency.

Psyllium: Concomitant intake of psyllium and riboflavin may decrease the absorption of riboflavin.

Vitamin E: Riboflavin may potentiate the antioxidant effect of Vitamin E.

FOODS
Concomitant intake of riboflavin with food enhances the absorption of riboflavin.

OVERDOSAGE
There are no reports of riboflavin overdosage in the literature.

DOSAGE AND ADMINISTRATION
Riboflavin and riboflavin 5^1-monophosphate are the principal forms of riboflavin supplements, with riboflavin being the major available form. Riboflavin is typically present in multivitamin, multivitamin/multimineral and B-complex preparations. Riboflavin is also available as a single ingredient supplement. Typical doses range from 1.7 to 10 milligrams daily. Pre- and postnatal supplements usually deliver riboflavin at a dose of 3.4 daily. In the migraine prophylaxis studies, 400 milligrams daily of riboflavin were used. Use of riboflavin for any medical indication must be

medically supervised. Doses of riboflavin greater than 30 milligrams should be taken in divided doses.

The Food and Nutrition Board of the Institute of Medicine of the National Academy of Sciences recommends the following dietary reference intakes (DRI) for riboflavin:

Infants	Adequate Intakes (AI)	
0-6 months	0.3 mg/day	0.04 mg/kg
7-12 months	0.4 mg/day	0.04 mg/kg

Children	Recommended Dietary Allowances (RDA)
1-3 years	0.5 mg/day
4-8 years	0.6 mg/day
Boys	
9-13 years	0.9 mg/day
14-18 years	1.3 mg/day
Girls	
9-13 years	0.9 mg/day
14-18 years	1.0 mg/day
Men	
19 years and older	1.3 mg/day
Women	
19 years and older	1.1 mg/day
Pregnancy	
14-50 years	1.4 mg/day
Lactation	
14-50 years	1.6 mg/day

The DV (Daily Value) for riboflavin (vitamin B$_2$), which is used for determining percentage of nutrient daily values on nutritional supplement and food labels, is 1.7 milligrams. This is based on the U.S. RDA for riboflavin.

LITERATURE
Akomporg T, Ghori N, Halder K. In vitro activity of riboflavin against the human malaria parasite Plasmodium faciparum. *Antimicrob Agents Chemother.* 2000; 44:88-96.

Boehnke C, Reuter U, Flach U, et al. High-dose riboflavin treatment is efficacious in migraine prophylaxis: an open study in a tertiary care centre. *Eur J Neurol.* 2004;11(7):475-477.

Christensen HN. Riboflavin can protect tissues from oxidative injury. *Nutr Rev.* 1998; 51:149-150.

Dietary Reference Intakes for Thiamin, Riboflavin, Niacin, Vitamin B$_6$, Folate, Vitamin B$_{12}$, Pantothenic Acid, Biotin, and Choline. Washington, DC: National Academy Press; 1998.

Dutta P, Pinto JT, Rivlin RS. Antimalarial effects of riboflavin deficiency. *Lancet.* 1985; 2:1040-1043.

Fraaije MW, van den Heuvel RH, van Berkel WJ, Mattevi A. Covalent flavinylation is essential for efficient redox catalysis in vanillyl-alcohol oxidase. *J Biol Chem*. 1999; 274:35514-35520.

Fraaije MW, Mattevi A. Flavoenzymes: diverse catalysts with recurrent features. *Trends Biochem Sci*. 2000; 25:126-132.

Fouty B, Frerman F, Reves R. Riboflavin to treat nucleoside analogue-induced lactic acidosis. *Lancet*. 1998; 352:291-292.

Huang S-N, Swaan PW. Involvement of a receptor-mediated component in cellular translocation of riboflavin. *J Pharmacol Exp Therap*. 2000; 294:117-125.

Hustad S, Ueland PM, Vollset SE, et al. Riboflavin as a determinant of plasma total homocysteine: effect modification by the methylenetetrahydrofolate reductase C677T polymorphism. *Clin Chem*. 2000; 468:1065-1071.

Kunsman GW, Levine B, Smith ML. Vitamin B_2 interference with TDx drugs-of-abuse assays. *J Forensic Sci*. 1998; 43:1225-1227.

Lakshmi AV, Ramalakshmi BA. Effect of pyridoxine or riboflavin supplementation on plasma homocysteine levels in women with oral lesions. *Natl Med J India*. 1998; 11:171-172.

Luzzati R, Del Bravo P, Di Perri G, et al. Riboflavine and severe lactic acidosis. *Lancet*. 1999; 353:901-902.

McCormick DB. Riboflavin. In: Shils ME, Olson JA, Shike M, Ross AC, eds. *Modern Nutrition in Health and Disease*. 9th ed. Baltimore, MD: Williams and Wilkins; 1999:391-399.

Munoz N, Hayashi M, Bang LJ, et al. Effect of riboflavin, retinol, and zinc on micronuclei of buccal mucosa and of esophagus: a randomized double-blind intervention study in China. *J Natl Cancer Inst*. 1987; 79:687-691.

Rivlin RS. Riboflavin. *Adv Exp Med Biol*. 1986; 206:349-355.

Rivlin RS, Dutta P. Vitamin B_2 (riboflavin). Relevance to malaria and antioxidant activity. *Nutrition Today*. 1995; 30:62-67.

Sándor PS, Áfra J, Ambrosini A, Schoenen J. Prophylactic treatment of migraine with beta-blockers and riboflavin: differential effects on the intensity dependence of auditory evoked cortical potentials. *Headache*. 2000; 40:30-35.

Schoenen J. [Anti-migraine treatment: present and future]. [Article in French]. *Rev Med Liege*. 1999; 54:79-86.

Schoenen J, Jacquy J, Lenaerts M. Effectiveness of high-dose riboflavin in migraine prophylaxis. A randomized controlled trial. *Neurology*. 1998; 50:466-470.

Thurnham DI, Zheng SF, Munoz N, et al. Comparison of riboflavin, Vitamin A, and zinc status of Chinese populations at high and low risk for esophageal cancer. *Nutr Canc*. 1985; 7:131-143.

Wahrendorf J, Munoz N, Lu JB, et al. Blood, retinol and zinc riboflavin status in relation to precancerous lesions of the esophagus: findings from a vitamin intervention trial in the People's Republic of China. *Cancer Res*. 1988; 48:2280-2283.

Royal Jelly

DESCRIPTION

Royal jelly, also known as gelee royale and RJ, is the milky-white gelatinous substance secreted from the cephalic glands of nurse worker bees *(Apis mellifera)* for apparently the sole purpose of stimulating the growth and development of the queen bee. Without royal jelly, the queen bee would be no different from the worker bees and would live about as long (seven to eight weeks). With royal jelly, the queen bee can live five to seven years. This fact explains the popular belief that royal jelly has rejuvenating qualities.

Royal jelly, however, has not lived up to expectations that it is an important anti-aging substance. But it is not without medical interest. Royal jelly consists of an emulsion of proteins, sugars, lipids and some other substances in a water base. Proteins make up about 13% of royal jelly. Most of the proteins comprise a family called major royal jelly proteins. One protein in royal jelly called royalsin possesses antibiotic properties against gram-positive, but not gram-negative, bacteria. About 11% of royal jelly is made up of sugars, such as fructose and glucose, similar to those found in honey. Lipids comprise about 5% of the substance and consist mainly of medium-chain hydroxy fatty acids, such as trans-10-hydroxy-2-decenoic acid, which is also thought to possess antimicrobial properties.

Royal jelly also contains vitamins, such as pantothenic acid, minerals and phytosterols. Neopterin, or 2-amino-6- (1,2,3-trihydroxypropyl)-4 (3H)-pteridinone, was initially isolated from royal jelly. Neopterin is also found in humans, and, although its precise role is not known, it appears to play an important role in the human immune system.

Melbrosia, a mixture of royal jelly and bee pollen, is sometimes used by menopausal women to manage climacteric symptoms.

ACTIONS AND PHARMACOLOGY

ACTIONS

Royal jelly may have hypolipidemic, antibacterial, anti-inflammatory and antiproliferative activities.

MECHANISM OF ACTION

The mechanism of actions of royal jelly is not known. The possible antibacterial activity of some royal jelly proteins, while of interest for topical use, is unlikely to be expressed when ingested.

PHARMACOKINETICS

There are no reported pharmacokinetic studies of royal jelly. Proteins, carbohydrates and lipids in royal jelly should be digested, absorbed and metabolized in the same way that other such substances found in food are digested, absorbed and metabolized.

INDICATIONS AND USAGE

Royal jelly may have favorable lipid effects, including cholesterol-lowering effects. There is very preliminary evidence that it may have some antibiotic, immunomodulatory, anti-inflammatory, wound-healing and anti-cancer effects.

RESEARCH SUMMARY

A meta-analysis of royal jelly's reported effects on serum lipids in experimental animals and in humans found significant, positive results. The substance significantly decreased serum and liver total lipids and cholesterol in rats and mice, and retarded the formation of atheromas in the aortas of rabbits fed hyperlipidemic diets. Meta-analysis of controlled human studies also showed significant reduction in total serum lipids and cholesterol, and, in those with hyperlipidemia, it normalized HDL- and LDL-cholesterol determined from decreases in beta/alpha lipoproteins. The author of this meta-analysis concluded: "The best available evidence suggests that royal jelly, at approximately 50 to 100 milligrams per day, decreased total serum cholesterol levels by about 14% and total serum lipids by about 10% in the group of patients studied."

One group of researchers has reported that a royal jelly extract has potent antibiotic effects against gram-positive bacteria, but not against gram-negative bacteria. Royal jelly has exhibited immunomodulating effects in an animal model, stimulating antibody production and immunocompetent cell proliferation.

It has been claimed, anecdotally, for some time that royal jelly has anti-inflammatory effects and wound-healing properties. These claims were given preliminary support in a study of streptozotocin-diabetic rats. The researchers were looking for a hypoglycemic effect from royal jelly; none was found, but the researchers noted that royal jelly showed some anti-inflammatory activity and that it shortened healing time in desquamated skin lesions.

There have been scattered reports that royal jelly and its constituent 10-hydroxy-2-decenoic acid might have anti-cancer effects. There was one report that both provided complete protection against transplantable mouse leukemia. Tumor growth inhibition of other cancers has been associated with royal jelly supplementation in other animal models. More research is needed.

CONTRAINDICATIONS, PRECAUTIONS, ADVERSE REACTIONS

CONTRAINDICATIONS

Royal jelly is contraindicated in those allergic or hypersensitive to any of its components.

PRECAUTIONS

Pregnant women and nursing mothers should avoid using royal jelly supplements.

ADVERSE REACTIONS

Adverse reactions have included eczema, rhinitis, urticaria and bronchospasm. There is one report of a woman developing hemorrhagic colitis following use of royal jelly for approximately one month. Acute asthma, anaphylaxis and, in one case, death secondary to royal jelly-induced asthma have also been reported.

OVERDOSAGE

No reported overdosage of royal jelly.

DOSAGE AND ADMINISTRATION

Those who use royal jelly take 50 to 100 milligrams daily. Royal jelly is also available in cosmetic formulations. Those who are allergic or hypersensitive to royal jelly may develop dermatitis conditions from topical use.

LITERATURE

Bullock RJ, Rohan A, Straatmans JA. Fatal royal jelly-induced asthma. *Med J Aust.* 1999; 160:44.

Fujii A, Kobayashi S, Kuboyama N. Augmentation of wound healing by royal jelly (RJ) in streptozoticin-diabetic rats. *Jpn J Pharmacol.* 1990; 53:331-337.

Fujiwara S, Imai J, Fujiwara M, et al. A potent antibacterial protein in royal jelly. Purification and determination of the primary structure of royalisin. *J Biol Chem.* 1990; 265:11333-11337.

Gene M, Aslan A. Determination of trans-10-hydroxy-2-decenoic acid content in pure royal jelly products by column liquid chromatography. *J Chromatogr.* 1999; 839:265-268.

Hamerlinck FF. Neopterin: a review. *Exp Dermatol.* 1999; 8:167-176.

Harwood M, Harding S, Beasley R, Frankish PD. Asthma following royal jelly. *N Z Med J.* 1996; 109:325.

Ishiwata H, Takeda Y, Yamada T, et al. Determination and confirmation of methyl p-hydroxybenzoate in royal jelly and other foods produced by the honey bee. *Food Addit Contam,* 1999; 12:281-285.

Leung R, Ho A, Chan J, et al. Royal jelly consumption and hypersensitivity in the community. *Clin Exp Allergy.* 1997; 27:333-336.

Orsolic SL, Tadic Z, Njari B, et al. A royal jelly as a new potential immunomodulator in rats and mice. *Comp Immunol Microbiol Infect Dis.* 1996; 19:31-38.

Shen X, Lu R, He G. [Effects of lyophilized royal jelly on experimental hyperlipidemia and thrombosis.] [Article in Chinese.] *Chung Hua Yu Fang I Hsueh Tsa Chih.* 1995; 29:27-29.

Szanto E, Gruber D, Sator M, et al. [Placebo-controlled study of melbrosia in treatment of climacteric symptoms.] [Article in German.] *Wien Med Wochenschr.* 1994; 144:130-134.

Tamura T, Fujii A, Kuboyama N. [Antitumor effects of royal jelly.] [Article in Japanese.] *Nippon Yakurigaku Zasshi.* 1987; 89:73-80.

Thien FC, Leung R, Baldo BA, et al. Asthma and anaphylaxis induced by royal jelly. *Clin Exp Allergy.* 1996; 26:216-222.

Vittek J. Effects of royal jelly on serum lipids in experimental animals and humans with atherosclerosis. *Experientia.* 1995; 51:927-935.

Yonei Y, Shibagaki K, Tsukada N, et al. Case report: hemorrhagic colitis associated with royal jelly intake. *J Gastroenterol Hepatol.* 1997; 12:495-499.

Rutin

DESCRIPTION

The flavonoid rutin is a flavonol glycoside comprised of the flavonol quercetin (see Quercetin) and the disaccharide rutinose. Rutin is found in many plants, especially the buckwheat plant *Fagopyrum esculentum* Moench, the flour of which is used to make pancakes. Other rich dietary sources of rutin include black tea and apple peels.

Rutin is a solid substance, pale yellow in appearance and only slightly soluble in water. It is, however, much more soluble in water than its aglycone quercetin. Rutin's molecular formula is $C_{27}H_{30}O_{16}$, its molecular weight is 610.53 daltons, and its structural formula is:

Rutin

The disaccharide moiety of rutin, rutinose, is comprised of the sugars rhamnose (6-deoxy-L-mannose) and glucose. Many names are used for rutin in the literature. They include rutoside, quercetin-3-rutinoside and sophorin. Also, 3, 3', 4', 5, 7-pentahydroxyflavone-3-rutinoside, 3-rhamnosyl-glucosyl quercetin and 3-[[6-O-(6-deoxy-alpha-L-mannopyranosyl)-beta-D-glucopyranosyl] oxy]-2-(3, 4-dihydroxyphenyl)-5,7-dihydroxy-4*H*-1-benzopyran-4-one.

ACTIONS AND PHARMACOLOGY

ACTIONS

Rutin may have antioxidant, anti-inflammatory, anticarcinogenic, antithrombotic, cytoprotective and vasoprotective activities.

MECHANISM OF ACTION

Many, if not most, of rutin's possible activities can be accounted for, in part, by rutin's antioxidant activity. Rutin is a phenolic antioxidant and has been demonstrated to scavenge superoxide radicals. Rutin can chelate metal ions, such as ferrous cations. Ferrous cations are involved in the so-called Fenton reaction, which generates reactive oxygen species. Rutin may also modulate the respiratory burst of neutrophils. The *in vivo* antioxidant activity of rutin is most likely due to its aglycone quercetin, to which it is metabolized following ingestion. Although most studies show rutin to inhibit lipid peroxidation, a few studies do not. Rutin may also help maintain levels of the biological antioxidant reduced glutathione. Importantly, under certain conditions, rutin or its metabolite quercetin may become a pro-oxidant. For example, nitrosation of rutin/quercetin may produce a pro-oxidant molecule that may have mutagenic potential.

PHARMACOKINETICS

The pharmacokinetics of rutin in humans is still under investigation. It appears that only about 17% of an ingested dose is absorbed. Absorption appears to occur mainly from the colon following the removal of the carbohydrate moiety by bacterial enzymes to form quercetin. Quercetin may undergo glucuronidation in the colonocytes. It is unclear to what extent there is absorption of quercetin glycosides. Quercetin and glucuronide conjugates of quercetin are transported to the liver via the portal circulation, where they undergo significant first pass metabolism. Metabolites may include isorhamnetin, kaempferol and tamarixetin. Quercetin itself may undergo glucuronidation and sulfation. Quercetin and its metabolites are distributed from the liver to various tissues in the body. Quercetin is strongly bound to albumin in the plasma.

INDICATIONS AND USAGE

Rutin may be useful in the management of venous edema. It may help strengthen capillaries, protect against some toxins and have anti-inflammatory effects, as well as some anti-cancer effects. It may also help prevent the oxidation of vitamin C and have some positive lipid effects.

RESEARCH SUMMARY

Some of the earliest research related to rutin found that, in daily doses of 200 to 600 mg, it is useful in treating some with conditions characterized by capillary fragility and attendant easy bruising. There was the suggestion in some of this early work that it might help decrease the incidence of cerebral hemorrhage, though no research was conducted to specifically confirm this. An early placebo-controlled study reported a significant reduction in mid-cycle menstrual bleeding in rutin-supplemented women.

Several placebo-controlled trials have demonstrated that rutin has significant efficacy in diminishing the venous edema that is an early sign of chronic venous disease of the leg.

Rutin's anti-inflammatory potential has been demonstrated in a number of animal studies. In experimentally induced colitis, both pre- and post-induction treatment with rutin conferred significant preventive and healing effects. Rutin was shown to increase colonic glutathione levels, thus reducing oxidative tissue damage in this inflammatory condition. It has also shown cytoprotective effects against ethanol injury in an animal model of ethanol-induced gastric lesions.

Rutin's radical-scavenging and, possibly, its iron-chelating abilities were said, in other animal studies, to significantly protect against asbestos-induced oxidative cellular injury.

Very preliminary animal research has found some evidence that rutin can inhibit some cancerous and pre-cancerous conditions, including chemically induced colonic neoplasia. Results, however, have been mixed. Far more research is required.

Although in most studies rutin has been found to inhibit lipid peroxidation, in one study rutin was not found to block cellular lipid peroxidation. However, according to the researchers, rutin may still potentially play a positive role in helping to prevent atherogenesis by inhibiting the depletion of cellular glutathione and ATP, thus perhaps reducing the cytotoxicity of oxidized LDL-cholesterol.

Finally, there is some evidence suggesting that rutin, taken with vitamin C, may help inhibit the oxidation of vitamin C and thus make it safer and more useful in some conditions. More research is needed to elucidate the relationship between the flavonoids and vitamin C.

CONTRAINDICATIONS, PRECAUTIONS, ADVERSE REACTIONS

CONTRAINDICATIONS
Rutin is contraindicated in those who are hypersensitive to any component of a rutin-containing product.

PRECAUTIONS
Pregnant women and nursing mothers should avoid using rutin supplements.

There is some suggestion that rutin may undergo nitrosation with, for example, nitrates and nitrites found in some processed meat products to form potentially mutagenic substances. Those who supplement with rutin should avoid using it concomitantly with such products.

ADVERSE REACTIONS
Rutin is generally well tolerated. Adverse reactions include gastrointestinal ones, such as nausea. There are rare reports of headache and mild tingling of the extremities.

INTERACTIONS

DRUGS
Quinolone antibiotics: Quercetin binds *in vitro* to the DNA gyrase site in bacteria. Therefore, theoretically, it can serve as a competitive inhibitor to the quinolone antibiotics, which also bind to this site.

NUTRITIONAL SUPPLEMENTS
Vitamin C: The interaction between flavonoids, such as rutin and quercetin, and vitamin C is unclear. It has been believed for some time that flavonoids work synergistically with vitamin C, enhancing the absorption of the vitamin and preventing it from oxidation. However, recent research indicates that flavonoids may actually inhibit the uptake of vitamin C into cells. More research is necessary in order to clarify this issue.

FOODS
Rutin may undergo nitrosation with nitrites and nitrates found in some processed meat products to form potentially mutagenic substances.

DOSAGE AND ADMINISTRATION
Typical doses used are 500 mg once or twice daily. Those with venous insufficiency/varicose veins often use 500 mg taken twice daily.

LITERATURE
Clement DL. Management of venous edema: insights from an international task force. *Angiology.* 2000; 51:13-17.

Cruz T, Galvez J, Ocete MA, et al. Oral administration of rutoside can ameliorate inflammatory bowel disease in rats. *Life Sci.* 1998; 62:687-695.

Deschner EE, Ruperto JF. Wong GY, Newmark HL. The effect of dietary quercetin and rutin on AOM-induced acute colonic epithelial abnormalities in mice fed a high-fat diet. *Nutr Cancer.* 1993; 20:199-204.

Drewa G, Schachtschabel DO, Palgan K, et al. The influence of rutin on the weight, metastasis and melanin content of B16 melanotic melanoma in C57BL/6 mice. *Neoplasma.* 1998; 45:266-271.

Galvez J, Cruz T, Crespo E, et al. Rutoside as mucosal protective in acetic acid-induced rat colitis. *Planta Med.* 1997; 63:409-414.

Kostyuk VA, Potapovich AI. Antiradical and chelating effects in flavonoid protection against silica-induced cell injury. *Arch Biochem Biophys.* 1998; 355:43-48.

Kostyuk VA, Potapovich AI, Speransky SD, Maslova GT. Protective effect of natural flavonoids on rat peritoneal macrophages injury caused by asbestos fiber. *Free Rad Biol Med.* 1996; 21:487-493.

Olthof MR, Hollman PC, Vree TB, Katan MB. Bioavailabilities of quercetin-3-glucoside and quercetin-4′-glucoside do not differ in humans. *J Nutr.* 2000; 130:1200-1203.

Park JB, Levine M. Intracellular accumulation of ascorbic acid is inhibited by flavonoids via blocking of dehydroascorbic acid and ascorbic acid uptakes in HL-60, U937 and Jurkat cells. *J Nutr.* 2000; 130:1297-1302.

Perez Guerrero C, Martin MG, Marhuenda E. Prevention by rutin of gastric lesions induced by ethanol in rats: role of endogenous prostaglandins. *Gen Pharmacol.* 1994; 25:575-580.

Rueff J, Gaspar J, Laires A. Structural requirements for mutagenicity of flavonoids upon nitrosation. A structure-activity study. *Mutagenesis.* 1995; 10:325-328.

Schmitt A, Savayre R, Delchambre J, Negre-Salvayre A. Prevention by alpha-tocopherol and rutin of glutathione and ATP depletion induced by oxidized LDL in cultured endothelial cells. *Br J Pharmacol.* 1995; 116:1985-1990.

Webster RP, Gawde MD, Bhattacharya RK, Protective effect of rutin, a flavonol glycoside, on the carcinogen-induced DNA damage and repair enzymes in rats. *Cancer Lett.* 1996; 109:185-191.

S-Adenosyl-L-Methionine (SAMe)

DESCRIPTION

S-adenosyl-L-methionine (SAMe) is a natural substance present in the cells of the body. It is a direct metabolite of the essential amino acid L-methionine. It is variously known as ademetionine, S-adenosylmethione, SAM, SAMe and SAM-e. It is represented structurally as:

S-Adenosylmethionine

SAMe is used as a drug in Europe for the treatment of depression, liver disorders, osteoarthritis and fibromyalgia. Recently, SAMe has been introduced into the United States as a dietary supplement for the support of bone and joint health, as well as mood and emotional well being.

ACTIONS AND PHARMACOLOGY

ACTIONS

SAMe plays a crucial biochemical role in the body by donating a one-carbon methyl group in a process called transmethylation. SAMe, formed from the reaction of L-methionine and adenosine triphosphate catalyzed by the enzyme S-adenosylmethionine synthetase, is the methyl-group donor in the biosynthesis of both DNA and RNA nucleic acids, phospholipids, proteins, epinephrine, melatonin, creatine and other molecules.

Supplemental SAMe may have antidepressant and hepatoprotective activities.

MECHANISM OF ACTION

The mechanism of action of supplemental SAMe is unclear. Much is known, however, of the mechanism of action of endogenous SAMe.

Methylation of DNA is critical in the biological phenomenon known as gene silencing. Gene silencing helps suppress genes that may give rise to cancer or those that may carry information for endogenous retroviruses. Methylation of RNA, particularly transfer RNA, is similarly important in safeguarding the form and function of these molecules in protein synthesis.

SAMe is the methyl donor to phosphatidylethanolamine in the formation of phosphatidylcholine (PC). PC is a major component of cell membranes and is vital for maintenance of cellular membrane fluidity, important in sustaining the bioenergetics and information-processing functions of cells.

SAMe is also involved in the methylation of histones, major elements in chromosomal structure. This methylation is believed to play a key role in the regulation of DNA transcription, the process by which RNA is formed. The carbon and nitrogen atoms of L-carnitine are derived from methylated lysine residues, which are formed by methylating certain proteins with SAMe's methyl group.

SAMe's importance in the body is further emphasized by the fact that it is also the methyl donor for the synthesis of epinephrine (adrenaline), creatine, melatonin, glutathione, the polyamines spermine and spermidine, and the amino acids L-cysteine and taurine, all of which play vital roles in human health.

PHARMACOKINETICS

SAMe is absorbed from the small intestine following oral intake. Absorption is better on an empty stomach, and enteric-coated tablets are better absorbed than non-enteric-coated varieties. Peak plasma concentrations obtained with enteric-coated tablet formulations are dose related, with a peak concentration of 0.5 to 1 mg/L achieved three to five hours after single doses in the range of 400 to 1,000 milligrams.

Limited trials in healthy volunteers show low bioavailability following oral intake of SAMe. This indicates significant first-pass metabolism in the liver. SAMe is mainly metabolized in the liver (about 50%).

SAMe is metabolized to S-adenosylhomocysteine, which in turn is metabolized to homocysteine. Homocysteine can either be metabolized to cystathionine and then cysteine or to methionine. The cofactor in the metabolism of homocysteine to cysteine is vitamin B_6. Cofactors for the metabolism of homocysteine to methionine are folic acid, vitamin B_{12} and trimethylglycine (betaine).

Orally administered SAMe follows the same metabolic pathways as the natural compound found in cells. SAMe crosses the blood-brain barrier with slow accumulation in the cerebrovascular fluid. It can also get into joint synovial fluid.

One study showed that 15% of a 200 milligram-dose of SAMe was excreted in urine within 48 hours and that an additional 23% was eliminated in feces within 72 hours. The remainder was believed to be incorporated in stable metabolic pools (phosphatidylcholine, DNA, RNA, proteins and creatine, among others).

The pharmacokinetics of SAMe are similar whether in healthy individuals or in those with chronic liver disease.

INDICATIONS AND USAGE

SAMe may be indicated for the promotion and support of mood and emotional well-being. It is being used by some for the treatment of depression. There is some indication it may be helpful in Alzheimer's disease. It may also be indicated for the support of joint health, mobility and joint comfort. It is used for the treatment of osteoarthritis; there is, as yet, little convincing evidence that it is useful in any other form of arthritis. It is also used in some liver conditions, including various forms of cirrhosis and cholestasis, and there is a very preliminary indication that it might be useful in lowering lipids.

RESEARCH SUMMARY

A number of studies have now demonstrated an association between various neuropsychiatric disorders and deficient SAMe metabolism. SAMe's possible influence on mono-amine neurotransmitter metabolism, in particular, has fo-cused attention on its possible role in depression. This has resulted in a series of small studies using oral and parenteral SAMe to treat depression. The results are preliminary but promising.

In a meta-analysis of the most significant clinical studies, SAMe's efficacy was shown to exceed that of placebo and to equal or slightly better that of tricyclic antidepressants. (There is no reliable data comparing SAMe with the selective serotonin reuptake inhibitors.) Parenteral administration was only slightly more effective than oral.

SAMe, unlike traditional antidepressants, has few side effects and a rapid onset of action (usually within one or two weeks compared with three to four weeks or longer for standard antidepressants). SAMe rarely produces the side effects common to many other antidepressants, such as insomnia, nervousness, nausea and sexual dysfunction. SAMe should only be used in bipolar disorder under strict medical supervision, if at all.

SAMe's possible role in ameliorating a number of other neurological disorders is suggested by some early research but is far from proved. These disorders include Alzheimer's dementia and other clinical dementia syndromes. SAMe has been shown to have some positive effect on mood and depression associated with Parkinson's disease and chronic epileptic seizures.

A recent paper suggested that SAMe might not be appropriate for Parkinson's disease since some mouse studies demonstrated adverse reactions. The same authors stated that these same adverse reactions might not occur in humans but that caution is advised, pending further research. Some others have worried that SAMe might also interfere with the activity of levodopa, often used in the treatment of Parkinson's. Fear has also been expressed that SAMe might potentiate the manic phase of bipolar disorder; use in subjects with this disorder may thus be contraindicated.

Some recent *in vitro* and animal studies have shown that SAMe supplementation may have the potential to favorably mediate glutathione S-transferase (GST) activity. Alzheimer's disease has been associated with reduced GST activity, diminished levels of S-adenosylmethionine (SAM) and increased s-adenosylhomocysteine (SAH). Diminished GST has been shown to result in increased oxidative species within brain tissues. Mice in some of these studies have shown reduced levels of SAM and increased levels of SAH, which, in turn, further inhibits SAM. Supplementing diet with SAMe has helped to correct these imbalances and might therefore, it has been postulated, be beneficial in those with Alzheimer's. Some dated studies suggested some benefit in mood and cognitive improvement among some early stage Alzheimer's patients taking SAMe. Much more recently, another study found that a "nutraceutical cocktail" containing vitamins and SAMe delayed cognitive decline and improved mood, again in early stage Alzheimer's subjects. This same cocktail was said to improve reaction time and cognitive performance among adults and elderly without dementia. These preliminary findings need follow-up.

SAMe is depleted in liver disease, and its replenishment through supplementation has been demonstrated in several studies. Its methylating properties promote the fluidity of liver lipid membranes. SAMe has been shown to improve functions measured by standard liver and liver-function tests, to increase hepatic glutathione levels in patients with both alcohol and non-alcoholic cirrhosis, to restore normal hepatic function in various forms of cholestasis and prevent or reverse hepatoxicity induced by drugs, alcohol and various chemicals.

Some dated studies indicated that SAMe is as effective as standard anti-inflammatory drugs in the treatment of osteoarthritis. More recently, a double-blind study pitted SAMe against celecoxib, a nonsteroidal anti-inflammatory drug. The latter produced more rapid effects, but SAMe seemed to match these effects over time. Lack of placebo control made results somewhat indefinite. More research is needed and warranted.

Again, some dated studies found SAMe helpful in cases of fibromyalgia. Most of these studies, however, used injectable SAMe. In one study using oral SAMe, 44 subjects with fibromyalgia were randomized to receive either 800 mg of SAMe daily or placebo for 8 weeks. By several measures—including mood, fatigue, and morning stiffness—the SAMe-supplemented subjects were judged to have enjoyed significant improvement, compared with placebo subjects, in whom no significant improvement was noted.

SAMe is used as a cytoprotective agent against liver toxicity and there hope that it might one day be used as a chemopreventive agent against liver tumors. Some animal experiments suggest the possibility that it could be useful for that purpose through its apparent ability to inhibit the expression of some oncogene functions.

There is a single study, apparently without follow-up, showing that SAMe might be an effective agent for lowering lipids in humans.

CONTRAINDICATIONS, PRECAUTIONS, ADVERSE REACTIONS

CONTRAINDICATIONS
Known hypersensitivity to a SAMe-containing product.

PRECAUTIONS
Sufferers of bipolar disorder (manic-depressive illness) should not use SAMe unless under medical supervision. Those who are taking antidepressant medications should confer with their physicians before taking SAMe in place of or in addition to those medications. They should continue to be monitored by their physician. SAMe is not recommended for use in children. It should only be used by pregnant women with a physician's approval and under a physician's supervision. Nursing mothers should avoid SAMe supplementation.

There is no evidence that SAMe is either mutagenic or carcinogenic. But since nucleic acid methylation patterns may change in those with cancer, the use of SAMe by cancer patients should be discussed with their physicians. SAMe may one day be shown to be effective in preventing and possibly even treating some forms of cancer but, in the meantime, because it is an active methylating agent, some caution is advised in those who have cancer.

Those undergoing gene therapy should avoid supplemental SAMe.

ADVERSE REACTIONS
Although classified and sold as a drug in Europe, SAMe is marketed in the United States as a dietary supplement. There are so far no reports of serious adverse events in those taking this supplement in doses up to 1,600 mg per day over long periods of time. Side effects that have been reported include mild gastrointestinal upsets (such as stomach pain, nausea, diarrhea and flatulence), anxiety, hyperactive muscle movement, insomnia and hypomania. When these side effects occur they often diminish with time or resolve with lower doses or cessation of use. There are no documented cases of allergies to SAMe.

INTERACTIONS
There are so far no reported adverse interactions with SAMe and other drugs, dietary supplements or foods.

OVERDOSAGE
No overdosage reported.

DOSAGE AND ADMINISTRATION
SAMe is highly unstable at temperatures above 0 degree C. Since the 1970s, certain salts of SAMe have become available that are stable at higher temperatures. These forms, which are clearly more desirable, include SAMe paratoluene sulfonates (SAMe tosyls). These more stable forms have been used in many of the SAMe studies, but they are not always the forms that are found in the supplement marketplace. Another temperature-stable form is SAMe 1,4 butanedisulfonate. Even these temperature-stable forms must be kept very dry since moisture can cause hydrolysis. Stable, enteric-coated tablets are recommended.

SAMe is most frequently available in 200 mg tablets. The usual oral dose for use in depression has been in the range of 400 to 1,600 milligrams daily in divided doses. For liver problems, usual doses reported are up to 1,600 mg daily in divided doses. For bone and joint health, the daily dose is typically 200 to 1,200 milligrams in divided doses. SAMe should always be taken on an empty stomach, i.e., one hour before meals or two hours after meals. It is often reported in the literature that these doses can usually be cut in half when a positive effect is achieved. Effects, if any, are usually evident within two weeks of starting supplementation.

It is advisable to take SAMe with supplemental B_6, B_{12}, folic acid and possibly trimethylglycine (particularly in those with elevated homocysteine levels). Some SAMe supplements come with B_6, B_{12} and folic acid. These other nutrients help metabolize homocysteine which, at elevated levels, increases the risk of cardiovascular disease and some other disorders.

LITERATURE

Almasio P, Bortolini M, et al. Role of S-adenosyl-l-methionine in the treatment of intrahepatic cholestasis. *Drugs.* 1990;40(Suppl 3):111-123.

Baldessarini RJ. Neuropharmacology of S-adenosyl-l-methionine. *Am J Med.* 1987;83 (Suppl 5A):95-105.

Bell KM, Plon L, Bunney Jr. WE, Potkin SG. S-adenosylmethionine treatment of depression: a controlled clinical trial. *Am J Psychiatry.* 1988;145:1110-1114.

Berger R, Nowak H. A new medical approach to the treatment of osteoarthritis. Report of an open phase IV study with ademetionine. *Am J Med.* 1987;83(Suppl 5A):84-88.

Bombardieri G, Pappalardo G, et al. Intestinal absorption of S-adenosyl-l-methionine in humans. *Int J Clin Pharm Ther Tox.* 1983;21:186-188.

Bottiglieri T, Godfrey P, et al. Cerebrospinal fluid S-adenosylmethionine in depression and dementia: effects of treatment with parenteral and oral S-adenosylmethionine. *J Neuro Neurosurg Psych.* 1990;53:1096-1098.

Bottiglieri T, Hyland K. S-adenosylmethionine levels in psychiatric and neurological disorders: a review. *Acta Neurol Scand.* 1994;(Suppl)154:19-26.

Bottiglieri T, Hyland K, Reynolds EH. The clinical potential of ademetionine (S-adenosylmethionine) in neurological disorders. *Drugs.* 1994;48(2):137-152.

Bradley JD, Flusser D, et al. A randomized double blind, placebo controlled trial of intravenous loading with S-adenosylmethionine (SAM) followed by oral SAMe therapy in patients with knee osteoarthritis. *J Rheumatol.* 1994;21:905-911.

Bressa GM. S-adenosyl-l-methionine (SAMe) as antidepressant: meta-analysis of clinical studies. *Acta Neurol Scand.* 1994;(Suppl)154:7-14.

Carney MWP, Toone BK, Reynolds EH. S-adenosylmethionine and affective disorders. *Am J Med.* 1987;83(Suppl 5A):104-106.

Caruso I, Pietrogrande V. Italian double-blind multicenter study comparing S-adenosylmethionine, naproxen and placebo in the treatment of degenerative joint disease. *Am J Med.* 1987;83(Suppl 5A):66-71.

Chawla RK, Bonkovsky HL, Galambos JT. Biochemistry and pharmacology of S-adenosyl-l-methionine and rationale for its use in liver disease. *Drugs.* 1990;40(Suppl 3):8-110.

Delle Chiaie R, Pancheri P, Scapicchio P. Efficacy and tolerability of oral and intramuscular S-adenosyl-L-methionine 1,4-butanedisulfonate (SAMe) in the treatment of major depression: comparison with imipramine in 2 multicenter studies. *Am J Clin Nutr.* 2002;76(5):1172S-1176S.

Di Padova C. S-adenosylmethionine in the treatment of osteoarthritis. Review of the clinical studies. *Am J Med.* 1987;83(Suppl 5A):60-65.

Fava M, Giannelli A, et al. Rapidity of onset of the antidepressant effect of parenteral S-adenosyl-l-methionine. *Psych Res.* 1995;56:295-297.

Fetrow CW, Avila JR. Efficacy of the dietary supplement S-adenosyl-L-methionine. *Ann Pharmacother.* 2001;35(11):1414-1425.

Frezza M. A meta-analysis of therapeutic trials with ademetionine in the treatment of intrahepatic cholestasis. *Ann Ital Med Int.* 1993;8:48S-51S.

Friedel HA, Goa KL, Benfield P. S-adenosyl-L-methionine. A review of its pharmacological properties and therapeutic potential in liver dysfunction and affective disorders in relation to its physiological role in cell membranes. *Drugs.* 1989;38(3):389-416.

Galeone F, Salvadorini F, et al. Effect of intravenous injection of CDP-choline, S-adenosylmethionine and citiolone in subjects with hyperlipidemia. *Artery.* 1979;5:157-169.

Hosea Blewett HJ. Exploring the mechanisms behind S-adenosylmethionine (SAMe) in the treatment of osteoarthritis. *Crit Rev Food Sci Nutr.* 2008;48(5):458-463.

Jacobsen S, Danneskiold-Samsoe B, Bach Andersen R. Oral S-adenosylmethionine in primary fibromyalgia. Double-blind clinical evaluation. *Scan J Rheumatol.* 1991;20:294-302.

Kagan BL, Sultzer MD, Rosenlicht N, et al. Oral S-adenosylmethionine in depression: a randomized double-blind, placebo-controlled trial. *Am J Psychiatry.* 1990;147:591-595.

Kaye GL, Blake JC, Burroughs AK. Metabolism of exogenous S-adenosyl-L-methionine in patients with liver disease. *Drugs.* 1990;40(Suppl 3):124-128.

Konig B. Long-term (two year) clinical trial with S-adenosylmethionine for the treatment of osteoarthritis. *Am J Med.* 1987;83(Suppl 5A):89-94.

Lieber CS. S-Adenosyl-L-methionine and alcoholic liver disease in animal models: implications for early intervention in human beings. *Alcohol.* 2002;27(3):173-177.

Lieber CS. S-adenosyl-L-methionine: its role in the treatment of liver disorders. *Am J Clin Nutr.* 2002;76(5):1183S-1187S.

Lieber CS, Packer L. S-Adenosylmethionine: molecular, biological, and clinical aspects—an introduction. *Am J Clin Nutr*. 2002;76(5):1148S-1150S.

Martínez-Chantar ML, García-Trevijano ER, Latasa MU, et al. Importance of a deficiency in S-adenosyl-L-methionine synthesis in the pathogenesis of liver injury. *Am J Clin Nutr*. 2002;76(5):1177S-1182S.

Muller-Fassbender H. Double-blind clinical trial of S-adenosylmethionine versus ibuprofen in the treatment of osteoarthritis. *Am J Med*. 1987;(Suppl 5A):81-83.

Najm WI, Reinsch S, Hoehler F, et al. S-adenosyl methionine (SAMe) versus celecoxib for the treatment of osteoarthritis symptoms: a double-blind cross-over trial. *BMC Musculoskelet Disord*. 2004;5:6.

Pascale RM, Marras V, et al. Chemoprevention of rat liver carcinogenesis by S-adenosyl-l-methionine: a long-term study. *Can Res*. 1992;52:4979-4986.

Salmaggi P, Bressa GM, et al. Double-blind, placebo-controlled study of S-adenosyl-l-methionine in depressed postmenopausal women. *Psychother Psychosom*. 1993;59:34-40.

Shea TB, Chan A. S-adenosyl methionine: a natural therapeutic agent effective against multiple hallmarks and risk factors associated with Alzheimer's disease. *J Alzheimers Dis*. 2008;13(1):67-70.

Stramentinoli G. Pharmacologic aspects of S-adenosylmethionine. *Am J Med*. 1987;83(Suppl 5A):35-42.

Tchantchou F, Graves M, Falcone D, et al. S-adenosylmethionine mediates glutathione efficacy by increasing glutathione S-transferase activity: implications for S-adenosyl methionine as a neuroprotective dietary supplement. *J Alzheimers Dis*. 2008;14(3):323-328.

Williams AL, Girard C, Jui D, et al. S-adenosylmethionine (SAMe) as treatment for depression: a systematic review. *Clin Invest Med*. 2005;28(3):132-139.

Secoisolariciresinol Diglycoside (SDG)

DESCRIPTION

Secoisolariciresinol diglycoside, or SDG, is a plant lignan most notably found in flaxseed (linseed). SDG is classified as a phytoestrogen since it is a plant-derived, nonsteroid compound that possesses estrogen-like activity. SDG has weak estrogenic activity. The level of SDG in flaxseed typically varies between 0.6% and 1.8%.

Lignans are one of the two major classes of phytoestrogens; the other class is the isoflavones. Plant lignans are polyphenolic substances derived from phenylalanine via dimerization of substituted cinnamic alcohols. Mammalian lignans are lignans derived from plant lignans. For example,

following ingestion, SDG is converted to the aglycone secoisolariciresinol, which is then metabolized to the mammalian lignans enterolactone and enterodiol. Most of the effects of oral SDG are mediated by enterolactone and enterodiol.

The molecular formula of SDG is $C_{32}H_{46}O_{16}$, and its molecular weight is 686.71 daltons. The aglycone of SDG is also known as 2, 3-bis (3-methoxy-4-hydroxybenzyl) butane-1, 4-diol. Enterolactone is also known as trans-2, 3-bis [(3-hydroxylphenyl) methyl]-butyrolactone. It is represented by the following structural formula:

Secoisolariciresinol diglycoside

See also Flaxseed Lignans.

ACTIONS AND PHARMACOLOGY

ACTIONS

SDG has estrogenic and antioxidant activities. It may also have antiestrogenic, anticarcinogenic, antiatherogenic and antidiabetic activities.

MECHANISM OF ACTION

SDG, as well as its mammalian lignan metabolites, enterolactone (EL) and enterodiol (ED), have weak estrogenic activity as measured in *in vivo* and *in vitro* assays.

SDG, EL and ED have a number of antioxidant activities, including inhibition of lipid peroxidation and scavenging of hydroxy radicals. SDG also has anti-platelet-activation factor (PAF) activity. PAF can induce the release of reactive oxygen species from neutrophils. SDG, via its metabolite EL, has been found to inhibit estrogen synthase (aromatase) and to stimulate the synthesis of sex hormone binding globulin (SHBG). Both of these actions could account for the possible anti-estrogen activity of SDG.

The possible anticarcinogenic, antiatherogenic and antidiabetic activities of SDG are thought to be due, in large part, to the antioxidant activities of its metabolites EL and ED.

PHARMACOKINETICS

SDG, following ingestion, is transported to the large intestine, where it is hydrolyzed by bacteria to the aglycone secoisolariciresinol. Secoisolariciresinol, in turn, is metabolized by bacteria in the large intestine to the mammalian lignans EL and ED. EL and ED are absorbed from the large intestine. Little is known about the distribution of EL and ED to the various tissues of the body. It is known that ED and EL undergo conjugation in the liver with glucuronate and sulfate. The glucuronide and sulfate conjugates of ED and EL are excreted in the urine and in the bile.

There appears to be considerable individual variation in the absorption and metabolism of the SDG metabolites ED and EL.

INDICATIONS AND USAGE

There is evidence in *in vitro* and animal research that SDG may have some ability to reduce cholesterol levels and protect against atherosclerosis; it may also have some anticancer and antidiabetic effects.

RESEARCH SUMMARY

Rabbits fed a high-cholesterol diet supplemented with flaxseed had 46% less atherosclerotic development than rabbits fed the same diet without flaxseed. Still better results were obtained (73% reduction in atherosclerosis) when the diet was supplemented with SDG instead of flaxseed. These effects were associated with reduced serum levels of cholesterol and LDL-cholesterol and increased levels of HDL-cholesterol.

SDG has exhibited a number of anticancer effects in *in vitro* and animal studies. SDG-treated rats were significantly protected against experimentally induced mammary cancer in one experiment. Subsequently, it was demonstrated that SDG significantly inhibited experimentally induced mammary tumor multiplicity in a dose-dependent fashion in rats, with more inhibition at higher doses. Flaxseed alone did not significantly affect tumor size, multiplicity or incidence in this study, but both flaxseed and SDG delayed progression of tumorigenesis. In another recent animal study, supplemental SDG decreased metastatic pulmonary melanoma tumor size in a dose-dependent fashion, compared with controls. Research continues.

In an animal model of human type 1 diabetes, SDG was said to significantly prevent this form of diabetes. Prevention was associated with a decrease in the serum and pancreatic lipid peroxidation product malondialdehyde. The researcher concluded that IDDM is mediated through oxidative stress and that SDG reduces this stress and thus helps prevent development of diabetes. In another experiment, SDG significantly prevented the development of streptozotocin-induced diabetes in rats. Clinical trials are needed.

CONTRAINDICATIONS, PRECAUTIONS, ADVERSE REACTIONS

CONTRAINDICATIONS

SDG is contraindicated in those who are hypersensitive to any component of an SDG-containing product.

PRECAUTIONS

Pregnant women and nursing mothers should avoid the use of SDG supplementation.

Women with estrogen receptor-positive tumors should discuss the advisability of the use of SDG-containing products with their physicians before deciding to use them.

Men with prostate cancer or benign prostatic hyperplasia (BPH) should discuss the advisability of the use of flax lignan supplements with their physician before deciding to use them.

OVERDOSAGE

There are no reports of overdosage.

DOSAGE AND ADMINISTRATION

Doses of 25 to 50 milligrams of SDG daily are frequently used.

Pills typically contain at least 35% SDG by weight.

SDG is present in flaxseed at levels of 0.6 to 1.8% and in much smaller amounts in flaxseed oil.

LITERATURE

Kitts DD, Yuan YV, Wijewickreme AN, et al. Antioxidant activity of the flaxseed lignan secoisolariciresinol diglycoside and its mammalian lignan metabolites enterodiol and enterolactone. *Mol Cell Biochem.* 1999;202:91-100.

Li D, Yee JA, Thompson LU, et al. Dietary supplementation with secoisolariciresinol diglycoside (SDG) reduces experimental metastasis of melanoma cells in mice. *Cancer Letters.* 1999;142:91-96.

Pool-Zobel BL, Adlercreutz H, Glei M, et al. Isoflavonoids and lignans have different potentials to modulate oxidative genetic damage in human colon cells. *Carcinogenesis.* 2000;21:1247-1252.

Prasad K. Hydroxyl radical-scavenging property of secoisolariciresinol diglucoside isolated from flax-seed. *Mol Cell Biochem.* 1997;168:117-123.

Prasad K. Oxidative stress as a mechanism of diabetes in diabetic BB prone rats: effect of secoisolariciresinol diglucoside (SDG). *Mol Cell Biochem.* 2000;209:89-96.

Prasad K. Reduction of serum cholesterol and hypercholesterolemic atherosclerosis in rabbits by secoisolariciresinol diglucoside isolated from flaxseed. *Circulation.* 1999;99:1355-1362.

Prasad K, Mantha SV, Muir AD, et al. Protective effect of secoisolariciresinol diglucoside against streptozotocin-induced diabetes and its mechanism. *Mol Cell Biochem.* 2000;206:141-150.

Schottner M, Spiteller G. Lignans interfering with 5alpha-dihydrotestosterone binding to human sex hormone-binding globulin. *J Nat Prod.* 1998;61:119-121.

Thompson LU, Seidl MM, Rickard SE, et al. Antitumorigenic effect of a mammalian lignan precursor from flaxseed. *Nutr Cancer.* 1996;26:159-165.

Selenium

DESCRIPTION

Selenium is an essential trace element in human and animal nutrition. It is involved in the defense against the toxicity of reactive oxygen species, in the regulation of thyroid hormone metabolism and the regulation of the redox state of cells. Recognition of the vital importance of selenium in human and animal nutrition was long impeded by its very real toxic potential and by fears that selenium might be carcinogenic, fears that have now been largely displaced by some evidence suggesting just the opposite–that selenium may provide protection against some cancers.

The amount of selenium in food is a function of the selenium content of the soil. Selenium enters the food chain through incorporation into plant proteins as the amino acids L-selenocysteine and L-selenomethionine. Selenium, like most trace elements and minerals, is not evenly distributed in the world's soil. Because of the uneven global distribution of selenium, disorders of both selenium deficiency and selenium excess are known. China has regions with both the lowest and highest selenium-containing soils in the world.

Marco Polo gave the first account of selenium toxicity, which he observed during his travels in western China in the 13th century. He linked the sloughing off of the hooves of horses to their consumption of certain plants in the regions. The soils of those areas are now known to contain the highest concentrations of selenium in the world. Soils rich in selenium are referred to as being seleniferous, and the condition of chronic selenium toxicity is known as selenosis. In the 1970s, a human cardiomyopathy endemic to certain areas of China was shown to be linked to dietary selenium deficiency. This disorder, known as Keshan disease, is endemic to those areas of China with some of the most selenium-poor soils in the world. Keshan disease is now treated and prevented by selenium supplementation.

Kashin-Beck disease, also known as "big joint disease," is an osteoarthropathy that is found in areas in China where the soil is selenium-poor. It is also linked to dietary selenium deficiency. Kashin-Beck disease is found in Tibet, Siberia and North Korea, also in areas where the soil is selenium-poor and in which dietary selenium-deficiency is endemic.

Selenium is a metalloid element with atomic number 34 and an atomic weight of 78.96 daltons. It belongs to the sulfur group of elements, which also includes oxygen, tellurium and polonium. Its atomic symbol is Se. Selenium was discovered in 1817 by Berzelius who named it after Selene, the Greek goddess of the moon.

The essentiality of selenium for animals was first reported in 1957. It was found that selenium administered to vitamin E-deficient rats prevented liver necrosis. Subsequently, it was found that selenium could prevent a number of disorders of farm animals. Isolated selenium deficiency in humans has not been described. Selenium deficiency appears to cause an illness or disorder in combination with a co-factor. In the case of Keshan disease, the co-factor appears to be the Coxsackievirus. It has been shown that infection of mice on a selenium-deficient diet with a nonvirulent Coxsackievirus selects a stable cardiovirulent strain. In the case of Kashin-Beck osteoarthropathy, the co-factor appears to be iodine deficiency.

Selenium is found in human and animal tissues as L-selenomethionine or L-selenocysteine. L-selenomethionine is incorporated randomly in proteins in place of L-methionine. These proteins are called selenium-containing proteins. Only a small fraction of L-methionine in proteins is present as L-selenomethionine. On the other hand, the incorporation of L-cysteine into proteins known as selenoproteins is not random. That is, in contrast to L-selenomethionine, which randomly substitutes for L-methionine, L-selenocysteine does not randomly substitute for L-cysteine. In fact, L-selenocysteine has its own triplet code and is considered to be the 21st genetically coded amino acid.

The selenoproteins are comprised of four selenium-dependent glutathione peroxidases (GSHPx-1, GSHPx-2, GSHPx-3 and GSHPx-4), three selenium-dependent iodothyronine deiodinases, three thioredoxin reductases, selenoprotein P, selenoprotein W and selenophosphate synthetase. The glutathione peroxidases, and possibly selenoprotein P and selenoprotein W, are antioxidant proteins. The selenium-dependent iodothyronine deiodinases convert thyroxine to triiodothyronine, thus regulating thyroid hormone metabolism. The thioredoxin reductases reduce intramolecular disulfide bonds and regenerate vitamin C from its oxidized state, among other things.

ACTIONS AND PHARMACOLOGY

ACTIONS

Selenium has antioxidant activity. Selenium may also have immunomodulatory, anticarcinogenic and anti-atherogenic activities. It may have activity in detoxification of some metals and other xenobiotics and activity in fertility enhancement in males.

MECHANISM OF ACTION

The antioxidant activity of selenium is mainly accounted for by virtue of its role in the formation and function of the selenium-dependent glutathione peroxidases (GSHPx). Glutathione peroxidases use reducing equivalents from glutathione to detoxify hydroperoxides. There are four different glutathione peroxidases. GSHPx-1 is present in most cells of the body. GSHPx-2 (originally known as GSHPx-GI) is mainly found in the cells of the gastrointestinal tract. GSHPx-3 is an extracellular glutathione peroxidase. GSHPx-4 is a membrane-bound hydroperoxide glutathione peroxidase. GSHPx-4 is also known as phospholipid hydroperoxide or PHGPx. GSHPx-4 can detoxify phospholipid hydroperoxides and, along with d-alpha-tocopherol, helps prevent oxidative damage to membranes. GSHPx-3, the extracellular glutathione peroxidase, eliminates peroxides in the extracellular fluid.

Glutathione peroxidases detoxify hydrogen peroxide and fatty acid-derived hydroperoxides. This is the antioxidant role of these enzymes. However, recent research indicates that reactive oxygen species play important roles in signal transduction processes. Therefore, by affecting the concentrations of reactive oxygen species in cells, the glutathione peroxidases may also be considered to play regulatory roles in signal transduction.

Antioxidant activity of selenium can also be accounted for by its role in the selenium-dependent thioredoxin reductases. These enzymes reduce intramolecular disulfide bonds and regenerate ascorbic acid from dehydroascorbic acid. Thioredoxin reductases can also affect the redox regulation of a variety of factors, including ribonucleotide reductase (the enzyme that converts ribonucleoside diphosphates to deoxyribonucleoside diphosphates), the glucocorticoid receptor and the transcription factors AP-1 and NF-KappaB.

Selenium deficiency appears to depress the effectiveness of various components of the immune system. In humans, selenium deficiency has been associated with depressed IgG and IgM antibody titers. In animal models, selenium deficiency has resulted in depressed neutrophil activity, decreased Candidacidal activity by neutrophils and depressed cellular immunity. Selenium supplementation in humans has resulted in increased natural killer cell activity. The possible immunomodulatory effects of selenium are not well understood. Selenium's antioxidant activity may play some role, perhaps a major one, in these possible effects. It is postulated that selenium's possible effect on boosting cellular immunity may be due to upregulation of the expression of the T-cell high-affinity interleukin (IL)-2 receptor, providing a vehicle for enhanced T-cell responses, as well as prevention of oxidative stress-induced damage to immune cells. Enhanced cellular immunity may explain the

possible stimulatory effects of selenium on antibody production.

The possible anticarcinogenic activity of selenium may be accounted, for, in part, by its antioxidant activity as well as its possible immune-enhancing activity. Selenium has been shown to upregulate apoptosis in tumor cells *in vitro* and increase macrophage killing and protect against oxidative DNA damage, again, *in vitro*. Animal studies suggest that selenium may have anti-angiogenic activity. A possible mechanism for selenium's possible anti-angiogenic activity is its inhibitory effect on the expression of vascular endothelial growth factors (VEGFs). This has been observed in some animal studies. Selenium, in cell culture, has also been found to inhibit the gelatinolytic activity of matrix metalloproteinase-2 (MMP-2).

Some epidemiological studies have shown an inverse relationship between coronary heart disease and selenium intake. The possible anti-atherogenic activity of selenium may be accounted for, in part, by its antioxidant activity. Glutathione peroxidase may protect low density lipoprotein (LDL) from oxidation. Oxidized-LDL is thought to be a crucial etiological factor in atherogenesis. Selenium may decrease platelet aggregation. Selenium deficiency results in lipoperoxide accumulation. Lipoperoxides impair prostacyclin synthesis and promote thromboxane synthesis, which can increase platelet aggregation.

Selenium has been demonstrated to antagonize the effects of a number of toxic metals, including cadmium and arsenic. Selenium inhibits the growth stimulatory effect of cadmium on human prostatic epithelium *in vitro*. The mechanism of the possible antagonistic action of selenium against various toxic metals and other xenobiotics is unclear. One possibility is that it forms inactive complexes with these substances.

Selenium may have fertility enhancing effects for males. Phospholipid hydroperoxide glutathione peroxidase (GSHPx-4), in addition to its antioxidant role in sperm, also appears to be responsible for maintaining the structure of sperm, at least in mouse sperm.

PHARMACOKINETICS

There are various forms of supplemental selenium, including high-selenium yeast, L-selenomethionine, sodium selenate and sodium selenite. High-selenium yeast contains L-selenomethionine in proteins. Proteins in high-selenium yeast are enzymatically digested in the small intestine to yield amino acids, oligopeptides and L-selenomethionine. L-selenomethionine is efficiently absorbed from the small intestine via a similar mechanism to that of L-methionine. L-selenomethionine is transported via the portal circulation to the liver where a fraction is extracted by the hepatocytes and the remaining amount is transported by the circulation to the various tissues of the body. L-selenomethionine enters the L-methionine pool in the hepatocytes and other cells of the body and shares the same metabolic fate of L-methionine until it is metabolized by the transsulfuration pathway. That is, L-selenomethionine participates in the synthesis of proteins and in the formation of seleno-adenosylmethionine (the selenium form of S-adenosylmethionine or SAMe), homoselenocysteine and L-selenocysteine, among other metabolites.

The metabolism of L-selenocysteine is different in several particulars from that of L-cysteine. L-selenocysteine is converted to hydrogen selenide via the enzyme selenocysteine beta-lyase. Hydrogen selenide can be metabolized to selenophosphate via selenophosphate synthetase or it can be methylated. The methylated metabolites are excreted in the urine. Selenophosphate is the precursor of L-selenocysteine in proteins or of selenium nucleosides in transfer RNA. The incorporation of L-selenocysteine in proteins is via seryl-transfer RNA. Selenocysteine synthase converts seryl-transfer RNA to selenocysteyl-transfer RNA. The L-selenocysteine residues found in all of the selenoproteins is derived from selenocysteyl-transfer RNA.

Free L-selenomethione is absorbed, distributed, and metabolized as described above. The inorganic forms of selenium, selenate and selenite, are also efficiently absorbed from the gastrointestinal tract. The fractional absorption of these inorganic forms is greater than 50%. Selenate or selenite is delivered to the liver via the portal circulation. A fraction is extracted by the hepatocytes and the rest is delivered via the systemic circulation to the various cells of the body. Within cells, these inorganic salts are converted to hydrogen selenide, and the further metabolism of hydrogen selenide is as described above.

Selenium homeostasis is achieved via regulation of its excretion by the kidneys. As selenium intake increases, urinary excretion of selenide metabolite increases. At very high intakes of selenium, volatile forms are exhaled. The odor of the exhaled forms of selenium is garlic-like. The excretory metabolites of selenium are mainly methylated metabolites of selenide. The principal urinary metabolites are methyselenol and trimethylselonium. Selenium excreted in the breath is mainly in the form of dimethylselenide.

INDICATIONS AND USAGE

Low dietary intake of selenium is associated with increased risk of some cardiomyopathies, ischemic heart disease and cardiovascular disease generally. Low intakes are also associated with increased incidence of some cancers, including prostate, lung, colorectal, gastric and skin cancers. Selenium supplementation has diminished these risks in some populations. There is the counterclaim that selenium supplementation might increase some cancers in some individuals. High levels of selenium have also recently been associated with increased risk of diabetes and higher mortality overall. Selenium's narrow therapeutic range makes toxicity a distinct possibility in some individuals. Selenium has demonstrated useful immune-enhancing effects in *in vitro*, animal and human studies. It is essential for healthy immune function. It may also have some anti-inflammatory benefits and could be useful in some with rheumatoid arthritis. It has the ability to detoxify some metals and xenobiotics. Selenium appears to play an important role in maintaining the viability of sperm cells, and supplemental selenium may thus be helpful in some infertile men. There is very preliminary evidence that high doses of selenium might promote modest weight gain. Reports that selenium can inhibit graying of hair are anecdotal.

RESEARCH SUMMARY

Epidemiological data indicate that low dietary intake of selenium is associated with increased incidence of several cancers, including lung, colorectal, skin and prostate cancers. There are *in vitro*, animal and human data showing that supplemental selenium can protect against some cancers. Much interest is now focusing on these findings, given gathering evidence that selenium intakes may actually be declining in some parts of the world, including some areas of the United States and the United Kingdom and other European countries.

There was one large cohort study, however, in which no significant selenium/cancer association was observed. Selenium in this study, however, was measured via selenium content in toenails. Some believe that this is not a reliable indicator of selenium status.

Studies to date indicate that diminished selenium status is not, in itself, carcinogenic but, rather, increases susceptibility to malignancy in the presence of carcinogens. Some studies have also shown that low selenium status predicts a poorer outcome in those who have some cancers. Findings however, are not entirely consistent.

In a recent well-controlled, large study conducted between 1983 and 1993, selenium supplementation (200 micrograms daily delivered via high-selenium brewer's yeast tablets) significantly diminished total cancer mortality (by 52% compared with controls). It did not significantly affect the incidence of basal and squamous cell carcinomas of the skin but did significantly reduce the incidence of lung, colorectal and prostate cancers. A total of 1,312 subjects (mostly men), aged 18-80 years, were enrolled in the study. Subjects had a history of basal cell or squamous cell carcinomas. Subjects, enrolled at seven dermatology clinics in the eastern United

States, were treated for a mean of 4.5 years and were followed up for 6.4 years.

Another long-term study, this one conducted in China, employed 200 micrograms of selenium daily over a four-year period. Those thus supplemented had a significantly lower incidence of primary liver cancer than did unsupplemented controls.

Some investigators have suggested that pharmacological doses of selenium, much higher than those used in typical supplements, might be effective in some established cancers. "Selenium compounds," one group has speculated, "that are able to generate a steady stream of methylated metabolites, in particular of the monomethylated species, are likely to have good chemopreventive potential."

Some now believe, however, that high-dose selenium could be dangerous and that in some susceptible individuals any selenium supplementation might be hazardous, increasing, rather than diminishing, cancer risk or progression. And the best available data suggest that dietary intake of selenium in the United States is on the high side, not the low side, as some previously speculated. A Nutritional Prevention of Cancer (NPC) trial, while finding some evidence for cancer prevention among some patients with lower selenium levels, additionally found a possible small increase in total cancer risk among participants with higher levels. A recent editorial in *The Annals of Internal Medicine* noted that "selenium has a narrow therapeutic range and may be toxic." On the positive side, the NPC study found a significant 49% reduction in prostate cancer risk among study subjects receiving a dietary supplement containing carotenoids, selenium and some other nutrients. Some large scale Phase III clinical trials are ongoing to further investigate the use of selenium in prostate and some other cancers. The World Cancer Research Fund and the American Institute for Cancer Research have both concluded that there is limited evidence suggestive of a selenium-protective effect in both prostate cancer and colorectal cancer. This, however, is not the same as saying there is convincing and conclusive evidence, which must still be sought.

In one recent study, serum selenium levels were measured in 13,887 adult participants in the Third National Health and Nutrition Examination Survey (NHANES III). Follow-up was for 12 years. Increasing selenium levels were associated with lower all-cause and cancer mortality up to a certain level. Thereafter, as levels increased higher so did all-cause and cancer mortality. There was no association between selenium levels and cardiovascular mortality in this study. The authors stated that their results should signal the need for caution in selenium supplementation but noted that "additional epidemiological studies are needed to establish

the levels of selenium associated with the lowest incidence of adverse health outcomes."

In both the NHANES III and the NPC trials discussed above, data emerged suggesting that selenium is not useful in diabetes and, in fact, may be harmful. High serum selenium levels were associated with a higher incidence of diabetes mellitus in the NHANES III study, and selenium supplementation was found to increase the risk of diabetes incidence in the NPC trial. Participants in the NPC trial received 200 micrograms of selenium daily for 7.7 years or placebo. This was the longest and largest experimental randomized, double-blind selenium trial to date comparing selenium with placebo. In view of these and other negative findings, editorialists writing in *The Annals of Internal Medicine* expressed the view that "until further randomized, controlled trials show that selenium supplementation does not cause diabetes or establish that the potential risk for diabetes is outweighed by yet unproven health benefits, people with diets that provide the Recommended Dietary Allowance for selenium should avoid selenium supplements, except in the context of experimental studies."

Keshan disease is a cardiomyopathy endemic in regions of China where selenium deficiency is prevalent. The Coxsackie viruses are co-factors with selenium deficiencies in this disease. A selenium-deficient environment in heart tissue appears to select for a cardiovirulent mutant of these viruses. *In vitro* animal and human data show that supplemental selenium can protect against this cardiomyopathy. Cardiomyopathies caused by long-term total parenteral nutrition (TPN) can also be prevented with adequate selenium supplementation.

Epidemiological data have demonstrated an inverse relationship between blood selenium levels and incidence of cardiovascular disease. Diminished selenium status has been associated with increased risk of myocardial infarction. Selenium has shown some ability to protect against oxidative damage to blood vessels. This damage is believed to play a role in the formation of atheromatous plaques. Selenium confers further protection by inhibiting peroxidation of some lipids. Still other heart benefits may accrue from selenium's demonstrated ability to inhibit platelet aggregation, modulate prostaglandin synthesis and protect against heavy metals.

Despite the foregoing positive evidence, large controlled prevention trials are still needed before selenium's preventive and therapeutic roles in cardiovascular disease can be properly assessed.

Selenium has been found to be essential for healthy immune function. Some viruses that are normally benign become pathogenic in those who are selenium deficient. This mechanism has been hypothesized by some to account for new mutant strains of influenza virus in China each year. Selenium has been shown to play important roles in T-cells and natural killer cells among other immune components. Deficiencies in selenium are associated with numerous adverse effects on immune function, including decreased CD4/ CD8 T-lymphocyte ratios and impaired phagocyte function.

Selenium supplementation has been shown to enhance T-cell responses, to stimulate antibody production and to partially reverse age-related cellular immunosuppression. Selenium supplementation has increased responsiveness to interleukin-2 (IL-2) in some studies. Supplementation also protects immune cells from oxidative damage in some instances. In one study, selenium supplementation reduced the incidence of hepatitis-B-induced hepatoma among those with low selenium status. Selenium status is predictive of survival time in some with AIDS, according to another study. Some have suggested that human immunodeficiency virus (HIV) may have been abetted in crossing the species barrier into humans in areas of Africa where selenium deficiency was prevalent. More research is needed and is ongoing with respect to supplemental selenium's role in immune function.

Selenium's anti-inflammatory effects are also related, at least in part, to its effects on immunity. Supplemental selenium can help protect some against Kashin-Beck Disease, a form of arthritis that afflicts many in selenium-deficient areas of China and other parts of Asia. There is some preliminary evidence that selenium, in combination with vitamin E, might alleviate articular pain and morning stiffness in some with arthritis.

In animal experiments, supplemental selenium has protected against some of the adverse effects of UV-radiation. In a mouse study, selenium significantly reduced the incidence of and mortality from non-melanoma skin cancers secondary to UV-exposure.

Selenium plasma levels have been found to be low in some infertile men. Selenium supplementation in these circumstances may improve sperm motility and enhance fertility. In a study of 64 infertile men living in an area of Scotland where low plasma levels of selenium are common, selenium supplementation over a two-year period significantly enhanced sperm motility compared with placebo. Five of the selenium-supplemented men fathered children; none of the men in the placebo group fathered children. There were 64 men in the study, including controls. Selenium appears to both protect sperm from oxidative damage and to help maintain the structural integrity of mature sperm. Follow-up is needed.

There is one report that selenium, in doses five times the recommended daily allowance (RDA) of this mineral, promoted modest weight gain among healthy men, aged 20 to 45. Supplementation continued for four months. The men all consumed the same diet, except for variations in selenium content. The diets were designed to maintain baseline body weight. The five men consuming the diet with high selenium content gained about 1.5 pounds. The six subjects consuming the diet low in selenium (providing about one fifth of the RDA) lost about 1 pound each. More research may be warranted.

CONTRAINDICATIONS, PRECAUTIONS, ADVERSE REACTIONS

CONTRAINDICATIONS

Selenium is contraindicated in those who are hypersensitive to any component of a selenium-containing preparation.

PRECAUTIONS

Pregnant women and nursing mothers should avoid selenium intakes greater than RDA amounts (60 and 70 micrograms daily, respectively).

ADVERSE REACTIONS

Intakes of selenium less than 900 micrograms daily (for adults) are unlikely to cause adverse reactions. Prolonged intakes of selenium of doses of 1,000 micrograms (or one milligram) or greater daily may cause adverse reactions.

The most frequently reported adverse reactions of selenosis or chronic selenium toxicity are hair and nail brittleness and loss. Other symptoms include skin rash, garlic-like breath odor, fatigue, irritability and nausea and vomiting. Perhaps the most famous example of selenium toxicity was reported in 1984. About 11 days after starting to take supplemental selenium, a 57-year-old female who was otherwise in good health noted marked hair loss which progressed over a two-month period to almost total alopecia. She also noted white horizontal streaking on one fingernail, as well as tenderness and swelling on the fingertips and purulent discharge from the fingernail beds. All of her fingernails eventually became involved and she lost the entire fingernail of the first digit affected. She also experienced episodes of nausea, vomiting, a sour-milk breath odor, and increase in fatigue. She learned a little over three months later that the selenium tablets she had taken were recalled by the distributor because they, in error, contained over 27 milligrams of selenium per tablet, 182 times higher than labeled. Others who took the same preparation suffered similar symptoms. Hair loss and fingernail changes (horizontal streaking, blackening, loss) were the most common symptoms.

Daily intake of 3.20 to 6.69 milligrams of selenium (average of 4 mg) by Chinese subjects in China produced loss of hair and nails, skin rash, garlic breath, fatigue, irritability and hyperreflexia. The same report described a 62-year-old man who took supplemental selenium in the form of sodium selenite; after two years he developed thickened, fragile nails and a garlic-like skin odor.

INTERACTIONS

DRUGS

There are no known interactions with drugs in clinical practice.

NUTRITIONAL SUPPLEMENTS

Iodine: Intake of selenium and iodide may have synergistic activity in the treatment of Kashin-Beck disease.

Vitamin C: Concomitant intake of selenium and the selenite form of selenium may decrease the absorption of selenium.

Vitamin E: Intake of vitamin E and selenium may produce synergistic beneficial effects.

OVERDOSAGE

Selenium overdosage has been reported in the literature. (See Adverse reactions).

DOSAGE AND ADMINISTRATION

Available forms of selenium supplements include high-selenium yeast, L-selenomethionine, sodium selenate and sodium selenite. Typical dosage ranges from 50 to 200 micrograms (as elemental selenium) daily. Se-methylseleno-cysteine is a predominant form of selenium found in garlic.

The average daily intake of selenium in the United States is about 100 micrograms.

The Food and Nutrition Board of the Institute of Medicine of the National Academy of Sciences has recommended the following Adequate Intake (AI) and Recommended Dietary Allowance (RDA) for selenium:

Infants	(AI)
0-6 months	15 micrograms/day
	(2.1 micrograms/kg)
7-12 months	20 micrograms/day
	(2.2 micrograms/kg)

Children	(RDA)
1-3 years	20 micrograms/day
4-8 years	30 micrograms/day

Boys	
9-13	40 micrograms/day
14-18 years	55 micrograms/day

Girls	
9-13 years	40 micrograms/day
14-18 years	55 micrograms/day

Men	
19-30 years	55 micrograms/day
31-50 years	55 micrograms/day
51-70 years	55 micrograms/day
Older than 70 years	55 micrograms/day

Women	
19-30 years	55 micrograms/day
31-50 years	55 micrograms/day
51-70 years	55 micrograms/day
Older than 70 years	55 micrograms/day

Pregnancy	
14-18 years	60 micrograms/day
19-30 years	60 micrograms/day
31-50 years	60 micrograms/day

Lactation	
14-18 years	70 micrograms/day
19-30 years	70 micrograms/day
31-50 years	70 micrograms/day

The Food and Nutrition Board has recommended the following Tolerable Upper Intake Levels (UL) for selenium:

Infants	(UL)
0-6 months	45 micrograms/day
7-12 months	60 micrograms/day

Children	
1-3 years	90 micrograms/day
4-8 years	150 micrograms/day
9-13 years	280 micrograms/day

Adolescents	
14-18 years	400 micrograms/day

Adults	
19 years and older	400 micrograms/day

Pregnancy	
14-18 years	400 micrograms/day
19-50 years	400 micrograms/day

Lactation	
14-18 years	400 micrograms/day
19-50 years	400 micrograms/day

The Lowest-Observed-Adverse-Effects-Level (LOAEL) for adults is about 900 micrograms daily.

The DV (Daily Value) for selenium, which is used for determining percentage of nutrient daily values on nutritional supplement and food labels, is 70 micrograms. The basis for the DV for selenium is the 1989 Estimated Safe and Adequate Daily Dietary Intake (ESADDI).

LITERATURE

Alaejos MS, Romero FJD, Romero CD. Selenium and cancer: some nutritional aspects. *Nutrition.* 2000;16:376-383.

Beck MA, Shi Q, Morris VC, Levander OA. Rapid genomic evolution of a non-virulent Coxsackievirus B3 in selenium-deficient mice results in selection of identical virulent strains. *Nature Med.* 1995;5:433-436.

Berry MJ, Banu L, Larsen PR. Type I iodothyronine deiodinase is a selenocysteine-containing enzyme. *Nature.* 1991;349:438-440.

Bleys J, Navas-Acien A, Guallar E. Selenium and diabetes: more bad news for supplements. *Ann Intern Med.* 2007;147(4):271-272.

Bleys J, Navas-Acien A, Guallar E. Serum selenium levels and all-cause, cancer, and cardiovascular mortality among US adults. *Arch Intern Med.* 2008;168(4):404-410.

Burk RF, ed. *Selenium in Biology and Human Health.* New York, NY: Springer-Verlag; 1994.

Burk RF, Levander OA. Selenium. In: Shils ME, Olson JA, Shike M, Ross AC, eds. *Modern Nutrition in Health and Disease.* Baltimore, MD: Williams and Wilkins; 1999:265-276.

Clark LC, Combs GF Jr, Turnbull BW, et al. Effects of selenium supplementation for cancer prevention in patients with carcinoma of the skin. *JAMA.* 1996;276:1957-1963.

Colditz GA. Selenium and cancer prevention. Promising results indicate further trials required (editorial). *JAMA.* 1996;276:1984-1985.

Dietary Reference Intakes for Vitamin C, Vitamin E, Selenium, and Carotenoids. Washington, DC: National Academy Press; 2000.

Diwadkar-Navsariwala V, Prins GS, Swanson SM, et al. Selenoprotein deficiency accelerates prostate carcinogenesis in a transgenic model. *Proc Natl Acad Sci USA.* 2006;103(21):8179-8184.

Dworkin BM. Selenium deficiency in HIV infection and the acquired immunodeficiency syndrome (AIDS). *Chem Biol Interact.* 1994;91:181-186.

Fleet JC. Dietary selenium repletion may reduce cancer incidence in people at high risk who live in areas with low soil selenium. *Nutr Rev.* 1997;55:277-279.

Flores-Mateo G, Navas-Acien A, Pastor-Barriuso R, et al. Selenium and coronary heart disease: a meta-analysis. *Am J Clin Nutr.* 2006;84(4):762-773.

Hendler SS. Micronutrition: vitamins, minerals, and trace elements. In: Newcomer VD, Young EM, eds. *Geriatric Dermatology. Clinical Diagnosis and Practical Therapy.* New York and Tokyo: Igaku-Shoin; 1989:365-393.

Huttunen JK. Selenium and cardiovascular diseases-an update. *Biomed Environ Sci.* 1997;10:220-226.

Ip C. Interaction of vitamin C and selenium supplementation in the modification of mammary carcinogenesis in rats. *J Natl Cancer Inst.* 1986;77:299-303.

Ip C. Lessons from basic research in selenium and cancer prevention. *J Nutr.* 1998;128:1845-1854.

Ip C, Thompson HJ, Zhu HJ, et al. In vitro and in vivo studies of methylseleninic acid: evidence that a monomethylated selenium metabolite is critical for cancer chemoprevention. *Cancer Res.* 2000;60:2882-2886.

Ip C, Zhu Z, Thompson HJ, et al. Chemoprevention of mammary cancer with Se-allylselenocysteine and other selenoaminoacids in the rat. *Anticancer Res.* 1999;19(4B):2875-2880.

Jiang C, Jiang W, Ip C, et al. Selenium-induced inhibition of angiogenesis in mammary cancer at chemopreventive levels of intake. *Mol Carcinog.* 1999;26:213-225.

Kardinaal AF, Kok FJ, Kohlmeier L, et al. Association between toenail selenium and risk of acute myocardial infarction in European men. The EURAMIC Study. European Antioxidant Myocardial Infarction and Breast Cancer. *Am J Epidemiol.* 1997;145:373-379.

Klein EA. Selenium and vitamin E cancer prevention trial. *Ann N Y Acad Sci.* 2004;1031:234-241.

Kohrle J. Thyroid hormone deiodinases—a selenoenzyme family acting as gate keepers to thyroid hormone action. *Acta Med Austriaca.* 1996;23:17-30.

Low SC, Berry MJ. Knowing when not to stop: selenocysteine incorporation in eukaryotes. *Trends Biochem Sci.* 1996;21:203-208.

Moreno-Reyes R, Suetens C, Mathieu F, et al. Kashin-Beck osteoarthropathy in rural Tibet in relation to selenium and iodine status. *N Engl J Med.* 1998;339:1112-1120.

Mukhopadhyay-Sardar S, Rana MP, Chatterjee M. Antioxidant associated chemoprevention by selenomethionine in murine tumor model. *Mol Cellul Biochem.* 2000;206:17-25.

Nadiminty N, Gao AC. Mechanisms of selenium chemoprevention and therapy in prostate cancer. *Mol Nutr Food Res.* Epub: 2008 Aug 22.

Navas-Acien A, Bleys J, Guallar E. Selenium intake and cardiovascular risk: what is new? *Curr Opin Lipidol.* 2008;19(1):43-49.

Olmsted L, Schrauzer GN, Flores-Arce M, Dowd J. Selenium supplementation of symptomatic human immunodeficiency virus infected patients. *Biol Trace Elem Res.* 1989;20:59-65.

Olson GE, Winfrey VP, Nagdas SK, et al. Selenoprotein P is required for mouse sperm development. *Biol Reprod.* 2005;73(1):201-211.

Peters U, Takata Y. Selenium and the prevention of prostate and colorectal cancer. *Mol Nutr Food Res.* Epub: 2008 Sep 2.

Rayman MP. Selenium in cancer prevention: a review of the evidence and mechanism of action. *Proc Nutr Soc.* 2005;64(4):527-542.

Reagan-Shaw S, Nihal M, Ahsan H, et al. Combination of vitamin E and selenium causes an induction of apoptosis of human prostate cancer cells by enhancing Bax/Bcl-2 ratio. *Prostate.* 2008;68(15):1624-1634.

Reilly C. Selenium: a new entrant into the functional food arena. *Trends Food Sci Technol.* 1998;9:114-118.

Schrauzer GN. Selenomethionine: a review of its nutritional significance, metabolism and toxicity. *J Nutr.* 2000;130:1653-1656.

Scott R, MacPherson A, Yates RWS, et al. The effect of oral selenium supplementation on human sperm motility. *J Urol.* 1998;82:76-80.

Selenium Intoxication-New York. *Morbidity and Mortality Weekly.* 1984; Report 33, No.12:157-158.

Stranges S, Marshall JR, Natarajan R, et al. Effects of long-term selenium supplementation on the incidence of type 2 diabetes: a randomized trial. *Ann Intern Med.* 2007;147(4):217-223.

Suadicani P, Hein HO, Gyntelberg F. Serum selenium concentration and risk of ischaemic heart disease in a prospective cohort study of 3,000 males. *Atherosclerosis.* 1992;96:33-42.

Thorpe JF, Jain S, Marczylo TH, et al. A review of phase III clinical trials of prostate cancer chemoprevention. *Ann R Coll Surg Engl.* 2007;89(3):207-211.

Ursini F, Heim S, Kiess M, et al. Dual function of the selenoprotein PHGPx during sperm maturation. *Science.* 1999;285:1393-1396.

Vunta H, Belda BJ, Arner RJ, et al. Selenium attenuates pro-inflammatory gene expression in macrophages. *Mol Nutr Food Res.* Epub: 2008 May 15.

Vunta H, Davis F, Palempalli UD, et al. The anti-inflammatory effects of selenium are mediated through 15-deoxy-Delta12,14-prostaglandin J2 in macrophages. *J Biol Chem.* 2007;282(25):17964-17973.

Yang G, Wang S, Zhou R, Sun S. Endemic selenium intoxication of humans in China. *Am J Clin Nutr.* 1988;37:872-881.

Yu MW, Horng IS, Hsu KH, et al. Plasma selenium levels and risk of hepatocellular carcinoma among men with chronic virus infection. *Am J Epidemiol.* 1999;150:367-374.

Yu SY, Zhu YJ, Li WG. Protective role of selenium against hepatitis B virus and primary liver cancer in Qidong. *Biol Trace Elem Res.* 1997;56:117-124.

Sesame Seed Lignans

DESCRIPTION

Sesame (*Sesamum indicum* L.) has a fascinating history. It is one of the oldest cultivated plants in the world and has been around for about 6,000 years. Sesame seed and its oil have been utilized as an important foodstuff and also for medicinal purposes, including providing energy and mental tranquility and preventing aging. It has also been used as an insecticide, for the preparation of mummies by the ancient Egyptians and as the fundamental body massage oil in Ayurvedic medicine. These days, bodybuilders use lignans from sesame seeds for supposed performance enhancement and weight loss. Recently, there has been a great deal of interest in studying sesame seed lignans for their biological effects and possible health benefits.

Sesame seed is one of the two major dietary sources of plant lignans, the other major source being flaxseed. The major sesame seed lignan is sesamin. Sesame seed contains about 0.4% sesamin in sesame oil or about 4 mg per gram. Sesame seed also contains about half as much of the lignan sesamolin and smaller amounts of sesamol, sesaminol, and the water-soluble lignans, sesaminol diglucoside and sesaminol triglucoside. (The aglycosides are lipid-soluble.) In addition, it contains small amounts of matairesinol, lariciresinol, pinoresinol and syringaresinol.

Sesamin, like all plant lignans, is a phenylpropanoid dimer. However, in contrast with the flaxseed lignan secoisolariciresinol diglucoside (see Flaxseed Lignans) and the spruce lignan 7-hydroxymatairesinol (see Spruce Lignans), which are of the dibenzylbutyrolactone structural type, sesamin is of the tetrahydrofuran, or furofuran structural type. The two major structural types of lignans in the plant kingdom are the dibenzylbutyrolactone and the tetrahydrofuran, or furofuran types. Sesamin and all of the sesame seed lignans are also classified as phytoestrogens.

The chemical names for sesamin are: 5,5'-(Tetrahydro-1*H*,3*H*-furo[3,4-*c*]furan-1,4-diyl)bis-1,3-benzodioxole; tetrahydro-1,4-bis[3,4-(methylenedioxy)phenyl]-1*H*,3*H*-furo[3,4-*c*]furan, and 2,6-bis(3,4-methylenedioxyphenyl)-3,7-dioxabicyclo[3.3.0]octane.

The molecular formula is $C_{20}H_{18}O_6$ and the molecular weight is 354.35. The CAS Registry Number for sesamin is 606-80-7. The sesamin preparation obtained as a by-product of the refining of edible sesame oil consists of a 1:1 ratio of sesamin and its epimer episesamin. Pure sesamin is available.

The chemical structures that follow are described within this monograph.

Sesamin

Enterolactone

ACTIONS AND PHARMACOLOGY

ACTIONS

Sesamin has possible anticancer, antihypertensive, antioxidant/pro-antioxidant/hepatoprotective, estrogenic/antiestrogenic, neuroprotective, lipid metabolism and hypocholesterolemic activities.

MECHANISM OF ACTION

Anticancer: Sesamin was shown to downregulate cyclin D1 protein expression in the human tumor cell line, MCF-7. Cyclin D1 belongs to a family of cyclin proteins that function as subunits of cyclin/cyclin-dependent kinase holoenzymes that regulate entry into and progression through the cell cycle. Overexpression of cyclin D1 may be involved in several cancers, including prostate, breast and colon cancer.

Sesamin was found to suppress the carcinogenic effect of 7, 12-dimethylbenz[a]anthracene (DMBA)-induced mammary carcinogenesis in female Sprague-Dawley rats. The mechanism of action of this effect is unclear. Possibilities include immunopotentiation and increased antioxidant activity.

Antihypertensive: The antihypertensive effect of sesamin has been demonstrated in three animal models of hypertension—the two kidney, one clip (2k,1c) renal hypertension rat model, the stroke-prone spontaneous hypertensive rat (SHR) model and the deoxycorticosterone acetate (DOCA) salt hypertensive rat model. The greatest antihypertensive activi-

ty was noted in the DOCA salt hypertensive rats. It is thought that the blood pressure-lowering effect of sesamin can be partly explained by its inhibitory effect on vascular superoxide production.

Blood pressure is regulated by arteriolar vascular tone. The endothelial bioavailability of endothelial nitric oxide (NO), produced by eNOS (endothelial nitric oxide synthase), is the major factor in the regulation of vascular tone. Superoxide anions react with NO-producing peroxynitrite, resulting in decreased endothelial bioavailability of vascular NO, arteriolar constriction and elevation of blood pressure. NADPH oxidase, a member of the NOX family of enzymes, produces superoxide anions, which is a major factor in the dysregulation of arteriolar tone. Inhibition of NADPH oxidase could play a major role in the maintenance of normal blood pressure. A recent paper (Nakano, et al., 2008) demonstrated suppression of aortic NADPH oxidase by administration of sesamin to DOCA hypertensive rats. More research and human studies are certainly warranted to determine if sesamin could have a role in the treatment of hypertension in humans.

Antioxidant/Pro-antioxidant: Sesamin itself does not appear to have antioxidant activity *in vitro*. Sesamin does not demonstrate radical scavenging effects on superoxide anions (O_2^-) or DPPH (2,2-diphenyl-2-picrylhydrazyl hydrate) radicals. Neither does it show inhibitory effects against lipid peroxidation. On the other hand, the minor sesame seed lignans that carry a phenolic hydroxyl group (sesamin does not)—sesaminol, episesaminol and sesamolinol—do exhibit antioxidant activity *in vitro*. It turns out that when sesamin was orally administered to rats, at least three compounds were formed via metabolism in the rats' livers, compounds that possessed phenolic hydroxyl groups and which did have strong superoxide anion (O_2^-) and hydroxyl radical (OH) scavenging activities. The methylenedioxyphenyl moiety in the structure of sesamin was shown to be converted into a methylenedihydrophenyl or catechol moiety. Sesamin has been shown to possess hepatoprotective activity against liver damage caused by ethanol or carbon tetrachloride. The mechanism of action of this hepatoprotective effect is most likely due to the antioxidant metabolites formed in the liver from sesamin.

In addition, sesamin is converted in the large intestine to the mammalian lignan, enterolactone (ENL), which is known to have antioxidant properties.

Prodrugs are drugs that are inactive but become active when they get metabolized. In this sense, sesamin can be considered a pro-antioxidant in that it does not have antioxidant activity until it is metabolized to active antioxidants.

Estrogen/Antiestrogen: In a study of postmenopausal women, it was found that ingestion of sesame seed caused an increase in sex hormone binding protein (SHBP) and also an increase in urinary 2-hydroxyestrone. This has also been seen in studies with flaxseed lignans and is possibly due to an estrogen/antiestrogen effect of an important metabolite of both sesame seed lignans and flaxseed lignans, the mammalian lignan, enterolactone. The amount of sesamin in the sesame seeds was approximately 250 mg and the total amount of lignans about 380 mg. An increase in the ratio of 2-hydroxyestrone over 16-hydroxyestrone is thought to favor a less mitogenic (carcinogenic) estrogen environment for women. Likewise, an increase in SHBP would result in a lower amount of free estrogen in the serum, also thought to create a less mitogenic estrogen environment for women. Much more work needs to be done in this area to in order to determine the role that sesamin might play in women's health.

Hypocholesterolemic: A few but not all animal studies have demonstrated cholesterol-lowering by sesamin, and a few human studies have done so as well. The mechanism of this possible cholesterol-lowering action is unclear and requires further research for elucidation. Possibilities offered have been inhibition of absorption of cholesterol and inhibition of the biosynthesis of cholesterol.

Lipid metabolism: Sesamin has been demonstrated to increase the activity and gene expression of enzymes involved in fatty acid oxidation in rat liver. This is thought to be through the activation of peroxisome proliferator activated receptor (PPAR)-alpha. Sesamin has also been demonstrated to lower the activity and gene expression of hepatic enzymes involved in fatty acid biosynthesis, through the downregulation of sterol regulatory element binding protein (SREBP)-1. Subsequent studies compared sesamin with the related sesamin lignan, sesamolin, and found that although sesamin was more effective in reducing serum and liver lipid levels in rats, sesamolin more strongly increased fatty acid oxidation. Because of these effects of sesamin on lipid metabolism, it has been speculated that sesamin might have an effect on adiposity. Studies of sesamin and related sesame lignans on hepatic fatty acid metabolism in humans are necessary and indicated, as are studies in humans on the possible effect of sesamin on weight control.

Neuroprotective: Neuroinflammation is a major factor in the pathogenesis of neurodegenerative diseases, including Alzheimer's disease, Parkinson's disease and multiple sclerosis. Microglia are macrophage-like cells that act as the first and main form of active immune defense in the central nervous system. Reactive oxygen and reactive nitrogen species (eg, nitric oxide, or NO) that are released from activated microglia may participate in neuroinflammatory and neurodegenerative processes. Bacterial lipopolysaccharide (LPS), cytokines and amyloid all rapidly cause the transcription and expression of inducible nitric oxide synthase (iNOS) in microglia. Activated microglia facilitate tumor necrosis factor (TNF)-alpha or NO-mediated neuronal cell death. Sesamin has been shown to suppress LPS-induced NO production in microglia via inhibition of signal transduction pathways or via inhibition of nuclear transcription factors.

Further investigation of this activity in a murine BV-2 microglial cell line indicated that sesamin inhibited LPS-induced IL (interleukin)-6 production by suppression of the p38 mitogen-activated protein kinase (MAPK) signal pathway and suppression of nuclear factor-kappaB (NF-kappaB) activation. The mechanism underlying this action is not clear and may have something to do with the antioxidant activity of sesamin.

PHARMACOKINETICS

The pharmacokinetics (PK) for sesamin and other sesame lignans in humans is incomplete and much work is yet to be performed in order to clarify the rather complex aspects of the absorption, distribution, metabolism and excretion of the sesame seed lignans. What follows is what we presently know about the PK of sesamin.

After ingestion, some sesamin is absorbed from the small intestine and some is converted by the intestinal microflora in the proximal or upper part of the large intestine to the mammalian lignan, enterolactone (ENT), and to a lesser degree to the mammalian lignan, enterodiol (END). Reports vary as to the extent of the conversion of sesamin to the mammalian lignans. Some sesamin is also absorbed in the small intestine and winds up in the liver where the methylenedioxyphenyl moiety of sesamin undergoes oxidative biotransformation and demethylation to form a number of hydroxylated catechol metabolites. In contrast to sesamin, which does not demonstrate antioxidant properties *in vitro,* the catechol metabolites are diphenols and do demonstrate antioxidant activity *in vitro.* There is evidence that some of the metabolism of sesamin takes place in the enterocytes of the small intestine before it gets to the liver. It appears that the major catechol metabolite of sesamin is a compound that goes by the cumbersome name of (1*R*,2*S*,5*R*,6*S*)-6-13, 4-dihydroxyphenyl)-2-(3,4-methylenedioxyphenyl)-3,7-dioxabiclo 3,7-[3,3,0]octane. This compound may be responsible for some of the biologic actions of sesamin, especially for the hepatoprotective activity of sesamin.

The catechol metabolites may get excreted in the bile and then get metabolized by the intestinal flora of the large intestine to ENT and ENL. It is unclear as to the amounts of END and ENL that are produced directly from the microflora metabolism of sesamin and from the catechol metabolites. The catechol metabolites form glucuronides and sulfates. The urinary excretion of the sesamin catechol metabolite described above ranges from about 22% to 39%, mostly in the glucuronide and sulfate forms.

INDICATIONS AND USAGE

Claims made for dietary lignans derived from sesame seeds include antioxidant, antihypertensive, anticarcinogenic, anti-thrombotic, cardioprotective and hepatoprotective effects. It has also been suggested that these lignans may help protect against type II diabetes and Alzheimer's disease, that they may have favorable immunomodulating effects and that they might be of benefit to postmenopausal women. The idea that the lignans might be beneficial in weight control has scant support.

RESEARCH SUMMARY

Sesame seed oil resists rancidification and heat degradation much better than many other oils, apparently owing primarily to the antioxidant properties of some of its lignans. The ancient Egyptians used sesame seed oil in the preservation of mummies, and, more recently, one group of Japanese researchers reported that sesame oil is considered best for deep-frying tempura because it excels at resisting heat-induced deterioration. In both *in vitro* and *in vivo* animal experiments, sesaminol significantly suppressed lipid peroxidation products. In one such experiment, it was found to be more effective in this regard than alpha-tocopherol and the lipid-lowering antioxidant agent probucol. *In vitro,* sesamin, on the other hand, shows little or no antioxidative effect. *In vivo,* however, there is evidence that sesamin, through various of its metabolites, also exerts significant antioxidative activity that may be beneficial. Sesamolin, another sesame lignan, resembles sesamin in that it, too, exhibits little antioxidant activity *in vitro* but seems to act as a prodrug *in vivo,* giving rise to derivatives that exert antioxidative activity that could have beneficial physiological effects.

Additionally, other research has suggested that the sesame lignans may synergize with and enhance the antioxidant properties of vitamins E and C. In one human study, elevated levels of vitamin E were attributed to daily feedings of muffins containing sesame seeds. In a rat study, sesaminol demonstrated a greater ability to elevate vitamin E than did sesamin. Other *in vitro* and animal studies also suggest that these lignans can potentiate vitamin E and synergize with it to reduce lipid peroxidation in the liver. Hairless mice exposed to ultraviolet irradiation suffered significantly less damage when treated with dietary compounds having vitamin E activity in combination with sesame lignans, when compared with controls. Another rat study indicates that dietary sesame seed and its lignans stimulate ascorbic acid

synthesis and, synergistically, thus boost the antioxidative activity of both sesame seed lignans and vitamin C.

Various researchers have now found that sesame seeds and sesame oil lower serum cholesterol concentrations and inhibit the absorption of cholesterol in lymph. Sesamin, similarly, has demonstrated the ability to lower serum cholesterol in normal rats and to do so, as well, in hypercholesterolemic, stroke-prone spontaneous hypertensive rats. *In vitro* studies have shown that sesaminol is useful in protecting against the damaging effects of LDL oxidation. Sesamin and vitamin E together exhibited favorable lipid effects in hypercholesterolemic human subjects in one of only a few relevant clinical trials. Antihypertensive effects have been observed in animal hypertension models treated with dietary sesamin. Antithrombotic effects have been observed, as well, in some preliminary *in vitro* investigations. Because of the experimental data, it is hoped that the sesame lignans may ultimately prove to have clinical significance as cardioprotective and anti-stroke agents through favorable effects on lipid metabolism, platelet aggregation and other pathways. In addition, owing to findings in rats that sesamin can significantly decrease serum triglycerides, upregulate fatty acid oxidation and downregulate the biosynthesis of fatty acids, it has been suggested that dietary sesame lignan supplementation might have some ability to suppress adiposity. Far more research would be required, however, to establish that the sesame lignans might have any benefit as weight control agents.

In terms of cancer protection, sesame lignans have shown some ability to suppress chemically-induced breast cancer in an animal model. In another study, the growth of human lymphoid leukemia cells was increasingly inhibited with increased concentrations of sesame lignan *in vitro*. A type of DNA fragmentation characteristic of apoptosis was observed. Sesaminol, in this experiment, was more effective than sesamin, sesamolin and episesamin. The lignans did not damage normal cells. More research on the anticarcinogenic potential of these lignans is warranted.

Liver function was said to be enhanced in a study of rats given large amounts of alcohol and fed sesamin. Enhanced ethanol metabolism, induced by sesamin, had previously been reported in mice. And human volunteers given whisky demonstrated ethanol resistance in another study in which the subjects were given 100 mg of sesamin daily for a week prior to the alcohol challenge. Alcohol decomposed more quickly in the sesamin supplemented volunteers than it did in control subjects who did not receive the lignan. Researchers have concluded that sesamin does not inhibit the absorption of alcohol but that it increases its decomposition in the liver and diminishes the toxicity of acetaldehyde, an oxidative product of alcohol.

There is very preliminary experimental evidence that the sesame lignans might be helpful in some immune disorders, possibly food allergy, through immunoregulatory activity, that they might be helpful in impeding Alzheimer's disease and oxidative stress-induced neuronal disorders and that they may exert hypoglycemic activity, which could be helpful in type II diabetes. Much more research is needed, and indicated, to further elucidate these possibilities.

Finally, sesamin has been reported to have estrogenic effects, possibly through its conversion by intestinal microflora to enterolactone. In a randomized, placebo-controlled study of 26 healthy postmenopausal women, the researchers concluded that the lignan, compared with placebo, conferred benefits upon the postmenopausal subjects by improving blood lipids and antioxidant status and by "possibly" improving sex hormone status. This study is inconclusive in terms of establishing any positive estrogenic effects in postmenopausal women.

CONTRAINDICATIONS, PRECAUTIONS, ADVERSE REACTIONS
CONTRAINDICATIONS
Sesame seed lignans are contraindicated in those who are hypersensitive to any component of a sesame seed lignan-containing product.

PRECAUTIONS
Pregnant women and nursing mothers should avoid the use of sesame lignan supplements pending long-term safety studies.

Men with prostate cancer or benign prostatic hyperplasia (BPH) should discuss the advisability of the use of sesame seed lignan supplements with their physicians before deciding to use them.

Women with estrogen receptor-positive tumors should exercise caution in the use of sesame lignan supplements and should only use them if they are recommended and monitored by a physician.

ADVERSE REACTIONS
None known.

INTERACTIONS
DRUGS
Antibiotics: Concomitant use with sesame seed lignans may decrease the production of the mammalian lignans enterolactone (ENT) and enterodiol (END) from sesame seed lignans.

Diclofenac: The sesame lignan sesamol has been shown to attenuate the acute gastric injury in rats caused by the diclofenac NSAID via its cyclooxygenase–independent antioxidant effect.

NUTRITIONAL SUPPLEMENTS
A single dose of the sesame seed lignans sesamin and sesamolin (136 mg) was found to reduce the urinary excretion of co-administered gamma-tocopherol in a human study. The sesame seed lignans sesamin and sesaminol were found to elevate the gamma-tocopherol concentrations in the tissues and serum of rats and to inhibit the formation of the gamma-tocopherol metabolite 2,7,8-trimethyl-2(2'-carboxyethyl)-6-hydroxychroman (gamma-CEHC) and its excretion in the urine via inhibition of the cytochrome P450-CYP3A-dependent metabolism of gamma-tocopherol.

Dietary sesamin, docosahexaenoic acid (DHA) and eicosapentaenoic acid (EPA) synergistically increased the gene expression of enzymes involved in hepatic peroxisomal fatty acid oxidation in rats, but not the gene expression of enzymes involved in mitochondrial fatty acid oxidation.

Vitamin E (alpha-tocopherol) and sesamin synergistically lowered blood pressure and decreased oxidative stress and cerebral thrombogenesis in stroke-prone spontaneous hypertensive rats (SHR).

Dietary tocotrienol was found to reduce UVB-induced skin damage in hairless mice, and sesamin was found to enhance the tocotrienol effect. In the study, tocotrienol was shown to protect the skin more strongly than D-alpha tocopherol. It was observed that sesamin produced higher alpha- and gamma-tocotrienols in the skin of rats fed diets containing alpha- and gamma-tocotrienols along with sesamin.

It has been demonstrated that the feeding of the sesame lignans sesamin and sesaminol to rats on a low D-alpha tocopherol diet or on a low gamma-tocopherol diet elevates alpha-tocopherol or gamma-tocopherol, respectively, in plasma, liver, kidney and brain. No change in either alpha-tocopherol or gamma-tocopherol levels was found when the sesame seed lignans were replaced by either the flaxseed lignan, secoisolariciresinol diglucoside (SDG), or the spruce lignan, 7-hydroxymatairesinol (HMR). Interestingly, both SDG and HMR are dibenzylbutyrolactone-type lignans, while the sesame lignans are tetrahydrofurofuran-type lignans.

FOODS
No known interactions.

HERBS
An extract of *Schisandra chinensis* berry, when combined with sesamin, was found to decrease blood viscosity and improve blood fluidity in a human clinical study.

OVERDOSAGE
There are no reports of flaxseed lignan overdosage.

DOSAGE AND ADMINISTRATION

Sesamin and other sesame seed lignans have been studied at doses of 300 mg to 400 mg daily for prolonged periods of time without any significant adverse events noted. However, the optimal dose for human consumption is not known.

The amount of sesamin in sesame seeds averages about 4 mg per gram.

Sesamin in capsules of 500 mg are available and used by bodybuilders for supposed weight reduction.

LITERATURE

Adlercreutz H. Lignans and human health. *Crit Rev Clin Lab Sci.* 2007;44(5-6):483-525.

Akimoto K, Kitagawa Y, Akamatsu T, et al. Protective effects of sesamin against liver damage caused by alcohol or carbon tetrachloride in rodents. *Ann Nutr Metab.* 1993;37(4):218-224.

Arachchige PG, Takahashi Y, Ide T. Dietary sesamin and docosahexaenoic and eicosapentaenoic acids synergistically increase the gene expression of enzymes involved in hepatic peroxisomal fatty acid oxidation in rats. *Metabolism.* 2006;55(3):381-390.

Ashakumary L, Rouyer I, Takahashi Y, et al. Sesamin, a sesame lignan, is a potent inducer of hepatic fatty acid oxidation in the rat. *Metabolism.* 1999;48(10):1303-1313.

Cooney RV, Custer LJ, Okinaka L, et al. Effects of dietary sesame seeds on plasma tocopherol levels. *Nutr Cancer.* 2001;39(1):66-71.

Frank J, Kamal-Eldin A, Traber MG. Consumption of sesame oil muffins decreases the urinary excretion of gamma-tocopherol metabolites in humans. *Ann N Y Acad Sci.* 2004;1031:365-367.

Fujiyama-Fujiwara Y, Umeda-Sawada R, Kuzuyama M, et al. Effects of sesamin on the fatty acid composition of the liver of rats fed N-6 and N-3 fatty acid-rich diet. *J Nutr Sci Vitaminol* (Tokyo). 1995;41(2):217-225.

Ghafoorunissa, Hemalatha S, Rao MV. Sesame lignans enhance antioxidant activity of vitamin E in lipid peroxidation systems. *Mol Cell Biochem.* 2004;262(1-2):195-202.

Gu JY, Wakizono Y, Dohi A, et al. Effect of dietary fats and sesamin on the lipid metabolism and immune function of Sprague-Dawley rats. *Biosci Biotechnol Biochem.* 1998;62(10):1917-1924.

Gu JY, Wakizono Y, Tsujita A, et al. Effects of sesamin and alpha-tocopherol, individually or in combination, on the polyunsaturated fatty acid metabolism, chemical mediator production, and immunoglobulin levels in Sprague-Dawley rats. *Biosci Biotechnol Biochem.* 1995;59(12):2198-2202.

Hirata F, Fujita K, Ishikura Y, et al. Hypocholesterolemic effect of sesame lignan in humans. *Atherosclerosis.* 1996;122(1):135-136.

Hirose N, Doi F, Ueki T, et al. Suppressive effect of sesamin against 7,12-dimethylbenz[a]-anthracene induced rat mammary carcinogenesis. *Anticancer Res.* 1992;12(4):1259-1265.

Hirose N, Inoue T, Nishihara K, et al. Inhibition of cholesterol absorption and synthesis in rats by sesamin. *J Lipid Res.* 1991;32(4):629-638.

Hou RC, Wu CC, Yang CH, et al. Protective effects of sesamin and sesamolin on murine BV-2 microglia cell line under hypoxia. *Neurosci Lett.* 2004;367(1):10-13.

Hou RC, Chen HL, Tzen JT, et al. Effect of sesame antioxidants on LPS-induced NO production by BV2 microglial cells. *Neuroreport.* 2003;14(14):1815-1819.

Hou RC, Huang HM, Tzen JT, et al. Protective effects of sesamin and sesamolin on hypoxic neuronal and PC12 cells. *J Neurosci Res.* 2003;74(1):123-133.

Ide T, Ashakumary L, Takahashi Y, et al. Sesamin, a sesame lignan, decreases fatty acid synthesis in rat liver accompanying the down-regulation of sterol regulatory element binding protein-1. *Biochim Biophys Acta.* 2001;1534(1):1-13.

Ide T, Hong DD, Ranasinghe P, et al. Interaction of dietary fat types and sesamin on hepatic fatty acid oxidation in rats. *Biochim Biophys Acta.* 2004;1682(1-3):80-91.

Ikeda S, Abe C, Uchida T, et al. Dietary sesame seed and its lignan increase both ascorbic acid concentration in some tissues and urinary excretion by stimulating biosynthesis in rats. *J Nutr Sci Vitaminol* (Tokyo). 2007;53(5):383-392.

Ikeda S, Kagaya M, Kobayashi K, et al. Dietary sesame lignans decrease lipid peroxidation in rats fed docosahexaenoic acid. *J Nutr Sci Vitaminol* (Tokyo). 2003;49(4):270-276.

Ikeda S, Tohyama T, Yamashita K. Dietary sesame seed and its lignans inhibit 2,7,8-trimethyl-2(2'-carboxyethyl)-6-hydroxychroman excretion into urine of rats fed gamma-tocopherol. *J Nutr.* 2002;132(5):961-966.

Ikeda T, Nishijima Y, Shibata H, et al. Protective effect of sesamin administration on exercise-induced lipid peroxidation. *Int J Sports Med.* 2003;24(7):530-534.

Jeng KC, Hou RC, Wang JC, et al. Sesamin inhibits lipopolysaccharide-induced cytokine production by suppression of p38 mitogen-activated protein kinase and nuclear factor-kappaB. *Immunol Lett.* 2005;97(1):101-106.

Kamal-Eldin A, Pettersson D, Appelqvist LA. Sesamin (a compound from sesame oil) increases tocopherol levels in rats fed ad libitum. *Lipids.* 1995;30(6):499-505.

Kiso Y. Antioxidative roles of sesamin, a functional lignan in sesame seed, and it's effect on lipid- and alcohol-metabolism in the liver: a DNA microarray study. *Biofactors.* 2004;21(1-4):191-196.

Kiso Y, Tsuruoka N, Kidokoro A, et al. Sesamin ingestion regulates the transcription levels of hepatic metabolizing enzymes for alcohol and lipids in rats. *Alcohol Clin Exp Res.* 2005;29(11 Suppl):116S-120S.

Kushiro M, Masaoka T, Hageshita S, et al. Comparative effect of sesamin and episesamin on the activity and gene expression of enzymes in fatty acid oxidation and synthesis in rat liver. *J Nutr Biochem.* 2002;13(5):289-295.

Kushiro M, Takahashi Y, Ide T. Species differences in the physiological activity of dietary lignan (sesamin and episesamin) in affecting hepatic fatty acid metabolism. *Br J Nutr.* 2004;91(3):377-386.

Lee CC, Chen PR, Lin S, et al. Sesamin induces nitric oxide and decreases endothelin-1 production in HUVECs: possible implications for its antihypertensive effect. *J Hypertens.* 2004;22(12):2329-2338.

Lim JS, Adachi Y, Takahashi Y, et al. Comparative analysis of sesame lignans (sesamin and sesamolin) in affecting hepatic fatty acid metabolism in rats. *Br J Nutr.* 2007;97(1):85-95.

Liu Z, Saarinen NM, Thompson LU. Sesamin is one of the major precursors of mammalian lignans in sesame seed (Sesamum indicum) as observed in vitro and in rats. *J Nutr.* 2006;136(4):906-912.

Matsumura Y, Kita S, Morimoto S, et al. Antihypertensive effect of sesamin. I. Protection against deoxycorticosterone acetate-salt-induced hypertension and cardiovascular hypertrophy. *Biol Pharm Bull.* 1995;18(7):1016-1019.

Matsumura Y, Kita S, Ohgushi R, et al. Effects of sesamin on altered vascular reactivity in aortic rings of deoxycorticosterone acetate-salt-induced hypertensive rat. *Biol Pharm Bull.* 2000;23(9):1041-1045.

Matsumura Y, Kita S, Tanida Y, et al. Antihypertensive effect of sesamin. III. Protection against development and maintenance of hypertension in stroke-prone spontaneously hypertensive rats. *Biol Pharm Bull.* 1998;21(5):469-473.

Miyahara Y, Komiya T, Katsuzaki H, et al. Sesamin and episesamin induce apoptosis in human lymphoid leukemia Molt 4B cells. *Int J Mol Med.* 2000;6(1):43-46.

Nakabayashi A, Kitagawa Y, Suwa Y, et al. alpha-Tocopherol enhances the hypocholesterolemic action of sesamin in rats. *Int J Vitam Nutr Res.* 1995;65(3):162-168.

Nakai M, Harada M, Nakahara K, et al. Novel antioxidative metabolites in rat liver with ingested sesamin. *J Agric Food Chem.* 2003;51(6):1666-1670.

Nakano D, Itoh C, Ishii F, et al. Effects of sesamin on aortic oxidative stress and endothelial dysfunction in deoxycorticosterone acetate-salt hypertensive rats. *Biol Pharm Bull.* 2003;26(12):1701-1705.

Nakano D, Itoh C, Takaoka M, et al. Antihypertensive effect of sesamin. IV. Inhibition of vascular superoxide production by sesamin. *Biol Pharm Bull.* 2002;25(9):1247-1249.

Nakano D, Kurumazuka D, Nagai Y, et al. Dietary sesamin suppresses aortic NADPH oxidase in DOCA salt hypertensive rats. *Clin Exp Pharmacol Physiol.* 2008;35(3):324-326.

Nakano D, Kwak CJ, Fujii K, et al. Sesamin metabolites induce an endothelial nitric oxide-dependent vasorelaxation through their antioxidative property-independent mechanisms: possible involvement of the metabolites in the antihypertensive effect of sesamin. *J Pharmacol Exp Ther.* 2006;318(1):328-335.

Namiki M. Nutraceutical functions of sesame: a review. *Crit Rev Food Sci Nutr.* 2007;47(7):651-673.

Nonaka M, Yamashita K, Iizuka Y, et al. Effects of dietary sesaminol and sesamin on eicosanoid production and immunoglobulin level in rats given ethanol. *Biosci Biotechnol Biochem.* 1997;61(5):836-839.

Ogawa H, Sasagawa S, Murakami T, et al. Sesame lignans modulate cholesterol metabolism in the stroke-prone spontaneously hypertensive rat. *Clin Exp Pharmacol Physiol Suppl.* 1995;22(1):S310-312.

Peñalvo JL, Heinonen SM, Aura AM, et al. Dietary sesamin is converted to enterolactone in humans. *J Nutr.* 2005;135(5):1056-1062.

Shimizu S, Akimoto K, Shinmen Y, et al. Sesamin is a potent and specific inhibitor of delta 5 desaturase in polyunsaturated fatty acid biosynthesis. *Lipids.* 1991;26(7):512-516.

Sirato-Yasumoto S, Katsuta M, Okuyama Y, et al. Effect of sesame seeds rich in sesamin and sesamolin on fatty acid oxidation in rat liver. *J Agric Food Chem.* 2001;49(5):2647-2651.

Suja KP, Jayalekshmy A, Arumughan C. Free radical scavenging behavior of antioxidant compounds of sesame (sesamum indicum L.) in DPPH(*) system. *J Agric Food Chem.* 2004;52(4):912-915.

Tsuruoka N, Kidokoro A, Matsumoto I, et al. Modulating effect of sesamin, a functional lignan in sesame seeds, on the transcription levels of lipid- and alcohol-metabolizing enzymes in rat liver: a DNA microarray study. *Biosci Biotechnol Biochem.* 2005;69(1):179-188.

Umeda-Sawada R, Fujiwara Y, Abe H, et al. Effects of sesamin and capsaicin on the mRNA expressions of delta6 and delta5 desaturases in rat primary cultured hepatocytes. *J Nutr Sci Vitaminol* (Tokyo). 2003;49(6):442-446.

Umeda-Sawada R, Ogawa M, Igarashi O. The metabolism and distribution of sesame lignans (sesamin and episesamin) in rats. *Lipids.* 1999;34(6):633-637.

Umeda-Sawada R, Ogawa M, Igarashi O. The metabolism and n-6/n-3 ratio of essential fatty acids in rats: effect of dietary arachidonic acid and a mixture of sesame lignans (sesamin and episesamin). *Lipids.* 1998;33(6):567-572.

Umeda-Sawada R, Ogawa M, Nakamura M, et al. Effect of sesamin on mitochondrial and peroxisomal beta-oxidation of arachidonic and eicosapentaenoic acids in rat liver. *Lipids.* 2001;36(5):483-489.

Umeda-Sawada R, Ogawa M, Okada Y, et al. Effect of sesamin on the composition of eicosapentaenoic acid in liver and on its lymphatic absorption in rats. *Biosci Biotechnol Biochem.* 1996;60(12):2071-2072.

Umeda-Sawada R, Takahashi N, Igarashi O. Interaction of sesamin and eicosapentaenoic acid against delta 5 desaturation and n-6/n-3 ratio of essential fatty acids in rat. *Biosci Biotechnol Biochem.* 1995;59(12):2268-2273.

Utsunomiya T, Chavali SR, Zhong WW, et al. Effects of sesamin-supplemented dietary fat emulsions on the ex vivo production of lipopolysaccharide-induced prostanoids and tumor necrosis factor alpha in rats. *Am J Clin Nutr*. 2000;72(3):804-808.

Utsunomiya T, Shimada M, Rikimaru T, et al. Antioxidant and anti-inflammatory effects of a diet supplemented with sesamin on hepatic ischemia-reperfusion injury in rats. *Hepatogastroenterology*. 2003;50(53):1609-1613.

Wu WH, Kang YP, Wang NH, et al. Sesame ingestion affects sex hormones, antioxidant status, and blood lipids in postmenopausal women. *J Nutr*. 2006;136(5):1270-1275.

Yamada Y, Obayashi M, Ishikawa T, et al. Dietary Tocotrienol Reduces UVB-Induced Skin Damage and Sesamin Enhances Tocotrienol Effects in Hairless Mice. *J Nutr Sci Vitaminol* (Tokyo). 2008;54(2):117-123.

Yamashita K, Iizuka Y, Imai T, et al. Sesame seed and its lignans produce marked enhancement of vitamin E activity in rats fed a low alpha-tocopherol diet. *Lipids*. 1995;30(11):1019-1028.

Yamashita K, Ikeda S, Obayashi M. Comparative effects of flaxseed and sesame seed on vitamin E and cholesterol levels in rats. *Lipids*. 2003;38(12):1249-1255.

Yamashita K, Kagaya M, Higuti N, et al. Sesamin and alpha-tocopherol synergistically suppress lipid-peroxide in rats fed a high docosahexaenoic acid diet. *Biofactors*. 2000;11(1-2):11-13.

Yamashita K, Nohara Y, Katayama K, et al. Sesame seed lignans and gamma-tocopherol act synergistically to produce vitamin E activity in rats. *J Nutr*. 1992;122(12):2440-2446.

Yamashita K, Yamada Y, Kitou S, et al. Hydroxymatairesinol and sesaminol act differently on tocopherol concentrations in rats. *J Nutr Sci Vitaminol* (Tokyo). 2007;53(5):393-399.

Yokota T, Matsuzaki Y, Koyama M, et al. Sesamin, a lignan of sesame, down-regulates cyclin D1 protein expression in human tumor cells. *Cancer Sci*. 2007;98(9):1447-1453.

Shark Cartilage

DESCRIPTION

Shark cartilage became popular as a nutritional supplement a number of years ago, based on the claim that sharks do not get cancer and that this substance must therefore be useful for the prevention and treatment of cancer. The fact is that sharks do get cancer. The claim that sharks do not, or rarely, get cancer originates from a 1992 book written by I. William Lane entitled *Sharks Don't Get Cancer*. In a 2004 review article published in *Cancer Research* and written by Gary Ostrander and his colleagues, both malignant and benign neoplasms of sharks and their relatives were described, including previously unreported cases from the Registry of Tumors in Lower Animals and two sharks with two cancers each. Although some components of cartilage, including shark cartilage, might have anticancer potential, the best scientific evidence to date supports neither the efficacy of

crude shark cartilage extracts nor the ability of possible effective components to reach and irradicate cancer cells.

Cartilage is a tissue that lacks blood vessels and rarely develops malignancies. Angiogenesis, the formation of new capillaries, is now known to be important in a number of pathological conditions, including solid tumors, proliferative retinopathy, neovascular glaucoma and rheumatoid arthritis. The process is also important in other physiological events as well, such as neovascularization following coronary artery occlusion.

In 1976, Judah Folkman and his colleagues reported on the isolation of a fraction from the scapular cartilage of calves that inhibited the growth of new blood vessels supporting implanted tumors in rabbits. It also stopped the growth of the tumors. Subsequent reports demonstrated a fraction in shark cartilage that also inhibited tumor neovascularization and growth.

The study of angiogenesis inhibitors has become a new field in cancer research. Since the earliest anti-angiogenesis substances discovered were derived from cartilage, research continues looking at cartilage to try to identify and characterize novel anti-angiogenic agents. Because sharks are an abundant source of cartilage, shark cartilage is being used by several research groups.

Sharks have an endoskeleton comprised entirely of cartilage, and while cartilage comprises less than 0.6% of the body weight of calves, it comprises about 6% of the body weight of sharks. Shark cartilage, like other forms of cartilage, is mainly composed of collagen, which participates in giving cartilage its tensile strength, and proteoglycans, themselves composed of a core protein to which is attached polysaccharides known as glycosaminoglycans or mucopolysaccharides. Proteoglycans impart resilience to cartilage. The main glycosaminoglycans in shark cartilage are the chondroitin sulfates. In addition to collagen and chondroitin sulfate, shark cartilage contains about 5 to 10% water, a large percentage of calcium and phosphate, low-molecular-weight proteins and polypeptides. A few low-molecular-weight proteins and polypeptides that appear to possess antiangiogenic activity have also been identified in shark cartilage. These substances are being researched as possible therapeutic candidates.

ACTIONS AND PHARMACOLOGY

ACTIONS

Shark cartilage has putative antitumor, antioxidant, anti-inflammatory and anti-atherogenic actions, although these putative actions are so far poorly supported by credible clinical research.

MECHANISM OF ACTION

The mechanism of the possible actions of shark cartilage is unclear. It appears that any possible therapeutic benefit derives mainly from low-molecular-weight protein molecules that are currently being researched. Some of these molecules possess anti-angiogenic activity and inhibit metalloproteinases and vascular endothelial growth factor (VEGF)-mediated signaling events, activities that could help explain any possible antitumor activity.

PHARMACOKINETICS

There is little known about the pharmacokinetics of shark cartilage.

INDICATIONS AND USAGE

Widespread claims are made for shark cartilage, including anticancer, anti-inflammatory, antiarthritic, antipsoriasis and antiatherosclerotic effects. At present there is no credible clinical data sufficient to support any of these claims.

RESEARCH SUMMARY

Shark cartilage has been heavily promoted as an anti-cancer agent. Some *in vitro* and animal studies show some anti-angiogenic properties. Inhibition of wound angiogenesis has recently been demonstrated in one study of human subjects given liquid shark cartilage extract, but there are no other human data related to shark cartilage's putative anti-angiogenic effects and certainly none that show this effect in cancer patients.

Shark cartilage was tested directly in human subjects with advanced cancers of various types. In this phase I/II trial of the safety and efficacy of shark cartilage in cancer treatment, the substance was found to be inactive "and had no salutary effect on quality of life." A more recent clinical trial was conducted to look at the impact of a popular shark cartilage dietary supplement in patients with advanced breast or colorectal cancer. The study was a two-arm randomized, placebo-controlled, double-blind, clinical trial. Data on a total of 83 evaluable patients were analyzed. There was no difference in overall survival between patients receiving standard care plus the shark cartilage product versus standard care plus placebo, and there was no improvement in quality of life for the patients receiving the shark cartilage compared with those receiving placebo. Some anti-inflammatory effects of shark cartilage have been demonstrated *in vitro* and in animal models, but no useful conclusion can yet be drawn from this very preliminary research.

CONTRAINDICATIONS, PRECAUTIONS, ADVERSE REACTIONS

CONTRAINDICATIONS

Shark cartilage is contraindicated in those who are hypersensitive to any component of a shark cartilage-containing product. It is also contraindicated in those with hypercalcemia (shark cartilage contains a high percentage of calcium).

PRECAUTIONS

Pregnant women and nursing mothers should avoid shark cartilage supplementation.

Those with renal failure or liver failure should exercise caution in the use of shark cartilage.

Those with cancer who wish to try shark cartilage must only do so under medical supervision.

ADVERSE REACTIONS

The major adverse reactions are gastrointestinal and include nausea and vomiting, bloating and constipation. Some find the taste of shark cartilage disagreeable. There is one report of hepatitis associated with the use of shark cartilage.

OVERDOSAGE

There are no reports of overdosage in the literature.

DOSAGE AND ADMINISTRATION

Shark cartilage supplements are available in powders, tablets and capsules. There are no typical doses.

LITERATURE

Ashar B, Vargo E. Shark cartilage-induced hepatitis. *Ann Intern Med.* 1996;125:780-781.

Bargahi A, Rabbani-Chadegani A. Angiogenic inhibitor protein fractions derived from shark cartilage. *Biosci Rep.* 2008;28(1):15-21.

Berbari P, Thibodeau A, Germain L, et al. Antiangiogenic effects of the oral administration of liquid cartilage extract in humans. *J Surg Res.* 1999;87:108-113.

Cho J, Kim Y. Sharks: a potential source of antiangiogenic factors and tumor treatments. *Mar Biotechnol (NY).* 2002;4(6):521-525.

Dupont E, Brazeau P, Juneau C, et al. Methods of using extracts of shark cartilage. United States Patent Number 6,028,118. Feb. 22, 2000.

Dupont E, Lachance Y, Lessard D, et al. Low molecular weight components of shark cartilage, processes for their preparation and therapeutic uses thereof. World patent WO004910A2. Feb. 3, 2000.

Dupont E, Savard PE, Jourdain C, et al. Antiangiogenic properties of a novel shark cartilage extract: potential role in the treatment of psoriasis. *J Cutan Med Surg.* 1998;2:146-152.

Felzenszwalb I, Pelielo de Mattos JC, Bernardo-Filho M, et al. Shark cartilage-containing preparation: protection against reactive oxygen species. *Food Chem Toxicol.* 1998;36:1079-1084.

Fontenele JB, Araujo GB, de Alencar JW, et al. The analgesic and anti-inflammatory effects of shark cartilage are due to a peptide molecule and are nitric oxide (NO) system dependent. *Biol Pharm Bull.* 1997;20:1151-1154.

Lee A, Langer R. Shark cartilage contains inhibitors of tumor angiogenesis. *Science.* 1983;221:1185-1187.

Loprinzi CL, Levitt R, Barton DL, et al. Evaluation of shark cartilage in patients with advanced cancer: a North Central Cancer Treatment Group trial. *Cancer.* 2005;104(1):176-182.

Miller DR, Anderson GT, Stark JJ, et al. Phase I/II trial of the safety and efficacy of shark cartilage in the treatment of advanced cancer. *J Clin Oncol.* 1998;16:3649-3655.

Oikawa T, Ashino-Fuse H, Shimamura M, et al. A novel angiogenic inhibitor derved from Japanese shark cartilage (I). Extraction and estimation of inhibitory activities toward tumor and embryonic angiogenesis. *Cancer Lett.* 1990;15:181-186.

Ostrander GK, Cheng KC, Wolf JC, et al. Shark cartilage, cancer and the growing threat of pseudoscience. *Cancer Res.* 2004;64(23):8485-8491.

Rabbani-Chadegani A, Abdossamadi S, Bargahi A, et al. Identification of low-molecular-weight protein (SCP1) from shark cartilage with anti-angiogenesis activity and sequence similarity to parvalbumin. *J Pharm Biomed Anal.* 2008;46(3):563-567.

Zheng L, Ling P, Wang Z, et al. A novel polypeptide from shark cartilage with potent anti-angiogenic activity. *Cancer Biol Ther.* 2007;6(5):775-780.

Silicon

DESCRIPTION

Silicon is a non-metallic element with atomic number 14 and symbol Si. In the periodic table, it is in the same group as carbon and is carbon's closest relative. Silicon is, next to oxygen, the most abundant element in the earth's crust and is found in plants, animals and in most living organisms.

Silicon is not currently considered an essential nutrient for humans. Silicon deficiency states have been reported in chicks and rats, and silicon is an essential nutrient for some plants. Chicks fed silicon-deficient diets are found to have abnormalities in their skulls and long bones. Abnormalities include poorly formed joints, defective endochondral growth and defective articular cartilage. Bone and cartilage abnormalities have also been found in rats fed silicon-deficient diets. In these animals, silicon appears to be involved in collagen and glycosaminoglycan formation. Silicon may play such a role in other animals, including humans, but this has not yet been established. Silicon has also been reported to inhibit experimental atheromas induced by an atheromatous diet in rabbits.

Daily dietary intake of silicon in the United States ranges from approximately 20 to 50 milligrams. The richest sources of silicon are cereal products and unrefined grains of high fiber content. Significant amounts of silicon in the diet occur in the form of silicon dioxide (silica), which is poorly absorbed. Animal foods are low in silicon.

Magnesium trisilicate is frequently used as an antacid, either alone or in combination products. In the stomach, magnesium trisilicate is converted to silicon dioxide and magnesium chloride.

ACTIONS AND PHARMACOLOGY

ACTIONS

The actions of supplemental silicon are not known.

PHARMACOKINETICS

Little is known about the pharmacokinetics of supplemental and dietary silicon in humans. There is great variability in the absorption of the various forms of silicon in the diet. Most forms of dietary silicon are poorly absorbed. Most of the silicon food additives are hardly absorbed at all. Silicon dioxide or silica is more poorly absorbed than orthosilic acid, which is formed by the hydration of silicon dioxide. The mechanisms of silicon absorption are unknown. Silicon is not bound in plasma, where it is believed to exist almost entirely as monomeric silicic acid. Most of the silicon in the body is found in connective tissues, such as in bone, tendons, the trachea, the aorta, skin, hair and nails. Absorbed silicon is mainly excreted in the urine.

INDICATIONS AND USAGE

There is, at present, insufficient evidence to support any indication for the use of supplemental silicon. A very preliminary animal study suggests that it might have some positive impact in atherosclerosis. There is very preliminary evidence suggesting that silicon supplementation might play a positive role in bone health.

RESEARCH SUMMARY

It has been hypothesized that lack of silicon may play a role in the etiology of atherosclerosis. Intravenous administration of silicon inhibited experimental atheromas in an animal model, making atheromatous plaques fewer in number and the lipid deposits more superficial. This research was conducted many years ago and needs follow-up.

Silicon deficiency has been associated with bone defects in various animals. Silicon supplementation has inhibited bone mass loss in ovariectomized rats. Little is known about the role of dietary silicon in bone health in humans. It has been reported, however, that dietary silicon correlated positively and significantly with bone mineral density at all hip sites in men and premenopausal (but not postmenopausal) women in a cross-sectional, population-based study involving 2,847 participants (Framingham Offspring cohort). This previously unrecognized association is being further explored in continuing research.

CONTRAINDICATIONS, PRECAUTIONS, ADVERSE REACTIONS

CONTRAINDICATIONS

Known hypersensitivity to a silicon-containing product.

PRECAUTIONS

There are reports of high doses of silicon intake, usually in the form of the antacid magnesium trisilicate, causing siliceous renal calculi. Those who form renal calculi should be cautious about the use of supplemental silicon.

ADVERSE REACTIONS

High doses of silicon have been reported to form siliceous renal calculi.

INTERACTIONS

Silicon may inhibit aluminum absorption.

OVERDOSAGE

No reports of overdosage.

DOSAGE AND ADMINISTRATION

There is not sufficient data to set dietary reference intakes (DRIs), including tolerable upper intake levels (UL), for silicon.

Silicon is available in multivitamin preparations, usually in the form of silicon dioxide or magnesium trisilicate, typically at doses of about 2 milligrams. Supplemental silicon is also available as orthosilicic acid. The stems of the herb horsetail (*Equisetum arvense*) are rich in silicon dioxide. *Equisetum* is also used as a homeopathic remedy. Silicon may be found in colloidal or liquid minerals.

LITERATURE

Calomme MR, Vandem Berghe DA. Supplementation of calves with stabilized orthosilicic acid. Effect on the Si, Ca, Mg, and P concentrations in serum and the collagen concentration in skin and cartilage. *Biol Trace Elem Res*. 1997;56:153-165.

Carlisle EM. Silicon as a trace nutrient. *Sci Total Environ*. 1988;73:95-106.

Carlisle EM. The nutritional essentiality of silicon. *Nutr Rev*. 1982;40:193-198.

Jugdaohsingh R, Tucker KL, Qiao N, et al. Dietary silicon intake is positively associated with bone mineral density in men and premenopausal women of the Framingham Offspring cohort. *J Bone Miner Res*. 2004;19(2):297-307.

Loeper J, Goy-Loeper J, Rozensztajn L, et al. The antiatheromatous action of silicon. *Atherosclerosis*. 1979;33:397-408.

Nielsen FH. Ultratrace minerals. In: Shils ME, Olson JA, Shike M, Ross AC, eds. *Modern Nutrition in Health and Disease*. 9th ed. Baltimore, MD: Williams and Wilkins; 199:283-303.

Reffitt DM, Ogston N, Jugdaohsingh R, et al. Orthosilicic acid stimulates collagen type 1 synthesis and osteoblastic differentiation in human osteoblast-like cells in vitro. *Bone*. 2003;32(2):127-135.

Rico H, Gallego-Lago JL, Hernandez ER, at al. Effect of silicon supplement on osteopenia induced by ovariectomy in rats. *Calcif Tissue Int*. 2000;66:53-55.

Schwarz K. A bound form of silicon in glycosaminoglycans and polyuronides. *Proc Nat Acad Sci*. 1973;70:1608-1612.

Schwarz K. Silicon, fibre, and atherosclerosis. *Lancet*. 1977;1:454-457.

Sodium Alginates and other Phyco-Polysaccharides

DESCRIPTION

The algal plants or seaweeds are classified into four principal groups: the green algae or *Chlorophyceae*, the blue-green algae or *Cyanophyceae*, the brown algae or *Phaeophyceae*, and the red algae or *Rodophyceae*. The study of algae is called phycology. The brown and red algae are important commercially because of their polysaccharide content. These phyco-polysaccharides have broad applications in foods, pharmaceuticals and cosmetics, and as nutritional supplements. Agar and carrageenan are extracted from various types of red seaweeds, and algin is derived from brown seaweeds.

Agar is comprised of two major polysaccharides, neutral agarose and charged agaropectin. Both of these polysaccharides are composed of linear chains of alternating beta-D-galactose and 3,6-anhydro-alpha-L-galactose residues. These polysaccharides are resistant to digestion by intestinal digestive enzymes. Agar is also known as agar-agar. Agar is marketed in flakes and powder form and is commonly used to replace gelatin in various recipes. Agar is sometimes used to promote bowel regularity.

Carrageenans are polysaccharides also derived from certain red seaweeds. They are polysulfated, straight-chain galactans comprised of residues of D-galactose and 3,6-anhydro-D-galactose. The principal carrageenans are called kappa-carrageenan, lambda-carrageenan and iota carrageenan. Carrageenans are also resistant to digestion by intestinal digestive enzymes. Carrageenans have been reported to lower cholesterol levels in animals and also to have antiviral activity against some membrane-containing viruses in culture.

Algin is a polysaccharide derived from the brown seaweeds or *Phaeophyceae*. Algin is present in these organisms as a mixed salt (sodium, potassium, calcium, magnesium) of alginic acid. Alginic acid is a high molecular polymer comprised of two types of uronic acid residues, beta-D-mannuronic acid and its C_5 epimer alpha-L-guluronic acid. The uronic acids are simple monosaccharides in which the primary hydroxyl group at C_6 has been oxidized to the corresponding carboxylic acid. For example, D-mannuronic acid is derived from D-mannose.

Algin is principally extracted from the giant kelp *Macrocystis pyrifera*. Its derivatives have wide application in the food industry (gelling, water-holding, emulsifying and stabilizing properties), in the cosmetic industry, and in medicine and dentistry (dental impressions). Calcium alginate, the calcium salt of alginic acid, is used as a wound dressing for the treatment of exudative wounds. Sailors have been treating their wounds with seaweed for hundreds of years. Sodium alginate, the sodium salt of alginic acid, is present in some antacid products and is effective for the treatment of gastroesophageal reflux disease or GERD. Sodium alginate reacts with gastric acid to form a viscous gel called the alginate raft. The alginate raft floats on top of the gastric contents and acts as a barrier to acid and food reflux.

Sodium alginate binds tightly to such substances as strontium, calcium, barium, cadmium and radium. Cows have been fed sodium alginate, which binds to radioactive strontium 90, causing it to pass out of the body without any of it getting absorbed. Sodium alginate has also been used to treat ouch-ouch or Itai-Itai-Byo disease. This disease has been found in Japan and is believed to be due to poisoning by cadmium-containing water used to irrigate rice. Painful joints are the major symptom of ouch-ouch disease.

Sodium alginate may be considered a soluble fiber. And, similar to other soluble fibers like pectin and psyllium, sodium alginate may have hypocholesterolemic and glycemic-regulatory activities.

ACTIONS AND PHARMACOLOGY

ACTIONS

Sodium alginate may have hypocholesterolemic and glycemic-regulatory activities. It may also have detoxification activity.

MECHANISM OF ACTION

Sodium alginate has been found to lower cholesterol in animal studies. It is speculated that this may be due to alginate-stimulated increase of fecal bile acid excretion.

Sodium alginate has also been demonstrated to lower glucose levels in diabetic animals. The mechanism of this activity is unknown.

Sodium alginate binds tightly to such substances as strontium, cadmium, radium and barium. It also binds to lead, but not as well. Sodium alginate's binding to these substances reduces their absorption.

PHARMACOKINETICS

There is little on the pharmacokinetics of sodium alginate in humans. It appears to be resistant to digestion by the digestive enzymes and is probably fermented, in part, by colonic bacteria to the short-chain fatty acids acetate, propionate and butyrate.

INDICATIONS AND USAGE

Sodium alginate may have some usefulness as a lipid-lowering agent, but the evidence for this possible indication is preliminary. Similarly, there is preliminary evidence that it may be of benefit in diabetes. It has demonstrated detoxifying effects and may be helpful in some with gastroesophageal reflux disease. Seaweed, rich in iodine, is used in many parts of the world to prevent and treat goiter. Carrageenans found in some red seaweeds have demonstrated some antiviral activity. Agar is used by some for regulating bowels. Calcium alginate has been used for wound healing, and sodium alginate has been effective in treating ouch-ouch disease. Some other polysaccharide components of seaweed have exhibited immunomodulating and anticarcinogenic effects in the laboratory. Folk remedy uses of seaweed products have included fever, eczema, gallstone and liver disease, gout, menstrual problems, hypertension, kidney disease and scabies. There is no credible research to support these folk uses.

RESEARCH SUMMARY

There are some preliminary animal studies in which sodium alginate and agar have been shown to reduce cholesterol levels. In one of these studies, sodium alginate enhanced cholesterol excretion into feces. It also inhibited blood glucose and insulin levels from rising 30 minutes after glucose administration. In another animal study, both algin and agar had favorable cholesterol effects but did not affect triglycerides. There are also preliminary reports that carrageenans derived from red seaweeds have some experimental cholesterol-lowering properties.

In a small human trial, consumption of 175 mg/kg/day of sodium alginate for seven days followed by consumption of 200 mg/kg/day for an additional 16 days resulted in no significant effects on hematological indices, plasma biochemistry and urinalysis parameters, blood glucose and plasma insulin concentrations, and breath hydrogen concentrations. No allergic responses were noted. There were only five subjects in this study—all with normal health at the outset.

Alginates have been used for heartburn and acid reflux for decades. Numerous *in vitro* and *in vivo* studies have demonstrated that alginate-based rafts effectively provide physical barriers to acidic gastric contents and can thus significantly reduce reflux episodes. Alginates are present in some over-the-counter antacids.

Calcium alginate is often used as a dressing for exudative wounds. It is an effective absorbable hemostatic and is often used to pack sinuses, bleeding wounds of various types and burns. Sodium alginate is also used for this purpose. In one study, the use of calcium alginate hemostatic swabs was credited with significantly reducing blood loss in various surgeries and with significantly reducing duration of operations. Calcium alginate was shown to be four times as absorbent per unit weight as gauze.

The alginates have been shown to bind tightly to strontium, barium, cadmium and radium so that these toxins pass out of the body with little or no absorption. It also binds with lead, but not as completely. Ouch-ouch disease, characterized by painful joints and believed to be caused by oral cadmium exposure, has been successfully treated with alginates in Japan. Reduction in the absorption of strontium has been noted in children given an alginate derivative. Retention of radioactive barium has been reduced in rats fed sodium alginate derivatives. In one human trial, 10 grams of sodium alginate ameliorated acute radiation effects due to exposure to radiation doses of 50 to 3,000 rads.

Calcium alginate has shown antiviral activity in some *in vitro* and animal studies. It is sufficiently effective that diagnostic laboratories caution against the use of calcium alginate swabs in some diagnostic sampling, owing to calcium alginate's toxicity to herpes viruses and chlamydia, among other infective agents.

The carrageenans, sulfated polysaccharides derived from red seaweeds like Irish moss, have inhibited both HSV1 and HSV2 *in vitro*. They also inhibit some other viruses, including HIV. The natural alginates, on the other hand, do not show antiherpetic or anti-HIV activity.

In one animal study, preparations from various edible seaweeds significantly reduced the incidence of chemically induced cancers, compared with controls that were unsupplemented with these preparations. In another animal study, an extract of the brown alga hijiki recently showed immuno-enhancing activity. The polysaccharide fraction of the extract, more than the nonpolysaccharide fraction, had immune-enhancing effects on the proliferative response of spleen cells. This response was associated with B-cell, but not T-cell, populations. More research is needed.

CONTRAINDICATIONS, PRECAUTIONS, ADVERSE REACTIONS
CONTRAINDICATIONS
Sodium alginate is contraindicated in those who are hypersensitive to any component of a sodium alginate-containing product.

PRECAUTIONS
Pregnant women and nursing mothers should avoid supplementation with sodium alginate unless it is recommended by their physicians.

ADVERSE REACTIONS
Gastrointestinal symptoms such as flatulence may occur with sodium alginate supplements.

INTERACTIONS
NUTRITIONAL SUPPLEMENTS
Sodium alginate may decrease the absorption of the carotenoids beta-carotene, lycopene and lutein if used concomitantly. It may also decrease the absorption of such minerals as calcium, zinc, manganese, chromium and magnesium if used concomitantly.

FOODS
Sodium alginate may reduce the absorption of food carotenoids, such as beta-carotene, lycopene and lutein and such minerals in foods as calcium, magnesium, zinc, manganese and chromium.

DOSAGE AND ADMINISTRATION
Sodium alginate supplements can be found in the marketplace, but there are no typical doses. Various algaes and seaweeds are available as supplements as well. Among algae or seaweeds often used as foods and supplements are hijiki, kombu, wakame and arame. These are all brown seaweeds or algae. The red seaweeds and some of their constituents are also widely used. These include nori, agar or agar-agar, dulse and Irish moss. There are no typical doses.

LITERATURE
Anderson DM, Brydon WG, Eastwood MA, Sedgwick DM. Dietary effects of sodium alginate in humans. *Food Addit Contam.* 1991; 8:237-248.

Carr TE, Harrison GE, Humphreys ER, Sutton A. Reduction in the absorption and retention of dietary strontium in man by alginate. *Int J Radiat Biol Relat Stud Phys Chem Med.* 1968; 14:225-233.

Harmuth-Hoene AE, Schelenz R. Effect of dietary fiber on mineral absorption in growing rats. *J Nutr.* 1980; 110:1774-1784.

Hendler SS. *The Doctors' Vitamin And Mineral Encyclopedia.* New York, NY: Simon and Schuster; 1990.

Kimura Y, Watanabe K, Okuda H. Effects of soluble sodium alginate on cholesterol excretion and glucose tolerance in rats. *J Ethnopharmacol.* 1996; 54:47-54.

Mandel KG, Daggy BP, Brodie DA, Jacoby HI. Review article: alginate-raft formulations in the treatment of heartburn and acid reflux. *Aliment Pharmacol Ther.* 2000; 14:669-690.

Ohta A, Taguchi A, Takizawa T, et al. The alginate reduce the postprandial glycaemic response by forming a gel with dietary calcium in the stomach of the rat. *Int J Vitam Nutr Res.* 1997; 67:55-61.

Okai Y, Higashi-Okai K, Ishizaka S, et al. Possible immunomodulating activities in an extract of edible brown alga, *Hijikia fusiforme* (Hijiki). *J Sci Food Agric.* 1998; 76:56-62.

Riedl J, Linseisen J, Hoffmann J, Wolfram G. Some dietary fibers reduce the absorption of carotenoids in women. *J Nutr.* 1989; 129:2170-2176.

Sayag J, Meaume S, Bohbot S. Healing properties of calcium alginate dressings. *J Wound Care*. 1996; 5:357-362.

Silva AJ, Fleshman DG, Shore B. The effects of sodium alginate on the absorption and retention of several divalent cations. *Health Phys*. 1970; 19:245-251.

Sutton A, Harrison GE, Carr TE, Barltrop D. Reduction in the absorption of dietary strontium in children by an alginate derivative. *Int J Radiat Biol Relat Stud Phys Chem Med*. 1971; 19:79-85.

Sutton A, Humphreys ER, Shepherd H, Howells GR. Reduction in the retention of radioactive barium in rats following the addition of sodium alginate derivatives to the diet. *Int J Radiat Biol Relat Stud Phys Chem Med*. 1972; 22:297-300.

Wu J, Peng SS. Comparison of hypolipidemic effect of refined konjac meal with several common dietary fibers and their mechanisms of action. *Biomed Environ Sci*. 1997; 10:27-37.

Soy Isoflavones

DESCRIPTION

Soy isoflavones are phytoestrogens (plant estrogens) found in soybeans. Phytoestrogens are plant-derived nonsteroidal compounds that possess estrogen-like biological activity. Soy isoflavones have both weak estrogenic and weak antiestrogenic effects. They have been found to bind to estrogen receptors-alpha (ER-alpha) and beta (ER-beta). They appear to bind better to ER-beta than to ER-alpha.

Soy isoflavones comprise three main isoflavones and their glycosylated forms. The three main isoflavones are the aglycones genistein, daidzein and glycitein. They can be represented by the following structural formulas:

Soy isoflavones

	R_1	R_2	R_3	R_4
Daidzein	H	H	OH	OH
Genistein	OH	H	OH	OH
Glycitein	H	OCH3	OH	OH

The glycosylated forms of genistein are genistin, 6″-O-malonylgenistin and 6″-O-acetylgenistin; those of daidzein are daidzin, 6″-O-malonyldaidzin and 6″-O-acetyldaidzin, and those of glycitein are glycitin, 6″-O-malonylglycitin and 6″-O-acetylglycitin. The malonyl glycosides of genistein are the major forms of the soy isoflavones that are found in

soybeans. Fermented soy foods, such as tempeh and miso, are rich in the soy isoflavone aglycones. The most abundant of the soy isoflavones in soybeans are the genistein glycosides (about 50%), followed by the daidzein glycosides (about 40%). The least abundant of the soy isoflavones in soybeans are the glycitein glycosides (about 5 to 10%). Soy protein derived from soybeans contains about 2 mg of genistin and daidzin per gram of protein. In soy germ, the order is different. Glycitein glycosides comprise about 40% of soy germ, daidzein glycosides about 50% and genistein glycosides about 10%.

Soy isoflavones, when marketed as nutritional supplements, are mainly present as the isoflavone glycosides genistin, daidzin and glycitin.

See also Daidzein, Equol, Genistein and Glycitein.

ACTIONS AND PHARMACOLOGY

ACTIONS

Soy isoflavones may have estrogenic, antiestrogenic and nonestrogenic activities. Soy isoflavones may also have antioxidant, anticarcinogenic, anti-atherogenic, vasoprotective and anti-osteoporotic activities. Soy isoflavones might also have activity for the treatment of menopausal hot flashes.

MECHANISM OF ACTION

Soy isoflavones have weak estrogenic activity. The order of activity in *in vivo* assays is glycitein greater than genistein greater than daidzein. They bind to estrogen receptors-alpha and beta. They appear to bind better to estrogen receptor-beta than to estrogen receptor-alpha.

The most studied of the soy isoflavones is genistein. Genistein has been found to have a number of antioxidant activities. It is a scavenger of reactive oxygen species and inhibits lipid peroxidation. It also inhibits superoxide anion generation by the enzyme xanthine oxidase. In addition, genistein, in animal experiments, has been found to increase the activities of the antioxidant enzymes superoxide dismutase, glutathionine peroxidase, catalase and glutathione reductase. Daidzein and glycitein also appear to have reactive oxygen scavenging activity. However, these isoflavones have not been studied as much as genistein has.

Regarding possible anticarcinogenic activity, again genistein has been the most studied of the soy isoflavones. Several mechanisms have been proposed for genistein's possible anticarcinogenic activity. These include upregulation of apoptosis, inhibition of angiogenesis, inhibition of DNA topoisomerase II and inhibition of protein tyrosine kinases. Genistein's weak estrogenic activity may be involved in its putative activity against prostate cancer. Other possible anti-prostate cancer mechanisms include inhibition of NF (nuclear factor)-kappa B in prostate cancer cells, downregulation of TGF (transforming growth factor)-beta and inhibition of EGF (epidermal growth factor)- stimulated growth. Genistein's anti-estrogenic action may be another possible mechanism to explain its putative activity against breast cancer. Additional possible anti-breast cancer mechanisms include inhibition of aromatase activity and stimulation of sex hormone binding globulin, both of which might lower endogenous estrogen levels.

The possible anti-atherogenic activity of soy isoflavones may be accounted for, in part, by their possible antioxidant activity, particularly with regard to inhibition of lipid peroxidation and oxidation of LDL. Oxidation of low density lipoprotein-cholesterol is thought to be a major factor in the pathogenesis of atherosclerosis. Soy isoflavones may have some cholesterol-lowering activity, but the mechanism of this possible effect is unclear. Soy isoflavones have been found to improve endothelial function independent of changes in blood pressure, lipid profile or glycemic control. The mechanism of this action is unclear (see Research Summary below).

Soy isoflavones' weak estrogenic effects may help protect against osteoporosis by preventing bone resorption and promoting bone density. However, the mechanism of this possible effect is entirely speculative at this time. Soy isoflavones' weak estrogenic actions may also aid in reducing hot flash symptoms.

PHARMACOKINETICS
See Genistein, Daidzein and Glycitein.

INDICATIONS AND USAGE
Soy isoflavones may be helpful in preventing and treating some forms of heart disease and cancer. They may ameliorate some menopausal symptoms (hot flashes) and may be beneficial in preventing osteoporosis. A recent clinical trial in patients with ischemic stroke demonstrated that a soy isoflavone supplement reversed endothelial dysfunction.

RESEARCH SUMMARY
Epidemiological data suggest that higher intakes of foods containing soy isoflavones are significantly correlated with reduced incidence of heart disease and some forms of cancer. Animal, in vitro and human studies have provided further support for the epidemiological findings. Soy proteins were shown to lower plasma levels of cholesterol in animal models of hypercholesterolemia, and, subsequently, a meta-analysis of human studies has more recently established that soy consumption is significantly associated with reduction in plasma cholesterol levels in humans, as well. These effects are attributed, in part, to the isoflavone components of soy.

Epidemiological data indicate that consumption of soy is particularly associated with reduced risk of breast, lung and prostate cancers, as well as leukemia. Here again, in vitro and animal research have further supported these observations.

Breast cancer incidence is reported to be four to seven times higher in women in the United States than among their counterparts in China or Japan. Dietary intake, especially intake of dietary soy, has been associated with this difference. Soy isoflavones have been shown to inhibit transcriptional factors involved in cancer metastasis, including vascular endothelial growth factor, which, in turn, is strongly associated with tumor angiogenesis, as noted in a recent editorial in the British Journal of Cancer. In a meta-analysis published in that journal on the epidemiology of soy exposures and breast cancer risk, researchers showed more clearly than had previously been demonstrated that a higher intake of soy isoflavones—20 mg per day or more, compared with a lower intake of about 5 mg per day—among Asian populations is associated with a consistent 29% reduction in the risk of developing breast cancer. Risk reduction was associated with higher soy intake in both pre- and postmenopausal women. And the greatest risk reduction was seen in females who had begun consuming more soy in adolescence, as opposed to those who only consumed high quantities after reaching adulthood. In the United States, the very low level of soy isoflavone intake (less than 1 mg per day) did not have any beneficial effect on breast cancer incidence. However, in the United States, another study has reported a reduction in all-cause and breast cancer-specific mortality among a cohort of breast cancer survivors who consumed higher levels of total flavonoids, particularly flavones, including soy isoflavones.

Recently, the relationship between soy isoflavones—and soy foods generally—and breast cancer has become a matter of some concern owing to in vitro and rodent data suggesting that isoflavones may stimulate the growth of existing estrogen-sensitive breast tumors. There is little evidence to suggest that soy isoflavones will increase breast cancer risk in healthy women or worsen the prognosis of breast cancer patients. Nor is there any evidence that soy isoflavone intake increases breast density in pre- or postmenopausal women or increases breast cell proliferation in postmenopausal women with or without a history of breast cancer. The majority of the epidemiology data suggest soy isoflavones to be neutral or to be protective against breast cancer, which is corroborated by recent human intervention study data.

In addition to the concern about a putative link between soy isoflavones and breast cancer, some are concerned that soy isoflavones might play a role in endometrial cancer. There is essentially no support for this notion. The endometrium is an estrogen-responsive tissue and rodent studies have shown that the uterus is responsive to high doses of soy isoflavones. However, these rodent studies did not find that soy isoflavones play any role in endometrial cancer. Endometrial cancer effects from consumption of soy isoflavones are not supported by most of the human trials, even those with duration of up to two years. One study of longer duration—five years—did find non-cancerous hyperplasia in 3.5% of the women tested; no cases of non-cancerous hyperplasia were found in the control group. This was surprising since the normal incidence of endometrial non-cancerous hyperplasia is approximately 5%, which is the incidence that one would have expected in the control group. Although there is little to no evidence supporting a connection between soy isoflavone consumption and breast and endometrial cancer, continued surveillance and monitoring for breast and endometrial cancer in women consuming soy isoflavones is wise and warranted.

Problems associated with menopause, including osteoporosis, appear to be favorably affected in some by higher intakes of soy products and by soy isoflavones specifically. A symptom that most perimenopausal women experience is the annoying feeling of intermittent intense heat, commonly known as a "hot flash." Hot flashes result from a vasomotor response to declining estrogen levels and can be very disruptive to one's life. While hormone replacement therapy (HRT) is an effective treatment for hot flashes, many women are concerned over potential adverse events of HRT. This concern became even greater following publication in 2002 of the results of The Women's Health Initiative (WHI) Estrogen plus Progestin Study, which was stopped on July 7, 2002 because of increased risk of breast cancer and cardiovascular disease in women taking active study pills, compared with those on placebo. Many women began using soy isoflavones, which some, but not all, studies suggested might help with hot flashes. A recent review of isoflavone-hot flash studies reported that studies that consistently reported a significant decrease in hot flash symptoms (intensity and frequency) all supplied more than 15 milligrams of the isoflavone genistein (calculated as aglycone equivalents) per treatment. These benefits have been demonstrated in randomized, double-blind studies.

Soy isoflavones have also been shown to prevent bone resorption and to help increase bone density in some *in vitro* and animal studies. The synthetic isoflavone ipriflavone (see Ipriflavone), the major metabolite of which is the soy isoflavone daidzein, has demonstrated a significant ability to prevent osteoporosis in both animal models and in humans.

However, recent studies have produced mixed results with respect to the soy isoflavones and their possible effects on bone density and other variables in postmenopausal women.

One recent randomized, controlled trial in which some of the healthy postmenopausal women received 25.6 grams of soy protein containing 99 mg of isoflavones daily for 12 months failed to reveal benefit in terms of improved bone mineral density, cognitive function or plasma lipids when started at the age of 60 or later. The researchers hypothesized, however, that younger postmenopausal women might benefit since, in a rat model, isoflavones were very effective in preventing bone loss when started soon after ovariectomy. Similarly, the researchers observed, estrogen has had the most favorable effects on cognitive function when administered in perimenopausal women, rather than in late post-menopausal women.

A recent randomized, double-blinded, placebo-controlled trial was performed to determine the effects of a soy isoflavone supplement on brachial flow-mediated dilatation (FMD) in patients with prior ischemic stroke. Compared with controls, FMD at 12 weeks was significantly greater in the isoflavone-treated patients. The vasoprotective effect of the isoflavones on brachial FMD was more pronounced in patients with more severe endothelial dysfunction. In addition, the isoflavone treatment resulted in a significant decrease in serum high-sensitivity-C-reactive protein levels. The researchers concluded that soy isoflavones may have an important role for secondary prevention in patients with cardiovascular disease, on top of conventional interventions.

One negative finding related to soy intake was reported recently. The authors of an epidemiological study based in Indonesia associated high intake of tofu by mainly elderly men with significantly poorer cognitive test performance, enlargement of ventricles and diminished brain weight. The study, however, was not able to control for many potentially important dietary and other variables that may have affected outcome. The British and Indonesian researchers themselves indicated that it was unclear whether the potential detrimental effects were due to the soy isoflavones or toxic additives like formaldehyde, which is used as a food preservative in Indonesia. The results of the study, while provocative, are too preliminary to support any definitive conclusions, although the toxic additive explanation appeared to be the more likely one. More research may be warranted.

CONTRAINDICATIONS, PRECAUTIONS, ADVERSE REACTIONS
CONTRAINDICATIONS
Soy isoflavones are contraindicated in those who are hypersensitive to any component of a soy isoflavone-containing product. Those who are allergic to birch pollen may also be hypersensitive to soy products.

PRECAUTIONS
Pregnant women and nursing mothers should avoid the use of soy isoflavone supplements pending long-term safety

studies. Men with prostate cancer should discuss the advisability of the use of soy isoflavones with their physicians before deciding to use them.

Women with estrogen receptor-positive tumors should exercise caution in the use of soy isoflavones and should only use them if they are recommended and monitored by a physician.

Those consuming soy isoflavones should ensure that they have an adequate intake of iodide (see Adverse Reactions).

ADVERSE REACTIONS

There is a theoretical concern based on *in vitro* and animal data that soy isoflavones may increase the risk of clinical hypothyroidism in individuals with compromised thyroid function and/or whose iodide intake is marginal. Therefore, those who use soy isoflavones should ensure that their intake of iodide is adequate. Several years ago, the National Center for Toxicological Research raised this concern because their scientists found that the soy isoflavones genistein and daidzein inhibited the activity of the enzyme thyroid peroxidase (TPO) in rats, both *in vitro* and *in vivo*. TPO catalyzes the iodination of thyroglobulin, the key metabolic step in the biosynthesis of thyroid hormone. The addition of iodide to the *in vitro* media completely abolished the inhibition of TPO. While iodide-deficient animals exhibit goitrogenic responses when consuming soy isoflavones, they have no effect on iodide-sufficient animals. With regard to human studies, in the hundreds of clinical trials conducted using soy isoflavones, there have been no reported adverse thyroid effects in any of the subjects participating in the trials. A recent review of 12 studies involving consumption of soy isoflavones reported that with the exception of one study that gave mixed results, none of the other studies showed statistically significant changes in the thyroid hormones TSH, T_4 and T_3.

DOSAGE AND ADMINISTRATION

Soy isoflavone supplements containing genistin, daidzin and glycitin are available with much smaller amounts of the aglycones genistein, daidzein and glycitein. The percentages of the soy isoflavones present in a standard soy isoflavone supplement reflect the percentages of these substances as found in soybeans and are: genistin, about 50%; daidzin, about 38%; and glycitin, about 12%. A 50-mg dose of soy isoflavones—a typical daily dose—delivers 25 mg of genistin, 19 mg of daidzin and about 6 mg of glycitin. Usually, 40% of the formula is comprised of soy isoflavones. Therefore, to get a dose of 50 milligrams of soy isoflavones, 125 mg daily of soy isoflavones are required. Various observational and epidemiological studies suggest 50 mg daily of soy isoflavones approximates the dose that may have health benefits.

Soy isoflavones are also available in some functional food products.

LITERATURE

Atmaca A, Kleerekoper M, Bayraktar M, et al. Soy isoflavones in the management of postmenopausal osteoporosis. *Menopause.* 2008;15(4 Pt 1):748-757.

Barnes S. Evolution of the health benefits of soy isoflavones. *Proc Soc Exp Biol Med.* 1998;217:386-392.

Casini ML, Marelli G, Papaleo E, et al. Psychological assessment of the effects of treatment with phytoestrogens on postmenopausal women: a randomized, double-blind, crossover, placebo-controlled study. *Fertil Steril.* 2006;85(4):972-978.

Chan YH, Lau KK, Yiu KH, et al. Reduction of C-reactive protein with isoflavone supplement reverses endothelial dysfunction in patients with ischaemic stroke. *Eur Heart J.* 2008 Sep 23. [Epub ahead of print]

Constantinou AI, Mehta RG, Vaughan A. Inhibition of N-methyl-N-nitrosourea-induced mammary tumors in rats by the soybean isoflavones. *Anticancer Res.* 1996;16:3293-3298.

Gammon MD, Fink BN, Steck SE, et al. Soy intake and breast cancer: elucidation of an unanswered question. *Br J Cancer.* 2008;98(1):2-3.

Goetzl MA, Van Veldhuizen PJ, Thrasher JB. Effects of soy phytoestrogens on the prostate. *Prostate Cancer Prostatic Dis.* 2007;10(3):216-223.

Grodstein F, Mayeux R, Stampfer MJ. Tofu and cognitive function: food for thought (Editorial). *J Am Coll Nutr.* 2000;19:207-209.

Klein KO. Isoflavones, soy-based infant formulas, and relevance to endocrine function. *Nutr Rev.* 1998;56:193-204.

Kreijkamp-Kaspers S, Kok L, Grobbee DE, et al. Dietary phytoestrogen intake and cognitive function in older women. *J Gerontol A Biol Sci Med Sci.* 2007;62(5):556-562.

Kreijkamp-Kaspers S, Kok L, Grobbee DE, et al. Effect of soy protein containing isoflavones on cognitive function, bone mineral density, and plasma lipids in postmenopausal women: a randomized controlled trial. *JAMA.* 2004;292(1):65-74.

Kurzer MS, Xu X. Dietary phytoestrogens. *Annu Rev Nutr.* 1997;17:353-381.

Merz-Demlov BE, Duncan AM, Wangen KE, et al. Soy isoflavones improve plasma lipids in normocholesterolemic premenopausal women. *Am J Clin Nutr.* 2000;71:1462-1469.

Messina M, Redmond G. Effects of soy protein and soybean isoflavones on thyroid function in healthy adults and hypothyroid patients: a review of the relevant literature. *Thyroid.* 2006;16(3):249-258.

Messina MJ, Wood CE. Soy isoflavones, estrogen therapy, and breast cancer risk: analysis and commentary. *Nutr J.* 2008;7:17.

Poulsen RC, Kruger MC. Soy phytoestrogens: impact on postmenopausal bone loss and mechanisms of action. *Nutr Rev.* 2008;66(7):359-374.

Rimbach G, Boesch-Saadatmandi C, Frank J, et al. Dietary isoflavones in the prevention of cardiovascular disease—a molecular perspective. *Food Chem Toxicol.* 2008;46(4):1308-1319.

Steiner C, Arnould S, Scalbert A, et al. Isoflavones and the prevention of breast and prostate cancer: new perspectives opened by nutrigenomics. *Br J Nutr.* 2008;99 E Suppl 1:ES78-108.

Third International Symposium on the Role of Soy in Preventing and Treating Chronic Disease. *J Nutr.* 2000;130:653S-711S.

Tikkanen MJ, Adlercreutz H. Dietary soy-derived isoflavone phytoestrogens. *Biochem Pharmacol.* 2000;60:1-5.

White LR, Petrovitch H, Ross GW, et al. Brain aging and midlife tofu consumption. *JAm Coll Nutr.* 2000;19:242-255.

Williamson-Hughes PS, Flickinger BD, Messina MJ, et al. Isoflavone supplements containing predominantly genistein reduce hot flash symptoms: a critical review of published studies. *Menopause.* 2006;13(5):831-839.

Wu AH, Yu MC, Tseng CC, et al. Epidemiology of soy exposures and breast cancer risk. *Br J Cancer.* 2008;98(1):9-14.

Soy Protein

DESCRIPTION

In October 1999, the Food and Drug Administration (FDA) approved a labeling health claim for dietary soy protein stating that it may reduce the risk of heart disease. The health claim that can be used on labels of products containing soy protein states: "Diets low in saturated fat and cholesterol that include 25 grams of soy protein a day may reduce the risk of heart disease." In order to carry the health claim, one serving of a product must contain at least 6.25 grams of soy protein and must also be low in total and saturated fat, cholesterol and sodium.

The substantive evidence underpinning the approval of the health claim came from a meta-analysis by James W. Anderson and his University of Kentucky colleagues, published in August 1995 in the *New England Journal of Medicine*. The article reported that regular consumption of soy protein lowered total cholesterol by 9.3%, LDL-cholesterol by 12.9%, triglycerides by 10.5% and raised HDL-cholesterol by 2.5%. The average daily soy protein intake by those included in the meta-analysis was 47 grams. Interestingly, those whose soy protein intake was 25 grams daily—the amount approved in the health claim—demonstrated only a 5% decrease in their LDL-cholesterol levels. Subsequent meta-analyses and clinical studies of the effects of soy protein intake on serum lipids reported LDL-cholesterol decreases ranging from 3 to 5.3%. One study found a 3% lowering of LDL-cholesterol at a soy protein intake of 36 grams daily. A review of 22 randomized clinical trials by the American Heart Association Nutrition Committee and published in 2005 reported that those consuming 50 grams daily of soy protein showed no higher than a 3% decrease in LDL-cholesterol and concluded that they could not support the use of soy protein to lower cholesterol. The FDA is reconsidering the soy protein health claim.

Soy protein isolates have become popular items in the nutritional supplement marketplace. Most of these supplements also contain the soy isoflavones genistin, daidzin and glycitin. (See Soy Isoflavones, Genistein, Daidzein and Glycitein.)

ACTIONS AND PHARMACOLOGY

ACTIONS

Soy protein has putative lipid-lowering, antiatherogenic, antioxidant, anticarcinogenic and antiosteoporotic activities.

MECHANISM OF ACTION

Diets rich in soy protein have been found to reduce serum levels of total cholesterol, LDL-cholesterol, triglycerides and apolipoprotein B (apo B). The mechanism of the possible lipid-lowering activity of soy protein is unclear. There are a few possible explanations. Soy protein is much richer in L-arginine than is animal protein, which is richer in L-lysine. Some animal studies indicate that dietary increases in L-arginine are accompanied by decreases in cholesterol levels. Further, some studies have demonstrated that, under certain conditions, e.g., hypercholesterolemia, high intakes of L-arginine could enhance endothelial-dependent vasodilation and nitric oxide or NO production (see L-Arginine). This could contribute to the possible antiatherogenic activity of soy protein.

The soy isoflavones may also contribute to the possible lipid-lowering activity of soy protein as well as its possible antiatherogenic activity. Most soy protein products contain the isoflavones genistin, daidzin and glycitin, which have weak estrogenic effects and also may have antiestrogenic activity (see Soy Isoflavones). Oral estrogens have been shown to decrease total cholesterol and LDL-cholesterol. The soy isoflavones may have similar actions.

Interestingly, a few studies have shown that when the isoflavones are removed from the soy protein, the protein itself has little hypocholesterolemic activity. Soy isoflavones themselves do not have the same hypocholesterolemic activity as the combination of soy protein and soy isoflavones. There are probably synergistic effects of these substances that are not understood at this time.

There are also other substances associated with soy protein, including saponins, trypsin inhibitor and bioactive peptides, which may also contribute to the lipid-lowering activity of soy protein. The soy isoflavones are antioxidants, and their antioxidant activity may contribute to the possible anti-atherogenic effect of soy protein. Recently, peptides in soybean protein hydrolysate produced by certain proteases have been reported to have hypocholesterolemic activity. Among the mechanisms suggested—blockage of bile acid and/or cholesterol absorption, inhibition of cholesterol synthesis and stimulation of low- density-lipoprotein receptor (LDL-R) transcription—the peptides appeared to stimulate LDL-R transcription. Stimulation of LDL-R transcription in the human liver cell line appeared to reduce serum cholesterol levels. Further research on the identity of the peptides and their mechanism of action is needed and warranted.

The possible antioxidant, anticarcinogenic and antiosteoporotic activities of soy protein are probably due, in large part, to the soy isoflavones (see Soy Isoflavones). Soy protein has been found to reduce intestinal mucosa polyamine levels in rats, which may be another anticarcinogenic mechanism. Also, a bioactive peptide has recently been isolated from soybeans and has been found to have potent antimitotic activity.

PHARMACOKINETICS

The digestion, absorption, distribution and metabolism of soy protein occur by normal physiological processes. See Soy Isoflavones, Genistein, Daidzein and Glycitein for the pharmacokinetics of these substances.

INDICATIONS AND USAGE

The FDA has allowed the following health claim for soy protein: "25 grams of soy protein a day, as part of a diet low in saturated fat and cholesterol, may reduce the risk of heart disease." The isoflavone constituents of soy protein may confer some additional benefits. The results of some recent reports, however, question the FDA-allowed health claim.

RESEARCH SUMMARY

The FDA-approved health claim—see Indications above—that soy protein, in adequate amounts, may help protect against heart disease is based upon numerous *in vitro*, animal, epidemiological and human studies. Evidence has accumulated over many decades showing that soy protein, but not animal protein, has significant cholesterol-lowering properties in animal studies. However, more recent results question some of the older evidence.

In a 1995 meta-analysis of clinical studies, most of them well-controlled, investigators concluded that soy protein significantly lowered serum concentrations of total cholesterol, LDL-cholesterol and triglycerides without significantly altering HDL-cholesterol concentrations.

Since the meta-analysis cited above was conducted, some, but not all, clinical research has continued to confirm the lipid-lowering ability of soy protein. One study demonstrated that administration for six weeks of as little as 20 grams of soy protein per day, in place of animal protein, achieved significant reductions of non-HDL-cholesterol and apolipoprotein (apo) B in moderately hypercholesterolemic men. However, the results of some more recent clinical studies and meta-analyses show much lower cholesterol-lowering activity of soy protein, and the FDA is reconsidering the allowed health claim for soy protein. However, even if the LDL-cholesterol-lowering activity of soy protein is much lower than what was originally thought, it may still be enough to confer some cardiovascular benefits. We know from prior studies that even a 1% reduction in LDL-cholesterol can result in a 2 to 4% percent reduced risk for heart disease and that could have enormous public health implications. Also, there may be other than LDL-cholesterol-lowering activities in soy protein that are also beneficial for cardiovascular health. Clearly, more high-quality clinical trials are needed and warranted to settle these important issues.

CONTRAINDICATIONS, PRECAUTIONS, ADVERSE REACTIONS
CONTRAINDICATIONS

Soy protein supplements are contraindicated in those who are hypersensitive to any component of a soy protein-containing product.

PRECAUTIONS

Pregnant women and nursing mothers should discuss the use of soy protein supplements with their physician before starting them.

Women with estrogen receptor-positive tumors should exercise caution in the use of soy protein supplements and should only use them if they are recommended and monitored by their physicians.

INTERACTIONS
NUTRITIONAL SUPPLEMENTS AND FOODS

Soy contains phytic acid, which may bind with certain minerals, such as calcium, magnesium, manganese, zinc, copper and iron, reducing their availability.

OVERDOSAGE

There are no reports of overdosage.

DOSAGE AND ADMINISTRATION

There are several soy protein supplements available. Typically the soy protein supplements contain soy isoflavones. Dosage is variable.

A total intake of 25 to 50 grams of soy protein and 50 milligrams of soy isoflavones daily may have cardiovascular and other health benefits. This can come from nutritional intake, as well as supplemental intake.

LITERATURE

Anderson JW, Johnstone BM, Cook-Newell ME. Meta-analysis of the effects of soy protein intake on serum lipids. *N Engl J Med.* 1995;333:276-282.

Aoyama T, Fukui K, Takamatsu K, et al. Soy protein isolate and its hydrolysate reduce body fat of dietary obese rats and genetically obese mice (yellow KK). *Nutrition.* 2000;16:349-354.

Carroll KK. Review of clinical studies on cholesterol-lowering response to soy protein. *J Am Diet Assoc.* 1991;91:820-827.

Carroll KK, Kurowska EM. Soy consumption and cholesterol reduction: review of animal and human studies. *J Nutr.* 1995;125(3Suppl):594S-597S.

Cho SJ, Juillerat MA, Lee CH. Cholesterol lowering mechanism of soybean protein hydrolysate. *J Agric Food Chem.* 2007;55(26):10599-10604.

Crouse JR III, Morgan T, Terry JG, et al. A randomized trial comparing the effect of casein with that of soy protein containing varying amounts of isoflavones on plasma concentrations of lipids and lipoproteins. *Arch Intern Med.* 1999;159:2070-2076.

Dewell A, Hollenbeck PL, Hollenbeck CB. Clinical review: a critical evaluation of the role of soy protein and isoflavone supplementation in the control of plasma cholesterol concentrations. *J Clin Endocrinol Metab.* 2006;91(3):772-780.

Erdman JW Jr. Control of serum lipids with soy protein (Editorial). *N Engl J Med.* 1995;333:313-315.

Gaddi A, Decovich GC, Noseda G, et al. Hypercholesterolemia treated by soybean protein diet. *Arch Dis Childhood.* 1987;62:274-278.

Galvez AF, deLumen BO. A soybean cDNA encoding a chromatin-binding peptide inhibits mitosis of mammalian cells. *Nat Biotechol.* 1999;17:495-500.

Greaves KA, Wilson MD, Rudel LL, et al. Consumption of soy protein reduces cholesterol absorption compared to casein protein alone or supplemented with an isoflavone extract or conjugated equine estrogen in ovariectomized cynomolgus monkeys. *J Nutr.* 2000;130:820.

Sacks FM, Lichtenstein A, Van Horn L, et al. Soy protein, isoflavones, and cardiovascular health: a summary of a statement for professionals from the American Heart Association Nutrition Committee. *Arterioscler Thromb Vasc Biol.* 2006;26(8):1689-1692.

Sacks FM, Lichtenstein A, Van Horn L, et al. Soy protein, isoflavones, and cardiovascular health: an American Heart Association Science Advisory for professionals from the Nutrition Committee. *Circulation.* 2006;113(7):1034-1044.

Teixeira SR, Potter SM, Weigel R, et al. Effects of feeding 4 levels of soy protein for 3 and 6 wk on blood lipids and apolipoproteins in moderately hypercholesterolemic men. *Am J Clin Nutr.* 2000;71:1077-1084.

Wang W, Higuch CM. Dietary soy protein is associated with reduced intestinal mucosal polyamine concentration in male Wistar rats. *J Nutr.* 2000;130:1815-1820.

Spirulina

DESCRIPTION

In its commercial use, Spirulina refers mainly to the dried biomass of the cyanobacterium *Arthrospira platensis.* *Arthrospira platensis* (*Spirulina platensis*) is a genus of the phylum *Cyanobacteria.* *Cyanobacteria* are classified as either blue-green algae or as blue-green bacteria. Spirulina is a popular food supplement in Japan and is marketed as a nutritional supplement in the United States. Spirulina, wheat grass, barley grass and chlorella are sometimes referred to as "green foods." There are several cyanobacteria species; however, Spirulina usually refers to only two of them, *Arthrospira platensis* (*Spirulina platensis*) and *Arthrospira maxima* (*Spirulina maxima*). The term Spirulina is commonly used for both the dietary supplement and the genus *Arthrospira.*

Spirulina used for the production of nutritional supplements is either grown in outdoor tanks or harvested from lakes in such places as Mexico, Central and South America, and Africa.

Spirulina is a rich source of protein. It also contains chlorophyll, carotenoids, minerals, gamma-linolenic acid (GLA) and some unique pigments. The pigments give Spirulina its bluish tinge. Phycocyanin is a blue, light-harvesting pigment in cyanobacteria. It belongs to a group of light-harvesting proteins, called phycobiliproteins. All phycobiliproteins are multi-chain holoproteins, comprised of apoproteins with covalently bound phycobilins. Phycobilins are open-chain tetrapyrolle chromophores. The three common phycobiliproteins are phycoerythrin, with phycoerythrobilin chromophores, and phycocyanin and allophycocyanin, with phycocyanobilin chromophores. Phycocyanorubin, a reduced form of phycocyanobilin, is similar in structure to the bile pigment bilirubin.

ACTIONS AND PHARMACOLOGY

ACTIONS

Spirulina has putative antiviral, hypocholesterolemic, antioxidant, hepatoprotective, antiallergic and immune-modulatory activities.

MECHANISM OF ACTION

A sulfated polysaccharide called calcium spirulan isolated from *Arthrospira platensis* (*Spirulina platensis*) was found to inhibit a number of membraned viruses. The viruses inhibited by the polysaccharide included herpes simplex virus 1 (HSV-1), cytomegalovirus, measles virus, mumps virus and HIV-1. Calcium spirulan appears to inhibit the penetration of these viruses into host cells. These studies were performed *in vitro*.

Spirulina has been shown to have hypocholesterolemic activity in experimental animals. The mechanism of this activity is unknown.

Phycocyanorubin, a reduced form of phycocyanobilin, is similar in structure to the bile pigment bilirubin. Those with borderline elevated bilirubin levels—for example, those with Gilbert's syndrome—have been noted to have a lower incidence of cardiovascular disease, reduced stroke prevalence and improved stroke outcomes, among other health benefits. Bilirubin has a number of antioxidant activities, including the inhibition of formation of superoxide anion radicals by NADPH oxidase. The antioxidant and radical scavenging activities of phycocyanin are well documented. The activities are mainly attributed to the phycocyanobilin moiety. Phycocyanorubin has also been demonstrated to have radical scavenging activity and might also possess NADPH oxidase inhibitory activity as well.

Phycocyanin has been found to protect against hepatotoxins in rats. The mechanism may be via its antioxidant activity. An extract of *Spirulina maxima* also protected against carbon tetrachloride hepatotoxicity in rats. The phycocyanin contained in the extract, as well as other antioxidants, probably account for the hepatoprotective effect.

Spirulina was found to inhibit mast-cell mediated immediate-type allergic reactions in rats. It is speculated that there are substances in Spirulina that may inhibit mast-cell degranulation, possibly by affecting the mast-cell membrane.

Spirulina platensis extracts have been demonstrated to enhance macrophage function in cats and to enhance humoral and cell-mediated immune functions in chickens. The mechanism of these effects is unknown.

It was shown that *in vitro* culture of Spirulina with human blood mononuclear cells modulated the production of some cytokines. Another study by the same group evaluated the impact of a Spirulina nutritional supplement on subjects with allergic rhinitis by assessing the production of the cytokines interleukin (IL)-4, interferon (IFN)-gamma and interleukin (IL)-2. These cytokines are critical to the regulation of immunoglobulin E-mediated allergic reactions. In a randomized, double-blinded, crossover study versus placebo, it was found that Spirulina modulated the Th (T-helper lymphocyte) profile in subjects with allergic rhinitis by suppressing the differentiation of Th2 cells, mediated, in part, by inhibiting the production of IL-4. Spirulina appeared not to be effective at modulating the secretion of the Th1 cytokines IFN-gamma and IL-2.

PHARMACOKINETICS

The pharmacokinetics of Spirulina in humans has not been studied. However, the proteins, lipids and carbohydrates in Spirulina should be digested, absorbed and metabolized by normal physiological processes.

INDICATIONS AND USAGE

Spirulina has shown some indication of having antiviral effects in preliminary *in vitro* and animal studies. There is also evidence of a preliminary nature that it might favorably affect some immune functions and have some hepatoprotective capability. It has shown some promise of inhibiting some allergic reactions in recent experimental studies. Hypocholesterolemic effects have been reported in some animal studies.

RESEARCH SUMMARY

An extract of Spirulina inhibited *in vitro* replication of HSV-1 simplex virus type 1. It also significantly prolonged survival time of HSV-1-infected hamsters. It seemed to act, not through direct virucidal effects, but rather through inhibition of viral penetration into cells. Subsequently, further experiments demonstrated that Spirulina extract significantly inhibited *in vitro* replication of several enveloped viruses, including human cytomegalovirus, measles virus, mumps virus, influenza A virus and HIV-1. Again, the mechanism of action was said to be selective inhibition of viral penetration into host cells.

More recently still, other researchers have focused specifically on the ability of a Spirulina extract to inhibit HIV-1 replication in human T-cell lines, peripheral blood mononuclear cells (PBMC) and Langerhans cells (LC). The researchers stated: "We conclude that aqueous *A platensis* extracts contain antiretroviral activity that may be of potential clinical interest."

Spirulina and some of its constituents have shown an ability to favorably affect various immune functions. In one animal experiment, it boosted phagocytic activity and increased natural killer (NK)-cell activity two-fold, compared with controls.

Spirulina has significantly inhibited chemically induced anaphylactic shock and serum histamine levels in rats, leading to the conclusion that Spirulina may inhibit mast-cell degranulation. In another animal experiment, Spirulina significantly inhibited local allergic reactions induced by anti-dinitrophenyl (DNP) IgE. It demonstrated, more specifically, a significant inhibitory effect on anti-DNP IgE-induced tumor necrosis factor-alpha production, leading the researchers to conclude that Spirulina inhibits mast-cell mediated immediate-type allergic reactions both *in vitro* and *in vivo*.

Finally, a constituent of Spirulina, administered intraperitoneally, significantly reduced the hepatotoxicity of a carbon tetrachloride challenge. A more recent study confirmed this finding.

CONTRAINDICATIONS, PRECAUTIONS, ADVERSE REACTIONS

CONTRAINDICATIONS

Spirulina is contraindicated in those who are hypersensitive to any component of a Spirulina-containing supplement.

PRECAUTIONS

Pregnant women and nursing mothers should avoid Spirulina-containing supplements.

Spirulina can accumulate heavy metals, such as mercury, from contaminated waters. Those who use Spirulina supplements should select reputable products that are free of any heavy metal contamination.

ADVERSE REACTIONS

Occasional gastrointestinal symptoms, such as nausea, have been reported. Also, there are a few reports of allergic reactions to Spirulina-containing supplements.

DOSAGE AND ADMINISTRATION

There are various forms of Spirulina supplements, including capsules, tablets, flakes and powders. Spirulina is also found in some functional foods and in combination "green food" products with barley grass, chlorella and wheat grass. Doses range from 250 mg to 5 grams daily.

LITERATURE

Ayehunie S, Belay A, Baba TW, et al. Inhibition of HIV-1 replication by an aqueous extract of Spirulina platensis (Arthrospira platensis). *J Acquir Immune Defic Synd Hum Retrovirol.* 1998;18:7-12.

Chamorro G, Salazar M, Favil L, et al. [Pharmacology and toxicology of Spirulina alga.] [Article in Spanish.] *Rev Invest Clin.* 1996;48:389-399.

Devi MA, Venkataraman LV. Hypocholesterolemic effect of blue-green algae *Spirulina platensis* in albino rats. *Ann Nutr Reports Int.* 1983;28:519-530.

Eriksen NT. Production of phycocyanin—a pigment with applications in biology, biotechnology, foods and medicine. *Appl Microbiol Biotechnol.* 2008;80(1):1-14.

Hayashi T, Hayashi K. Calcium spirulan, an inhibitor of enveloped virus replication, from a blue-green alga *Spirulina platensis*. 1996;59:83-87.

Hayashi K, Hayashi T, Morita N, et al. An extract from Spirulina platensis is a selective inhibitor of herpes simplex virus type 1 penetration into HeLa cells. *Phytotherapy Res.* 1993;7:76-80.

Johnson PE, Shubert LE. Accumulation of mercury and other elements by spirulina (cyanophyceae). *Nutr Rep Intl.* 1986;34:1063-1071.

Kim HM, Lee EH, Cho HH, et al. Inhibitory effect of mast cell-mediated immediate-type allergic reactions in rats by spirulina. *Biochem Pharmacol.* 1998;55:1071-1076.

Lissi EA, Pizarro M, Aspee A, et al. Kinetics of phycocyanine bilin groups destruction by peroxyl radicals. *Free Rad Biol Med.* 2000;28:1051-1055.

Mao TK, Van de Water J, Gershwin ME. Effects of a Spirulina-based dietary supplement on cytokine production from allergic rhinitis patients. *J Med Food.* 2005;8(1):27-30.

McCarty MF. Clinical potential of Spirulina as a source of phycocyanobilin. *J Med Food.* 2007;10(4):566-570.

McCarty MF. Iatrogenic Gilbert syndrome—a strategy for reducing vascular and cancer risk by increasing plasma unconjugated bilirubin. *Med Hypotheses.* 2007;69(5):974-994.

Miranda MS, Cintra RG, Barros SB, et al. Antioxidant activity of the microalga Spirulina maxima. *Braz J Med Biol Res.* 1998;31:1075-1079.

Perlstein TS, Pande RL, Beckman JA, et al. Serum total bilirubin level and prevalent lower-extremity peripheral arterial disease: National Health and Nutrition Examination Survey (NHANES) 1999 to 2004. *Arterioscler Thromb Vasc Biol.* 2008;28(1):166-172.

Quereshi MA, Ali RA. Spirulina platensis exposure enhances macrophage phagocytic function in cats. *Immunopharmacol Immunotoxicol.* 1996;18:457-463.

Quereshi MA, Garlich JD, Kidd MT. Dietary Spirulina platensis enhances humoral and cell-mediated functions in chickens. *Immunopharmacol Immunotoxicol.* 1996;18:465-476.

Romay C, Armesto J, Ramirez D, et al. Antioxidant and anti-inflammatory properties of C-phycocyanin from blue-green algae. *Inflamm Res.* 1998;47:36-41.

Torres-Durán PV, Miranda-Zamora R, Paredes-Carbajal MC, et al. Studies on the preventive effect of *Spirulina maxima* on fatty liver development induced by carbon tetrachloride. *J Ethnopharmacol.* 1999;64:141-147.

Watanabe F, Katsura H, Takenaka S, et al. Pseudovitamin B_{12} is the predominant cobamide of an algal health food, spirulina tablets. *J Agric Food Chem.* 1999;47:4736-4741.

Yang H-N, Lee E-H, Kim H-M. *Spirulina platensis* inhibits anaphylactic reaction. *Life Sciences.* 1997;61:1237-1244.

Spruce Lignans (7-hydroxymatairesinol)

DESCRIPTION

Lignans are phenylpropanoid dimers widely distributed in the plant kingdom. Flaxseed and sesame seed are two of the richest sources of dietary lignans. (See Flaxseed Lignans and Sesame Seed Lignans.) One of the richest sources of lignans in the plant kingdom is the Norway spruce tree (*Picea abies* L. Karst). Lignans are found in high concentrations in the heartwood (wood that has died) of branches and knots (branch stubs) of the Norway spruce. Norway spruce knots comprise a portion of side branches embedded in the wood of stems or larger branches. Spruce knots consist of 6% to 16% of lignans, the major lignan being 7-hydroxymatairesinol (HMR). HMR represents 65% to 80% of the total lignan content found in spruce knots. HMR may be the most abundant lignan in nature.

HMR is a dibenzylbutyrolactone. This is one of the two major structural types of plant lignans. The plant lignan secoisolariciresinol diglucoside (SDG), found in flaxseed, also possesses this type of chemical structure. The other major chemical type is the tetrahydrofuran type found in the sesame seed lignans, sesamin and sesaminol. The chemical structure of HMR is closely related to the structure of matairesinol, a lignan found in small amounts in flaxseed and sesame seed. Because of the chiral carbon center at position 7, HMR is composed of two stereoisomers—*allo*-HMR and HMR. HMR itself refers to the mixture of both diastereomers of 7-hydroxymatairesinol. The stereoisomers are usually present in a 1:9 ratio. HMR, the major isomer, is also known as (7S,8R,8'R)-(–)-7-hydroxymatairesinol, and *allo*-HMR, the minor isomer, is also known as (7R,8R,8'R)-(–)-*allo*-hydroxymatairesinol. The HMR product used for supplementation is usually 7-hydroxymatairesinol potassium acetate. The potassium acetate adduct is generated during the purification process. The biphenolic nature of SDG resembles many of the substances known to exert estrogenic action or to block estrogen receptor sites.

HMR is converted mainly to enterolactone (ENL) by the intestinal microflora in the proximal part of the large intestine. ENL is not itself a plant lignan and is classified as a mammalian lignan or an enterolignan. ENL is also known as *trans*-dihydro-3,4-bis[(3-hydroxyphenyl)methyl]-2(3H)-Furanone and has a molecular weight of 298. It is thought that ENT may be responsible for many of the biological actions of HMR.

The chemical structures below are described within this monograph.

7-hydroxymatairesinol

Enterolactone

ACTIONS AND PHARMACOLOGY

ACTIONS

7-hydroxymatairesinol (HMR) has possible antioxidant, estrogenic, antiestrogenic, chemopreventive, anticancer and cardiovascular protective actions.

MECHANISM OF ACTION

HMR was shown to inhibit lipid peroxidation and LDL oxidation and to scavenge superoxide anions produced by xanthine oxidase and peroxyl radicals, in all cases *in vitro*.

The estrogenicity of HMR and ENL in comparison to estradiol (E2) was evaluated by measuring their effects on growth and apoptotic markers in the human estrogen-sensitive cell line, MCF-7. It was concluded that both HMR and ENL do have estrogenic activity, although much less potent and efficacious than that of E2. However, not all studies have shown estrogenic activity of HMR. In a study looking at the effect of HMR on growing tumors in a rat dimethyl-ben[a]anthracene (DMBA)-induced mammary tumor model, HMR decreased the number of growing tumors and increased the proportion of regressing and stabilized tumors, but was not found to exert estrogenic or antiestrogenic activity in the uterine growth test in immature rats. Nor did HMR show antiandrogenic effects in the growth of accessory sex glands in adult male rats.

HMR showed chemopreventive activity in the adenomatous polyposis coli multiple intestinal neoplasia (APC)[Min] mouse model. The mean number of adenomas in the small intestine was significantly lower in those mice fed HMR. In addition, HMR resulted in normalization of beta-catenin levels in adenoma tissue, suggesting that the effect was mediated via the Apc-beta-catenin pathway. More research is necessary and warranted in order to elucidate the mechanism of HMR's possible chemopreventive activity.

The effect of HMR on uterine carcinogenesis was studied in adult Donryu rats. The rats were treated with the carcinogen N-ethyl-N′-nitro-N-nitrosoguanidine (ENNG) followed by a range of doses of HMR. Treatment with HMR significantly lowered the incidence of uterine adenocarcinoma in the rats. The mechanism of this effect was unclear. It was speculated that the decrease in uterine adenocarcinoma was due to an antiestrogen effect, such as inhibition of the aromatase enzyme. Further studies are warranted to verify and elucidate the action and mechanism of the possible chemopreventive action of HMR in uterine carcinogenesis.

HMR was administered to athymic nude male mice implanted with LNCaP (human prostate cancer cells) xenografts. Mice treated with HMR had smaller tumor volume, lower tumor take rate, increased proportion of nongrowing tumors, higher cell apoptotic index compared with controls and a reduced cell proliferation index. Again, the mechanism of action of this anticancer effect was unclear. Possibilities include endocrine modulation, inhibition of the androgen-mobilizing enzymes 5-alpha reductase, hydroxysteroid oxidoreductase and aromatase, decreasing the binding of sex hormone binding protein (SHBP), thus accelerating the metabolic clearance of endogenous androgens, and binding to estrogen receptors alpha and beta. Other possibilities may also exist and, again, further studies are necessary and warranted to help elucidate the mechanism of this possible anticancer effect.

Both HMR and ENL were found to reduce the growth and metastasis of solid AH109A hepatomas in rats. Again, the mechanism of action of this effect was unclear.

In an epidemiological study with Finnish men, high serum ENL concentrations were associated with a decrease in mortality caused by cardiovascular disease. Since HMR is metabolized to ENT, clinical trials are warranted to see if administration of HMR might have a cardiovascular protective effect.

PHARMACOKINETICS

The pharmacokinetics for 7-hydroxymatairesinol (HMR) in humans is incomplete. After ingestion, HMR is metabolized to the mammalian lignan enterolactone (ENT) and, to a much smaller extent, to hydroxyenterolactone, by intestinal bacteria. Both SDG and ENT are absorbed from the intestine and are found in the serum and later in the urine, mainly in their conjugated forms—glucuronides and sulfates.

INDICATIONS AND USAGE

Claims for the plant lignan 7-hydroxyhydroxymatairesinol (HMR) derived from the Norway spruce include antioxidant and anticancer activities, as well as estrogenic effects that could be useful in controlling some post-menopausal complaints. Claims related to menopausal symptoms have no clinical basis at this time.

RESEARCH SUMMARY

HMR demonstrates antioxidant effects in some *in vitro* and animal studies. Similarly, several studies using various animal cancer models have revealed that HMR has some anticancer potential. In one study, focusing on chemically induced mammary cancer in rats, administration of HMR in the diet, started prior to chemical induction, resulted in reduced tumor volume and reduced tumor growth. There was, however, no significant reduction in the number of tumors per animal. The growth of established tumors was also inhibited when HMR administration began after chemical induction of the cancer. Since there was no increase in uterine weight in this study, the researchers concluded that the mode of action was not estrogenic in character and suggested that further studies are needed to clarify both the effects and the underlying mode of action.

Other animal studies have shown positive HMR effects on uterine carcinogenesis, hepatomas, prostate malignancies and colon cancer. In the uterine cancer study, HMR helped prevent and diminish the incidence of chemically induced uterine adenocarcinomas. Significant reduction was achieved in a dose-dependent fashion. Similarly, dietary HMR significantly inhibited growth and metastasis of hepatocellular carcinoma in rats. In the first study of HMR in prostate cancer, a mouse model subcutaneously injected with human prostate cancer xenografts demonstrated positive effects. Mice administered HMR in the diet had smaller tumor volume, lower tumor take rate, increased proportion of nongrowing tumors and higher quantifiable tumor cell death rates when compared with controls that did not receive HMR. Another mouse study has suggested that dietary HMR might also have protective effects against colon cancer.

Clinical data is so far lacking and will be needed to establish whether the spruce lignan and its derivatives may have any anticancer efficacy in humans. Such studies are warranted.

Some have hypothesized that spruce lignan might have estrogenic effects sufficient to significantly reduce some of the troublesome symptoms, such as "hot flushes," that occur in post-menopausal women. A human pilot study claimed to find some efficacy in this regard, but the study was not published in a peer-reviewed journal and cannot be evaluated. In one *in vitro* study, utilizing a human estrogen-sensitive cell line, HMR demonstrated effects that led the researchers to conclude that dietary supplementation with the lignan might result in mild estrogenic activity in humans. At this point it appears doubtful that HMR could become an alternative treatment sufficient in potency to supplant standard estrogen replacement therapy in post-menopausal women—but further investigation may be indicated.

CONTRAINDICATIONS, PRECAUTIONS, ADVERSE REACTIONS

CONTRAINDICATIONS

7-hydroxyhydroxymatairesinol (HMR) is contraindicated in those who are hypersensitive to any component of an HMR-containing product.

PRECAUTIONS

Consumption of HMR is not recommended for children.

Pregnant women and nursing mothers should avoid the use of HMR supplements.

Men with prostate cancer should discuss the advisability of the use of HMR supplements with their physicians before deciding to use them.

Women with estrogen receptor-positive tumors should exercise caution in the use of HMR supplements and should only use them if they are recommended and monitored by a physician.

ADVERSE REACTIONS
None known.

INTERACTIONS

DRUGS
Antibiotics may decrease the production of ENL from HMR.

NUTRITIONAL SUPPLEMENTS
None known.

FOODS
No known interactions.

HERBS
None known

OVERDOSAGE

There are no reports of HMR overdosage.

DOSAGE AND ADMINISTRATION

The major manufacturer of HMR recommends a daily dose of 50 mg of HMR.

LITERATURE

Bylund A, Saarinen N, Zhang JX, et al. Anticancer effects of a plant lignan 7-hydroxymatairesinol on a prostate cancer model in vivo. *Exp Biol Med* (Maywood). 2005;230(3):217-223.

Cosentino M, Marino F, Ferrari M, et al. Estrogenic activity of 7-hydroxymatairesinol potassium acetate (HMR/lignan) from Norway spruce (Picea abies) knots and of its active metabolite enterolactone in MCF-7 cells. *Pharmacol Res*. 2007;56(2):140-147

Kangas L, Saarinen N, Mutanen M, et al. Antioxidant and antitumor effects of hydroxymatairesinol (HM-3000, HMR), a lignan isolated from the knots of spruce. *Eur J Cancer Prev*. 2002;11 Suppl 2:S48-S57.

Katsuda S, Yoshida M, Saarinen N, et al. Chemopreventive effects of hydroxymatairesinol on uterine carcinogenesis in Donryu rats. *Exp Biol Med* (Maywood). 2004;229(5):417-424.

Lina B, Korte H, Nyman L, et al. A thirteen week dietary toxicity study with 7-hydroxymatairesinol potassium acetate (HMR lignan) in rats. *Regul Toxicol Pharmacol*. 2005;41(1):28-38.

Miura D, Saarinen NM, Miura Y, et al. Hydroxymatairesinol and its mammalian metabolite enterolactone reduce the growth and metastasis of subcutaneous AH109A hepatomas in rats. *Nutr Cancer*. 2007;58(1):49-59.

Oikannen SI, Pajari AM, Mutanen M. Chemopreventative activity of crude hydroxymatairesinol (HMR) extract in Apc(Min) mice [corrected]. *Cancer Lett*. October 2000;159(2):183-187. Erratum in: *Cancer Lett* 2000;161(2):251.

Oikarinen SI, Pajari A, Mutanen M. Chemopreventive activity of crude hydroxsymatairesinol (HMR) extract in Apc(Min) mice. *Cancer Lett*. 2000;161(2):253-258.

Saarinen NM, Huovinen R, Wärri A, et al. Uptake and metabolism of hydroxymatairesinol in relation to its anticarcinogenicity in DMBA-induced rat mammary carcinoma model. *Nutr Cancer*. 2001;41(1-2):82-90.

Saarinen NM, Wärri A, Mäkelä SI, et al. Hydroxymatairesinol, a novel enterolactone precursor with antitumor properties from coniferous tree (Picea abies). *Nutr Cancer*. 2000;36(2):207-216.

Vanharanta M, Voutilainen S, Rissanen TH, et al. Risk of cardiovascular disease-related and all-cause death according to serum concentrations of enterolactone: Kuopio Ischaemic Heart Disease Risk Factor Study. *Arch Intern Med*. 2003;163(9):1099-1104.

Wolterbeek AP, Roberts A, Korte H, et al. Prenatal developmental toxicity study with 7-hydroxymatairesinol potassium acetate (HMR lignan) in rats. *Regul Toxicol Pharmacol*. 2004;40(1):1-8.

Yamashita K, Yamada Y, Kitou S, et al. Hydroxymatairesinol and sesaminol act differently on tocopherol concentrations in rats. *J Nutr Sci Vitaminol* (Tokyo). 2007;53(5):393-399.

Yamauchi S, Sugahara T, Nakashima Y, et al. Radical and superoxide scavenging activities of matairesinol and oxidized matairesinol. *Biosci Biotechnol Biochem*. 2006;70(8):1934-1940.

Squalene

DESCRIPTION

Squalene, a 30-carbon isoprenoid, is a lipid found in large quantities in shark liver oil and in smaller amounts (0.1 to 0.7%) in olive oil, wheat germ oil, rice bran oil and yeast. It is a key intermediate in the biosynthesis of cholesterol. Squalene is an all-trans isoprenoid containing six isoprene units. Chemically, it is known as (all-E)-2, 6, 10, 15, 19, 23-Hexamethyl-2, 6, 10, 14, 18, 22-tetracosahexaene. It is represented structurally as:

Squalene

It is also known as spinacene and supraene. Squalene is also found in human sebum. Squalene has the ability to absorb oxygen. However, the amount of oxygen absorbed would be physiologically significant only for the shark.

ACTIONS AND PHARMACOLOGY

ACTIONS

Squalene has demonstrated proliferative activity in animal cancer studies; to date no human data are available. Squalene may have some radioprotective effects, but, again, there are no human data. Animal work suggests that squalene may also have a cholesterol-lowering effect, but this has not been tested in humans.

MECHANISM OF ACTION

Squalene is a key precursor in the biosynthesis of cholesterol. It inhibits 3-hydroxy-3-methylglutaryl coenzyme A reductase activity, thus reducing farnesyl pyrophosphate availability for prenylation of the ras oncogene, an activity that could account for its anti-proliferative effect in some animal cancer models. Apoptosis inhibition may also play a role in the anti-tumor effects of squalene in animals. The mechanism of the radioprotective effect of squalene is unknown.

PHARMACOKINETICS

Over 60% of ingested squalene is absorbed from the small intestine; from there it is carried in the lymph in the form of chylomicrons into the systemic circulation. In the blood, squalene is carried mainly in very-low-density lipoproteins and distributed to the various tissues of the body. A large percentage of squalene gets distributed to the skin. Squalene is metabolized to cholesterol.

INDICATIONS AND USAGE

Animal work suggests that indications could one day emerge for squalene in the prevention and treatment of some cancers, for immune enhancement and possibly for lowering cholesterol. It is not indicated for gastritis, joint pain and inflammation or to improve lung function.

RESEARCH SUMMARY

Squalene is being investigated as an adjunctive therapy in some cancers. In animal models, it has proved effective in inhibiting lung tumors. It has also demonstrated chemopreventive effects against colon cancer in animal models. Supplementation of squalene in mice has produced enhanced immune function and, in other animal studies, it has reduced cholesterol levels, prompting one researcher to suggest that it might be used to potentiate cholesterol-lowering drugs.

A mouse study showed squalene to confer radioprotection against lethal whole-body radiation.

CONTRAINDICATIONS, PRECAUTIONS, ADVERSE REACTIONS

CONTRAINDICATIONS

Known hypersensitivity to a squalene-containing product.

PRECAUTIONS

Squalene supplementation should be avoided in infants, children, pregnant women and nursing mothers.

ADVERSE REACTIONS

Those taking squalene supplements may have mild gastrointestinal symptoms such as diarrhea.

INTERACTIONS

None known.

OVERDOSAGE

There have been no reports of overdosage.

DOSAGE AND ADMINISTRATION

Squalene is a liquid that is available in capsules for oral use. Doses of 500 milligrams to 4 grams are used; the higher doses are used by some cancer sufferers. The source of squalene is usually from shark liver oil and sometimes from olive oil.

Squalene should not be confused with squalamine, which is an unusual steroid found in the dogfish shark and which has antibiotic properties.

LITERATURE

Kelly GS. Squalene and its potential clinical uses. *Altern Med Rev.* 1999; 4:29-36.

Newmark HL, Squalene, olive oil, and cancer risk: a review and hypothesis. *Cancer Epidemiol Biomarkers Prev.* 1997; 6:1101-1103.

Rao CV, Newmark HL, Reddy BS. Chemopreventive effect of squalene on colon cancer. *Carcinogenesis.* 1998; 19:287-290.

Smith TJ, Yank GY, Seril DN, et al. Inhibition of 4-(methylnitrosamino)-1-(3-pyridyl)-1-butanone-induced lung tumorogenesis by dietary olive oil and squalene. *Carcinogenesis.* 1998; 19:703-706.

Storm HM, Oh SY, Kimler BF, Norton S. Radioprotection of mice by dietary squalene. *Lipids.* 1993; 28:555-559.

Sulforaphane

DESCRIPTION

Sulforaphane is the aglycone breakdown product of the glucosinolate glucoraphanin, also known as sulforaphane glucosinolate (SGS). Glucosinolates are beta-thioglucoside-N-hydroxysulfates and are primarily found in cruciferous vegetables (cabbage, broccoli, broccoli sprouts, brussels sprouts, cauliflower, cauliflower sprouts, bok choy, kale, collards, arugula, kohlrabi, mustard, turnip, red radish and watercress). Young broccoli sprouts and young cauliflower sprouts are especially rich in glucoraphanin.

Sulforaphane may have cancer chemopreventive activity. However, glucosinolates themselves typically have low anticancer activity. Sulforaphane is produced from sulforaphane glucosinolate via the action of the enzyme myrosinase (thioglucoside glucohydrolase), an enzyme present in cruciferous vegetables that is activated upon maceration of the vegetables.

Sulforaphane is also classified as an isothiocyanate. Its molecular formula is $C_6H_{11}NOS_2$, and its molecular weight is 177.29 daltons. It is also known as 4-methylsulfinylbutyl isothiocyanate and (-)-1-isothiocyanato-4(R)-(methylsulfinyl) butane. Sulforaphane glucosinolate (glucoraphanin) is also known as 4-methylsufinylbutyl glucosinolate. The structural formula is:

Sulforaphane

ACTIONS AND PHARMACOLOGY

ACTIONS

Sulforaphane may have anticarcinogenic activity.

MECHANISM OF ACTION

Sulforaphane's possible anticarcinogenic activity is accounted for by its ability to induce phase II detoxication enzymes, such as glutathione S-transferase and quinone reductase [NAD(P)H: (quinone-acceptor) oxidoreductase]. These enzymes may afford protection against certain carcinogens and other toxic electrophiles, including reactive oxygen species.

PHARMACOKINETICS

Little is presently known about the pharmacokinetics of sulforaphane in humans. Some preliminary studies indicate that sulforaphane is absorbed and that it is metabolized by first undergoing conjugation with reduced glutathione to form a dithiocarbamate. The dithiocarbamate is then converted sequentially to conjugates with cysteinylglycine, cysteine and N-acetylcysteine.

INDICATIONS AND USAGE

Experimental data suggest that sulforaphane may have anticarcinogenic effects.

RESEARCH SUMMARY

Sulforaphane has significantly reduced the incidence, multiplicity and rate of development of chemically induced mammary tumors in rats. It has demonstrated an ability to detoxify a number of carcinogens and thus might have the ability to protect against a variety of cancers. It has been shown that dietary supplementation with sulforaphane enhances glutathione S-transferase (GST) enzyme activity, which is known to detoxify many carcinogens.

One group of researchers has reported that three-day-old sprouts of certain broccoli and cauliflower cultivars contain 10 to 100 times higher levels of glucoraphanin, the glucosinolate of sulforaphane, than do mature broccoli and cauliflower sprouts. Thus they have concluded that "small quantities of crucifer sprouts may protect against the risk of cancer as effectively as much larger quantities of mature vegetables of the same variety." Additionally they have noted that the indole glucosinates that are prevalent in mature broccoli, for example, are present in only small quantities in the sprouts. One report suggested that the degradation products (e.g., indole-3-carbinol) of these glucosinates might themselves promote tumorigenesis, but several other investigators have not confirmed this.

CONTRAINDICATIONS, PRECAUTIONS, ADVERSE REACTIONS

CONTRAINDICATIONS

Sulforaphane is contraindicated in those who are hypersensitive to any component of a sulforaphane-containing product.

PRECAUTIONS

Pregnant women and nursing mothers should avoid sulforaphane supplementation pending long-term safety data.

ADVERSE REACTIONS

No adverse reactions reported.

DOSAGE AND ADMINISTRATION

Sulforaphane is available in a few different formulations, usually in combination with other dietary phytochemicals. There are no typical doses.

Sulforaphane, in the form of its glucosinolate glucoraphanin, is abundant in three-day old broccoli sprouts, which are available in the marketplace. The levels of glucoraphanin in three-day old broccoli sprouts are from 10 to 100 times greater than in mature broccoli.

LITERATURE

Fahey JW, Talalay P. Antioxidant functions of sulforaphane: a potent inducer of Phase II detoxification enzymes. *Food Chem Toxicol.* 1999; 37:973-979.

Fahey JW, Zhang Y, Talalay P. Broccoli sprouts: an exceptionally rich source of inducers of enzymes that protect against chemical carcinogens. *Proc Natl Acad Sci USA.* 1997; 94:10367-10372.

Faulkner K, Mithen R, Williamson G. Selective increase of the potential anticarcinogen 4-methylsulphinylbutyl glucosinolate in broccoli. *Carcinogenesis.* 1998; 19:605-609.

Singletary K, MacDonald C. Inhibition of benzo[a]pyrene- and 1, 6-dinitropyrene-DNA adduct formation in human mammary epithelial cells by dibenzoylmethane and sulforaphane. *Cancer Letters.* 2000; 155:47-54.

Zeligs MA. Diet and estrogen status: the cruciferous connection. *J Med Food.* 1998; 1:67-82.

Zhang Y. Role of glutathione in the accumulation of anticarcinogenic isothiocyanates and their glutathione conjugates by murine hepatoma cells. *Carcinogenesis.* 2000; 21:1175-1182.

Zhang Y. Talalay P, Cho CG, Posner GH. A major inducer of anticarcinogenic protective enzymes from broccoli: isolation and elucidation of structure. *Proc Natl Acad Sci USA.* 1992; 89:2399-2403.

Supplemental Enzymes

DESCRIPTION

Enzymes are biological catalysts. Until recently, it was thought that all enzymes were protein in nature. It is now known that ribonucleic acids and other non-protein substances can have enzymatic activity, as well. Enzymes have important roles in medicine. They are used for the rapid lysis of blood clots (streptokinase, tissue plasminogen activator or TPA, urokinase) and for the treatment of Gaucher's disease (glucocerebrosidase), among other things. Enzymes are also used in the treatment of pancreatic insufficiency secondary to such disorders as cystic fibrosis and chronic alcoholic pancreatitis. Enzymes, in addition to being used therapeutically, are marketed as nutritional supplements. They are principally used as digestants. Some enzymes, in particular proteolytic enzymes, have putative anti-inflammatory and anticarcinogenic activities. The enzymes marketed for supplemental use are derived from animal, plant and fungal sources. The following describes the enzymes that are available in the nutritional supplement market place.

ALPHA-GALACTOSIDASE

Alpha-galactosidase is an enzyme that is derived from selected strains of the fungus *Aspergillus niger*. Alpha-galactosidase catalyzes the hydrolysis of the alpha-1→6 linkages in such carbohydrates as the disaccharide melibiose, the trisaccharide raffinose, the tetrasaccharide stachyose and the nonsaccharide verbascose. These oligosaccharides are widely found in legumes and cruciferous vegetables, including beans, peas, broccoli, brussels sprouts and cabbage. These carbohdyrates are gas productive in some. Hydrolysis of melibiose yields D-galactose and D-glucose; hydrolysis of raffinose yields D-galactose and sucrose; hydrolysis of stachyose yields D-galactose and sucrose; and verbascose yields D-galactose, D-glucose and D-fructose. The activity of alpha galactosidases is expressed in galactose units or GalU. A tablet of alpha-galactosidase typically contains 150 GalU.

AMYLASE

Amylases are enzymes that catalyze the hydrolysis of alpha-1, 4-glycosidic linkages of polysaccharides to yield dextrins, oligosaccharides, maltose and D-glucose. Amylases are derived from animal, fungal and plant sources. Pancreatin and pancrelipase contain amylase derived from the pancreas of animals, usually porcine pancreas. Amylase is also derived from barley malt and the fungus *Aspergillus oryzae*. There are a few different amylases. These enzymes are classified according to the manner in which the glysosidic bond is attacked. Alpha-amylases hydrolyze alpha-1, 4-glycosidic linkages, randomly yielding dextrins, oligosaccharides and monosaccharides. Alpha-amylases are endo-amylases. Exoamylases hydrolyze the alpha-1, 4-glycosidic linkage only from the non-reducing outer polysaccharide chain ends. Exoamylases include beta-amylases and glucoamylases (gamma-amylases, amyloglucosidases). Beta-amylases yield beta-limit dextrins and maltose. Gamma-amylases yield glucose. Amylases are used as digestants. Amylase activity is expressed as Dextrinizing Units or DU.

BROMELAIN

Bromelain refers to proteolytic enzymes which are derived from the ripe and unripe fruit, as well as the stem and leaves, of the pineapple plant, *Ananas comosus (Ananas sativus)*.

Bromelain is comprised of several proteolytic enzymes which differ in their specificities. These enzymes hydrolyze proteins to form oligopeptides and amino acids. Bromelain is used as a digestive aid. It also has putative anti-inflammatory activity. The activity of bromelain may be expressed in bromelain units or BU. The assay is based on a 60-minute proteolytic hydrolysis of casein at pH 6.0 and 40°C. One BU is defined as that quantity of enzyme that liberates the equivalent of one microgram of L-tyrosine per hour. The bromelain proteolytic enzymes are cysteine proteinases. There are at least four distinct bromelain cysteine proteinases. The activity of bromelain may also be expressed in gelatin dissolving units (GDU) or milk clotting units (MCU). One GDU is equivalent to about 1.5 MCU.

CELLULASE

Cellulase is an enzyme derived from the fungi *Aspergillus niger* and *Trichoderma longbrachiatum* or other sources. Cellulose is an indigestible plant polysaccharide. It is the principal constituent of the cell wall of plants. Cellulase has cellulolytic activity, meaning that it hydrolyzes cellulose. Cellulase hydrolyzes the beta-D-1, 4-glycosidic bonds of cellulose. Cellulase derived from *Trichoderma longbrachiatum* is comprised of an enzyme complex consisting of cellulase, a glucosidase, cellobiohydrolase and a glucanase. This complex converts cellulose to beta-dextrins and ultimately to D-glucose. Cellulase is used as a digestive aid, particularly in animals, and for the management of flatulence. The activity of cellulase is expressed in cellulose units or CU.

CHYMOTRYPSIN

Chymotrypsin is a proteolytic enzyme that is principally derived from ox pancreas. Chymotrypsin is a serine proteinase, referring to the fact that serine and histidine residues at the active site are involved in catalysis. Trypsin, also a serine proteinase, and chymotrypsin have similar tertiary structures although very different substrate specificities. Trypsin hydrolyzes peptides at Lys/Arg residues while chymotrypsin recognizes large hydrophobic residues. Chymotrypsin is found in pancreatic preparations, such as pancreatin and pancrelipase. It is used in ophthalmology for the dissection of the zonule of the lens. It is also used as a digestant and it has putative anti-inflammatory activity.

LACTASE

Lactase or beta-galactosidase is an enzyme that is derived from the fungus *Kluyveromyces lactis* (formerly known as *Saccharomyces lactis*) or from the fungus *Aspergillus oryzae*. Lactase hydrolyzes the lactose beta-D-galactoside linkage, yielding D-galactose and D-glucose. Lactase may be helpful to those with lactose or milk sugar intolerance. The activity of lactase supplements is expressed in acid lactase units or ALU. A regular strength lactase caplet typically contains 4,500 ALU. Lactase derived from *Kluyveromyces lactis* is used to pretreat milk for use by those with lactose intolerance. The activity of lactase in milk is expressed in neutral lactase units or NLU. The maximum recommended dose of lactase in milk is 3,000 NLU per liter.

PANCREATIN

Pancreatin is a pancreatic enzyme preparation derived from hog pancreas. Pancreatin is comprised of the pancreatic enzymes trypsin, amylase and lipase. Pancreatin and pancrelipase are similar except that pancrelipase has relatively more lipase activity than does pancreatin. Trypsin hydrolyzes proteins to oligopeptides, amylase hydrolyzes starch to oligosaccharides and the disaccharide maltose, and lipase hydrolyzes triglycerides to fatty acids and glycerol. Pancreatin is a digestant that is used in the treatment of pancreatic insufficiency as pancreatic enzyme replacement. A typical 500-milligram tablet of pancreatin contains 12,500 USP units of trypsin, 12,500 USP units of amylase and 1,000 USP units of lipase.

PANCRELIPASE

Pancrelipase is a standardized preparation of porcine pancreas that principally contains the pancreatic enzymes lipase, trypsin and amylase. Pancrelipase is similar to pancreatin except that it has relatively more lipase activity than pancreatin. Lipase hydrolyzes triglycerides to fatty acids and glycerol. Amylase hydrolyzes starch to oligosaccharides and the disaccharide maltose, and trypsin hydrolyzes proteins to oligopeptides. Pancrelipase is a digestant. It is used in the treatment of steatorrhea secondary to pancreatic insufficiency such as occurs in cystic fibrosis or in chronic alcoholic pancreatitis. A typical capsule of pancrelipase contains 4,500 USP (United States Pharmacopoeia) units of lipase, 25,000 USP units of trypsin and 20,000 USP units of amylase.

PAPAIN

Papain is a mixture of proteolytic enzymes derived from the juice of the unripe fruit of the tropical plant *Caroica papaya*, commonly known as papaya. Papain hydrolyzes proteins to form oligopeptides and amino acids. Papain also contains the proteolytic enzyme chymopapain which differs from papain in electrophoretic mobility, solubility and substrate specificity. The molecular weight of chymopapain is approximately 27,000 daltons. Papain is used as a digestive aid. It is also used as a meat tenderizer. Papain has putative anti-inflammatory activity. The activity of papain is expressed in papain units or PU. The assay of papain activity is based on the hydrolysis of casein.

PEPSIN

Pepsin is a proteolytic enzyme which is secreted by the stomach where it hydrolyzes proteins to polypeptides and oligopeptides. Pepsin that is derived from animal tissue is sometimes used in combination with dilute hydrochloric acid or betaine hydrochloride as an adjunct in the management of gastric hypochlorhydria.

TRYPSIN

Trypsin is a proteolytic enzyme which is principally derived from porcine pancreas. It is a serine proteinase, referring to the fact that serine and histidine residues at the active site are involved in catalytic activity. Chymotrypsin, also a serine proteinase, and trypsin have similar tertiary structures, although very different substrate specificities. Trypsin hydrolyzes peptides at Lys/Arg residues, while chymotrypsin recognizes large hydrophobic residues. Trypsin is found in pancreatic preparations, such as pancreatin and pancrelipase;

it has been used for the debridement of wounds. It is used as a digestant and it has putative anti-inflammatory activity.

SUPEROXIDE DISMUTASE
Superoxide dismutases are enzymes that play major roles in the protection of cells against oxidative damage. The two major forms of superoxide dismutase (SOD) in humans are the mitochondrial manganese SOD and the cytosolic copper/zinc SOD. A copper/zinc SOD, isolated from beef liver, has been used intra-articularly for degenerative joint disorders as an anti-inflammatory agent. SOD is also marketed as a nutritional supplement. Oral SOD has putative anti-inflammatory activity.

WOBE-MUGOS/WOBENZYME
Wobe-Mugos and Wobenzyme are proprietary enzyme preparations that have putative anti-inflammatory and anticarcinogenic activities. Wobe-Mugos contains the proteolytic enzymes papain, trypsin and chymotrypsin. The papain is derived from the fruit of the papaya plant. Trypsin and chymotrypsin are derived from bovine pancreas. Wobenzyme contains pancreatin, papain, bromelain, trypsin and chymotrypsin. Pancreatin, which contains amylase, trypsin and lipase, is derived from porcine pancreas. Bromelain is derived from the pineapple plant. The activity of the proteolytic enzymes in Wobe-Mugos and Wobenzyme is expressed in FIP units. The FIP unit is the measurement of enzyme activity according to the test methods of the Federation Internationale Pharmaceutique. Wobe-Mugos (papain, trypsin and chymotrypsin) is an orphan drug for the treatment of multiple myeloma.

ACTIONS AND PHARMACOLOGY
ACTIONS
Alpha-galactosidase, amylase, bromelain, cellulase, chymotrypsin, lactase, pancreatin, pancrelipase, papain and pepsin have digestant activities. Bromelain, chymotrypsin, papain, and trypsin have putative anti-inflammatory activity. Superoxide dismutase has putative anti-inflammatory activity. Wobe-Mugos and Wobenzyme have putative anti-inflammatory and anticarcinogenic activities.

MECHANISM OF ACTION
Alpha-galactosidase hydrolyzes melibiose to D-galactose, and D-glucose; raffinose to D-galactose and sucrose; stachyose to D-galactose; and sucrose and verbascose to D-galactose, D-glucose and D-fructose. Amylase hydrolyzes starch to oligosaccharides and maltose. Bromelain hydrolyzes proteins to oligopeptides and amino acids. Cellulase hydrolyzes cellulose to D-glucose. Chymotrypsin hydrolyzes proteins to oligopeptides. Lactase hydrolyzes lactose to D-galactose and D-glucose. Pancreatin and pancrelipase hydrolyze triglycerides to fatty acids and glycerol, proteins to oligopeptides and starch to oligosaccharides and maltose.

Papain hydrolyzes proteins to oligopeptides and amino acids. Pepsin hydrolyzes proteins to polypeptides and oligopeptides. Trypsin hydrolyzes proteins to oligopeptides.

The mechanism of the putative anti-inflammatory activity of the proteolytic enzymes bromelain, chymotrypsin, papain and trypsin is not well understood. It is believed that a fraction of these proteolytic enzymes is absorbed, probably via the enteropancreatic circulation. It is speculated that the putative anti-inflammatory activity of these enzymes may be accounted for, in part, by their activation of plasmin production from plasminogen and by their reduction of kinin via inhibition of the conversion of kininogen to kinin. Degradation of circulating immune complexes may be another possible mechanism.

The putative anti-inflammatory and anticarcinogenic activities of Wobe-Mugos and Wobenzyme are also open to speculation. Possibilities include a decrease of circulating immune complexes, disruption of adhesion molecules on tumor and endothelial cells, degradation of cytokines and cytokine receptors and possible immunomodulatory effects. Bromelain is speculated to play a role in differentiation of malignant cells.

The mechanism of the putative anti-inflammatory activity of superoxide dismutase is unknown.

PHARMACOKINETICS
The fungal- and plant-derived enzymes appear more resistant to inactivation and denaturation by stomach acid than are the animal-derived enzymes. Pancreatin and pancrelipase require enteric coating to prevent denaturation and inactivation by stomach acid. In the small intestine, a fraction of the enzymes may be absorbed via the enteropancreatic circulation. Much is unknown regarding the pharmacokinetics of oral enzymes in humans.

INDICATIONS AND USAGE
Supplemental enzymes (alpha-galactosidase, chymotrypsin lactase, pancreatin, pancrelipase, papain and pepsin) are used as digestive aids in some circumstances. Some (bromelain, superoxide dismutase, chymotrypsin, papain and trypsin) are said to have some anti-inflammatory activity. There is some evidence that Wobe-Mugos and Wobenzyme may have some anti-inflammatory and anticarcinogenic activities.

RESEARCH SUMMARY
Supplemental enzymes have been used for some time as digestive aids with various degrees of efficacy. Those with digestive disorders, however, should not use digestive enzymes unless they are approved by their physicians. Pancreatin is used pharmaceutically in some with pancreatic insufficiency secondary to such disorders as cystic fibrosis and chronic alcoholic pancreatitis. It is used in this context as

pancreatic enzyme replacement therapy. Pancrelipase is used in the treatment of steatorrhea secondary to pancreatic insufficiency related, again, to such disorders as cystic fibrosis and chronic alcoholic pancreatitis.

Pepsin, in combination with dilute hydrochloric acid has been used as an adjunctive treatment of gastric hypochlorhydria. Papain is used as a digestant. Lactase is effective in some with milk sugar (lactose) intolerance, and cellulase has reportedly been of benefit in some with flatulence. Amylases have been used as digestants, as has chymotrypsin and bromelain. Alpha-galactosidase is used to manage flatulence in those who develop "gas" from the consumption of certain foods, such as beans. Superoxide dismutase, used intra-articularly, has reportedly shown some anti-inflammatory effects in animals, but clinical studies are lacking.

More studies have been done on bromelain, Wobe-Mugos and Wobenzyme. Bromelain is a major constituent of Wobenzyme, which also includes pancreatin, papain, trypsin and chymotrypsin. Wobe-Mugos contains papain, trypsin and chymotrypsin. These enzyme preparations have demonstrated some anti-inflammatory and anticarcinogenic activity. Wobe-Mugos is an orphan drug for use in the treatment of multiple myeloma.

Wobe-Mugos and Wobenzyme have shown an ability to clear circulating immune complexes from the body, in both animal and human experiments. These antibody/antigen complexes have been implicated in some inflammatory processes, including those related to rheumatoid arthritis and some other autoimmune diseases. Antigen-induced experimental arthritis in rabbits was inhibited by these enzyme preparations in one experiment. Wobenzyme reportedly improved the condition of patients with chronic polyarthritis in another study. No side effects were noted. Recently, significant pain reduction was associated with use of these proteolytic enzyme preparations in subjects with osteoarthritis of the knee and periarthritis of the shoulder.

Long-term rectal administration of Wobe-Mugos has been reported to inhibit growth of solid tumors and development of experimental metastases in mice inoculated with B16 melanoma cells. In another recent study, Wobe-Mugos significantly increased survival time in mice with Lewis lung carcinoma. In a recent randomized trial, Wobe-Mugos was said to significantly reduce the acute sequelae of radiation in head and neck cancers.

There is a report in which Wobe-Mugos was tested in comparison with acyclovir in subjects with herpes zoster. The enzyme preparation was said to be as efficacious as acyclovir in alleviating pain. Effects on skin lesions were largely equal. More study is needed.

CONTRAINDICATIONS, PRECAUTIONS, ADVERSE REACTIONS

CONTRAINDICATIONS

Supplemental enzymes are contraindicated in those hypersensitive to any component of an enzyme-containing preparation.

PRECAUTIONS

The use of digestive enzymes for the treatment of pancreatic insufficiency requires medical supervision.

Those who wish to use supplemental enzymes for any indication should first discuss their use with their physicians.

Pregnant women and nursing mothers should avoid supplemental enzymes unless prescribed by their physicians.

Galactosemics should avoid the use of alpha-galactosidase. D-galactose is one of the substances formed via the action of alpha-galactosidase.

Those on anticoagulants or antithrombotic agents should be cautious in the use of bromelain. Bromelain may have blood-thinning activity in some.

ADVERSE REACTIONS

Alpha-galactosidase: Gastrointestinal symptoms such as cramping and diarrhea have been reported. Allergic-type reactions, including rash and pruritis, have also been reported.

Amylase: Allergic-type reactions, including rash and pruritis, have been reported.

Bromelain: Gastrointestinal symptoms such as nausea and vomiting, diarrhea and cramping, have been reported. Metrorrhagia and menorrhagia have been occasionally reported. Hypersensitivity reactions have been reported, including rashes and exacerbation of asthma.

Pancreatin: The most frequently reported adverse reactions are gastrointestinal and include diarrhea, abdominal pain, nausea and vomiting. Hyperuricemia has been reported with the use of pancreatin products.

Pancrelipase. The most frequently reported adverse reactions are gastrointestinal and include diarrhea, abdominal pain, nausea and vomiting, constipation, melena and perianal irritation. Hyperuricemia and hyperuricosuria have been reported with the use of pancrelipase products, primarily with non-enteric coated formulations. Cases of fibrosing colonopathy have been reported primarily in cystic fibrosis patients.

Wobe-Mugos/Wobenzyme: The most frequently reported adverse reactions are gastrointestinal and include diarrhea, abdominal pain, nausea and vomiting. There is a report of an anaphylactic reaction in a woman receiving intramuscular injections of Wobe-Mugos. There is a report of circulatory shock in a woman receiving injections and suppositories of Wobe-Mugos, as well as Wobenzyme tablets.

INTERACTIONS

DRUGS

Acarbose: Concomitant intake of enzyme preparations (containing amylase, pancreatin, pancrelipase) and acarbose may decrease the efficacy of acarbose.

Anticoagulants (e.g., warfarin): Bromelain may enhance the anticoagulant activity of such drugs as warfarin.

Antithrombotic agents (e.g., aspirin): Bromelain may enhance the antithrombotic activity of such drugs as aspirin.

NUTRITIONAL SUPPLEMENTS

Folic acid: Pancreatic enzymes (pancreatin, pancrelipase) have been reported to decrease the absorption of folic acid if taken concomitantly. However, this has not been substantiated.

Soy oligosaccharides: Concomitant intake of alpha-galactosidase and soy oligosaccharide prebiotics may inactivate the prebiotic activity of the soy oligosaccharides.

DOSAGE AND ADMINISTRATION

Supplemental enzymes are available in the nutritional supplement marketplace; pancreatin and pancrelipase are available as pharmaceutical agents for the treatment of pancreatic insufficiency. Supplemental enzymes that are available include alpha-galactosidase, alpha-amylase, amyloglucosidase, bromelain, cellulase, chymotrypsin, hemicellulase, lactase, lipase, pepsin, protease, superoxide dismutase, trypsin and Wobenzyme. A plant-derived analogue of pancreatin is also available. Those who wish to use supplementary enzymes should first discuss their use, as well as dosage, with their physicians.

LITERATURE

Anthony H, Collins CE, Davidson G, et al. Pancreatic enzyme replacement therapy in cystic fibrosis: Australian guidelines. *J Pediatr—Child Health.* 1999; 35:125-129.

Billigmann P. [Enzyme therapy—an alternative in treatment of herpes zoster. A controlled study of 192 patients]. [Article in German]. *Fortschr Med.* 1995; 113:43-48.

Bock U, Kolac C, Borchard G, et al. Transport of proteolytic enzymes across Caco-2 cell monolayers. *Pharm Res.* 1998; 15:1393-1400.

Coenen TMM, Bertens AMC, De Hoog SCM, Verspeek-Rip CM. Safety evaluation of a lactase enzyme preparation derived from *Kluyveromyces lactis. Food Chem Toxicol.* 2000; 38:671-677.

de Smet PA, Pegt GW, Meyboom RH. [Acute circulatory shock following administration of the non-regular enzyme preparation Wobe-Mugos]. [Article in Dutch]. Ned Tijdschr *Geneeskd.* 1991; 135:2341-2344.

Dominguez-Munoz JE, Birckelbach U, Glassbrenner B, et al. Effect of oral pancreatic enzyme administration on digestive function in healthy subjects: comparison between two enzyme preparations. *Aliment Pharmacol Ther.* 1997; 11:403-408.

Eckert K, Grabowska E, Stange R, et al. Effects of oral bromelain administration on the impaired immunocytotoxicity of mononuclear cells from mammary tumor patients. *Oncol Rep.* 1999; 6:1191-1199.

Farkas G, Takacs T, Baradnay G, Szasz Z. [Effect of pancreatin replacement on pancreatic function in the postoperative period after pancreatic surgery]. [Article in Hungarian]. *Orv Hetil.* 1999; 140:2751-2754.

Greenberger NJ. Enzymatic therapy in patients with chronic pancreatitis. *Gastrenterol Clin North Am.* 1999; 28:687-693.

Kaul R, Mishra BK, Sutrador P, et al. The role of Wobe-Mugos in reducing acute sequelae of radiation in head and neck cancers—a clinical phase-III randomized trial. *Indian J Cancer.* 1999; 36:141-148.

Kiessling WR. [Anaphylactic reaction in enzyme therapy of multiple sclerosis]. [Article in German]. *Fortschr Neurol Psychiatr.* 1987; 55:385-386.

Klein G, Kullich W. [Reducing pain by oral enzyme therapy in rheumatic diseases]. [Article in German]. *Wien Med Wochenschr.* 1999; 149:577-580.

Rowan AD, Buttle DJ, Barrett AJ. The cysteine proteinases of the pineapple plant. *Biochem J.* 1990; 266:869-875.

Stauder G, Ransberger K, Streichhan P, et al. The use of hydrolytic enzymes as adjuvant therapy in AIDS/ARC/LAS patients. *Biomed Pharmacother.* 1988; 42:31-34.

Steffen C, Menzel J. [Enzyme breakdown of immune complexes]. [Article in German]. *Z Rheumatol.* 1983; 42:249-255.

Steffen C, Smolen J, Miehlke K, et al. [Enzyme therapy in comparison with immune complex determinations in chronic polyarthritis]. [Article in German]. *Z Rheumatol.* 1985; 44:51-56.

Wald M, Olejár T, Pouková P, Zadinova M. Proteinases reduce metastatic dissemination and increase survival time in C57B16 mice with the Lewis lung carcinoma. *Life Sciences.* 1998; 63:PL237-243.

Wald M, Závadová E, Pouková P, et al. Polyenzyme preparation Wobe-Mugos inhibits growth of solid tumors and development of experimental metastases in mice. *Life Sciences.* 1998; 62:PL43-48.

Wolf M, Ransberger K. [Effect of proteolytic enzymes on the reciprocal growth modification of normal and tumor tissues]. [Article in German]. *Arch Geschwulstforsch.* 1968; 31:317-331.

Synbiotics

DESCRIPTION

Synbiotics refer to combination nutritional supplements comprised of probiotics and prebiotics. Probiotics (see Probiotics) are live microbial food supplements that beneficially affect the host by improving its intestinal microflora balance. Prebiotics (see Prebiotics) are nondigestible dietary substances, typically oligosaccharides and disaccharides, that beneficially affect the host by selectively stimulating the growth and/or activity of a limited number of bacterial species already resident in the large intestine.

Synbiotics could improve the survival of the probiotic organism by providing the specific substrate to the probiotic organism for its fermentation.

Synbiotic supplements that are currently available, include combinations of bifidobacteria and fructo-oligosaccharides (FOS), *Lactobacillus* GG and inulins and bifidobacteria and lactobacilli and FOS or inulins.

ACTIONS AND PHARMACOLOGY

ACTIONS

Synbiotics may have antimicrobial, anticarcinogenic, immunomodulatory, antidiarrheal, antiallergenic, hypolipidemic and hypoglycemic activities. They may also have activity in improving mineral absorption and balance and may have anti-osteoporotic activity.

MECHANISM OF ACTION

The antimicrobial activity of the synbiotics can be accounted for by the probiotic component of these substances. The bacteria can reinforce the barrier function of the intestinal mucosa, helping in the prevention of the attachment of pathogenic bacteria to the intestinal wall, essentially by crowding them out. These bacteria may also produce antimicrobial substances and stimulate antigen specific and nonspecific immune responses.

The possible anticarcinogenic activity of synbiotics is not well understood. The prebiotic oligosaccharides are fermented by the probiotic bacteria, as well as other bacteria that reside in the colon, to butyrate and other short-chain fatty acids. Butyrate may induce growth arrest and cell differentiation and may also upregulate apoptosis, three activities which could be significant for the possible anticarcinogenic activity of butyrate. The prebiotic oligosaccharides may also aid in increasing the concentrations of calcium and magnesium in the colon. Elevated concentrations of these cations in the colon may help to control the rate of cell turnover. Elevated concentrations of calcium in the colon may also help to control the formation of insoluble bile or salts of fatty acids. This might reduce the potential damaging effects of bile or fatty acids on colonocytes. The probiotic bacteria may bind to and inactivate some carcinogens and may directly inhibit the growth of some tumors as well as some bacteria that may convert precarcinogens into carcinogens.

The probiotic bacteria may increase levels of circulating immunoglobulin A (IgA) and enhance nonspecific immune mechanisms, such as increasing phagocytic activity.

Probiotics that colonize the colon may be helpful in the management of some with food allergies, helping to reinforce the barrier function of the intestinal mucosa, thus possibly preventing aberrant absorption of intraluminal antigens.

The prebiotics may lower triglyceride levels in some. The mechanism of this possible effect is unclear. Decreased hepatocyte *de novo* synthesis of triglycerides is one hypothetical possibility. The prebiotics may also lower total cholesterol and LDL-cholesterol levels in some. Again, the mechanism of this possible effect is unclear. Propionate, a product of prebiotic oligosaccharide fermentation in the colon, may inhibit HMG-CoA reductase.

The mechanism of the possible effect of the prebiotic oligosaccharides on modulating serum levels glucose is not well understood, but could be accounted for in a few ways. The oligosaccharides may delay gastric emptying and/or shorten small-intestinal tract transit time. This may be via the short-chain fatty acids produced from the oligosaccharides in the colon. Short-chain fatty acids may also stimulate contractions of the ileum and shorten ileal emptying. In addition, propionate may inhibit gluconeogenesis, reduce serum levels of free fatty acids and enhance glycolysis.

The oligosaccharides may bind/sequester such minerals as calcium and magnesium in the small intestine. The short-chain fatty acids formed from the bacterial fermentation of the oligosaccharides may facilitate the colonic absorption of calcium and, possibly, also magnesium ions. This could be beneficial in the prevention of osteoporosis.

PHARMACOKINETICS

The effectiveness of probiotics is related to their ability to survive in the acid stomach environment and the alkaline conditions in the duodenum as well as to their ability to adhere to the intestinal mucosa of the large intestine and to colonize the colon. After passage through the stomach and the small intestine, those probiotics that do survive become established transiently in the colon.

Following ingestion, the prebiotic oligosaccharides reach the colon with little of them being digested in the upper gastrointestinal tract. The oligosaccharides are fermented by bifidobacteria, lactobacilli and some other bacteria in the colon to produce the short-chain fatty acids acetate, propionate and butyrate; the gases hydrogen, hydrogen sulfide, carbon dioxide and methane; and lactate, pyruvate, succinate and formate. Acetate, propionate and butyrate that are not metabolized in colonocytes are absorbed from the colon and transported via the portal circulation to the liver. These short-chain fatty acids are extensively metabolized in hepatocytes. Acetate, propionate and butyrate that are not metabolized in hepatocytes are transported by the circulation to various tissues where they undergo further metabolism. Butyrate is an important respiratory fuel for colonocytes.

INDICATIONS AND USAGE

Synbiotics are useful for the same indications as prebiotics and probiotics. Some may protect against intestinal pathogens and ameliorate the severity of some inflammatory bowel diseases. Some may be helpful in antibiotic associated diarrhea, as well as some infectious and viral diarrheas. They may have some immune-enhancing, anticarcinogenic, antiosteoporotic, glucose-modulating and lipid-modulating effects.

RESEARCH SUMMARY

See Probiotics and Prebiotics.

CONTRAINDICATIONS, PRECAUTIONS, ADVERSE REACTIONS

CONTRAINDICATIONS

Synbiotics are contraindicated in those who are hypersensitive to any component of a synbiotic-containing supplement.

PRECAUTIONS

Pregnant women and nursing mothers should only use synbiotic supplementation if prescribed by their physicians.

ADVERSE REACTIONS

The most common adverse reaction to synbiotics is flatulence.

INTERACTIONS

NUTRITIONAL SUPPLEMENTS

Minerals (calcium, magnesium): Concomitant intake of calcium or magnesium supplements and synbiotics may enhance the colonic absorption of these minerals.

FOODS

Synbiotics, via their prebiotic oligosaccharides, may enhance the colonic absorption of calcium and magnesium in foods.

DOSAGE AND ADMINISTRATION

Synbiotic supplements that are currently available include combinations of bifidobacteria and fructo-oligosaccharides (FOS), Lactobacillus GG and inulins and bifidobacteria and lactobacilli and FOS or inulins. New combinations are currently being developed.

Probiotic intake typically ranges from one to ten billion colony-forming units a few times a week. Doses of prebiotics, in the form of synbiotics, are variable.

LITERATURE

Collins MD, Gibson GR. Probiotics, prebiotics, and synbiotics: approaches for modulating the microbial ecology of the gut. *Am J Clin Nutr.* 1999; 69(suppl):1052S-1057S.

Macfarlane GT, Cummings JH. Probiotics and prebiotics: can regulating the activities of intestinal bacteria benefit health? *West J Med.* 1999; 17:187-191.

Roberfroid MB. Prebiotics and synbiotics: concepts and nutritional properties. *Br J Nutr.* 1998; 80:S197-S202.

For additional Literature, see Prebiotics and Probiotics.

Tangeretin

DESCRIPTION

Tangeretin is a member of the polymethoxylated flavone, or polymethoxyflavone, family of flavones. Flavones themselves comprise a subclass of the large class of plant substances, the flavonoids. Polymethoxylated flavones (PMFs) exist almost exclusively in the *Citrus* genus, particularly in the peels and tissues of sweet oranges (*Citrus sinensis*), the peels and tissues of bitter oranges (*Citrus aurantium* L.) and, especially, in the peels and tissues of tangerines (*Citrus reticulata* Blanco), including Dancy and Cleopatra tangerines and clementines. The two most common PMFs found in citrus peels and tissues are nobiletin (see Nobiletin) and tangeretin. Sinensetin is the third most common PMF found in the peels and tissues of citrus fruits. Only trace amounts of tangeretin, at best, are found in lemons (*Citrus limon*) and grapefruits (*Citrus paradisi*).

Tangeretin, like other flavonoids, is a plant secondary metabolite. Plant secondary metabolites comprise the defense system of plants against fungi, predators and pests, among other things. Tangeretin possesses activity against certain fungal diseases, such as mal seco, an often fatal disease of horses in Argentina. However, tangeretin is not nearly as potent in this regard as is nobiletin (see Nobiletin).

Tangeretin has been studied for its possible lipid-lowering activity, as well as for its possible anticancer activity.

Tangeretin is chemically described as 5,6,7,8-tetramethoxy-2-(4-methoxyphenyl)-4H-1-benzopyran-4-one. It is also known as 4′,5,6,7,8-pentamethoxyflavone, and ponkanetin (ponkan is the conventional name for *Citrus reticulata*). Its CAS number is 481-53-8. Its empirical formula is $C_{20}H_{20}O_7$ and its molecular weight is 372.37. The major chemical difference between tangeretin and nobiletin is the absence of a 3′-methoxy group on the flavone skeleton in tangeretin and the presence of a 3′- methoxy group on the flavone skeleton in nobiletin.

The following chemical structures are described within this monograph.

Tangeretin

Flavone Skeleton

Flavonoid Skeleton

ACTIONS AND PHARMACOLOGY

ACTIONS

Tangeretin has antifungal activity against some citrus pathogenic fungi. Tangeretin has possible anticancer and hypolipidemic activities.

MECHANISM OF ACTION

Anticancer activity: Tangeretin was found to induce cell-cycle G1 arrest in human colorectal carcinoma COLO 205 cells, inhibiting the growth of these cells. The polymethoxylated flavone was demonstrated to inhibit the activities of cyclin-dependent kinases 2 (Cdk2) and 4 (Cdk4). In addition, the Cdk inhibitors p21 and p27 were also shown to be elevated with the tangeretin treatment. Tangeretin possibly exerted its growth inhibitory effect either via modulation of the activities of several key G1 regulatory proteins (Cdk2, Cdk4) or via mediating the increase of Cdk inhibitors (p21, p27). More research is needed to understand this growth inhibitory effect of tangeretin.

Tangeretin was demonstrated to inhibit the growth of human mammary cells. In estradiol-primed human T47D mammary cancer cells, it was observed that tangeretin inhibited extracellular signal-regulated kinases 1/2 (ERK1/2) phosphorylation. It was thought that this kinase inhibitory action accounted, in part, for the inhibition of mammary cell growth.

Antifungal: The antifungal mechanism of action of tangeretin is not entirely clear.

Hypolipidemic: Apolipoprotein B (apoB) is the primary apolipoprotein of low-density lipoprotein (LDL), which is responsible for carrying cholesterol to tissues. The role of tangeretin on the regulation of apoB and lipid metabolism was studied in the human hepatoma cell line HepG2. It was found that tangeretin significantly lowered apoB secretion and decreased intracellular synthesis of cholesteryl esters, free cholesterol and triacylglycerol (TAG). The suppression of TAG synthesis went along with lowered activity of diacylglycerol (DAG) acyltransferase (DGAT) and microsomal triglyceride transfer protein (MTP). Tangeretin was also found to activate the peroxisome proliferator-activated receptor (PPAR). PPAR is a transcription factor that has a positive regulatory impact on fatty acid oxidation and TAG availability.

Citrus polymethoxylated flavones (PMFs), especially tangeretin, were found to significantly lower total cholesterol, very low-density lipoprotein (VLDL) and LDL-cholesterol in hamsters with diet-induced hypercholesterolemia. The PMFs reduced or tended to reduce serum triglyceride levels, as well. High-density lipoprotein cholesterol (HDL) was not affected. The mechanism of this lipid-lowering effect is unclear.

The hypolipidemic effect of tangeretin in human HepG2 cells along with its hypocholesterolemic effect in hamsters warrants further study as well as human trials to determine if tangeretin might have a role in the management of hyperlipidemia.

PHARMACOKINETICS

The pharmacokinetics (PK) of tangeretin is incomplete. Almost all of the PK studies of tangeretin have been performed in animals. Tangeretin is absorbed across the small intestine to some degree. Tangeretin has very low solubility in water, but its permeability is quite high, which ultimately contributes to fair bioavailability for this citrus flavone. Tangeretin, following absorption, most likely enters first into the lymphatics and is transported to the systemic circulation, which transports it to various tissues and organs, including the liver. It has been reported that tangeretin crosses the blood-brain barrier and, in a rat study, it was found in the hypothalamus, the striatum and the hippocampus. In contrast to polyphenolic flavonoids, tangeretin itself is not glucuronidated by UDP-glucuronosyltransferase to a glucuronide. Nor does it get sulfated by sulfotransferases to a sulfate. This is because the hydroxyl groups are methylated.

However, when the methoxy groups get demethylated, phenolic hydroxyl groups open up, which can be glucuronidated or sulfated. Metabolites of tangeretin that have been found in rat urine include monohydroxytetramethoxy flavone, dihydroxytrimethoxy flavone and glucuronide conjugates of the flavones.

INDICATIONS AND USAGE

Clinical evidence in support of the claim that the citrus flavonoid tangeretin is therapeutic in breast and some other cancers is lacking. There is very preliminary nonclinical data suggesting that tangeretin might have beneficial lipid-lowering effects, antidiabetic effects and neuroprotective effects.

RESEARCH SUMMARY

There was hope that tangeretin might be an effective anticancer treatment because, in numerous *in vitro* studies, it inhibited proliferation of cancer cells without inducing cell death (apoptosis), leaving open the possibility that it would thus spare normal cells, in contrast with so many other highly toxic cancer therapies. Most notably in these *in vitro* studies, tangeretin proved cytostatic in both human breast and colon cancer cells lines. Other *in vitro* research showed positive results in human lung carcinoma cells.

In a study using the hamster cheek pouch model, however, tangeretin and three other flavonoids (hesperetin, neohesperidin and nobiletin) all failed to inhibit chemically induced cancer. (Two flavonoids derived from grapefruit—naringin and naringenin—did, however, exert significant anticancer effects in this study.)

Several researchers have reported finding that tangeretin is not effective in inhibiting breast cancer *in vivo*, and that, in fact, it neutralizes the effects of the selective estrogen receptor modulator (SERM) tamoxifen, often used to reduce the risk of breast cancer. In a study of mice with mammary cancer, one group of mice was given water with tamoxifen, another group water with tangeretin added, another both tamoxifen and tangeretin and a fourth group water alone (control group). The group receiving only tamoxifen had significantly enhanced survival time. The tangeretin group did not; neither did the combination tangeretin/tamoxifen group, indicating that the flavonoid had neutralized the drug's beneficial effect. Another group of researchers has reported that tangeretin reduces the number of natural killer cells *in vivo* and that this may explain why its positive *in vitro* effects are abolished *in vivo*. One group cautions that those using tamoxifen should avoid tangeretin supplements or any tangeretin-fortified products. Fruit juices that do not include pulped peel are thought to be safe for those taking tamoxifen.

Given that there are other flavonoids that show more promise as potential cancer therapies, an indication for further research on tangeretin in this context is debatable.

One group has reported that formulations containing citrus PMFs, primarily tangeretin, show some promise as cholesterol- and triacylglycerol-lowering agents. These conclusions were based upon both *in vitro* and animal studies. One of the same researchers, in collaboration with others, has also reported that PMFs ameliorate fructose-induced hyperglyceridemia and other metabolic abnormalities associated with insulin resistance in hamsters. More research is needed and warranted to determine whether tangeretin and related substances can be of benefit in lipid and glucose metabolism and thus, possibly, in heart disease and diabetes.

Finally, there is one report in which tangeretin was found to exert a neuroprotective effect in a rat model of Parkinson's disease. After 28 days of oral administration of tangeretin, significant levels of tangeretin were found in the brains of these animals, producing the first evidence that it can cross the brain-blood barrier. Study data showing that the supplement has protective effects on dopaminergic neurons suggest that tangeretin should be investigated to confirm and further explain its possible beneficial activity in this context.

CONTRAINDICATIONS, PRECAUTIONS, ADVERSE REACTIONS

CONTRAINDICATIONS

Tangeretin is contraindicated in those who are hypersensitive to any component of a tangeretin-containing product.

PRECAUTIONS

Women who are under tamoxifen treatment should avoid excessive consumption of tangeretin-containing citrus products and supplements while under treatment.

Those who wish to try tangeretin for the support of any health condition should first discuss its use with his or her physician.

ADVERSE REACTIONS

None known.

INTERACTIONS

DRUGS

Midazolam: Midazolam is a member of the benzodiazepine family of drugs and has anxiolytic and sedative activities. Midazolam is metabolized by the cytochrome P450-3A4 (CYP3A4) enzyme. Naringin, a flavonoid found in grapefruit and grapefruit juice, is a potent inhibitor of CYP3A4 and can cause a number of interactions with drugs and dietary supplements, some that are not at all desirable. Naringin is an inhibitor of the metabolism of CYP3A4. On the other hand, tangeretin has been found to stimulate the catalytic activity of CYP3A4. Studies have found that besides slightly delaying the absorption of midazolam in fasting volunteers, ingestion of tangerine juice along with an oral dose of midazolam had no influence on the pharmacokinetics of midazolam, including its metabolism. It was concluded from these studies that neither tangeretin nor tangerine juice was likely to have much of an effect on CYP3A4-mediated drug metabolism in humans, very unlike the situation with the citrus flavonoid, naringin.

Tamoxifen: When tangeretin was added to the drinking water of a tumor-bearing mouse line (MCF 7/6), it was found to neutralize the tumor-suppressing effect of the drug tamoxifen. Tamoxifen is a selective estrogen receptor modulator (SERM) used to reduce the risk of breast cancer. Tangeretin has also been found to downregulate lymphokine activation of natural killer (NK) cells. NK cells are cytotoxic-type lymphocytes that play a major role in innate immunity.

NUTRITIONAL SUPPLEMENTS, FOODS, HERBS
None known.

OVERDOSAGE
There are no reports of overdosage.

DOSAGE AND ADMINISTRATION
The optimal dose of tangeretin for health benefits is not known.

Tangeretin is found in high concentrations in some tangerine juices (approximately 3.7 mg per liter) and in some tangerine peel oils (approximately 1.86 grams per liter). The highest concentrations of tangeretin are found in the tangerines *Citrus kinokuni* or kishu (27.9 mg per gram of dry weight) and *Citrus depressa* or shiikuwasha (26.7 mg per gram of dry weight). Shiikuwasha is a cross between a tangerine and a lime and found mainly in Okinawa, Japan. Clementines (*Citrus clementina*) contain about 2.6 mg per gram of dry weight. Only trace amounts of tangeretin, at best, are found in lemons (*Citrus limon*) and grapefruits (*Citrus paradisi*). Tangerines (mandarins) are the richest source of tangeretin.

At present, only one dietary supplement containing a mixture of polymethoxylated flavones (PMFs), including tangeretin, is being marketed in the U.S. In addition, the supplement contains tocotrienols and ascorbyl palmitate. The PMF/tocotrienol mixture contains a total of 150 mg per capsule and those using this supplement take about two capsules per day.

It is expected that other tangeretin dietary supplements will enter the dietary supplement marketplace.

LITERATURE

Backman JT, Mäenpää J, Belle DJ, et al. Lack of correlation between in vitro and in vivo studies on the effects of tangeretin and tangerine juice on midazolam hydroxylation. *Clin Pharmacol Ther*. 2000;67(4):382-390.

Bracke ME, Depypere HT, Boterberg T, et al. Influence of tangeretin on tamoxifen's therapeutic benefit in mammary cancer. *J Natl Cancer Inst*. 1999;91(4):354-359.

Bracke ME, Vyncke BM, Van Larebeke NA, et al. The flavonoid tangeretin inhibits invasion of MO4 mouse cells into embryonic chick heart in vitro. *Clin Exp Metastasis*. 1989;7(3):283-300.

Canivenc-Lavier MC, Brunold C, Siess MH, et al. Evidence for tangeretin O-demethylation by rat and human liver microsomes. *Xenobiotica*. March 1993;23(3):259-66. Erratum in: *Xenobiotica* 1993;23(6):717.

Chaumontet C, Bex V, Gaillard-Sanchez I, et al. Apigenin and tangeretin enhance gap junctional intercellular communication in rat liver epithelial cells. *Carcinogenesis*. 1994;15(10):2325-2330.

Chaumontet C, Droumaguet C, Bex V, et al. Flavonoids (apigenin, tangeretin) counteract tumor promoter-induced inhibition of intercellular communication of rat liver epithelial cells. *Cancer Lett*. 1997;114(1-2):207-210.

Chen KH, Weng MS, Lin JK. Tangeretin suppresses IL-1beta-induced cyclooxygenase (COX)-2 expression through inhibition of p38 MAPK, JNK, and AKT activation in human lung carcinoma cells. *Biochem Pharmacol*. 2007;73(2):215-227.

Depypere HT, Bracke ME, Boterberg T, et al. Inhibition of tamoxifen's therapeutic benefit by tangeretin in mammary cancer. *Eur J Cancer*. 2000;36 Suppl 4:S73.

Hirano T, Abe K, Gotoh M, et al. Citrus flavone tangeretin inhibits leukaemic HL-60 cell growth partially through induction of apoptosis with less cytotoxicity on normal lymphocytes. *Br J Cancer*. 1995;72(6):1380-1388.

Kurowska EM, Manthey JA. Hypolipidemic effects and absorption of citrus polymethoxylated flavones in hamsters with diet-induced hypercholesterolemia. *J Agric Food Chem*. 2004;52(10):2879-2886.

Kurowska EM, Manthey JA, Casaschi A, et al. Modulation of HepG2 cell net apolipoprotein B secretion by the citrus polymethoxyflavone, tangeretin. *Lipids*. 2004;39(2):143-151.

Martínez Conesa C, Vicente Ortega V, Yáñez Gascón MJ, et al. Treatment of metastatic melanoma B16F10 by the flavonoids tangeretin, rutin, and diosmin. *J Agric Food Chem*. 2005;53(17):6791-6797.

Morley KL, Ferguson PJ, Koropatnick J. Tangeretin and nobiletin induce G1 cell cycle arrest but not apoptosis in human breast and colon cancer cells. *Cancer Lett*. 2007;251(1):168-178.

Nielsen SE, Breinholt V, Cornett C, et al. Biotransformation of the citrus flavone tangeretin in rats. Identification of metabolites with intact flavane nucleus. *Food Chem Toxicol*. 2000;38(9):739-746.

Nogata Y, Sakamoto K, Shiratsuchi H, et al. Flavonoid composition of fruit tissues of citrus species. *Biosci Biotechnol Biochem*. 2006;70(1):178-192.

Pan MH, Chen WJ, Lin-Shiau SY, et al. Tangeretin induces cell-cycle G1 arrest through inhibiting cyclin-dependent kinases 2 and 4 activities as well as elevating Cdk inhibitors p21 and p27 in human colorectal carcinoma cells. *Carcinogenesis*. 2002;23(10):1677-1684.

Van Slambrouck S, Parmar VS, Sharma SK, et al. Tangeretin inhibits extracellular-signal-regulated kinase (ERK) phosphorylation. *FEBS Lett*. 2005;579(7):1665-1669.

Walle T. Methoxylated flavones, a superior cancer chemopreventive flavonoid subclass? *Semin Cancer Biol*. 2007;17(5):354-362.

Taurine

DESCRIPTION

Taurine is a nonprotein amino acid. It is an end product of L-cysteine metabolism and the principal free intracellular amino acid in many tissues of humans and other animal species. Taurine is present in high amounts in the brain, retina, myocardium, skeletal and smooth muscle, platelets and neutrophils. It is classified as a conditionally essential amino acid because it is necessary to be supplied in the diet of infants for normal retinal and brain development.

Research of taurine was greatly stimulated by the finding that it is an essential nutrient for cats. Taurine deficiency in cats can result in a variety of clinical abnormalities, including central retinal degeneration, dilated cardiomyopathy and platelet function abnormalities. Shortly after the discovery that dietary taurine deficiency leads to retinal degeneration in cats, it was observed that infants who were fed formulas lacking taurine had lower plasma levels of this amino acid than did infants fed human milk. Further, it was discovered that children receiving total parenteral nutrition not containing taurine had abnormal electroretinograms, as well as low plasma taurine levels. Taurine has been added to most human infant formulas since the mid-1980s.

Taurine is produced in the body from L-cysteine. The first reaction in the pathway is the formation of cysteine sulfinic acid. Cysteine sulfinic acid (CSA) is converted to hypotaurine via the enzyme CSA-decarboxylase, and taurine is formed from hypotaurine. Cats have low activity of CSA-decarboxylase. Dietary taurine mainly comes from animal food. Taurine is present in very low levels in plant foods. Taurine is found in seaweeds.

The most understood role of taurine in humans is its involvement in the formation of taurine bile acid conjugates in the liver, which are essential for micelle formation and fat absorption. Taurine is involved in the pre-and post-natal development of the central nervous system and visual system, although the details of its involvement in these processes are unclear. Taurine also has antioxidant and membrane-stabilizing activities. Much remains to be learned about the role of taurine in human physiology.

Taurine is different from most biological amino acids in a few particulars. It is a sulfonic acid rather than a carboxylic acid; it is a beta-amino acid rather than an alpha-amino acid and it does not have a chiral center. Taurine is also known as 2-aminoethane sulfonic acid. Its molecular formula is $C_2H_7NO_3S$, and its molecular weight is 215.15 daltons.

ACTIONS AND PHARMACOLOGY

ACTIONS

Taurine has antioxidant activity. It has putative hypocholesterolemic, hypotensive, antiatherogenic and detoxifying activities. It may also have steatorrhea-reducing activity in those with cystic fibrosis and has putative antidiabetic, inotropic and antiseizure activities.

The major antioxidant activity of taurine derives from its ability to scavenge the reactive oxygen species hypochlorite, which is generated in neutrophils during respiratory-burst activity of these cells. Taurine reacts with excess hypochlorite produced in the process of phagocytosis to form the relatively harmless N-chlorotaurine. N-chlorotaurine is then reduced to taurine and chloride. This activity may protect against collateral tissue damage that can occur from the respiratory burst of neutrophils. Taurine may also suppress peroxidation of membrane lipoproteins by other reactive oxygen species. It is thought that this effect is not due to taurine's scavenging of these reactive oxygen species, but rather to taurine's membrane-stabilizing activity, which confers greater resistance to the membrane lipoproteins against lipid peroxidation.

Taurine has been demonstrated to reduce cholesterol levels in animals, but results in humans have been contradictory. The hypocholesterolemic effect of taurine in animals is thought to be due, in large part, to the stimulation of bile acid synthesis and enhancement of cholesterol 7 alpha-hydroxylase activity. Taurine has been found to have antiatherogenic activity in animals, but there is less evidence that it does in humans. The antiatherogenic activity of taurine in animals is thought to be due, in large part, to its hypocholesterolemic activity.

Taurine has been found to normalize blood pressure in spontaneous hypertensive rats, and there is some evidence from human studies that it also has hypotensive activity in hypertensive, but not normotensive, individuals. It is speculated that the hypotensive effect of taurine may result from the normalization of increased sympathetic activity in hypertensive individuals.

Taurine has been found to ameliorate bleomycin-induced lung fibrosis in hamsters and also to ameliorate the side effects of some nitrogen mustards. It is thought that the possible antioxidant and membrane-stabilizing activities of taurine may account for these detoxifying actions.

Some studies have shown decreased steatorrhea in cystic fibrosis patients receiving taurine. It is though that the mechanism of this effect is taurine's stimulation of bile acid formation resulting in increased fat absorption in these individuals.

Again in animals, but not in humans, taurine has been found to have antidiabetic activity. The mechanism of this effect is unclear. It is thought that taurine may decrease insulin resistance.

Cats who are deficient in taurine develop dilated cardiomyopathy and congestive heart failure. Taurine has an inotropic effect when given to these animals. Some studies suggest that taurine has an inotropic effect in humans with congestive heart failure. The mechanism of this possible effect is unclear. It is thought that taurine may modulate the calcium current.

The mechanism of taurine's putative antiseizure activity is unknown.

PHARMACOKINETICS

Following ingestion, taurine is absorbed from the small intestine via the beta-amino acid or taurine transport system, a sodium- and chloride-dependent carrier system that serves gamma-aminobutyric acid and beta-alanine, as well as taurine. This carrier system is located in the apical membrane of intestinal mucosa cells. Taurine is transported to the liver via the portal circulation, where much of it forms conjugates with bile acids. Taurocholate, the bile salt conjugate of taurine and cholic acid, is the principal conjugate formed via the action of the enzyme choloyl-CoA N-acyltransferase. The taurine conjugates are excreted via the biliary route. Taurine that is not conjugated in the liver is distributed via the systemic circulation to various tissues in the body. Taurine is not usually completely reabsorbed from the kidneys, and some fraction of an ingested dose of taurine is excreted in the urine.

INDICATIONS AND USAGE

Taurine may be helpful in some with congestive heart failure and hypertension. It has demonstrated some antiatherogenic effects in both animal and human studies. There is the suggestion, mostly from animal data, that taurine might improve glucose tolerance and protect against some toxins. Some older studies suggest if might have some antiseizure activity. There is preliminary evidence that it might be helpful in some with cystic fibrosis.

RESEARCH SUMMARY

In a study of 24 subjects with congestive heart failure, administration of 2 grams of taurine, twice a day, resulted in clinical improvement in 19 patients. Roentgenographic data helped confirm the improvement. These positive results were subsequently confirmed in a double-blind, randomized, crossover, placebo-controlled study in which taurine was added to conventional treatment for a four-week period. Compared with placebo, taurine produced significant improvement as evaluated by a number of measures, including chest films. In still another study, supplemental taurine, but not coenzyme Q10, was said to have significant benefit in patients with congestive heart failure secondary to ischemic or idiopathic dilated cardiomyopathy. This was a double-blind study using 3 grams of taurine daily.

Taurine has demonstrated hypotensive effects in some animal studies. In humans, it has lowered blood pressure in borderline hypertensive patients using 6 grams of taurine daily for seven days. Lipid-lowering effects have been seen in animals, but human data are few and contradictory. There is some preliminary evidence from one small study that 0.4 to 1.6 grams of taurine daily for eight days inhibited platelet aggregation in a dose-dependent manner. Supplementation with 1.5 grams of taurine daily decreased platelet aggregation in subjects with type 1 diabetes. Insulin sensitivity was significantly improved by taurine supplementation in a rat model of spontaneous type 2 diabetes. Serum cholesterol and triacylglycerol were decreased in the supplemented animals. Taurine was also effective in another animal model of insulin resistance.

Taurine has exerted some detoxifying effects in animal experiments. It helped prevent bleomycin-induced lung injury and fibrosis in mice. It also appeared to have protective effects, as measured by changes in memory and lipid peroxidation levels in the brain, in rats exposed to ozone. Additionally, it has inhibited ethanol-induced elevation of plasma acetaldehyde in other animal studies. In one of these, it prevented the development of ethanol-induced hypertension in rats.

In some older studies, taurine demonstrated some preliminary ability to suppress some epileptic seizures. Follow-up is needed.

Finally, taurine was shown to be of benefit in a study of 22 Canadian children with cystic fibrosis and documented steatorrhea. They were given taurine (30 mg/kg/day) and placebo during separate six-month periods. Severity of fat malabsorption was significantly reduced in most of the subjects, especially in those with the most severe steatorrhea. A more recent study, however, failed to note these benefits, but significant differences in the two study groups may account for this discrepancy. A second study by the Canadian group showed positive effects of taurine on fat absorption in cystic fibrosis patients. Again, those with the greatest malabsorption at baseline seemed to benefit the most.

CONTRAINDICATIONS, PRECAUTIONS, ADVERSE REACTIONS

CONTRAINDICATIONS

Taurine is contraindicated in those hypersensitive to any component of a taurine-containing nutritional supplement.

PRECAUTIONS

Pregnant women and nursing mothers should avoid taurine supplements unless recommended by their physicians. Those with congestive heart failure should only use taurine under medical supervision.

ADVERSE REACTIONS

No reports of adverse reactions.

INTERACTIONS

DRUGS

In animal studies, taurine was found to ameliorate the pulmonary side effects (pulmonary fibrosis) of bleomycin.

DOSAGE AND ADMINISTRATION

Doses are variable and range from 500 mg to 3 grams daily.

LITERATURE

Azuma J, Sawamura A, Awata N, et al. Therapeutic effect of taurine in congestive heart failure: a double-blind, crossover trial. *Clin Cardiol.* 1985; 8:267-282.

Azuma J, Sawamura Z, Awata N. Usefulness of taurine in congestive heart failure and its prospective application. *Jpn Circ J.* 1992; 56:95-99.

Barbeau A, Donaldson J. Taurine in epilepsy. *Lancet.* 1973; 2(7825):387.

Chesney RW. Taurine: its biological role and clinical implications. Advances in Pediatrics. 1985:22:1-42.

Chesney RW. Taurine: is it required for infant nutrition? *J Nutr.* 1988; 118:6-10.

Darling PB, Lepage G, Leroy C, et al. Effect of taurine supplements on fat absorption in cystic fibrosis. *Pediatr Res.* 1985; 19:578-582.

Geggel HS, Ament ME, Heckenlively JR, et al. Nutritional requirement for taurine in patients receiving long-term parenteral supplementation. *N Engl J Med.* 1985; 312:142-146.

Gurujeyalakshmi G, Wang Y, Giri SN. Taurine and niacin block lung injury and fibrosis by down-regulating bleomycin-induced activation of transcription nuclear factor-kappa B in mice. *J Pharmacol Exp Ther.* 2000; 293:82-90.

Hayes KC, Carey RE. Retinal degeneration associated with taurine deficiency in the cat. *Science.* 1975; 188:949-951.

Hayes KC, Sturman JA. Taurine in metabolism. *Ann Rev Nutr.* 1981; 1:401-425.

McCarty MF. The reported clinical utility of taurine in ischemic disorders may reflect a down-regulation of neutrophil activation and adhesion. *Med Hypothesis.* 1999; 53:290-299.

Murakami S, Kondo Y, Tomisawa K, Nagate T. Prevention of atherosclerotic lesion development in mice by taurine. *Drugs Exp Clin Res.* 1999; 25:227-234.

Nakamura T, Ogasawara M, Koyama I, et al. The protective effect of taurine on the biomembrane against damage produced by oxygen radicals. *Biol Pharm Bull.* 1993; 16:970-972.

Niitynen L, Nurminen M-L, Korpela R, et al. Role of arginine, taurine and homocysteine in cardiovascular diseases. *Ann Med.* 1999; 31:318-326.

Pierson HF, Fisher JM, Rabinovitz M. Modulation by taurine of the toxicity of taumustine, a compound with antitumor activity. *J Natl Canc Inst.* 1985; 75:905-909.

Pion PD, Kittleson MD, Rogers QR, Morris JG. Myocardial failure in cats associated with low plasma taurine: a reversible cardiomyopathy. *Science.* 1987; 237: 764-767.

Rivas-Arancibia S, Dorado-Martínez C, Borgonio-Pérez G, et al. Effects of taurine on ozone-induced memory deficits and lipid peroxidation in brains of young, mature, and old rats. *Environ Res.* 2000; 82:7-17.

Stipanuk MH. Homocysteine, Cysteine, and Taurine. In: Shils ME, Olson JA, Shike M, Ross AC, eds. *Modern Nutrition in Health and Disease*, 9th ed. Baltimore, MD: Williams and Wilkins; 1999:543-558.

Wang Q, Giri SN, Hyde DM, Nakashima JM. Effects of taurine on bleomycin-induced lung fibrosis in hamsters. *Proc Soc Exp Biol Med.* 1989; 190:330-338.

Thiamin (Vitamin B₁)

DESCRIPTION

In 1911, the chemist Casimir Funk isolated a substance from rice bran extracts which he thought was the anti-beriberi factor. Because the substance was an amine and because he thought the substance had a vital dietary function, he named it vitamine. As it turned out, Funk's vitamine was not the anti-beriberi factor which was subsequently isolated and called thiamin or vitamin B₁. Nevertheless, Funk did coin the term vitamin and the concept that vitamins are essential dietary factors.

Thiamin is a water-soluble vitamin. Structurally it consists of a substituted pyrimidine ring joined by a methylene bridge to a substituted thiazole ring. The free vitamin is a base. The thiazolium salts of thiamin, thiamin hydrochloride and thiamin mononitrate, are the forms of thiamin which are typically used in nutritional supplements and for food fortification. In addition to being known as vitamin B₁, thiamin is known as thiamine, aneurin and 3-[(4-amino-2-methyl-5-pyrimidinyl)   methyl]-5-(2-hydroxyethyl)-4-methyl-thiazonium. The structural formula of thiamin follows:

Thiamin

The classic deficiency state of thiamin is beriberi. An analogous disorder in fowl is called polyneuritis. The term beriberi is derived from the Sinhalese word meaning extreme weakness. Beriberi was very common during the early part of the last century in those whose diets consisted principally of highly polished rice. Interestingly, those who ate parboiled rice—partially boiled rice—did not develop beriberi. Milling removes the husk, which contains most of the thiamin, while parboiling the rice before husking disperses thiamin throughout the grain. Beriberi still occurs in those whose diet mainly consists of polished rice. Thiamin deficiency is also associated with alcoholism and occurs in some cases of malnutrition, those receiving total parenteral nutrition without thiamin, malabsorption syndromes, increased carbohydrate intake, major catabolic and physiologic stress states, acute infection, folate deficiency, thyrotoxicosis and those on long-term loop diuretics (furosemide, ethacrynic acid, bumetanide). Subclinical thiamin deficiency may not be uncommon.

There are three types of beriberi: dry beriberi, wet beriberi and cerebral beriberi or Wernicke-Korsakoff syndrome. Dry or neurologic beriberi occurs when thiamin deficiency affects the peripheral nervous system resulting in peripheral neuropathy. The peripheral neuropathy is characterized by a bilateral, symmetric impairment of sensory, motor and reflex functions involving predominantly the lower extremities. Symptoms and signs of dry beriberi, include paresthesias of the toes, burning of the feet, calf muscle tenderness and cramps, difficulty in rising from a squatting position, a decrease in the vibratory sensation in the toes, loss of ankle and knee jerks and footdrop and toedrop. Wet or cardiovascular beriberi involves the heart and circulatory system. Cardiovascular manifestations of thiamin deficiency are characterized by peripheral vasodilatation with increased cardiac output, sodium and water retention and myocardial failure. The most extreme form of wet beriberi is shoshin beriberi. Shoshin is Japanese for damage to the heart and is characterized by global heart failure with lactic acidosis in the context of blood tests showing thiamin deficiency. Shoshin beriberi, if not promptly treated, is rapidly fatal. Alcoholics who present with unexplained lactic acidosis, a hyperdynamic state and high output failure, or cardiogenic shock without evidence of a myocardial infarction, are unlikely to have anything but Shoshin beriberi.

Alcoholism is the major cause of thiamin deficiency in Wernicke-Korsakoff syndrome or cerebral beriberi. Wernicke-Korsakoff syndrome is characterized by abnormal ocular motor signs, ataxia and derangement of mental functions. The ocular motor signs include paresis of abduction which is accompanied by horizontal diplopia, strabismus and nystagmus. Derangement of mental functions include a global-confusional apathetic state and amnesia. Wernicke-Korsakoff syndrome represents the full-blown clinical state of cerebral beriberi. Wernicke's disease itself is characterized by abnormal ocular motor signs and ataxia without an evident amnesic state. Korsakoff's psychosis itself is characterized by the mental derangements mentioned above.

Thiamin occurs in cells principally in its active coenzyme form called thiamin pyrophosphate (TPP, cocarboxylase). Thiamin, in the form of thiamin pyrophosphate, plays an essential role as a cofactor in key reactions in carbohydrate metabolism. It is also involved in the metabolism of branched-chain amino acids and may have non-coenzyme (non-cofactor) roles in excitable cells. TPP is a coenzyme in the oxidative decarboxylation of pyruvate to acetyl-coenzyme A (acetyl-CoA), of alpha-ketoglutarate to succinyl-CoA, and of the oxidative decarboxylation of the branched-chain alpha-keto acids, which are metabolites of the branched-chain amino acids L-leucine, L-isoleucine and L-valine. TPP is also a cofactor in the reversible transketolase reactions in the phosphogluconate pathway, also know as the pentose phosphate pathway and the hexose monophosphate shunt. The two transketolase reactions are the reversible conversions of D-xylulose 5-phosphate and D-ribose 5-phosphate to D-sedoheptulose 7-phosphate and D-glyceraldehyde 3-phosphate, and D-xylulose-5-phosphate and D-erythrose-4-phosphate to D-fructose 6-phosphate and D-glyceraldehyde 3-phosphate. The first of these two reactions represents the pathway for the non-oxidative production of ribose.

The total metabolic pool of thiamin in the body is approximately 30 milligrams. The predominant form of thiamin in the body is thiamin pyrophosphate (TPP, also known as thiamin diphosphate or TDP and cocarboxylase). Approximately 80% of thiamin in blood is present in erythrocytes as TPP. About 50% of total body thiamin is present in skeletal muscles. Thiamin is also found in heart, liver kidneys and brain. Other forms of thiamin present in the body include, thiamin triphosphate (TTP, about 10%), thiamin monophosphate (TMP) and free thiamin. TMP and free thiamin comprise about 10% of total body thiamin. The most reliable method of evaluating thiamin status is the measurement of erythrocyte transketolase activity and the percentage enhancement of the transketolase activity resulting from added thiamin pyrophosphate.

All plant and animal foods contain thiamin. Good dietary sources of the vitamin, include whole-grain products, brown rice, meat products, vegetables, fruits, legumes and seafood.

ACTIONS AND PHARMACOLOGY

ACTIONS

Thiamin may have antioxidant, erythropoietic, cognition-and mood-modulatory, antiatherosclerotic and detoxification activities. It has putative ergogenic activity.

MECHANISM OF ACTION

Thiamin has been found to protect against lead-induced lipid peroxidation in rat liver and kidney. Thiamin deficiency results in selective neuronal death in animal models. The neuronal death is associated with increased free radical production, suggesting that oxidative stress may play an important early role in brain damage associated with thiamin deficiency. The mechanism of the possible antioxidant activity of thiamin is unknown.

Even though anemia is not one of the consequences of thiamin deficiency, there is a type of anemia, called thiamin-responsive megaloblastic anemia, that responds well to large doses of thiamin. It is thought that those with thiamin-responsive megaloblastic anemia may actually be thiamin-deficient secondary to reduced thiamin transport and absorption, and to impaired intracellular thiamin pyrophosphorylation.

Thiamin deficiency is associated with cognitive and emotional changes. For example, Korsakoff's psychosis is characterized by the inability to form new memories, the poorly organized retrieval of remote memories, apathy and emotional blandness. The treatment of Korsakoff's patients with thiamin often results in significant improvement in these symptoms. Marginal thiamin deficiency may also result in cognitive and emotional changes. There are a few studies suggesting that high-dose thiamin supplementation may have a positive effect on mood and cognition in those with marginal deficiency, and even adequate status, of the vitamin. In one study with female subjects, improved thiamin status was associated with improved mood, and a decline in thiamin status associated with poorer mood. In another study, again with female subjects, those taking 50 milligrams of thiamin daily for 20 months were found to have improvement in thiamin status associated with reports of being more clearheaded, composed and energetic. Reaction times were also faster. The study was placebo-controlled and performed in subjects whose thiamin status was adequate. The mechanism of the neurophysiological actions of thiamin are not well understood. Thiamin may play a role in neurophysiology independent of its coenzyme function. Thiamin is located in nerve cell membranes and phosphorylated forms of thiamin are associated with sodium channel proteins. It is thought that phosphorylated forms of thiamin may play roles in the control of sodium conductance at axonal membranes and in other neurological processes.

Migration and proliferation of arterial smooth muscle cells are thought to play an important role in the development of atherosclerosis. Glucose and insulin have been found to have an additive effect on the proliferation of infragenicular arterial smooth muscle cells *in vitro*. Thiamin has been found to inhibit human infragenicular arterial muscle cell proliferation induced by high glucose and insulin, in cell culture. Thiamin plays a key role in intracellular glucose metabolism and it is thought that thiamin inhibits the effect of glucose and insulin on arterial smooth muscle cell proliferation. However, the mechanism of this *in vitro* effect is not well understood. Inhibition of endothelial cell proliferation may also promote atherosclerosis. Endothelial cells in culture have been found to have a decreased proliferative rate and delayed migration in response to hyperglycemic conditions. Thiamin has been shown to inhibit this effect of glucose on endothelial cells. It is thought that the mechanism of action of thiamin on endothelial cells is related to a reduction in intracellular protein glycation by redirecting the glycolytic flux. Atherosclerosis and peripheral artery disease are significant problems in those with type 2 diabetes mellitus. Further study of the possible anti-atherosclerotic activity of thiamin, particularly in those with type 2 diabetes, is warranted.

Some animal studies have found that high doses of thiamin block some of the toxic symptoms from orally administered lead. Thiamin may protect against lead toxicity by inhibiting lead-induced lipid peroxidation.

There are few studies investigating the effect of large doses of thiamin as an aid to exercise performance. In one such study, carbohydrate-loaded mice administered very high doses of thiamin demonstrated an improvement in swim time to exhaustion. In another study, experienced cyclists administered 900 milligram daily of thiamin for three days were found to have lower exercise heart rates, blood glucose and blood lactate concentrations. In still another study, thiamin supplementation at 100 milligram/day was found to decrease exercise-induced fatigue in male athletes. A recent study, however, using a thiamin derivative, thiamin tetrahydrofurfuryl disulfide, which is better absorbed than thiamin, showed no effect on high-intensity exercise performance. There is insufficient evidence to suggest that thiamin may have exercise performance-enhancing activity. The possible mechanism of this putative effect is unknown.

PHARMACOKINETICS

Thiamin is absorbed from the lumen of the small intestine—mainly the jejunum—by active transport and passive diffusion mechanisms. At lower amounts, absorption from the small intestine is by an active, carrier-mediated process that is energy-dependent as well as sodium-dependent. Passive diffusion occurs with higher amounts of thiamin. Absorption of thiamin appears to be limited by a saturable rate-limiting transport mechanism. Only a small percentage of a high dose of thiamin is absorbed. Certain lipid-soluble thiamin derivatives known as allithiamins, do not appear to be subject to the rate-limiting transport mechanism. Thiamin is transported by the portal circulation to the liver and by the systemic circulation to various tissues in the body. Thiamin is metabolized to thiamin monophosphate (TP, TMP), thiamin pyrophosphate (TPP, cocarboxylase, thiamin diphosphate, TDP) and thiamin triphosphate (TTP). Thiamin is phosphorylated directly to thiamin pyrophosphate by thiamin diphosphokinase and thiamin pyrophosphate is dephosphorylated to thiamin monophosphate via thiamin diphosphatase. Approximately 80% of thiamin in blood is present in erythrocytes as TPP. The transport of thiamin into erythrocytes appears to occur by facilitated diffusion; it enters other cells by an active process. Total thiamin content in the adult body is about 30 milligrams. Thiamin and its metabolites are mainly excreted by the kidneys.

INDICATIONS AND USAGE

Frank and marginal thiamin deficiency may not be uncommon and may be a particular problem among alcoholics, the elderly and the chronically ill. Thiamin supplementation may be useful in these subgroups, among others. There is evidence that supplemental thiamin can help protect against some of the metabolic imbalances caused by heavy alcohol consumption. It may help protect against Wernicke's encephalopathy and some other forms of brain damage seen in some alcoholics, some with HIV-disease, some with anorexia nervosa and others. It may be helpful in alcohol withdrawal. It is needed in those who receive total parenteral nutrition, particularly to prevent lactic acidosis due to thiamin deficiency. It may increase glucose tolerance and may help prevent atherosclerosis, particularly in diabetics. It has been used in congestive heart failure with benefit under certain circumstances and may be helpful in some other forms of heart disease. There is preliminary evidence that it can improve mood and cognition in some. Data are in short supply and results mixed with respect to claims that thiamin can enhance exercise performance and increase energy. Thiamin's use in cancer might be ill-advised, as there is evidence that it may promote tumor-cell proliferation.

RESEARCH SUMMARY

Alcoholics are at particularly high risk of thiamin deficiency. Alcohol interferes with the absorption of thiamin and its storage in tissue. It also inhibits conversion of thiamin to its active form. In addition, alcoholics generally have unbalanced diets low in thiamin. Some alcoholics suffer from frank beriberi, which, among other things, can lead to congestive heart failure. More frequently, alcoholics suffer from such beriberi symptoms as mental confusion, visual disturbances and staggering gait. Beriberi can be prevented and, in some cases, successfully treated with high doses of thiamin (up to 100 milligrams daily).

Thiamin can also help prevent some cases of Wernicke's encephalopathy, a potentially fatal disorder that occurs in some who consume very large amounts of alcohol. Symptoms include double vision, mental confusion, muscle weakness and disturbed gait. Untreated, this disorder can result in permanent brain damage and memory impairment. In extreme cases it leads to coma and death. It is often reversible with prompt thiamin treatment. Some use thiamin as part of alcohol-withdrawal therapy.

Others at higher than average risk of Wernicke's encephalopathy include those suffering from anorexia nervosa, typically young women. Older people are also at higher risk. So are people with HIV disease. Thiamin deficiency was found in 23% of HIV patients in one study, and brain lesions characteristic of those found in sufferers of Wernicke's encephalopathy have been seen in some with HIV-disease. Some researchers have recommended dietary thiamin supplementation in all newly diagnosed cases of HIV-disease.

It is now recognized that thiamin deficiency may occur with total parenteral nutrition (TPN). Several cases of lactic acidosis have been reported in TPN patients not receiving thiamin. Administration of thiamin has resolved the acidosis with attendant clinical improvement. Researchers stress that thiamin deficiency should always be included in the differential diagnosis of lactic acidosis. A recent shortage of multivitamin preparations for TPN is said to have resulted in a number of cases of lactic acidosis due to thiamin deficiency. A previous shortage led to several TPN-related deaths.

Thiamin deficiency is associated with abnormal glucose tolerance, and there is some evidence that supplemental thiamin may, in some cases, help correct the abnormality. In a recent *in vitro* study, thiamin inhibited accelerated proliferation of arterial smooth muscle cells. This proliferation contributes to atherosclerosis and preferentially affects the infragenicular vasculature in patients with diabetes mellitus. High insulin and glucose levels demonstrate additive effects in this process *in vitro*. This research gives some preliminary indication that thiamin may help prevent or delay atherosclerotic complications in some diabetics.

Thiamin supplementation has improved left ventricular function in patients with congestive heart failure being administered long-term furosemide therapy and, as noted above, supplemental thiamin can help prevent and treat heart disease related to beriberi. In addition, intravenous injection of thiamin proved helpful in an animal model of myocardial infarction, increasing strength of contractions and decreasing oxygen demand. Russian researchers have reported similar results in humans. Thiamin pyrophosphate (cocarboxylase) was used in these heart attack experiments. Research is needed to see whether thiamin itself might be beneficial.

Thiamin was found to have positive effects on mood and cognitive functioning in a recent study of 120 young females. In a previous study, females receiving a multivitamin supplement for three months were said to have improved mood compared with controls who received placebo. Using biochemical indices, an association was made between thiamin status and improved mood. These same measures did not support an association between any of eight other vitamins and elevated mood.

In this recent study, focus was on thiamin alone among the vitamins. All but one of the 120 women had normal thiamin levels at baseline. They were randomized to receive 50 milligrams of thiamin daily or placebo. After two months, the thiamin group significantly improved (more than doubled) their scores on the clear-headedness and mood subsets of the bipolar profile of mood states psychological test. There was no change in these measures in the placebo group. The thiamin group also showed nonsignificant improvement in feelings of confidence, composure and elation. The researchers considered their findings remarkable given that they were obtained in a group which, as measured by transketolase activation, had normal thiamin nutrition. More research is warranted.

Thiamin and a thiamin derivative have not shown any effect on exercise performance in two studies. High-dose thiamin (100 milligrams daily) was found to be helpful in preventing or accelerating recovery from exercise-induced fatigue in a third study. This trial tested thiamin in 16 male volunteer athletes using bicycle ergometer exercises. Followup is needed.

Finally, a group of researchers have recently called thiamin supplementation "a double-edged sword" in cancer patients. Like other seriously ill patients, cancer sufferers may benefit from improved thiamin status in terms of general nutrition, but, as these researchers observed, there is some evidence that thiamin may also, in effect, nourish some cancers. There is some indication that high-dose thiamin supplementation may promote tumor cell proliferation. More research is needed to help clarify this issue.

CONTRAINDICATIONS, PRECAUTIONS, ADVERSE REACTIONS

CONTRAINDICATIONS

Thiamine is contraindicated in those hypersensitive to any component of a thiamin-containing product.

PRECAUTIONS

The use of thiamin for the treatment of a thiamin-deficiency state, lactic acidosis secondary to thiamin-deficiency, Wernicke-Korsakoff syndrome, Wernicke's encephalopathy, Korsakoff's psychosis or any medical condition must only be undertaken under medical supervision.

A typical dose of thiamin used in pre- and postnatal multivitamin/multimineral supplements is three milligrams daily. Pregnant women and nursing mothers should avoid intakes of thiamin greater than this amount unless higher doses are prescribed by their physicians.

Those who are treated with parenteral thiamin for thiamin deficiency, should be given the thiamin prior to receiving parenteral glucose. Administration of intravenous glucose prior to receiving thiamin could result in severe lactic acidosis.

ADVERSE REACTIONS

Oral thiamin is well tolerated even at doses up to 200 milligrams daily or higher. There have been occasional reports of serious and even fatal responses to parenteral thiamin. These have probably been anaphylactic reactions. There are also reports of less serious allergic reactions to parenteral thiamin.

There is some animal evidence that high doses of parenteral thiamin may promote tumor growth.

INTERACTIONS

DRUGS

Loop diuretics (furosemide, ethacrynic acid, bumetanide): Chronic use of loop diuretics may result in thiamin deficiency. Chronic use of furosemide for the treatment of congestive heart failure has been reported to result in thiamin deficiency. Thiamin repletion in such patients can improve left ventricular function.

FOODS

Substances in food that inactivate thiamin are called antithiamin factors.

Sulfites: Concomitant intake of thiamin and foods and beverages containing sulfites may inactivate thiamin.

Tea, coffee and decaffeinated coffee: Concomitant intake of these beverages and thiamin may inactivate thiamin. Tannic acid is most likely the substance in tea that inactivates thiamin by forming a tannin-thiamin adduct.

OVERDOSAGE

Overdosage of thiamin has not been reported in the literature.

DOSAGE AND ADMINISTRATION

Thiamin is available in nutritional supplements in the form of thiamin hydrochloride and thiamin nitrate. These are also the forms used for food fortification. Thiamin pyrophosphate or cocarboxylase may also be available in some products. Supplemental doses of thiamin are variable and range from the U.S. RDA amount of 1.5 milligrams/day to 10 milligrams/day or higher. There is a rapid decline in absorption that occurs at oral doses above five milligrams. Thiamin is typically found in the form of multivitamin, multivitamin/multimineral or B-complex preparations. Single ingredient thiamin supplements are also available. Pre- and postnatal supplements typically deliver a thiamin dose of 3 milligrams daily.

Lipid-soluble thiamin derivatives called allithiamins are also available. These forms are better absorbed at higher intakes than is thiamin.

The Food and Nutrition Board of the Institute of Medicine of the National Academy of Sciences recommends the following dietary reference intakes (DRIs) for thiamin:

Infants	Adequate Intakes (AI)	
0-6 months	0.2 mg/day	0.03 mg/kg
7-12 months	0.3 mg/day	0.03 mg/kg

	Recommended Dietary Allowances (RDA)
Children	
1-3 years	0.5 mg/day
4-8 years	0.6 mg/day
Boys	
9-13 years	0.9 mg/day
14-18 years	1.2 mg/day
Girls	
9-13 years	0.9 mg/day
14-18 years	1.0 mg/day
Men	
19 years and older	1.2 mg/day
Women	
19 years and older	1.1 mg/day
Pregnancy	
14-50 years	1.4 mg/day
Lactation	
14-50 years	1.4 mg/day

The DV (Daily Value) for thiamin (vitamin B_1), which is used for determining percentage of nutrient daily values on nutritional supplement and food labels, is 1.5 mg. This is based on the U.S. RDA for thiamin.

LITERATURE

Avena R, Arora S, Carmody BJ, et al. Thiamin (vitamin B_1) protects against glucose- and insulin-mediated proliferation of human infragenicular arterial smooth muscle cells. *Ann Vasc Surg.* 2000; 14:37-43.

Bakker SJL, Hoogeveen EK, Nijpels G, et al. The association of dietary fibres with glucose tolerance is partly explained by concomitant intake of thiamin: The Hoorn Study. *Diabetologia.* 1998; 41:1168-1175.

Benton D, Griffiths R, Haller J. Thiamin supplementation mood and cognitive functioning. *Psychopharmacol.* 1997; 129:66-71.

Bettendorff L. A non-cofactor role of thiamin derivatives in excitable cells? *Arch Physiol Biochem.* 1996; 104:745-751.

Blanc P, Boussuges A. [Cardiac beriberi]. [Article in French]. *Arch Mal Coeur Vaiss.* 2000; 93:371-379.

Boros LG. Population thiamine status and varying cancer rates between western, Asian and African countries. *Anticancer Res.* 2000; 20(3B):2245-2248.

Boros LG, Brandes JL, Lee WN, et al. Thiamine supplementation to cancer patients: a double edge sword. *Anticancer Res.* 1998; 18(1B):595-602.

Boros LG, Comin B, Boren J, et al. Over-expression of transketolase: a mechanism by which thiamine supplementation promotes cancer growth. *Am Assoc Cancer Res.* 2000; 41:66(Ab #4234).

Butterworth RF, Gaudreau C, Vincelette J, et al. Thiamin deficiency and Wernicke's encephalopathy in AIDS. *Metab Brain Dis.* 1991; 6:207-212.

Dietary Reference intakes for Thiamin, Riboflavin, Niacin, Vitamin B_6, Folate, Vitamin B_{12}, Pantothenic Acid, Biotin, and Choline. Washington, DC: National Academy Press; 1998.

Frank T, Bitsch R, Maiwald J, Stein G. High thiamine diphosphate concentrations in erythrocytes can be achieved in dialysis patients by oral administration of benfotiamine. *Eur J Clin Pharmacol.* 2000; 56:251-257.

Härdig L, Daae C, Dellborg M, et al. Reduced thiamine phosphate, but not thiamine diphosphate, in erythrocytes in elderly patients with congestive heart failure treated with furosemide. *J Int Med.* 2000; 247:597-600.

La Selva M, Beltramo E, Pagnozzi F, et al. Thiamine corrects delayed replication and decreases production of lactate and advanced glycation end-products in bovine retinal and human umbilical vein endothelial cells cultured under high glucose conditions. *Diabetologia.* 1996; 39:1263-1268.

Muri RM, Von Overbeck J, Furrer J, Ballmer PE. Thiamin deficiency in HIV-positive patients: evaluations by erythrocyte transketolase activity and thiamin pyrophosphate effect. *Clin Nutr.* 1999; 18:375-378.

Pekovich SR, Martin PR, Singleton CK. Thiamine deficiency decreases steady-state transketolase and pyruvate dehydrogenase but not alpha-ketoglutarate dehydrogenase mRNA levels in three human cell types. *J Nutr.* 1998; 128:683-687.

Romanski SA, McMahon MM. Metabolic acidosis and thiamine deficiency. *Mayo Clin Proc.* 1999; 74:259-263.

Sato Y, Nakagawa M, Higuchi I, et al. Mitochondrial myopathy and familial thiamine deficiency. *Muscle Nerve.* 2000; 23:1069-1075.

Senapati SK, Dey S, Dwivedi SK, et al. Effect of thiamine hydrochloride on lead induced lipid peroxidation in rat liver and kidney. *Vet Hum Toxicol.* 2000; 42:236-237.

Shimon I, Almog S, Vered Z, et al. Improved left ventricular function after thiamine supplementation in patients with congestive heart failure receiving long-term furosemide therapy. *Am J Med.* 1995; 98:485-490.

Suter PM, Haller J, Hany A. Diuretic use: a risk for subclinical thiamine deficiency in elderly patients. *J Nutr Health Aging.* 2000; 4:69-71.

Suzuki M, Itokawa Y. Effects of thiamine supplementation on exercise-induced fatigue. *Metab Brain Dis.* 1996; 11:95-106.

Tanphaichitr V. Thiamin. In: Shils ME, Olson JA, Shike M, Ross AC, eds. *Modern Nutrition in Health and Disease.* 9th ed. Baltimore, MD: Williams and Wilkins; 1999:381-389.

Todd K, Butterworth RF. Mechanisms of selective neuronal cell death due to thiamine deficiency. *Ann NY Acad Sci.* 1999; 893:404-411.

Webster MJ. Physiological and performance responses to supplementation with thiamin and pantothenic acid derivatives. *Eur J Appl Physiol Occup Physiol.* 1998; 77:486-491.

Webster MJ, Scheett TP, Doyle MR, Branz M. The effect of a thiamin derivative on exercise performance. *Eur J Appl Physiol.* 1997; 75:520-524.

Tin

DESCRIPTION

Tin is a metallic element with atomic number 50 and symbol Sn. It is a heavy metal. Tin is not considered an essential nutrient for humans. A tin-deficiency state has been reported in rats.

Rats fed a diet low in tin showed poor growth, alopecia and lowered response to sound compared with rats fed a tin-rich diet. Abnormalities in mineral status were also noted in the tin-deficient rat group. At least for rats tin, may serve as an essential nutrient.

The typical daily dietary intake of tin ranges from about 1 to 40 milligrams. Tin intake is essentially dependent on food stored in tin cans. Higher intakes of tin are obtained from foods preserved in unlacquered tin cans than from foods preserved in lacquered tin cans.

Regarding potential drug applications of tin, an organotin compound, tin protoporphyrin or Sn-P, a potent inhibitor of heme oxygenase and bilirubin formation, is being studied as a treatment for controlling severe hyperbilirubinemia in full-term breast-fed newborns with high bilirubin levels after birth. It is also being studied as a treatment for neuropathic and incisional pain.

ACTIONS AND PHARMACOLOGY

ACTIONS

The actions and pharmacology of dietary tin are not known.

INDICATIONS AND USAGE

There is no evidence that supplemental tin has immune-enhancing activity in humans; nor is there any evidence that it has anticarcinogenic activity in humans.

RESEARCH SUMMARY

It has been hypothesized that the thymus gland secretes tin-containing substances that possess immune-enhancing properties. There are some animal studies suggesting that tin may have immune-modulating activity and may also have anti-proliferative activity. There is no evidence that tin has these activities in humans. Such studies are needed, especially if the animal studies have any validity.

CONTRAINDICATIONS, PRECAUTIONS, ADVERSE REACTIONS

CONTRAINDICATIONS

Tin supplementation is not recommended for anyone.

PRECAUTIONS

Given our present state of knowledge regarding tin, supplemental tin is not recommended for anyone.

DOSAGE AND ADMINISTRATION

No recommended dosage. Tin may be found in colloidal or liquid mineral preparations. It is also found in some multivitamin preparations, typically at a dose of about 10 micrograms.

LITERATURE
Arakawa Y. [Biological activity of tin and immunity.] [Article in Japanese.] *Sangyo Eiseigaku Zasshi.* 1997; 39:1-20

Biego GH, Joyeux M, Hartemann P, Debry G. Determination of tin intake in an adult French citizen. *Arch Environ Contam Toxicol.* 1999; 36:227-232.

Cardarelli N. Tin and the thymus gland: a review. *Thymus.* 1990; 15:223-231.

Martinez JC, Garcia HO, Otheguy LE, et al. Control of severe hyperbilirubinemia in full-term newborns with the inhibitor of bilirubin production Sn-mesoporphyrin. *Pediatrics.* 1999; 103:1-5.

Nielsen FH. Ultratrace minerals. In: Shils ME, Olson JA, Shike M, Ross AC, eds. *Modern Nutrition in Health and Disease.* 9th ed. Baltimore, MD: Williams and Wilkins; 1999; 283-303.

Pekelharing HL, Lemmens AG, Beynan AC. Iron, copper and zinc status in rats fed on diets containing various concentrations of tin. *Br J Nutr.* 1994; 71:103-109.

Yokoi K, Kimura M, Itokawa Y. Effect of dietary tin deficiency on growth and mineral status in rats. *Biol Trace Elem Res.* 1990; 223-231.

Tiratricol (TRIAC)

FDA warns against consuming dietary supplements containing Tiratricol.

DESCRIPTION

Tiratricol is an orphan drug for use in combination with levothyroxine to suppress thyroid stimulating hormone (TSH) in patients with well-differentiated thyroid cancer who are intolerant to adequate doses of levothyroxine alone. Tiratricol is a metabolite of the thyroid hormone triiodothyronine (T_3) and has thyroid hormone activity.

Tiratricol is also marketed as a dietary supplement for weight-loss purposes. In November 2000, the Food and Drug Administration (FDA) warned against consuming dietary supplements containing tiratricol. This was based on reports of individuals using tiratricol developing side effects, such as fatigue, lethargy, profound weight loss and severe diarrhea. They were also found to have abnormal thyroid function tests. Further action by the FDA is being considered.

Tiratricol is also known as triiodothyroacetic acid, TRIAC, 3,5,3'-triiodothyroacetic acid and [4-(4-hydroxy-3-iodophenoxy)-3,5-di-iodophenyl]acetic acid. Its molecular formula is $C_{14}H_9I_3O_4$, and its molecular weight is 621.9 daltons.

ACTIONS AND PHARMACOLOGY

ACTIONS

Tiratricol has thyroid hormone activity, including various metabolic effects. It also inhibits the secretion of thyroid-stimulating hormone (TSH) by the pituitary gland. Tiratricol is a product of triiodothyronine or T_3 metabolism, derived by deamination and oxidative decarboxylation of the alanine chain. In humans, tiratricol production by the liver and other tissues accounts for about 14% of T_3 metabolism and is increased under certain physiological conditions, such as fasting. Tiratricol may play a role in regulating energy balance.

MECHANISM OF ACTION

The mechanism by which thyroid hormones exert their various actions has not been completely elucidated. Tiratricol is known to act as a feedback inhibitor of TSH secretion by the pituitary gland.

PHARMACOKINETICS

Much is unknown about the pharmacokinetics of tiratricol in humans. The pharmacokinetics of tiratricol appears to be similar to those of thyroxine and triiodothyronine. Tiratricol is absorbed from the small intestine following ingestion. Distribution of tiratricol in the body has not been fully elucidated. Most of this substance appears to be bound to serum proteins, including thyroxine-binding protein and albumin. It appears to be less firmly bound to serum proteins than are T_4 and T_3. The liver appears to be the major site of degradation of tiratricol. Tiratricol appears to be conjugated with glucuronic acid and sulfuric acid and excreted in the bile. Mainly because it is less tightly bound to serum proteins, tiratricol has a shorter half-life than T_4 or T_3.

INDICATIONS AND USAGE

The FDA has warned consumers not to purchase tiratricol-containing dietary supplements due to risk of serious health consequences, including heart attacks and strokes. Tiratricol should be used only under a physician's supervision. Tiratricol is currently used by some as a supplement to burn fat. The doses required to achieve this effect pose significant health risks.

RESEARCH SUMMARY

Tiratricol is an orphan drug. The FDA has determined that it should not be used as a dietary supplement due to serious potential health risks including heart attack and stroke.

CONTRAINDICATIONS, PRECAUTIONS, ADVERSE REACTIONS

CONTRAINDICATIONS

Tiratricol is contraindicated in those with untreated thyrotoxicosis of any etiology and in those with uncorrected adrenal insufficiency. Thyroid hormones increase tissue demands for adrenocortical hormones and may thereby precipitate acute adrenal crisis. Tiratricol is also contraindicated in those who are hypersensitive to any component of a tiratricol-containing product. FDA warns against consuming dietary supplements containing tiratricol.

PRECAUTIONS

Tiratricol should only be used for specific approved indications and only under strict medical supervision. Tiratricol should not be used as a treatment for obesity. Tiratricol should be used with extreme caution in those with cardiovascular disorders (including angina, coronary artery disease and hypertension) and in the elderly who have a greater likelihood of occult cardiac disease. Concomitant use of tiratricol and sympathomimetic agents in those with coronary artery disease may increase the risk of coronary insufficiency. Use of tiratricol in those with concomitant diabetes mellitus, diabetes insipidus or adrenal cortical insufficiency may aggravate the intensity of their symptoms.

FDA warns against consuming dietary supplements containing tiratricol.

ADVERSE REACTIONS

Reported adverse reactions include fatigue, lethargy, profound weight loss and severe diarrhea. Tiratricol has also been reported to cause abnormal thyroid function tests.

INTERACTIONS

DRUGS

Anticoagulants (oral). The hypoprothrombinemic effect of anticoagulants, such as warfarin, may be potentiated.

Sympathomimetic agents. There is a possible increased risk of coronary insufficiency in those with coronary artery disease.

Thyroid drugs (levothyroxine, triiodothyronine, thyroid). Concomitant use of tiratricol with these thyroid drugs is likely to produce additive effects.

LABORATORY TESTS

Tiratricol is likely to alter thyroid function tests, including TSH, T_4 and T_3.

OVERDOSAGE

There have been no reports of overdosage with tiratricol. Excessive doses of tiratricol theoretically may result in a hypermetabolic state indistinguishable from thyrotoxicosis.

DOSAGE AND ADMINISTRATION

Tiratricol is not recommended for use as a dietary supplement.

LITERATURE

Anon. FDA warns against consuming dietary supplements containing tiratricol. *FDA Talk Paper.* Nov. 21, 2000.

Bracco D, Morin O, Schutz Y, et al. Comparison of the metabolic effects of 3,5,3'-triiodothyroacetic acid and thyroxine. *J Clin Endocrin Met.* 1993;77:221-228.

Darendeliler F, Ba F. Successful therapy with 3,5,3'-triiodothyroacetic acid (TRIAC) in pituitary resistance to thyroid hormone. *J Pediatr Endocrinol Metab.* 1997;10(5):535-538.

Iglesias P, Díez JJ. [Therapeutic possibilities in patients with selective pituitary resistance to thyroid hormones.] [In Spanish.] *Med Clin (Barc).* 2008;130(9):345-350.

Medina-Gomez G, Calvo RM, Obregon MJ. Thermogenic effect of triiodothyroacetic acid at low doses in rat adipose tissue without adverse side effects in the thyroid axis. *Am J Physiol Endocrinol Metab.* 2008;294(4):E688-697.

Pisarev MA, Brenta G, Schnitman M, et al. [Triiodothyroacetic acid in euthyroid goiter. New data on its mechanisms of action. Comparison with L-thyroxin.] [In French.] *Bull Acad Natl Med.* 2007;191(8):1705-1715; discussion 1715.

Radetti G, Persani L, Molinaro G, et al. Clinical and hormonal outcome after two years of triiodothyroacetic acid treatment in a child with thyroid hormone resistance. *Thyroid.* 1997;7:775-778.

Takeda T, Suzuki S, Liu RT, et al. Triiodothyroacetic acid has unique potential for therapy of resistance to thyroid hormone. *J Clin Endocrinol Metab.* 1995;80:2033-2040.

Tocotrienols

DESCRIPTION

Tocotrienols comprise one of the two groups of molecules belonging to the vitamin E family, the other group being the tocopherols. Tocotrienols and tocopherols are sometimes collectively called tocols. Just as there are four natural tocopherols, alpha-, beta-, gamma- and delta-tocopherol, there are also four natural tocotrienols, alpha-, beta-, gamma- and delta-tocotrienol. The tocotrienols differ from the tocopherols in the chemical nature of the side chain or tail. Tocopherols have a saturated phytyl side chain, whereas tocotrienols have an unsaturated isoprenoid or farnesyl side chain possessing three double bonds.

The major source of tocotrienols are plant oils, and the richest sources are palm oil, rice bran oil, palm kernel oil and coconut oil. Tocotrienols are also found in such cereal grains as oat, barley and rye. Vegetable oils, such as those from canola, cottonseed, olive, peanut, safflower, soybean and sunflower, contain little to no tocotrienols. However, those oils do contain tocopherols. Corn oil has small amounts of tocotrienols.

All of the natural tocotrienols are fat-soluble, water-insoluble oils. The tocotrienols, as well as the tocopherols, possess chain-breaking, peroxyl radical scavenging activities. In contrast to tocopherols, tocotrienols inhibit the rate-limiting enzyme of the cholesterol biosynthetic pathway beta-hydroxy-beta-methylglutaryl-coenzyme A (HMG-CoA) reductase.

The four natural tocotrienols are characterized by the number of methyl groups and their position in the chromanol ring. Alpha-tocotrienol has three methyl groups located on positions 5, 7 and 8 of the chromanol ring; beta-tocotrienol has two methyl groups located on positions 5 and 8 of the ring; gamma-tocotrienol has two methyl groups located on positions 7 and 8 of the ring and delta-tocotrienol has one methyl group located on position 8 of the ring.

While tocopherols have three chiral centers, tocotrienols have only one chiral center. Therefore, each tocotrienol has two stereoisomeric possibilities in comparison with eight such possibilities for each of the tocopherols. The natural tocotrienols exist as d-stereoisomers: d-alpha-tocotrienol, d-beta-tocotrienol, d-gamma-tocotrienol and d-delta-tocotrienol. The chiral center in the tocotrienol structure is at the point where the isoprenoid side chain bonds to the chromanol ring, the 2 position of the ring. The natural tocotrienols are E, E in reference to the geometric configuration of the double bonds of the side chain.

D-Alpha-tocotrienol is also known as 2R, 3′E, 7′E-alpha tocotrienol and is abbreviated alpha-T_3; d-beta-tocotrienol is known as 2R, 3′E, 7′E-beta-tocotrienol and abbreviated beta-T_3; d-gamma-tocotrienol is known as 2R, 3′E, 7′E-gamma-tocotrienol and abbreviated gamma-T3; delta-tocotrienol is known as 2R, 3′E, 7′E-delta-tocotrienol and abbreviated delta-T_3. Tocotrienols are presently available in nutritional supplement form as mixed tocotrienols. Typically, the gamma form is the most abundant one in the mixture.

Occasionally tocotrienol is used in the singular but refers to the entire group of natural tocotrienols.

ACTIONS AND PHARMACOLOGY

ACTIONS

Tocotrienols have antioxidant activity. They may also have hypocholesterolemic, anti-atherogenic, antithrombotic, anticarcinogenic and immunomodulatory actions.

MECHANISM OF ACTION

All the tocotrienols are lipid soluble, chain-breaking, peroxyl radical scavengers. As such, they can protect polyunsaturated fatty acids (PUFAs) within membrane phospholipids as well as PUFAs within plasma lipoproteins, such as low density lipoproteins, from lipid peroxidation. Which of the tocols have the highest antioxidant activity is still open to debate. For many years, alpha-tocopherol was thought to be the most potent antioxidant in the vitamin E family. Some studies have shown tocotrienols to be more effective inhibitors of both lipid peroxidation and protein oxidation than alpha-tocopherol. In these same studies, the order of antioxidant potency was gamma-tocotrienol followed by the alpha and delta tocotrienol homologues. Gamma-tocopherol is a peroxynitrite scavenger, and gamma-tocotrienol may be, as well. The possible greater antioxidant activity of the tocotrienols, compared with alpha-tocopherol, may be accounted for by a more efficient interaction of the chromanol ring with reactive oxygen species, a higher recycling efficiency of the chromanoxyl radicals of the tocotrienols and a more uniform distribution of the tocotrienols in cellular membranes. In any case, alpha-tocopherol is the dominant tocol in human plasma and tissue, and, therefore, would be expected to be the dominant antioxidant form, as well.

Tocotrienols inhibit the rate-limiting enzyme of the cholesterol biosynthetic pathway, beta-hydroxy-beta-methlyglutaryl-coenzyme A (HMG-CoA) reductase. Tocopherols do not have this activity. This hypocholesterolemic effect of tocotrienols is accounted for by the tocotrienol isoprenoid side-

chain's ability to increase the concentration of cellular farnesol. Farnesol is derived from mevalonate, the product of the HMG-CoA reductase reaction. Farnesol, post-transcriptionally, suppresses HMG-CoA reductase synthesis and enhances the proteolytic catabolism of this enzyme. This mechanism is different from that of the statin hypocholesterolemic drugs (atorvastatin, cerivastatin, fluvastatin, lovastatin and pravastatin) which are competitive inhibitors of the enzyme. Gamma-tocotrienol and delta-tocotrienol are significantly more active than alpha-tocotrienol in suppressing HMG-CoA reductase activity.

The possible anti-atherogenic activity of tocotrienols can be accounted for by a few mechanisms. These include inhibition of LDL oxidation, suppression of HMG-CoA reductase activity and inhibition of platelet aggregation. Additional possible mechanisms include tocotrienol-mediated reduction of plasma apolipoprotein B-100 (apoB) levels, reduction of lipoprotein (a) [Lp (a)] plasma levels and inhibition of adhesion molecule (e.g., ICAM-1 and VCAM-1) expression and monocyte cell adherence. High plasma levels of apoB as well as Lp (a) are considered risk factors for coronary artery disease.

Tocotrienols' possible antithrombotic effect may be due to tocotrienols' (especially gamma-tocotrienol's) inhibition of thromboxane B_2 synthesis, as well as their suppression of plasma levels of platelet factor 4.

Tocotrienols have been found to inhibit the growth of several tumor cell lines in culture, including both estrogen receptor-negative and estrogen receptor-positive human breast cancer cells. The mechanism of this effect is unclear, but there is some speculation about it. Tocotrienols may upregulate apoptosis in these lines. Another possible mechanism may relate to tocotrienols' post-transcriptional suppression of HMG-CoA reductase. The suppression of mevalonate synthesis depletes tumor tissues of farnesyl pyrophosphate and geranylgeranylpyrophosphate. These intermediates in the cholesterol biosynthetic pathway play important roles in growth control-associated proteins. Suppressing the production intermediates could result in suppression of prenylation of the oncogene ras protein. Post-translational farnesylation of Ras is required for the cytoplasmic localization of the active Ras p21 to the cell membrane, enabling this oncogene to stimulate growth and induce malignant transformation.

PHARMACOKINETICS

The efficiency of absorption of tocotrienol is low and variable. Absorption from the lumen of the small intestine is lower on an empty stomach than with meals. Prior to their absorption, tocotrienols are emulsified with the aid of bile salts and form micelles with dietary fats and products of lipid hydrolysis. Tocotrienols, after absorption into the enterocytes, are secreted by these cells into the lymphatics in the form of chylomicrons. The chylomicrons are transported by the lymphatics to the circulation where they are metabolized to chylomicron remnants. Some tocotrienols are transferred to various tissues, including adipose tissue, muscle and possibly the brain. Chylomicrons transfer tocotrienols to HDL, which, in turn, transfers them to LDL and VLDL. These remnants can also acquire apolipoprotein E, which directs them and the tocotrienols they contain to the liver for further metabolism.

Chylomicron remnants are taken up by the liver. Tocotrienols do not bind very well to the hepatic alpha-tocopherol transfer protein. It is this protein that is involved in the secretion from the liver of alpha-tocopherol in VLDLs. Very little tocotrienol is secreted by the liver to the circulation in VLDLs.

Some tocotrienol is metabolized, and the metabolites are excreted in the urine. Fecal excretion is the main route of exertion of oral tocotrienols. Fecal excretion products include non-absorbed tocotrienols and tocotrienols that may be excreted by the biliary route.

INDICATIONS AND USAGE

Indications and uses of the tocotrienols are, generally, the same as those of vitamin E. (See Vitamin E.) The tocotrienols may, in some conditions, be more potent and, in others, less potent than vitamin E, but research related to this issue is preliminary. There are some data suggesting that tocotrienols may have greater hypolipidemic effects than the tocopherols. The tocotrienols show some promise in inhibiting breast cancer and some other malignancies, though this work, too, is preliminary. Tocotrienols were reported, in one recent animal study, to promote healing of ethanol-induced gastric lesions.

RESEARCH SUMMARY

There is evidence, in animal models, that tocotrienols decrease serum cholesterol levels. Both total and LDL-cholesterol levels have been significantly reduced in swine, 44% and 60% respectively. Serum cholesterol levels were lowered 29% in hypercholesterolemic chickens fed a tocotrienol-enriched diet. In some animal studies, it has also inhibited platelet aggregation.

In some small, case-controlled human trials, tocotrienol preparations showed an ability to reduce cholesterol, principally LDL-cholesterol, while leaving HDL-cholesterol essentially unchanged. Despite good results in these studies and in animal and *in vitro* studies, coupled with epidemiological data suggesting that high tocotrienol status confers protection against cardiovascular disease, some recent, small studies have not been quite as promising.

In one randomized, placebo-controlled trial of 50 subjects with cerebrovascular disease (including carotid stenosis), a daily supplement containing 64 milligrams of alpha-tocopherol and 160 milligrams of gamma-tocotrienol failed to produce any positive lipid effects. The lack of effect persisted even when the dose was boosted to 96 milligrams of alpha-tocopherol and 240 milligrams of gamma-tocotrienol.

But, even though there was no lipid-lowering effect, the treated group showed improvement, compared with controls receiving placebo in terms of ultrasonigraphically measured rate of progression and, in some cases, regression of carotid stenosis. It was hypothesized that the treatment might have inhibited protein kinase C stimulation and may thus have prevented proliferation of smooth muscle cells among other possible mechanisms of action.

More recently, another randomized, double-blind, placebo-controlled study found no lipid effects from a supplement containing 35 milligrams of tocotrienols and 20 milligrams of alpha-tocopherol in 20 men with slightly elevated lipid concentrations. Larger studies, perhaps using higher doses of tocotrienols in subjects with more pronounced hyperlipidemia, are needed.

In one small, double-blind, crossover study of hypercholesterolemic subjects, 200 milligrams of a tocotrienol-enriched fraction of palm oil daily for four weeks significantly lowered total cholesterol, LDL-cholesterol, Apo B, thromboxane, platelet factor 4 and glucose. The crossover confirmed these findings.

Subsequently, both gamma-tocotrienol and the same tocotrienol-enriched fraction of palm oil described above were tested in more hypercholesterolemic subjects. Both supplements produced significant cholesterol reduction in these subjects. Gamma tocotrienol (200 milligrams daily) was more effective than the palm oil preparation (which contained 40 milligrams of alpha-tocotrienol and 60 milligrams of delta-tocotrienol).

Gamma and delta-tocotrienols, but not alpha- and gamma-tocopherols, have shown significant tumor-inhibition activity in several *in vitro* studies. In one of these, a tocotrienol-rich fraction of palm oil significantly inhibited the growth of a human breast cancer cell line, whereas alpha-tocopherol did not. Additional *in vitro* studies have demonstrated that tocotrienols inhibit the growth of human breast cancer cells in culture irrespective of the estrogen receptor status of the cells. It has been suggested by some researchers that tocotrienols might productively be combined with tamoxifen as a breast cancer treatment. The efficacy and safety of such a combination have not been tested, but the potential for such a treatment might be considerable, particularly with respect to treating hormone-responsive breast cancer that has become resistant to tamoxifen and other antiestrogens.

Tocotrienols have shown experimental activity against a number of other cancers. Research continues.

Recently, a tocotrienol-enriched fraction of palm oil was found to enhance the healing of ethanol-induced gastric mucosal lesions in rats. It was not, however, able to prevent such injuries. It was hypothesized that tocotrienols may abet healing through inhibition of lipid peroxidation. Further study is needed.

CONTRAINDICATIONS, PRECAUTIONS, ADVERSE REACTIONS

CONTRAINDICATIONS

Tocotrienols are contraindicated in those with known hypersensitivity to these substances.

PRECAUTIONS

Those on warfarin should be cautious in using doses of tocotrienols greater than 100 milligrams daily and, if they do so, they should have their INRs carefully monitored and their warfarin dose appropriately adjusted if indicated. Likewise, those with vitamin K deficiencies, such as those with liver failure, should be cautious in using doses of tocotrienols greater than 100 milligrams daily. Tocotrienols should also be used with caution in those with lesions with a propensity to bleed (e.g., bleeding peptic ulcers), those with a history of hemorrhagic stroke and those with inherited bleeding disorders (e.g., hemophilia).

High dose tocotrienol supplementation (greater than 100 milligrams daily) should be stopped about one month before surgical procedures and may be resumed following recovery from the procedure.

Those taking iron supplements should not take tocotrienols and iron at the same time.

ADVERSE REACTIONS

Tocotrienol supplements have only recently been introduced in the nutritional supplement marketplace. No adverse reactions have been reported.

INTERACTIONS

DRUGS

Antiplatelet drugs, such as aspirin, dipyridamole, eptifibatide, clopidogrel, ticlopidine, tirofiban and abciximab: Tocotrienol supplementation may potentiate the effects of these antiplatelet drugs.

Cholestyramine: may decrease tocotrienol absorption.

Colestipol: may decrease tocotrienol absorption.

Isoniazid: may decrease tocotrienol absorption.

Mineral oil: may decrease tocotrienol absorption.

Neomycin: may impair utilization of tocotrienols.

Orlistat: is likely to inhibit tocotrienol absorption.

Statins: atorvastatin, cerivastatin, fluvastatin, lovastatin, pravastatin: The possible cholesterol-lowering action of tocotrienols may be additive to that of the statins.

Sucralfate: may interfere with tocotrienol absorption.

Warfarin: Tocotrienol doses greater than 100 milligrams daily may enhance the anticoagulant response of warfarin. Monitor INRs and appropriately adjust warfarin dose if necessary.

NUTRITIONAL SUPPLEMENTS

Desiccated ox bile: may increase the absorption of tocotrienols.

Iron: Most iron supplements contain the ferrous form of iron. This form can oxidize tocotrienols, marketed in their unesterified forms, to their pro-oxidant forms if taken concomitantly.

Medium-chain triglycerides: may enhance absorption of tocotrienols if taken concomitantly.

Phytosterols and phytostanols, including beta-sitosterol and beta-sitostanol: may lower plasma tocotrienol levels.

FOOD

Olestra: is likely to inhibit the absorption of tocotrienols. Alpha-tocopherol is the only member of the vitamin E family that is added to olestra.

HERBS

Some herbs, including ginkgo and garlic, possess antithrombotic activity, and tocotrienols, if taken concomitantly with these herbs, may enhance their antithrombotic activity.

OVERDOSAGE

Tocotrienol overdosage has not been reported in the literature.

DOSAGE AND ADMINISTRATION

Presently marketed forms of tocotrienols contain mixed tocotrienols in their unesterified forms. These products typically contain d-alpha-tocotrienol, d-gamma-tocotrienol and d-delta-tocotrienol. Gamma-tocotrienol is usually the major tocotrienol in these preparations, which are marketed in the form of softgel capsules (tocotrienol is an oil).

Doses of 200 to 300 milligrams daily, with food, have been used in clinical trials studying possible cholesterol-lowering activity of tocotrienol.

The unesterified forms of tocotrienols, as well as tocopherols, are susceptible to oxidation and should therefore be stored in tightly closed, opaque containers in a cool, dry place. Tocotrienols should not be taken concomitantly with iron supplements.

LITERATURE

Elson CE. Suppression of mevalonate pathway activities by dietary isoprenoids: protective roles in cancer and cardiovascular disease. *J Nutr.* 1995; 125(6 Suppl):1666S-1672S.

Guthrie N, Gapor A, Chambers AF, Carroll KK. Inhibition of proliferation of estrogen receptor-negative MDA-MB-435 and—positive MCF-7 human breast cancer cells by palm oil tocotrienols and tamoxifen, alone and in combination. *J Nutr.* 1997; 127:544S-548S.

Kamat JP, Devasagayam TP. Tocotrienols from palm oil as inhibitors of lipid peroxidation and protein oxidation in rat brain mitochondria. *Neurosci Lett.* 1995; 195:179-182.

Kamat JP. Sarma HD, Devasagayam TPA, et al. Tocotrienols from palm oil as effective inhibitors of protein oxidation and lipid peroxidation in rat liver microsomes. *Mol Cell Biochem.* 1997; 170:131-137.

Mc Intyre BS, Briski KP, Tirmenstein MA, et al. Antiproliferative and apoptotic effects of tocopherols and tocotrienols on normal mouse mammary epithelial cells. *Lipids.* 2000; 35:171-180.

Mensink RP, van Houwelingen AC, Kromhout D, Hornstra G. A vitamin E concentrate rich in tocotrienols had no effect on serum lipids, lipoproteins, or platelet function in men with mildly elevated serum lipid concentrations. *Am J Clin Nutr.* 1999; 69:213-219.

Nesaretnam K, Guthrie N, Chambers AF, Carroll KK. Effects of tocotrienols on the growth of a human breast cancer cell line in culture. *Lipids.* 1995; 30:1139-1143.

Nesaretnam K, Stephen R, Dils R, Dabre P. Tocotrienols inhibit the growth of human breast cancer cells irrespective of estrogen receptor status. *Lipids.* 1998; 33:461-469.

Parker RA, Pearce BC, Clark RW, et al. Tocotrienols regulate cholesterol production in mammalian cells by post-transcriptional suppression of 3-hdroxy-3-methylglutaryl-coenzyme A reductase. *J Biol Chem.* 1993; 268:11230-11238.

Pearce BC, Parker RA, Deason ME, et al. Inhibitors of cholesterol biosynthesis. 2. Hypocholesterolemic and antioxidant activities of benzopyran and tertrahydronaphthalene analogues of the tocotrienols. *J Med Chem.* 1994; 37:526-541.

Quereshi AA, Bradlow BA, Manganello J, et al. Response of hypercholesterolemic subjects to administration of tocotrienols. *Lipids.* 1995; 30:1171-1177.

Quereshi AA, Pearce BC, Nor RM, et al. Dietary alpha-tocopherol on hepatic 3-hydroxy-3-methlyglutaryl coenzyme A reductase activity in chickens. *J Nutr.* 1996; 126:389-394.

Quereshi AA, Quereshi N, Hasler-Rapacz JO, et al. Dietary tocotrienols reduce concentrations of plasma cholesterol, apolipoprotein B, thromboxane B2 and platelet factor 4 in pigs with inherited hyperlipidemica. *Am J Clin Nutr.* 1991; 53(Suppl):1042S-1046S.

Serbinova E, Khwaja S, Catudioc J, et al. Palm oil vitamin E protects against ischemia reperfusion injury in the isolated perfused Langendorff heart. *Nutr Res.* 1992; 12(Suppl 1):S203-S215.

Theriault A, Chao J-T, Wang Q, et al. Tocotrienol: a review of its therapeutic potential. *Clinic Biochem.* 1999; 32:309-319.

Theriault A, Wang Q, Gapor A, Adeli K. Effects of gamma-tocotrienol on ApoB synthesis, degradation, and secretion in Hep G2 cells. *Arterioscler Thromb Vasc Biol.* 1999; 19:704-712.

Tomeo AC, Geller M, Watkins TR, et al. Antioxidant effects of tocotrienols in patients with hyperlipidemia and carotid stenosis. *Lipids.* 1995; 30:1179-1183.

Wang Q, Theriault A, Gapor A, Adeli K. Effects of tocotrienol on the intracellular translocation and degradation of apolipoprotein B: possible involvement of a proteasome independent pathway. *Biochem Biophys Res Commun.* 1998; 246:640-643.

Watkins T, Lenz P, Gapor A, et al. Gamma-tocopherol as a hypocholesterolemic and antioxidant agent in rats fed atherogenic diets. *Lipids.* 1993; 28:1113-1118.

Transgalacto-Oligosaccharides

DESCRIPTION

Transgalacto-oligosaccharides (TOS), also known as galactooligosaccharides (GOS), are a mixture of oligosaccharides consisting of D-glucose and D-galactose. Transgalacto-digosaccharides are produced from D-lactose via the action of the enzyme beta-galactosidase obtained from *Aspergillus oryzae*.

TOS are not normally digested in the small intestine. They are, however, fermented by a limited number of colonic bacteria. This could lead to changes in the colonic ecosystem in favor of some bacteria, such as bifidobacteria, which may have health benefits, including protection against certain cancers and lowering of cholesterol levels. TOS and other non-digestible oligosaccharides are sometimes referred to as bifidogenic factors.

Substances such as TOS that promote the growth of beneficial bacteria in the colon are called prebiotics. Prebiotics are typically non-digestible oligosaccharides.

ACTIONS AND PHARMACOLOGY

ACTIONS

Transgalacto-oligosaccharides may have antitumor, antimicrobial, hypolipidemic and hypoglycemic actions. They may also help improve mineral absorption and balance.

MECHANISM OF ACTION

The possible antitumor activity of TOS might be accounted for by the possible antitumor action of butyrate, one of the substances produced from TOS in the colon. Butyrate, the anion of the naturally occurring short-chain fatty acid butyric acid, is produced by bacterial fermentation of TOS in the colon. Studies suggest that butyrate induces growth arrest and cell differentiation and may upregulate apoptosis, three activities that could be significant for antitumor activity. Interestingly, butyrate also appears to inhibit vascular smooth muscle cell proliferation, at least in the rat, an activity that could have relevance with regard to a possible antiatherogenic role. TOS may promote the growth of favorable bacterial populations, such as bifidobacteria, in the colon. Bifidobacteria may inhibit the growth of pathogenic bacteria, such as *Clostritium perfringens* and diarrheogenic strains of *Escherichia coli*.

There is evidence, again from rat studies, that butyrate may suppress cholesterol synthesis in the liver and intestine. Propionate, another short-chain fatty acid produced from the bacterial fermentation of TOS in the colon, may reduce plasma free fatty acids. This might be good for blood glucose and insulin sensitivity in the long term, since high levels of plasma free fatty acids lower tissue glucose utilization and induce insulin resistance. Propionate may also aid in lowering cholesterol levels in some by possibly inhibiting HMG-CoA reductase.

TOS, similar to dietary fiber, may bind/sequester such minerals as calcium and magnesium in the small intestine. The short-chain fatty acids (acetate, propionate, butyrate) formed from the bacterial fermentation of TOS may facilitate the colonic absorption of calcium and magnesium ions. This could have both bone- and cardiovascular-health benefits.

PHARMACOKINETICS

Under normal conditions, following ingestion of TOS, no digestion of these oligosaccharides takes place in the small intestine. A small amount of TOS may undergo some acid hydrolysis in the stomach. TOS are fermented in the colon by bifidobacteria and some other bacteria to produce the short-chain fatty acids acetate, propionate and butyrate. Lactate is also produced. Acetate, propionate and butyrate that are not metabolized in colonocytes are absorbed from the colon and transported via the portal circulation to the liver. These short-chain fatty acids are extensively metabolized in hepatocytes. Acetate, propionate and butyrate that are not metabolized in hepatocytes are transported by the circulation to various tissues, where they undergo further metabolism. Butyrate is an important respiratory fuel for the colonocytes and is metabolized in them to CO_2 and H_2O. Energy is produced (ATP) from the catabolism of butyrate. Those with ileostomies may have a microbial population colonizing their ileums. In those cases, TOS could be fermented by some of the bacteria to short-chain fatty acids and lactic acid.

INDICATIONS AND USAGE

Transgalacto-oligosaccharides are being investigated for possible protective effects against colorectal cancer and infectious bowel diseases, for modulation of lipids and prevention of bone loss. Animal research suggests a role for TOS in those situations, but there is still little substantial clinical research.

RESEARCH SUMMARY

TOS, through their stimulation of bifidobacteria, have shown some protective effects against colorectal cancer and infectious bowel diseases in animal and *in vitro* experiments. TOS inhibit putrefactive bacteria (*Clostridium perfringens*) and pathogenic bacteria, such as *Escherichia coli*, *salmonella*, *listeria* and *shigella*.

A recent human study showed that supplemental TOS (in doses of 7.5 and 10 grams daily) are completely fermented in the human colon but that they did not, in this study, beneficially change the composition of the intestinal microflora. Another study, however, did show some alteration in the fermentative activity of colonic flora in humans given 10 grams of TOS per day for 21 days.

TOS have demonstrated some preliminary positive effects on calcium absorption and lipid metabolism in animal studies. Reduced serum triglyceride levels have been noted. A significant TOS hypocholesterolemic effect was observed in ovariectomized rats that had elevated total cholesterol at baseline. This same study also demonstrated a significant positive TOS effect on calcium absorption and prevention of bone loss in these animals. The stimulatory effect of TOS on calcium absorption has been observed in additional studies. Research continues.

CONTRAINDICATIONS, PRECAUTIONS, ADVERSE REACTIONS

CONTRAINDICATIONS

Transgalacto-oligosaccharides are contraindicated in those who are hypersensitive to any component of a TOS-containing product.

PRECAUTIONS

Because of absence of long-term safety studies, pregnant women and nursing mothers should exercise caution in the use of TOS supplements.

Those with lactose intolerance should be cautious in the use of TOS supplements.

ADVERSE REACTIONS

Doses of 10 grams daily are well tolerated. Higher doses may cause some gastrointestinal symptoms, such as flatulence, bloating and diarrhea.

INTERACTIONS

NUTRITIONAL SUPPLEMENTS

TOS may enhance the colonic absorption of calcium and magnesium supplements if used concomitantly with them.

Probiotics. The possible beneficial effects of TOS may be enhanced if used in combination with probiotics.

FOODS

TOS may enhance the colonic absorption of calcium and magnesium in foods.

DOSAGE AND ADMINISTRATION

Transgalacto-oligosaccharides are available in Japan and Europe as nutritional supplements and as functional foods. They are also expected to enter the U.S. marketplace. Typical dosage is about 10 grams daily, usually taken in divided doses.

LITERATURE

Bouhnik Y, Flourié B, D'Agay-Abensour L, et al. Administration of transgalacto-oligosaccharides increases fecal bifidobacteria and modifies colonic fermentation metabolism in healthy humans. *J Nutr.* 1997; 127:444-448.

Chonan O, Matsumoto K, Watanuki M. Effect of galactooligosaccharides on calcium absorption and preventing bone loss in ovariectomized rats. *Biosci Biotechnol Biochem.* 1995; 59:236-239.

Chonan O, Watanuki M. Effect of galactooligosaccharides on calcium absorption in rats. *J Nutr Sci Vitaminol (Tokyo).* 1995; 11:95-104.

Ito M, Deguchi Y, Matsumoto K, et al. Influence of galactooligosaccharides on the human fecal microflora. *J Nutr Sci Vitaminol (Tokyo).* 1993; 39:635-640.

Vanadium

DESCRIPTION

Vanadium is a metallic element with atomic number 23 and atomic symbol V. Vanadium is a transition element that exists in several oxidation states, including +2, +3, +4 and +5. Vanadium compounds are striking for their varied colors. For this reason, vanadium was first named panchromium. The element chromium, another colorful element, is vanadium's next-door neighbor to the left in the periodic table. Vanadium is widely found in nature in the form of minerals, as well as in living matter, such as the human body. In living matter, vanadium is found mainly as the tetravalent vanadyl cation and the pentavalent vanadate form.

Nutritional essentiality for humans has not been established for vanadium. Vanadium-deficiency states have been reported in some animals. Goats fed diets deficient in vanadium had an elevated spontaneous abortion rate and depressed milk production, and approximately 40% of kids from these goats died between days 7 and 91 of life, with some deaths preceded by convulsions. Only 8% of kids from vanadium-supplemented goats died during the same period. Rats fed vanadium-deficient diets were found to have decreased growth.

Vanadyl and vanadate compounds act as insulin-mimetics and are being studied as potentially orally active replacements for insulin. However, these substances are poorly absorbed from the gastrointestinal tract, and the amounts needed for an effective oral dose are likely to be toxic. Vanadium-containing compounds are being developed for the treatment of diabetes with higher therapeutic-to-toxicity ratios. Such compounds include peroxovanadiums, bis(picolinato) oxovanadium and the vanadium ligand L-glutamic acid gamma-monohydroxamate.

Typical diets supply less than 30 micrograms of vanadium daily. The average daily dietary intake of vanadium is approximately 15 micrograms. Foods rich in vanadium include black pepper, mushrooms, shellfish, parsley, dill seed and some prepared foods. Foods low in vanadium include fresh fruits and vegetables, oils and beverages.

Tetravalent vanadium compounds are sometimes designated as vanadium (IV) and pentavalent vanadium compounds are designated as vanadium (V).

ACTIONS AND PHARMACOLOGY

ACTIONS

Vanadium salts have insulin-mimetic activity, and vanadium compounds are being studied as potentially orally active replacements for insulin. The doses of supplemental vanadium that may affect blood glucose levels are potentially toxic, and supplemental vanadium is not recommended for the management of diabetes, hyperglycemia, hypoglycemia or insulin resistance.

MECHANISM OF ACTION

Vanadium salts mimic most of the effects of insulin *in vitro* and also induce normoglycemia and improve glucose homeostasis in insulin-deficient and insulin-resistant diabetic rodents *in vivo*. Vanadium salts appear to have these effects via alternative pathways not involving insulin receptor tyrosine kinase activation or phosphorylation of insulin receptor substrate. Vanadium's mechanisms of action appear to involve inhibition of protein-phosphotyrosine phosphatase and activation of nonreceptor protein-tyrosine kinases.

PHARMACOKINETICS

The absorption of dietary vanadium and supplemental vanadium (usually vanadyl sulfate) is poor, and most ingested vanadium is excreted in the feces. It is estimated that less than 5% of dietary vanadium is absorbed. Most ingested vanadium appears to be converted to tetravalent vanadyl in the stomach. Any absorbed vanadate is converted to cationic vanadyl in the blood. The vanadyl cation complexes with transferrin and ferritin in plasma and other body fluids. Vanadium is removed from the plasma and is found in highest amounts in the kidney, liver, testes, bone and spleen. Absorbed vanadium is mainly excreted in the urine in both high- and low-molecular weight complexes. Some absorbed vanadium may be excreted via the bile.

INDICATIONS

The use of supplemental vanadium is not indicated for any purpose at this time. Vanadium is showing promise in the treatment of both type 1 and type 2 diabetes, but this work is still preliminary and utilizes pharmacological doses of vanadium with unknown long-term safety consequences. Claims that vanadium increases muscle mass have no research support.

RESEARCH SUMMARY

Both experimental and clinical trials indicate that vanadium has significant insulin-mimetic properties in pharmacological doses. *In vitro*, vanadium salts have most of the major effects of insulin itself on insulin-sensitive tissues. Favorable results are seen, as well, in animal models of insulin deficiency, where vanadium significantly reduces blood glucose levels, and in insulin-resistant diabetic animals, where vanadium improves glucose homeostasis.

In *in vivo* animal studies examining the relationship between hyperinsulinemia, insulin resistance and hypertension, vanadium compounds produce significant, sustained decreases in both plasma insulin concentration and blood pressure. Restoring plasma insulin levels reversed the blood-pressure effect.

Clinical trials with vanadium compounds have produced some benefits in both type 1 and type 2 diabetic patients. Results have been better, however, in type 2 patients. Six type 2 diabetic subjects treated with 100 milligrams of vanadyl sulfate daily for four weeks had significant reductions in fasting plasma glucose; beneficial effects on insulin sensitivity persisted for up to four weeks after vanadium treatment ended.

However, a recent systematic review of vanadium oral supplements for glycemic control in type 2 diabetes concluded, "There is no rigorous evidence that oral vanadium supplementation improves glycemic control in type 2 diabetes. The routine use of vanadium cannot be recommended. A large-scale randomized controlled trial is needed to address this clinical question."

Recently, new vanadium compounds have been developed that are reportedly less toxic and more effective. Animal studies are underway, and clinical trials are planned.

Reports that vanadium promotes muscle-mass development are refuted by research.

CONTRAINDICATIONS, PRECAUTIONS, ADVERSE REACTIONS

CONTRAINDICATIONS

Known hypersensitivity to a vanadium-containing product.

PRECAUTIONS

Those with diabetes or hyperglycemia are cautioned not to use supplemental vanadium to manage their diabetes or hyperglycemia. Those with hypoglycemia should avoid using vanadium supplements.

ADVERSE REACTIONS

The amount of vanadium in typical diets (less than 30 micrograms daily) appears to have low toxicity. In one study, 12 subjects were given 13.5 milligrams of vanadium daily for two weeks, followed by 22.5 milligrams daily for five months, Five subjects experienced gastrointestinal symptoms (nausea, vomiting, diarrhea, cramps) and five subjects developed green tongues. In another study, six subjects receiving daily doses of 4.5 to 18 milligrams of vanadium for six to 10 weeks developed green tongues, diarrhea and cramps at the higher doses.

INTERACTIONS

Chromium, ferrous ion, chloride, aluminum hydroxide and EDTA may decrease absorption of vanadium.

OVERDOSAGE

Overdosage with supplemental vanadium in humans has not been reported.

DOSAGE AND ADMINISTRATION

No recommended dosage. Vanadium, usually as the tetravalent vanadyl sulfate, is available in some vitamin and mineral preparations. Doses range from 10 micrograms to about 10 milligrams (expressed as vanadium). Tetravalent bis (maltolato) oxovanadium (BMOV) is available in some nutritional supplements as is bis-glycinato oxovanadium (BGOV). Colloidal or liquid vitamins also may contain vanadium.

The Food and Nutrition Board of the U.S. National Academy of Sciences has published the following Dietary Reference Intakes (DRI) for vanadium. A summary of DRIs for various age groups and conditions is as follows:

DRI values (milligrams/day)

	UL
Infants	
0-6 months	ND
7-12 months	ND

Children
1-3 years	ND
4-8 years	ND

Boys
9-13 years	ND
14-18 years	ND

Girls
9-13 years	ND
14-18 years	ND

Men
19-30 years	1.8
31-50 years	1.8
51-70 years	1.8
Older than 70 years	1.8

Women
19-30 years	1.8
31-50 years	1.8
51-70 years	1.8
Older than 70 years	1.8

Pregnancy
14-18 years	ND
19-30 years	ND
31-50 years	ND

Lactation
14-18 years	ND
19-30 years	ND
31-50 years	ND

There are no Recommended Dietary Allowances (RDA), Estimated Average Requirements (EAR) or Adequate Intake levels established for vanadium.

The UL is the Tolerable Upper Intake Level and usually represents the total intake from food, water and supplements.

ND = Not determinable. The value is not determinable because of the lack of data on adverse effects in these groups and concern regarding the lack of ability to handle excess amounts. To prevent high levels of intake, the only source of vanadium for these groups should be from food.

LITERATURE

Badmaev V, Prakash S, Majeed M. Vanadium: a review of its potential role in the fight against diabetes. *J Altern Complement Med.* 1999;5:273-291.

Boden G, Chen X, Ruiz J, et al. Effects of vanadyl sulfate on carbohydrate and lipid metabolism in patients with non-insulin dependent diabetes mellitus. *Metabolism.* 1996;45:1130-1135.

Clarkson PM, Rawson ES. Nutritional supplements to increase muscle mass. *Crit Rev Food Sci Nutr.* 1999;39:317-328.

Goldwaser I, Li J, Gershonov E, et al. L-glutamic acid gamma-monohydroxamine. A potentiator of vanadium-evoked glucose metabolism *in vitro* and *in vivo. J Biol Chem* 1999;274:26617-26624.

Institute of Medicine, Food and Nutrition Board. Dietary Reference Intakes for vitamin A, vitamin K, arsenic, boron, chromium, copper, iodine, iron, manganese, molybdenum, nickel, silicon, vanadium, and zinc. Washington, DC: National Academy Press, 2001.

Meyerovitch J, Rothenberg P, Schechter Y, et al. Vanadate normalizes hyperglycemia in two mouse models of non-insulin-dependent diabetes mellitus. *J Clin Invest.* 1991;87:1286-1294.

Nielsen FH. Ultratrace minerals. In: Shils ME, Olson JA, Shike M, Ross AC, eds. *Modern Nutrition in Health and Disease.* 9th ed. Baltimore, MD: Williams and Wilkins;1999:283-303.

Pepato MT, Magnani MR, Kettelhut IC, Bruneti IL. Effect of oral vanadyl sulfate treatment on serum enzymes and lipids of streptzotocin-diabetic young rats. *Mol Cell Biochem.* 1999;198:157-161.

Smith DM, Pickering RM, Lewith GT. A systematic review of vanadium oral supplements for glycaemic control in type 2 diabetes mellitus. *QJM.* 2008;101(5):351-358.

Thompson KH. Vanadium and diabetes. *Biofactors.* 1999;10:43-51.

Verma S, Cam MC, Mac Neill JH. Nutritional factors that can favorably influence the glucose/insulin system: vanadium. *J Amer Col Nutr.* 1998;17:11-18.

Vinpocetine

DESCRIPTION

Vinpocetine is a semi-synthetic derivative of vincamine. Vincamine is an alkaloid derived from the plant *Vinca minor* L., a member of the periwinkle family. Vinpocetine, as well as vincamine, are used in Europe, Japan and Mexico as pharmaceutical agents for the treatment of cerebrovascular and cognitive disorders. In the United States, vinpocetine is marketed as a dietary supplement. It is sometimes called a nootropic, meaning cognition enhancer, from the Greek *noos* for mind.

Vinpocetine is also known as ethyl apovincaminate; ethyl apovincaminoate; eburnamenine-14-carboxylic acid ethyl ester; 3 alpha, 16 alpha-apovincaminic acid ethyl ester; ethyl apovincamin-22-oate; and cavinton, which is sometimes used generically for a branded product with that name. Another vinca alkaloid called vinconate is also being researched as a possible cognition enhancer. The structural formula of vinpocetine is:

Vinpocetine

ACTIONS AND PHARMACOLOGY

ACTIONS

Vinpocetine has several possible actions, including increasing cerebral blood flow and metabolism, anticonvulsant, cognition enhancement, neuroprotection and antioxidant. Vincamine, the parent compound of vinpocetine, is believed to be a cerebral vasodilator.

MECHANISM OF ACTION

Several mechanisms have been proposed for the possible actions of vinpocetine. Vinpocetine has been reported to have calcium-channel blocking activity, as well as voltage-gated sodium channel blocking activity. It has also been reported to inhibit the acetylcholine release evoked by excitatory amino acids (for example, glutamate) and to protect neurons against excitotoxicity. In addition, vinpocetine has been shown to inhibit a cyclic GMP phosphodiesterase, and it is speculated that this inhibition enhances cyclic GMP levels in the vascular smooth muscle, leading to reduced resistance of cerebral vessels and increase of cerebral flow. In some studies, vinpocetine has demonstrated antioxidant activity equivalent to that of vitamin E.

PHARMACOKINETICS

Vinpocetine is absorbed from the small intestine, from whence it is transported to the liver via the portal circulation. From the liver via the systemic circulation, it is distributed to various tissues in the body, including the brain. Absorption of vinpocetine is significantly higher when given with food and can be up to about 60% of an ingested dose. On an empty stomach, absorption of an ingested dose can be as low as 7%. Peak plasma levels are obtained one to one and a half hours after ingestion. Extensive metabolism to the inactive apovincaminic acid occurs in the liver. Only small amounts of unmetabolized vinpocetine are excreted in the urine, the major route of excretion of apovincaminic acid. Most of a dose is excreted within 24 hours as this metabolite. The elimination half-life of vinpocetine following ingestion is one to two hours.

INDICATIONS AND USAGE

The primary claim made for vinpocetine is that it decreases fatality and dependency in ischemic stroke. Research results are mixed. Vinpocetine has not been helpful in Alzheimer's disease, but there is some suggestion that it might help some with other dementias and cerebral dysfunction. Very preliminary research additionally suggests that vinpocetine may help protect the eye and ear from injuries caused by trauma (and, in the case of the eye, from infection) and that it might be gastroprotective, ameliorate symptoms of motion sickness and help prevent atherosclerosis.

RESEARCH SUMMARY

Several small studies, in both animals and humans, have reported significant vinpocetine-associated protective effects in ischemic stroke. A review of these studies, however, found only one positive study of truly randomized, unconfounded clinical trials that compared the effect of vinpocetine to either placebo or another reference treatment for acute stroke where treatment started no later than 14 days after stroke onset. A recent Cochrane Database Systematic Review update concluded that there is not enough evidence to evaluate the effect of vinpocetine on survival or dependency in patients with acute ischemic stroke. Further research is needed.

There is some evidence vinpocetine may be useful in some other cerebral maladies. In one multi-center, double-blind, placebo-controlled study lasting 16 weeks, 203 patients described as having mild to moderate psychosyndromes, including primary dementia, were treated with varying doses of vinpocetine or placebo. Significant improvement was achieved in the vinpocetine-treated group as measured by 'global improvement' and cognitive performance scales. Three 10-milligram doses daily were as effective as, or more effective than, three 20-milligram doses daily. Similarly good results were found in another double-blind clinical trial testing vinpocetine versus placebo in elderly patients with cerebrovascular and central nervous system degenerative disorders. Studies of Alzheimer's disease, however, have shown no vinpocetine benefit.

Some preliminary research suggests that vinpocetine may have some protective effects in both sight and hearing. One study of patients with mild burn trauma in the eyes showed that vinpocetine enhanced healing, most likely as a result of increased blood flow to the damaged tissue. Vinpocetine has also been associated with improvements seen in retinas damaged by hepatitis B virus. Damage from acoustic trauma has similarly been reduced by vinpocetine treatment.

Vinpocetine gastroprotective effects have been reported in animal models challenged with noxious agents. There are anecdotal reports that vinpocetine is protective against some of the gastric and neurological toxicity of excessive alcohol consumption.

There are some reports that vinpocetine may be an effective motion sickness preventative and some early findings in animals that it may exert some anti-atherosclerotic effects through a reported ability to decalcify cholesterol-induced atherosclerotic lesions.

CONTRAINDICATIONS, PRECAUTIONS, ADVERSE REACTIONS

CONTRAINDICATIONS

Vinpocetine is contraindicated in those hypersensitive to any component of a vinpocetine-containing product.

PRECAUTIONS

Pregnant women and nursing mothers should avoid vinpocetine supplements. The use of vinpocetine for any health condition should first be discussed with one's physician. Those with a history of allergic reactions or hypersensitivity reactions during treatment with other vinca alkaloids, such as vinblastine and vincristine, should avoid vinpocetine. Those on warfarin are advised to have their INRs (international normalized ratios) regularly monitored when using vinpocetine supplements (see Interactions). Those with hypotension or orthostatic hypotension should be cautioned that prolonged use of vinpocetine may lead to slight reductions in systolic and diastolic blood pressure.

ADVERSE REACTIONS

Reported adverse reactions include nausea, dizziness, insomnia, drowsiness, dry mouth, transient hypotension, transient tachycardia, pressure-type headache and facial flushing. Slight reductions in both systolic and diastolic blood pressure with prolonged use of vinpocetine have been reported, as well as slight reductions in blood glucose.

INTERACTIONS

Warfarin: Slight changes in prothrombin time have been noted in those adding vinpocetine to warfarin dosing. The changes appear minimal. However, regular monitoring of INR is advised in those using warfarin and vinpocetine concomitantly. There are no other known drug or nutritional supplement, herb or food interactions.

OVERDOSAGE

There are no reports of vinpocetine overdosage.

DOSAGE AND ADMINISTRATION

Vinpocetine is available as an individual supplement and in combination products. Typical doses for supplement use are 5 to 10 milligrams daily with food. Some take up to 20 milligrams daily. Higher doses are not advised.

LITERATURE

Bereczki D, Fekete I. Vinpocetine for acute ischaemic stroke. *Cochrane Database Syst Rev.* 2008 Jan 23;(1):CD000480. Review.

Bereczki D, Fekete I. A systematic review of vinpocetine therapy in acute ischaemic stroke. *Eur J Clin Pharmacol.* 1999;55:349-352.

Bukanova YV, Solntseva EI. Nootropic agent vinpocetine blocks delayed rectified potassium currents more strongly than high-threshold calcium currents. *Neurosci Behav Physiol* 1998;28:116-120.

Cholnoky E, Domok LI. Summary of safety tests of ethyl apovincaminate. *Arzneimittelforschung.* 1976;26(10a):1938-1944.

Gulyas B, Halldin C, Karlsson P, et al. Brain uptake and plasma metabolism of [11C] vinpocetine: a preliminary PET study in a cynomolgus monkey. *J Neuroimaging.* 1999;9:217-222.

Hindmarch I, Fuchs HH, Erzigkeith H. Efficacy and tolerance of vinpocetine in ambulant patients suffering from mild to moderate organic psychosyndromes. *Int Clin Psychopharmacol.* 1991;6:31-43.

Kiss B, Karpati E. [Mechanism of action of vinpocetine.] [Article in Hungarian.] *Acta Pharm Hung.* 1996;66:213-224.

Lakics V, Sebestyén MG, Erdö SL. vinpocetine is a highly potent neuroprotectant against veratridine-induced cell death in primary cultures of rat cerebral cortex. *Neurosci Lett.* 1995;185:127-130.

Miskolczi P, Vereczkey L, Szalay L, Gondoc C. Effect of age on the pharmacokinetics of vinpocetine (Cavinton) and apovincaminic acid. *Eur J Clin Pharmacol.* 1987;33:185-189.

Nosalova V, Machova J, Babulova A. Protective action of vinpocetine against experimentally induced gastric damage in rats. *Arzneimittelforschung.* 1993;43:981-985.

Pudleiner P, Vereczkey L. Study of the absorption of vinpocetine and apovincamic acid. *Eur J Drug Metab Pharmacokinet.* 1993;18:317-321.

Subhan Z, Hindmarch I. Psychopharmacological effects of vinpocetine in normal healthy volunteers. *Eur J Clin Pharmacol.* 1985;28:567-571.

Szakall S, Boros I, Balkay L, et al. Cerebral effects of a single dose of intravenous vinpocetine in chronic stroke patients: a PET study. *J Neuroimaging.* 1998;8:197-204.

Thal LJ, Salmon DP, Lasker B, et al. The safety and lack of efficacy of vinpocetine in Alzheimer's disease. *J Am Geriatr Soc.* 1989;37:515-520.

Vereczkey L, Czira G, Tamas J, et al. Pharmacokinetics of vinpocetine in humans. *Arzneimittelforschung.* 1979;29:957-960.

Vitamin A

DESCRIPTION

Vitamin A refers to a group of fat-soluble substances that are structurally related to and possess the biological activity of the parent substance of the group called all-*trans* retinol or retinol. Vitamin A plays vital roles in vision, epithelial differentiation, growth, reproduction, pattern formation during embryogenesis, bone development, hematopoiesis and brain development. It is also important for the maintenance of the proper functioning of the immune system. Certain carotenoids, such as beta-carotene alpha-carotene and beta-cryptoxanthin, are dietary precursors of vitamin A. Collectively, these substances are called provitamin A. (See Beta-Carotene). The term retinoids refers to retinol and its metabolites, such as retinoic acid, as well as to synthetic analogues that are structurally similar to retinol but may not have the same biological activities as retinol.

Vitamin A deficiency can result in night blindness (defective vision at low illumination), xerosis of the conjunctiva and cornea (destruction of the cornea secondary to vitamin A deficiency or xerophthalmia is a major cause of blindness in children), keratinization of the lung, gastrointestinal tract and urinary tract epithelia, growth retardation, follicular hyperkeratosis of the skin, increased susceptibility to infections and death. Children are particularly susceptible to the effects of vitamin A deficiency. Deficiency of the vitamin is a serious public health issue in developing countries.

Vitamin A deficiency was probably the first nutritional deficiency to be recognized. The ancient Egyptians and Greeks apparently treated the corneal changes due to deficiency of the vitamin and night blindness by the topical application and the feeding of liver, a rich source of vitamin A. In addition to liver, other rich sources of vitamin A are fish liver oils (e.g., cod liver oil), egg yolks, butter and cream. Vitamin A occurs naturally in the form of fatty acid esters, such as vitamin A palmitate (retinyl palmitate).

Vitamin A deficiency occurs under certain conditions. These include inadequate dietary intake of vitamin A or provitamin A, malabsorption syndromes (cystic fibrosis, Whipple's disease, Crohn's disease, ulcerative colitis, short bowel syndrome), pancreatic disease and chronic liver disease (e.g., cirrhosis).

The effects of vitamin A are mediated by two different mechanisms. The eye illustrates both of these mechanisms. Vitamin A (all-*trans* retinol) is converted in the retina to the 11-*cis*-isomer of retinaldehyde or 11-*cis*-retinal. 11-*cis*-retinal functions in the retina in the transduction of light into the neural signals necessary for vision. 11-*cis*-retinal, while attached to opsin in rhodopsin is isomerized to all-*trans*-retinal by light. This is the event that triggers the nerve impulse to the brain which allows for the perception of light. All-*trans*-retinal is then released from opsin and reduced to all-*trans*-retinol. All-*trans*-retinol is isomerized to 11-*cis*-retinol in the dark, and then oxidized to 11-*cis*-retinal. 11-*cis*-retinal recombines with opsin to re-form rhodopsin. Night blindness or defective vision at low illumination

results from a failure to resynthesize 11-*cis* retinal rapidly. This is a consequence of vitamin A deficiency. Vitamin A deficiency results in the depletion of the vitamin A storage pool (retinyl ester) in the retinal pigment epithelial cells.

The normal differentiation of the cells of the cornea and conjunctiva is dependent on another metabolite of vitamin A, retinoic acid. Retinoic acid acts as a hormone and is involved in signal transduction. Retinoic acid signaling and signaling by other retinoids are mediated by two classes of nuclear receptors, retinoic acid receptors (RAR-alpha, -beta and -gamma) and retinoid X receptors (RXR-alpha, -beta and -gamma). The RARs and RXRs belong to the superfamily of nuclear hormone receptors. Members of this family, which, in addition to retinoic acid, include receptors for small hydrophobic hormones, such as steroids, the biologically active form of vitamin D, thyroid hormones and metabolites of long-chain fatty acids, associate with DNA response elements in the promoter region of target genes and act either to activate or repress transcription. The response elements to which retinoic acid and other retinoids bind to are called retinoid response elements. The role of vitamin A in epithelial differentiation, as well as in other physiological processes, is thought to be mediated via retinoic acid's hormonal activity.

High-dose vitamin A has been used in the management of various skin disorders, including acne; Darier's disease or keratosis follicularis, an autosomal dominant disorder of keratinization; pityriasis rubra pilaris, an abnormality of follicular keratinization; Kyrle's disease, a focal derangement of orientation of keratinization and xerosis. None of the above uses are FDA approved. FDA-approved retinoids, include tretinoin (all-trans-retinoic acid), which is used topically for acne vulgaris; isotretinoin (13-*cis*-retinoic acid), for cystic acne; etretinate, a synthetic analog of retinoic acid ethyl ester, for psoriasis; and acitretin, a metabolite of etretinate, also for psoriasis. FDA-approved retinoids used for the treatment of malignancies, include alitretinoin (9-*cis*-retinoic acid), a topical treatment for Kaposi's sarcoma; all-*trans*-retinoic acid, for acute promyelocytic leukemia; and bexarotene, for refractory cutaneous T-cell lymphoma.

The parent compound of the vitamin A family is all-*trans*-retinol. It is also the most abundant dietary form of vitamin A. All-*trans*-retinol occurs naturally in the form of fatty acid esters, such as vitamin A palmitate (retinyl palmitate). Vitamin A palmitate and vitamin A acetate (retinyl acetate) are the principal forms used as nutritional supplements. All-*trans*-retinol, as is the case of all forms of vitamin A, is a derivative of beta-ionone. All-*trans*-retinol is also known as retinol, vitamin A_1, anti-infective vitamin, vitamin A alcohol and (all-*E*)-3, 7-dimethyl-9- (2, 6, 6-trimethyl-1-cyclohexen-1-y1)-2, 4, 6, 8-nonatetraen-1-o1. Its molecular formula is

$C_{20}H_{30}O$ and its molecular weight is 286.46 daltons. Its structural formula is:

Vitamin A

Other naturally occurring forms of vitamin A, include retinal (retinaldehyde, retinene, vitamin A_1 aldehyhde), retinoic acid (vitamin A_1 acid), retinoyl-beta-glucuronide (vitamin A_1 beta-glucuronide), retinyl phosphate (vitamin A_1 phosphate), 3-dehydroretinol (vitamin A_2), 11-*cis*-retinal (11-*cis*-retinal-dehyde, 11-*cis* or neo b vitamin A_1 aldehyde), 5, 6-epoxyretinol (5, 6-epoxy vitamin A_1 alcohol), anhydroretinol (anhydro vitamin A_1) and 4-ketoretinol (4-keto-vitamin A_1 alcohol). Except for all-*trans*-retinol, retinyl palmitate and retinyl acetate, all the other above-mentioned forms are minor dietary components.

Amounts of vitamin A are expressed in four ways: international units (IU), United States Pharmacopeia (USP) units, micrograms and retinol equivalents. One IU is equal to one USP unit. One IU of vitamin A activity is defined as either equal to 0.30 micrograms of all-*trans* retinol or to 0.60 micrograms of the provitamin A, all-*trans*-beta-carotene. One retinol equivalent (RE) is defined as one microgram of all-*trans* retinol, six micrograms of all-*trans*-beta-carotene or 12 micrograms of other provitamin A carotenoids.

ACTIONS AND PHARMACOLOGY

ACTIONS

Vitamin A may prevent loss of vision or restore lost vision. Vitamin A may have anticarcinogenic, immunomodulatory and antioxidant activities.

MECHANISM OF ACTION

Vitamin A deficiency can result in night blindness and blindness due to the destruction of the cornea (xerophthalmia). The ability of vitamin A to prevent these two visual problems and its mechanism of action in doing so is well known (see Description). There are a couple of recent reports that suggest vitamin A may affect some visual problems in those who are not vitamin A-deficient. Sorsby's fundus dystrophy (SFD) is an autosomal dominant retinal degeneration disorder which, among other things, can result in night blindness. SFD, both clinically and histopathologically, shares similarities with age-related macular degeneration, the most common cause of loss of vision in the elderly. In an SFD family, it was found that vitamin A at 50,000 IU daily resolved night blindness within a week in those members of the family who were at early stages of the disease. The

mechanism of this effect is not clear. The researchers hypothesized that the abnormally thickened Bruch's membrane, with its lipid deposits, acts as a barrier to the diffusion of vitamin A presented from the choroidal vasculature, essentially causing vitamin A deficiency in the retina. According to this hypothesis, large doses of vitamin A override the reduced transport efficiency of retinol across the defective Bruch's extracellular matrix. Direct or indirect effects of retinol on retinal pigment epithelial (RPE) cells are other possibilities. Vitamin A is known to modulate RPE cellular function and behavior. In another study, an oral retinoid was found to restore visual pigment and function in a mouse model of childhood blindness. Leber's congenital amaurosis (LCA) is an autosomal recessive mitochondrial disease which results in retinal degeneration. It is a rare variant of the more common disease, retinitis pigmentosum. Researchers found that administration of the vitamin A form 9-*cis*-retinal to the mice led to signs of visual improvement. The researchers hypothesized that 9-*cis*-retinal bypassed the biochemical block in the retina caused by the disease. Human studies are needed. It must be noted, however, that high doses of vitamin A have the potential for serious side effects.

Vitamin A and retinoids have been found to inhibit tumor development, especially those of epithelial origin, in a variety of *in vitro* studies. All-*trans*-retinol has been demonstrated to suppress the malignant behavior of cultured cells transformed by radiation, chemicals or viruses, to delay the development of transplanted tumors and to prevent malignancy in animals exposed to various potent carcinogens. It is thought that the anticarcinogenic effect of preformed vitamin A (all-*trans*-retinol) in these cases are mediated by its conversion to retinoic acid. Retinoic acid, via its binding to nuclear receptors (retinoic acid receptors, retinoid X receptors), may induce cell differentiation, inhibit proliferation and/or induce apoptosis. Many of these results were obtained using doses of all-*trans*-retinol that were very high and that would be too toxic for general, preventive use. Further, it is unclear whether sufficient conversion of all-*trans*-retinol to retinoic acid occurs to make a significant anticarcinogenic impact. A recent two-year study (EUROSCAN) of high-dose retinyl palmitate showed no benefit—in terms of survival, event-free survival, or secondary primary tumors—for patients with head and neck cancer or with lung cancer, most of whom were previous or current smokers.

Some retinoids, however, have shown anticancer effects in certain situations. All-*trans*-retinoic acid is an approved drug for the treatment of acute promyelocytic leukemia (APL). The mechanism of action of all-*trans*-retinoic acid in the treatment of APL is not fully understood. Those with APL possess an abnormal gene for retinoic acid receptor-alpha

(RAR-alpha). Treatment with all-*trans*-retinoic acid induces expression of the remaining normal RAR-alpha allele, which may rebalance the receptor system toward normal differentiation. Bexarotene is a synthetic retinoid analogue which is approved for the treatment of cutaneous T-cell lymphoma. The mechanism of action of bexarotene is unknown. It is known to activate retinoid X receptors (RXR), which pair with other cellular receptors to control the expression of genes involved in cellular differentiation and growth. The use of retinoids in the treatment of cancer is known as differentiation therapy.

Vitamin A deficiency results in decreased resistance to infection. Vitamin A deficiency affects both cell-mediated and antibody-mediated immune responses. Nonspecific immune responses involving neutrophils, macrophages and natural killer cells, are also affected by vitamin A deficiency. It is thought that vitamin A's participation in the immune response is via signal transduction pathways which are necessary for the normal functioning of the immune system. Retinol may also stimulate the immune response in animals and humans who are not vitamin A deficient. High doses of retinyl palmitate have been found to stimulate the nonspecific immune system in animals. Retinol and retinoic acid have also been found to enhance the antibody response to specific antigens, again, in animals. In surgery patients treated with high doses of vitamin A for seven days after surgery, lymphocyte proliferation did not differ from the control group after one day, but was significantly greater after seven days. The mechanism of action of the possible immunomodulatory effect of vitamin A is not well understood. Further, the studies of immunomodulation in animals that were not vitamin A-deficient used vitamin A doses that would be toxic in humans.

Vitamin A deficiency has been found to cause oxidative damage to liver mitochondria in rats. In these animals, a deficit of Vitamin A produced an increase in oxidized glutathione, malondialdehyde, 8-oxo-deoxyguanosine, a drop in the mitochondrial membrane potential and an 80% decrease in the reduced glutathione to oxidized glutathione ratio. Vitamin A has also been found to protect against lipid peroxidation induced by doxorubicin in heart and brain membrane lipids and to inhibit chemiluminescence and lipid peroxidation in isolated rat liver microsomes and mitochondria. The antioxidant mechanism of vitamin A is thought to be due, in part, to the hydrophobic chain of polyene units, which can quench singlet oxygen, neutralize thiyl radicals and stabilize and combine with peroxyl radicals.

PHARMACOKINETICS
Preformed vitamin A is present in food in the form of retinyl esters. The principal nutritional supplement forms of preformed vitamin A are retinyl palmitate and retinyl acetate.

Retinyl palmitate is also used in food fortification. Preformed vitamin A is efficiently absorbed from the small intestine. The efficiency of absorption ranges from 60%-90%. Vitamin A absorption requires bile salts, pancreatic enzymes and dietary fat. Vitamin A is delivered to the enterocytes in the form of micelles. Prior to its absorption, the retinyl esters are hydrolyzed by a pancreatic hydrolase. Long-chain retinyl esters, such as retinyl palmitate, appear to be hydrolyzed by a hydrolyase which is a component of the brush border. Within the enterocytes, all-*trans*-retinol is re-esterified to retinyl esters and the retinyl esters are secreted by the enterocytes into the lymphatics in the form of chylomicrons.

The chylomicrons enter the circulation via the thoracic duct. Chylomicrons undergo metabolism in the circulation via lipoprotein lipase to form chylomicron remnants. Most of the retinyl esters in chylomicron remnants are rapidly taken up into liver parenchymal cells. Within the liver parenchymal cells, retinyl esters are again hydrolyzed to all-*trans*-retinol and fatty acids. All-*trans*-retinol may be stored in the liver as retinyl esters or may be transported in the circulation bound to serum retinol binding protein (RBP). RBP delivers retinol to the various tissues. Approximately 50%-85% of the total body vitamin A content is stored in the liver. Greater than 95% of serum retinol is present in its unesterified form.

Serum retinol binding (RBP) protein is the principal carrier of all-*trans*-retinol, which comprises over 90% of serum vitamin A. RBP is found in serum in association with a cotransport protein called transthyretin or prealbumin. The mechanism of the transport of retinol into target cells is not known. Within cells, retinol and its metabolites are bound to retinoid-binding proteins in the cytosol and nucleus. The cytosolic retinoid-binding proteins are: cellular retinol-binding protein I (CRBP-I), cellular retinol-binding protein II (CRBP-II), cellular retinoic acid-binding protein I (CRABP-I) and cellular retinoic acid-binding protein II (CRABP-II). The nuclear retinoid-binding proteins are: retinoic acid receptor-alpha (RAR-alpha), retinoic acid receptor-beta (RAR-beta), retinoic acid receptor-gamma (RAR-gamma), retinoid X receptor-alpha (RXR-alpha), retinoid X receptor-beta (RXR-beta) and retinoid X receptor-gamma (RXR-gamma). The cytosolic retinoid-binding proteins limit the amounts of unbound or free retinoids and channel them to specific enzymes responsible for their metabolism. The nuclear retinoid-binding proteins bind retinoids and regulate the activities of retinoid-responsive genes.

All-trans retinol is oxidized to retinal via retinol dehydrogenase: retinal is metabolized to retinoic acid via retinal dehydrogenase. All-*trans*-retinol is delivered to the cornea via the tears and by diffusion through eye tissue. Retinol and retinoic acid form a number of oxidized metabolites. The metabolites of retinol and retinoic acid undergo glucuronidation, glucosylation and amino acylation and are excreted mainly via the biliary route. Some excretion of retinol and its metabolites occurs via the kidneys.

INDICATIONS AND USAGE

A major role has emerged for vitamin A in the treatment of malnourished children, principally in developing countries. It is credited with significantly reducing mortality and the incidence of blindness, diarrhea, measles and some other infections in these populations. Vitamin A appears to have many positive effects in the immune system and may have some anti-cancer effects. It can help with some skin conditions and may be useful in some with Sorsby's fundus dystrophy. There is emerging evidence that vitamin A plays crucial roles in embryonic development, and some believe it will eventually be used to prevent teratogenesis under some circumstances. Pregnant women, however, should not use doses of vitamin A greater than the U.S. RDA (5,000 IU/day) without a physician's recommendation and supervision.

RESEARCH SUMMARY

Several large, well-controlled, double-blind intervention trials have shown that intermittent high-dose vitamin A supplementation in malnourished children can significantly reduce mortality and the incidence of blindness, diarrhea, measles and some other infections. In one of these trials, there was a significant 27% relative reduction in mortality from all causes in children who received vitamin A supplementation. In another study, this one involving 11,200 children in Indonesia, there was a 30% lower mortality in supplemented children. Six of eight such intervention studies have shown significant reductions in mortality.

Other studies have shown significant reduction in morbidity in similar populations supplemented with vitamin A. Significant reductions in xerophthalmia, blindness, measles, diarrhea and some parasitic infections have been reported. Less dramatic effects have been seen in respiratory infections. The World Health Organization estimates that there are 250 million preschool-age children worldwide whose health may be compromised by vitamin A deficiency. For some years, WHO and some other health organizations have recommended administering large doses of vitamin A to at-risk children at the time they are vaccinated for measles. This practice caused concern when one study suggested that the vitamin A dose was interfering with seroconversion to live measles vaccine in infants with maternal antibodies. A more recent study, however, has refuted this finding to the satisfaction of many. The researchers concluded that "there is no indication that simultaneous administration of measles vaccine and vitamin A supplements has a negative effect on measles immunity."

Vitamin A's effects on immunity generally appear to be broad. It was demonstrated some years ago that high-dose vitamin A can significantly protect against some of the immune-depressing effects of radiation and cancer chemotherapy. Animal and *in vitro* work, as well as some human work, has shown that vitamin A can protect immune function by helping to maintain the integrity of epithelial barriers to infection and by activating phagocytes and cytotoxic T-cells, among other activities.

There is some evidence that vitamin A can stimulate and otherwise favorably affect the immune system even in the absence of frank or marginal vitamin A deficiency. Such effects have been demonstrated in a number of animal models.

An *in vitro* experiment showed that a form of vitamin A found in breast milk inhibits herpes simplex virus-1. And vitamin A, administered to surgical patients in large daily doses (90 to 135 milligrams) for seven days, significantly increased lymphocyte proliferation. Research on the immune-modulating effects of vitamin A continues. Many *in vitro* and some animal studies have shown that vitamin A can inhibit malignant activity in various types of cells adversely affected by radiation, chemicals and viruses. The vitamin variously delayed or prevented malignancy in animals exposed to several different carcinogens. Drug derivatives of vitamin A have demonstrated efficacy against some cancers and pre-cancerous lesions, including oral leucoplakia, myelodysplastic syndrome, cutaneous T-cell lymphoma and cervical cancer. Retinoids have been shown to help regulate the expression of some proto-oncogenes and protein growth factors. And retinoic acid has demonstrated an ability to inhibit proliferation of some tumor cells and to promote differentiation of some other cancer cells *in vitro*.

On the other hand, vitamin A, in combination with beta-carotene, showed no anti-cancer efficacy in an aborted intervention study of smokers, former smokers and workers exposed to asbestos. There was a statistically non-significant increase in incidence of lung cancer and mortality in the treated group. (See Beta-Carotene.)

Vitamin A and its drug derivatives have been used with significant success in the treatment of several skin disorders, including cystic acne, acne vulgaris, psoriasis and photoaged skin. High-dose vitamin A and theses drugs require careful medical supervision and must not be used during pregnancy, owing to risk of birth defects.

One study has shown that high-dose vitamin A (50,000 IU per day) significantly reversed night blindness in some with Sorsby's fundus dystrophy, a rare autosomal retinal degeneration disorder that is clinically similar to age-related macular degeneration. Lower doses (5,000 IU daily) had no effect, but it was suggested that lower doses begun early in disease progression might be helpful. Testing with intermediate doses was also proposed.

Recently, research has suggested that vitamin A might be helpful in preventing some birth defects—surprising to some, since high-dose vitamin A supplementation is itself associated with risk of birth defects. But so is vitamin A deficiency. Current research shows that retinoic acid signaling is crucial for proper development of the early embryonic mesoderm. There are further suggestions that impaired retinoid signaling could have negative effects not only on the embryo but later in life, as well, in terms of neurologic and behavioral development and function. Even schizophrenia, some researchers believe, may be promoted by retinoid defects. Obviously, much more research will be required before any possible strategies for safely and effectively utilizing vitamin A for the prevention of birth defects emerge.

CONTRAINDICATIONS, PRECAUTIONS, ADVERSE REACTIONS

CONTRAINDICATIONS

Doses of vitamin A above 5,000 IU are contraindicated in pregnant women.

Vitamin A is contraindicated in those hypersensitive to any component of a vitamin A-containing product.

Vitamin A is contraindicated in those with hypervitaminosis A.

PRECAUTIONS

The use of vitamin A for the treatment of vitamin A deficiency requires medical supervision.

The use of vitamin A or any retinoid for the treatment of any medical condition must be prescribed and supervised by a physician.

Nursing mothers should avoid doses of vitamin A great than the U.S. RDA (5,000 IU daily), unless prescribed by a physician.

Supplemental vitamin A may add to the toxicity of retinoids or retinoid analogues which are used pharmaceutically. These include acitretin, all-*trans*-retinoic acid, bexarotene, etretinate and isotretinoin. Those taking any of these drugs should avoid the use of supplemental vitamin A.

Too little or too much vitamin A may increase the risk of osteoporosis. Further research into the relationship between vitamin A and the risk of osteoporosis is needed and warranted. For now, doses higher than the DV or U.S. RDA (5,000 IU) should not be used except if medically indicated and prescribed and monitored by a physician.

ADVERSE REACTIONS

High intakes of vitamin A may cause acute or chronic toxicity. (see overdosage for acute toxicity). Symptoms and signs of chronic toxicity include dry rough skin, cracked lips, sparse coarse hair and alopecia of the eyebrows. These are early signs. Late symptoms and signs include irritability, headache, pseudotumor cerebri (benign intracranial hypertension), elevated serum liver enzymes, reversible noncirrhotic portal hypertension, hepatic fibrosis and cirrhosis. There are a few reports of death secondary to liver failure.

Supplemental doses of 10,000 IU of vitamin A daily or greater have been reported to increase the risk of birth defects when used by pregnant women.

Subjects in the EUROSCAN study were given 300,000 IU/day of vitamin A for one year followed by 150,000 IU/day for the second year. Typical side effects were mucocutaneous ones (dryness, desquamation, itching, bleeding and hair loss).

Hepatotoxicity has been reported in one patient who took 25,000 IU/day of vitamin A over a six-year period.

INTERACTIONS

DRUGS

Cholestyramine: Concomitant intake of cholestyramine and vitamin A may reduce the absorption of vitamin A.

Colestipol: Concomitant intake of colestipol and vitamin A may reduce the absorption of vitamin A.

Mineral Oil: Concomitant intake of mineral oil and vitamin A may reduce the absorption of vitamin A.

Oral Contraceptives: Oral contraceptives may increase serum retinol.

Orlistat: Orlistat may decrease the absorption of vitamin A.

Retinoid Drugs (acitretin, all-trans-retinoic acid, bexarotene, etretinate and isotretinoin): Supplemental vitamin A may add to the toxicity of these drugs (see Precautions).

NUTRITIONAL SUPPLEMENTS

Vitamin K: Intake of large doses of vitamin A may decrease the absorption of vitamin K.

FOODS

Olestra: The fat substitute olestra inhibits the absorption of vitamin A as well as the other fat-soluble vitamins D, E and K. These vitamins are added to olestra to compensate for this. Olestra contains 170 IU of vitamin A per gram (51 retinol equivalents per gram).

OVERDOSAGE

Acute toxicity in infants or children can occur with a single dose of 25,000 IU per kilogram of body weight. Vomiting, increased intracranial pressure and death may occur. A dose of 2,000,000 IU or greater in adults, can cause a similar clinical picture. Some Arctic explorers have ingested several million units of vitamin A from eating polar bear or seal liver, two of the richest sources of vitamin A. The Arctic explorers developed irritability, drowsiness, headache and vomiting. There are few reports of fatalities with such high doses of vitamin A.

DOSAGE AND ADMINISTRATION

The two principal forms of vitamin A supplements are retinyl acetate and retinyl palmitate. Multivitamin preparations contain vitamin A in one of these forms, a combination of vitamin A and beta-carotene (provitamin A) or beta-carotene alone. Rarely are doses higher than 5,000 IU of vitamin A exceeded in these formulas. Supplemental doses of vitamin A greater than 10,000 IU daily are not recommended. Many take beta-carotene for vitamin A supplementation (see Beta-Carotene). Vitamin A is also available in the form of cod liver oil.

Dietary Reference Intake (DRI) values for Vitamin A

DRI values—microgram Retinol Activity Equivalent (RAE)/day

Infants	Adequate Intake (AI)
0-6 months	400 (1,333 IU)
7-12 months	500 (1,667 IU)

Children	Recommended Daily Allowance (RDA)
1-3 years	300 (1,000 IU)
4-8 years	400 (1,333 IU)

Boys	
9-13 years	600 (2,000 IU)
14-18 years	900 (3,000 IU)

Girls	
9-13 years	600 (2,000 IU)
14-18 years	700 (2,333 IU)

Men	
19-30 years	900 (3,000 IU)
31-50 years	900 (3,000 IU)
51-70 years	900 (3,000 IU)
Older than 70 years	900 (3,000 IU)

Women	
19-30 years	700 (2,333 IU)
31-50 years	700 (2,333 IU)
51-70 years	700 (2,333 IU)
Older than 70 years	700 (2,333 IU)

Pregnancy	
14-18 years	750 (2,500 IU)
19-30 years	770 (2,567 IU)
31-50 years	770 (2,567 IU)

Lactation	
14-18 years	1,200 (4,000 IU)
19-30 years	1,300 (4,333 IU)
31-50 years	1,300 (4,333 IU)

The following summarizes the Tolerable Upper Intake Level (UL) for various age groups and conditions:

Children	(UL)
1-3 years	600 (2,000 IU)
4-8 years	600 (2,000 IU)
9-13 years	1,700 (5,660 IU)

Adolescents	
14-18 years	2,800 (9,300 IU)

Adults	
19 years and older	3,000 (10,000 IU)

Pregnancy	
14-18 years	2,800 (9,300 IU)
19 years and older	3,000 (10,000 IU)

Lactation	
14-18 years	2,800 (9,300 IU)
19 years and older	3,000 (10,000 IU)

RAE-Retinol activity equivalent. 1 microgram RAE = 1 microgram retinol, 12 micrograms beta carotene, and 24 micrograms alpha-carotene or beta-cryptoxanthin. The RAE for dietary provitamin A carotenoids in foods is twofold greater than retinol equivalents (RE), whereas the RAE for preformed vitamin A in foods is the same as the RE.

The UL for Vitamin A applies only to preformed vitamin A. It does not apply to Vitamin A derived from carotenoids.

One IU or one USP unit equals 0.30 micrograms of all-*trans*-retinol, 0.344 micrograms of retinyl acetate or 0.55 micrograms of retinyl palmitate.

The U.S. RDA is different than the customary RDAs. The U.S. RDA, which is used on nutritional supplement labels and food labels, is usually the highest RDA value. In the case of vitamin A, the U.S. RDA is 5,000 IU, which is slightly higher than the highest RDA value (4,333) for the vitamin.

The DV (Daily Value) for vitamin A, which is used for determining percentage of nutrient daily values on nutritional supplement and food labels, is 5,000 IU (International Units). The basis for the DV for vitamin A is the U.S. RDA.

LITERATURE

Acott TS, Weleber RG. Vitamin A megatherapy for retinal abnormalities. *Nature Med.* 1995;1:884-885.

Barber T, Borrás E, Torres L, et al. Vitamin A deficiency causes oxidative damage to liver mitochondria in rats. *Free Rad Biol Med.* 2000;29:1-7.

Barreto ML, Santos LMP, Assis AMO, et al. Effect of vitamin A supplementation on diarrhoea and acute lower-respiratory-tract infections in young children in Brazil. *Lancet.* 1994;344:228-231.

Bates CJ. Vitamin A. *Lancet.* 1995;345:31-35.

Benn CS, Aaby P, Balé C, et al. Randomized trial of effect of vitamin A supplementation on antibody response to measles vaccine in Guinea-Bissau, West Africa. *Lancet.* 1997;350:101-105.

Chiang M-Y, Misner D, Kempermann G, et al. An essential role for retinoid receptors RARbeta and RXRgamma in long-term potentiation and depression. *Neuron.* 1998;21:1353-1361.

Collins MD, Mao GE. Teratology of retinoids. *Annu Rev Pharmacol Toxicol.* 1999;39:399-430.

Futoryan T, Gilchrest BA. Retinoids and the skin. *Nutr Rev.* 1994;52:299-310.

Gilchrest B. Anti-sunshine vitamin A. *Nature Med.* 1999;5:376-377.

Hadi H, Stoltzfus RJ, Dibley MJ, et al. Vitamin A supplementation selectively improves the linear growth of Indonesian preschool children: results from a randomized controlled trial. *Am J Clin Nutr.* 2000;71:507-513.

Humphrey JH, Rice AL. Vitamin A supplementation of young infants. *Lancet.* 2000;356:422-424.

Institute of Medicine, Food and Nutrition Board. Dietary Reference Intakes for vitamin A, vitamin K, arsenic, boron, chromium, copper, iodine, iron, manganese, molybdenum, nickel, silicon, vanadium, and zinc. Washington, DC: National Academy Press, 2001.

Jacobson SG, Cideciyan AV, Regunath G, et al. Night blindness in Sorsby's fundus dystrophy reversed by vitamin A. *Nature Gen.* 1995;11:27-32.

Kowalski TE, Falestiny M, Furth E, Malet PF. Vitamin A hepatotoxicity: a cautionary note regarding 25,000 IU supplements. *Am J Med.* 1994;97:523-528.

Lee M-O, Han S-Y, Jiang S, et al. Differential effects of retinoic acid on growth and apoptosis in human colon cancer cell lines associated with the induction of retinoic acid receptor beta. *Biochem Pharmacol.* 2000;59:485-496.

Ribaya-Mercado, JD, Blumberg JB. Vitamin A: is it a risk factor for osteoporosis and bone fracture? *Nutr Rev.* 2007;65(10):425-438.

Ross AC. Vitamin A and retinoids. In: Shils ME, Olson JA, Shike M, Ross AC, eds. *Modern Nutrition in Health and Disease.* 9th ed. Baltimore, MD: Williams and Wilkins;1999:305-327.

Ross AC, Stephensen CB. Vitamin A and retinoids in antiviral responses. *FASEB J.* 1996;10:979-985.

Rothman KJ, Moore LL, Singer MR, et al. Teratogenicity of high vitamin A intake. *N Engl J Med.* 1995;333:1369-1373.

Russell RM. The vitamin A spectrum: from deficiency to toxicity. *Am J Clin Nutr.* 2000;71:878-884.

Sohlenius-Sternbeck A-K, Appelkvist E-L, De Pierre JW. Effects of vitamin A deficiency on selected xenobiotic-metabolizing enzymes and defenses against oxidative stress in mouse liver. *Biochem Pharmacol.* 2000;59:377-383.

Underwood BA, Arthur P. The contribution of vitamin A to public health. *FASEB J.* 1996;10:1040-1048.

Van Hooser JP, Aleman TS, He Y-G, et al. Rapid restoration of visual pigment and function with oral retinoid in a mouse model of childhood blindness. *Proc Natl Acad Sci USA.* 2000;97:8623-8628.

Varani J, Warner RL, Gharaee-Kermani M, et al. Vitamin A antagonizes decreased cell growth and elevated collagen-degrading matrix metalloproteinases and stimulates collagen accumulation in naturally aged human skin. *J Invest Dermatol.* 2000;114:480-486.

Wang Z, Boudjelal M, Kang S, et al. Ultraviolet irradiation of human skin causes functional vitamin A deficiency, preventable by all-*trans* retinoic acid pre-treatment. *Nature Med.* 1999;5:418-422.

West KP Jr, Pokhrel RP, Katz J, et al. Efficacy of vitamin A in reducing preschool child mortality in Nepal. *Lancet.* 1991;338:67-71.

Wolf G. A history of vitamin A and retinoids. *FASEB J.* 1996; 10:1102-1107.

Wolf G. A regulatory pathway of thermogenesis in brown fat through retinoic acid. *Nutr Rev.* 1995;53:230-231.

Wolf G. Vitamin A functions in the regulation of the dopaminergic system in the brain and pituitary gland. *Nutr Rev.* 1998; 56:354-358.

Vitamin B$_6$

DESCRIPTION

Vitamin B$_6$ is the collective term for a group of three related compounds, pyridoxine (PN), pyridoxal (PL) and pyridox-amine (PM), and their phosphorylated derivatives, pyridox-ine 5'-phosphate (PNP), pyridoxal 5'-phosphate (PLP) and pyridoxamine 5'-phosphate (PMP). Although all six of these vitamers should technically be referred to as vitamin B$_6$, the term vitamin B$_6$ is commonly used interchangeably with just one of the vitamers, pyridoxine. Vitamin B$_6$, principally in the form of the coenzyme pyridoxal 5'-phosphate, is involved in a wide range of biochemical reactions, including the metabolism of amino acids and glycogen, the synthesis of nucleic acids, hemogloblin, sphingomyelin and other sphingolipids, and the synthesis of the neurotransmitters serotonin, dopamine, norepinephrine and gamma-aminobutyric acid (GABA).

Food sources of vitamin B_6, include meat, poultry, fish, eggs, white potatoes and other starchy vegetables, noncitrus fruits, fortified ready-to-eat cereals and fortified soy-based meat substitutes. The principal forms of vitamin B_6 in animal products are pyridoxal 5'-phosphate and pyridoxamine 5'-phosphate. In plant-derived foods, the major forms of vitamin B_6 are pyridoxine, pyridoxine 5'-phosphate and pyridoxine glucosides. Glycosylated forms of pyridoxine range from approximately 5% to 75% of the total vitamin B_6 content in fruits, vegetables and grains, with little to none in animal products. Pyridoxine appears to be the only glycosylated form of vitamin B_6. The major glycosylated form of pyridoxine in most plant-derived foods is pyridoxine 5'-beta-D-glucoside. Pyridoxine hydrochloride is the form of vitamin B_6 most commonly used for fortification of foods and in nutritional supplements.

The classical symptoms and signs of vitamin B_6 deficiency are a microcytic, hypochromic anemia, seizure activity, seborrheic dermatitis, confusion and depression. Vitamin B_6-deficiency states in infants and children primarily result in electroencephalogram abnormalities and seizure activity, while in adults, vitamin B_6 deficiency primarily results in cheilosis (chapping and fissuring of the lips), glossitis (inflammation of the tongue), stomatitis (inflammation of the oral mucosa), anemia, irritability, confusion and depression. Many of these signs are not specific for vitamin B_6 deficiency and may be due to deficiencies of other vitamins or result from other causes. Vitamin B_6 deficiency may result from the use of certain drugs, including isoniazid (isonicotinic acid hydrazide or INH), penicillamine, cycloserine, ethionamide, hydralazine and theophylline. Subclinical vitamin B_6 deficiency frequently occurs in those with malabsorption syndromes, uremia, cancer, heart failure and cirrhosis, and in alcoholics, the elderly and adolescent females and during pregnancy. In the elderly and in those with malabsorption syndromes, clinical deficiency of the vitamin may occur.

In addition to vitamin B_6 deficiency conditions, vitamin B_6-dependency conditions exist. Certain inborn errors of metabolism exist in which a vitamin B_6-dependent enzyme is defective in the coenzyme (pyridoxal 5'-phosphate) binding site, and the enzyme only has significant activity when the tissue concentration of pyridoxine 5'-phosphate, the biologically active form of vitamin B_6, is much higher than normal.

These vitamin B_6-dependent conditions, which may be responsive to treatment with large doses of the vitamin, include convulsions of the newborn secondary to glutamate decarboxylase (GAD) deficiency, cystathionuria secondary to cystathionase deficiency, gyrate atrophy with ornithinuria secondary to ornithinine-delta-aminotransferase deficiency, homocystinuria secondary to cystathionine beta-synthase deficiency, primary hyperoxaluria type 1 secondary to peroxisomal alanine-glyoxylate transaminase deficiency, sideroblastic anemia secondary to delta-aminolevulinate synthase deficiency and xanthurenic aciduria secondary to kynureninase deficiency. These genetic disorders are all rare.

Vitamin B_6 in the form of pyridoxal 5'-phosphate is a coenzyme for over 100 enzymes. Most of these enzymes are involved in amino acid metabolism and include aminotransferases (transaminases), decarboxylases. Pyridoxal 5'-phosphate is sometimes referred to as codecarboxylase. The basic chemistry accounting for the broad range of reactions of B_6 is Schiff's base formation. Schiff's bases are reaction products of aldehyde and amino groups. In the resting state of the above enzymes, the aldehyde group of pyridoxal 5'-phosphate is covalently linked to the epsilon-amino group of a lysine residue at the active site of the enzyme. Upon binding of the amino acid substrate, the lysine is exchanged for the alpha-amino group of the substrate, forming a Schiff's base with the aldehyde group of pyridoxal 5'-phosphate. A quinonoid intermediate follows the formation of the Schiff's base, which in turn is followed by the formation of the reaction products. Schiff's base chemistry is the mechanism of almost all of the reactions in which pyridoxal 5'-phosphate participates. One exception is the glycogen phosphorylase reaction. Glycogen phosphorylase catalyzes the breakdown of the storage polysaccharide glycogen to yield glucose 1-phosphate. Much of the total pyridoxal 5'-phosphate in the body is found in muscle bound to glycogen phosphorylase. In glycogen phosphorylase, the phosphate group of pyridoxal 5'-phosphate, rather than its aldehyde group, participates in the catalytic role of the enzyme.

Vitamin B_6 is involved in several key biological processes. Pyridoxal 5'-phosphate is the coenzyme for delta-aminolevulinate synthase, the first step in the synthesis of porphyrins. Heme is derived from protoporphyrin IX. Heme is the iron-containing prosthetic group that is an essential component of such proteins as hemoglobin, myoglobin and the cytochromes. Homocysteine is an intermediate in methionine metabolism and may undergo one of two metabolic fates, remethylation to L-methionine or further metabolism, leading to the synthesis of L-cysteine. The pathway leading to the synthesis of cysteine is known as the transsulfuration pathway. This pathway has two pyridoxal 5'-phosphate-dependent enzymes: cystathionine beta-synthase and cysta-thionase. The conversion of tryptophan to niacin also requires pyridoxal-5'-phosphate, this time as a cofactor for the pyridoxal 5'-phosphate-dependent enzyme kynureninase. And, via its role in transamination, pyridoxal 5'-phosphate is involved in the production of energy.

Decarboxylation of amino acids yields amines, including gamma-aminobutyrate, dopamine, norepinephrine, epinephrine and serotonin, which play important roles as neurotransmitters or hormones. The amino acid decarboxylases are also pyridoxal 5'-phosphate-dependent enzymes. Pyridoxal 5'-phosphate plays a role in the regulation of steroid hormone activity: Physiological levels of pyridoxal 5'-phosphate interact with glucocorticoid receptors to downregulate their activity. Pyridoxal 5'-phosphate has also been shown to negatively modulate steroid-dependent gene expression induced by progesterone, androgen and estrogen hormones. Finally, serine hydroxymethyltransferase is a pyridoxal 5'-phosphate-dependent enzyme that catalyzes the interconversion of serine and glycine, both of which are major sources of one-carbon units necessary for the *de novo* synthesis of purine nucleotides, including thymidylate. Purine nucleotides are precursors of DNA and RNA, and thymidylate is a precursor of DNA.

The vitamers comprising the vitamin B6 family are pyridine derivatives. Specifically, they are derivatives of 3-hydroxy-5-hydroxymethyl-2-methyl pyridine. The vitamers differ by the nature of the chemical group occupying the 4 position of the parent compound. In the case of pyridoxine, the 4 position is occupied by an hydroxymethyl group. Pyridoxine is also known as 5-hydroxy-6-methyl-3, 4-pyridinedimethanol, 2-methyl-3-hydroxy-4,5-bis(hydroxymethyl)pyridine and pyridoxol. Its molecular formula is $C_8H_{11}NO_3$ and its molecular weight is 169.17 daltons. Pyridoxine hydrochloride is the principal form of vitamin B6 used in nutritional supplements and for food fortification.

Pyridoxal is also known as 3-hydroxy-5-(hydroxymethyl)-2-methyl-4-pyridinecarboxaldehyde and 2-methyl-3-hydroxy-4-formyl-5-hydroxymethylpyridine. In the case of pyridoxal, the 4 position of the parent compound is occupied by a formyl group. The molecular formula of pyridoxal is $C_8H_9NO_3$ and its molecular weight is 167.16 daltons. Pyridoxamine has an aminomethyl group occupying the 4 position of the parent structure. Pyridoxamine is also known as 4-(aminomethyl)-5-hydroxy-6-methyl-3-pyridinemethanol and 2-methyl-3-hydroxy-4-aminomethyl-5-hydroxymethyl-pyridine. Its molecular formula is $C_8H_{12}N_2O_2$ and its molecular weight is 168.18.

ACTIONS AND PHARMACOLOGY
ACTIONS
Vitamin B6 has antineurotoxic activity and may have activity in a number of inborn errors of metabolism, including pyridoxine-dependent seizures in infants, sideroblastic anemia, primary hyperoxaluria, homocystinuria and cystathioninuria. Vitamin B6 has putative antiatherogenic, immunomodulatory, anticarcinogenic and mood-modulatory activities.

MECHANISM OF ACTION
Vitamin B6 is used in the prophylaxis and treatment of vitamin B6 deficiency and peripheral neuropathy in those receiving isoniazid (isonicotinic acid hydrazide, INH). The antituberculosis drug isoniazid reacts non-enzymatically with pyridoxal 5'-phosphate to form a metabolically inactive hydrazone. This can result in vitamin B6 deficiency and peripheral neuropathy. It may also result in pellagra. The formation of niacin from tryptophan is catalyzed by, among other enzymes, kynureninase. Kynureninase is a vitamin B6-dependent enzyme. Therefore, vitamin B6 deficiency resulting from isoniazid, particularly in the context of marginal or clinical niacin deficiency, may lead to the niacin deficiency disorder pellagra. The peripheral neuropathy resulting from isoniazid does not appear to be due to vitamin B6 deficiency, but to isoniazid itself. The antineurotoxic effect of vitamin B6 in the case of isoniazid appears to be accounted for by the reaction of the vitamin with the drug, thus lowering its tissue level and its neurotoxicity.

High theophylline levels may cause seizures. It is thought that this is due to reaction of theophylline with pyridoxal 5'-phosphate, leading to lowered plasma levels of the vitamin. Pyridoxal 5'-phosphate is involved in the metabolism of gamma-aminobutyric acid (GABA). GABA is a major inhibitory neurotransmitter in the central nervous system. When the concentration of GABA in the brain decreases to below a threshold level, seizures and other neurological disorders may occur. The concentration of GABA in the brain is controlled by two pyridoxal 5'-phosphate-dependent enzymes, glutamate decarboxylase (GAD) and GABA transaminase (GABA-T). A decrease in the levels of GABA in the brain secondary to decreased levels of pyridoxal 5'-phosphate can lead to seizures. It has been found that the administration of vitamin B6 to mice treated with theophylline reduced the number of seizures, and the vitamin administered to rabbits reversed electroencephalogram changes caused by high doses of theophylline.

Seven inborn errors of metabolism are known in which a vitamin B6-dependent enzyme has a defect in the coenzyme (pyridoxal 5'-phosphate) binding site, and the enzyme only has significant activity when the tissue concentration of pyridoxine 5'-phosphate is much higher than normal. The disorders and their enzyme defects are pyridoxine-dependent seizures in infants (glutamate decarboxylase deficiency resulting in decreased CNS levels of GABA), pyridoxine-responsive sideroblastic anemia (delta-aminolevulinate synthase deficiency resulting in decreased synthesis of hemogloblin), primary hyperoxaluria type 1 (peroxisomal alanine-glyoxylate transaminase deficiency), homocystinuria (cystathionine beta-synthase deficiency), cystathioninuria (gamma-cystathionase deficiency), xanthurenic aciduria (kynureninase deficiency) and gyrate atrophy of the choroid and retina (ornithine-delta-aminotransferase deficiency). These disorders may be responsive to high doses of vitamin B_6, which increase tissue levels of pyridoxal 5'-phosphate.

The putative antiatherogenic activity of vitamin B_6 may be accounted for by a few different mechanisms. Hyperhomocysteinemia is a risk factor for atherosclerosis, coronary heart disease and stroke. L-homocysteine is a sulfur amino acid that is an intermediate in the metabolism of L-methionine. It is either remethylated to L-methionine via methionine synthase, which requires 5-methyl-tetrahydrofolate as a methyl donor, and methylcobalamin (a biologically active form of vitamin B_{12}) as a cofactor for its enzymatic activity, or, via the transsulfuration pathway, is converted to L-cysteine. Two pyridoxal 5'-phosphate-dependent enzymes are involved in the conversion of homocysteine to L-cysteine: cystathionine beta-synthase and gamma-cystathionase. Cystathionine beta-synthase catalyzes the reaction of homocysteine and serine to produce cystathionine, and gamma-cystathionase hydrolyzes cystathionine to form L-cysteine and alpha-ketobutyrate. Under physiological conditions, there is a balance between homocysteine formation and degradation. Elevation of plasma total homocysteine is associated with increased cardiovascular risk and over the past two decades a number of large prospective studies have shown that hyperhomocysteinemia is predictive for an increased relative risk of coronary events, stroke, venous thromboembolism, cognitive impairment and death. Recently it was shown that feeding mice a diet deficient in the B-vitamins pyridoxal 5'-phosphate (vitamin B_6), folic acid and cyanocobalamin (vitamin B_{12}) caused hyperhomocysteinemia and vascular cognitive impairment. The hypothesis that hyperhomocysteinemia is a cardiovascular risk factor first arose from clinical and pathological observations in children and young adults with the rare disease hereditary homocysteinemia. (Mutations in cystathionine beta-synthase are the most common cause of hereditary hyperhomocysteinemia.) Those with this affliction, if untreated, develop severe hyperhomocysteinemia with plasma homocysteine levels greater than 100 micromoles per liter (normal levels are from 5 to 15 micromoles per liter), which can lead to thromboembolic events, vascular lesions and death. The treatment is high doses of vitamin B_6, vitamin B_{12}, folic acid and betaine,

and restriction of dietary methionine. However, several intervention trials have failed to show any clinical benefit of homocysteine-lowering therapy with B-vitamins. Interestingly, most of these trials were performed in subjects with relatively mild homocysteinemia (plasma levels between 10 and 30 micromoles per liter). Explanations for these negative trials range from insufficient statistical power of the trials, which would exclude a small clinical benefit, to concluding that mild hyperhomocysteinemia is not a causative risk factor. Clearly, further studies are needed and warranted.

Vitamin B_6, in the form of pyridoxine hydrochloride, has been found to lower systolic and diastolic blood pressure in a small group of subjects with essential hypertension. Hypertension is another risk factor for atherosclerosis and coronary heart disease. The mechanism of action of the antihypertensive effect of vitamin B_6 is unknown. Another study showed pyridoxine hydrochloride to inhibit ADP- or epinephrine-induced platelet aggregation and to lower total cholesterol levels and increase HDL-cholesterol levels, again in a small group of subjects. The mechanisms of action of the possible platelet and lipid effects of vitamin B_6 are unknown. Vitamin B_6, in the form of pyridoxal 5'-phosphate, was found to protect vascular endothelial cells in culture from injury by activated platelets. Endothelial injury and dysfunction are critical initiating events in the pathogenesis of atherosclerosis. The mechanism of the possible endothelial-protective effect of vitamin B_6 is unclear. It is thought that vitamin B_6 plays a role in the maintenance of endothelial integrity. Vitamin B_6 has been shown to have singlet oxygen quenching activity *in vitro*. Single oxygen is a reactive oxygen species and oxidative stress is thought to play a major role in the pathogenesis of atherosclerosis. Finally, vitamin B_6 is involved in the metabolism of (n-3) polyunsaturated fatty acids from alpha-linoleic acid to eicosapentaenoic acid (EPA) and docosahexaenoic acid (DHA). This may play some role in the putative antiatherogenic activity of vitamin B_6.

Both animal and human studies have demonstrated that vitamin B_6 deficiency affects cellular and humoral responses of the immune system. Vitamin B_6 deficiency results in altered lymphocyte differentiation and maturation, reduced delayed-type hypersensitivity (DTH) responses, impaired antibody production, decreased lymphocyte proliferation and decreased interleukin (IL)-2 production, among other immunologic activities. Those at risk for vitamin B_6 deficiency and associated immunological dysfunction are the elderly, those with uremia and those with HIV (human immunodeficiency virus) disease. Repletion of vitamin B_6 in those with vitamin B_6 deficiency can correct immunological dysfunctions. Supplementation of the vitamin in those who are vitamin B_6 sufficient, has not to date shown immune-enhancing or immunomodulatory effects. The mechanism through which vitamin B6 deficiency alters immune responses is not well understood. Vitamin B6 deficiency appears to impair nucleic acid synthesis. The impaired nucleic acid synthesis is associated with altered one-carbon metabolism, particularly the activity of serine hydroxymethyltransferase. Serine hydroxymethyltransferase is a pyridoxal 5'-phosphate-dependent enzyme which catalyzes the interconversion of serine and glycine, both of which are major sources of one-carbon units necessary for the synthesis of purine nucleotides and thymidylate. Impairment of purine nucleotide and thymidylate synthesis would impair the synthesis of nucleic acids. Serine hydroxymethyltransferase activity appears to be low in resting lymphocytes. Antigenic or mitogenic stimulation of immune cells triggers their proliferation. Serine hydroxymethyltransferase activity increases in immune cells under the influence of antigenic or mitogenic stimulation, thus supplying the increased demand for nucleic acid synthesis during an immune response. Since vitamin B6 is involved in the synthesis of nucleic acids, via serine hydromethyltransferase, deficiency of the vitamin would result in decreased DNA replication, with consequent decreases in RNA and protein synthesis and immune cell proliferation.

Pyridoxal has been found to inhibit the growth of human malignant melanoma cells *in vitro*. It has also been found to inhibit the growth of melanoma cells injected into mice. There is one report of topical vitamin B6 inducing lesion regression in two patients with melanoma. The mechanism of the putative anticarcinogenic activity of vitamin B6 is unknown. A recent Scottish large case-control observational study reported a moderately strong inverse association between vitamin B6 intake and incidence of colorectal cancer. The mechanism of action of this possible anticancer effect is unclear.

Vitamin B6 may be useful in managing the depressive symptoms in some women with premenstrual dysphoric disorder (PMDD), also known as premenstrual syndrome (PMS). However, the evidence for this comes mainly from poor-quality trials. The mechanism of this putative effect may be accounted for, in part, by the participation of pyridoxal 5'-phosphate as a coenzyme in the synthesis of the neurotransmitters serotonin and dopamine. Modulation of steroid-dependent gene expression, by the vitamin, may also play some role in this putative effect.

PHARMACOKINETICS

The major forms of vitamin B6 from animal products are pryridoxal 5'-phosphate and pyridoxamine 5'-phosphate. The major forms of vitamin B6 from plant-derived foods are pyridoxine, pyridoxine 5'-phosphate and pyridoxine glucosides. Pyridoxine hydrochloride is the principal form of

vitamin B6 used for food fortification and in nutritional supplements. Pyridoxal 5'-phosphate is also available as a nutritional supplement.

The phosphorylated forms of vitamin B6 undergo hydrolysis in the small intestine via alkaline phosphatase, and the nonphosphorylated forms of the vitamin are absorbed by a nonsaturable passive diffusion process, mainly in the jejunum. The efficacy of absorption of vitamin B6 is high and even extremely high doses of vitamin B6 are well absorbed. The pyridoxine glucosides are less efficiently absorbed than the other vitamin B6 forms. The pyridoxine glucosides are deconjugated by a mucosal glucosidase. A fraction of the pyridoxine glucosides is absorbed intact and hydrolyzed in various tissues.

Some vitamin B6 is converted to pyridoxal 5'-phosphate in the enterocytes where it is used in various metabolic reactions. Most of the absorbed vitamin B6 is transported via the portal circulation to the liver. In the liver, pyridoxine, pyridoxal and pyridoxamine are metabolized to pyridoxine 5'-phosphate, pyridoxal 5'-phosphate and pyridoxamine 5'-phosphate, by pyridoxal 5'-phosphate kinase. Pyridoxal 5'-phosphate is secreted by the liver and transported by the systemic circulation to the various tissues of the body. Pyridoxal 5'-phosphate is the primary form of vitamin B6 in the circulation and is bound to serum albumin.

The major body pool of vitamin B6 is in muscle, where most of the vitamin is present as pyridoxal 5'-phosphate bound to glycogen phosphorylase. The principal catabolite of vitamin B6 is 4-pyridoxic acid which is the primary form of the vitamin excreted in the urine. 4-Pyridoxic acid, which is principally formed in the liver, accounts for approximately 50% of the vitamin B6 compounds in the urine. At very high doses of vitamin B6, which is mainly in the form of pyridoxine, much of the dose is excreted unchanged in the urine.

INDICATIONS AND USAGE

INDICATIONS

Vitamin B6 is used for the treatment of vitamin B6 deficiency and for the prophylaxis of isoniazid-induced peripheral neuropathy. It may also be helpful in treatment of convulsions of the newborn secondary to glutamate decarboxylase deficiency, sideroblastic anemia secondary to delta-aminolevulinate synthase deficiency, primary hyperoxaluria type 1 secondary to peroxisomal alanine-glyoxylate transaminase deficiency, homocystinuria secondary to cystathionine beta-synthase deficiency, cystathioninuria secondary to gamma-cystathionase deficiency, xanthurenic aciduria secondary to kynureninase deficiency and gyrate atrophy of choroid and retina secondary to ornithinine-delta-aminotransferase deficiency.

Vitamin B_6 may be helpful in some women with premenstrual dysphoric disorder (PMDD), also known as premenstrual syndrome (PMS), and may be useful in some cases of gestational diabetes and for protection against metabolic imbalances associated with the use of some oral contraceptives. Results are mixed and largely negative with the respect to claims that vitamin B_6 is an effective treatment of carpal tunnel syndrome. There is very preliminary evidence that vitamin B_6 may help protect against atherosclerosis, that it might show some activity against melanoma and that it might be helpful in some neurologic conditions. It has some immune stimulating properties. It is an anti-emetic in some circumstances. There is little evidence to support claims that vitamin B_6 is an effective treatment for depression (other than, possibly, the depression associated with premenstrual syndrome), autism, schizophrenia, atopic dermatitis, alcoholism, diabetic peripheral neuropathy, Down's syndrome, dental caries, Huntington's chorea or steroid-dependent asthma.

RESEARCH SUMMARY

A recent review of randomized, double-blind, placebo-controlled trials of vitamin B_6 in the treatment of premenstrual syndrome (PMS) concluded that the treatment appeared to relieve overall premenstrual and premenstrual-associated depressive symptoms. Doses ranged between 50 milligrams and 600 milligrams of vitamin B_6 daily. Only one of 940 subjects included in these studies reported symptoms suggestive of sensory neuropathy, the principal adverse reaction of high dose vitamin B_6. Premenstrual symptoms appeared to be relieved by 100 milligrams of vitamin B_6 daily (typically in divided 50 milligram doses). There was less evidence of efficacy at a 50 milligram daily dose. Though the review authors found methodological flaws in many of the studies, several of which were of poor quality, they have stated that the available evidence warrants a large-scale multicenter clinical trial. Vitamin B_6's apparent efficacy in PMS has been speculatively attributed, in part, to its role as a cofactor in the synthesis of serotonin and dopamine, deficits in the availability and function of which may play a part in the pathogenesis of PMS.

There are reports that vitamin B_6 supplementation can help normalize disturbances in the metabolism of tryptophan associated with the use of some oral contraceptives. Studies suggest that 5 to 50 milligrams daily are adequate for this purpose. Improved glucose tolerance has been reported in some of these studies. Some other studies, however, have shown no vitamin B_6 effect on the nausea, vomiting, dizziness and irritability sometimes associated with the use of oral contraceptives. Evidence is conflicting and inconclusive with respect to vitamin B_6's impact on depression linked to the use of oral contraceptives.

Claims that vitamin B_6 is useful in improving glucose tolerance in diabetics in general is poorly supported except in gestational diabetes where the evidence is somewhat better, though still far from conclusive. More research is needed.

Studies on the use of vitamin B_6 in the treatment of carpal tunnel syndrome have produced mixed results which, on balance, suggest little benefit. Some open trials have found that vitamin B_6 is helpful, but most double-blind, placebo-controlled trials have reported no benefit. Until larger, better-designed studies are conducted, no useful conclusion can be reached with respect to vitamin B_6's role, if any, in treating carpal tunnel syndrome.

A lingering question is whether or not vitamin B_6 possesses antiatherogenic activity. Hyperhomocysteinemia is a risk factor for atherosclerosis, coronary heart disease and stroke. Results have been mixed on the ability of supplemental vitamin B_6 per se to lower homocysteine levels. Vitamin B_6, along with vitamin B_{12} and folic acid, lowers homocysteine levels in those with severe hyperhomocysteinemia, such as is found in the rare genetic disorder hereditary homocysteinemia, thus decreasing the risk of atherosclerosis, coronary heart disease, stroke and death in those individuals. Vitamin B_6 lowers homocysteine levels in pyridoxine-responsive homocystinuria and in patients with severe vitamin B_6 deficiencies. However, several intervention trials have failed to show any clinical benefit for homocysteine-lowering therapy with B-vitamins, including vitamin B_6, in subjects with relatively mild homocysteinemia. There is one uncontrolled report associating supplemental vitamin B_6 use with reduced incidence of acute cardiac chest pain and myocardial infarction. And there is a study showing a significant protective effect of vitamin B_6 on function and integrity of vascular endothelium subjected to experimental injury by activated platelets. There are also preliminary reports that supplemental vitamin B_6 can reduce hypertension in some. This work needs confirmation. A recent report of a large prospective study of middle-aged Japanese found a significant inverse association between vitamin B_6 intake and the risk of coronary heart disease, primarily myocardial infarction (MI). An approximately 40 to 50% reduction was found among individuals who consumed the highest quintile of dietary vitamin B_6 (median intake of 1.6 mg daily) compared with those at the lowest quintile of intake (median intake of 1.3 mg daily). A significant inverse association with MI was also found for vitamin B_{12}; the inverse association with MI was marginal for folate. The mechanism of action of the vitamin B_6 effect was unclear. It is clear, however, that further research is needed and warranted before the lingering question whether or not vitamin B_6 possesses antiatherogenic activity can be satisfactorily answered.

There was a report in 1985 that a topical application of pyridoxal produced significant regression in the metastatic melanoma of two patients. Greater than 50% regression of lesions was noted after two weeks of treatment. Untreated lesions did not regress. This preliminary report needs follow-up.

Vitamin B6 is an effective treatment for seizures in infants caused by a specific inborn metabolic disorder. Deficiencies in vitamin B6 have been associated with a number of neurologic and behavioral disorders, but interventive data are largely lacking. There is a study of Egyptian mothers and their infants significantly relating the vitamin B6 nutritional status of the mother to infant behavior. Some studies have indicated that, even in the United States, a significant percentage of women of child-bearing age, as well as pregnant and lactating women, may have vitamin B6 intakes below the recommended dietary allowance.

Studies are needed to determine the effects of low maternal vitamin B6 intake on neurologic and behavioral development in offspring: Experiments with vitamin B6-deficient maternal rats have demonstrated effects that might impair developmental processes related to learning and memory in offspring.

Vitamin B6 plays an active role in the immune system. Even marginal deficiency, such as is found in many of the elderly, may result in some immune deficits. Chronically ill patients, notably those with HIV-disease, also often exhibit marginal or frank vitamin B6 deficiency. Both humoral and cell-mediated immune responses have been shown to be impaired in those with vitamin B6 deficiencies. Supplementation to normal levels generally restores immune function due to deficiency. Higher doses have not been reported to further stimulate or modulate the immune system.

In one study, approximately one-third of a healthy elderly population had marginal vitamin B6 deficiency. Supplementation with the vitamin in elderly subjects has produced significant improvement in immune function as determined by a number of laboratory measures, including lymphocyte proliferative responses to both T- and B-cell mitogens. Percentages of CD3+ and CD4+ (but not CD8+) cells increased significantly in elderly subjects receiving 50 milligrams of vitamin B6 daily.

Vitamin B6 has been used with some success as an anti-emetic in a dose range of 50-200 milligrams daily. It has been effective in treating nausea subsequent to radiotherapy and nausea associated with pregnancy ("morning sickness"). In one double-blind trial, vitamin B6 alleviated the severe nausea and significantly reduced the vomiting of those who received the vitamin in 25 milligram doses every eight hours for three days.

CONTRAINDICATIONS, PRECAUTIONS, ADVERSE REACTIONS

CONTRAINDICATIONS

Vitamin B6 is contraindicated in those hypersensitive to any component of a vitamin B6-containing product.

PRECAUTIONS

Pre- and postnatal vitamin/mineral supplements typically deliver vitamin B6 (as pyridoxine) at a dose of between 2 to 20 milligrams daily. Pregnant women and nursing mothers should avoid doses of vitamin B6 greater than these doses, unless higher doses are prescribed by their physicians.

Those who are being treated with levodopa without concurrently taking carbidopa should avoid doses of vitamin B6 of 5 milligrams or greater daily.

The use of vitamin B6 for the treatment of vitamin B6 deficiency, for the prophylaxis of isoniazid-induced peripheral neuropathy, for the treatment of vitamin B6-dependency disorders (see Indications) or for the treatment of any other medical condition requires medical supervision.

ADVERSE REACTIONS

Doses of vitamin B6, typically in the form of pyridoxine, of up to 200 milligrams daily are generally well tolerated. One report showed severe sensory neuropathy in seven adults after pyridoxine intakes that started at 50 to 100 milligrams/day and were steadily increased to 2 to 6 grams/day over 2 to 40 months. None of the subjects in the report showed sensory neuropathy at doses of pyridoxine of less than 2 grams/day. There is one report of a woman who had been taking 200 milligrams/day of pyridoxine for 2 years without showing sensory neuropathy who developed sensory neuropathy after she increased her pyridoxine dose to 500 milligrams/day. There are rare reports of sensory neuropathy occurring at pyridoxine doses in the range of 100 to 200 milligrams/day. The Food and Nutrition Board of the Institute of Medicine of the U.S. National Academy of Sciences has concluded that reports and studies showing sensory neuropathy at doses of pyridoxine less than 200 milligrams/day are weak and inconsistent, with the weight of evidence indicating that sensory neuropathy is unlikely to occur in adults taking pyridoxine at doses less than 500 milligrams/day.

Other adverse reactions reported with high doses of pyridoxine, include nausea, vomiting, abdominal pain, loss of appetite and breast soreness. Rare cases of pyridoxine-induced photosensitivity have been reported.

INTERACTIONS

DRUGS

Amiodarone: Concomitant use of vitamin B6 and amiodarone may enhance amiodarone-induced photosensitivity reactions. Doses of vitamin B_6 greater than 5-10 milligrams/day should be avoided by those taking amiodarone.

Carbamazepine: Chronic use of carbamazepine may result in a significant decrease in plasma pyridoxal 5'-phosphate levels.

Cycloserine: Cycloserine may react with pyridoxal 5'-phosphate to form a metabolically inactive oxime, which may result in a functional vitamin B_6 deficiency.

Ethionamide: The use of ethionamide may increase vitamin B_6 requirements.

Fosphenytoin: High doses of vitamin B_6 may lower plasma levels of phenytoin. Fosphenytoin is a prodrug of phenytoin.

Hydralazine: The use of hydralazine may increase vitamin B_6 requirements.

Isoniazid: (isonicotinic acid, INH). Isoniazid reacts with pyridoxal 5'-phosphate to form a metabolically inactive hydrazone, which may result in functional vitamin B_6 deficiency.

Levodopa: Concomitant use of levodopa and vitamin B_6 in doses of 5 milligrams or more daily may reverse the therapeutic effects of levodopa. Vitamin B_6 does not reverse the therapeutic effects of levodopa if levodopa is taken concurrently with the levodopa decarboxylase inhibitor carbidopa. Levodopa is typically administered as a combination product with carbidopa.

Oral contraceptives: The use of oral contraceptives may increase vitamin B_6 requirements. This was more the case with the older oral contraceptive agents with high-dose estrogen/progestin. It appears to be less the case with the newer low-dose estrogen/progestin products.

Penicillamine: Penicillamine may react with pyridoxal 5'-phosphate to form a metabolically inactive thiazolidine, which may result in a functional vitamin B_6 deficiency.

Phenelzine: Phenelzine may react with pyridoxal 5'-phosphate to yield a metabolically inactive hydrazone compound.

Phenobarbital: High doses of vitamin B_6 may lower plasma levels of phenobarbital.

Phenytoin: High doses of vitamin B_6 may lower plasma levels of phenytoin.

Theophylline: Theophylline may react with pyridoxal 5'-phosphate leading to low plasma levels of the coenzyme. This may increase the risk of theophylline-induced seizures.

Valproic acid: Chronic use of valproic acid may result in a significant decrease in plasma pyridoxal 5'-phosphate levels.

FOODS

Alcoholic beverages: Alcohol may increase the catabolism of pyridoxal 5'-phosphate. Chronic and excessive use of alcoholic beverages can result in vitamin B_6 deficiency.

OVERDOSAGE

No reports.

DOSAGE AND ADMINISTRATION

Vitamin B_6 is available in nutritional supplements principally in the form of pyridoxine hydrochloride. Pyridoxal 5'-phosphate is also available as a nutritional supplement. Pyridoxine hydrochloride is available in multivitamin and multivitamin/multimineral products as well as products that, in addition to vitamins and minerals, contain other nutritional substances. Single ingredient pyridoxine products are also available. Some products are available which contain mixtures of pyridoxine hydrochloride and pyridoxal 5'-phosphate. Typical doses of pyridoxine used for nutritional supplementation range from 2 to 20 milligrams/day.

Those who use pyridoxine for the management of premenstrual syndrome, typically use doses ranging from 50 to 100 milligrams/day. Those who use pyridoxine for the management of carpal tunnel syndrome, typically use doses ranging from 100 to 200 milligrams/day.

The Food and Nutrition Board of the Institute of Medicine of the National Academy of Sciences has recommended the following Dietary Reference Intakes (DRI) for vitamin B_6:

Infants	Adequate Intakes (AI)
0 through 6 months	0.1mg/day ~ 0.014 mg/Kg
7 through 12 months	0.3 mg/day ~ 0.033 mg/Kg

Children	Recommended Dietary Allowances (RDA)
1 through 3 years	0.5 mg/day
4 through 8 years	0.6 mg/day

Boys	
9 through 13 years	1.0 mg/day
14 through 18 years	1.3 mg/day

Girls	
9 through 13 years	1.0 mg/day
14 through 18 years	1.2 mg/day

Men	
19 through 50 years	1.3 mg/day
51 through 70 years	1.7 mg/day
Older than 70 years	1.7 mg/day

Women	
19 through 50 years	1.3 mg/day
51 through 70 years	1.5 mg/day
Older than 70 years	1.5 mg/day

Pregnancy

14 through 50 years	1.9 mg/day
Lactation	2.0 mg/day

The DV (Daily Value) for vitamin B_6 (pyridoxine and related compounds), which is used for determining the percentage of nutrient daily values on nutritional supplement and food labels, is 2.0 mg. This is based on the U.S. RDA for vitamin B_6.

The Food and Nutrition Board has identified a Lowest-Observed-Adverse-Effect Level (LOAEL) for vitamin B_6 of 500 milligrams/day (See Adverse Reactions) and a No-Observed-Adverse-Effect Level (NOAEL) of 200 milligrams/day. Based on the NOAEL and an uncertainty factor of 2, the Food and Nutrition Board has recommended the following Tolerable Upper Intake Levels (UL) for vitamin B_6:

Infants	UL
0 through 12 months	ND

Children

1 through 3 years	30 mg/day of vitamin B_6 as pyridoxine
4 through 8 years	40 mg/day of vitamin B_6 as pyridoxine
9 through 13 years	60 mg/day of vitamin B_6 as pyridoxine
Adolescents	80 mg/day of vitamin B_6 as pyridoxine

Pregnancy

14 through 18 years	80 mg/day of vitamin B_6 as pyridoxine
19 years and older	100 mg/day of vitamin B_6 as pyridoxine

Lactation

14 through 18 years	80 mg/day of vitamin B_6 as pyridoxine
19 years and older	100 mg/day of vitamin B_6 as pyridoxine

Adults

19 years and older	100 mg/day of vitamin B_6 as pyridoxine

ND = Not Determinable

LITERATURE

Albert CM, Cook NR, Gaziano JM, et al. Effect of folic acid and B vitamins on risk of cardiovascular events and total mortality among women at high risk for cardiovascular disease: a randomized trial. *JAMA*. 2008;299(17):2027-2036.

Aybak M, Sermet A, Ayylidiz MO, et al. Effect of oral pyridoxine hydrochloride supplementation on arterial blood pressure in patients with essential hypertension. *Arzneimittelforschung*. 1995;45:1271-1273.

Balk EM, Raman G, Tatsioni A, et al. Vitamin B_6, B_{12}, and folic acid supplementation and cognitive function: a systematic review of randomized trials. *Arch Intern Med*. 2007;167(1):21-30.

Bender DA. Non-nutritional uses of vitamin B_6. *Br J Nutrition*. 1999;81:7-20.

Bendich A, Cohen M. Vitamin B_6 safety issues. *Ann NY Acad Sci*. 1990;585:321-330.

Bernstein AL. Vitamin B_6 in clinical neurology. *Ann NY Acad Sci*. 1990;585:250-260.

Bernstein AL, Dinesen JS. Brief communication: effect of pharmacologic doses of vitamin B_6 on carpal tunnel syndrome, electroencephalographic results, and pain. *J Am Coll Nutr*. 1993;12:73-76.

Bilski P, Li MY, Ehrenshaft M, et al. Vitamin B_6 (pyridoxine) and its derivatives are efficient singlet oxygen quenchers and potential fungal antioxidants. *Photochem Photobiol*. 2000;71:129-134.

Bleie ø, Semb AG, Grundt H, et al. Homocysteine-lowering therapy does not affect inflammatory markers of atherosclerosis in patients with stable coronary artery disease. *J Intern Med*. 2007;262(2):244-253.

Candito M, Rivet R, Herbeth B, et al. Nutritional and genetic determinants of vitamin B and homocysteine metabolisms in neural tube defects: a multicenter case-control study. *Am J Med Genet A*. 2008 May 1;146A(9):1128-1133.

Chang S-J. Vitamin B_6 protects vascular endothelial injury by activated platelets. *Nutr Res*. 1999;19:1613-1624.

Dakshinamurti, K, ed. *Vitamin B_6*. New York, NY: The New York Academy of Sciences; 1990.

DiSorbo DM, Wagner R Jr, Nathanson L. In vivo and in vitro inhibition of B_{16} melanoma growth by vitamin B_6. *Nutr Cancer*. 1985;7:43-52.

Ebbing M, Bleie ø, Ueland PM, et al. Mortality and cardiovascular events in patients treated with homocysteine-lowering B vitamins after coronary angiography: a randomized controlled trial. *JAMA*. 2008;300(7):795-804.

Ellis J, Folkers K, Watanabe T, et al. Clinical results of a cross-over treatment with pyridoxine and placebo of the carpal tunnel syndrome. *Am J Clin Nutr*. 1979;32:2040-2046.

Ellis JM, McCully KS. Prevention of myocardial infarction by vitamin B_6. *Res Commun Mol Pathol Pharmacol*. 1995;89:208-220.

Figueiredo JC, Levine AJ, Grau MV, et al. Vitamins B2, B6, and B12 and risk of new colorectal adenomas in a randomized trial of aspirin use and folic acid supplementation. *Cancer Epidemiol Biomarkers Prev*. 2008;17(8):2136-2145.

Franzblau A, Rock CL, Werner RA, et al. The relationship of vitamin B_6 status to median nerve function and carpal tunnel syndrome among active industrial workers. *J Occup Environ Med.* 1996;38:485-491.

Gregory JF III. Nutritional properties and significance of vitamin glycosides. *Annu Rev Nutr.* 1998;18:277-296.

Gridley DS, Schultz TD, Stickney DR, et al. In vivo and in vitro stimulation of cell-mediated immunity by vitamin B_6. *Nutr Res.* 1988;8:201-207.

Guilarte TR. Vitamin B_6 and cognitive development: recent research findings from human and animal studies. *Nutr Rev.* 1993;51:193-198.

Institute of Medicine. Food and Nutrition Board. Dietary Reference Intakes for thiamin, riboflavin, niacin, vitamin B_6, folate, vitamin B_{12}, pantothenic acid, biotin, and choline. Washington, DC: National Academy Press, 1998.

Ishihara J, Iso H, Inoue M, et al. JPHC Study Group. Intake of folate, vitamin B_6 and vitamin B_{12} and the risk of CHD: the Japan Public Health Center-Based Prospective Study Cohort I. *J Am Coll Nutr.* 2008;27(1):127-136.

Kashanian M, Mazinani R, Jalalmanesh S. Pyridoxine (vitamin B_6) therapy for premenstrual syndrome. *Int J Gynaecol Obstet.* 2007;96(1):43-44.

Khatami M. Role of pyridoxal phosphate/pyridoxine in diabetes. Inhibition of nonenzymatic glycosylation. *Ann N Y Acad Sci.* 1990;585:502-504.

Laso Guzman FJ, Gonzalez-Buitrago JM, de Arriba F, et al. Carpal tunnel syndrome and vitamin B_6. *Klin Wochenschr.* 1989;67:38-41.

Leklem JE. Vitamin B_6. In: Shils ME, Olson JA, Shike M, Ross AC, eds. *Modern Nutrition in Health and Disease.* 9th ed. Baltimore, MD: Williams and Wilkins; 1999;413-421.

Lerner V, Miodownik C, Kaptsan A, et al. Vitamin B_6 treatment for tardive dyskinesia: a randomized, double-blind, placebo-controlled, crossover study. *J Clin Psychiatry.* 2007;68(11):1648-1654.

Lonn E. Homocysteine-lowering B vitamin therapy in cardiovascular prevention—wrong again? *JAMA.* 2008;299(17):2086-2087.

Lonn E, Yusuf S, Arnold MJ, et al. Heart Outcomes Prevention Evaluation (HOPE) 2 Investigators. Homocysteine lowering with folic acid and B vitamins in vascular disease. *N Engl J Med.* 2006;354(15):1567-1577.

Maksymowych AB, Robertson NM, Litwack G. Efficacy of pyridoxal treatment in controlling the growth of melanomas in cell culture and an animal pilot study. *Anticancer Research.* 1993;13:1925-1937.

Ntaios GC, Savopoulos CG, Chatzinikolaou AC, et al. Vitamins and stroke: the homocysteine hypothesis still in doubt. *Neurologist.* 2008;14(1):2-4.

Okada H, Moriwaki K, Kanno Y, et al. Vitamin B_6 supplementation can improve peripheral polyneuropathy in patients with chronic renal failure on high-flux haemodialysis and human recombinant erythropoietin. *Nephrol Dial Transplant.* 2000;15:1410-1413.

Perry C, Yu S, Chen J, et al. Effect of vitamin B_6 availability on serine hydroxymethyltransferase in MCF-7 cells. *Arch Biochem Biophys.* 2007;462(1):21-27.

Piazzini DB, Aprile I, Ferrara PE, et al. A systematic review of conservative treatment of carpal tunnel syndrome. *Clin Rehabil.* 2007;21(4):299-314.

Rall LC, Meydani SN. Vitamin B_6 and immune competence. *Nutr Rev.* 1993;51:217-225.

Rimland B, Calloway E, Dreyfus P. The effects of high doses of vitamin B_6 on autistic children: a double-blind crossover study. *Am J Psychiatry.* 1978;135:472-475.

Rodionov RN, Lentz SR. The homocysteine paradox. *Arterioscler Thromb Vasc Biol.* 2008;28(6):1031-1033.

Schaumburg H, Kaplan J, Windebank A, et al. Sensory neuropathy from pyridoxine abuse. *N Engl J Med.* 1983;309:445-448.

Schneider G, Kàck H, Lindquist Y. The manifold of vitamin B_6 dependent enzymes. *Structure.* 2000;8:R1-R6.

Scott K, Zeris S, Kothari MJ. Elevated B6 levels and peripheral neuropathies. *Electromyogr Clin Neurophysiol.* 2008;48(5):219-223.

Sermet A, Aybak M, Ulak G, et al. Effect of oral pyridoxine hydrochloride supplementation on *in vitro* platelet sensitivity to different agonists. *Arzneimittelforschung.* 1995;45:19-21.

Seto T, Inada H, Kobayashi N, et al. [Depression of serum pyridoxal levels in theophylline-related seizures]. [Article in Japanese]. *No To Hattatsu.* 2000;32:295-300.

Shane B. Folate and vitamin B_{12} metabolism: overview and interaction with riboflavin, vitamin B_6, and polymorphisms. *Food Nutr Bull.* 2008;29(2 Suppl):S5-16; discussion S17-9.

Shimizu T, Maeda S, Arakawa H, et al. Relation between theophylline and circulating vitamin levels in children with asthma. *Pharmacology.* 1996;53:384-389.

Shimizu T, Maeda S, Mochizuki H, et al. Theophylline attenuates circulating vitamin B_6 levels in children with asthma. *Pharmacology.* 1994;49:392-397.

Spence JD. Homocysteine-lowering therapy: a role in stroke prevention? *Lancet Neurol.* 2007;6(9):830-838.

Spooner GR, Desai HB, Angel JF, et al. Using pyridoxine to treat carpal tunnel syndrome. Randomized control trial. *Can Fam Physician.* 1993;39:2122-2127.

Stern F, Berner YN, Polyak Z, et al. [Nutritional status and vitamin B_6 supplementation in the institutionalized elderly]. [Article in Hebrew]. *Harefuah.* 2000;139:97-102,167,166.

Stransky M, Rubin A, Lava NS, et al. Treatment of carpal tunnel syndrome with vitamin B_6: a double-blind study. *South Med J.* 1989;82:841-842.

Tai WP, Yue H, Hu PJ. Coma caused by isoniazid poisoning in a patient treated with pyridoxine and hemodialysis. *Adv Ther.* Epub: 2008 Sep 20.

Theodoratou E, Farrington SM, Tenesa A, et al. Dietary vitamin B6 intake and the risk of colorectal cancer. *Cancer Epidemiol Biomarkers Prev.* 2008;17(1):171-182.

Trabetti E. Homocysteine, MTHFR gene polymorphisms, and cardio-cerebrovascular risk. *J Appl Genet.* 2008;49(3):267-282.

Troen AM, Shea-Budgell M, Shukitt-Hale B, et al. B-vitamin deficiency causes hyperhomocysteinemia and vascular cognitive impairment in mice. *Proc Natl Acad Sci U S A.* 2008;105(34):12474-12479.

Ubbink JB, Hayward Vermaak WJ, Delport R, et al. The relationship between vitamin B6 metabolism, asthma, and theophylline therapy. *Ann NY Acad Sci.* 1990;585:285-294.

Wierzbicki AS. Homocysteine and cardiovascular disease: a review of the evidence. *Diab Vasc Dis Res.* 2007;4(2):143-150.

Wyatt K, Dimmock P, Jones P. Poor-quality studies suggest that vitamin B(6) use is beneficial in premenstrual syndrome. *West J Med.* 2000;172(4):245.

Wyatt KM, Dimmock PW, Jones PW, et al. Efficacy of vitamin B6 in the treatment of premenstrual syndrome: systemic review. *Br Med J.* 1999;318:1375-1381.

Vitamin B12

DESCRIPTION

The term vitamin B_{12} (cobalamin) is used in two different ways. Vitamin B_{12}, a member of the B-vitamin family, is a collective term for a group of cobalt-containing compounds known as corrinoids. The principal cobalamins are cyanocobalamin, hydroxocobalamin and the two coenzyme forms of vitamin B_{12}, methylcobalamin and 5-deoxyadenosylcobalamin (adenosylcobalamin). The term vitamin B_{12} is more commonly used to refer to only one of these forms, cyanocobalamin. Cyanocobalamin is the principal form of the vitamin used for fortification of foods and in nutritional supplements. In this monograph, vitamin B_{12} will be used in both ways. The meaning will be clear from its context. The cobalamins are comprised of a nucleotide (base, ribose and phosphate) attached to a corrin ring. The corrin ring is made up of four pyrrole groups and an atom of cobalt in its center. The cobalt atom attaches to a methyl group, a deoxyadenosyl group, a hydroxyl group or a cyano group, to yield the four cobalamin forms mentioned above.

Vitamin B_{12} is the most chemically complex of all the vitamins. It is also one of the most biologically interesting ones. Because of the striking dark red color of its crystals, vitamin B_{12} has been called "nature's most beautiful cofactor." Its close relatives hemoglobin, chlorophyll and the cytochromes are also brightly colored complex organometallic substances, which, along with vitamin B_{12} and some others derived from the parent molecule called uroporphyrinogen III, have led to their being known as the pigments of life. Vitamin B_{12} works in close partnership with folate in the synthesis of the building blocks for DNA and RNA synthesis as well as the synthesis of molecules important for the maintenance of the integrity of the genome. It is also essential for the maintenance of the integrity of the nervous system and for the synthesis of molecules which are involved in fatty acid biosynthesis and the production of energy. The human body does all of this with just two to three milligrams of the vitamin, which is much less than the weight of a tenth of a drop of water. It is even speculated that B_{12} was mainly responsible for the origin of the DNA world from the RNA world.

Deficiency of vitamin B_{12} results in hematological, neurological and gastrointestinal effects. The hematological effects of the deficiency are identical to that of folate deficiency and are caused by interference with DNA synthesis. The hematologic symptoms and signs of B_{12} deficiency, include hypersegmentation of polymorphonuclear leukocytes, macrocytic, hyperchromic erythrocytes, elevated mean corpuscular volume (MCV), elevated mean corpuscular hemoglobin concentration (MCH, MCHC), a decreased red blood cell count, pallor of the skin, decreased energy and easy fatigability, shortness of breath and palpitations. The resulting anemia of B_{12} deficiency, as is the case of the anemia of folate deficiency, is a megaloblastic macrocytic anemia. However, in the context of a simultaneous iron deficiency anemia, which is a microcytic one, anemia secondary to B_{12} deficiency may not result in macrocytic erythrocytes.

The neurological effects of the vitamin deficiency may occur even in the absence of anemia. This is particularly true in those who are over 60 years old. Vitamin B_{12} deficiency principally affects the peripheral nerves, and in later stages, the spinal cord. The symptoms and signs of the neurological effects of B_{12} deficiency, include tingling and numbness in the extremities (particularly the lower extremities), loss of vibratory and position sensation, abnormalities of gait, spasticity, Babinski's responses, irritability, depression and cognitive changes (loss of concentration, memory loss, dementia). Visual disturbances, impaired bladder and bowel control, insomnia and impotence may also occur. Gastrointestinal effects of B_{12} deficiency, include intermittent diarrhea and constipation, abdominal pain, flatulence and burning of the tongue (glossitis). Anorexia and weight loss are general symptoms of B_{12} deficiency. Recently, age-related hearing loss has been associated with poor vitamin B_{12} and folate status. Poor B_{12} status has also been associated with Alzheimer's disease.

Pernicious anemia is the most common cause of clinical B_{12} deficiency in temperate regions. Pernicious anemia is the result of an autoimmune process in which parietal cell autoantibodies against the gastric H^+/K^+-adenosine triphosphatase (the gastric proton pump) cause loss of gastric parietal cells. The loss of parietal cells results in diminished production of the intrinsic factor. The intrinsic factor is necessary for B_{12} absorption (see Pharmacokinetics). Deficiency of intrinsic factor results in B_{12} deficiency. Inadequate B_{12} intake is another cause of B_{12} deficiency. Breastfed infants of vegan mothers are particularly at risk for B_{12} deficiency. Total gastrectomy results in B_{12} deficiency secondary to lack of intrinsic factor. Pancreatic insufficiency and atrophic gastritis result in B_{12} deficiency secondary to inability to digest dietary protein-bound B_{12}. Small bowel disorders, including ileal resection or bypass, Crohn's disease, malignancy, tropical sprue, celiac sprue (gluten-induced enteropathy) and amyloidosis result in B_{12} deficiency secondary to decreased absorption of the vitamin. Bacterial overgrowth of the small intestine results in B_{12} deficiency secondary to bacterial competition for uptake of the vitamin. Certain drugs, including proton pump inhibitors can interfere with absorption of the vitamin (see Interactions). Nitrous oxide anesthesia can cause a functional B_{12} deficiency via degradation of B_{12} coenzymes (see Interactions). Rare congenital disorders such as transcobalamin II deficiency and defective intrinsic factor production result in B_{12} deficiency. Finally, infestation with the tapeworm *Diphyllobothrium latum* can cause B_{12} deficiency secondary to competition for uptake of B_{12} by the parasite. In this regard, in the early 1900s, B_{12} deficiency was common in Jewish women in the United States who prepared their own gefilte fish. They used fresh-water fish, including pike, pickeral and carp, which hosted the wormlike larvae of the parasite. The women would sample the fish, by tasting it, from the time it was quite raw until it was well cooked. Although their children totally enjoyed the prepared gefilte fish, the Jewish mothers wound up with forty-foot parasites in their digestive tracts and B_{12} deficiencies.

The two coenzyme forms of vitamin B_{12} are methylcobalamin and 5'-deoxyadenosylcobalamin (adenosylcobalamin). Methylcobalamin is a cofactor for the enzyme methionine synthase, while adenosycobalamin is a cofactor for the enzyme L-methylmalonyl coenzyme A (methylmalonyl-CoA) mutase. Methionine synthase is one of the key enzymes in intermediary metabolism. It catalyzes the conversion of homocysteine to methionine. Its folate partner in the reaction is 5-methyltetrahydrofolate (intracellular folates are present in their polyglutamate forms). This is the only reaction in the body in which folate and B_{12} coparticipants. In addition to forming methionine, 5-methyltetrahydrofolate is converted to tetrahydrofolate. The reactions occur in the following manner: methylcobalamin transfers its methyl group to homocysteine yielding methionine and 5-methyltetrahydrate transfers its methyl group to cobalamin reconverting it to methylcobalamin. Methionine is converted to S-adenosylmethionine (SAMe), the major donor of methyl groups in transmethylation reactions, including reactions that are involved in the synthesis of basic myelin basic protein.

Tetrahydrofolate is converted to 5,10-methylenetetrahydrofolate via the action of the enzyme serine hydroxymethyltransferase. 5,10-Methylenetetrahydrofolate is presented with three metabolic opportunities. It can be converted to 5-methyltetrahydrofolate—the folate cofactor of the methionine synthase reaction—via the enzyme 5,10-methylenetetrahydrofolate reductase; it can transfer its one-carbon residue to deoxyuridylic acid to form thymidylic acid or it can be converted to 5-formyltetrahydrofolate, which is a one-carbon donor in the *de novo* synthesis of purine nucleotides.

The hematological effects of B_{12} deficiency are accounted for as follows: B_{12} deficiency leads to reduced synthesis of tetrahydrofolate as well as methionine. Decreased tetrahydrofolate results in decreased 5,10-methylenetetrahydrofolate which in turn, results in decreased conversion of deoxyuridylate to thymidylate and decreased *de novo* synthesis of purine nucleotides. In addition, because of decreased synthesis of methionine and S-adenosylmethionine, the enzyme 5,10-methylenetetrahydrofolate reductase converts most of the 5,10-methylenetetrahydrofolate to 5-methyltetrahydrofolate, the so-called methyl trap. To summarize, decreased B_{12} results in a decrease in the nucleotide precursor pool for DNA synthesis (thymidylic acid, purine nucleotides) which results in decreased DNA replication and cell division and finally to a megaloblastic anemia. Since the megaloblastic anemia induced by B_{12} deficiency is caused by a functional cellular folate deficiency, it is not surprising that it can be corrected with administration of folate. On the other hand, the neurological deficits of vitamin B_{12} deficiency can not be corrected with folate administration. Further, high doses of folate administered to those with an undiagnosed B_{12} deficiency can cause progression of neurological symptoms.

The neurological effects of B_{12} deficiency are accounted for as follows: Consequences of B_{12} deficiency, in addition to those mentioned above, include increased serum levels of homocysteine, decreased levels of methionine and S-adenosylmethionine and a decreased ratio of S-adenosylmethionine to S-adenosylhomocysteine, the product of S-adenosylmethionine methyltransferase reactions. Decreased S-adenosylmethionine in the central nervous system results in decreased methylation reactions and an overall state of hypomethylation. Transmethylation reactions are important in the synthesis of a number of substances in the central nervous system, including myelin basic protein which is involved in the process of myelination. Much research is needed to better elucidate the mechanism of the neurological effects of B_{12} deficiency.

In addition to methionine synthase, B_{12} is a cofactor in the methylmalonyl-CoA mutase reaction. In this reaction, the coenzyme form of B_{12} is adenosylcobalamin. A number of substances, including the branched-chain amino acids isoleucine and valine, as well as methionine, threonine, thymine and odd-chain fatty acids are metabolized via methylmalonyl semialdehyde or propionyl-CoA to methylmalonyl-CoA. Methylmalonyl-CoA mutase converts methylmalonyl-CoA to succinyl-CoA. This occurs in the mitochondria. Succinyl-CoA can be metabolized in the tricarboxylic acid cycle to produce energy and it is also involved in the synthesis of fatty acids. Methylmalonic acid is elevated in the serum and urine in those with B_{12} deficiency.

Animal products are the principal food sources of vitamin B_{12}. B_{12} cannot be made by plants or by animals. It is thought that only bacteria (eubacteria, archaebacteria) manufacture the vitamin. The B_{12} in animal products is derived from bacterial B_{12} sources. The richest dietary sources of cobalamin are the liver, brain and kidney. Other sources, include egg yolk, clams, oysters, crabs, sardines, salmon and heart. Lower amounts of cobalamin are found in fish, beef, lamb, pork, chicken, cheese and milk. Plant foods are generally devoid of B_{12}. Some fermented plant products, e.g., tempeh, may have some vitamin B_{12}. Pseudovitamin B_{12} refers to B_{12}-like substances which are found in certain organisms, such as *Spirulina* spp. (blue-green algae, cyanobacteria). However, these substances do not have B_{12} biological activity for humans. Food-form B_{12} is comprised of protein-bound methylcobalamin and adenosylcobalamin.

Vitamin B_{12}, B_{12} and cobalamin are terms that are used interchangeably. Vitamin B_{12} most commonly refers to one of the cobalamin forms, cyanocobalamin. Cyanocobalamin is also known as 5,6-dimethylbenzimidazolyl cyanocobamide. Its molecular formula is $C_{63}H_{88}CoN_{14}O_{14}P$ and its molecular weight is 1355.38 daltons. The structural formula is:

Vitamin B_{12}

ACTIONS AND PHARMACOLOGY

ACTIONS

Vitamin B_{12} is used in the treatment of B_{12} deficiency states, including megaloblastic anemia. It may have antiatherogenic, neuroprotective, anticarcinogenic and detoxifying activities. B_{12} has putative anti-allergic and mood-modulatory activities.

MECHANISM OF ACTION

Vitamin B_{12}, in the form of methylcobalamin, is a cofactor in the methionine synthase reaction. The enzyme converts homocysteine to methionine. Folate, in the form of 5-methyltetrahydrofolate (as the pentaglutamate) is the other cofactor in the reaction. In addition to methionine, tetrahydrofolate (again, as the pentaglutame) is also formed. Tetrahydrofolate is converted to 5,10-methylenetetrahydrofolate which is a cofactor in the formation of thymidylic acid from deoxyuridylic acid and which is also converted to 5-formyltetrahydrofolate, a one-carbon donor in the *de novo* synthesis of purine nucleotides. B_{12} deficiency results in decreased formation of thymidylic acid and purine nucleotides, precursors of DNA synthesis and which are necessary for normal cell division. Megaloblastic anemia is the consequence of this and administration of B_{12}, which yields the B_{12} cofactor for methionine synthase, corrects this problem. Methionine is a precursor of S-adenosylmethionine

(SAMe). SAMe is the principal transmethylating agent and is involved in, among many other things, the synthesis of myelin basic protein. Abnormal myelin basic protein resulting in defective myelination, is thought to be responsible for many of the neurological effects of B_{12} deficiency. The neurological effects may or may not be corrected with administration of B_{12} in those with B_{12} deficiency. Whether the neurological effects are reversible after treatment depends on their duration.

Hyperhomocysteinemia is thought to be an independent risk factor for coronary heart disease and other vascular disorders. B_{12} works in concert with folate in the methionine synthase reaction, which metabolizes homocysteine to methionine. This is a key reaction in the maintenance of low serum homocysteine levels. The mechanism by which elevated homocysteine levels might increase the risk of developing vascular disease is unclear. It has been shown that homocysteine increases platelet adhesiveness, promotes the growth of smooth muscle cells and causes endothelial dysfunction. Homocysteine may also promote oxidative stress resulting in, among other things, the oxidation of low-density lipoproteins (LDL) to oxidized-LDL. All of these possible activities of homocysteine can play roles in atherogenesis.

B_{12} deficiency can result in a number of neurological effects, including peripheral neuropathy and cognitive changes, including memory loss and dementia. Administration of B_{12} successfully reverses mild memory impairment and peripheral neuropathy, if not advanced neurological deficits, in most elderly subjects deficient in the vitamin. The mechanism by which B_{12} deficiency causes neurological effects and by which B_{12} administration may reverse them is not well understood. B_{12} and folate are cofactors in the conversion of homocysteine to methionine and methionine is the precursor of the transmethylating agent S-adenosylmethionine (SAMe). SAMe is involved in the synthesis of myelin basic protein which can become defective in the context of B_{12} deficiency. Defective myelin basic protein and resultant defective myelination can account, in large part, for the peripheral neuropathy of B_{12} deficiency. Hyperhomocysteinemia, another consequence of B_{12} deficiency, may also contribute to the neurological effects of deficiency of the vitamin. Elevated homocysteine levels may cause cerebrovascular effects which could lead to cognitive changes. Decreased brain levels of SAMe may result in disturbances in certain neurotransmitters. SAMe is involved in key methylation reactions in catecholamine synthesis and metabolism in the brain. These neurotransmitters are known to be important in maintaining the affective state. In the elderly, depression often presents as cognitive changes, including dementia.

Vitamin B_{12} deficiency has been associated with Alzheimer's disease, at least in some with this neurodegenerative disorder. It is hypothesized that the altered B_{12} status that may occur in those with the disorder is due, in part, to a defect in the protein megalin. Megalin is a member of the low-density lipoprotein receptor family, and mediates the ileal uptake of the cubulin-bound B_{12}-intrinsic factor complex (see Pharmacokinetics). The low-density lipoprotein receptors include receptors that bind apolipoprotein E, amyloid precursor protein and alpha$_2$-macroglobulin, substances that have been linked to Alzheimer's disease. Impaired transport of B_{12} to the central nervous system may, in part, account for the pathogenesis of the disorder.

There is some evidence, mainly epidemiological, that B_{12} may protect against certain types of cancer. A couple of clinical studies have shown that a combination of B_{12} and folic acid significantly reduces the number of abnormal bronchial cells thought to be cancer cell precursors. The mechanism of the possible anticarcinogenic effect of B_{12} is unclear. B_{12} deficiency results in decreased levels of SAMe and thymidylic acid, as discussed above. SAMe, among other things, is involved in DNA methylation which results in regulation of its genetic expression via a process known as gene silencing. Abnormal DNA methylation patterns are characteristic of neoplastic cells. Decreased SAMe and thymidylic acid levels may also lead to increased errors in DNA replication, increased DNA strand breaks and defective DNA repair.

Hydroxocobalamin is used in conditions which are associated with cyanide toxicity, such as may occur with sodium nitroprusside therapy and Leber's optic atrophy. Hydroxocobalamin is used parenterally in these cases; it combines with cyanide to form cyanocobalamin. Clearly, cyanocobalamin is not the right form of B_{12} for use in these conditions. B_{12} can also combine with sulfite and has been found to be effective in the management of sulfite-induced hypersensitivity conditions in some preliminary studies. The studies used cyanocobalamin. Perhaps better results could have been obtained with hydroxocobalamin. There is no evidence that B_{12} has any effect in the management of other hypersensitive or allergic conditions.

Vitamin B_{12} may have mood-modulatory activity in some, e.g., the elderly, who are B_{12} deficient. There is no evidence that B_{12} has mood-modulatory activity in those who are not deficient in the vitamin. As discussed above, SAMe is involved in key methylation reactions in catecholamine synthesis in the brain and these neurotransmitters are known to be important in maintaining the affective state.

PHARMACOKINETICS

Vitamin B_{12} is found naturally in food sources (principally animal products) in protein-bound forms. Cyanocobalamin is the principal form of vitamin B_{12} used in nutritional supplements and for fortification of foods. Methylcobalamin is also available for nutritional supplementation and hydroxocobalamin is available for parenteral administration.

Naturally found B_{12} is dissociated from proteins in the stomach via the action of acid and the enzyme pepsin. The forms of B_{12} released by this process are methylcobalamin and adenosylcobalamin. All forms of B_{12} bind to proteins called haptocorrins or R proteins, which are secreted by the salivary glands and the gastric mucosa. This binding occurs in the stomach. Pancreatic proteases partially degrade the B_{12}-haptocorrin complexes in the small intestine where the B_{12} that is released then binds to intrinsic factor (IF). Intrinsic factor is a glycoprotein which is secreted by gastric parietal cells. The B_{12}-intrinsic factor complex is absorbed from the terminal ileum into the ileal enterocytes via a process that first requires the complex to bind to a receptor called cubilin. Within the enterocytes, B_{12} is released from the B_{12}-IF complex and then binds to another protein called transcobalamin II which delivers it to the portal circulation. The portal circulation transports B_{12} to the liver which takes up about 50% of the vitamin; the reminder is transported to the other tissues of the body via the systemic circulation.

Vitamin B_{12} in the circulation is bound to the plasma proteins transcobalamin I (TCI), transcobalamin II (TCII) and transcobalamin III (TCIII). Approximately 80% of plasma B_{12} is bound to TCI. TCII is the principal B_{12} binding protein for the delivery of B_{12} to cells, via specific receptors for TCII. This B_{12} binding protein (TCII) is identical to the one that delivers B_{12} from the enterocytes to the portal circulation (see above).

Total absorption increases with increased intake of the vitamin. However, the absorption efficacy of the vitamin decreases with increased dosage. Studies with cyanocobalamin found that 50% of the vitamin was absorbed at a dose of one microgram, 20% at a dose of 5 micrograms and about 5% at a dose of 25 micrograms. Significantly, very large doses of B_{12} are absorbed with an absorption efficiency of about one percent. This occurs via passive diffusion even in the absence of intrinsic factor. Thus, large oral doses may be given for the treatment of B_{12} deficiency instead of using the parenteral route (usually, intramuscularly). There are now several studies confirming this. The absorption efficiency of B_{12} from foods is approximately 50%.

The vitamin B_{12}-transcobalamin II complex is degraded intracellularly via lysosomal proteases to yield cobalamin (cyanocobalamin, methylcobalamin, adenosylcobalamin, hydroxocobalamin). Cobalamin is metabolized to methylcobalamin in the cytosol and to adenosylcobalamin in the mitochondria. Methylcobalamin is the principal circulating form of cobalamin. Adenosylcobalamin comprises more than 70% of cobalamin in the liver, erythrocytes, kidney and brain. The total body content of cobalamin ranges from two to three milligrams, with approximately 50% of it residing in the liver.

Vitamin B_{12} is secreted in the bile and reabsorbed via the enterohepatic circulation. Some of the B_{12} secreted in the bile is excreted in the feces. Also, oral B_{12} that is not absorbed is excreted in the feces. Reabsorption of B_{12} via the enterohepatic circulation requires the intrinsic factor. If the circulating level of B_{12} exceeds the B_{12} binding capacity of the blood, a situation that usually occurs following parenteral administration of the vitamin, the excess is excreted in the urine.

INDICATIONS AND USAGE

Vitamin B_{12} is of such vital nutritional importance that some authorities have recently called for mandatory fortification of some foods with this vitamin. Vitamin B_{12} is indicated in those with vitamin B_{12} deficiency. It is especially important for the elderly and for those who have had gastric surgery. Both groups are at high risk for vitamin B_{12} deficiency. There is evidence that it may be beneficial in some others with low vitamin B_{12} status and in some with malabsorption of B_{12}, including some who are chronically ill, as well as some vegetarians, among others. There is some preliminary indication that vitamin B_{12} may be helpful in inhibiting a pre-cancerous condition in the lungs of smokers, that it might help ameliorate the symptoms of some neuropsychiatric disorders and that it might be useful in some with chronic fatigue and HIV disease. It has been suggested that vitamin B_{12} might help prevent some vascular diseases and breast cancer, based upon epidemiological and theoretical considerations. Claims that it is a general "energizer" are anecdotal. There is some evidence that vitamin B_{12} can protect against hypersensitivity to sulfites. Earlier open trials suggested that methylcobalamin was effective in the management of sleep-wake rhythm disorders. However, a recent double-blind controlled trial with this form of B_{12} failed to confirm this. A recent study has associated low vitamin B_{12} status with brain atrophy/shrinkage and subsequent cognitive impairment in the elderly.

RESEARCH SUMMARY

Clinically, overt vitamin B_{12} deficiency manifests as megaloblastic anemia and neurologic dysfunction. There are more clinically silent and subtle forms of cobalamin deficiency which are also reversible with vitamin B_{12} therapy. In addition, mild deficiency may be present in a number of populations, including, most significantly, the elderly. It is estimated that 10-15% of those over 60 have vitamin B_{12} deficiency, due, principally, to decreased absorption of naturally occurring vitamin B_{12} caused by an age-related atrophic gastritis that diminishes the acid-pepsin secretions that normally release free vitamin B_{12} from food proteins.

An editorial in the *American Journal of Clinical Nutrition* recently suggested that the time may be fast approaching when mandatory fortification of some foods with vitamin B_{12} will be deemed appropriate. The editorialists note that data from the U.S. National Health and Nutrition Examination Survey (NHANES) "indicate that the function of vitamin B_{12} deteriorates as serum folate status increases in persons who are deficient in vitamin B_{12}. More seriously, the data show that persons with both low vitamin B_{12} and high folate concentrations were at particularly high risk of memory impairment and anemia." Thus a very significant proportion of the elderly could be at high risk of cognitive impairment because of an imbalance between folate and vitamin B_{12}. This is of special concern because since 1998 mandatory folic acid fortification has been in effect in the United States, Canada and more than 50 other countries, largely for the purpose of reducing the incidence of neural tube defects in the unborn. Folate fortification is useful, but if it creates a harmful imbalance with respect to vitamin B_{12}, the editorialists argue, then the need for concurrent mandatory vitamin B_{12} fortification becomes more urgent. They also point out that whereas neural tube defects are a relatively rare event in pregnancies (1 per 1,000), the negative sequelae of vitamin B_{12} deficiency are comparatively enormous, including not only increased cognitive dysfunction but also increased incidence of anemia, breast cancer and possibly diabetes in the offspring, among others. There is also the problem, they point out, that folic acid can mask vitamin B_{12} deficiency by preventing anemia but not neurological damage. Irrespective of folic acid fortification, they suggest that vitamin B_{12} fortification will benefit vegetarians, breastfed infants and the elderly, all of whom are at high risk for deficiencies. So why not do this right now, they ask? And they answer by suggesting that the following investigations first be undertaken:

1) Dose-response studies in persons with low vitamin B_{12} status due to food-cobalamin malabsorption, the most common cause of low cobalamin status in the elderly.

2) Evidence of benefit from randomized trials using low-dose vitamin B_{12} with clinical outcomes; current trial evidence, even from high-dose trials, is far from unequivocal.

3) Evidence of a lack of adverse effects in large-scale trials; thus far, studies have not been designed to assess such effects. Observational studies that have reported an associa-

tion of B_{12} status or intake with an increased risk of cancer should not be ignored.

4) Cyanocobalamin is rather unstable and may form cobalamin analogues that interfere with normal cobalamin metabolism and transport.

5) Before fortification is introduced, a coherent plan should be developed to document changes in vitamin B_{12} status; to monitor the effects on NTD births, on cognition, and anemia in the elderly; and to assess the possible occurrence of untoward effects on the population.

6) While waiting for a decision on vitamin B_{12} fortification, authorities urgently need to consider how to manage the newly discovered large-scale problem of those with low vitamin B_{12} status and high folate status in countries that have fortified with folic acid.

All of this takes on added urgency in view of an important recent study in which an association was made between low vitamin B_{12} status and rate of brain volume loss/shrinkage in the elderly. This was a prospective study of 107 community-dwelling volunteers aged 61 to 87 without cognitive impairment at enrollment. The subjects were evaluated annually for five years by clinical examination, MRI scans and cognitive tests. The association observed remained significant after adjustment for age, sex, initial brain volume and several other relevant variables. Confidence in the result was boosted by the fact that this study measured markers of vitamin B_{12} status more sensitive than those used in previous studies, most of which merely measured total plasma vitamin B_{12}. The researchers hypothesized that vitamin B_{12} might help diminish inflammation in the brain and help preserve the integrity of brain myelin. Larger trials are needed to further confirm and expand these findings.

Neurologic symptoms of vitamin B_{12} deficiency can occur, contrary to what was previously believed, in the absence of predecessor hematologic abnormalities. Among neurologic abnormalities noted are those involving the spinal cord, peripheral nerves, optic nerves and cerebrum. Sensory disturbances, such as paresthesias in the extremities, are considerably more common than motor disturbances. Neuropathies and myelopathies can occur alone or in combination. Cognitive impairment and mood changes are more common than dementia, psychosis, paranoia and violent behavior. There are rare instances of visual impairment. Age-related hearing loss has been associated with B_{12} and folate deficiency in the elderly. Researchers stress the need for prompt treatment. These conditions, if left untreated, often become irreversible.

Those with mild deficiency usually suffer only from neuropathy and modest memory impairment. Some immunologic deficits are also sometimes noted, but it is not known if these are caused by the deficiency. Supplemental vitamin B_{12} successfully reverses mild memory impairment and neuropathy in most elderly subjects deficient in this vitamin.

The Food and Nutrition Board has recommended that elderly people obtain 2.4 micrograms of vitamin B_{12} daily—from verifiable sources, e.g., either from eating fortified foods, such as cereals, that clearly identify the amount of vitamin B_{12} per serving and/or from vitamin B_{12} supplements. And some researchers, again noting the danger of irreversibility of neurologic symptoms that go untreated, have recently recommended regular periodic screening of the elderly for detection of vitamin B_{12} deficiency at an early stage.

A high prevalence of vitamin B_{12} deficiency has also been reported in those who have had gastric surgery. A recent study detected this deficiency in 31% of those who had undergone this type of surgery, compared with 2% of controls of similar age and race. Previous studies had noted an incidence of vitamin B_{12} deficiency of 1%-20% in gastric surgery patients, but the most recent study used more metabolic variables to detect the deficiency and tested an older patient sample. It also looked for the deficiency over a longer period of time. Median age of subjects in this study was 67 years.

These researchers found that vitamin B_{12} deficiency is often undetected in post-gastric surgery patients whose subsequent neurologic symptoms are often misdiagnosed. Most had not been advised, after surgery, to be monitored for vitamin B_{12} deficiency. These researchers stress the need for regular vitamin B_{12} screening in all gastric surgery patients, no matter how many years elapsed since the surgery. They point out that vitamin B_{12} deficiency may develop many years after surgery.

Vitamin B_{12} deficiencies have been reported in some chronically ill populations. Vitamin B_{12} has been found to be malabsorbed in some with HIV disease. There have also been reports of vitamin B_{12} deficiency in individuals with chronic fatigue of various etiologies. There are anecdotal reports that supplemental vitamin B_{12} is helpful in these disorders. Controlled trials are lacking.

Two placebo-controlled trials have shown that a combination of vitamin B_{12} and folic acid inhibited a precursor of bronchial squamous cell cancer of the lung in humans. In one of these studies, supplementation with 10 milligrams of folic acid daily, combined with 500 micrograms of vitamin B_{12} daily, for four months, produced a significant reduction in the number of subjects, all heavy smokers, who exhibited the abnormal bronchial cells said to be cancer precursors.

Many researchers have noted that diminished vitamin B_{12} status is strongly associated with hyperhomocysteinemia, a significant risk factor for cardiovascular disease. Two researchers have noted that, "although folate deficiency is a far more common cause of elevated homocysteine levels than are vitamin B_{12} and vitamin B_6 deficiencies, an elevated homocysteine value in an older person should not be considered due to folate deficiency alone. Because elderly people may have elevated homocysteine levels due to vitamin B_{12} deficiency, lowering serum total homocysteine levels to reduce the high incidence of vascular disease among the elderly by supplying adequate amounts of all three vitamins may become an important public health issue."

Recently, diminished vitamin B_{12} status has been identified as an additional nutritional risk factor for breast cancer among post-menopausal women. This preliminary finding needs follow-up before its significance, if any, can be assessed.

Claims that vitamin B_{12} can enhance exercise performance and that it is an "energizer" have not been tested and are based upon anecdotal accounts.

There is evidence that some who are on strict vegetarian or macrobiotic diets may need supplemental vitamin B_{12}. Children and the elderly who are on these diets may, in particular, have need of this supplementation. Some have claimed that miso, tamari, tempeh and other soy products can provide adequate B_{12} in the absence of meats and dairy products. This has not been demonstrated. Nor has the claim that adequate B_{12} can be obtained from spirulina, sea weeds and other sea vegetables. Even unpasteurized miso, claimed to be an excellent source of B_{12}, appears to have very little to none of the vitamin. Nor can vegetarians get adequate B_{12} from brewer's yeast, grains, cereals or mushrooms. Some sea vegetables are said to contain significant amounts of vitamin B_{12}, but accumulating evidence suggests that, instead, these foods contain vitamin B_{12} analogues (pseudovitamin B_{12}) that do not confer the functions and protection of vitamin B_{12} itself.

Again, vitamin B_{12} supplementation is highly advised for vegetarians, especially children who are vegetarians. Vegetarians whose diets allow for the regular use of eggs and dairy products can generally obtain enough vitamin B_{12} from their diets. Vegetarians consume certain foods (garlic, onions) that contain certain substances (e.g., inulins) which stimulate the growth of certain bacteria (e.g., *lactobacillus*) in the colon. These bacteria produce B_{12} and may supply some of the vitamin to the body. However, this needs to be proven.

Finally, there is evidence that vitamin B_{12} can protect some from allergy to the sulfites that are added to some foods and wines. In one study, 2,000 micrograms of sublingual vitamin B_{12} significantly prevented reactions to sulfites in 17 of 18 sulfite-sensitive subjects challenged with sulfites. Subsequent placebo-controlled trials confirmed this protective effect.

CONTRAINDICATIONS, PRECAUTIONS, ADVERSE REACTIONS

CONTRAINDICATIONS

Vitamin B_{12} (cyanocobalamin, hydroxocobalamin, methylcobalamin) is contraindicated in those hypersensitive to any component of a vitamin B_{12}-containing product.

PRECAUTIONS

The use of vitamin B_{12} to treat vitamin B_{12} deficiency or to treat any medical condition requires medical supervision.

Cyanocobalamin should not be used in those with Leber's optic atrophy. This is a congenital disorder associated with chronic cyanide intoxication (e.g., from tobacco smoke). Decreased levels of B_{12} have been associated with reduced ability to detoxify the cyanide in exposed individuals and cyanocobalamin may increase the risk of irreversible neurological damage from optic atrophy in those affected with the disorder. Hydroxocobalamin can aid in the detoxification of cyanide. This form of B_{12} is an acceptable form for B_{12} supplementation in those with this disorder.

A typical dose of B_{12} (cyanocobalamin) in nutritional supplements used by pregnant women and nursing mothers is 12 micrograms daily. Pregnant women and nursing mothers should only use doses higher than this if recommended by their physicians.

Administration of doses of vitamin B_{12} greater than 10 micrograms daily may produce a hematological response in those with anemia secondary to folate deficiency.

ADVERSE REACTIONS

Oral vitamin B_{12} is well tolerated even at high doses. There are occasional reports of hypersensitivity reactions (urticaria, rash, pruritus) in those receiving parenteral B_{12}. Those who have experienced hypersensitivity reactions from use of parenteral B_{12} may experience similar reactions from oral B_{12}, although there are very few reports of this occurring.

INTERACTIONS

DRUGS

Antibiotics: The use of antibiotics may alter the intestinal microflora and may decrease the possible contribution of B_{12} by certain inhabitants of the microflora (e.g., *Lactobacillus* species) to the body's requirement for the vitamin. This may particularly be a problem for vegetarians. Garlic, onions, leeks, bananas, asparagus and artichokes, among other vegetables and fruits, contain inulins which promote the growth of certain colonic bacteria, including *Lactobacillus* species (see Inulins).

Cholestyramine: Cholestyramine may decrease the enterohepatic reabsorption of B_{12}.

Colchicine: Colchicine may cause decreased absorption of B_{12}.

Colestipol: Colestipol may decrease the enterohepatic reabsorption of B_{12}.

H₂ blockers (cimetidine, famotidine, nizatidine, ranitidine): Chronic use of H_2 blockers may result in decreased absorption of vitamin B_{12} naturally found in food sources. They are unlikely to affect the absorption of supplemental B_{12}.

Metformin: Metformin may decrease the absorption of vitamin B_{12}. This possible effect may be reversed with oral calcium supplementation.

Nitrous oxide: Inhalation of the anesthetic agent nitrous oxide (not to be confused with nitric oxide) can produce a functional vitamin B_{12} deficiency. Nitrous oxide forms a complex with cobalt in methylcobalamin, the cofactor for methionine synthase, resulting in inactivation of the enzyme.

Para-aminosalicylic acid: Chronic use of the anti-tuberculosis drug may decrease the absorption of B_{12}.

Potassium chloride: It has been reported that potassium chloride may decrease the absorption of dietary B_{12} in some.

Proton pump inhibitors (lansoprazole, omeprazole, pantoprazole, rabeprazole): Chronic use of proton pump inhibitors may result in decreased absorption of vitamin B_{12} naturally found in food sources. They are unlikely to affect the absorption of supplemental B_{12}.

NUTRITIONAL SUPPLEMENTS

Calcium: Calcium supplementation may reverse the possible metformin-induced decrease of B_{12} absorption.

Folate: Folic acid may work synergistically with vitamin B_{12} in lowering homocysteine levels.

Vitamin B_6: Vitamin B_6 may work synergistically with vitamin B_{12} and folate in lowering homocysteine levels.

Vitamin C: Low serum B_{12} levels reported in those receiving large doses of vitamin C were artifacts of the effect of ascorbate on the radioisotope assay for B_{12}. There are no known interactions between vitamin C and vitamin B_{12}.

OVERDOSAGE

There are no reports of vitamin B_{12} overdosage in the literature.

DOSAGE AND ADMINISTRATION

The principal form of B$_{12}$ used in nutritional supplements is cyanocobalamin. Methylcobalamin is also available for nutritional supplementation. Hydroxocobalamin is presently only available for parenteral use.

Cyanocobalamin is available as a single ingredient product and in multivitamin, multivitamin/multimineral and B complex products. Lozenges of cyanocobalamin and methylcobalamin are also available. Prenatal and postnatal vitamin/mineral formulas typically deliver a dose of 12 micrograms of B$_{12}$ daily. A general range of B$_{12}$ dosage is 3 to 30 micrograms daily. Some use much higher doses. Absorption of naturally occurring B$_{12}$ decreases with age. Because of this, the Food and Nutrition Board advises that those older than 50 years should consume foods fortified with B$_{12}$ or take a vitamin B$_{12}$-containing nutritional supplement in order to meet the RDA (2.4 micrograms daily).

Those with B$_{12}$ deficiency may be managed with high doses of oral B$_{12}$. However, this requires prescription and management by a physician.

The Food and Nutrition Board of the Institute of Medicine of the National Academy of Sciences has recommended the following Dietary Reference Intakes (RDI) for vitamin B$_{12}$:

Infants	Adequate Intakes (AI)
0 through 6 months	0.4 micrograms/day ~ 0.05 micrograms/Kg
7 through 12 months	0.5 micrograms/day ~ 0.05 micrograms/Kg
Children	Recommended Dietary Allowance (RDA)
1 through 3 years	0.9 micrograms/day
4 through 8 years	1.2 micrograms/day
Boys	
9 through 13 years	1.8 micrograms/day
14 through 18 years	2.4 micrograms/day
Girls	
9 through 13 years	1.8 micrograms/day
14 through 18 years	2.4 micrograms/day
Men	
19 years and older	2.4 micrograms/day
Women	
19 years and older	2.4 micrograms/day
Pregnancy	
14 through 50 years	2.6 micrograms/day
Lactation	
14 through 50 years	2.8 micrograms/day

The DV (Daily Value) for vitamin B$_{12}$ (cobalamin), which is used for determining the percentage of nutrient daily values on nutritional supplement and food labels, is 6 micrograms. This is based on the U.S. RDA for vitamin B$_6$.

LITERATURE

Adachi S, Kawamoto T, Otsuka M, et al. Enteral vitamin B$_{12}$ supplements reverse postgastrectomy B$_{12}$ deficiency. *Ann Surg.* 2000;232:199-201.

Baik HW, Russell RM. Vitamin B$_{12}$ deficiency in the elderly. *Annu Rev Nutr.* 1999;19:357-377.

Battersby AR. How nature builds the pigments of life: The conquest of vitamin B$_{12}$. *Science.* 1994;264:1551-1557.

Bauman WA, Shaw S, Jayatilleke E, et al. Increased intake of calcium reverses vitamin B$_{12}$ malabsorption induced by metformin. *Diabetes Care.* 2000;23:1227-1231.

Bottiglieri T. Folate, vitamin B$_{12}$, and neuropsychiatric disorders. *Nutr Rev.* 1996;54:382-390.

Butzkueven H, King JO. Nitrous oxide myelopathy in an abuser of whipped cream bulbs. *J Clin Neurosci.* 2000;7:73-75.

Carmel R. Subtle cobalamin deficiency. *Ann Intern Med.* 1996;124:338-339.

Carmel R, Gott PS, Waters CH, et al. The frequency of low cobalamin levels in dementia usually signify treatable metabolic, neurologic and electrophysiologic abnormalities. *Eur J Haematol.* 1995;54:245-253.

Choi S-W. Vitamin B$_{12}$ deficiency: A new risk factor for breast cancer? *Nutr Rev.* 1999;57:250-253.

Clarke R, Smith AD, Jobst KA, et al. Folate, vitamin B$_{12}$, and serum total homocysteine levels in confirmed Alzheimer's disease. *Arch Neurol.* 1998;55:1449-1455.

Dagnelie PC, van Staveren WA, van den Berg H. Vitamin B$_{12}$ from algae appears not to be bioavailable. *Am J Clin Nutr.* 1991;53:695-697.

Delpre G, Stark P, Niv Y. Sublingual therapy for cobalamin deficiency as an alternative to oral and parenteral cobalamin supplementation. *Lancet.* 1999;354:740-741.

Dietary Reference Intakes for Thiamin, Riboflavin, Niacin, Vitamin B$_6$, Folate, Vitamin B$_{12}$, Pantothenic Acid, Biotin, and Choline. Washington, DC: National Academy Press; 1998:306-356.

Drennan CL, Huang S, Drummond JT, et al. How a protein binds B$_{12}$: A 3.0 A X-ray structure of B$_{12}$-binding domains of methionine synthase. *Science.* 1994;266:1669-1674.

Elia M. Oral or parenteral therapy for B$_{12}$ deficiency (commentary). *Lancet.* 1998;352:1721-1722.

Ellenbogen L. Vitamin B$_{12}$. In: Machlin LJ, ed. *Handbook of Vitamins.* New York, NY: Marcel Dekker, Inc; 1984:497-547.

Farquharson J, Adams JF. Conversion of hydroxo(aquo)co-balamin to sulfitocobalamin in the absence of light: a reaction of importance in the identification of the forms of vitamin B$_{12}$, with possible clinical significance. *Am J Clin Nutr.* 1977;30:1617-1622.

Fata FT, Herzlich BC, Schiffman G, et al. Impaired antibody responses to pneumcoccal polysaccharide in elderly patients with low serum vitamin B$_{12}$ levels. *Ann Intern Med.* 1996;124:299-304.

Funada U, Wada M, Kawata T, et al. Changes in CD4+CD8+/ CD4-CD8+ ratio and humoral immune functions in vitamin B$_{12}$-deficient rats. *Int J Vitam Nutr Res.* 2000;70:167-171.

Harriman GR, Smith PD, Horne MK, et al. Vitamin B$_{12}$ malabsorption in patients with acquired immunodeficiency syndrome. *Arch Intern Med.* 1989;149:2039-2041.

Hazra A, Kraft P, Selhub J, et al. Common variants of FUT2 are associated with plasma vitamin B(12) levels. *Nat Genet.* 2008;40(10):1160-1162.

Heimburger DC, Alexander CB, Birch R, et al. Improvement in bronchial squamous metaplasia in smokers treated with folate and vitamin B$_{12}$. Report of a preliminary randomized, double-blind intervention trial. *JAMA.* 1988;259:1525-1530.

Higginbottom MC, Sweetman L, Nyhan WL. A syndrome of methylmalonic aciduria, homocystinuria, megaloblastic anemia and neurological abnormalities in a vitamin B$_{12}$-deficient breast-fed infant of a strict vegetarian. *N Engl J Med.* 1978;299:317-323.

Houeto P, Hoffman JR, Imbert M, et al. Relation of blood cyanide to plasma cyanocobalamin concentration after a fixed dose of hydroxycobalamin in cyanide poisoning. *Lancet.* 1995;346:605-608.

Houston DK, Johnson MA, Nozza RJ, et al. Age-related hearing loss, vitamin B$_{12}$, and folate in elderly women. *Am J Clin Nutr.* 1999;69:564-571.

Jacobsen DW, Simon RA, Singh M. Sulfite oxidase deficiency and cobalamin protection in sulfite sensitive asthmatics. *J Allergy Clin Immunol.* 1984;73(Suppl):135.

Kaptan K, Beyan C, Ural AU, et al. Helicobacter pylori—is it a novel causative agent in Vitamin B$_{12}$ deficiency? *Arch Int Med.* 2000;160:1349-1353.

Kozyraki R, Fyfe J, Kristiansen M, et al. The intrinsic factor-vitamin B$_{12}$ receptor, cabilin, is a high-affinity apolipoprotein A-1 receptor facilitating endocytosis of high-density lipoprotein. *Nat Med.* 1999;5:656-661.

Kristiansen M, Kozyraki R, Jacobsen C, et al. Molecular dissection of the intrinsic factor-vitamin B$_{12}$ receptor, cubilin, discloses regions important for membrane association and ligand binding. *J Biol Chem.* 1999;274:20540-20544.

Kuzuminski AM, Del Giacco EJ, Allen RH, et al. Effective treatment of cobalamin deficiency with oral cobalamin. *Blood.* 1998;92:1191-1198.

Laine L, Ahnen D, McClain C, et al. Review article: potential gastrointestinal effects of long-term acid suppression with proton pump inhibitors. *Aliment Pharmacol Ther.* 2000;14:651-668.

Langdon FW. Nervous and mental manifestations of pre-pernicious anemia. *JAMA.* 1905;45:1635-1638.

Lindenbaum J, Healton EB, Savage DG, et al. Neuropsychiatric disorders caused by cobalamin deficiency in the absence of anemia or macrocytosis. *N Engl J Med.* 1988;318:1720-1728.

Lindstedt G. [Nitrous oxide can cause cobalamin deficiency. Vitamin B$_{12}$ is a simple and cheap remedy]. [Article in Swedish]. *Lakartidningen.* 1999;96:4801-4805.

McCaddon A, Kelly CL. Familial Alzheimer's disease and vitamin B$_{12}$ deficiency. *Age Ageing.* 1994;23:334-337.

Nilsson-Ehle H. Age-related changes in cobalamin (vitamin B$_{12}$) handling. Implications for therapy. *Drugs Aging.* 1998;12:277-292.

Okawa M, Takahashi K, Egashira K, et al. Vitamin B$_{12}$ treatment for delayed sleep phase syndrome. *Psychiatry Clin Neurosci.* 1997;51:275-279.

Ostreicher DS. Vitamin B$_{12}$ supplements as protection against nitrous oxide inhalation. *NY State Dent J.* 1994;60:47-49.

Refsum H, Smith AD. Are we ready for mandatory fortification with vitamin B-12? *Am J Clin Nutr.* 2008;88(2):253-254.

Robertson J, Iemolo F, Stabler SP, et al. Vitamin B$_{12}$, homocysteine and carotid plaque in the era of folic acid fortification of enriched cereal grain products. *CMAJ.* 2005;172(12):1569-1573.

Rosener M, Dichgans J. Severe combined degeneration of the spinal cord after nitrous oxide anaesthesia in a vegetarian. *J Neurol Neurosurg Psychiatry.* 1996;60:354.

Salom IL, Silvis SE, Doscherholmen A. Effect of cimetidine on the absorption of vitamin B$_{12}$. *Scan J Gastroenterol.* 1982;17:129-131.

Scalabrino G, Tredici G, Buccellato FR, et al. Further evidence for the involvement of epidermal growth factor in the signaling pathway of vitamin B$_{12}$ (cobalamin) in the rat central nervous system. *J Neuropathol Exp Neurol.* 2000;59:808-814.

Selhub J, Morris MS, Jacques PF. In vitamin B$_{12}$ deficiency, higher serum folate is associated with increased total homocysteine and methylmalonic acid concentrations. *Proc Natl Acad Sci USA.* 2007;104(50):19995-20000.

Stubbe J. Binding site of nature's most beautiful cofactor. *Science.* 1994;266:1663-1664.

Sumner AE, Chin MM, Abrahm JL, et al. Elevated methylmalonic acid and total homocysteine levels show high prevalence of vitamin B$_{12}$ deficiency after gastric surgery. *Ann Intern Med.* 1996;124:469-476.

van Asselt DZ, Blom HJ, Zuiderent R, et al. Clinical significance of low cobalamin levels in older hospital patients. *Neth J Med.* 2000;57:41-49.

Vogiatzoglou A, Refsum H, Johnston C, et al. Vitamin B$_{12}$ status and rate of brain volume loss in community-dwelling elderly. *Neurology.* 2008;71(11):826-832.

Warren MJ. Finding the final pieces of the vitamin B$_{12}$ biosynthetic jigsaw. *Proc Natl Acad Sci USA*. 2006;103(13):4799-4800.

Watanabe F, Katsura H, Takenaka S, et al. Pseudovitamin B$_{12}$ is the predominant cobamide of an algal health food, spirulina tablets. *J Agric Food Chem*. 1999;47:4736-4741.

Weir DG, Scott JM. Brain function in the elderly: role of vitamin B$_{12}$ and folate. *Br Med Bull*. 1999;55:669-682.

Weir DG, Scott JM. Vitamin B$_{12}$ "Cobalamin." In: Shils ME, Olson JA, Shike M, Ross AC, eds. *Modern Nutrition in Health and Disease*. 9th ed. Baltimore, MD; Williams and Wilkins; 1999:447-458.

Wolters M, Ströhle A, Hahn A. Cobalamin: a critical vitamin in the elderly. *Prev Med*. 2004;39(6):1256-1266.

Vitamin C

DESCRIPTION

The term vitamin C applies to substances that possess antiscorbutic activity and includes two compounds and their salts: L-ascorbic acid, commonly called ascorbic acid, and L-dehydroascorbic acid. Ascorbic acid is the major dietary form of vitamin C. The terms vitamin C, ascorbic acid, L-ascorbic acid, L-ascorbate and ascorbate are commonly used interchangeably.

Vitamin C is a hexose derivative, similar in structure to the six-carbon sugar glucose. It is an essential nutrient for humans, and, as pointed out by Linus Pauling in 1970, "differs from other nutrients in that it is required in the diet by only a few species of animals—man, other primates, the guinea pig, an Indian fruit-eating bat, and the red-vented barbul and some related species of Passeriform birds." It is also an essential nutrient for Coho salmon, rainbow trout, carp and some insects. Most other animals, all higher plant species and probably all algal classes can synthesize vitamin C from glucose or other sugars. Molecules similar to ascorbic acid are made by some fungi but not by bacteria. All vitamin C requiring animals lack the enzyme L-gulano-gamma-lactone oxidase, the final step in the synthesis of ascorbic acid from glucose. Plants produce large amounts of ascorbic acid to facilitate resistance to the oxidative stresses associated with the myriad biotic and abiotic challenges inherent to photosynthesis.

The major deficiency syndrome of vitamin C is scurvy. Symptoms of scurvy include inflamed and bleeding gums, petechiae, ecchymosis, follicular hyperkeratosis, coiled hairs, perifollicular hemorrhages, impaired wound healing, dry eyes and mouth (Sjögren's syndrome), arthralgia, joint effusions, muscle weakness, myalgia, fatigue, depression, frequent infections, anemia, anorexia, diarrhea, and pulmo-nary and kidney problems that can lead to coma and death. All systems of the body are affected by scurvy.

The antiscorbutic factor was isolated from the ox adrenal cortex in 1927 by the Hungarian biochemist and Nobel laureate Albert Szent-Györgyi and his colleagues, although at the time Szent-Györgyi didn't know that it was the antiscorbutic factor. In fact, his interest then was not in vitamins at all but in biological oxidation and reduction, and he was looking for reducing substances in extracts of the adrenal cortex. What was later to be known as ascorbic acid, Szent-Györgyi called "C XII" since it was the 12th substance prepared and examined in his work on tissue oxidation and the function of the adrenal cortex. He later discovered that C XII was indeed vitamin C, the antiscorbutic factor, that its empirical formula was $C_6H_8O_6$ and that the molecule was a carbohydrate, most likely a sugar derivative. He submitted a paper on his discovery, which he named Ignose (from "ignosco"—"I don't know" in Latin—and "-ose" to indicate that it was a member of the sugar family). However, the editor of the journal rejected that name and also the next one that Szent-Györgyi came up with, "Godnose." The editor suggested "hexuronic acid" to indicate that it had six carbons and was a sugar acid similar to glucuronic acid. Szent-Györgyi gave in and accepted that name, which shortly was to change to ascorbic acid. Szent-Györgyi actually didn't know the exact structure of ascorbic acid, which explains Ignose and Godnose. It was the chemist and also Nobel laureate Walter Haworth who actually deciphered the structure. Szent-Györgyi found a rich source of ascorbic acid in the fruit of the Hungarian red pepper or paprika (*Capsicum annuum*). He also found some other interesting reducing agents in paprika. He called these substances vitamin P. They were the first flavonoids identified. In 1932, the American biochemist Glen King and his colleagues isolated ascorbic acid from lemon juice, which is where the vitamin C story first began. Well, actually lime juice, but close enough.

Many of the symptoms of scurvy, particularly those having to do with connective tissue, can be explained by the known biochemical roles of vitamin C, particularly its role as a cofactor for prolyl and lysyl hydroxylase, enzymes important in the formation of collagen. Collagen synthesized in the absence of ascorbic acid—as occurs in scurvy—cannot properly form fibers, resulting in blood-vessel fragility, among other defects. In the prolyl and lysyl hydroxylase reactions, as well as in most of the biochemical reactions ascorbic acid participates in, it acts as a reducing agent. In these reactions, the vitamin reduces ferric and cupric ions to their ferrous and cuprous states, forms which are required for the reactions to proceed.

Ascorbic acid is also involved in the biosynthesis of other connective-tissue components, including elastin, fibronectin, proteoglycans, bone matrix and elastin-associated fibrillin. It also appears to play a role in collagen gene expression and cellular procollagen secretion.

The fatigue and weakness of scurvy may be due to L-carnitine deficiency. Ascorbic acid is a cofactor for crucial reactions in the carnitine biosynthetic pathway.

Ascorbic acid is involved in modulating iron absorption, transport and storage. It aids in the intestinal absorption of iron by reducing ferric iron to ferrous iron and may stimulate ferritin synthesis to promote iron storage in cells. It is involved in the biosynthesis of corticosteroids and aldosterone, the conversion of cholesterol to bile acids and it functions as a reducing agent for mixed-function oxidases.

For all of this, ascorbic acid is best known for its antioxidant properties and its possible role in the prevention of certain chronic degenerative disorders, such as coronary heart disease and cancer. In fact, ascorbic acid may be the most important water-soluble antioxidant in the body.

The daily dietary intake of vitamin C necessary to prevent scurvy is about 5 to 10 milligrams. Scurvy is rare in developed countries, since most people living in these countries typically consume much more than this amount.

About 90% of vitamin C in the average diet comes from fruits and vegetables. Peppers—sweet green and red peppers and hot red and green chili peppers—are especially rich in vitamin C. Other good sources include citrus fruits and juices, brussels sprouts, cauliflower, cabbage, kale, collards, mustard greens, broccoli, spinach and strawberries. Nuts and grains contain very little vitamin C. Cooking destroys vitamin C activity.

About 5% to 10% of the total vitamin C content of fresh fruits and vegetables is comprised of dehydroascorbic acid. In the case of processed foods, dehydroascorbic acid makes up about 30% of the vitamin C content. D-ascorbic acid (erythorbic acid or isoascorbic acid), the epimer of L-ascorbic acid, is frequently added to food as an antioxidant preservative. Erythorbic acid has very low vitamin C activity.

In addition to being known as ascorbic acid and L-ascorbic acid, vitamin C is also known as 2, 3-didehydro-L-*threo*-hexano-1, 4-lactone, 3-oxo-L-gulofuranolactone, L-*threo*-hex-2-enonic acid gamma-lactone, L-3-keto-*threo*-hexuronic acid lactone, L-*xylo*-ascorbic acid and antiscorbutic vitamin. It is abbreviated AA. Ascorbic acid is a crystalline, water-soluble substance with a pleasant (to some), sharp acidic taste. Its molecular weight is 176.13 daltons, and its

molecular formula is $C_6H_8O_6$. The structural formula of vitamin C is represented as follows:

Vitamin C

The other form of vitamin C is the oxidation product of L-ascorbic acid, L-dehydroascorbic acid or DHA.

VITAMIN C WITH BIOFLAVONOIDS

Vitamin C with bioflavonoids is a mixture of vitamin C, either as ascorbic acid or as an ascorbate, with flavonoids. Typically, the flavonoids are citrus flavonoids and are derived from lemons, oranges and grapefruits. It is believed that flavonoids work synergistically with vitamin C. This belief originates from the work and writings of the Hungarian biochemist Albert Szent-Györgyi, the co-discoverer of ascorbic acid. Szent-Györgyi also isolated substances from citrus fruits and Hungarian paprika which he called vitamin P. Vitamin P is now referred to as bioflavonoids or flavonoids. Flavonoids are not vitamins.

Szent-Györgyi believed that bioflavonoids and vitamin C worked synergistically to maintain blood capillary health and prevent capillary fragility. There is some *in vitro* evidence that flavonoids and vitamin C do work synergistically. One study showed that ascorbic acid acts synergistically with the flavonoid quercetin to protect cutaneous tissue cells in culture against oxidative damage induced by glutathione deficiency. However, there is, as yet, no good evidence that vitamin C and flavonoids work synergistically *in vivo*. A recent study, in cell culture, suggested that flavonoids may even inhibit the uptake of vitamin C into cells.

Flavonoids have biological effects independent of any interaction with vitamin C. (See various monographs on flavonoids.) Flavonoids from grapefruit include quercetin, naringenin and kaempferol. Lemon flavonoids include hesperidin (hesperitin 7-0-beta-rutinoside) and eriocitrin (eriodictyol 7-0-beta-rutinoside). These flavonoids, along with rutin and others, may be found in vitamin C/bioflavonoid supplements. Some formulations use flavonoids from the sour orange *Citrus aurantium.*

EFFERVESCENT VITAMIN C

Effervescent vitamin C is comprised of L-ascorbic acid, citric acid and sodium bicarbonate. It is similar to Alka Seltzer with ascorbic acid added. When the tablet is placed in water, the citric acid reacts with sodium bicarbonate to form sodium citrate and carbon dioxide. Also, some sodium bicarbonate reacts with ascorbic acid to form some sodium ascorbate. Some find effervescent C a more tolerable supplement than ascorbic acid.

ACEROLA VITAMIN C

Acerola vitamin C is vitamin C derived from acerola fruit. Acerola is the fruit of the small tree or shrub known as *Malphighia glabra* L. *Malphighia glabra* is native to the Antilles and northern South America. Acerola is also known as Barbados cherry, Antilles cherry, West Indies cherry, Puerto Rican cherry, cereso, cereja-das-antilhas and cereja-do-para. In 1945, the Barbados cherry was analyzed by researchers at the School of Medicine, University of Puerto Rico, and was found to be very rich in vitamin C. Interestingly, the analysis was inspired by the use of the fruit for colds by the local people.

Acerola is one of the richest sources of vitamin C in the world. The vitamin C content of the fruit depends on ripeness, seasons, climates and localities. Content is highest when the fruit is still green and lowest when ripe. The vitamin C content of unripe fruits can range up to 4.7 grams per 100 grams of fruit or 4.7% and is about 2 grams per 100 grams or 2% in very ripe fruit. For comparison, the vitamin C content of a peeled orange is 0.05% or 50 milligrams per 100 grams. Acerola also contains flavonoids, other vitamins, such as thiamin, riboflavin, niacin, pantothenic acid and beta carotene, and minerals, such as magnesium and potassium.

Malphighia glabra has also shown active anti-fungal properties. Folk medicine uses of acerola include treatment of liver ailments, diarrhea, dysentery, coughs, colds and sore throats.

ROSE HIP VITAMIN C

Rose hips are the fruit of roses. The rose hip is the swollen ovary of the flower which produces seed after the petals of a blossom wither and fall. Once the petals have fallen off a rose all that remains attached to the stem is the rose hip. Rose hips are rich sources of Vitamin C. In fact, one species, *Rosa rugosa* Thunb, contains the highest amount of vitamin C of any organism in the world. *Rosa rugosa* Thunb rose hips can contain up to 7 grams of vitamin C per 100 grams of rose hips or 7%. Acerola, the next richest source of natural vitamin C produces up to 4.7% vitamin C, and, for comparison, the peeled orange contains 0.05% vitamin C.

During World War II, England, Norway and Sweden were faced with a scurvy crisis. Since the war had restricted normal shipping, the British could not obtain enough citrus fruit for vitamin C. Children began showing the symptoms of early scurvy. The British discovered rose hips to be an excellent source of vitamin C and made the fruit of the rose into teas, soups and syrups. The children received these supplements daily, and this prevented any problem with scurvy.

Rose hips are the major source of natural vitamin C. A few species are used to obtain the vitamin, including *Rosa canina*, *Rosa mosqueta* and *Rosa rugosa* Thunb. In addition to vitamin C, rose hips contain such carotenoids as beta-carotene, lycopene, zeaxanthin, rubixanthin, gazaniaxanthin, beta cryptoxanthin, gamma-carotene, lutein, violaxanthin, and antheraxanthin. They also contain flavonoids, catechins, polyphenols, procyanidins and pectins.

Rose hips have other applications. The oil extracted from its seeds is included in many cosmetic preparations for its high content of alpha-linolenic acid (45%-50%) and linoleic acid (40%). The fruit has been used as food, mainly for preparing jams, teas and alcoholic beverages.

REDUCED-ACIDITY VITAMIN C

Reduced-acidity vitamin C consists of a mixture of 50% ascorbic acid and 50% sodium ascorbate. Some find this form of vitamin C a more tolerable supplement than ascorbic acid. Since the first pKa of ascorbic acid is 4.2, the pH of the mixture dissolved in water would be 4.2. Reduced-acidity vitamin C is also known as buffered vitamin C.

NON-ACID VITAMIN C

Non-acid vitamin C consists of an ascorbate salt of sodium or calcium which has a neutral pH when dissolved in water. The calcium salt consists of two molecules of ascorbate and one atom of calcium. The molecular formula is $C_{12}H_{14}CaO_{12}$. Calcium ascorbate is freely soluble in water. The sodium salt consists of one molecule of ascorbate and one atom of sodium. The molecular formula is $C_6H_7NaO_6$. Some find sodium ascorbate and calcium ascorbate more acceptable forms for vitamin C supplementation.

ASCORBATE AND VITAMIN C METABOLITES

Ascorbate and vitamin C metabolites refer to marketed vitamin C supplements containing vitamin C in a salt form, typically as calcium ascorbate, and vitamin C metabolites. Vitamin C metabolites can include the aldonic acids L-threonic acid, L-xylonic acid and L-lyxonic acid. Typically, the vitamin C metabolite present in these products is L-threonic acid, also known as 2, 3, 4-trihydroxy- [threo] butanoic acid. L-threonic acid is usually also present as the calcium salt or calcium L-threonate, and the percentage of calcium L-threonate in the product is usually 1% of the amount of ascorbate. That is, a tablet supplying 500 milligrams of ascorbate would supply 5 milligrams of L-threonate.

Ascorbate and vitamin C metabolites are sometimes referred to as metabolite-supplemented ascorbate. Some *in vitro* studies have shown that the addition of L-threonate to ascorbate enhances the transfer efficiency of ascorbate into cells. Animal studies have reported increased absorption and higher retention of vitamin C when the animals were supplemented with ascorbate plus threonate than when supplemented with ascorbate alone. One cell-culture study showed that the addition of threonate to ascorbate enhanced the production of collagenous protein and mineralized tissue when compared with ascorbate alone. The authors concluded that this finding could have relevance with respect to wound healing and bone regeneration.

Although the *in vitro* and animal studies appear interesting, what is wanting are well-designed and well-executed clinical trials in humans to determine if vitamin C metabolites, such as L-threonate, positively affect vitamin C status.

ACTIONS AND PHARMACOLOGY

ACTIONS

Vitamin C has antioxidant activity. It may also have anti-atherogenic, anticarcinogenic, antihypertensive, antiviral, antihistaminic, immunomodulatory, ophthalmoprotective and airway-protective actions. Vitamin C may aid in the detoxification of some heavy metals, such as lead and other toxic chemicals.

MECHANISM OF ACTION

Vitamin C is arguably the most important water-soluble biological antioxidant. It can scavenge both reactive oxygen species and reactive nitrogen species. Ascorbic acid or, more specifically, L-ascorbate is an excellent reducing agent, and it acts as a cofactor in various biochemical reactions to reduce the transition metals, iron and copper.

Ascorbate can be oxidized by most reactive oxygen and nitrogen species thought to play roles in tissue injury associated with various diseases. These species include superoxide, hydroxyl, peroxyl and nitroxide radicals, as well as such non-radical reactive species as singlet oxygen, peroxynitrite and hypochlorite. By virtue of this scavenging activity, ascorbate inhibits lipid peroxidation, oxidative DNA damage and oxidative protein damage.

Ascorbate is oxidized by reactive oxygen and nitrogen species to the semidehydroascorbate radical that is either reconverted to ascorbate via the enzyme NADH semidehydroascorbate reductase or is converted to dehydroascorbate. Dehydroascorbate in turn can be converted back to ascorbate via glutathione-dependent enzymes or catabolized.

Ascorbate can act as a secondary antioxidant. At least *in vitro*, ascorbate regenerates the major lipid antioxidant alpha-tocopherol from the alpha-tocopheroxyl radical form. Ascorbate may also participate in regenerating and sparing alpha-tocopherol *in vivo*, though this has not been clearly demonstrated. Vitamin C does preserve intracellular reduced glutathione concentrations.

The possible anti-atherogenic activity of vitamin C may be explained in a few ways. Oxidation of low-density lipoprotein (LDL) is thought to be a key early step in atherogenesis. Vitamin C protects against LDL peroxidation by scavenging peroxyl radicals in the aqueous phase. Vitamin C may enhance endothelial function by promoting the synthesis of nitric oxide (also known as NO and EDRF for endothelium-derived relaxing factor) or by preventing its inactivation by scavenging superoxide radicals. Superoxide reacts with nitric oxide to form peroxynitrite. High concentrations of vitamin C are required to prevent the interaction of superoxide with nitric oxide, extracellularly. Although such high plasma concentrations are feasible if vitamin C is given parenterally, they are likely not to occur with oral administration of vitamin C.

As noted above, vitamin C helps preserve intracellular reduced glutathione concentrations. This activity likely helps maintain nitric oxide levels and potentiates its vasoactive effects. Oral vitamin C can reach high enough concentrations intracellularly to scavenge superoxide radicals. Thus, intracellular sources of superoxide that impair nitric oxide may be scavenged by oral vitamin C. Recently, it has been found that ascorbic acid enhances nitric oxide synthase activity by increasing intracellular tetrahydrobiopterin.

Vitamin C may modulate prostaglandin synthesis to favor the production of eicosanoids with antithrombotic and vasodilatory activity. The possible sparing and regeneration of alpha-tocopherol by vitamin C could be yet another factor in the vitamin's possible anti-atherogenic action.

Vitamin C's possible anticarcinogenic effects may be accounted for, in part, by its ability to detoxify carcinogens, as well as its ability to block carcinogenic processes through its antioxidant activity. Vitamin C can prevent the formation of such carcinogens as nitrosamines in foods and in the gastrointestinal tract and can detoxify such chemical mutagens and carcinogens as anthracene, benzo[a]pyrene, organochlorine pesticides and heavy metals. High concentrations of ascorbic acid in gastric juice may reduce the risk of gastric cancer by inhibiting, as noted, the formation of carcinogenic N-nitroso compounds. Additionally, increased oxidative stress to the gastric mucosa has been reported in *Helicobacter pylori*-associated gastritis, a condition that predisposes to gastric cancer. There is preliminary evidence that vitamin C can inhibit growth of *Helicobacter pylori*.

Evidence appears to suggest that vitamin C may have cancer-preventive activity, at least for certain types of cancer. However, the role of vitamin C, if any, in the treatment of cancer remains very unclear. A cell-culture study of human breast carcinoma lines showed vitamin C to improve the antineoplastic activity of doxorubicin, cisplatin and paclitaxel. The mechanism of the effect may be pro-oxidant, not antioxidant, activity of the vitamin in potentiating the effects of these chemotherapeutic agents. Another study suggests that the pro-oxidant form of vitamin C may upregulate some of the enzymes involved in DNA repair. This possible activity may play some anticarcinogenic role. Recently, it has been found that ascorbic acid enhances arsenic trioxide-induced cytotoxicity in multiple myeloma cells. Again, this may be attributed to a pro-oxidant effect of vitamin C. Increasing reduced glutathione (GSH) levels attenuates arsenic trioxide-induced cytotoxicity. Decreases in GSH have been associated with ascorbic acid metabolites. Arsenic trioxide is an anticancer drug with multiple actions.

Vitamin C may have anti-hypertensive activity in some. The mechanism of this possible effect is a matter of speculation. Some *in vitro* studies show that vitamin C increases the synthesis of the vasodilatory prostaglandin PGE_1. However, this may not have relevance in the regulation of vascular tone in humans. As observed above, vitamin C may help maintain nitric oxide levels and potentiate its vasoactive effects. There is an indication that vitamin C may improve endothelial-dependent vasodilation in those with essential hypertension, as well as in those with hypercholesterolemia, and may help restore nitric oxide-mediated flow-dependent vasodilation in those with congestive heart failure.

There is some evidence that vitamin C inhibits the replication of human immunodeficiency virus 1 (HIV-1) *in vitro*. One study showed upregulation of the expression of glucose transporter 1 (Glut1) in HIV-infected cells Glut1 is one of the transport proteins for ascorbic acid. Increased cellular concentrations of ascorbate may be toxic to HIV-infected cells due to degradation of the viral nucleic acid by the action of the pro-oxidant form of vitamin C. The mechanism of the anti-HIV effect of the vitamin *in vitro*, however, is unclear, as is the relevance of this finding to HIV-positive individuals.

There is no evidence that vitamin C affects the replication of the viruses that cause the common cold *in vivo*. There is some evidence that vitamin C supplementation decreases the incidence, severity and duration of common cold symptoms in some. It is thought that this is due, at least in part, to antihistaminic activity of vitamin C.

The possible immunomodulatory activity of vitamin C may also be due, in part, to an antihistaminic effect of the vitamin. Vitamin C may enhance neutrophilic chemotaxis indirectly by reducing immunosuppressive effects of histamine. Some studies have shown that vitamin C, *in vitro*, enhances mitogen-stimulated lymphocyte proliferation, de-layed-type hypersensitivity (DTH) response to skin antigens, natural killer cell activity and neutrophil chemotaxis. However, other studies have shown no effect of the vitamin on these and other indices of immune function.

Some studies suggest a protective effect of vitamin C supplementation against cataracts. Age-related lens opacities are thought to be due to oxidative stress. Ocular tissue concentrates vitamin C, and the antioxidant action of the vitamin could account for its possible effect in protection against cataracts.

Vitamin C may protect against asthma and other obstructive pulmonary diseases, as well as protect the airways against the effects of allergens, viral infections and irritants in some. Allergens, viruses and irritants, including ozone, nitrogen oxides and sulfur oxides, subject the airways to increased oxidative stress which can lead to bronchoconstriction. The possible protective action of vitamin C appears clearly due to its antioxidant properties.

The antioxidant properties of vitamin C can also account for its role in protecting against the tissue-damaging effect of some toxic chemicals and heavy metals. High serum levels of ascorbic acid have been reported to be associated with a decreased prevalence of elevated blood lead levels. The mechanism of the possible lead-lowering action of vitamin C is unclear. One study compared the chelating properties of ascorbic acid and the known lead-chelating agent EDTA and found them to have equivalent activity with respect to lead.

PHARMACOKINETICS

Absorption of vitamin C from the lumen of the small intestine depends on the amount of dietary intake. At a dietary intake of 30 milligrams daily, the vitamin is nearly completely absorbed from the lumen of the small intestine into the enterocytes. At an intake of 30 to 180 milligrams daily, about 70% to 90% is absorbed. About 50% of a single dose of 1 to 1.5 grams is absorbed. The percentage of a single dose absorbed decreases with increasing amounts. For example, only 16% of a single dose of 12 grams is absorbed. Maximum vitamin C absorption of large doses is attained by ingestion of several spaced doses throughout the day rather than by a single large dose. Further, sustained-release forms of large doses will give a higher efficiency of absorption than an equivalent dose that is not sustain-released. The type of food consumed does not appear to affect the absorption of supplemental vitamin C or vitamin C found in food.

The intestinal absorption of vitamin C from foods and from supplements, up to about 500 milligrams, occurs via a sodium-dependent active transport process. At doses higher than 500 milligrams, diffusion processes come into play. The major intestinal vitamin C transporter is SVCT1 (sodium-dependent vitamin C transporter 1). Some ascorbic acid may be oxidized to dehydroascorbic acid and transported into enterocytes via glucose transporters. Dietary dehydroascorbic acid is absorbed from the lumen of the small intestine into the enterocytes in such a manner. All dehydroascorbic acid within the enterocytes is reduced to ascorbic acid via reduced glutathione, and ascorbic acid leaves the enterocytes to enter, first, the portal and, subsequently, the systemic circulation. Ascorbic acid is distributed to the various tissues of the body.

Higher levels of ascorbic acid are found in the pituitary gland, the adrenal glands, the various white blood cells and the brain. Ascorbic acid itself cannot cross the blood-brain barrier. In order to enter the brain, ascorbic acid is first oxidized to dehydroascorbic acid or DHA. DHA is then transported across the blood-brain barrier by facilitative diffusion via glucose transporter 1 (GLUT1). DHA is next transported through GLUT1 at the surface of the blood-brain barrier endothelial cells. DHA is transported out of the endothelial cells through GLUT1. DHA in the brain is reduced to ascorbic acid. Ascorbic acid, once formed, is essentially trapped in the brain since it cannot be transported through GLUT1.

Ascorbic acid appears to be transported into intestinal cells, liver cells and kidney cells by a sodium-dependent active transport process via SVCT1 (sodium-dependent vitamin C transporter 1). The transporter SVCT2 (sodium-dependent vitamin C transporter 2) appears to aid in the transport of vitamin C into the aqueous humor of the eyes. Uptake of ascorbic acid into neutrophils appears to be by facilitative diffusion via GLUT1.

Regarding the metabolism of ascorbic acid, it is oxidized to dehydroascorbic acid which can either be reduced back to ascorbic acid or hydrolyzed to diketogulonate. Other metabolites include oxalic acid, threonic acid, L-xylose and ascorbate-2-sulfate. The principal route of excretion of ascorbic acid and its metabolites is via the kidney. In order to maintain ascorbic acid homeostasis, very little unmetabolized ascorbate is excreted with dietary intakes up to about 80 milligrams daily. Renal excretion of ascorbate increases proportionately with higher doses. As mentioned earlier, as the dose of supplemental ascorbic acid increases, the percentage of its absorption proportionately decreases. Consequently, there is significant fecal excretion of ascorbic acid with high supplemental intakes of the vitamin.

INDICATIONS AND USAGE

Vitamin C may be helpful in chronic diseases characterized by oxidative damage to biological molecules. Though vitamin C also has a pro-oxidant potential under some circumstances, fears raised in that regard in recent years appear overblown. There is currently no credible evidence

for *oral* vitamin C pro-oxidant damage in humans except, possibly, in rare circumstances involving iron overload.

Vitamin C's antioxidant activity, on the other hand, is well established, and that activity may be helpful in the prevention of some cancers and cardiovascular disease. Vitamin C may also be helpful in protecting against some of the lipid oxidation caused by smoking. Vitamin C's demonstrated ability to reduce some forms of oxidative DNA damage and indications that it may also reduce protein oxidation under some circumstances further suggest that it may be of benefit in smokers and some with chronic stress and disease, in general. Considerable excitement has attended recent *in vitro* and *in vivo* animal research findings that *injected* vitamin C may have potent anticancer effects in a number of established malignancies, renewing interest in vitamin C not only as a possible cancer preventive but also as a potentially potent cancer interventive. These same findings have suggested that Vitamin C may also have some anti-infective potential greater than previously acknowledged.

Vitamin C may also be useful as an immune stimulator and modulator in some circumstances. Claims that it is a "cure" for common colds are unsubstantiated, although several studies have shown that vitamin C can significantly reduce the duration and severity of colds in some and reduce incidence in others. There is also preliminary evidence that vitamin C can be useful in ameliorating some other respiratory infections.

Vitamin C may help prevent cataracts.

Recently it was demonstrated that vitamin C can inhibit growth of *Helicobacter pylori* and may thus be protective against some ulcers and gastric carcinomas. There is also the suggestion in a recent report that low serum levels of ascorbic acid may be associated with a higher incidence of gall bladder disease in women. In another recent report, vitamin C supplementation was associated with reduced risk of reflex sympathetic dystrophy after wrist fracture. It may be of benefit in some burn victims and may be helpful, generally, in promoting wound healing and gum health

Vitamin C has previously shown some benefit in some individuals with asthma, although a recent review concluded that the vitamin C asthma data remain inconclusive. Whether it might also be useful in some other airway disorders/impairment, such as those present in cystic fibrosis, remains unclear and largely untested. There is a preliminary indication that it might be helpful in Charcot-Marie-Tooth disease, the most common hereditary peripheral neuropathy. There is no convincing evidence that it is useful in Alzheimer's disease. A strong inverse association between plasma vitamin C levels and type 2 diabetes mellitus risk has been noted recently. Effects on muscle and endurance performance are unclear.

RESEARCH SUMMARY

Vitamin C's antioxidant effects are well established. It has been reported to protect plasma lipids from oxidative damage. It also significantly protects DNA and protein from various oxidative processes, as demonstrated in numerous studies.

There is still controversy around claims that vitamin C can be a dangerous pro-oxidant in humans. These claims are now generally discounted, and the research that led to these fears has been widely challenged as being flawed in a number of respects. One researcher recently reviewed this controversy and concluded: "there is nothing in current data to worry members of the public who take ascorbate supplements."

Other researchers have also recently reviewed this controversy, noting that in vitro observations of DNA damage arising in the presence of vitamin C and redox-active transition metal ions are unlikely to have relevance in vivo. The damaging effect demonstrated in vitro, these researchers point out, "requires the availability of free, redox-active metal ions and a low ratio of vitamin C to metal ion, conditions unlikely to occur in vivo under normal circumstances. Furthermore, it was shown recently that in biological fluids such as plasma, vitamin C acts as an antioxidant toward lipids even in the presence of free, redox-active iron . . . there is no convincing evidence for a pro-oxidant effect of vitamin C in humans." However, although this is the case for orally administered vitamin C, the vitamin may indeed have a pro-oxidant effect when administered parenterally (see below).

On the other hand, vitamin C's antioxidant activity is marked and appears to play an important role in its possible cardioprotective activity. Several studies have shown that vitamin C, either alone, or in combination with other nutrients significantly inhibits LDL-cholesterol oxidation. This effect is most consistent when vitamin C is combined with vitamin E and/or beta-carotene, but it has also been observed when vitamin C is used alone. In the latter case, some hypothesize that it works by sparing or recycling vitamin E, an activity that has been observed in vitro. Results have been mixed in smokers in whom lipid oxidation is a serious problem. One of the better designed studies, utilizing a particularly sensitive measure of lipid oxidation, found that heavy smokers benefited from 2,000 milligrams of vitamin C administered for only five days, as measured by a significant reduction in a specific lipid oxidation marker, the F2 isoprostane 8-epi-PGF$_2$-alpha.

Where there have been discrepancies in results from lipid (and other) biomarkers studies, some researchers attribute these, in part, to the failure of some investigators to differentiate between subjects whose tissues are already saturated with vitamin C at baseline and those whose tissues are not thus saturated. Even dietary, non-supplemental, vitamin C intake, they argue, can readily result in saturation sufficient to rule out further reductions in oxidative damage, no matter what supplemental dose is administered.

Vitamin C supplementation has also been reported, in some studies, to significantly reduce total serum cholesterol. Some others have not shown this benefit. And there have been several observational reports associating high plasma vitamin C concentrations with higher levels of HDL-cholesterol.

Platelet aggregation has been reduced in two studies utilizing 2,000-3,000 milligrams of vitamin C daily for one to six weeks. No effect was noted on platelets in another study using 250 milligrams of vitamin C daily for eight weeks. Leukocyte adhesion to endothelium, an activity implicated in atherogenesis, was significantly inhibited in smokers receiving 2,000 milligrams of vitamin C daily for 10 days.

Several studies have shown that vitamin C has positive effects on hypertension. Here, too, there have been some conflicting results, but the preponderance of evidence suggests a positive effect. Epidemiological studies also consistently show that lower vitamin C intake is associated with hypertension. In one recent randomized, double-blind, placebo-controlled study, hypertensive patients received placebo or 500 milligrams of vitamin C daily for 30 days. Vitamin C resulted in a 13 mmHg reduction in systolic blood pressure. Placebo had no effects.

Several other studies have shown that both oral administration (1,000-2,000 milligrams) and intra-arterial infusion with vitamin C can exert significant, positive effects on vasodilation in coronary artery disease patients. Similar benefits have been found in several other test groups, including smokers and those with both type 1 and type 2 diabetes.

Vitamin C's potential impact on incidence of heart attack, stroke and death related to cardiovascular disease may be quite significant according to the findings of several epidemiological studies. In an analysis of findings from the First National Health and Nutrition Examination Survey, researchers found that "the relation of the standardized mortality ratio (SMR) for all causes of death to increasing vitamin C intake is strongly inverse for males and weakly inverse for females." Among males with the highest vitamin C intake, SMRs were 0.65 for all causes, 0.78 for all cancers and 0.58 for all cardiovascular disease. Among females with the highest vitamin C intake, SMRs were 0.90 for all causes, 0.86 for all cancers and 0.75 for all cardiovascular disease. Comparisons were made relative to the U.S. white population, for which the SMR was defined as 1.00.

In a 20-year follow-up study of a cohort of randomly selected elderly people in Britain, Scotland and Wales, mortality from stroke was highest in those with the lowest vitamin C status, as measured by dietary intake and plasma ascorbic acid concentration. Adjustments were made for age, sex and established cardiovascular risk factors. The association noted was independent of social class and other dietary variables. No association was found in this study between vitamin C status and risk of death from coronary artery disease, but the researchers noted this may have been due to the age of their observed population. "Factors that may predict premature death from coronary heart disease may become less important when measured in a population of elderly survivors," they noted. The subjects in this cohort were 65-74 years of age.

Recently, a five-year prospective population study of 1,605 Finnish men aged 42-60, who were free of atherosclerotic heart disease at baseline, concluded with these results: risk of myocardial infarction was considerably higher among those with the lowest baseline plasma vitamin C concentrations than among those with higher levels; 13.2% of those with the lowest levels suffered MIs versus 3.8% of those with higher levels.

What made this study particularly significant was its finding that increased risk of MI, in relation to plasma vitamin C concentrations, was confined to that group of subjects who were frankly deficient in vitamin C. In men with normal to high concentrations, there was no increased risk. This may have significance for some other studies that found no benefit from vitamin C in reducing cardiovascular disease risk.

It has been established by prior research that the Finnish population suffers high mortality from coronary heart disease and that many Finnish men have low plasma ascorbate concentrations. A reviewer of the Finnish study thus concluded that the finding in this study "that only individuals who are vitamin C-deficient are at increased risk may explain to some extent why no significant relationship was observed in many studies of relatively well-nourished populations."

This observation might apply, some believe, to the Nurses' Health Study and the Health Professionals' Study, both follow-up investigations that showed a relationship between increased vitamin E intake and reduced coronary heart disease risk but no similar relationship with respect to vitamin C.

As the reviewer further observed: "Both of these studies involved generally health-conscious study subjects. The vast majority of antioxidant-disease studies, even controlled intervention studies, involve generally healthy, well-nour-

ished populations, primarily because these populations are much easier to study. The Finnish study results, therefore, provide a special perspective that may help us to understand the mixed results from past studies and better plan future studies."

Vitamin C has, experimentally, demonstrated an ability to protect against various cancers, most likely through its ability to inhibit DNA oxidation, through reactive nitrogen species scavenging and other antioxidant actions, as well as through its possible effects on the immune system, among other activities. There are numerous epidemiological and case-control studies showing a consistent relationship between higher dietary intakes of vitamin C and lower incidence of cancer, particularly colorectal, stomach, lung, breast, esophageal, oral cavity and larynx-pharynx cancers. In one review of 75 epidemiologic studies, 54 found significant evidence of reduced cancer risk in those with higher dietary vitamin C intake.

Several *in vitro* and animal studies have demonstrated benefits. Results of some animal studies suggested that vitamin C therapy could reduce the toxicity and/or increase the effectiveness of some standard cancer therapies. Currently some researchers have expressed fear that vitamin C might reduce the effectiveness of some radiation and cancer chemotherapies by reducing their toxicity in cancer cells, as well as in normal ells. This idea has neither been confirmed nor refuted in animal or human studies and requires further investigation. Meanwhile, other researchers have expressed doubts about this hypothesis. They point out, as noted above, that several experimental studies indicate that high doses of vitamin C not only protect normal cells from toxic cancer therapies but may simultaneously fight the cancer cells, as well.

Many population studies have found evidence of a vitamin C protective effect against some cancers. Some other studies, however, have been negative. One group of researchers reported a significant 29% reduction in risk of all cancer in males consuming 113 milligrams or more of vitamin C daily, compared with males consuming less than 82 milligrams daily. Another found that consumption of 300 milligrams of vitamin C daily, derived from diet and from supplementation, was associated with a 21% reduction in risk from all cancers in men compared with daily consumption of less than 49 milligrams daily.

In a review of many of the epidemiological studies, the authors noted: "Interestingly, virtually all of the studies in which vitamin C intakes were greater than 87 milligrams a day in the lowest intake group (quantile) found no or nonsignificant effects on cancer risk reduction with higher intakes of vitamin C . . . . More studies investigating cancer risk in persons with lower vitamin C intakes are warranted."

Studies of those using higher dose vitamin C supplements have generally not shown protective effects against cancer, "possibly," these reviewers observed, "because the dietary intake of vitamin C was already sufficient for tissue saturation." Intervention trials with high dose vitamin C have also been mostly negative.

At present, there is evidence that vitamin C helps protect against a number of cancers. Generally amounts sufficient to exert preventive activity can be obtained from a diet that includes several servings of fruits and vegetables daily and/or through low-dose vitamin C supplementation.

Recently evidence has emerged that vitamin C may also have a potent *interventive* potential in cancer—but not via diet/supplementation but, rather, via injection. A few years ago, several researchers from various branches of the National Institutes of Health conducted an *in vitro* study, the results of which surprised many in the research world. These researchers exposed human Burkitt's lymphoma cells to concentrations of ascorbic acid equal to what they determined could be achieved through injection (but not through oral administration). They cited pharmacokinetics studies that had demonstrated that 10 grams of ascorbic acid given intravenously can produce at least a 25-fold higher plasma concentration than can the same dose given orally. Their results demonstrated that the much higher levels achievable through the intravenous route effectively killed cancer but not normal cells, acting as a pro-drug to deliver extracellular hydrogen peroxide as the selective killing agent. Why the hydrogen peroxide generated by the ascorbate does not affect normal cells remains unknown. The cancer cell death occurred by apoptosis and pyknosis/necrosis. The researchers hypothesized that the hydrogen peroxide might target cancer cellular membrane lipids forming hydroperoxides or reactive intermediates that are quenched/repaired in normal cells but not in cancer cells. In any case, the researchers concluded that these findings have "major therapeutic implications" and not only for cancer but also possibly for numerous infections that have been shown to be susceptible to hydrogen peroxide attack. (Among these: some viruses, including hepatitis C.) They pointed as well to a possible therapeutic application of vitamin C in patients with chronic granulomatous disease—again via injection, not oral administration.

Very recently, some of these same researchers generated headlines around the world when they extended their *in vitro* observations to *in vivo* animal cancer models, again with notable positive results. In these experiments, the researchers delivered pharmacologic parenteral doses of ascorbate to mice bearing aggressive tumor xenografts. Single doses of the ascorbate produced significant, sustained ascorbate radical and hydrogen peroxide formation selectively within interstitial fluids of tumors but not in blood. Daily administration of ascorbate significantly reduced growth rates of established ovarian, pancreatic and glioblastoma tumors in the mice. The researchers showed as well that the same pharmacologic concentrations of ascorbate were easily achieved via vitamin C injection in humans. They concluded that ascorbate as a pro-drug may have benefits in cancers "with poor prognosis and limited therapeutic options." Clearly further research is indicated and warranted.

Vitamin C has shown a variety of activities in the immune system. It has been shown, in animal and *in vitro* studies, to favorably modulate lymphocytes and phagocytes. It can regulate natural killer cells under some circumstances and affect production of cytokines, antibodies and complement components.

Because supplemental vitamin C was not shown, in several studies, to reduce the incidence of the common cold, many concluded that it was of no use whatever in colds. That is still the impression of some physicians, but it is probably an erroneous one. First, a few studies have, in fact, shown a reduction in incidence of colds. Most studies have been done in normally nourished subjects in western countries; these have, typically, shown no effect on incidence. But in three trials of subjects under acute physical stress, vitamin C supplementation resulted in a 50% reduction in common cold incidence. And in four British trials, there was an average 30% reduction in incidence among those receiving vitamin C. Dietary vitamin C intake is known to be low in the UK.

Placebo-controlled trials have consistently found that supplemental vitamin C, in doses of 1 gram or greater daily, alleviated the duration and severity of cold symptoms. In several of these studies, the alleviation has been significant. For unexplained reason, there seems to be a greater effect in children than in adults and possibly, a greater effect in males than in females. The best results have been obtained with 2-gram (or greater) daily doses. There was a 6% median reduction in cold duration in five studies in which adults were administered 1 gram of vitamin C daily. There was a median decrease of 26% in two studies of children given 2 grams of vitamin C daily. A recent review found no consistent evidence for vitamin C reducing the incidence of colds in the normal population, but it did find a strong positive effect among those exposed to brief periods of strenuous physical exercise and/or cold environments. An analysis of six trials involving a total of 642 skiers, marathon runners and soldiers on sub-arctic exercises indicated that vitamin C supplementation cut the risk of colds in half. The reviewers called for more therapeutic trials to further clarify the vitamin's potential in treating/preventing/shortening colds.

Vitamin C has also been found to be of benefit in patients with pneumonia and bronchitis. Incidence of pneumonia was significantly reduced in three controlled vitamin C studies, and substantial vitamin C treatment benefit was noted in elderly UK patients hospitalized with pneumonia or bronchitis.

There is evidence that supplemental vitamin C can inhibit the growth of *Helicobacter pylori* in both *in vitro* and animal studies. Thus it might have the potential to reduce the incidence of *H. pylori*-induced ulcers and subsequent gastric carcinoma. *In vitro*, high concentrations of vitamin C inhibited up to 90% of *H. pylori* growth. There was also significant inhibition of growth in animal experiments using oral administration of vitamin C.

High intake of vitamin C is strongly associated with reduced incidence of cataracts, according to the findings of case-control studies. In one study, intake of 300 milligrams or more per day was associated with a 70% reduction in risk. Another study found a 75% reduction in risk with daily intake of 490 milligrams or more per day, compared with intakes less than 125 milligrams per day. An intervention study using 120 milligrams of vitamin C daily produced a nonsignificant reduction in cataract risk of 22%, but a significant 36% reduction was observed in the same trial in subjects who consumed a multivitamin/mineral supplement.

Laboratory work has shown that vitamin C can slow chemical reactions that lead to cataracts by causing various lens proteins to aggregate. This has been demonstrated in animal work and in the human eye.

In a study of women who took vitamin C for at least ten years, incidence of cataracts was significantly reduced compared with controls who did not take vitamin C. The vitamin C-supplemented women were only 23% as likely to develop cataracts compared with the women who did not take supplements. In women not taking supplements, mean daily dietary intake of vitamin C was 130 milligrams per day, about twice the recommended intake but still less than one-third the average of women taking supplements.

Recently, serum ascorbic acid levels were found to be inversely related to prevalence of gall bladder disease among women but not among men. Previously, it was shown that vitamin C-deficient guinea pigs have a high incidence of gallstones. Further clinical investigation is warranted.

In another recent study, this one a double-blind, placebo-controlled trial of vitamin C in patients with conservatively treated wrist fractures, treatment with 500 milligrams of vitamin C daily for 50 days significantly reduced the incidence of reflex sympathetic dystrophy (RSD). Follow-up continued for one year. The researchers proposed that "this simple and cheap means of prevention could also be useful in the prophylaxis of RSD after other injuries, such as trauma of the foot or ankle, talar and calcaneal fractures, or crural fractures."

It was the use of vitamin C as an antioxidant therapy in dermal burns that led the researchers to believe that an antioxidant therapy might also be of benefit in preventing post-traumatic dystrophy (after wrist fracture). Researchers have found that vitamin C helps protect endothelial cells and reduces capillary permeability by reducing lipid peroxidation after burns. Some of these same mechanisms apparently account for reported beneficial effects of vitamin C in a variety of wounds, in addition to burns. There is some evidence that supplemental vitamin C may decrease permeability of gum surface tissue and may, by that and other mechanisms, help protect against periodontal gum disease.

Some studies have indicated that vitamin C can be of benefit in alleviating some of the symptoms of asthma. In one of these studies, a 500-milligram dose of vitamin C taken 90 minutes before exercise reduced bronchial spasms in some asthma sufferers. In another study, 1 gram of ascorbate daily reduced airway reactivity to various harmful inhalants in asthmatics. A recent review of the vitamin C asthma literature, however, found no convincing evidence (from randomized control trials) that the vitamin has an established role in the treatment of this disorder. The authors concluded that the data gathered to date are insufficient upon which to base any conclusion.

There is no evidence that vitamin C is helpful in Alzheimer's disease. Vitamin C's role in muscle metabolism and any possible benefit in endurance training remain to be delineated or demonstrated. In one recent study, oral administration of vitamin C was said to decrease muscle mitochondrial biogenesis and hamper training-induced adaptations in endurance performance in a small clinical trial. Oral doses of 1 gram daily were administered over an eight-week training period. Some of the findings of this study were derived from a concurrent animal study. Again, these data are insufficient for reaching any meaningful conclusion.

Recently, a strong inverse association was noted between plasma vitamin C levels and the risk of new-onset type 2 diabetes mellitus. Fruit and vegetable intake, to a lesser degree, was also inversely associated with this risk.

Finally, an intriguing study has suggested that ascorbic acid might be helpful in the treatment of Charcot-Marie-Tooth disease, the most common hereditary peripheral neuropathy, affecting 1 in 2,500 people. The only other treatments for this disease are physical rehabilitation and corrective surgery. This is a disease characterized by abnormal myelination of the peripheral nerves with consequent progressive weakness and atrophy of the distal muscles of the limbs. In this mouse model of the disease, ascorbate, a known promoter of myelination, substantially ameliorated the condition, reducing the expression of what is believed to be the responsible gene to a level below that required to induce the disease phenotype. The researchers, noting the absence of good alternatives, concluded that vitamin C "offers an immediate therapeutic possibility for patients with the disease."

CONTRAINDICATIONS, PRECAUTIONS, ADVERSE REACTIONS

CONTRAINDICATIONS

Vitamin C is contraindicated in those with known hypersensitivity to the substance or to any ingredient in a vitamin C-containing product.

Rose hip vitamin C

Rose hip vitamin C is contraindicated in those with known hypersensitivity to rose hips. There are reports of allergic reactions in those working with rose hips.

PRECAUTIONS

Although oxalic acid is formed when ascorbic acid is metabolized, this is highly unlikely to cause renal problems in healthy individuals without preexisting renal problems or who are not predisposed to increased crystal aggregation. Those with preexisting kidney stone disease or a history of renal insufficiency, defined as serum creatine greater than 2 and/or creatinine clearance less than 30, should exercise caution in the use of higher than RDA amounts of vitamin C (see Dosage and Administration).

Ascorbic acid is involved in modulating iron absorption and transport. It is highly unlikely that healthy individuals who take supplemental vitamin C will have any problem with iron overload. On the other hand, those with hemochromatosis, thalassemia, sideroblastic anemia, sickle cell anemia and erythrocyte G6PD deficiency might have such a problem if they use large amounts of vitamin C.

Pregnant women and nursing mothers should avoid using supplemental doses of vitamin C higher than RDA amounts.

ADVERSE REACTIONS

In healthy adults, oral doses up to 3 grams daily of vitamin C are unlikely to cause adverse reactions. The most common adverse reaction in those who take oral doses greater than 3 grams daily are gastrointestinal and include nausea, abdominal cramps, diarrhea and flatulent distention. These reactions are attributed to the osmotic effect of unabsorbed vitamin C passing through the intestine. Some advocates of megadose vitamin C use recommend titrating the daily dose of vitamin C to what they refer to as "bowel tolerance", i.e., the point at which the user begins experiencing diarrhea. This is not recommended.

Rare adverse reactions have been reported in healthy individuals taking high oral doses of vitamin C. These include elevation of serum glucose in an adult male taking 4.5 grams daily, a gastrointestinal obstruction in a 66-year-old woman taking 4.5 grams daily of ascorbic acid and esophagitis in one person taking a single 500 milligram dose. Daily ingestion of high-dose vitamin C is generally regarded as largely innocuous. However, vitamin C-induced hyperoxaluria, although rare, has been reported. It was reported (July 2008) that a patient admitted to a hospital in New Zealand developed acute renal failure secondary to vitamin C-induced hyperoxaluria, from which the patient died.

INTERACTIONS

DRUGS

Aluminum-containing antacids: The intake of large doses of vitamin C used at the same time as aluminum-containing antacids has been reported to increase urinary aluminum excretion, suggesting increased aluminum absorption from these antacids. However, this is not well documented.

Aspirin: Chronic use of high dose aspirin may lead to impaired vitamin C status.

Chemotherapeutic agents: Vitamin C may potentiate the antineoplastic activity of cisplatin, doxorubicin and paclitaxel. It may also help ameliorate the cardiotoxic effect of doxorubicin and the nephrotoxic effect of cisplatin. This is based on *in vitro* and animal studies. There is a concern by some researchers that supplemental doses of vitamin C may diminish the efficacy of some chemotherapeutic agents. Ascorbic acid has been found to enhance arsenic trioxide-induced cytotoxicity in multiple myeloma cells. It has also been found to overcome drug resistance in myeloma and to significantly increase the anti-myeloma effects of both arsenic trioxide and melphalan in cell culture models and in animal models. Arsenic trioxide is an anticancer drug with multiple actions, and a number of clinical studies are examining the possible synergistic effect that vitamin C may have when administered along with arsenic trioxide. In all of these cases, vitamin C is given parenterally and not orally.

However, a recent report found that vitamin C may antagonize the cytotoxic effects of a number of antineoplastic drugs, including doxorubicin, vincristine, methotrexate, cisplatin and imatinib mesylate. This was based on a preliminary *in vitro* study and requires follow-up before any conclusions can be drawn.

Estrogen: Ascorbic acid may enhance 17 beta-estradiol inhibition of oxidized LDL formation.

Propranolol: Ascorbic acid may affect both the absorption process and the first pass metabolism of propranolol. Heart rate has been found to decrease less when propranolol was administered with ascorbic acid, when compared to controls. The interaction has little biological importance.

Vitamin C/Bioflavonoid combinations and drugs that inhibit cytochrome P-450 3A4: Preparations containing grapefruit flavonoids may interact with some drugs. Some drugs have up to a three-fold greater bioavailability when coadministered with grapefruit juice. It is thought that the grapefruit flavonoid naringenin plays some role in this effect. Naringenin and/or other substances found in grapefruit juice inhibit cytochrome P-450 3A4 (CYP 3A4). Drugs affected include the calcium channel blocker felodipine, as well as carbamazepine, cyclosporine, lovastatin, simvastatin, saquinavir and nisoldipine. Those taking these drugs need to exercise some caution in the use of any grapefruit products.

NUTRITIONAL SUPPLEMENTS
Copper: One study showed that high doses of vitamin C negatively affected copper status in men. Other studies have not shown such effects.

Flavonoids: Vitamin C may act synergistically with various flavonoids. This is the basis of combining flavonoids with vitamin C in some supplements. However, it is not known if any synergism occurs to any extent in humans. There is a report that the vitamin acts synergistically with the flavonoid quercetin to protect cutaneous cells against oxidative damage. The study was performed with cells in culture. There are other reports, again from cell culture studies, that certain flavonoids such as quercetin and hesperetin may inhibit the uptake of vitamin C into cells.

Glutathione: Ascorbic acid may help maintain reduced glutathione levels in cells.

Iron: Vitamin C used concomitantly with nonheme iron supplements may increase the uptake of iron. This may cause problems in those with high iron stores or with propensity for iron overload, such as those with hemochromatosis, sideroblastic anemia, sickle cell anemia, thalassemia and erythrocyte G6PD deficiency.

Selenium: One animal study reported that the protective effect of selenite in tumorogenesis was nullified by vitamin C. The chemopreventive action of selenomethionine, a form of selenium derived from foods, was not affected by the vitamin. Selenite may be reduced by vitamin C to a form that is not available for uptake by tissue.

Vitamin E: Vitamin C may regenerate or spare d-alpha-tocopherol. However, this is based on *in vitro* and animal studies. It is not yet known if this occurs in humans and, if it does, to what extent.

LABORATORY TESTS
Bilirubin assay: High intakes of vitamin C may cause falsely elevated bilirubin values.

Creatinine assay: Large intakes of vitamin C may cause falsely elevated urine and serum creatinine levels. However, this is not well documented.

Glucose assay: Large intakes of vitamin C may cause false positive glucose readings measured by copper reduction methods (e.g., Clinitest) and false negative glucose results as measured by the oxidase methods (e.g., Clinistix and Tes-Tape).

Guaiac assay for occult blood: Intakes of vitamin C greater than 1 gram daily may cause a false negative guaiac test.

OVERDOSAGE
There are no reports of vitamin C overdosage in the literature.

DOSAGE AND ADMINISTRATION
A dose of 200 milligrams daily is almost enough to maximize plasma and lymphocyte levels. Doses of vitamin C vary from those equivalent to the RDAs up to 5 to 10 grams daily and, in some, even higher. Typical doses used range from 500 milligrams to 2 grams daily. Some increase their dose to 4 to 5 grams daily when coming down with a cold. Such doses may have antihistaminic-like action. A dose of vitamin C of 5 grams daily for 4 weeks was found to significantly inhibit *Helicobacter pylori* in one report. Although a dose of 200 milligrams daily is almost enough to maximize plasma and lymphocyte levels, high doses may aid in detoxifying some carcinogens in the stomach prior to absorption of the vitamin.

Absorption of supplemental vitamin C is most efficient if spaced throughout the day or if taken in time-release form.

The DV (Daily Value) for vitamin C, which is used for determining percentage of nutrient daily values on nutritional supplement and food labels, is 60 mg. This is based on the U.S. RDA for vitamin C.

In the United States, the average intake of vitamin C is about 95 milligrams for women and 107 milligrams for men. Children between the ages of one to five consume about 83 milligrams daily.

The most recent (2,000) dietary reference intakes (DRI) for vitamin C are as follows:

Infants	Adequate Intake (AI)	Tolerable Upper Intake Level (UL)
0-6 months	40 milligrams daily or 6mg/kg	ND
7-12 months	50 milligrams daily or 6mg/kg	ND

	Recommended Dietary Allowances (RDA)	Tolerable Upper Intake Level (UL)
Children		
1-3 years	15 mg daily	400 mg daily
4-8 years	25 mg daily	650 mg daily
Boys		
9-13 years	45 mg daily	1,200 mg daily
14-18 years	75 mg daily	1,800 mg daily
Girls		
9-13 years	45 mg daily	1,200 mg daily
14-18 years	65 mg daily	1,800 mg daily
Men		
19-30 years	90 mg daily	2,000 mg daily
31-50 years	90 mg daily	2,000 mg daily
51-70 years	90 mg daily	2,000 mg daily
Older than 70 years	90 mg daily	2,000 mg daily
Women		
19-30 years	75 mg daily	2,000 mg daily
31-50 years	75 mg daily	2,000 mg daily
51-70 years	75 mg daily	2,000 mg daily
Older than 70 years	75 mg daily	2,000 mg daily
Pregnancy		
14-18 years	80 mg daily	1,800 mg daily
19-30 years	85 mg daily	2,000 mg daily
31-50 years	85 mg daily	2,000 mg daily
Lactation		
14-18 years	115 mg daily	1,800 mg daily
19-30 years	120 mg daily	2,000 mg daily
31-50 years	120 mg daily	2,000 mg daily
Smokers		
Men	125 mg daily	NR
Women	110 mg daily	NR

ND = Not determinable

NR = Not reported

A LOAEL (Lowest-Observed-Adverse-Effect Level) of 3 grams daily has been established for vitamin C for adults. Based on this LOAEL, a Tolerable Upper Level Intake (UL) for the vitamin has been set at 2 grams daily for men and women 19 years and older.

LITERATURE

Aguirre R, May JM. Inflammation in the vascular bed: importance of vitamin C. *Pharmacol Ther.* 2008;119(1):96-103.

Agus DB, Gambhir SS, Pardridge WM, et al. Vitamin C crosses the blood-brain barrier in the oxidized form through the glucose transporters. *J Clin Invest.* 1997;100:2842-2848.

Antunes LMG, Darin JDC, Bianchi MDLP. Protective effects of vitamin C against cisplatin-induced nephrotoxicity and lipid peroxidation in adult rats: a dose-dependent study. *Pharmacol Res.* 2000;41:405-411.

Audera C, Patulny RV, Sander BH, et al. Mega-dose vitamin C in treatment of the common cold: a randomised controlled trial. *Med J Aust.* 2001;175(7):359-362.

Boothby LA, Doering PL. Vitamin C and vitamin E for Alzheimer's disease. *Ann Pharmacother.* 2005;39(12):2073-2080.

Bors W, Michel C, Schikora S. Interaction of flavonoids with ascorbate and determination of their univalent redox potentials: a pulse radiolysis study. *Free Rad Biol Med.* 1995;19:45-52.

Bush MJ, Verlangieri AJ. An acute study on the relative gastro-intestinal absorption of a novel form of calcium ascorbate. *Res Commun Chem Pathol Pharmacol.* 1987;57:137-140.

Carr A, Frei B. Does vitamin C act as a pro-oxidant under physiological conditions? *FASEBJ.* 1999;13:1007-1024.

Carr AC, Tijerina T, Frei B. Vitamin C protects against and reverses specific hypochlorous acid- and chloramine-dependent modifications of low-density lipoprotein. *Biochem J.* 2000;346 Pt 2:491-496.

Chen Q, Espey MG, Krishna MC, et al. Pharmacologic ascorbic acid concentrations selectively kill cancer cells: action as a pro-drug to deliver hydrogen peroxide to tissues. *Proc Natl Acad Sci USA.* 2005;102(38):13604-13609.

Chen Q, Espey MG, Sun AY, et al. Ascorbate in pharmacologic concentrations selectively generates ascorbate radical and hydrogen peroxide in extracellular fluid in vivo. *Proc Natl Acad Sci USA.* 2007;104(21):8749-8754.

Chen Q, Espey MG, Sun AY, et al. Pharmacologic doses of ascorbate act as a prooxidant and decrease growth of aggressive tumor xenografts in mice. *Proc Natl Acad Sci USA.* 2008;105(32):11105-11109.

Cooke MS, Evans MD, Podmore ID, et al. Novel repair action of vitamin C upon in vivo oxidative DNA damage. *FEBS Lett.* 1998;439:363-367.

Douglas RM, Hemilä H, Chalker E, et al. Vitamin C for preventing and treating the common cold. *Cochrane Database Syst Rev.* 2007;(3):CD000980.

Duarte TL, Lunec J. Review: When is an antioxidant not an antioxidant? A review of novel actions and reactions of vitamin C. *Free Radic Res.* 2005;39(7):671-686.

Duconge J, Miranda-Massari JR, Gonzalez MJ, et al Pharmacokinetics of vitamin C: insights into the oral and intravenous administration of ascorbate. *P R Health Sci J*. 2008;27(1):7-19.

Duffy SJ, Gokce N, Holbrook M, et al. Treatment of hypertension with ascorbic acid. *Lancet*. 1999;354:2048-2049.

Enstrom JE, Kanim LE, Klein MA. Vitamin C intake and mortality among a sample of the United States population. *Epidemiology*. 1992;3:194-202.

Fan X, Monnier VM. Vitamin C-mediated Maillard reaction in the lens probed in a transgenic-mouse model. *Ann N Y Acad Sci*. 2008;1126:194-200.

Fan X, Reneker LW, Obrenovich ME, et al. Vitamin C mediates chemical aging of lens crystallins by the Maillard reaction in a humanized mouse model. *Proc Natl Acad Sci USA*. 2006;103(45):16912-16917.

Fay MJ, Bush MJ, Verlangieri AJ. Effect of aldonic acids on the uptake of ascorbic acid by 3T3 mouse fibroblasts and human T lymphoma cells. *Gen Pharmacol*. 1994;25:1465-1469.

Fay MJ, Verlangieri AJ. Stimulatory action of calcium L-threonate on ascorbic acid uptake by a human T-lymphoma cell line. *Life Sci*. 1991;49:1377-1381.

Fischer H, Schwarzer C, Illek B. Vitamin C controls the cystic fibrosis transmembrane conductance regulator chloride channel. *Proc Natl Acad Sci USA*. 2004;101(10):3691-3696.

Frei B, Lawson S.Vitamin C and cancer revisited. *Proc Natl Acad Sci USA*. 2008;105(32):11037-11038.

Friedman PA, Zeidel ML. Victory at C. *Nature Med*. 1999;5:620-621.

Gamble J, Grewal PS, Gartside IB. Vitamin C modifies the cardiovascular and microvascular responses to cigarette smoke inhalation in man. *Clin Science*. 2000;98:455-460.

Giovannoni JJ. Completing a pathway to plant vitamin C synthesis. *Proc Natl Acad Sci USA*. 2007;104(22):9109-9110.

Gomez-Cabrera MC, Domenech E, Romagnoli M, et al. Oral administration of vitamin C decreases muscle mitochondrial biogenesis and hampers training-induced adaptations in endurance performance. *Am J Clin Nutr*. 2008;87(1):142-149.

Gonzalez JP, Valdivieso A, Calvo R, et al. Influence of vitamin C on the absorption and first pass metabolism of propranolol. *Eur J Clin Pharmacol*. 1995;48(3-4):295-297.

Grad JM, Bahlis NJ, Reis I, et al. Ascorbic acid enhances arsenic trioxide-induced cytotoxicity in multiple myeloma cells. *Blood*. 2001;98(3):805-813.

Halliwell B. Vitamin C: poison, prophylactic or panacea? *Trends Biochem Sci*. 1999;24:255-259.

Harakeh S, Jariwalla RJ, Pauling L. Suppression of human immunodeficiency virus replication by ascorbate in chronically and acutely infected cells. *Proc Natl Acad SciUSA*. 1990;87:7245-7249.

Harding AH, Wareham NJ, Bingham SA, et al. Plasma vitamin C level, fruit and vegetable consumption, and the risk of new-onset type 2 diabetes mellitus: the European prospective investigation of cancer—Norfolk prospective study. *Arch Intern Med*. 2008;168(14):1493-1499.

Harding JJ, Hassett PC, Rixon KC, et al. Sugars including erythronic and threonic acids in the human aqueous humor. *Curr Eye Res*. 1999;19:131-136.

Heaney ML, Gardner JR, Karasavvas N, et al. Vitamin C Antagonizes the Cytotoxic Effects of Antineoplastic Drugs. *Cancer Research*. 2008;68:8031-8038.

Hemilä H, Douglas RM. Vitamin C and acute respiratory infections. *Int J Tuberc Lung Dis*. 1999;3:756-761.

Hemilä H, Koivula TT. Vitamin C for preventing and treating tetanus. *Cochrane Database Syst Rev*. 2008;(2):CD006665.

Hemilä H, Louhiala P. Vitamin C for preventing and treating pneumonia. *Cochrane Database Syst Rev*. 2007;(1):CD005532.

Hodison T, Socaciu C, Ropan I, et al. Carotenoid composition of *Rosa canina* fruits determined by thin-layer chromatography and high performance liquid chromatography. *J Pharmaceut Biomed Anal*. 1997;16:521-528.

Hornero-Méndez D, Minguez-Mosquera MI. Carotenoid pigments in *Rosa mosqueta* hips, an alternative carotenoid source for foods. *J Agric Food Chem*. 2000;48:825-828.

Hwang J, Peterson H, Hodis HN, et al. Ascorbic acid enhances 17 beta-estradiol-mediated inhibition of oxidized low density lipoprotein formation. *Atherosclerosis*. 2000;150:275-284.

Institute of Medicine, Food and Nutrition Board. *Dietary Reference Intakes for vitamin C, vitamin E, Selenium, and Carotenoids*. Washington, DC: National Academy Press, 2000.

Ip C. Interaction of vitamin C and selenium supplementation in the modification of mammary carcinogenesis in rats. *J Nat Cancer Inst*. 1986;77:299-303.

Jacob RA. Vitamin C In: Shils ME, Olson JA, Shike M, Ross AC, eds. *Modern Nutrition in Health and Disease*. 9th ed. Baltimore, MD: William and Wilkins; 1999:467-483.

Jarosz M, Dzieniszewski J, Dabrowska-Ufniarz E, et al. Effects of high dose vitamin C treatment on Helicobacter pylori ingestion and total vitamin C concentration in gastric juice. *Eur J Cancer Prev*. 1998;7:449-454.

Kelly RP, Poo Yeo K, Isaac HB, et al. Lack of effect of acute oral ingestion of vitamin C on oxidative stress, arterial stiffness or blood pressure in healthy subjects. *Free Radic Res*. 2008;42(5):514-522.

Koc M, Imik H, Odabasoglu F. Gastroprotective and Anti-oxidative Properties of Ascorbic Acid on Indomethacin-induced Gastric Injuries in Rats. *Biol Trace Elem Res*. Epub: 2008 Aug 23.

Kurbacher CM, Wagner U, Kolster B, et al. Ascorbic acid (vitamin C) improves the antineoplastic activity of doxorubicin, cisplatin, and paclitaxel in human breast carcinoma cells in vitro. *Cancer Letters*. 1996;103:183-189.

Kwaselow A, Rowe M, Sears-Ewald D, Ownby D. Rose hips: a new occupational allergen. *J Allergy Clin Immunol*. 1990;85:704-708.

Loizidis T, Sioga A, Economou L, et al. The role of ascorbic acid and exercise in chronic ischemia of skeletal muscle in rats. *J Appl Physiol*. 2007;102(1):321-330.

Lykkesfeldt J, Christen S, Wallock LM, et al. Ascorbate is depleted by smoking and repleted by moderate supplementation: a study in male smokers and nonsmokers with matched dietary intakes. *Am J Clin Nutr*. 2000;71:530-536.

Markham RG. Compositions and methods for administering vitamin C. United States Patent Number 4, 822, 816. April 18, 1989.

Mathew D, Nair CK, Jacob JA, et al. Ascorbic acid monoglucoside as antioxidant and radioprotector. *J Radiat Res* (Tokyo). 2007;48(5):369-376.

McHugh GJ, Graber ML, Freebairn RC. Fatal vitamin C-associated acute renal failure. *Anaesth Intensive Care*. 2008;36(4):585-588.

Miura S, Ishida-Nakajima W, Ishida A, et al. Ascorbic acid protects the newborn rat brain from hypoxic-ischemia. *Brain Dev*. Epub: 2008 Aug 3.

Moertel CG, Fleming TR, Creagan ET, et al. High-dose vitamin C versus placebo in the treatment of patients with advanced cancer who had no prior chemotherapy. A randomized double-blind comparison. *N Engl J Med*. 1985; 312:137-141.

Montel-Hagen A, Kinet S, Manel N, et al. Erythrocyte Glut1 triggers dehydroascorbic acid uptake in mammals unable to synthesize vitamin C. *Cell*. 2008;132(6):1039-1048.

Mowat C, Carswell A, Wirz A, et al. Omeprazole and dietary nitrate independently affect levels of vitamin C and nitrite in gastric juice. *Gastroenterology*. 1999;116:813-822.

Nefié H. Anticlastogenic effect of Vitamin C on cisplatin induced chromosome aberrations in human lymphocyte cultures. *Mutat Res*. 2001;498(1-2):89-98.

Nefié H. The genotoxicity of vitamin C in vitro. *Bosn J Basic Med Sci*. 2008;8(2):141-146.

Ness AR, Chee D, Elliot P. Vitamin C and blood pressure—an overview. *J Hum Hypertens*. 1997;11:343-350.

Padayatty SJ, Sun H, Wang Y, et al. Vitamin C pharmacokinetics: implications for oral and intravenous use. *Ann Intern Med*. 2004;140(7):533-537.

Panda K, Chattopadhyay R, Ghosh MK, et al. Vitamin C prevents cigarette smoke induced oxidative damage of proteins and increased proteolysis. *Free Rad Biol Med*. 1999;27:1064-1079.

Park JB, Levine M. Intracellular accumulation of ascorbic acid is inhibited by flavonoids via blocking of dehydroascorbic acid and ascorbic acid uptakes in HL-60, U937 and Jurkat cells. *J Nutr*. 2000;130:1297-1302.

Passage E, Norreel JC, Noack-Fraissignes P, et al. Ascorbic acid treatment corrects the phenotype of a mouse model of Charcot-Marie-Tooth disease. *Nat Med*. 2004;10(4):396-401.

Pauling L. Evolution and the need for ascorbic acid. *Proc Natl Acad SciUSA*. 1970;67:1643-1648.

Pauling L. The significance of the evidence about ascorbic acid and the common cold. *Proc Natl Acad SciUSA*. 1971;68:2678-2681.

Podmore ID, Griffiths HR, Herbert KE, et al. Vitamin C exhibits pro-oxidant effects. *Nature*. 1998;392:559.

Raitakari OT, Adams MR, McCredie RJ, et al. Oral vitamin C and endothelial function in smokers: short-term improvement, but no sustained beneficial effect. *J Amer Coll Cardiol*. 2000;35:1616-1621.

Ram FS, Rowe BH, Kaur B. Vitamin C supplementation for asthma. *Cochrane Database Syst Rev*. 2004;(3):CD000993.

Rehman A, Collis CS, Yang M, et al. The effects of iron and vitamin C co-supplementation on oxidative damage to DNA in healthy volunteers. *Biochem Biophys Res Commun*. 1998;246:293-298.

Rivas CI, Vera JC, Guaiquil VH, et al. Increased uptake and accumulation of Vitamin C in human immunodeficiency virus 1-infected hematopoietic cell lines. *J Biol Chem*. 1997;272:5814-5820.

Rowe DJ, Ko S, Tom XM, et al. Enhanced production of mineralized nodules and collagenous proteins in vitro by calcium ascorbate supplemented with vitamin C metabolites. *J Periodontol*. 1999;70:992-999.

Sakagami H, Satoh K, Hakeda Y, et al. Apoptosis-inducing activity of vitamin C and vitamin K. *Cell Mol Biol*. 2000;46:129-143.

Simon JA, Hudes ES. Relationship of ascorbic acid to blood lead levels. *JAMA* 1999;281:2289-2293.

Simon JA, Hudes ES. Serum ascorbic acid and gallbladder disease prevalence among US adults. The Third National Health and Nutrition Examination Survey (NHANES III). *Arch Intern Med*. 2000;160:931-936.

Skaper SD, Fabris M, Ferrari V, et al. quercetin protects cutaneous tissue-associated cell types including sensory neurons from oxidative stress induced by glutathione depletion: cooperative effects of ascorbic acid. *Free Rad Biol Med*. 1997;22:669-678.

Taddei S, Virdis A, Ghiadoni L, et al. Vitamin C improves endothelium-dependent vasodilation by restoring nitric oxide activity in essential hypertension. *Circulation*. 1998;97:2222-2229.

Tecklenburg SL, Mickleborough TD, Fly AD, et al. Ascorbic acid supplementation attenuates exercise-induced bronchoconstriction in patients with asthma. *Respir Med*. 2007;101(8):1770-1778.

Toohey JI. Dehydroascorbic acid as an anti-cancer agent. *Cancer Lett*. 2008;263(2):164-169.

Tsukaguchi H, Tokui T, Mackenzie B, et al. A family of mammalian Na+-dependent L-ascorbic acid transporters. *Nature*. 1999;399:70-75.

Valkonen MM, Kuusi T. Vitamin C prevents the acute atherogenic effects of passive smoking. *Free Rad Biol Med.* 2000;28:428-436.

Verlangieri AJ, Fay MJ, Bannon AW. Comparison of L-ascorbic acid and Ester C in the non-ascorbate synthesizing Osteogenic Disorder Shionogi (ODS) rat. *Life Sci.* 1991;48:2275-2281.

Wang Y, Mackenzie B, Tsukaguchi H, et al. Human vitamin C (L-ascorbic acid) transporter SVCT1. *Biochem Biophys Res Commun.* 2000;267:488-494.

Zhang HM, Wakisaka N, Maeda O, et al. Vitamin C inhibits the growth of a bacterial risk factor for gastric carcinoma: Helicobacter pylori. *Cancer.* 1997;80:1897-1903.

Zollinger PE, Tuinebreijer WE, Kreis RW, et al. Effect of vitamin C on frequency of reflex sympathetic dystrophy in wrist fractures: a randomized trial. *Lancet.* 1999;354:2025-2028.

Vitamin D

DESCRIPTION

The term vitamin D refers to the secosterols ergocalciferol or vitamin D_2 and cholecalciferol or vitamin D_3 as well as to the metabolites and analogues of these substances. All forms of vitamin D possess antirachitic activity. Vitamin D is different from all of the other vitamins in human nutrition because it is the only vitamin that is a conditional one. Vitamin D_3 is synthesized in the skin from 7-dehydrocholesterol via photochemical reactions using ultraviolet B (UV-B) radiation from sunlight. However, there are conditions where the synthesis of vitamin D_3 in the skin is not sufficient to meet physiological requirements. Humans who are not exposed to sufficient sunlight due to reason of geography, shelter or clothing, require dietary intake of vitamin D. Under these conditions, vitamin D is an essential nutrient. Vitamin D without a subscript refers to either vitamin D_2 or vitamin D_3.

Vitamin D is the principal regulator of calcium homeostasis in the body. It is particularly important in skeletal development and bone mineralization. Vitamin D is a prohormone. That is, it has no hormone activity itself, but is converted to a molecule which does.

The active form of vitamin D is 1alpha, 25-dihydroxyvitamin D or 1,25(OH_2)D (again, when D is used without a subscript it refers to either D_2 or D_3). The vitamin D hormone 1,25 (OH_2)D mediates its actions via binding to vitamin D receptors (VDRs) which are principally located in the nuclei of target cells. 1,25(OH_2)D enhances the efficiency of calcium absorption, and, to a much lesser extent, phosphorus absorption, from the small intestine. Vitamin D deficiency is characterized by inadequate mineralization or demineraliza-

tion of the skeleton. Inadequate mineralization of the skeleton is the cause of rickets in children (vitamin D is also known as the antirachitic factor), while demineralization of the skeleton results in osteomalacia in adults. Further, vitamin D deficiency in adults can lead to osteoporosis. This results from a compensatory increase in the production of parathyroid hormone resulting in resorption of bone.

Very few foods are natural sources of vitamin D. Foods that do contain vitamin D include fatty fish, fish liver oils (e.g., cod liver oil) and eggs from hens that have been fed vitamin D. Nearly all the vitamin D intake from foods comes from fortified milk products and other foods, such as breakfast cereals, which have been fortified with vitamin D. Vitamin D is a fat-soluble vitamin and therefore its absorption is adversely affected in those with malabsorption disorders. Those with chronic liver disease, cystic fibrosis, Crohn's disease, Whipple's disease and sprue are prone to vitamin D deficiency. Others at risk for vitamin D deficiency, include those that do not drink milk and who do not receive much sunlight, those who live in regions where they receive little natural light, and alcoholics. The elderly are at risk for vitamin D deficiency for several reasons, including inadequate exposure to sunlight, consumption of low amounts of vitamin D-containing foods and the use of certain drugs, which interfere with the absorption and/or metabolism of vitamin D (see Interactions). In addition, older adults need higher amounts of vitamin D than younger adults because of decreased absorption of the vitamin. The use of sunscreens is another factor that can negatively affect vitamin D status. However, those who spend time in the sun without using a sunscreen put themselves at risk for skin cancers.

Over the last several years, studies have indicated that vitamin D may play beneficial roles in a wide range of diseases and disorders, including osteoporosis, cancer, multiple sclerosis, heart disease, psoriasis and Alzheimer's disease. We are also gaining greater insight into the mechanism of the various actions of the vitamin/prohormone. As mentioned above, it appears the active form of vitamin D, 1,25 $(OH_2)D_3$, mediates its actions via binding to the vitamin D receptor (VDR). The VDR is a high-affinity receptor, which acts as a ligand-activated transcription factor. Ligand binding results in obligate VDR heterodimerization with the retinoid X receptor (RXR). This receptor is a common partner for nuclear receptors. The activated heterodimer binds with strong affinity to vitamin D response elements (VDREs) in the promotion of target genes, close to the basic transcriptional machinery. The process is associated with the recruitment and assembly of several nuclear proteins serving as positive or negative coregulators, ultimately altering the rate of gene transcription. VDR, like other nuclear receptors, recruits in the nucleus co-regulators with either histone acetyltransferase or histone deacetylase activities. Histone acetylation results in a more relaxed chromatin structure associated with greater levels of gene transcription. On the other hand, histone deacetylation results in a less relaxed chromatin structure associated with lesser levels of gene transcription. Thus, VDR function is directly linked to epigenetic events. Importantly, the global tissue distribution of VDR underscores the ability of 1,25 $(OH_2)D_3$ to regulate cellular processes not directly related to mineral and skeletal homeostasis.

The two forms of vitamin D used for nutritional supplementation are the secosterols ergocalciferol (vitamin D_2) and cholecalciferol (vitamin D_3). Secosterols or secosteroids are derived from the cyclopentanoperhydrophenanthrene ring structure, the basic structure of all steroids. The cyclopentanoperhydrophenanthrene structure is comprised of four rings (A, B, C and D). Secosterols or secosteroids are steroids in which one of the rings has been broken. In the case of vitamin D, the bond between carbons 9 and 10 of ring B is broken, and this is indicated by the inclusion of "9, 10-seco" in the chemical name of the molecule. Seco is from the Greek word for split.

Vitamin D_2 is derived from fungal and plant sources. It is usually produced by the ultraviolet irradiation of the fungal sterol ergosterol. Vitamin D_2 is also known as ergocalciferol. Its chemical names are 9, 10-seco (5Z, 7E)-5, 7, 10(19), 22-ergostatetraene-3beta-ol and (3 beta, 5Z, 7E, 22E)-9, 10-secoergosta-5, 7, 10(19), 22-tetraen-3-ol. Its molecular formula is $C_{28}H_{44}O$ and its molecular weight is 396.66 daltons. The configuration of the double bonds are notated *E* for entgegen (from the German, meaning to stand opposite to) or *trans*, and *Z* for zusammen (from the German, meaning together) or *cis*. Vitamin D_2 is represented by the following structural formula:

Vitamin D_2

Vitamin D_3 is derived from animal sources. Vitamin D_3 is also known as cholecalciferol and calciol. Its chemical names are 9, 10-seco (5Z, 7E)-5, 7, 10(19) cholestatriene-3beta-ol and (3beta, 5Z, 7E)-9, 10-secocholesta-5, 7, 10(19)-trien-3-ol. Its molecular formula is $C_{27}H_{44}O$, and its molecular weight is 384.65 daltons. The only structural difference between vitamin D_2 and vitamin D_3 is in their side chains. The side chain of vitamin D_2 contains a double bond between carbons 22 and 23 and a methyl group on carbon 24. The structural formula of vitamin D_3 can be represented as follows:

Vitamin D_3

Pharmaceutical forms of vitamin D include calcitriol (1alpha, 25-dihydroxycholecalciferol), doxercalciferol and calcipotriene. Calcitriol and doxercalciferol are used to treat certain metabolic disorders; calcipotriene is used topically for the treatment of psoriasis.

Vitamin D analogues called deltanoids are being developed as chemopreventive agents. These analogues separate desirable antiproliferative and pro-differentiation activities from the undesirable hypercalcemic activity of vitamin D. High doses of vitamin D can result in hypercalcemia.

ACTIONS AND PHARMACOLOGY
ACTIONS
Vitamin D may have anti-osteoporotic, antituberculosis, anti-inflammatory (immunomodulatory), anticarcinogenic, antipsoriatic, antioxidant and mood-modulatory activities.

MECHANISM OF ACTION
Antiosteoporotic activity: Osteoporosis results from an imbalance between bone resorption and bone formation. Decreased vitamin D levels result in decreased production of the active form of vitamin D, 1,25-dihydroxyvitamin D (1,25$(OH)_2$ D). 1,25 $(OH)_2$ D enhances the efficiency of

calcium absorption. Chronic vitamin D deficiency results in decreased calcium absorption and secondary hyperparathyroidism. Increased bone resorption may be a consequence of vitamin D deficiency, resulting from secondary hyperparathyroidism. Therefore, vitamin D supplementation might be expected to protect against osteoporosis and fractures in those with occult vitamin D deficiency. Vitamin D may also be effective in the treatment of corticosteroid-induced osteoporosis by virtue of its stimulation of calcium absorption from the small intestine and its inhibition of the secretion and production of parathyroid hormone.

Antituberculosis activity: In the prechemotherapy era, tuberculosis (TB) was treated with good nutrition, vitamin D-containing cod-liver oil, rest, sunlight (especially sunlight) and fresh air. This regimen was the basis of the sanatorium movement for the treatment of tuberculosis. Those who are familiar with Thomas Mann's *The Magic Mountain* know that the setting of the novel is a tuberculosis sanatorium in Davos in the Swiss Alps. The first sanatorium in the United States was established in Saranac Lake, New York, in the heart of the Adirondack Mountains. Well over a century ago, it was thought that sunlight could treat tuberculosis.

In 1903, the Danish physician Niels Ryberg Finsen was awarded the Nobel Prize in Physiology or Medicine "in recognition of his contribution to the treatment of diseases, especially lupus vulgaris (tuberculosis of the skin), with concentrated light radiation, whereby he has opened a new avenue for medical science." Unfortunately, he could not attend the award ceremony, since he was very ill from a progressive hereditary disorder, Niemann-Pick disease. The philosopher Jacob Bronowski held that the greatest discoveries in science are made when the scientist tries to answer a very personal question. For Finsen, that question was how to treat his serious and disabling disease. In his 20s, he began to believe that, since he lived in a house facing the north, he would feel better if he received more sun. He began to collect observations about animals seeking the sun and he became more and more convinced that the sun had useful and important effects on the organism. In simple experiments, he found that the most refractive rays from the sun or from an electric arc had a stimulating effect on tissue. He eventually exposed patients with lupus vulgaris to high-intensity light produced from an electric arc lamp. The exposure of a small area of affected skin to the intense light, comprised of both ultraviolet and infrared rays, produced a moderate sunburn, leading to the peeling away of the superficial skin layers and leaving normal, healthy skin. He discovered that this phototherapeutic treatment cured or substantially improved tuberculosis of the skin in approximately 95% of those affected with this disorder. By the 1920s, sun exposure for the treatment of pulmonary tuberculosis had become routine. It also became clearer why sanatoria located in the Swiss Alps, the Adirondacks, or other places where the absorption of the sun's rays by the atmosphere was small had a good success rate with their tuberculosis patients. Sadly, the concentrated chemical light ray therapy did not stop the progression of Finsen's Niemann-Pick disease, and he died at the age of 43.

It is only recently that the mechanism of the antituberculosis effect of sunlight has become clearer. It appears that sunlight, by stimulating the synthesis of vitamin D, upregulates the expression of a microbe-fighting peptide known as LL-37 (cathelicidin). Sunlight, especially its UVB rays, induces the synthesis within the skin of vitamin D_3 (cholecalciferol) from 7-dehydrocholesterol (7-DHC). Vitamin D_3 is converted successively to 25-hydroxyvitamin D_3 and then to 1,25-dihydroxyvitamin D_3 within the skin keratinocytes. Sunlight also induces the expression of the vitamin D receptor (VDR). Together, 1,25-dihydroxyvitamin D_3 and the VDR induce the expression of the gene encoding the human antimicrobial peptide LL-37. Human LL-37 is a 37 aminoacid peptide that belongs to the cathelicidin family of antimicrobial peptides. (LL-37 is also referred to as cathelicidin, its family name.) The above pathway for the production of the antimicrobial peptide LL-37 is located in the skin. There is yet another pathway for the production of LL-37 that is located in the circulating monocytes-macrophages. That pathway begins with vitamin D_3 entering the systemic circulation where it is transported to the liver to be converted to 25-hydroxyvitamin D_3. Circulating monocytes are activated by toll-like receptor2/1 (TLR2/1) agonists present on specific microbes. The genes encoding VDR and CYP27B1 are induced. CYP27B1 converts 25-hydroxyvitamin D_3 to 1,25-dihydroxyvitamin D_3, which joins with the VDR and activates the gene encoding LL-37, leading to an increase in cellular LL-37 and enhanced microbicidal activity of the phagocytes.

Immunomodulatory/anti-inflammatory activities: Vitamin D has been found to modulate nuclear factor-kappa B (NF-kappaB) activation and to modulate the canonical Wnt signaling pathway. Increased NF-kappaB activity was noted in fibroblasts derived from VDR$^{-/-}$ mice, probably due to a loss of both VDR-mediated stabilization of IkappaBalpha, a potent NF-kappaB inhibitor, by 1,25 (OH)$_2$ D_3, and physical interaction between VDR and the p65 subunit of NF-kappaB. Vitamin D was found to upregulate IkappaBalpha levels in murine macrophage cells by increasing mRNA stability and decreasing IkappaBalpha phosphorylation, all molecular events that led to blunting of NF-kappaB activity. The vitamin D-VDR mediated effects on the NF-kappaB signaling pathway, a major proinflammatory pathway, provide a strong mechanistic rationale for the well-documented anti-inflammatory/immunomodulatory role of vitamin D.

Vitamin D deficiency has long been suspected to increase the susceptibility to tuberculosis. The active form of vitamin D, 1,25 (OH)$_2$ D, has been found to enhance the ability of mononuclear phagocytes to suppress the intracellular growth of *Mycobacterium tuberculosis*. 1,25(OH)$_2$D has demonstrated beneficial effects in animal models of such autoimmune diseases as rheumatoid arthritis. It has also been found to induce monocyte differentiation and to inhibit lymphocyte proliferation and production of cytokines, including interleukin (IL)-1 and IL-2, as well as to suppress immunoglobulin secretion by B lymphocytes. These effects are thought to be mediated by vitamin D receptors (VDRs) which are expressed constitutively in monocytes but induced upon activation of T and B lymphocytes. 1,25(OH)$_2$D has also been found to enhance the activity of some vitamin D-receptor positive immune cells and to enhance the sensitivity of certain target cells to various cytokines secreted by immune cells. Vitamin D appears to demonstrate both immune-enhancing and immunosuppressive effects.

Anticarcinogenic activity: 1,25-dihydroxyvitamin D has been found to induce differentiation, to inhibit cell proliferation and to induce apoptosis in a number of malignant cell lines, including human prostate cancer cells. 1,25-dihydroxyvitamin D suppresses the *in vivo* growth of human cancer (colon cancer, malignant melanoma) solid tumor xenografts. It has been demonstrated in various cancer cell lines that 1,25-dihydroxyvitamin D causes a dose-dependent inhibition of cell proliferation and switches cellular activity from proliferation to differentiation. 1,25-dihydroxyvitamin D has also been demonstrated to inhibit the growth of renal cell carcinoma cells in culture, to inhibit the growth of retinoblastoma in mice and to be antiproliferative and pro-differentiating for leukemia cells. The anticarcinogenic activity of the active form of vitamin D appears to be correlated with cellular vitamin D receptor (VDR) levels. Vitamin D receptors belong to the superfamily of steroid-hormone zinc-finger receptors. VDRs selectively bind 1,25-dihydroxyvitamin D and retinoic acid X receptor (RXR) to form a heterodimeric complex that interacts with specific DNA sequences known as vitamin D-responsive elements. VDRs are ligand-activated transcription factors. The receptors activate or repress the transcription of target genes upon binding their respective ligands. For example, the binding of 1,25-dihydroxyvitamin D to the VDR in intestinal cells activates the transcription of the calcium-binding protein which enhances the absorption of calcium. It is thought that the anticarcinogenic effect of vitamin D is mediated via VDRs in cancer cells.

The mechanism of action of the anticarcinogenic activity of vitamin D, however, is not fully understood. A recurring observation is that one of the key antiproliferative actions of vitamin D is upregulation of members of the Cip/Kip family of inhibitors of cell cycle progression, such as p21[waf1/cip1], a regulatory action on the cell cycle that vitamin D shares with the tumor suppressor protein p53. It has been shown that the tumor p21 gene has at least three vitamin D-responsive promoter regions, in two of which p53 also colocalizes. 1,25-dihydroxyvitamin D has been found to induce apoptosis of cancer cells *in vitro* and *in vivo*. It downregulates the antiapoptotic bcl-2 protein and upregulates p53 expression, resulting in active cell death. It also upregulates clusterin and cathepsin B. 1,25-dihydroxyvitamin D has also been shown to have antiangiogenesis activity. *In vitro*, it was found to inhibit vascular endothelial growth factor (VEGF)-induced endothelial sprouting and elongation and to have a significant inhibitory effect on VEGF-induced endothelial cell proliferation. *In vivo*, it was found to produce tumors that were less vascularized than tumors formed in mice treated with vehicle alone.

Antipsoriatic activity: 1,25-dihydroxyvitamin D and its analogues have been found to be effective in the treatment of psoriasis when applied topically. Psoriasis is a cutaneous disorder involving abnormal cellular proliferation and differentiation. The mechanism of action of 1,25-dihydroxyvitamin D and its analogues in the treatment of psoriasis is accounted for by their antiproliferative activity for keratinocytes and their stimulation of epidermal cell differentiation.

Antioxidant activity: Vitamin D$_3$ has been found to inhibit lipid peroxidation in rat hepatocytes *in vivo*, to inhibit iron-dependent lipid peroxidation in liposomes and to modulate cellular antioxidant defense in lymphoma-bearing mice. The mechanism of the antioxidant effect of vitamin D is unknown.

Mood modulating activity: Vitamin D$_3$, in two human studies, was found to significantly enhance positive affect and possibly reduce negative affect. The mechanism of this possible mood-modulating effect is unclear. It is speculated that vitamin D may affect brain serotonin levels.

PHARMACOKINETICS

Vitamin D is principally absorbed in the small intestine. It is absorbed from the lumen of the small intestine into the enterocytes by passive diffusion. Vitamin D is delivered to the enterocytes in micelles formed from bile acids and other substances. The efficiency of absorption of vitamin D is high. Approximately 50% to 80% of ingested vitamin D is absorbed. Vitamin D is secreted by the enterocytes into the lymphatics in the form of chylomicrons. It enters the circulation via the thoracic duct. Vitamin D is transported in the blood bound to an alpha-globulin vitamin D binding protein. This protein is also known as the vitamin D-binding protein (DBP) and the group-specific component (Gc) protein. A large faction of circulating vitamin D is extracted by the hepatocytes. It is metabolized to 25-hydroxyvitamin D (25(OH)D) or calcidiol in the hepatocytes, via the enzyme vitamin D 25-hydroxylase. 25(OH)D is the major circulating form of vitamin D. This metabolite of vitamin D, however, is not biologically active under physiological conditions. The biologically active hormone form of vitamin D, 1,25-dihydroxyvitamin D (1,25(OH)$_2$ D) or calcitriol, is produced in the kidney via the enzyme 25-hydroxyvitamin D1-alpha-hydroxylase. This enzyme is a cytochrome P450 mixed function oxygenase also known as CYP27B1. 25(OH)D and 1,25(OH)$_2$ D may undergo hydroxylation catalyzed by the enzyme cytochrome P450C24 (CYP24), also a cytochrome P450 mixed function oxygenase, to form 24, 25-dihydroxyvitamin D (24, 25(OH)$_2$ D) and 1,24,25-trihydroxyvitamin D (1,24,25(OH)$_3$ D), respectively. Deactivation of 1,25(OH)$_2$ D and 25 (OH) D occurs via hydroxylation at C-24 catalyzed by CYP24. Other metabolites of 1,25 (OH)$_2$ D include calcitroic acid and the lactone 1alpha, 25R(OH)$_2$-26,23S-lactone cholecalciferol. Vitamin D and its metabolites are excreted primarily via the biliary route. The final degradation product of 1, 25 (OH)$_2$ D$_3$ is calcitroic acid, which is excreted by the kidney.

INDICATIONS AND USAGE

In recent years, it can be argued, no major nutrient has garnered as much research attention as vitamin D, nor produced as many significant positive results. Once a dowdy backbencher in the supplement marketplace, vitamin D now appears to be reaching for superstar supplement status, partly due to the findings that most of us do not get adequate amounts of this crucial vitamin, either from diet or sun exposure, and that this deficit can result in serious negative health consequences. Since the first edition of this *PDR* appeared, evidence of vitamin D's benefit in bone health has expanded and solidified considerably. It appears to reduce bone loss in aging men and in postmenopausal women, and to significantly reduce the risk of falls among the aging. Some have calculated that in this context alone increased vitamin D intake could save the economy billions of dollars a year in avoidable medical costs. It also helps ensure normal bone development in infants and toddlers. Evidence is mounting that demonstrates significant anticancer and cardioprotective effects of vitamin D. Some researchers have concluded that *half* of all colorectal cancers in the United States might be prevented through increased vitamin D intake. Some 28,000 deaths from this cancer alone might thus be prevented, say these researchers. Other research suggests that vitamin D is useful in breast, prostate and ovarian cancers, among others.

Research is intensifying with respect to vitamin D's role in heart health as a result, in part, of recent findings that vitamin D levels are associated with all-cause and cardiovascular mortality. Indeed, some recent research observations suggest that vitamin D supplementation might have an antimortality effect generally. Vitamin D has immunomodulating activity and may be helpful in some autoimmune disorders, including multiple sclerosis. It has antimicrobial properties and may be useful, for example, in tuberculosis. It shows some promise in both type 1 and type 2 diabetes. It may be neuroprotective and shows very preliminary promise of impeding cognitive decline in those with Alzheimer's disease. It may have some positive impact in some forms of mental depression and may be radioprotective. Additionally, it may be of benefit in seizure, bilateral cochlear deafness, sick sinus syndrome and some forms of infertility. Its hoped-for usefulness in chronic kidney disease remains unproven.

RESEARCH SUMMARY

Vitamin D is an important prohormone derived from diet, from supplements and from our skin's ability to synthesize it with the help of sunlight. Since it is naturally available in very few foods (principally in fatty fish), a number of foods, especially milk and some cereals, have been fortified with it in an effort to provide greater intake. Though principally known for its important role in calcium metabolism and skeletal mineralization, it is widely present in many organs/tissues of the body where it plays varied and complex roles, which are only gradually beginning to be more fully understood. Various recent studies indicate that most of us get inadequate vitamin D either in our diets or via exposure to sunlight. How significant is this inadequacy? One study suggested that a majority of us are getting less than half of the currently recommended amount of this vitamin.

Other studies indicate that at least 40% of elderly men and women are frankly vitamin D deficient. Why is this? In our distant history, it has been pointed out, we were largely unclothed and exposed to much more sunlight and to sunlight, moreover, that was not attenuated by the prevalent air pollution we experience globally today. Given the much shorter life spans of that early human history, the development of skin cancers later in life was not the issue that it is today. Prevalent use of sunscreens and concern about skin cancer and aging have today further reduced our exposure to sunlight and thus to endogenous vitamin D production via skin synthesis. Increasingly, researchers are thus recommending supplementation with vitamin D "to at least 800 IU of vitamin D, per day" (*New England Journal of Medicine*). The National Academy of Sciences has set 2,000 IU daily as the safe upper intake level. Obtaining even 800 IU through diet is almost impossible unless one eats large amounts of oily fish or spends inordinate amounts of time, unprotected, in sunlight—not advised. Considerably higher doses of Vitamin D pose toxicity issues and should be avoided. (See Dosage and Administration for more-detailed recommendations.)

It has long been known that vitamin D deficiencies can lead to rickets and other bone problems in the young. Now the importance of this vitamin in the bone health of the elderly is becoming clearer. Most of the case control studies that have addressed this issue have found an inverse relationship between vitamin D levels and fracture in elderly men and postmenopausal women. There are, however, some inconsistencies in the data and the association is strongest for white, postmenopausal women. Functional bone health outcomes, such as the effect of falls, are the best-investigated aspect of this emerging picture. In a meta-analysis of vitamin D's effect on falls, a reduction of 22% in the risks attending these falls was reported among ambulatory or institutionalized older individuals with stable health. Only double-blind, randomized trials were included in the analysis—and the positive effect reported was said to be independent of calcium supplementation and several other important variables. The favorable result seen here was attributed in large part to the binding of a vitamin D metabolite to a highly specific nuclear receptor in muscle tissue (an action reported in several other research inquiries), resulting in enhanced muscle function which, in turn, it was hypothesized, helped prevent falls. This effect helps reduce the so-called "body sway" often observed in the aging. In some of the studies, doses in the 400 IU daily range were said to be insufficient to exert a significant effect, whereas 800 IU daily did exert significant effect. Given the high morbidity, mortality and economic cost of falls among the elderly, the authors of this meta-analysis stated that the case for supplementation in this population is "compelling." Other data established a clear relationship between low serum levels of vitamin D and incidence of osteoarthritis and bone fracture. The progression of osteoarthritis of the knee was associated with low dietary intake of vitamin D in the Framingham study.

A high incidence of occult vitamin D deficiency was found in a group of postmenopausal women who had suffered hip fractures. The researchers suggested that "repletion of vitamin D and suppression of parathyroid hormone at the time of fracture may reduce future fracture risk and facilitate hip fracture repair." They added that "supplements of about 800 IU of vitamin D per day and calcium may be necessary to attenuate bone loss in the winter and to reduce fractures."

Some have doubted that supplemental vitamin D would have much direct impact on osteoporosis and bone fracture. Vitamin D deficiency has not been shown to be a direct cause of osteoporosis. It produces osteomalacia, a defect in bone mineralization, rather than the reduction in bone mass that characterizes osteoporosis. Nonetheless, osteomalacia itself may predispose to bone fracture. Others have observed that vitamin D deficiency, now known to be considerably more prevalent in elderly populations than previously suspected, can also result in muscle weakness, another possible contributor to falls and fractures. And recently at least one function of vitamin D in osteoblasts associated with the development of clinical osteoporosis has been found.

Some studies have, in fact, failed to find any benefit from supplemental vitamin D in the prevention and treatment of osteoporosis. The majority of studies, however, have reported significant benefits, evidenced by a review of 23 studies. Positive outcomes, measured primarily by increase in bone density, were associated, in this review, with higher doses, longer duration of use and more sensitive methods of measuring bone mass.

Some of the best results have been obtained in studies using considerably higher than the typical 400 IU doses daily and administering calcium simultaneously. Response also appears sensitive to the subject population. More geriatric and infirm populations that are indoors more tend to have lower vitamin D levels and greater suppression of serum parathyroid hormone levels, and these populations seem to show greater response to vitamin D therapy.

In a three-year study, supplemental vitamin D was given at a dose of 800 IUs daily in combination with a calcium supplement. The population group included nursing home residents who were indoors most of the time. The vitamin D-calcium combination was found to significantly protect against hip fracture in this randomized, double-blind, placebo-controlled study.

In another recent three-year double-blind, placebo-controlled study, a combination of vitamin D (700 IUs daily) and calcium (500 milligrams daily) was tested for its effects on nonvertebral fracture incidence and bone mass maintenance in 389 men and women older than 65. The researchers concluded that this combination "led to a positive change in biochemical markers related to bone turnover, slowed the rate of bone loss and significantly decreased fracture incidence."

There is evidence from *in vitro*, animal and clinical research that supplemental vitamin D, administered during pregnancy in appropriate circumstances and under a physician's supervision, can be of benefit to the neonate, helping to ensure healthy osteogenesis and to prevent low-birth weight. There is also evidence that supplemental vitamin D enhances lactational performance in some. Again, supplemental vitamin D in greater than U.S. RDA amounts should be used during pregnancy and breast feeding only with the recommendation and monitoring of a physician.

There is an abundance of epidemiological data establishing an inverse relationship between vitamin D levels and cancer incidence, particularly with respect to colorectal, breast, prostate and ovarian cancers. It should be noted that black populations have lower levels of vitamin D than do white populations. These levels, in fact, are about half the levels seen in white populations. Some studies have shown that some black populations have higher incidences of some cancers, and researchers, in some instances, have associated these higher incidences to lower vitamin D levels. It has been noted for some time that age-adjusted death rates for colon cancer are higher in areas with low levels of winter sunlight and lower in areas with high levels of winter sunlight. Lower circulating levels of vitamin D are similarly—and highly— correlated with higher incidences of colon cancer. There is a markedly greater risk of colon cancer in the Northeast and lower risks in the South, West and Southwest. One research group recently concluded that intake of 1,000 IU of vitamin D daily is associated with a 50% reduction in risk of colorectal cancer. This was the research group that also concluded that half of the 145,000 new cases of colorectal cancer per year in the U.S. could be prevented with intakes of vitamin D in the 1,000 IU daily range. Another suggests 2,000 IU daily in order to achieve, they estimate, a 50% reduction in colorectal cancer incidence in the U.S. Still another research group, noting a relationship between low levels of vitamin D and digestive-system cancers, has recommended 1,500 IU daily of vitamin D as a preventive for that subset of cancers.

Breast cancer rates are also higher in low-sunlight areas, and observational studies again establish that women with the lowest levels of vitamin D may be at as much as five times the risk of getting breast cancer as those with the highest levels. Supplementing animals with vitamin D, sometimes in combination with calcium, has significantly decreased mammary malignancy in those animal models. Incidence of prostate cancer is three to six times higher, as measured in various studies, in men with low levels of vitamin D, compared to those with high levels. Similar findings apply to ovarian cancer. One group of reviewers has recently stated that it will require doses of 3,500 IU of vitamin D daily to achieve a 50% reduction in breast cancer incidence in the U.S. That dose should be taken only if a medical doctor recommends it and provides monitoring. Worldwide, this group estimates that 250,000 cases of colorectal cancer and 350,000 cases of breast cancer could be prevented with adequate vitamin D intake.

Recently, the results of a four-year population-based, double-blind, placebo-controlled trial revealed a substantially reduced all-cancer risk in postmenopausal women attributable, the researchers concluded, to enhanced calcium and vitamin D nutrition. The amount of vitamin D used in this study was 1,100 IU daily.

Some other recent studies have suggested that higher levels of vitamin D are associated with lower mortality in general, not only with respect to cancer. A meta-analysis of 18 independent, randomized, controlled trials involving 57,311 participants discerned a significant anti-mortality effect associated with vitamin D supplementation. Another group has similarly reported recently that, among 13,331 subjects included in the Third National Health and Nutrition Examination Survey (NHANES III), those with the lowest levels of vitamin D had the highest incidence of all-cause mortality. The subject population was considered representative of the general U.S. population.

The mechanisms by which vitamin D may inhibit mortality overall remain to be clarified; some of the mechanisms by which it inhibits cancer have been partially delineated. There is evidence that it inhibits tumor angiogenesis and exerts antiproliferative effects through enhancement of intercellular communication. It has been shown to inhibit mitosis of breast epithelial cells and to induce apoptosis in various cancer cell lines. It exerts antimetastatic and antiproliferative effects on prostate cells. There is some evidence that vitamin D may be useful in preventing prostate cancer but that vitamin D analogs may be required to effectively treat it once established.

Vitamin D is found in vascular smooth muscle, endothelium and cardiomyocytes. Its favorable role in heart health is suggested by the repeated observation that low serum vitamin D levels are associated with greater prevalence of peripheral arterial disease in the general U.S. population, as well as in many other populations around the world. In *in vitro* experiments, vitamin D exhibits anticoagulant activity and exhibits other properties that might be favorable to cardiovascular health. In animal studies it inhibits the renin-angiotensin system as well as myocardial cell hypertrophy. The results of a nested case-control study in 18,225 men aged 40 to 75 in the Health Professionals Follow-up Study indicated that low levels of vitamin D are associated with higher risk of heart attack, even after controlling for factors known to be contributive to coronary artery disease. And recently the authors of a prospective cohort study of 3,258 consecutive male and female patients scheduled for coronary angiography at a single center concluded that vitamin D levels are independently associated with all-cause and cardiovascular mortality. The intervention trials needed to establish a definite causal relationship have yet to be conducted, but are needed and warranted.

Preliminary evidence that vitamin D might be able to improve glucose tolerance in some diabetics began to emerge several years ago. Recently, the author of a case report stated that regular doses of vitamin D, up to 2,000 IU daily, showed some efficacy in reducing the risk of developing type 1 diabetes and that vitamin D intervention had improved glycemic control and insulin sensitivity in both type 1 and type 2 diabetics, as well as in normal individuals. This author cited earlier reports that low vitamin D levels have been associated with insulin resistance and obesity. In the case studies cited by this author, reversal of vitamin D deficiency resulted in changes favorable in those with diabetes. Insulin sensitivity has reportedly been improved more by vitamin D administration than by either metformin or troglitazone in one study. Follow-up was too brief in this study, however, to allow for meaningful conclusions. In another study, supplementation with 500 mg of calcium and 700 IU of vitamin D prevented a rise in fasting glucose and slowed the progression of insulin resistance over a three-year period, compared with placebo, in patients with impaired fasting glucose. Three Asian patients exhibited reduced glycemic control after receiving vitamin D_2. Unknown metabolites in vitamin D_2, it was suggested, might be responsible for the adverse effect seen in that study. Different vitamin D receptor genotypes in various ethnic groups have also been seen to be variable determinants of insulin secretory capacity. Given the overall suggestion of benefit in these preliminary studies, and the fact that prior research has found that vitamin D can help prevent islet cell death and can help improve the survival of islet cell grafts, further study is clearly warranted.

Vitamin D exhibits a number of immunomodulating abilities that may be involved in observed positive effects in some autoimmune disorders, in some infections and, as previously noted, in some cancers. Research conducted some years ago suggested that it increases the potency of cytokines and enhances phagocyte activity and antibody-dependent cytotoxicity of macrophages, and that it boosts natural killer cell activity and helps regulate T cells, among other things. Vitamin D-deficient subjects given supplemental vitamin D have reportedly had significantly fewer infections. One researcher has observed that vitamin D is a "flexible" bidirectional immunomodulator that, in some circumstances, can also dampen immune activity in favorable ways. It has been reported, for example, to improve joint symptoms caused by autoimmune psoriatic arthritis. Animal experiments suggest efficacy in some other disorders with autoimmune components, such as multiple sclerosis and rheumatoid arthritis. It has also shown some preliminary ability to control graft rejection and thus may prove helpful in transplantation. Some have suggested that vitamin D and its analogs may be superior to cyclosporine in suppressing transplant rejection and without the serious side effects of that drug. A vitamin D analog's antiproliferative and immunomodulating activities may account for some of its early reported success in treating some with psoriasis. Vitamin D itself has not exhibited this ability in that condition.

Much attention has been given to Vitamin D as a possible adjunctive immunotherapy in tuberculosis, a major public health hazard. In the 1800s and early 1900s, sunlight and vitamin D-rich cod-liver oil were the treatments of choice for tuberculosis. With the advent of antimycobacterial drugs, those once effective treatments were set aside and largely forgotten. Then *in vitro* tests reminded researchers that vitamin D can inhibit the growth of *Mycobacterium tuberculosis*. It has been demonstrated that human macrophages require activated vitamin D to kill TB bacilli. It has also recently been shown that vitamin D upregulates the expression of a microbe-fighting peptide. With tuberculosis resurgent again and often very difficult to treat with available drugs, vitamin D is being re-examined anew in this context, particularly as a possible preventive among at-risk populations. A recent review of this issue suggested that vitamin D might have the potential to shorten treatment, reduce infectivity and improve response in drug-resistant TB to other interventives. These reviewers have called for clinical trials to further assess the safety and efficacy of vitamin D in the treatment and prevention of tuberculosis, particularly in conjunction with other substances.

There is emerging evidence that vitamin D has some neuroprotective properties and that it may help inhibit neurocognitive decline and dysfunction, including, possibly, Alzheimer's disease. A recent review of the research literature concluded that vitamin D has neuroprotective effects attributable to its antioxidative, immunomodulating, nerve conducting and detoxifying properties. The vitamin D receptor and catalytic enzymes, these researchers report, have been localized in brain areas related to complex planning and processing and to new memory formation. They concede that the extent to which vitamin D and cognitive function are related remains indefinite but conclude that "the biological plausibility of this relationship is well supported." Quoting studies that show that elderly populations worldwide are 40-100% vitamin D deficient, and that age-related dementia is an enormous and growing public health problem, they conclude that "the need for well designed longitudinal investigations of vitamin D and cognitive function are critical." Some have estimated the national direct and indirect costs of dementia to be in the neighborhood of $100 billion annually. And the U.S. Census Bureau has estimated that nearly 19 million Americans will be age 85 by 2050 and that more than half of these will have some form of dementia.

In a recent cross-sectional study, researchers examined serum levels and Mini-Mental State Examination (MMSE) test scores of 225 older outpatients diagnosed with probable Alzheimer's disease. The vitamin D-sufficient patients were found to have significantly higher MMSE scores compared with vitamin D-insufficient patients. Vitamins B_1, B_6 and B_{12} were also examined in this study, but no correlation was observed between levels of these nutrients and MMSE performance. More-definitive studies will be needed—and are warranted—to determine a definite causal relationship between the vitamin and enhanced cognition in Alzheimer's patients.

A relationship between season and frequency of multiple sclerosis (MS) lesions has been observed. Investigators have postulated that vitamin D levels, whether enhanced by diet, supplementation or sunlight, contribute to diminished MS lesion activity. They concluded: "The impressive correlation also supports the need for proper clinical trials to test whether vitamin D nutrition can reduce formation of CNS lesions and slow the progression of MS."

Recently, a large population-based study revealed a strong relationship between low serum vitamin D levels/increased parathyroid hormone levels and depression (and severity of depression) in older adults. The finding persisted after adjusting for age, sex, smoking status, BMI, health status, level of urbanization and level of physical activity. Low levels of vitamin D cause an increase in serum parathyroid hormone levels, and primary hyperparathyroidism has been associated with minor depressive disorders. Improvement in mood is commonly seen with successful treatment of hyperparathyroidism. Some previous studies yielded conflicting results with regard to vitamin D's possible role in major depressive disorders; there was some indication in one study it might be helpful in seasonal-related depression. Vitamin D receptor distribution has been reported particularly dense in the human hypothalamus, in areas implicated in the pathogenesis of depression. More pathophysiologic research is needed to further explore this finding. It has been suggested that some future large-scale vitamin D intervention studies on, for example, osteoporosis, might usefully include mood as one of the outcome measures.

Additionally, vitamin D has shown some positive effects on spermatogenesis and benefit in some cases of bilateral cochlear deafness; there is a case study in which it seemed to obliterate the symptoms of sick sinus syndrome, a disorder of sinus node function that is generally treated with antiarrhythmia drugs. In one recent *in vitro* study, a vitamin D derivative (calcitriol) protected keratinocytes from deleterious effects of ionizing radiation. A recent meta-analysis found that vitamin D compounds do not consistently benefit those with chronic kidney disease.

CONTRAINDICATIONS, PRECAUTIONS, ADVERSE REACTIONS

CONTRAINDICATIONS

Vitamin D is contraindicated in those with hypercalcemia and in those with evidence of vitamin D toxicity. Vitamin D is contraindicated in those with hypersensitivity to any component of a vitamin D-containing product.

PRECAUTIONS

Pregnant women and nursing mothers should avoid vitamin D supplemental intakes greater than U.S. RDA amounts of the vitamin unless higher amounts are prescribed by their physicians. The U.S. RDA for vitamin D is 400 IU or 10 micrograms daily.

Pharmaceutical use of vitamin D must only be undertaken under medical supervision.

Supplemental vitamin D should be used cautiously in those on digoxin or any cardiac glycoside. Hypercalcemia in those on digoxin may precipitate cardiac arrhythmias. Supplemental doses of vitamin D greater that upper limit intake levels (UL) should only be used if medically prescribed and should be avoided by those on digoxin or other cardiac glycoside. The UL for adults is 2,000 IU or 50 micrograms daily.

Concomitant use of thiazides and pharmacologic doses of vitamin D may cause hypercalcemia in some.

ADVERSE REACTIONS

Dosage of vitamin D up to 60 micrograms (2,400 IU)/day in healthy individuals rarely causes adverse reactions. Chronic dosage of 95 micrograms (3,800 IU)/day or greater in healthy individuals may cause hypercalcemia. Early symptoms of hypercalcemia, include nausea and vomiting, weakness, headache, somnolence, dry mouth, constipation, metallic taste, muscle pain and bone pain. Late symptoms and signs of hypercalcemia, include polyuria, polydipsia, anorexia, weight loss, nocturia, conjunctivitis, pancreatitis, photophobia, rhinorrhea, pruritus, hyperthermia, decreased libido, elevated BUN, albuminuria, hypercholesterolemia, elevated ALT (SGPT) and AST (SGOT), ectopic calcification, nephrocalcinosis, hypertension and cardiac arrhythmias.

INTERACTIONS

DRUGS

Cholestyramine: Concomitant intake of cholestyramine and vitamin D may reduce the absorption of vitamin D.

Colestipol: Concomitant intake of colestipol and vitamin D may reduce the absorption of vitamin D.

HIV protease inhibitors: The HIV protease inhibitors ritonavir, indinavir and nelfinavir may impair vitamin D bioactivation to 1,25-dihydroxyvitamin D. This is based on *in vitro* studies conducted in human hepatocyte and monocyte cell lines. Ritonavir had the most potent inhibitory effect.

Ketoconazole: Ketoconazole may inhibit the biosynthesis and catabolism of 1,25-dihydroxyvitamin D. Reductions in serum 1,25-dihydroxyvitamin D concentrations have been observed following the administration of 300 to 1,200 milligrams daily of ketoconazole to healthy men for seven days.

Mineral Oil: Concomitant use of mineral oil and vitamin D may reduce the absorption of vitamin D.

Orlistat: Orlistat may decrease the absorption of vitamin D.

Phenobarbital and Phenytoin: Phenobarbital and phenytoin may reduce plasma levels of 25-hydroxyvitamin D by inhibiting vitamin D 25-hydroxylase activity in the liver.

NUTRITIONAL SUPPLEMENTS
Calcium: Concomitant intake of calcium and vitamin D may be more effective than no therapy or calcium alone in corticosteroid-induced osteoporosis.

FOODS
Olestra: The fat substitute olestra inhibits the absorption of vitamin D as well as the other fat-soluble vitamins A, E and K. Vitamins A, D, E (alpha-tocopherol) and K are added to olestra to compensate for this. Olestra contains 12 IU (0.3 micrograms) of vitamin D per gram.

OVERDOSAGE

Hypercalcemia can result either from excess intakes of prescribed forms of vitamin D or from consumption of high amounts of vitamin D_2 or vitamin D_3. The hypercalcemia associated with hypervitaminosis D may cause multiple debilitating effects. Anorexia, nausea and vomiting have been observed in hypercalcemic individuals treated with 1,250 to 5,000 micrograms (50,000 to 200,000 IU)/day of vitamin D. Hypercalcemia can result in a loss of the urinary concentrating mechanism of the kidney tubule, resulting in polyuria and polydipsia. The prolonged ingestion of excessive amounts of vitamin D and the accompanying hypercalcemia can result in metastatic calcification of soft tissues, including the kidney, blood vessels, heart and lungs. Typically, chronic ingestion of 50,000 to 100,000 IU/day of vitamin D is required to produce hypercalcemia. Since vitamin D stores in fat may be substantial, vitamin D intoxication may persist for weeks after vitamin D ingestion is terminated. The elimination half-life of vitamin D is about 20 to 29 days.

DOSAGE AND ADMINISTRATION

Supplemental vitamin D is available as vitamin D_2 (ergocalciferol) or vitamin D_3 (cholecalciferol). Typical dosage is 200 to 400 IU (5 to 10 micrograms) daily. Pre- and postnatal multi-vitamin, multi-mineral supplements typically deliver a dose of 400 IU daily. Vitamin D_2, which comes from the UV irradiation of ergosterol obtained from yeast, has been used for the prevention and treatment of vitamin D deficiency in children and adults for over 80 years and has been considered to be equally as effective as vitamin D_3 for bone health. However, a couple of reports suggest that vitamin D_2 is less effective than vitamin D_3 in maintaining vitamin D status. A recent study, though, found that a 1,000 IU dose of vitamin D_2 daily was as effective as 1,000 IU of vitamin D_3 in maintaining serum 25-hydroxyvitamin D levels.

Although it is not commonly done, it would be a wise to have one's serum vitamin D level checked by a physician. In fact, recognizing that adequate vitamin D levels might save millions of dollars for the healthcare industry, it would be a good idea to have vitamin D levels as part of a regular blood panel. Serum 25-hydroxyvitamin D_3 is the major circulating form of vitamin D. It has been suggested by some of the leading vitamin D researchers that a beneficial level of serum 25-hydroxyvitamin D_3 should be at least 30 nanograms per milliliter (30 ng/ml), but not more than 150 ng/ml. For some, this may require 2,000 to 3,000 IU a day, or higher, to reach that goal. Consult your physician before exceeding 2,000 IU daily.

Pharmaceutical preparations containing 50,000 IU (1,250 micrograms) of vitamin D_2 are used in the treatment of vitamin D deficiency in the elderly and in those with malabsorption syndromes, nephrotic syndrome and hepatic failure. Dosage used is 50,000 IU once weekly for eight weeks. This must be done under medical supervision.

The Food and Nutrition Board of the Institute of Medicine of the U.S. National Academy of Sciences has recommended the following adequate intakes (AI) for vitamin D (the biological activity of one microgram of vitamin D_2 or vitamin D_3 is 40 IU [international units]):

Infants	(AI)
0 through 12 months	5.0 micrograms (200 IU)/day

Children	
1 through 8 years	5.0 micrograms (200 IU)/day

Boys	
9 through 18 years	5.0 micrograms (200 IU)/day

Girls	
9 through 18	5.0 micrograms (200 IU)/day

Men	
19 through 50 years	5.0 micrograms (200 IU)/day
51 through 70 years	10.0 micrograms (400 IU)/day
Older than 70 years	15.0 micrograms (600 IU)/day

Women

19 through 50 years	5.0 micrograms (200 IU)/day
51 through 70 years	10.0 micrograms (400 IU)/day
Older than 70 years	15.0 micrograms (600 IU)/day

Pregnancy

14 through 50 years	5.0 micrograms (200 IU)/day

Lactation

14 through 50 years	5.0 micrograms (200 IU)/day

The LOAEL (lowest-observed-adverse-effect level) for vitamin D is set at 95 micrograms (3,800 IU)/day. The adverse effect referenced is hypercalcemia which is defined as a serum calcium level above 2.75 mmoles per liter or 11 milligrams per deciliter. The NOAEL (no observed-adverse-effect level) for vitamin D is set at 60 micrograms (2,400 IU)/day.

The Food and Nutrition Board of the Institute of Medicine has recommended the following tolerable upper limit intake levels (UL) for vitamin D:

Infants	(UL)
0 through 12 months	25 micrograms (1,000 IU)/day

Children

1 through 18 years	50 micrograms (2,000 IU)/day

Adults

Older than 18 years	50 micrograms (2,000 IU)/day

Pregnancy

14 through 50 years	50 micrograms (2,000 IU)/day

Lactation

14 through 50 years	50 micrograms (2,000 IU)/day

The DV (Daily Value) for vitamin D, which is used for determining the percentage of nutrient daily values on nutritional supplement and food labels, is 400 IU. This is based on the U.S. RDA for vitamin D.

LITERATURE

Aloia JF, Patel M, Dimaano R, et al. Vitamin D intake to attain a desired serum 25-hydroxyvitamin D concentration. *Am J Clin Nutr.* 2008;87(6):1952-1958.

Amin S, La Valley MP, Simms RW, et al. The role of vitamin D in corticosteroid-induced osteoporosis. A meta-analytic approach. *Arthritis Rheum.* 1999;42:1740-1751.

Ashcroft DM, Po ALW, Williams HC, et al. Systemic review of comparative efficacy and tolerability of calcipotriol in treating chronic plaque psoriasis. *Br Med J.* 2000;320:963-967.

Autier P, Gandini S. Vitamin D supplementation and total mortality: a meta-analysis of randomized controlled trials. *Arch Intern Med.* 2007;167(16):1730-1737.

Barger-Lux MJ, Heaney RP, Dowell S, et al. Vitamin D and its major metabolites: serum levels after graded oral dosing in healthy men. *Osteoporosis Int.* 1998;8:222-230.

Basha B, Rao DS, Han Z-H, et al. Osteomalacia due to vitamin D depletion: a neglected consequence of intestinal malabsorption. *Am J Med.* 2000;108:296-300.

Bishop N. Rickets today—children still need milk and sunshine (editorial). *N Engl J Med.* 1999;341:602-603.

Blutt SE, Weigel NL. Vitamin D and prostate cancer. *Proc Soc Exp Biol Med.* 1999;221:89-98.

Bodyak N, Ayus JC, Achinger S, et al. Activated vitamin D attenuates left ventricular abnormalities induced by dietary sodium in Dahl salt-sensitive animals. *Proc Natl Acad Sci USA.* 2007;104(43):16810-16815.

Bouillon R, Carmeliet G, Verlinden L, et al. Vitamin D and Human Health: Lessons from Vitamin D Receptor Null Mice. *Endocr Rev.* 2008 Aug 11. 2008;29(6):726-776.

Brannon PM, Yetley EA, Bailey RL, et al. Overview of the conference "Vitamin D and Health in the 21st Century: an Update". *Am J Clin Nutr.* 2008;88(2):483S-490S.

Buell JS, Dawson-Hughes B. Vitamin D and neurocognitive dysfunction: Preventing "D"ecline? *Mol Aspects Med.* Epub: 2008 May 13.

Bushinsky DA, Silver J. Nutritional vitamin D: the benefits of supplementation. *Curr Opin Nephrol Hypertens.* 2008;17(4):345-347.

Cauley JA, Lacroix AZ, Wu L, et al. Serum 25-hydroxyvitamin D concentrations and risk for hip fractures. *Ann Intern Med.* 2008;149(4):242-250.

Chapuy MC, Arlot ME, Duboeuf F, et al. Vitamin D_3 and calcium to prevent hip fractures. *N Engl J Med.* 1992;327:1637-1642.

Cianferotti L, Cox M, Skorija K, et al. Vitamin D receptor is essential for normal keratinocyte stem cell function. *Proc Natl Acad Sci USA.* 2007;104(22):9428-9433.

Cozzolino M, Vidal M, Arcidiacono MV, et al. HIV-protease inhibitors impair vitamin D bioactivation to 1,25-dihydroxy vitaminD. *AIDS.* 2003;17(4):513-520.

Davis CD. Vitamin D and cancer: current dilemmas and future research needs. *Am J Clin Nutr.* 2008;88(2):565S-569S.

De Luca HF, Zierold C. Mechanisms and functions of vitamin D. *Nutr Rev.* 1998;56:S4-S10.

Dobnig H, Pilz S, Scharnagl H, et al. Independent association of low serum 25-hydroxyvitamin d and 1,25-dihydroxyvitamin d levels with all-cause and cardiovascular mortality. *Arch Intern Med.* 2008;168(12):1340-1349.

Embry AF, Snowden LR, Vieth R. Vitamin D and seasonal fluctuations of gadolinium-enhancing magnetic resonance imaging lesions in multiple sclerosis. *Ann Neurol.* 2000;48:271-272.

Fleet JC. Vitamin D receptors: not just in the nucleus anymore (review). *Nutr Rev.* 1999;57:60-62.

Fraser DR. Vitamin D. *Lancet*. 1995;345:104-107.

Freedman DM, Looker AC, Chang SC, et al. Prospective study of serum vitamin D and cancer mortality in the United States. *J Natl Cancer Inst*. 2007;99(21):1594-1602.

Fujita T. Vitamin D in the treatment of osteoporosis. *Proc Soc Exp Biol Med*. 1992;199:394-399.

Garland CF, Garland FC, Gorham ED, et al. The role of vitamin D in cancer prevention. *Am J Public Health*. 2006;96(2):252-261.

Garland CF, Gorham ED, Baggerly CA, et al. Re: Prospective study of vitamin D and cancer mortality in the United States. *J Natl Cancer Inst*. 2008;100(11):826-827.

Garland CF, Gorham ED, Mohr SB, et al. Vitamin D and prevention of breast cancer: pooled analysis. *J Steroid Biochem Mol Biol*. 2007;103(3-5):708-711.

Garland CF, Grant WB, Mohr SB, et al. What is the dose-response relationship between vitamin D and cancer risk? *Nutr Rev*. 2007;65(8 Pt 2):S91-S95.

Giovannucci E. Can vitamin D reduce total mortality? *Arch Intern Med*. 2007;167(16):1709-1710.

Giovannucci E, Liu Y, Hollis BW, et al. 25-hydroxyvitamin D and risk of myocardial infarction in men: a prospective study. *Arch Intern Med*. 2008;168(11):1174-1180.

Giovannucci E, Liu Y, Rimm EB, et al. Prospective study of predictors of vitamin D status and cancer incidence and mortality in men. *J Natl Cancer Inst*. 2006;98(7):451-459.

Gissel T, Rejnmark L, Mosekilde L, et al. Intake of vitamin D and risk of breast cancer-A meta-analysis. *J Steroid Biochem Mol Biol*. 2008;111(3-5):195-199.

Glorieux FH, Feldman D, eds. *Vitamin D*. San Diego, CA: Academic Press; 1997.

Gloth FM III, Gundberg CM, Hollis BW, et al. Vitamin D deficiency in homebound elderly persons. *JAMA*. 1995;274:1683-1686.

Gordon CM, Feldman HA, Sinclair L, et al. Prevalence of vitamin D deficiency among healthy infants and toddlers. *Arch Pediatr Adolesc Med*. 2008;162(6):505-512.

Gorham ED, Garland CF, Garland FC, et al. Vitamin D and prevention of colorectal cancer. *J Steroid Biochem Mol Biol*. 2005;97(1-2):179-194.

Heaney RP. Vitamin D in Health and Disease. *Clin J Am Soc Nephrol*. 2008;3(5):1535-1541.

Holick MF. Vitamin D deficiency. *N Engl J Med*. 2007;357(3):266-281.

Holick MF. Vitamin D: importance in the prevention of cancers, type 1 diabetes, heart disease, and osteoporosis. *Am J Clin Nutr*. 2004;79(3):362-371.

Holick MF. Vitamin D In: Shils ME, Olson JA, Shike M, Ross AC, eds. *Modern Nutrition in Health and Disease*. 9th ed Baltimore, MD: Williams and Wilkins; 1999:329-345.

Holick MF, Biancuzzo RM, Chen TC, et al. Vitamin D2 is as effective as vitamin D3 in maintaining circulating concentrations of 25-hydroxyvitamin D. *J Clin Endocrinol Metab*. 2008;93(3):677-681.

Hoogendijk WJ, Lips P, Dik MG, et al. Depression is associated with decreased 25-hydroxyvitamin D and increased parathyroid hormone levels in older adults. *Arch Gen Psychiatry*. 2008;65(5):508-512.

Institute of Medicine, Food and Nutrition Board. Dietary Reference Intakes for calcium, phosphorous, magnesium, vitamin D, and fluoride. Washington, DC: National Academy Press, 1997.

Kato S. The function of vitamin D receptor in vitamin D action. *J Biochem*. 2000;127:717-722.

Kensler TW, Dolan PM, Grange SJ, et al. Conceptually new deltanoids (vitamin D analogues) inhibit multistage skin tumorigenesis. *Carcinogenesis*. 2000;21:1341-1345.

Kreiter SR, Schwartz RP, Kirkman HN Jr., et al. Nutritional rickets in African American breast-fed infants. *J Pediatr*. 2000;137:153-157.

Lal H, Pandey R, Aggarwal SK. Vitamin D: non-skeletal actions and effects on growth. *Nutr Res*. 1999;19:1683-1718.

Lamprecht SA, Lipkin M. Chemoprevention of colon cancer by calcium, vitamin D and folate: molecular mechanisms. *Nat Rev Cancer*. 2003;3(8):601-614.

Landsdowne ATG, Provost SC. Vitamin D3 enhances mood in healthy subjects during winter. *Psychopharmacol*. 1998;135:319-323.

Lane NE, Gore L, Cummings SR, et al. Serum vitamin D levels and incident changes of radiographic osteoarthritis. *Arthritis Rheum*. 1999;42:854-860.

Langberg M, Rotem C, Fenig E, et al. Vitamin D protects keratinocytes from deleterious effects of ionizing radiation. *Br J Dermatol*. Epub: 2008 Aug 19.

Lappe JM, Travers-Gustafson D, Davies KM, et al. Vitamin D and calcium supplementation reduces cancer risk: results of a randomized trial. *Am J Clin Nutr*. 2007;85(6):1586-1591.

LeBoff MS, Kohlmeier L, Hurwitz S, et al. Occult vitamin D deficiency in postmenopausal US women with acute hip fracture. *JAMA*. 1999;281:1505-1511.

Li M, Hener P, Zhang Z, et al. Topical vitamin D3 and low-calcemic analogs induce thymic stromal lymphopoietin in mouse keratinocytes and trigger an atopic dermatitis. *Proc Natl Acad Sci USA*. 2006;103(31):11736-11741.

Lipkin M, Lamprecht SA. Mechanisms of action of vitamin D: recent findings and new questions. *J Med Food*. 2006;9(2):135-137.

Lips P, Graafmans WC, Ooms ME, et al. Vitamin D supplementation and fracture incidence in elderly persons. A randomized, placebo-controlled clinical trial. *Ann Intern Med*. 1996;124:400-406.

Liu PT, Stenger S, Li H, et al.Toll-like receptor triggering of a vitamin D-mediated human antimicrobial response. *Science.* 2006;311(5768):1770-1773.

Lowe KE, Norman AW. Vitamin D and psoriasis. *Nutr Rev* 1992;50:138-142.

Maalouf J, Nabulsi M, Vieth R, et al. Short- and long-term safety of weekly high-dose vitamin D3 supplementation in school children. *J Clin Endocrinol Metab.* 2008;93(7):2693-2701.

Malloy PJ, Feldman D. Vitamin D resistance. *Am J Med.* 1999;106:355-370.

Malloy PJ, Pike JW, Feldman D. The vitamin D receptor and the syndrome of hereditary 1,25-dihydroxyvitamin D-resistant rickets. *Endocrine Reviews.* 1999;20:156-188.

Manolagas SC, Provvedini DM, Tsoukas CD. Interactions of 1,25-dihydroxyvitamin D_3 and the immune system. *Mol Cell Endocrinol.* 1985;43:113-122.

Mantell DJ, Owens PE, Bundred NJ, et al. 1alpha, 25-Dihydroxyvitamin D_3 inhibits angiogenesis in vitro and in vivo. *Circ Res.* 2000;87:214-220.

McAlindon TE, Felson DT, Zhang Y, et al. Relation of dietary intake and serum levels of vitamin D to progression of osteoarthritis of the knee among participants in the Framingham study. *Ann Intern Med.* 1996;125:353-359.

Melamed ML, Michos ED, Post W, et al. 25-hydroxyvitamin D levels and the risk of mortality in the general population. *Arch Intern Med.* 2008;168(15):1629-1637.

Melamed ML, Muntner P, Michos ED, et al. Serum 25-hydroxyvitamin D levels and the prevalence of peripheral arterial disease: results from NHANES 2001 to 2004. *Arterioscler Thromb Vasc Biol.* 2008;28(6):1179-1185.

Moan J, Porojnicu AC, Dahlback A, et al. Addressing the health benefits and risks, involving vitamin D or skin cancer, of increased sun exposure. *Proc Natl Acad Sci USA.* 2008;105(2):668-673.

Mukhopadhyay S, Singh M, Chatterjee M. Vitamin D_3 as a modulator of cellular antioxidant defense in murine lymphoma. *Nutr Res.* 2000; 20:91-102.

Nehring JA, Zierold C, DeLuca HF. Lithocholic acid can carry out in vivo functions of vitamin D. *Proc Natl Acad Sci USA.* 2007;104(24):10006-10009.

Ng K, Meyerhardt JA, Wu K, et al. Circulating 25-hydroxyvitamin d levels and survival in patients with colorectal cancer. *J Clin Oncol.* 2008;26(18):2984-2991.

O'Brien KO. Combined calcium and vitamin D supplementation reduces bone loss and fracture incidence in older men and women. *Nutr Rev.* 1998;56(5 Pt 1):148-150.

Oudshoorn C, Mattace-Raso FU, van der Velde N, et al. Higher serum vitamin D3 levels are associated with better cognitive test performance in patients with Alzheimer's disease. *Dement Geriatr Cogn Disord.* 2008;25(6):539-543.

Palmer SC, McGregor DO, Macaskill P, et al. Meta-analysis: vitamin D compounds in chronic kidney disease. *Ann Intern Med.* 2007;147(12):840-853.

Prabhala A, Garg R, Dandona P. Severe myopathy associated with vitamin D deficiency in Western New York. *Arch Intern Med.* 2000;160:1199-1203.

Raghuwanshi A, Joshi SS, Christakos S. Vitamin D and multiple sclerosis. *J Cell Biochem.* 2008;105(2):338-343.

Ralph AP, Kelly PM, Anstey NM. L-arginine and vitamin D: novel adjunctive immunotherapies in tuberculosis. *Trends Microbiol.* 2008;16(7):336-344.

Richards JB, Valdes AM, Gardner JP, et al. Higher serum vitamin D concentrations are associated with longer leukocyte telomere length in women. *Am J Clin Nutr.* 2007;86(5):1420-1425.

Sardar S, Chakraborty A, Chatterjee M. Comparative effectiveness of vitamin D_3 and dietary vitamin E on peroxidation of lipids and enzymes of the hepatic antioxidant system in Sprague-Dawley rats. *Int J Vitam Nutr Res.* 1996;66:39-45.

Sato Y, Asoh T, Oizumi K. High prevalence of vitamin D deficiency and reduced bone mass in elderly women with Alzheimer's disease. *Bone.* 1998;23:555-557.

Shah N, Bernardini J, Piraino B. Prevalence and correction of 25(OH) vitamin D deficiency in peritoneal dialysis patients. *Perit Dial Int.* 2005;25(4):362-366.

Takasu H, Sugita A, Uchiyama Y, et al. c-Fos protein as a target of anti-osteoclastogenic action of vitamin D, and synthesis of new analogs. *J Clin Invest.* 2006;116(2):528-535.

Tonelli M. Vitamin D in patients with chronic kidney disease: nothing new under the sun. *Ann Intern Med.* 2007;147(12):880-881.

Tsoukas CD, Watry D, Escobar SS, et al. Inhibition of interleukin-1 production by 1,25-dihydroxyvitamin D_3. *J Clin Endocrinol Metabolism.* 1989;69:127-133.

Vieth R. Vitamin D supplementation, 25-dihydroxyvitamin D concentrations and safety. *Am J Clin Nutr.* 1999;69:842-856.

Wang TJ, Pencina MJ, Booth SL, et al. Vitamin D deficiency and risk of cardiovascular disease. *Circulation.* 2008;117(4):503-511.

Wilkinson RJ, Llewelyn M, Toossi Z, et al. Influence of vitamin D deficiency and vitamin D receptor polymorphisms on tuberculosis among Gujarati Asians in west London: a case-control study. *Lancet.* 2000;355:618-621.

Yu S, Cantorna MT. The vitamin D receptor is required for iNKT cell development. *Proc Natl Acad Sci USA.* 2008;105(13):5207-5212.

Vitamin E

DESCRIPTION

Vitamin E is the collective term for a family of chemical substances that are structurally and, in some cases, biologically related to the best known member of this family, alpha-tocopherol. Vitamin E is a fat-soluble vitamin and an essential nutrient for humans. However, in contrast with the other vitamins present in human nutrition, its exact biochemical role remains unknown.

Vitamin E does not appear to play roles in reproduction and lactation in humans as it does in such animals as rats, and overt deficiency states of this vitamin are rare. Deficiency states of vitamin E, however, do exist in humans, and suboptimal nutriture of the vitamin may increase the risk of certain degenerative disorders, such as coronary heart disease, Alzheimer's disease and cancer.

Vitamin E deficiency occurs as a result of rare genetic abnormalities affecting the alpha-tocopherol transfer protein (alpha-TTP), as a result of various malabsorption syndromes and as a result of protein-energy malnutrition. Alpha-TTP is a protein found in the liver, heart, cerebellum and retina. Alpha-TTP selectively recognizes alpha-tocopherol and is believed to mediate the secretion of alpha-tocopherol taken up by the liver cells into the circulation. It may also function in delivering alpha-tocopherol to the cerebellum and retina.

Genetic defects in alpha-TTP are associated with a characteristic syndrome, ataxia with vitamin E deficiency or AVED, previously called familial isolated vitamin E (FIVE) deficiency. AVED patients suffer from neurologic symptoms that are characterized by progressive peripheral neuropathy.

Vitamin E deficiency can also be caused by genetic defects in lipoprotein synthesis. Lipoproteins containing apolipoprotein (apo-B) are necessary for absorption and transport of vitamin E. Those with homozygous hypobetalipoproteinemia have a defect in the apo-B gene and those with abetalipoproteinemia have genetic defects in the microsomal triglyceride-transfer protein. Homozygous hypobetalipoproteinemics and abetalipoproteinemics become vitamin E-deficient and develop the progressive peripheral neuropathy characteristic of vitamin E deficiency.

Fat malabsorption syndromes can result in vitamin E deficiency. Since vitamin E requires biliary and pancreatic secretions, as well as an intact and healthy intestine for its absorption, a wide range of hepatobiliary, pancreatic and intestinal disorders can lead to deficiency of the vitamin. These disorders include cholestatic hepatobiliary disease in children, cystic fibrosis, primary biliary cirrhosis, chronic pancreatitis, short bowel syndromes, Crohn's disease, celiac disease, mesenteric vascular thrombosis, blind loop syndrome, intestinal pseudo-obstruction, intestinal lymphangiectasia, Whipple's syndrome and sclerodermal bowel disease. In adults with these disorders, the development of the neurological symptoms of vitamin E deficiency takes many years. In children, the deficiency symptoms of vitamin E deficiency can be reversed by supplementation with vitamin E but only if it is provided before irreversible neurological injury occurs.

The primary syndrome of vitamin E deficiency, whether genetic or secondary to fat malabsorption syndromes or protein-calorie malnutrition, is peripheral neuropathy. This neuropathy is characterized by the degeneration of the large-caliber axons in the sensory neurons. The cardinal neuropathological changes consist of marked dying back-type degeneration of the posterior columns of the spinal cord. In addition, spinocerebellar ataxia, skeletal myopathy and pigmented retinopathy have been observed in vitamin E deficiency in humans. Vitamin E-deficiency anemia may also occur in premature infants as a result of peroxidation damage to red blood-cell membranes.

The vitamin E family of molecules can be divided into two groups, the tocopherols and the tocotrienols. Vitamin E occurs naturally in eight different forms: four tocopherols, alpha-, beta-, gamma- and delta-tocopherol and four tocotrienols, alpha-, beta, gamma- and delta-tocotrienol. All of these forms consist of a substituted hydroxylated ring system (the chromanol ring or head group) with a long phytyl side chain or tail. The phytyl tail is bonded to the chromanol ring at the 2 position of the ring. It is the hydroxyl group of the chromanol ring that confers antioxidant activity to vitamin E.

Tocopherols differ from tocotrienols in that tocopherols have three chiral centers, (at positions 2, 4' and 8') while the tocotrienols have only one chiral center (at position 2) and three double bonds in the tail. That is, tocotrienols possess polyunsaturated phytyl side chains. The chiral center of the tocotrienols is located at the point where the phytyl side chain bonds to the chromanol ring (the 2 position of the ring).

The various natural tocopherols and tocotrienols are characterized by the number of methyl groups and the pattern of methylation in the chromanol ring. Alpha-tocopherol and tocotrienol have three methyl groups, beta- and gamma-tocopherol and tocotrienol have two methyl groups and delta-tocopherol and tocotrienol have one methyl group.

Of the eight naturally occurring forms of vitamin E, it appears that only alpha-tocopherol is maintained in human plasma. This is most likely due to the fact that alpha-tocopherol transfer protein (alpha-TTP) selectively recognizes alpha-tocopherol and is believed to mediate the secretion of alpha-tocopherol taken up by the liver cells into the circulation. This does not rule out possible important roles for the other natural forms of vitamin E. It does, however, indicate that alpha-tocopherol is probably the most important member of the vitamin E family in human physiology.

Alpha-tocopherol is commonly known as d-alpha-tocopherol. Chemically, this implies that alpha-tocopherol has only one chiral center. In fact, alpha-tocopherol has three chiral centers. Its correct name is RRR-alpha-tocopherol or 2, 5, 7, 8-tetramethyl-2R- (4'R, 8'R, 12' trimethyltridecyl)-6-chromanol. Since alpha-tocopherol has 3 chiral centers, it can have 2^3 or eight stereoisomeric forms. d-alpha-tocopherol is represented by the following chemical structure:

d-Alpha-Tocopherol

Synthetic vitamin E, which is produced by coupling trimethylhydroquinone with racemic isophytol, does contain all eight stereoisomers of alpha-tocopherol in equal amounts Synthetic alpha-tocopherol is commonly known as dl-alpha-tocopherol. This would be correct if alpha-tocopherol had only one chiral center, but since it has three, this nomenclature is incorrect. Synthetic alpha-tocopherol is correctly called *all racemic*-or *all rac*-alpha-tocopherol. It is also known as (2RS)-2,5,7,8-tetramethyl-2-(4,8,12-trimethyltridecyl)-6-chromanol. *All rac*-alpha-tocopherol consists of four 2R-stereoisomers: RRR-alpha-tocopherol, RSR-alpha-tocopherol, RRS-alpha-tocopherol and RSS-alpha-tocopherol and four 2S-stereoisomers: SRR-alpha-tocopherol, SSR-alpha-tocopherol, SRS-alpha-tocopherol and SSS-alpha-tocopherol. 2R and 2S refer to the configuration of the phytyl tail at the point it meets the chromanol ring or the 2 position of the ring.

The only forms of alpha-tocopherol that are maintained in human plasma are the 2R-stereoisomers. The 2S-stereoisomers of alpha-tocopherol are not maintained in human plasma or tissue. Therefore, the only forms of alpha-tocopherol maintained in human plasma are the natural RRR-alpha-tocopherol and the four 2R synthetic stereoisomers.

Vitamin E is found in plants, animals and in some green, brown and blue/green algae. The richest sources of the vitamin are found in unrefined edible vegetable oil, including wheat germ, safflower, sunflower, cottonseed, canola and olive oils. In these oils, approximately 50% of the tocopherol content is in the form of alpha-tocopherol. Soybean and corn oils contain about ten times as much gamma-tocopherol as

they do alpha-tocopherol. Palm, rice bran and coconut oils are rich sources of tocotrienols. Alpha-tocopherol is the major form of vitamin E in animal products and is found mainly in the fatty portion of the meat. Other foods containing vitamin E include unrefined cereal grains, fruits, nuts and vegetables.

Most of the marketed supplemental RRR-alpha-tocopherol (d-alpha-tocopherol) is derived from unrefined soy oil. Since soy oil contains mainly gamma-tocopherol, a synthetic process is necessary to convert the gamma-tocopherol to the alpha-tocopherol. Therefore, alpha-tocopherol derived from soy oil is a semi-synthetic product for which reason it is called natural-source alpha-tocopherol, rather than natural alpha-tocopherol.

D-ALPHA-TOCOPHERYL ACETATE

d-Alpha-tocopheryl acetate is the acetate ester of natural-source d-alpha-tocopherol. Its molecular weight is 472.75 daltons. It is obtained by the vacuum steam distillation and acetylation of edible vegetable oil products. It is found in nutritional supplement products either as a light brownish yellow, nearly odorless, clear viscous oil or as a water-dispersible solid substance with a melting point of 25° centigrade. The water-dispersible solid form of d-alpha-tocopheryl acetate is about 96 to 100% d-alpha-tocopheryl acetate, while the typical oil supplement is comprised of about 40-50% d-alpha-tocopheryl acetate.

d-Alpha-tocopheryl acetate is also known as RRR-alpha-tocopheryl acetate and 2R, 4', 8'R-d-alpha-tocopheryl acetate.

d-Alpha-tocopheryl acetate, in addition to being available as a nutritional supplement, is used in topical skin care products. It appears that it can diffuse into skin cells where it is converted to d-alpha-tocopherol. The acetate itself does not have antioxidant activity. d-alpha-tocopherol may protect skin against ultraviolet damage and is also a skin moisturizer. Some are hypersensitive to topical d-alpha-tocopherol and may develop dermatitis from its use.

DL-ALPHA-TOCOPHERYL ACETATE

dl-alpha-tocopheryl acetate is an all-synthetic form of alpha-tocopherol. It is produced by coupling racemic isophytol with trimethylhydroquinone to form dl-tocopherol. This product is then acetylated to produce dl-alpha-tocopheryl acetate. Since alpha-tocopherol has three chiral centers, eight stereoisomers are formed in the coupling reaction in equal amounts, four 2R-stereoisomers and four 2S-stereoisomers. 2R and 2S refer to the configuration of the phytyl tail at the point it bonds to the chromanol ring, the 2 position of the ring. The four 2R-stereoisomers are RRR-alpha tocopherol, RRS-alpha-tocopherol, RSS-alpha-tocopherol and RSR-alpha tocopherol. The four 2S-stereoisomers are SRR-alpha-tocopherol, SSR-alpha-tocopherol, SRS-alpha-tocopherol and SSS-alpha-tocopherol.

The 2R-stereoisomers are the only forms of alpha-tocopherol that are maintained in human plasma and tissue. The activity of natural or natural-source alpha-tocopherol (RRR alpha-tocopherol), on an equal weight basis, is at least twice as high as synthetic alpha-tocopherol. This is mainly because half of the stereoisomers of synthetic alpha-tocopherol are not maintained in human plasma and are, therefore, not bioavailable.

Although synthetic alpha-tocopheryl acetate is commonly referred to as dl-alpha-tocopheryl acetate, this is not chemically correct. Chemically correct names are *all-racemic-* or *all-rac*-alpha-tocopheryl acetate and 2, 5, 7, 8-tetramethyl-2RS-(4'RS, 8'RS, 12' trimethyldecyl)- 6-chromanol hydrogen acetate.

D-ALPHA-TOCOPHEROL SUCCINATE
d-Alpha-tocopherol succinate is the succinate ester of natural-source d-alpha-tocopherol. It is a white to off-white crystalline powder with a molecular weight of 530.79 daltons. d-Alpha-tocopherol succinate is obtained by the vacuum steam distillation and succinylation of edible vegetable oil. It is insoluble in water, but is water-dispersible.

d-Alpha-tocopheryl succinate is also known as RRR-alpha-tocopheryl succinate and 2R, 4', 8'R-alpha-tocopheryl succinate. It is sometimes called "dry" vitamin E, referring to its solid nature.

Some cell culture studies show that d-alpha-tocopheryl succinate can enter into cells as the intact ester and is then hydrolyzed intracellularly to d-alpha-tocopherol. Most ingested d-alpha-tocopheryl succinate is hydrolyzed to d-alpha-tocopherol prior to absorption from the lumen of the small intestine into enterocytes. A small percentage of ingested d-alpha-tocopheryl succinate may enter enterocytes as the ester and is subsequently hydrolyzed to d-alpha-tocopherol within the enterocytes. d-Alpha-tocopheryl succinate itself has no antioxidant activity.

DL-ALPHA-TOCOPHERYL SUCCINATE
dl-Alpha-tocopheryl succinate is an all-synthetic form of alpha-tocopherol. It is produced by coupling racemic isophytol with trimethylhydroquinone to form dl-tocopherol. The dl-tocopherol product is then succinylated to dl-alpha-tocopheryl succinate. Since alpha-tocopherol has three chiral centers, eight stereoisomers are formed in the coupling reaction in equal amounts, four 2R-stereoisomers and four 2S-stereoisomers. 2R and 2S refer to the configuration of the phytyl tail at the point it bonds to the chromanol ring, the 2 position of the ring. The four 2R- stereoisomers are RRR-alpha-tocopherol, RRS-alpha-tocopherol, RSS-alpha-tocopherol and RSR-alpha-tocopherol. The four 2S-stereoisomers: SRR-alpha-tocopherol, SSR-alpha-tocopherol, SRS-alpha-tocopherol and SSS-alpha-tocopherol. dl-Alpha-tocopheryl succinate is not a commercial product. The major reason for its lack of commercial availability is that it does not crystallize well but forms a paste. However, it is available for research purposes.

The 2R-stereoisomers are the only forms of alpha-tocopherol that are maintained in human plasma and tissue. The activity of natural or natural-source alpha-tocopherol (RRR-alpha-tocopherol), on an equal weight basis, is at least twice as high as synthetic alpha-tocopherol. This is due to the fact that 50% of the stereoisomers of synthetic alpha-tocopherol are not maintained in human plasma.

Although synthetic alpha-tocopheryl succinate is commonly referred to as dl-alpha-tocopheryl succinate, this is not chemically correct. Chemically correct names for this substance are *all-racemic-* or *all-rac*-alpha-tocopheryl succinate and 2, 5, 7, 8-tetramethyl-2RS- (4' RS, 8'RS, 12'trimethyldecyl)-6-chromanol hydrogen succinate.

MIXED TOCOPHEROLS
Mixed tocopherols consist of mixtures of the natural tocopherol homologues: d-alpha-tocopherol, d-beta-tocopherol, d-gamma-tocopherol and d-delta-tocopherol. These tocopherols are present in their unesterified forms. Mixed tocopherols are obtained by the vacuum steam distillation of edible vegetable oil products.

There are two types of mixed tocopherol products available for nutritional supplementation: high-alpha-mixed-tocopherols and low-alpha-mixed-tocopherols. High-alpha-mixed-tocopherols contain mainly d-alpha-tocopherol with much smaller amounts of beta-, gamma- and delta-tocopherol. Low-alpha-mixed-tocopherols typically contain gamma-tocopherol as the major tocopherol homologue. High-alpha-mixed-tocopherols are labeled to indicate the milligrams of d-alpha-tocopherol present, as well as the milligrams of total tocopherols present. Low-alpha-mixed-tocopherols are usually labeled to indicate the total amount of tocopherols and sometimes tocotrienols-present, as well as the amounts of gamma-, beta- and delta-tocopherols. Mixed tocopherols occur as brownish-red to red, clear viscous oils.

ACTIONS AND PHARMACOLOGY
ACTIONS
Vitamin E has antioxidant activity. It may also have anti-atherogenic, antithrombotic, anticoagulant, neuroprotective, antiproliferative, immunomodulatory, cell membrane-stabilizing and antiviral actions.

MECHANISM OF ACTION

All forms of vitamin E possess antioxidant activity. However, the only forms maintained in human plasma and tissue are the 2R-alpha forms, including the natural RRR-alpha-tocopherol, commonly known as d-alpha-tocopherol. Vitamin E is the principal antioxidant of the lipid domains of the body, such as cellular membranes. It is a chain-breaking antioxidant that prevents the propagation of free radical activities. It is a peroxyl radical scavenger and especially protects the polyunsaturated fatty acids (PUFAs) within membrane phospholipids and in plasma lipoproteins (LDL) against oxidation. The hydroxyl group of the chromanol ring reacts with an organic peroxyl radical to form the corresponding organic hydroperoxide and the tocopheroxyl radical. The tocopheroxyl radical is the pro-oxidant form of vitamin E and is thought to be regenerated to the antioxidant form by a network of other antioxidants, including vitamin C and glutathione.

The relative antioxidant activity of the tocopherols with regard to peroxyl radical scavenging is alpha > beta > gamma > delta. The order is similar among the tocotrienols. Interestingly, this order also parallels the relative order of their biological activities as determined by the classical rat fetal gestation-resorption assay.

This is the case, though, only for the natural tocopherols. All eight stereoisomers of the synthetic all rac-alpha-tocopherol, commonly known as dl-alpha-tocopherol, have equivalent peroxyl radical scavenging activity but different activities in the rat fetal resorption assay. And, alpha-tocotrienol has about one-third the activity of alpha-tocopherol in this assay but is a better peroxyl radical scavenger than alpha-tocopherol.

It can be concluded that antioxidant activity of vitamin E is not sufficient to explain the vitamin's biological activity. Recently, it has been demonstrated that vitamin E has activity against reactive nitrogen species (peroxyl radicals are reactive oxygen species). In this regard, gamma-tocopherol inhibits peroxynitrite-induced lipid peroxidation more effectively than alpha-tocopherol (see Gamma-Tocopherol).

Several mechanisms have been proposed to account for vitamin E's possible anti-atherogenic activity. Oxidation of LDL is believed to be a key early step in atherogenesis. It is thought that oxidation of LDL triggers a number of events which lead to the formation of atherosclerotic plaque. These events include uptake of oxidized (ox) LDL by monocytes leading to foam cell formation, promotion of apoptosis by oxLDL, induction of endothelial-cell damage and stimulation of cytokine and growth factor release from cells in the artery wall. LDL contains alpha-tocopherol and smaller amounts of gamma-tocopherol. Alpha-tocopherol inhibits the oxidation of LDL and the accumulation of oxLDL in the arterial wall. It, as well as gamma-tocopherol, also appears to reduce oxLDL-induced apoptosis in human endothelial cells.

A non-antioxidative mechanism of vitamin E is its inhibition of protein kinase C (PKC) activity. PKC is involved in smooth muscle cell proliferation, and, consequently, inhibition of PKC results in inhibition of smooth muscle cell proliferation. Smooth muscle cell proliferation is involved in atherogenesis. PKC inhibition by alpha-tocopherol is, in part, attributable to its attenuating effect on the generation of membrane-derived diacylglycerol, a lipid that facilitates PKC translocation thus increasing its activity. Mitogen-activated protein kinase (MAPK) is also involved in smooth muscle proliferation, and both alpha-tocopherol and gamma-tocopherol inhibit this activity.

Vitamin E enrichment of endothelial cells in culture downregulates the expression of intracellular cell adhesion molecule(ICAM)-1 and vascular cell adhesion molecule(VCAM)-1, both induced by exposure to oxLDL, thereby decreasing the adhesion of blood-cell components to the endothelium. Vitamin E also upregulates the expression of cytosolic phospholipase A_2 and cyclooxygenase (COX)-1. The enhanced expression of these two rate-limiting enzymes in the arachidonic acid cascade appears to explain the observation that vitamin E, in a dose-dependent fashion, enhances the release of prostacyclin, a vasodilating factor and inhibitor of platelet aggregation in humans.

Vitamin E appears to inhibit platelet adhesion, aggregation and platelet release reactions. Enhancing the release of prostacyclin may play a role in these effects. Also, it is known that platelet aggregation is mediated by a common mechanism that involves the binding of fibrinogen to the glycoprotein IIb/IIIa (GPIIb/ IIIa) complex of platelets. GPIIb/IIIa is the major membrane receptor protein that is central to the role of the platelet aggregation response. Glycoprotein IIb (GPIIb) is the alpha-subunit of this platelet membrane protein. It has been shown in tissue culture that alpha-tocopherol downregulates, in a dose-dependent manner, GPIIb promoter activity. This could result in reduction of GPIIb protein expression and decreased platelet aggregation.

Vitamin E has also been found in culture to decrease plasma production of thrombin, a protein which binds to platelets and induces aggregation. A metabolite of vitamin E called vitamin E quinone or alpha-tocopheryl quinone (TQ) is a potent anticoagulant. This metabolite inhibits vitamin K-dependent carboxylase, which is a major enzyme in the coagulation cascade.

A number of mechanisms are proposed to account for the possible neuroprotective effects of high doses of vitamin E.

Oxidative stress is thought to be a factor in the pathogenesis of many disorders of the nervous system. Since the nervous system is rich in lipids and since vitamin E is the principal lipid antioxidant, the vitamin has become attractive as a possible preventive, as well as therapeutic agent, for nervous system disorders. Also, the primary syndrome of overt deficiency of this vitamin is peripheral neuropathy.

Vitamin E may play a special role in the cerebellum because concentrations of the vitamin are the lowest in this part of the brain, and the vitamin is more quickly depleted in the cerebellum than in other parts of the brain during vitamin E deficiency. Electrophysiologic investigations in vitamin E-deficient humans show signs of a distal "dying-back" axonal neuropathy, especially in the posterior columns and the gracile and cuneate nuclei.

Vitamin E may also be involved in signal-transduction. Vitamin E may play a number of roles associated with neuronal cell membranes and other lipids in the nervous system. However, a specific and unique mechanism of action of the vitamin in the nervous system has not been elucidated.

Several animal and human studies have shown that vitamin E can improve the immune response in aged animals and humans. *In vitro*, alpha-tocopherol increases mitogenic response of T lymphocytes from aged mice. The mechanism of this response by vitamin E is not well understood. It has been suggested that vitamin E itself may have mitogenic activity independent of its antioxidant activity. All four homologues of tocopherol, alpha-, beta-, gamma- and delta-tocopherol, were found to enhance both spontaneous and mitogen-stimulated lymphocyte proliferation in mouse splenocytes in culture.

Alpha-tocopherol was reported to have potent activity against human immunodeficiency virus (HIV)-1. Oxidative stress is thought to contribute to HIV-1 pathogenesis, as well as to the pathogenesis of other viral infections. The anti-HIV-1 activity may be due, in part, to alpha-tocopherol's antioxidant activity. Vitamin E also affects membrane integrity and fluidity. HIV-1 is a membraned virus. Altering membrane fluidity of HIV-1 may interfere with its ability to bind to cell-receptor sites, thus decreasing its infectivity. It is unclear, however, how much vitamin E would bind to HIV-1 if administered *in vivo*, since vitamin E can bind to several different sites including alpha-tocopherol transfer protein (alpha-TTP) and LDL.

In conclusion, oxidative stress appears to play a major role in the pathogenesis of many chronic degenerative disorders, and, as the principal lipophilic antioxidant in the body, vitamin E may play a significant role in the prevention, as well as treatment of these disorders. Vitamin E may also have roles independent of its antioxidant action. The action

and mechanisms of action of this vitamin are a work in progress.

PHARMACOKINETICS

The precise rate of vitamin E absorption is not known with certainty. The absorption of this vitamin is typically low and variable. The absorption of one form of vitamin E, d-alpha-tocopheryl polyethylene glycol 1000 succinate or vitamin E TPGS, is different (see d-Alpha-Tocopheryl Polyethylene Glycol 1000 Succinate).

Reported rates of absorption of vitamin E following intake with food have varied from as high as 51% to 86% to as low as 21% to 29%. It is likely the higher values are an overestimation and that the lower numbers represent a truer picture. Absorption is significantly lower on an empty stomach and may be somewhat higher with the esterified acetate and succinate delivery forms of vitamin E. However, some studies show that the free and esterified tocopherols have similar absorption efficiency. All forms of vitamin E, including all of the tocopherol and tocotrienol homologues, are absorbed in a similar manner.

Vitamin E is absorbed from the lumen of the small intestine into the enterocytes by passive diffusion. Prior to its absorption, vitamin E is emulsified together with dietary lipids. Bile acids and salts secreted by the liver aid in the emulsification process. Lipolysis and emulsification of the formed lipid droplets lead to the spontaneous formation of mixed micelles. Esterified forms of vitamin E, alpha-tocopheryl acetate and succinate, undergo hydrolysis via esterases secreted by the pancreas. The micelles containing vitamin E are absorbed at the brush border of the intestinal mucosa in the enterocytes. There is some recent evidence that the Niemann-Pick C1-like 1 (NPC1L1) transporter may help mediate the uptake of alpha-tocopherol. Vitamin E is secreted by the enterocytes into the lymphatics in the form of chylomicrons. The chylomicrons contain the various forms of vitamin E, including alpha-, beta-, gamma-, and delta-tocopherol, alpha-, beta-, gamma- and delta-tocotrienol and, if consumed either in supplement form or in fortified foods, all eight stereoisomers of *all rac*-alpha-tocopherol (d1-alpha-tocopherol).

Chylomicrons undergo metabolism in the circulation via lipoprotein lipase to form chylomicron remnants. During this process, some vitamin E, including all the above-cited forms, is transferred to various tissues, such as adipose tissue, muscle and possibly the brain. Lipoprotein lipase appears to be required for the transfer of vitamin E to these tissues. Chylomicron remnants can transfer tocopherols to high density lipoproteins (HDL), which, in turn, can transfer tocopherols to LDL and very low density lipoproteins (VLDL). Chylomicron remnants can also acquire apolipoprotein E (apoE), which directs them to the liver for metabolism. The remnants are taken up by the liver, which, in turn, secretes vitamin E in VLDLs.

The secretion by the liver of vitamin E in VLDLs is, arguably, the most important singular event in the biochemistry of vitamin E. The only forms of the vitamin secreted by the liver are the natural RRR-alpha-tocopherol and the four 2R forms of synthetic tocopherol. The four 2S synthetic forms of *all rac*-alpha-tocopherol are not secreted by the liver in VLDLs, and only very small amounts of the other tocopherol and tocotrienol homologues are secreted. It is this step that discriminates between all the various forms of vitamin E; the reason for this is that hepatic alpha-tocopheryl transfer protein (alpha-TTP) is selective for the binding of RRR-alpha-tocopherol and the 2R forms of alpha-tocopherol. The secretion of RRR-alpha-tocopherol in VLDLs by the liver is also the mechanism that maintains the plasma concentration of vitamin E. Following secretion of VLDL in the circulation, lipoprotein lipase and triglyceride lipase convert VLDL to LDL. Alpha-tocopherol is transported in the plasma mainly in LDL and also in HDL. Alpha-tocopherol is distributed to the central nervous system (CNS) via LDL. Newly absorbed vitamin E slowly accumulates in the CNS. Sebaceous gland secretion is a major route of vitamin E delivery to the skin.

Alpha-tocopherol can be oxided to the tocopheroxyl radical, which is the pro-oxidant form of this molecule. Reduction back to the antioxidant form is thought to take place with the help of such reducing agents as vitamin C and glutathione. Alpha-tocopherol, vitamin C, glutathione and alpha-lipoic acid are major components of the so-called antioxidant network. Metabolites of alpha-tocopherol include alpha-tocopheryl quinone, alpha-tocopheryl hydroquinone and 2, 5, 7, 8-tetramethyl-2- (2^9 -carboxyethyl)-6-hydroxychroman (alpha-CEHC). A gamma-tocopherol metabolite is 2, 7, 8-trimethyl-2- (2^9-carboxyethyl)-6-hydroxychroman (gamma-CEHC).

Fecal excretion is the major route of excretion of oral vitamin E. Fecal excretion of the vitamin includes non-absorbed vitamin E, as well as vitamin E forms not utilized. For example, the forms not secreted by the liver, such as the 2S alpha-tocopherol forms and the beta-, gamma- and delta-tocopherol homologues, are excreted via the biliary route.

Vitamin E metabolites, such as alpha-CEHC and gamma-CEHC, are excreted via the urinary route. About three times as much *all rac*-alpha-tocopherol, compared with RRR-alpha-tocopherol, is excreted as alpha-CEHC. Alpha-CEHC is the major urinary metabolite of alpha-tocopherol.

INDICATIONS AND USAGE

Vitamin E is a widely recognized fat soluble vitamin essential for human health and notable for some of its antioxidant properties. Claims that it is an effective treatment for established cardiovascular disease continue to be controversial and unsettled. The evidence for prevention of cardiovascular disease is somewhat better. It may have anticancer effects and favorable immunomodulating activity. The evidence that vitamin E has meaningful neuroprotective effects is equivocal. There is the suggestion of limited vitamin E benefit in some patients with asthma and rheumatoid arthritis. It may be protective to some extent against some forms of air pollution and other toxins. It may be of some benefit in some eye disorders, in some forms of diabetes and in premenstrual syndrome. It may help protect against ultraviolet irradiation. Claims that it boosts male fertility, sexual prowess and exercise performance and that it reverses skin aging are poorly supported. It may have some benefit in muscle cramps. There is very preliminary evidence that it might be helpful in treating non-alcoholic steatohepatitis (NASH).

RESEARCH SUMMARY

The results of a very large number of studies, including *in vitro* and animal studies, epidemiological and intervention trials, support a role for vitamin E in the prevention of cardiovascular disease. Recently, however, some large intervention trials have raised some doubts about that role; concurrently, controversy has erupted over the design of these trials. The situation, in some ways, parallels that of the conflicting evidence related to beta-carotene's possible role in preventing lung cancer. (See Beta-Carotene.) Vitamin E has been shown to inhibit the oxidation of LDL-cholesterol in various *in vitro*, animal and human experiments. Other *in vitro*, animal and some human studies demonstrate that vitamin E also acts on coagulation, platelet aggregation and endothelial relaxation, among other factors, in ways that may reduce cardiovascular risk.

In one study of hyperlipidemic rabbits, supplemental vitamin E significantly reduced oxidation of LDL-cholesterol and surface area of atherosclerotic lesions. In male monkeys, 108 IUs of vitamin E daily decreased progression (and produced some regression) of atherosclerosis over a three-year study period. Rabbits on high cholesterol diets given supplemental vitamin E or beta-carotene exhibited aortas with normal endothelial function, compared with controls receiving only the high-cholesterol diet. A number of animal studies have consistently shown that supplemental vitamin E can reduce formation of atheromas by 25% to 50%.

In humans supplemented with vitamin E, their LDL-cholesterol was subsequently shown to contain elevated amounts of the vitamin. Concurrently, increased oxidation resistance was measured in these LDL samples.

Many epidemiological studies have associated low-vitamin E status with significantly increased risk of cardiovascular disease. Angina sufferers, in some case-control studies, were found to have lower vitamin E levels than controls. In a much larger case-control study, results were obtained suggesting that higher concentrations of vitamin E in adipose tissue indirectly helped protect against myocardial infarction through vitamin E's favorable effects on beta-carotene.

Among prospective cohort studies examining the possible role of vitamin E in cardiovascular disease, The Nurses' Health Study has yielded some significant findings. In a cohort of 87,000 of these nurses, all free of cardiovascular disease at baseline, there was a 34% reduction in coronary heart disease risk among those women in the highest versus the lowest quintile of vitamin E intake after adjustment for age, smoking and other relevant variables. Dietary intake alone did not show this significant inverse relationship, but total intake (diet plus supplementation) did. The nurses were followed for eight years. In nurses in the highest quintile of vitamin E intake from supplementation extending for at least two years, risk reduction was even greater: 46%. Similar risk reduction was seen in a large cohort of men free of heart disease at baseline (the Health Professionals Follow-Up Study). Almost all of the benefit was restricted to those men who took daily supplements of vitamin E in doses of 100 IUs or greater for at least two years.

Several other smaller cohort studies have similarly reported significant evidence of vitamin E's protective role in cardiovascular disease. High dietary intake alone (without supplementation) has also been associated with significantly reduced risk in some of these studies.

A number of other studies have correlated blood levels of vitamin E with risk of cardiovascular disease. In many, but not all, of these, high levels of the vitamin have correlated with reduced risk. Additionally, there are angiography and ultrasound studies that provide some further evidence that vitamin E helps protect the arteries.

Some small clinical intervention trials have found supplemental vitamin E to be beneficial in some with intermittent claudication and angina. More recently, however, the large Alpha-Tocopherol Beta-Carotene Cancer Prevention (ATBC) study of 29,000 Finnish male smokers failed to find any overall significant cardiovascular benefit from low dose (50 milligrams daily) vitamin E (synthetic). However, a subsequent analysis showed some slight benefit from vitamin E among those smokers who had no history of myocardial infarction. After a median follow-up of 6.1 years, there was an observed 4% reduction in primary major coronary events

in this subset. Vitamin E decreased the incidence of fatal coronary heart disease by 8%. These findings were statistically non-significant. There was also a significant increase in fatal hemorrhagic stroke in the vitamin E group, although use of the vitamin was associated with a reduction in ischemic stroke, and, overall, there was no statistically significant difference in stroke between those taking the vitamin and those not taking it.

This study has been criticized for using doses of vitamin E significantly lower than those generally shown to have positive preventive effects. Additionally this study involved subjects who had been smoking, in many cases, for decades and thus, some argued, posed a far greater challenge for antioxidant therapy.

Much was made, by some, of the small but statistically significant increase in hemorrhagic stroke associated with vitamin E supplementation in this study. Others, however, have pointed out that some other long-term studies, using considerably higher doses of vitamin E, found no increased risk. There was a statistically non-significant reduction in risk of ischemic stroke in the vitamin E-supplemented subjects in the Nurses' Health Study. There was also a statistically non-significant reduction in cerebrovascular mortality in the vitamin E-supplemented group in the large interventive Linxian China study. And there was a statistically non-significant reduction in total stroke incidence among those receiving vitamin E in the recently concluded GISSI-Prevenzione trial.

In the Cambridge Heart Antioxidant Study (CHAOS), 2002 subjects with cardiovascular disease confirmed by angiography were given 400-800 IUs of natural source vitamin E daily or placebo. A significant 77% reduction in risk of nonfatal myocardial infarction was reported after 510 days of vitamin E administration. There was, however, no effect on cardiovascular death or total mortality.

There was, in fact, a small statistically non-significant increase in cardiovascular death in the vitamin E group. This was a group with serious cardiovascular disease at baseline, and there were considerably more deaths in the early stages of the study, at a point when vitamin E had been used for a relatively short period of time, than at later stages. Thus, there was little concern that the vitamin itself was contributing to an increase in death. Additionally, a recent further analysis has shown that most of these deaths occurred in subjects who were non-compliant with the vitamin E regimen.

The study's reliability has been questioned by some due to purported design flaws, small size and short duration. Defenders of the study, however, say that its results are all the more dramatic, given that the subjects who benefited were already beset with advanced cardiovascular disease. Moreover, the benefit came in relatively short order. This suggested, they said, that the vitamin might be affecting more than just lipid oxidation in these subjects.

One reviewer, commenting on this possibility, has noted that in subgroup analyses of the Cholesterol Lowering Atherosclerosis Study (CLAS), vitamin E supplementation, in doses greater than 100 IUs daily, was shown to reduce the rate of angiographic progression of mild-to-moderate lesions over a two-year period. On the other hand, some critics of the CHAOS trial said the reported results were improbable in so short a study period, and they concluded that the results occurred by chance alone rather than owing to any real vitamin E effect.

In the Linxian China study, supplemental beta-carotene (15 milligrams daily), synthetic vitamin E (30 IUs daily) and selenium (50 micrograms daily) significantly protected against total mortality and total cancer (which was the primary focus of the study) and non-significantly protected against cerebrovascular disease. The vitamin E dose used in this study was even smaller than that used in the ATBC study. In both cases, synthetic alpha-tocopherol was used.

In the GISSI-Prevenzione trial, 11,324 Italian survivors of myocardial infarction were given 300 milligrams of synthetic vitamin E daily or a mixture of n-3 polyunsaturated fatty acids (PUFA) in a combination of docosahexaenoate (DHA) and eicosapentaenoate (EPA), or both the vitamin E and the n-3 PUFA combination, or neither. The primary end points were nonfatal myocardial infarction, stroke and death. Comparing each treatment against no treatment, the n-3 PUFA combination achieved a statistically significant 15% reduction in primary endpoint risk, while vitamin E achieved a statistically non-significant 11% reduction in the same risks. Vitamin E produced a non-significant reduction in risk of stroke, while the n-3 PUFA combination non-significantly increased risk of stroke.

The GISSI researchers noted that "a possible beneficial effect of vitamin E" was suggested "in the secondary analyses of the individual components of cardiovascular death of the combined endpoints, for which the increasing benefit (from 20% for all cardiovascular deaths to 35% for sudden death) is similar to the picture for n-3 PUFA. The absence of a difference in the rate of non-fatal cardiovascular events between vitamin E and the control group is also similar to the findings related to n-3 PUFA." They added: "The significant decrease of cardiovascular deaths . . . cannot be easily dismissed."

The multi-center GISSI study has been criticized by some for not being placebo-controlled and for dispensing with independent monitors at each participating center. One reviewer

noted that synthetic vitamin E was used in this study, reducing the potency of the 300 milligram daily doses, he said, to the equivalent of 150 milligrams of natural-source vitamin E. The greater potency of natural-source vitamin E is widely recognized, and some studies have indicated that natural-source alpha-tocopherol is at least twice as bioavailable as synthetic vitamin E.

Some other researchers said the GISSI trial made too little of the reduction in deaths apparently attributable to vitamin E. Two researchers stated that "cardiovascular mortality was significantly reduced by vitamin E in GISSI, and the effect on overall survival showed a very favorable trend." Others argued that a longer follow-up period was needed. The GISSI trial lasted for 3.5 years.

One of the CHAOS researchers commented on the GISSI trial: "Whether patients who have an MI despite a lifetime of Mediterranean diet and are subsequently treated with a statin would be expected to benefit from vitamin E is not clear, especially since many of the complications of MI depend more on the state of the myocardium than of the coronary arteries." Since the Mediterranean diet is generally higher in vitamin E than the English diet consumed in the CHAOS study, this researcher suggested that the English subjects might be more responsive to vitamin E supplementation.

In this same commentary, the CHAOS researcher observed that investigators in that trial have reported that the English patients had a 3.5-fold increased frequency for a polymorphism in the gene for endothelial nitric oxide synthase (eNOS). Vascular endothelial function is reduced in such individuals, and he speculated that vitamin E may thus have worked in these subjects through an avenue other than the inhibition of LDL-cholesterol oxidation. Conceivably this might help explain the more rapid activity of vitamin E seen in the CHAOS study and might explain why some other populations (with possibly lower frequency of the eNOS gene) are less responsive. More research is needed to clarify these issues.

Recently, results of the Heart Outcomes Prevention Evaluation (HOPE) study were released. This study of 2,545 women and 6,996 men 55 years and older with cardiovascular disease or diabetes tested 400 IUs of natural-source vitamin E against placebo (it also tested the angiotensin-converting-enzyme inhibitor ramipril against placebo) and found no significant protective effect for vitamin E with respect to either primary or secondary endpoints: myocardial infarction, stroke and death from cardiovascular causes, unstable angina, congestive heart failure, revascularization or amputation, death from any cause, complications of diabetes and cancer. Neither did it find any adverse vitamin E effects. Subjects were supplemented for a mean of 4.5 years.

If there was an inconsistency in this study it was that, in contrast with the previous large intervention trials, it appeared to consistently show virtually no vitamin E activity, positive or negative.

The HOPE researchers hypothesized that this lack of activity could be due, in part, to the moderate duration of the trial, to the characteristics of the population studied and/or to the fact that vitamin E was used by itself without some of the co-factors found in some other studies to potentiate its effects. They noted that some trials in which vitamin E is used with some other antioxidants are now in progress. Clearly, these and other studies may be needed before vitamin E's role in various populations with various forms and stages of cardiovascular disease can be adequately evaluated. Some do not expect antioxidants to have notable effects in established disease and say their real strength is in preventing disease in healthy populations.

Unfortunately, in the years since these controversial studies were published, subjected to multiple analyses and, in some cases, modified by the original authors, still more controversy—and very little clarity—has accrued with respect to vitamin E's possible role as a cardioprotectant or interventive in cardiovascular disease. The HOPE study, for example, was extended to the so-called HOPE-TOO trial, the TOO standing for The Ongoing Outcomes. HOPE-TOO looked at long-term vitamin E (400 IU daily) on cardiovascular events and cancer. The subjects, as in the HOPE trial, had cardiovascular disease and/or diabetes mellitus. Again, no benefit was seen and, in fact, the authors noted that vitamin E, in these patients, might be associated with increased risk for heart failure. The authors concluded that "vitamin E supplements should not be used in patients with vascular disease or diabetes mellitus." The study was again criticized by some who pointed out that many of the participants in the original study did not agree to continue in the extended study, that all were suffering from disease and were often on multiple medications and that the observation related to increased heart failure risk could have been due to chance. Indeed, the authors conceded that the latter finding "cannot be confirmed at this time by other trials." That said, the trial nonetheless provided some evidence that vitamin E is not likely to have significant efficacy in treating established cardiovascular disease, at least in the dose tested. It does not address the issue of prevention.

About the same time that the HOPE-TOO results were published, another group published a meta-analysis suggesting that dosages of vitamin E 400 IU or greater daily may increase all-cause mortality "and should be avoided." This meta-analysis involved 19 clinical trials, nine of them with vitamin E alone and 10 with vitamin E in combination with other vitamins and minerals. Considerable criticism of this meta-analysis ensued, emanating from individual researchers and from some major research groups around the world. One critic noted that 12 clinical trials that were among those with the lowest reported deaths were excluded from the meta-analysis. Others said that the inconsistent use of the various vitamin E isoforms, as well as the large variability in patient conditions, dosages, trial designs and end-point analyses, were so significant that comparisons became "difficult and fallacious." The combination of vitamin E with various other substances also presented difficulties in terms of drawing meaningful conclusions. The authors of the DATATOP trial took exception to the analysis of their data included in the meta-analysis. In the DATATOP trial, 800 patients with early Parkinson's disease were randomly administered 2,000 IU of vitamin E daily or seligilene (399 received vitamin E). This study used the highest dose of vitamin E of any of the studies included in the meta-analysis and might thus have been expected to provide the best evidence of increased mortality if such an effect was real. The DATATOP authors stated that the authors of the meta-analysis did not adequately analyze their data and that, in fact, "after adjustment for age and sex in a logistic regression, there was no excess mortality in the group assigned to vitamin E." They further concluded: "We found no evidence of increased mortality in DATATOP related to 2.6 years of high-dosage vitamin E exposure through 13 years of observation." Researchers at another university center called the increased mortality finding an artifact of a flawed analytical design and added: "We also question the applicability of the data to the general population." They pointed out that most of the subjects included in the meta-analysis were suffering from cardiovascular disease. They also stated they were "surprised by the lack of emphasis on the benefits of reduction of all-cause mortality by doses of vitamin E below 400 IU, an effect that reached statistical significance if vitamin E alone was considered." These critics pointed to their own double-blind, placebo-controlled study of vitamin E supplementation (200 IU daily for one year) in patients in nursing homes. No difference was noted in this study in all-cause mortality between controls and experimentals. Benefit was observed in the vitamin E group in terms of significantly reduced group-acquired upper respiratory tract infections, particularly the common cold, a significant health problem in the aging population. Numerous other criticisms were mounted by other researchers.

Mixed results continue to accumulate. One research group recently reported that, in contrast with some other clinical trials that failed to find a vitamin E benefit in cardiovascular disease, they found benefit in subgroups with increased oxidative stress, specifically in individuals with both type 2 diabetes mellitus and the haptoglobin 2-2 genotype. Myocardial infarction, stroke and cardiovascular death were significantly reduced in vitamin E-supplemented (400 IU daily) subjects compared with controls in this prospective double-blinded trial. In another recent study, vitamin E supplementation was judged to have beneficial effects on endothelial complications in type 2 diabetes mellitus patients who underwent coronary artery bypass graft. Also, recently, researchers using data from the ATBC cohort study concluded that higher circulating concentrations of alpha-tocopherol within the normal range are associated with significantly lower total and cause-specific mortality in older male smokers. In the HDL Atherosclerosis Treatment Study (HATS), subjects with low HDL-cholesterol levels benefited from treatment with simvastatin and niacin. Angiographically confirmed stenosis regressed in the simvastatin-niacin group but progressed in a group given simvastatin-niacin along with a combination of antioxidants that included vitamin E, suggesting that the antioxidant combination might actually attenuate the benefits of simvastatin and niacin in coronary disease. If this is true it may provide a clue as to why some antioxidants may not be of benefit in established cardiovascular disease. In a recent review of the vitamin E literature, however, a study is cited in which transplant-associated atherosclerosis was prevented by supplementation with combined vitamin E and C. In this double-blind prospective trial, 40 patients (0-2 years after cardiac transplant) were randomly assigned vitamin C (500 mg) plus vitamin E (400 IU) or placebo. After one year of treatment, disease progression was significantly inhibited in the vitamin group but not in the placebo group. Various other clinical studies conducted in recent years have demonstrated both positive and negative effects of vitamin E on atherosclerotic progression. Some of these have used vitamin E alone and others have used vitamin E in combination with other antioxidants without consistent results.

Some review authors have tried to address the hypothesis that vitamin E may be useful as a preventive but not as an interventive in cardiovascular disease. They found some evidence of adverse interactions between vitamin E and other substances used to treat disease that might explain an adverse vitamin E effect, particularly in severe disease states requiring significant medication. Their conclusion may be the most persuasive based on current knowledge: "In summary, the often neutral outcome of secondary prevention studies suggests that vitamin E supplementation is not an effective therapy against pre-existing cardiovascular disease, but rather may play a preventive role as evidenced in the more positive outcome seen in primary prevention and epidemiologic studies."

Another useful conclusion may have been drawn by the authors of the recent study, using the ATBC cohort data, in which they reported that higher serum concentrations of vitamin E are associated with lower total and cause-specific mortality in older male smokers. "Because supplemental vitamin E has not been shown to reduce mortality in randomized trials, efforts to improve vitamin E status through dietary means (e.g., through increased consumption of foods rich in vitamin E, including nuts, seeds, whole grains and dark-green leafy vegetables) may be warranted." Though part of this statement is contradicted by other studies (some randomized trials *have* shown reduced mortality, as discussed above), the dietary recommendation may be well-founded.

Though it has long been assumed that vitamin E's starring role would be in heart disease, it may turn out to have as big a part to play in preventing and treating some cancers. The same study that dealt a blow to claims that beta-carotene supplementation prevents lung cancer raised hopes that vitamin E might effectively help prevent prostate cancer. In the ATBC study of Finnish smokers, low-dose synthetic vitamin E (50 milligrams daily) reduced the incidence of prostate cancer by a significant 32% and prostate cancer deaths by a significant 41%. This unexpected result was sufficiently impressive that the National Cancer Institute continues to follow up via the ongoing Selenium and Vitamin E Cancer Prevention Trial (SELECT), the largest ever prostate cancer prevention trial.

Reduction in prostate cancer incidence became evident in the ATBC study within two years of beginning supplementation. Some believe there is the suggestion in this and other research that vitamin E blocks the progression of latent prostate cancer, particularly important, if verified, because latent prostate cancer cannot be detected clinically, and many deaths occur because of this. There is often little or no warning of the transition from latent to aggressive disease. A lesser reduction in colon cancer associated with vitamin E supplementation was also seen in this study.

In the Linxian China study, another randomized long-term intervention study, administration of synthetic vitamin E, in combination with selenium and beta-carotene, resulted in a significant reduction in total mortality and total cancer incidence. Only this combination of nutrients, among four regimens tested, was effective with respect to these endpoints. The combination was particularly protective against esophageal and stomach cancers. This was the only regimen tested that included vitamin E. Dosage was low—30 IUs daily.

In a recent further analysis of data from the ATBC study, researchers found that "higher serum alpha-tocopherol status is associated with reduced lung cancer risk; this relationship appears stronger among younger persons and among those with less cumulative smoke exposure. These findings suggest that high levels of alpha-tocopherol, if present during the early critical stages of tumorigenesis, may inhibit lung cancer development." Those in the highest versus the lowest quintile of serum vitamin E concentrations had a 19% reduction in incidence of lung cancer in this study. The researchers further noted that "There was a stronger inverse association among younger men .... And possibly among men receiving supplementation."

Did vitamin E supplementation, then, help protect against lung cancer? The conclusion in the original study report was that it did not. Secondary analyses of the ATBC trial, however, suggested that study subjects who supplemented with vitamin E for the longest periods of time experienced a 10-15% reduction in lung cancer risk in this cohort of smokers. Supplementation was low-dose (50 milligrams daily of synthetic alpha-tocopherol).

In the serum vitamin E analysis, the researchers further concluded that there was "synergism between usual intake and the controlled intervention." Those who had higher pre-trial serum levels of vitamin E did better than those with lower pre-trial serum levels, and still better results were seen in those with higher pre-trial serum levels who also received vitamin E supplements during the trial. Thus there is the suggestion that epidemiology may coincide here with intervention.

The researchers concluded that "while it is tempting, based on the present data, to speculate that the administration of greater quantities of alpha-tocopherol might have produced a substantial reduction in lung cancer incidence in the ATBC study, only future studies, and controlled trials in particular, can shed light on this question."

Numerous epidemiological studies have associated higher vitamin E status with reduced cancer, including lung, colorectal, prostate, colon, stomach, reproductive organs, upper gastrointestinal tract, bladder, breast, cervix, mouth, pharynx and thyroid cancer. Reduced serum vitamin E levels are also associated with a higher incidence of lymphoma and leukemia in some populations. Not all epidemiological studies have shown an inverse relationship between vitamin E status and cancer risk, but the majority have.

Vitamin E has shown significant activity against various cancers *in vitro* and in experimental animal models of carcinogenesis. In a review of animal work, results overall strongly indicated that vitamin E significantly reduced the incidence of a variety of cancers. Vitamin E has shown significant anti-cancer activity in these experiments when used alone and when used in combination with vitamin C and/or selenium, among other antioxidant companions. Mammary tumors have been significantly inhibited in rat experiments using vitamin E and selenium. Chemically induced skin cancers in mice were inhibited with vitamin E and beta-carotene.

In one intervention trial, neither beta-carotene, vitamin C, nor vitamin E reduced the incidence of colorectal adenoma recurrence in subjects who had undergone removal of colorectal adenoma prior to entering this study. Supplementation continued for four years. Critics of the study said far longer supplementation would be required to have any impact on this problem.

Vitamin E (400 IUs twice daily for 24 weeks) achieved clinical improvement (disappearance of at least 50% of lesions) in 20 of 43 patients with oral leukoplakia. In a randomized, double blind, placebo-controlled study, a topical preparation of vitamin E completely resolved the oral lesions of subjects with chemotherapy-induced mucositis.

The HOPE-TOO trial, discussed earlier, did not find evidence of reduced cancer in the patients it studied with vascular disease and/or diabetes mellitus. In a further amplification of the ATBC cancer findings, researchers have reported that participants in that study who had higher concentrations of the major vitamin E fractions had significantly lower prostate cancer risk. This association held both before supplementation was given and afterwards (when the effect was accentuated). The authors of a recent mini-review of the vitamin E cancer data concluded that different vitamin E isomers and analogs have different anticancer potencies and activities. Their findings persuaded them that more research is needed and warranted to determine which of these substances, either singly or in various combinations, are most likely to serve as possible adjuvant chemotherapeutic agents in a variety of cancers. They believe that alpha-tocopherol itself may not be capable of effective tumor cell apoptosis (in contrast with some of the other isomers and analogs) but that it might still be effective, primarily through its antioxidative properties.

High plasma vitamin E levels have been associated with greater resistance to infection in some, but not all, epidemiological studies. Some of these have shown a stronger protective effect in the elderly. *In vitro* and animal studies have demonstrated that vitamin E can enhance some immune functions. In animals, there is evidence that supplemental vitamin E increased resistance to a number of pathogens including *Escherichia coli* and *Pneumoccocus pneumonia* type I. Influenza viral lung titers were significantly reduced in elderly mice supplemented with vitamin E, compared with unsupplemented controls who were also infected and who consumed normal amounts of vitamin E in their diets. A number of immunologic studies have tested vitamin E alone and in combination with other nutrients in humans. The number of CD4 and CD8 T cells were high and lymphocyte proliferative response to mitogen was significantly enhanced in elderly subjects given supplemental vitamins A, E and C for four weeks, compared with those given placebo. In some other human studies, supplementation with vitamin E alone or in combination with vitamin C, beta-carotene and some other nutrients has favorably affected T-cell counts, lymphocyte response, levels of interleukin-2 and natural killer cell activity.

One reviewer of the vitamin E literature concluded: "Evidence from animal and human studies indicates that vitamin E plays an important role in the maintenance of the immune system. Even a marginal vitamin E deficiency impairs the immune response, while supplementation with higher than recommended dietary levels of vitamin E enhances humoral and cell-mediated immunity."

In one double-blind, placebo-controlled study, 88 healthy elderly subjects were randomized to receive 60, 200 or 800 milligrams of synthetic vitamin E daily or placebo for 235 days. The objective was to determine the effects, if any, of these varying doses of vitamin E on various measures of cell-mediated immunity. Some older healthy people have been shown to have an impaired ability to produce an effective delayed-type hypersensitivity skin response (DTH), which, in turn, has been associated with greater mortality. Decreased DTH appears to be indicative of diminished capacity to deal with infectious and neoplastic challenges and prolonged illness.

Subjects receiving 200 milligrams of vitamin E daily in this study had a significant 65% increase in DTH and a six-fold increase in antibody titer to hepatitis B, compared with subjects receiving placebo. Subjects receiving the 200 milligram dose also had significant increases in antibody titer to tetanus vaccine, compared with controls. Supplementation did not affect antibody titer to diphtheria, immunoglobulin levels or levels of T and B cells. Nor was there any observed effect on antibody levels.

The 60 milligram dose did not produce statistically significant results in some of the parameters measured. The 200 milligram dose generally produced better results than the 800 milligram dose. Thus the researchers concluded that there may be a threshold level for vitamin E's observed immunostimulatory effects and that the 200 milligram dose, pending possible different findings in future research, appears to be the optimal dose for healthy elderly individuals seeking to preserve immune function. Very high doses of vitamin E have been associated with adverse effects on immunity in some studies. Subjects given 1,600 milligrams of vitamin E daily for one week, for example, were shown to have diminished polymorphonuclear leukocyte bactericidal activity.

Finally, with respect to immunity, there have been some reports that vitamin E may be helpful in some with HIV-disease. In a study of 311 HIV-infected individuals followed over a period of nine years, those with the highest blood levels of vitamin E were 34% less likely than those with low levels to progress to fully-developed AIDS. The higher vitamin E status was also associated in this study with higher T helper lymphocyte counts.

In another study, there was the suggestion that low vitamin E status might be associated with elevated immunoglobulin E (IgE) levels and consequent increased inflammation in HIV-infected individuals. This inflammation is postulated to increase HIV replication.

And in an animal model of AIDS, vitamin E supplementation reportedly helped restore some T cell functions and reduced production of inflammation-promoting interleukin-6 and tumor necrosis factor.

Results of an additional study showed that vitamin E, in combination with erythropoietin and interleukin-3, increased survival and weight of fetuses in pregnant rats administered AZT. Thus it has been suggested that vitamin E might help protect against some of the toxic effects of AZT and similar drugs. Research continues.

As for autoimmune disorders, here too there is epidemiological evidence linking low vitamin E status with a higher incidence of rheumatoid arthritis. In one small interventive trial, 1,200 IUs of vitamin E daily reportedly reduced pain in rheumatoid arthritis patients but not inflammation, compared with subjects receiving placebo. Other studies have also reported significant pain reduction.

Vitamin E has been used with benefit in some with asthma. Lung function measures were significantly improved in one double-blind, placebo-controlled study of asthmatic volunteers exposed to ozone and sulfur dioxide who received 400 IUs of vitamin E and 500 milligrams of vitamin C daily for five weeks.

Various animal and human experiments have demonstrated that supplemental vitamin E can protect against some of the toxic effects of cigarette smoke and smog. In a recent study of Dutch bicyclists, 100 milligrams of vitamin E and 500 milligrams of vitamin C daily for 15 weeks significantly protected measures of lung function against effects of ozone, compared with controls receiving placebo.

Vitamin E (50 milligrams daily) did not have any effect on the recurrence or incidence of chronic obstructive bronchopulmonary diseases in the ATBC study of Finnish smokers. Higher dietary intake of vitamin E, however, was associated in this study with lower incidence of chronic bronchitis and dyspnea.

Supplemental vitamin E has shown some positive activity in neurological disorders. In a well-designed double-blind, multicenter, placebo-controlled study, 2,000 IUs of synthetic vitamin E daily, alone or in combination with the drug selegiline (10 milligrams daily), were administered to subjects with moderate Alzheimer's disease over a two-year period. Primary endpoints were death, severe dementia, loss of ability to perform everyday tasks and need of institutionalization. Those receiving vitamin E alone had a 53% reduction in risk of reaching any of these endpoints, while those on selegiline had a 43% reduction in risk, and those taking both vitamin E and selegiline had a 31% reduction. There was an increase of 230 days in the time it took on vitamin E to reach a primary endpoint, compared to those on placebo. Partly because of this study, the American Psychiatric Association updated its treatment guidelines for Alzheimer's disease. Those guidelines include the use of vitamin E in newly diagnosed, mildly impaired and moderately impaired victims of this disease and some other diseases that also cause dementia.

Unfortunately, a follow-up to the study cited above did not yield similarly positive effects. In this study, subjects with risk for progression to Alzheimer's were randomly assigned to receive 2,000 IU vitamin E daily or the drug donepezil or placebo for three years. The donepezil showed some small effect, which was abolished after the first year. Vitamin E was no better than placebo in inhibiting the onset of cognitive impairment. In another trial, 160 patients with Alzheimer's got no benefit from 5,000 IU of vitamin E daily based on cognitive measures taken after 18 months of follow-up.

In another trial, selegiline but not vitamin E was shown to significantly delay the need for levodopa in patients with Parkinson's disease (a benefit that was not sustained during follow-up).

Results have been mixed with respect to vitamin E's effects on tardive dyskinesia. In one study, the vitamin significantly out-scored placebo at 400-800 IUs daily. In a more recent randomized, multicenter, placebo-controlled study, vitamin E (1,600 IUs daily) showed no effect in the treatment of tardive dyskinesia over a two-year supplementation period.

In a study of 3,385 elderly men, age 71 to 93 years, use of either vitamin E or vitamin C supplements, ascertained by questionnaire, was significantly associated with better cognitive test performance and protection against vascular dementia.

Pre-treatment and post-treatment with vitamin E enhanced neurologic recovery after experimental spinal cord compression injury in cats. Four weeks post-injury, treated cats recovered 72% of pre-injury function, compared with 20% recovery in untreated controls.

Epidemiological associations have been made between high blood levels of vitamin E and reduced incidence of cataract. In a study of 764 elderly subjects, those taking vitamin E supplements had a 50% reduced risk that their cataracts would progress over a 4-5 year period. Multivitamin use was associated with a 33% reduction in the same risk. Vitamin E supplementation has prevented cataract development and significantly inhibited its progression in several animal models.

Results of a population-based study of 2,584 French subjects recently showed that high plasma vitamin E levels are associated with decreased risk of late age-related macular degeneration (AMD). The risk of late AMD was reduced by 82% in those individuals in the highest vitamin E quintile compared with the lowest quintile. There was also a lesser but still significant reduction in risk of early signs of AMD associated with high vitamin E status. The study adjusted for smoking and factors related to cardiovascular disease including diabetes, all of which are associated with increased AMD risk. No association was found between reduced risk of AMD and plasma retinol, ascorbic acid levels or with red blood cell glutathione values.

The controlled, clinical intervention trial that could demonstrate supplemental vitamin E's possible benefit in the treatment of AMD has yet to be conducted, but, as several researchers have noted, such a study is clearly warranted.

Through its possible cardiovascular-protective effects, vitamin E is hypothesized by some to be beneficial in some cases of diabetes. Additionally, in animal studies, vitamin E has exerted various effects in the kidneys, eyes and nerves that may be helpful in combating some of the damage of diabetes. Vitamin E did not show any benefit with respect to incidence of complications of diabetes in the HOPE study previously discussed. Some said the follow-up was of insufficient duration to show and any effect.

A recent report indicated serum vitamin E concentrations at baseline, in a case-control study nested within a 21-year follow-up study, were inversely associated with insulin-dependent diabetes mellitus incidence 4-14 years later. Risk was diminished 85% among those with the highest vitamin E status versus those with the lowest. This reduced risk persisted after adjustment for serum cholesterol levels.

Recently, researchers reported that supplemental oral vitamin E normalized retinal hemodynamic abnormalities and improved renal function in type 1 diabetic patients of short disease duration. This was a randomized, double-blind, placebo-controlled crossover trial of eight months duration. Vitamin E dose was 1,800 IUs daily.

In another recent double-blind, placebo-controlled study 1,600 IUs of vitamin E daily did not improve postulated receptor-specific vascular endothelial dysfunction in subjects with type 2 diabetes mellitus. Vitamin E has, however, been shown to prevent and reverse some of the vascular complications of diabetes in *in vitro*, animal and human studies. Vitamin E has demonstrated an ability to inhibit hyperglycemia-induced activation of protein kinase C (PKC) and to also inhibit diacylglycerol (DAG) levels. Both PKC and DAG have been implicated in diabetic complications, and inhibition of PKC has reversed some of the vascular dysfunctions in retina, kidney and cardiovascular systems caused by hyperglycemia or diabetes.

In a recent pilot study, vitamin E treatment (300 mg daily for six months) resulted in a reduction in biochemical markers and oxidative stress associated with nonalcoholic steatohepatitis. A subsequent study similarly suggested a possible role for vitamin E in the treatment of this disease.

Preliminary research has indicated that supplemental vitamin E might be helpful in some with premenstrual syndrome (PMS). In a double-blind, placebo-controlled trial, vitamin E (in doses of 150, 300 or 600 IUs daily administered for two months) significantly outperformed placebo. It reportedly significantly improved three of four classes of PMS symptoms. A subsequent double-blind, placebo-controlled study found significant improvement in some affective and physical symptoms of PMS in subjects treated with 400 IUs of vitamin E daily for three menstrual cycles. The same research group conducted both of these studies in the 1980s. They need follow-up.

There is evidence from *in vitro* and animal studies that both oral and topically applied vitamin E can help protect against UV light-induced skin changes and protect against skin cancer. In animals and humans, studies have shown that UV irradiation diminishes both skin and plasma levels of various nutrients, including vitamin E.

In one experiment, the UVB irradiation that is considered to be the most carcinogenic suppressed immune functions in the skin of mice. This suppression was blocked with vitamin E. *In vitro*, vitamin E has also blocked some of the immune-suppressing effects UVA radiation has on human cells. Topically applied vitamin E prevented UVB-induced skin tumors in an animal model.

Some studies in humans have demonstrated that topical vitamin E can protect skin against photo-damage and subsequent wrinkling. In one placebo-controlled study, topically applied vitamin E, more than placebo, reportedly reduced eyelid wrinkling over a four-week period. And, in another human study, a patented cream containing, among other things, vitamin E and C, reportedly produced significant improvement in wrinkling. An oral preparation of vitamin E and C had no effect. Placebos were used. Treatment continued for 18 months. More rigorous follow-up studies are required before vitamin E's ability, if any, to reverse photo-damage is established.

In a recent double-blind study, vitamin E ointment did not improve the cosmetic appearance of surgical scars. Application of topical vitamin E was associated with contact dermatitis in 33% of the subjects.

It has been claimed that supplemental vitamin E increases male sexual performance and enhances male fertility. There is no evidence that supplemental vitamin E has any effect on sexual performance in either males of females. An Israeli research group has reported that 200 milligrams of oral vitamin E daily for one month apparently helped two men overcome their long-term infertility. Both had very high levels of lipid peroxidation as measured by elevated levels of malondialdehyde prior to beginning vitamin E supplementation. Within one month of starting vitamin E supplementation, the malondialdehyde levels dropped significantly. Both men were able to impregnate their wives.

A combination of vitamin E and selenium seemed to improve sperm motility and morphology in one group of men. Similar results were obtained in a second study, this one using 600 IUs of vitamin E daily. It is possible that these changes might enhance male fertility, but that endpoint was not investigated in these studies.

More recently, a more rigorous randomized placebo-controlled, double-blind study found no improvement in semen parameters in infertile men supplemented with 1,000 milligrams of vitamin C and 800 milligrams of vitamin E for 56 days. Semen parameters studied included semen volume, sperm concentration and motility, sperm count and viability.

Also poorly supported are claims that vitamin E can enhance exercise/athletic performance. There is some evidence that supplemental vitamin E can reduce some measures of oxidative stress in some exercisers but no evidence that it enhances performance.

Notable relief from persistent nocturnal cramps of legs and feet was seen in 82% of 125 subjects taking 300 IUs or less of vitamin E daily.

CONTRAINDICATIONS, PRECAUTIONS, ADVERSE REACTIONS
CONTRAINDICATIONS
Vitamin E is contraindicated in those with known hypersensitivity to any component of a vitamin E-containing product.

PRECAUTIONS

Those on warfarin should be cautious in using high doses of vitamin E (i.e., doses greater than 100 milligrams daily of d-alpha-tocopherol or 200 milligrams daily of dl-alpha-tocopherol), and if they do use such doses, they should have their INRs monitored and their warfarin dose appropriately adjusted if indicated. Likewise, those with vitamin K deficiencies, such as those with liver failure, should be cautious in using high doses of vitamin E. Vitamin E should be used with extreme caution in those with any lesions that have a propensity to bleed (e.g., bleeding peptic ulcers), those with a history of hemorrhagic stroke and those with inherited bleeding disorders (e.g., hemophilia).

Supplemental doses of vitamin E higher than RDA amounts should be avoided by pregnant women and nursing mothers.

High dose vitamin E supplementation should be stopped about one month before surgical procedures and may be resumed following recovery from the procedure. Use of supplemental vitamin E in low birth weight premature infants must be undertaken with extreme caution and only by trained medical personnel.

ADVERSE REACTIONS

The risk of adverse reactions to vitamin E supplementation (in doses up to one gram daily of alpha-tocopherol) generally appears to be very low. A large randomized trial, the Alpha-Tocopherol Beta Carotene (ATBC) Cancer Prevention Study, the subjects of which were Finnish male smokers, reported that subjects consuming 50 milligrams daily of dl-alpha-tocopherol for 6 years had a 50% increase in mortality from hemorrhagic stroke. The numbers were 66 versus 44 strokes in the supplemented versus the control groups. This result was statistically significant. Interestingly, an increase in hemorrhagic stroke has not been observed in other large, long-term studies using much higher doses of the vitamin. The overall stroke rate between the two groups was not statistically significant in the ATBC study. In their most recent report (April, 2000) on vitamin E, the National Research Council comments "The unexpected finding in the ATBC study was considered preliminary and provocative, but not convincing until it can be corroborated or refuted in further large-scale clinical trials."

Adverse reactions reported for vitamin E supplementation include fatigue, breast soreness, emotional disturbances, thrombophlebitis, retinuria, gastrointestinal disturbances, altered serum lipid levels and thyroid problems. These adverse reactions were rare and none of these has been reported in controlled studies. An increased incidence of necrotizing enterocolitis has been reported in premature, very-low birth weight infants receiving 200 milligrams daily of alpha-tocopheryl acetate.

The meta-analysis discussed earlier suggested that vitamin E at 400 IU daily and above may increase all-cause mortality. There was also much criticism of this meta-analysis.

INTERACTIONS

DRUGS

Amiodarone: Alpha-tocopherol may ameliorate some of the adverse side effects of this drug. This is based on the results of cell culture studies.

Anticonvulsants such as phenobarbital, phenytoin and carbamazepine: Anticonvulsants may lower plasma vitamin E levels.

Antiplatelet drugs such as aspirin, dipyridamole, eptifibatide, clopidogrel, ticlopidine HCI, tirofiban and abciximab: High doses of vitamin E may potentiate the effects of these antiplatelet drugs.

Cholestyramine: may decrease vitamin E absorption.

Colestipol: may decrease vitamin E absorption.

Cyclosporin: Based on cell culture studies, alpha-tocopherol may help to ameliorate the renal side effects of cyclosporin.

Ezetimibe: may inhibit the intestinal absorption of alpha-tocopherol.

Isoniazid: may decrease vitamin E absorption.

Mineral oil: may decrease vitamin E absorption.

Multidrug-resistance (MDR) modifying agents: Based on cell culture studies, alpha-tocopherol is reported to antagonize the multidrug-resistance (MDR)-modifying activity of the chemosensitizing agents cyclosporin A, verapamil, clofazimine, GF120918 and B669 to both doxorubicin and vinblastine.

Neomycin: may impair utilization of vitamin E.

Orlistat: inhibits vitamin E absorption. Absorption of a vitamin E acetate supplement was inhibited by approximately 60% by orlistat.

Sucralfate: interferes with vitamin E absorption.

Warfarin: Vitamin E may enhance anticoagulant response. Monitor INRs and appropriately adjust dose of warfarin if necessary.

Zidovudine: Vitamin E may ameliorate myelosuppressive side effects of zidovudine.

NUTRITIONAL SUPPLEMENTS

Beta-carotene: Some studies have suggested that oral supplements of beta-carotene may cause a decrease in serum levels of alpha-tocopherol. However, more recent and much larger and longer studies have demonstrated that supplementation with beta-carotene does not alter serum concentrations of vitamin E.

Desiccated ox bile: Desiccated ox bile may increase the absorption of vitamin E.

Dietary fiber: Dietary fiber supplementation may decrease the antioxidative effect of a supplement containing alpha-tocopherol and carotenoids.

Iron: Most iron supplements contain the ferrous form of iron. This cation can oxidize unesterified vitamin E to its pro-oxidant form if taken concomitantly. This does not occur with esterified vitamin E (alpha-tocopheryl acetate and succinate).

Medium–chain triglycerides: Medium-chain triglycerides, if taken concomitantly with vitamin E, may enhance its absorption.

Phytosterols and phytostanols, including beta-sitosterol and beta-sitostanol: Phytosterols and phytostanols may lower plasma vitamin E levels.

Plant phenolic compounds and flavonoids: These substances may participate in redox cycling reactions and help maintain levels of reduced vitamin E.

Polyunsaturated fatty acids (PUFAs): Supplementary PUFAs, including alpha-linolenic acid (in flaxseed oil and perilla oil), gamma-linolenic acid (in borage oil, blackcurrant oil, evening primrose oil), docosahexaenoic acid, eicosapentaenoic acid and conjugated linoleic acid may increase vitamin E requirements. In most cases this can be satisfied by supplemental use of either at least 15 milligrams daily of d-alpha-tocopherol or 30 milligrams daily of d1-alpha-tocopherol.

Selenium: Selenium may function synergistically with vitamin E.

Vitamin C: Vitamin C may spare vitamin E. It, along with other antioxidants, such as glutathione, alpha-lipoic acid and coenzyme Q_{10}, are thought to be involved in a so-called antioxidant network which helps to regenerate reduced alpha-tocopherol from the tocopheroxyl radical.

FOOD

Dietary polyunsaturated fat: High polyunsaturated fatty acid intakes should be accompanied by increased vitamin E intakes to prevent their oxidation.

Olestra: The fat substitute olestra inhibits the absorption of vitamin E, as well as the other fat-soluble vitamins A, D and K, carotenoids and flavonoids. Vitamins A, D, E (alpha-tocopherol) and K are added to olestra to partly compensate for this.

HERBS

Some herbs, including garlic and ginkgo, possess antithrombotic activity. High doses of vitamin E used at the same time as these herbs may enhance their antithrombotic activity.

OVERDOSAGE

There are no reports of overdosage with vitamin E in any form.

DOSAGE AND ADMINISTRATION

There are several forms of vitamin E available commercially. These are available as nutritional supplements or in functional and fortified foods. The following table lists these forms and their common names.

Vitamin E Forms

Correct Name	Common Name
RRR-alpha-tocopherol	d-alpha-tocopherol
RRR-alpha-tocopheryl acetate	d-alpha-tocopheryl acetate
RRR-alpha-tocopheryl succinate	d-alpha-tocopheryl succinate
all-rac-alpha-tocopherol	dL-alpha-tocopherol
all-rac-alpha-tocopheryl acetate	dl-alpha-tocopheryl acetate
all-rac-alpha-tocopheryl succinate	d1-alpha-tocopheryl succinate (Available for research purposes only)
gamma-tocopherol	gamma-tocopherol
mixed tocopherols	mixed tocopherols
RRR-alpha-tocopheryl polyethylene glycol 1000 succinate	TPGS
all-rac-alpha-tocopheryl nicotinate	dL-alpha-tocopheryl nicotinate
mixed tocotrienols	mixed tocotrienols

For the purpose of defining dietary reference intakes (RDI) for vitamin E, the National Research Council, in its most recent report, restricted vitamin E activity to only one of the homologues of the tocopherol family, *RRR*-alpha-tocopherol. Therefore, the term alpha-tocopherol, when referring to vitamin E activity, includes only the naturally occurring form, *RRR*-alpha-tocopherol, commonly, but incorrectly, called d-alpha-tocopherol, and four out of the eight forms of synthetic alpha-tocopherol, *all-rac*-alpha-tocopherol, commonly, but incorrectly, known as d1-alpha-tocopherol. The four included forms are the 2*R* structures: *RRR*-, *RSR*-, *RRS*- and *RSS*-alpha-tocopherol. *RRR*-alpha-tocopherol, natural alpha-tocopherol (called "natural-source" alpha-tocopherol when sold commercially), has approximately twice the availability of the *all-rac* (synthetic) alpha-tocopherol and is probably the better form for supplementation. Natural-source vitamin E supplements are called natural source rather than natural, since *RRR*-alpha-tocopherol is produced from natural gamma-tocopherol via a synthetic step.

The new RDA for alpha-tocopherol for both men and women is 15 milligrams a day. This is for natural or natural-source alpha-tocopherol (*RRR*-alpha-tocopherol). Since only four out of the eight stereoisomers of the *all-rac*-alpha-tocopherol have vitamin E activity, 30 milligrams daily of *all-rac*-alpha-tocopherol are needed to supply the RDA for the vitamin.

To estimate milligrams of 2*R*-alpha-tocopherol in a vitamin E supplement labeled in internationals units, multiply the dose by 0.45 mg/IU if the supplement is *all-rac*-alpha-tocopherol (synthetic) or by 0.67 mg/IU if the supplement is *RRR*-alpha-tocopherol (natural or natural source). Natural and natural source forms, include d-alpha-tocopherol, d-alpha-tocopheryl acetate and d-alpha-tocopheryl succinate. Synthetic forms, include dl-alpha-tocopherol, dl-alpha-tocopheryl acetate and dl-alpha-tocopheryl succinate. The same conversion factor (0.67 mg/IU) is used for all forms of natural and natural source vitamin E (alpha-tocopherol, d-alpha-tocopheryl acetate and d-alpha-tocopheryl succinate), and the same conversion factor (0.45 mg/IU) is used for all forms of *all-rac*-alpha-tocopherol (dl-alpha-tocopherol, dl-alpha-tocopheryl acetate and dl-alpha-tocopheryl succinate). One will note that the term *RRR*-alpha-tocopherol is used in this section interchangeably with d-alpha-tocopherol, and the term *all-rac*-alpha-tocopherol is used interchangeably with dl-alpha-tocopherol. The reason for this is because the incorrect terms d-alpha-tocopherol and dl-alpha-tocopherol are still the more commonly used terms. One day they won't be.

Regarding doses, vitamin E-deficiency conditions need to be managed by medical personnel.

Recommended doses for supplementation range from 100 to 400 IU daily. Supplemental vitamin E is best taken with meals.

The average intake of *RRR*-alpha-tocopherol derived from various dietary surveys ranges from about 7.5 to 10.3 milligrams daily for men and 5.4 to 7.3 milligrams daily for women. It is believed that these intake estimates may be low due to underreporting of fat and caloric intake and uncertainties about the particular fats or oils consumed. It is thought that an average daily intake of about 15 milligrams may be closer to reality, but this is not clear. The principal vitamin E form in the American diet is gamma-tocopherol. Vitamin E is present in fortified foods as the *all-rac* form.

The Food and Nutrition Board of the National Academy of Sciences has recently issued its report on dietary reference intakes (RDI) for vitamin E, as well as for some other antioxidant nutrients. In establishing the Recommended Dietary Allowance (RDA) for vitamin E, only *RRR*-alpha-tocopherol was taken into account. Other naturally occurring forms of vitamin E (beta-, gamma-, and delta-tocopherol and alpha-, beta-, gamma- and delta-tocotrienols) were not considered to meet the vitamin E requirement since they are not converted to alpha-tocopherol in humans and have significantly lower binding affinities to the alpha-tocopherol transfer protein. For establishing RDAs of vitamin E, alpha-tocopherol is defined as the natural *RRR*-alpha-tocopherol and the 2*R*-stereoisomers of synthetic vitamin E (found in supplements and fortified foods), *RRR*-, *RSR*-, *RRS*-, and *RSS*-alpha-tocopherols. The 2*S*-stereoisomers are excluded by this definition. All forms of supplemental vitamin E are included in calculating the Tolerable Upper Intake Level (UL).

The new RDA for vitamin E (again, defined as only *RRR*-alpha-tocopherol) for both men and women is 15 milligrams daily. To convert *RRR*-alpha-tocopherol from milligrams to International Units (IU), the conversion factor is 1.49. Therefore, 15 milligrams of *RRR*-alpha-tocopherol is equal to 22.4 IU. The UL for vitamin E is 1,000 milligrams or 1,490 IU/day expressed as *RRR*-alpha-tocopherol.

The following summarizes the DRIs for various age groups and conditions:

Infants	Adequate Intake (AI)	
0-6 months	4 mg/day	0.6 mg/kg
7-12 months	5 mg/day	0.6 mg/kg

	Recommended Daily Allowance (RDA)
Children	
1-3 years	6 mg/day
4-8 years	7 mg/day
Boys	
9-13 years	11 mg/day
14-18 years	15 mg/day
Girls	
9-13 years	11 mg/day
14-18 years	15 mg/day
Men	
19-30 years	15 mg/day
31-50 years	15 mg/day
51-70 years	15 mg/day
Older than 70 years	15 mg/day

Women

19-30 years	15 mg/day
31-50 years	15 mg/day
51-70 years	15 mg/day
Older than 70 years	15 mg/day

Pregnancy

14-18 years	15 mg/day
19-30 years	15 mg/day
31-50 years	15 mg/day

Lactation

14-18 years	19 mg/day
19-30 years	19 mg/day
31-50 years	19 mg/day

The DV (Daily Value) for vitamin E, which is used for determining percentage of nutrient daily values on nutritional supplement and food labels, is 30 IU (International Units). This is based on the U.S. RDA for vitamin E.

The following summarizes the Tolerable Upper Intake Level (UL) for various age groups and conditions:

Children	(UL)
1-3 years	200 mg/day
4-8 years	300 mg/day
9-13 years	600 mg/day

Adolescents	
14-18 years	800 mg/day

Adults	
19 years and older	1,000 mg/day

Pregnancy	
14-18 years	800 mg/day
19 years and older	1,000 mg/day

Lactation	
14-18 years	800 mg/day
19 years and older	1,000 mg/day

D-ALPHA-TOCOPHEROL

d-Alpha-tocopherol is available as a stand-alone supplement and in the form of mixed tocopherols. d-Alpha-tocopherol is unesterified and thus much more susceptible to oxidation. It should be stored in a tightly closed, opaque bottle and in a cool, dry place. Typical doses for supplementation range from 100 to 400 IU daily. d-Alpha-tocopherol is also available for cosmetic application as an antioxidant and moisturizer. Some are hypersensitive to topical d-alpha-tocopherol and may develop dermatitis from its use. To convert from International Units (IU) of d-alpha-tocopherol to milligrams, multiply by 0.67. To convert from milligrams of d-alpha-tocopherol to IU, multiply by 1.49.

D-ALPHA-TOCOPHERYL ACETATE

d-Alpha-tocopheryl acetate is available as a stand-alone supplement and in multivitamin preparations. Since the acetate group protects the hydroxyl group of the chromanol ring against oxidation, it is a more stable form than d-alpha-tocopherol, the free or unesterified form.

Typical doses for supplementation range from 100 to 400 IU daily (as d-alpha-tocopherol). To convert from International Units (IU) of d-alpha-tocopheryl acetate to milligrams, multiply by 0.67. To convert milligrams of d-alpha-tocopheryl acetate to IU, multiply by 1.49.

DL-ALPHA-TOCOPHERYL ACETATE

dl-Alpha-tocopheryl acetate is available as a stand-alone supplement and in combination products. Typical doses for supplementation range from 100 to 400 IU daily (as alpha-tocopherol). To convert from International Units (IU) of dl-alpha-tocopheryl acetate to milligrams, multiply by 0.45.

D-ALPHA-TOCOPHERYL SUCCINATE

d-Alpha-tocopheryl succinate is available as a stand-alone supplement and in combination vitamin preparations. Since the succinate group protects the hydroxyl group of the chromanol ring against oxidation, it is a more stable form than d-alpha-tocopherol, the free or unesterified form.

Typical doses for supplementation range from 100 to 400 IU daily (as d-alpha-tocopherol). To convert from International Units (IU) of d-alpha-tocopheryl succinate to milligrams, multiply by 0.67. To convert milligrams of d-alpha-tocopheryl succinate to IU, multiply by 1.49.

D1-ALPHA-TOCOPHERYL SUCCINATE

dl-Alpha-tocopheryl succinate is not available as a nutritional supplement. The reason for this is that it does not crystallize well but forms a paste. However, it is available for research purposes.

MIXED TOCOPHEROLS

Typical doses for supplementation of high-alpha-mixed-tocopherols range from 50 to 250 milligrams daily, determined as d-alpha-tocopherol. Typical doses for supplementation of low-alpha-mixed-tocopherols are around 200 milligrams daily, determined as d-gamma-tocopherol.

Since the tocopherols are present in their unesterified forms, forms which are much more susceptible to oxidation than esterified forms, mixed tocopherols should be stored in a tightly closed, opaque bottle and in a cool, dry place.

LITERATURE

Adler LA, Rotrosen J, Edson R, et al. Vitamin E treatment for tardive dyskinesia. *Arch Gen Psychiatry.* 1999;56:836-841.

Age-Related Eye Disease Study Research Group. A randomized, placebo-controlled, clinical trial of high-dose supplementation with vitamins C and E and beta carotene for age-related cataract and vision loss:AREDS report no. 9. *Arch Ophthalmol.* 2001;119(10):1439-1452.

Ahn J, Moslehi R, Weinstein SJ, et al. Family history of prostate cancer and prostate cancer risk in the Alpha-Tocopherol, Beta-Carotene Cancer Prevention (ATBC) Study. *Int J Cancer.* 2008;123(5):1154-1159.

Aiub CA, Pinto LF, Felzenszwalb I. DNA-repair genes and vitamin E in the prevention of N-nitrosodiethylamine mutagenicity. *Cell Biol Toxicol.* Epub: 2008 Jun 26.

Anderson DK, Waters TR, Means ED. Pretreatment with alpha-tocopherol enhances neurologic recovery after experimental spinal cord compression injury. *J Neurotrauma.* 1998;5:61-67.

Asleh R, Blum S, Kalet-Litman S, et al. Correction of HDL dysfunction in individuals with Diabetes and the Haptoglobin2-2 genotype. *Diabetes.* 2008;57(10):2794-2800.

Atkinson J, Epand RF, Epand RM.Tocopherols and tocotrienols in membranes: a critical review. *Free Radic Biol Med.* 2008;44(5):739-764.

Baumann LS, Spencer J. The effects of topical vitamin E on the cosmetic appearance of scars. *Dermatol Surg.* 1999;25:311-315.

Bjelakovic G, Nikolova D, Gluud LL, et al. Mortality in randomized trials of antioxidant supplements for primary and secondary prevention: systematic review and meta-analysis. *JAMA.* 2007;297(8):842-857.

Blot WJ, Li JY, Taylor PR, et al. Nutrition intervention trials in Linxian, China: supplementation with specific vitamin/mineral combinations, cancer incidence, and disease-specific mortality in the general population. *J Natl Cancer Inst.* 1993;85(18):1483-1492.

Blumberg JB, Frei B. Why clinical trials of vitamin E and cardiovascular diseases may be fatally flawed. Commentary on "The relationship between dose of vitamin E and suppression of oxidative stress in humans". *Free Radic Biol Med.* 2007;43(10):1374-1376.

Boaz M, Smetana S, Weinstein T, et al. Secondary prevention with antioxidants of cardiovascular disease in endstage renal disease (SPACE): randomised placebo-controlled trial. *Lancet.* 2000;356(9237):1213-1218.

Bozbuga M, Izgi N, Canbolat A. The effects of chronic alpha-tocopherol administration on lipid peroxidation in an experimental model of acute spinal cord injury. *Neurosurg Rev.* 1998;21:36-42.

Brigelius-Flohe R, Traber MG. Vitamin E: function and metabolism. *FASEB J.* 1999;13:1145-1155.

Brown BG, Crowley J. Is there any hope for vitamin E? *JAMA.* 2005;293(11):1387-1390.

Brown BG, Zhao XQ, Chait A, et al. Simvastatin and niacin, antioxidant vitamins, or the combination for the prevention of coronary disease. *N Engl J Med.* 2001;345(22):1583-1592.

Bursell S-E, King GL. Can protein kinase C inhibition and vitamin E prevent the development of diabetic vascular complications? *Diabetes Res Clin Pract.* 1999;45:169-182.

Burton GW, Traber MG, Acuff RV, et al. Human plasma and tissue alpha-tocopherol concentrations in response to supplementation with deuterated natural and synthetic vitamin E. *Am J Clin Nutr.* 1998;67:669-684.

Cheung MC, Zhao XQ, Chait A, et al. Antioxidant supplements block the response of HDL to simvastatin-niacin therapy in patients with coronary artery disease and low HDL. *Arterioscler Thromb Vasc Biol.* 2001(8):1320-1326.

Christen WG, Glynn RJ, Chew EY, et al. Vitamin E and age-related cataract in a randomized trial of women. *Ophthalmology.* 2008;115(5):822-829.

Chylack LT Jr, Brown NP, Bron A, et al. The Roche European American Cataract Trial (REACT): a randomized clinical trial to investigate the efficacy of an oral antioxidant micronutrient mixture to slow progression of age-related cataract. *Ophthalmic Epidemiol.* 2002(1):49-80.

Clarke MW, Burnett JR, Croft KD. Vitamin E in human health and disease. *Crit Rev Clin Lab Sci.* 2008;45(5):417-450.

Constantinou C, Papas A, Constantinou AI. Vitamin E and cancer: An insight into the anticancer activities of vitamin E isomers and analogs. *Int J Cancer.* 2008;123(4):739-752.

Cuddihy SL, Ali SS, Musiek ES, et al. Prolonged alpha-tocopherol deficiency decreases oxidative stress and unmasksalpha-tocopherol-dependent regulation of mitochondrial function in the brain. *J Biol Chem.* 2008;283(11):6915-6924.

de Gaetano G; Collaborative Group of the Primary Prevention Project. Low-dose aspirin and vitamin E in people at cardiovascular risk: a randomized trial in general practice. Collaborative Group of the Primary Prevention Project. *Lancet.* 2001;357(9250):89-95.

De la Fuente M, Hernanz A, Guayerbas N, et al. Vitamin E ingestion improves several immune functions in elderly men and women. *Free Radic Res.* 2008;42(3):272-280.

Delcourt C, Cristol J-P, Tessier F, et al. Age-related macular degeneration and antioxidant status in the POLA study. *Arch Opthalmol.* 1999;117:1384-1390.

Dong LF, Low P, Dyason JC, et al. Alpha-tocopheryl succinate induces apoptosis by targeting ubiquinone-binding sites in mitochondrial respiratory complex II. *Oncogene.* 2008;27(31):4324-4335.

Dowd P, Zheng ZB. On the mechanism of the anticlotting action of vitamin E quinone. *Proc Natl Acad Sci USA.* 1995;92:8171-8175.

Friedrich MJ. To "E" or not to "E," vitamin E's role in health and disease is the question. *JAMA.* 2004;292(6):671-673.

Girodon F, Galan P, Monget AL, et al. Impact of trace elements and vitamin supplementation on immunity and infectionsin institutionalized elderly patients: a randomized controlled trial. *Arch Intern Med.* 1999;159(7):748-754.

GISSI-Prevenzione Investigators. Dietary supplementation with n-3 polyunsaturated fatty acids and vitamin E after myocardial infarction: results of the GISSI-Prevenzioni trial. *Lancet.* 1999;354:447-455.

Gogu SR, Lertora JJL, George WJ, et al. Protection of zidovudine-induced toxicity against murine erythroid progenitor cells by vitamin E. *Exp Hematol.* 1999;19:649-652.

Greenberg ER. Vitamin E supplements: good in theory, but is the theory good? *Ann Intern Med.* 2005;142(1):75-76.

Greenberg ER, Baron JA, Tosteson TD, et al. A clinical trial of antioxidant vitamins to prevent colorectal adenoma. Polyp Prevention Study Group. *N Engl J Med.* 1994;331(3):141-147.

Grundman M. Vitamin E and Alzheimer's disease: the basis for additional clinical trials. *Am J Clin Nutr.* 2000;71:630S-636S.

Guallar E, Hanley DF, Miller ER 3rd. An editorial update: Annus horribilis for vitamin E. *Ann Intern Med.* 2005;143(2):143-145.

Hacquebard M, Vandenbranden M, Malaisse WJ, et al. Vitamin e transfer from lipid emulsions to plasma lipoproteins: mediation by multiple mechanisms. *Lipids.* 2008;43(7):663-671.

Hamblin M, Smith HM, Hill MF. Dietary supplementation with vitamin E ameliorates cardiac failure in type I diabetic cardiomyopathy by suppressing myocardial generation of 8-iso-prostaglandin F2alpha and oxidized glutathione. *J Card Fail.* 2007;13(10):884-892.

Hamdy NM, Suwailem SM, El-Mesallamy HO. Influence of vitamin E supplementation on endothelial complications in type 2 diabetes mellitus patients who underwent coronary artery bypass graft. *J Diabetes Complications.* Epub: 2008 Jan 3.

Heart Protection Study Collaborative Group. MRC/BHF Heart Protection Study of antioxidant vitamin supplementation in 20,536 high-risk individuals: a randomised placebo-controlled trial. *Lancet.* 2002;360(9326):23-33.

Heinonen OP, Albanes D, Virtamo J, et al. Prostate cancer and supplementation with alpha-tocopherol and beta-carotene: incidence and mortality in a controlled trial. *J Natl Cancer Inst.* 1998;90:440-446.

Hendler SS, Sanchez R. Tocopherol-based antiviral agents and method of using same. United States Patent Number 5, 114, 957. 1992.

Huebbe P, Schaffer S, Jofre-Monseny L, et al. Apolipoprotein E genotype and alpha-tocopherol modulate amyloid precursor protein metabolism and cell cycle regulation. *Mol Nutr Food Res.* 2007;51(12):1510-1517.

Huey K, Fiscus G, Richwine AF, et al. In vivo vitamin E administration attenuates IL-6 and IL-1β responses to an acute inflammatory insult in mouse skeletal and cardiac muscle. *Exp Physiol.* Epub: 2008 Jun 27.

Institute of Medicine, Food and Nutrition Board. *Dietary Reference Intakes for vitamin C, vitamin E, Selenium, and Carotenoids.* Washington, DC: National Academy Press, 2000.

Isaac MG, Quinn R, Tabet N. Vitamin E for Alzheimer's disease and mild cognitive impairment. *Cochrane Database Syst Rev.* 2008;(3):CD002854.

Jacobs EJ, Thun MJ. Low-dose aspirin and vitamin E: challenges and opportunities in cancer prevention. *JAMA.* 2005;294(1):105-106.

Jatoi A, Kahanic SP, Frytak S, et al. Donepezil and vitamin E for preventing cognitive dysfunction in small cell lung cancer patients: preliminary results and suggestions for future study designs. *Support Care Cancer.* 2005;13(1):66-69.

Jia L, Yu W, Wang P, et al. In vivo and in vitro studies of anticancer actions of alpha-TEA for human prostate cancer cells. *Prostate.* 2008;68(8):849-860.

Kawanaka M, Mahmood S, Niiyama G, et al. Control of oxidative stress and reduction in biochemical markers by Vitamin E treatment in patients with nonalcoholic steatohepatitis: a pilot study. *Hepatol Res.* 2004;29(1):39-41.

Kayden HJ, Traber M. Absorption, lipoprotein transport and regulation of plasma concentrations of vitamin E in humans. J Lipid Res. 1993;34:343-358.

Knekt P, Reunanen A, Marniemi J, et al. Low vitamin E status is a potential risk factor for insulin-dependent diabetes mellitus. *J Intern Med.* 1999;245:99-102.

Kottschade L, Loprinzi C, Rao R. Vitamin e for the prevention of chemotherapy-induced peripheral neuropathy: rationale for an ongoing clinical trial. *Support Cancer Ther.* 2007;4(4):251-253.

Lee I-K, Koya D, Ishi H, et al. Alpha-tocopherol prevents the hyperglycemia induced activation of diacylglycerol (DAG)-protein kinase C (PKC) pathway in vascular smooth muscle cell by an increase of DAG kinase activity. *Diabetes Res Clin Pract.* 1999;45:189-190.

Lee IM, Cook NR, Gaziano JM, et al. Vitamin E in the primary prevention of cardiovascular disease and cancer: the Women's Health Study: a randomized controlled trial. *JAMA.* 2005;294(1):56-65.

Lee IM, Gaziano JM, Buring JE. Vitamin E in the prevention of prostate cancer: where are we today? *J Natl Cancer Inst.* 2006;98(4):225-227.

Levy AP, Blum S. Pharmacogenomics in prevention of diabetic cardiovascular disease: utilization of the haptoglobin genotype in determining benefit from vitamin E. *Expert Rev Cardiovasc Ther.* 2007;5(6):1105-1111.

Li JY, Taylor PR, Li B, et al. Nutrition intervention trials in Linxian, China: multiple vitamin/mineral supplementation, cancer incidence, and disease-specific mortality among adults with esophageal dysplasia. *J Natl Cancer Inst.* 1993;85(18):1492-1498.

Lonn E, Bosch J, Yusuf S, et al. HOPE and HOPE-TOO Trial Investigators. Effects of long-term vitamin E supplementation on cardiovascular events and cancer: a randomized controlled trial. *JAMA.* 2005;293(11):1338-1347.

Lonn E, Yusuf S, Hoogwerf B, Pogue J, et al. HOPE Study; MICRO-HOPE Study. Effects of vitamin E on cardiovascular and microvascular outcomes in high-risk patients with diabetes: results of the HOPE study and MICRO-HOPE substudy. *Diabetes Care.* 2002;25(11):1919-1927.

McNeil JJ, Robman L, Tikellis G, et al. Vitamin E supplementation and cataract: randomized controlled trial. *Ophthalmology.* 2004;111(1):75-84.

Meydani SN, Leka LS, Fine BC, et al. Vitamin E and respiratory tract infections in elderly nursing home residents: a randomized controlled trial. *JAMA.* 2004;292(7):828-836.

Meydani SN, Meydani M, Blumberg JB, et al. Vitamin E supplementation and in vivo immune response in healthy elderly subjects. *JAMA.* 1997;277:1380-1386.

Miller ER 3rd, Pastor-Barriuso R, Dalal D, et al. Meta-analysis: high-dosage vitamin E supplementation may increase all-cause mortality.*Ann Intern Med.* 2005;142(1):37-44.

Milman U, Blum S, Shapira C, et al. Vitamin E supplementation reduces cardiovascular events in a subgroup of middle-aged individuals with both type 2 diabetes mellitus and the haptoglobin 2-2 genotype: a prospective double-blinded clinical trial. *Arterioscler Thromb Vasc Biol.* 2008;28(2):341-347.

Minamiyama Y, Takemura S, Bito Y, et al. Supplementation of alpha-tocopherol improves cardiovascular risk factors via the insulin signalling pathway and reduction of mitochondrial reactive oxygen species in type II diabetic rats. *Free Radic Res.* 2008;42(3):261-271.

Mortality in DATATOP: a multicenter trial in early Parkinson's disease. Parkinson Study Group. *Ann Neurol.* 1998;43(3):318-325.

Munteanu A, Zingg JM. Cellular, molecular and clinical aspects of vitamin E on atherosclerosis prevention. *Mol Aspects Med.* 2007;28(5-6):538-590.

Narushima K, Takada T, Yamanashi Y, et al. Niemann-pick C1-like 1 mediates alpha-tocopherol transport. *Mol Pharmacol.* 2008;74(1):42-49.

Paolisso G, Gambardella A, Giugliano D, et al. Chronic intake of pharmacological doses of vitamin E might be useful in the therapy of elderly patients with coronary heart disease. *Am J Clin Nutr.* 1995;61:848-852.

Peralta EA, Brewer AT, Louis S, et al. Vitamin E Increases Biomarkers of Estrogen Stimulation When Taken With Tamoxifen. *J Surg Res.* Epub: 2008 Apr 22.

Petersen RC, Thomas RG, Grundman M, et al; Alzheimer's Disease Cooperative Study Group. Vitamin E and donepezil for the treatment of mild cognitive impairment. *N Engl J Med.* 2005;352(23):2379-2388.

Pryor WA. Vitamin E and heart disease: basic science to clinical intervention trials. Free *Rad Biol Med.* 2000;28:141-164.

Rapola JM, Virtamo J, Ripatti S, et al. Effects of alpha-tocopherol and beta-carotene supplements on symptoms, progression, and prognosis of angina pectoris. *Heart.* 1998;79:454-458.

Reagan-Shaw S, Nihal M, Ahsan H, et al. Combination of vitamin E and selenium causes an induction of apoptosis of human prostate cancer cells by enhancing Bax/Bcl-2 ratio. *Prostate.* 2008;68(15):1624-1634.

Redberg RF. Vitamin E and cardiovascular health: does sex matter? *JAMA.* 2005;294(1):107-109.

Rimm EB, Stampfer MJ, Ascherio A, et al. Vitamin E consumption and the risk of coronary heart disease in men. *N Engl J Med.* 1993;328:1450-1456.

Rode S, Rubic T, Lorenz RL. alpha-Tocopherol disturbs macrophage LXRalpha regulation of ABCA1/G1 and cholesterol handling. *Biochem Biophys Res Commun.* 2008;369(3):868-872.

Sano M, Ernesto C, Thomas RG, et al. A controlled trial of selegiline, alpha-tocopherol, or both as treatment for Alzheimer's disease. *N Engl J Med.* 1997; 336:1216-1222.

Schwenke DC. Nutrition and metabolism: alpha-tocopherol to prevent cardiovascular disease–deficiency, dose, delivery, and developing context. *Curr Opin Lipidol.* 2008;19(2):203-207.

Selman C, McLaren JS, Mayer C, et al. Lifelong alpha-tocopherol supplementation increases the median life span of C57BL/6 mice in the cold but has only minor effects on oxidative damage. *Rejuvenation Res.* 2008;11(1):83-96.

Shim M, Eling TE. Vitamin E succinate induces NAG-1 expression in a p38 kinase-dependent mechanism. *Mol Cancer Ther.* 2008;7(4):961-971.

Shirpoor A, Salami S, Khadem-Ansari MH, et al. Cardioprotective effect of vitamin E: rescues of diabetes-induced cardiac malfunction, oxidative stress, and apoptosis in rat. *J Diabetes Complications.* Epub: 2008 Apr 2.

Shoulson I. DATATOP: a decade of neuroprotective inquiry. Parkinson Study Group. Deprenyl and tocopherol antioxidative therapy of Parkinsonism. *Ann Neurol.* 1998; 44(3 Suppl 1): S160-S166.

Singh M, Kaur P, Sandhir R, et al. Protective effects of vitamin E against atrazine-induced genotoxicity in rats. *Mutat Res.* 2008;654(2):145-149.

Stahl W, Heinrich U, Jungmann H, et al. Carotenoids and carotenoids plus vitamin E protect against ultraviolet light-induced erythrema in humans. *Am J Clin Nutr.* 2000;71:795-798.

Stampfer MJ, Hennekens CH, Manson JE, et al. Vitamin E consumption and the risk of coronary disease in women. *N Engl J Med.* 1993;328:1444-1449.

Steinberg D, Parthsarathy S, Carew TE, et al. Beyond cholesterol: modifications of low-density lipoprotein that increases its atherogenicity. *N Engl J Med.* 1989;320:915-924.

Steiner M. Vitamin E, a modifier of platelet function: rationale and use in cardiovascular disease. *Nutr Rev.* 1999;57:306-309.

Stephens NG, Parsons A, Schofield PM, et al. Randomized controlled trial of vitamin E in patients with coronary disease: Cambridge Heart Antioxidant Study (CHAOS). *Lancet.* 1996;347:781-786.

Stone WL, Pappas AM. Tocopherols and the etiology of colon cancer. *J Natl Cancer Inst.* 1997;89:1006-1014.

Takanami Y, Iwane H, Kawai Y, Shimomitsu T. Vitamin E supplementation and endurance exercise: are there benefits? *Sports Med.* 2000;29:73-83.

The Alpha-Tocopherol Beta-Carotene Cancer Prevention Study Group. The effect of vitamin E and beta-carotene on the incidence of lung cancer and other cancers in male smokers. *N Engl J Med.* 1994; 330:1029-1035.

The effect of vitamin E and beta carotene on the incidence of lung cancer and other cancers in male smokers. The Alpha-Tocopherol, Beta Carotene Cancer Prevention Study Group. *N Engl J Med.* 1994;330(15):1029-1035.

The Heart Outcomes Prevention Evaluation Study Investigators. Vitamin E supplementation and cardiovascular events in high-risk patients. *N Engl J Med.* 2000;342:154-160.

Traber MG. How much vitamin E? . . . Just enough! *Am J Clin Nutr.* 2006;84(5):959-960.

Traber MG. Vitamin E. In: Shils ME, Olson JA, Shike M, Ross AC, eds. *Modern Nutrition in Health and Disease.* 9th ed. Baltimore, MD: Williams and Wilkins; 1999:347-362.

Traber MG, Arai H. Molecular mechanisms of vitamin E transport. *Annu Rev Nutr.* 1999;19:343-355.

Traber MG, Frei B, Beckman JS. Vitamin E revisited: do new data validate benefits for chronic disease prevention? *Curr Opin Lipidol.* 2008;19(1):30-38.

Trevithick JR, Xiong H, Lee S, et al. Topical tocopheryl acetate reduces post-UVB, sunburn-associated erythema, edema, and skin sensitivity in hairless mice. *Arch Biochem Biophys.* 1992;296:575-582.

Vatassery GT, Bauer T, Dysken M. High doses of vitamin E in the treatment of the central nervous system in the aged. *Amer J Clin Nutr.* 1999;70:793-801.

Vejux A, Guyot S, Montange T, et al. Phospholipidosis and down-regulation of the PI3-K/PDK-1/Akt signalling pathway are vitamin E inhibitable events associated with 7-ketocholesterol-induced apoptosis. *J Nutr Biochem.* Epub: 2008 May 19.

Violi F, Cangemi R. Statin treatment as a confounding factor in human trials with vitamin E. *J Nutr.* 2008;138(6):1179-1181.

Virtamo J, Pietinen P, Huttunen JK, et al; ATBC Study Group. Incidence of cancer and mortality following alpha-tocopherol and beta-carotene supplementation: a postintervention follow-up. *JAMA.* 2003;290(4):476-485.

Wadleigh RG, Redman RS, Graham ML, et al. Vitamin E in the treatment of chemotherapy-induced mucositis. *Ann J Med.* 1992;92:481-484.

Waters DD, Alderman EL, Hsia J, et al. Effects of hormone replacement therapy and antioxidant vitamin supplements on coronary atherosclerosis in postmenopausal women: a randomized controlled trial. *JAMA.* 2002;288(19):2432-2440.

Woodson K, Tangrea JA, Barrett MJ, et al. Serum alpha-tocopherol and subsequent risk of lung cancer among male smokers. *J Natl Cancer Inst.* 1999;91;1738-1743.

Wright ME, Lawson KA, Weinstein SJ, et al. Higher baseline serum concentrations of vitamin E are associated with lower total and cause-specific mortality in the Alpha-Tocopherol, Beta-Carotene CancerPrevention Study. *Am J Clin Nutr.* 2006;84(5):1200-1207.

Wu D, Meydani M, Beharka AA, et al. In vitro supplementation with different tocopherol homologues can affect the function of immune cells in old mice. *Free Rad Biol Med.* 2000;28:643-651.

Wu D, Meydani SN. Age-associated changes in immune and inflammatory responses: impact of vitamin E intervention. *J Leukoc Biol.* 2008;84(4):900-914.

Wu XX, Kakehi Y, Jin XH, et al. Induction of Apoptosis in Human Renal Cell Carcinoma Cells by Vitamin E Succinate in Caspase-independent Manner. *Urology.* Epub: 2008 Aug 8.

Yamaoka S, Kim HS, Ogihara T, et al. Severe Vitamin E deficiency exacerbates acute hyperoxic lung injury associated with increased oxidative stress and inflammation. *Free Radic Res.* 2008;42(6):602-612.

Yokota T, Uchihara T, Shiojiri T, et al. Postmortem study of ataxia with retinitis pigmentosa by mutation of the alpha-tocopherol transfer protein gene. *J Neurol Neurosurg Psychiatry.* 2000;68:521-525.

You WC, Chang YS, Heinrich J, et al. An intervention trial to inhibit the progression of precancerous gastric lesions: compliance, serum micronutrients and S-allyl cysteine levels, and toxicity. *Eur J Cancer Prev.* 2001;10(3):257-263.

Yu W, Jia L, Wang P, Lawson KA, et al. In vitro and in vivo evaluation of anticancer actions of natural and synthetic vitamin E forms. *Mol Nutr Food Res.* 2008;52(4):447-456.

Yusuf S, Dagenais G, Pogue J, et al. Vitamin E supplementation and cardiovascular events in high-risk patients. The Heart Outcomes Prevention Evaluation Study Investigators. *N Engl J Med.* 2000;342(3):154-160.

Zureik M, Galan P, Bertrais S, et al. Effects of long-term daily low-dose supplementation with antioxidant vitamins and minerals on structure and function of large arteries. *Arterioscler Thromb Vasc Biol.* 2004;24(8):1485-1491.

Vitamin E Phosphate

DESCRIPTION

Vitamin E phosphate is the phosphate ester of d-alpha-tocopherol. It was one of the first vitamin E derivatives studied, in the 1940s, but it garnered little attention until recently, when it entered the dietary supplement marketplace as one of the available forms of vitamin E (See Vitamin E).

Vitamin E phosphate is chemically described as [(2R)-2,5,7,8-tetramethyl-2-[(4R,8R)-4,8,12-trimethyltridecyl]chroman-6-yl] dihydrogen phosphate. It is also known as RRR-alpha-tocopheryl phosphate, alpha-tocopherol phosphate, alpha-tocopheryl phosphate, alpha-tocopherylphosphate, tocopherol phosphate, tocopheryl phosphate, all-rac-tocopherol phosphate and alpha-tocopherol-6-O-phosphate. Its molecular weight is 510.69, its molecular formula is $C_{29}H_{51}O_5P$ and its CAS registry number is 38976-17-9. Vitamin E Phosphate is represented by the following chemical structure.

Tocopherol phosphate

In 1942, it was reported that administration of vitamin E phosphate, but not alpha-tocopherol, to dystrophic rabbits, restored to normal the excessive *in vitro* oxygen consumption and excessive metabolic rate of muscle tissue of the rabbits. This was the first experimental evidence that vitamin E played a role in cellular respiration. It appeared that vitamin E was required to be in the phosphorylated form for this effect to occur. This would make it similar to other vitamins that enter into biological oxidation, and it was speculated that the mechanism of the vitamin E phosphate action might be one that involved its dephosphorylation. That vitamin E phosphate had an effect on vitamin E-deficient muscle slices, *in vitro*, which alpha-tocopherol did not, raised the question whether vitamin E was naturally present in tissues as its phosphate ester. However, when others tried to repeat these studies with vitamin E phosphate, they found that the addition of vitamin E *in vitro* had no significant effect on the respiration of muscle strips or slices, either from normal or dystrophic animals. By the end of the 1940s, vitamin E phosphate went out of favor as a form of vitamin E to explore.

Recently, there have been reports that vitamin E phosphate exists naturally in the tissues of plants and animals, including humans. Small amounts of vitamin E phosphate have been reported in wheat germ, chocolate and cheeses such as cheddar and brie. The reason given for not having detected vitamin E phosphate in plant and animal tissue previously is that vitamin E phosphate is a water-soluble substance that is resistant to both acid and alkaline hydrolysis and that the standard analytical methods for detection and assay of alpha-tocopherol would not have detected vitamin E phosphate. Using techniques such as electrospray mass spectrometry (ESMS), high-performance liquid chromatography (HPLC), liquid chromatography mass spectrometry (LCMS), liquid chromatography tandem mass spectrometry (LCMS/MS and gas chromatography mass spectrometry (GCMS) appeared to be necessary in order to identify vitamin E phosphate as a natural form of vitamin E. These techniques were not available to those researchers of the 1940s who believed that vitamin E phosphate was a natural form of vitamin E.

One of the big mysteries in nutritional biochemistry is what the unique biological role of vitamin E is. To date, that mystery has not been solved. There are some who believe that vitamin E phosphate may help to do so.

ACTIONS AND PHARMACOLOGY

ACTIONS

Vitamin E phosphate has possible antioxidant activity. It may also have possible apoptotic, antiatherogenic, cardioprotective and UVB-protective activities. Vitamin E phosphate may also have activity as a transdermal delivery form for insulin and other biological molecules.

MECHANISM OF ACTION

Antiatherogenic activity: Both vitamin E acetate and vitamin E phosphate, but more so vitamin E phosphate, were reported to have atherosclerotic-preventing effects in rabbits fed with a high-cholesterol diet. Vitamin E phosphate was also found to be more potent than vitamin E acetate in downregulating the expression of CD36. CD36 is an integral membrane protein found on the surface of many cell types. It is a member of the class B scavenger receptor family of cell surface proteins. CD36 is thought to be involved in atherosclerosis, among other disorders.

The mechanism of the possible antiatherogenic effect of vitamin E phosphate is not clear.

Antioxidant activity: Vitamin E is the principal antioxidant of the lipid domains of the body, such as cellular membranes. It is a chain-breaking antioxidant that prevents the propagation of free radical activities. It is a peroxyl radical scavenger and especially protects the polyunsaturated fatty acids (PUFAs) within membrane phospholipids and in plasma lipoproteins against oxidation. This antioxidant activity depends on the free hydroxyl group of the chromanol ring, which reacts with an organic peroxyl radical to form the corresponding organic hydroperoxide and the tocopheroxyl radical. The tocopheroxyl radical is the pro-oxidant form of vitamin E and is thought to be regenerated to the antioxidant form by a network of other antioxidants, including vitamin C and glutathione.

When the phenolic hydroxyl group is in its esterified form—for example, vitamin E acetate or vitamin E succinate—it no longer can inhibit lipid peroxidation until it is converted back to its unesterified form. One therefore would expect that vitamin E phosphate would also be unable to inhibit lipid peroxidation unless converted to its unesterified form. It has now been reported that, unlike vitamin E acetate and vitamin E succinate, vitamin E phosphate per se inhibits lipid peroxidation. The mechanism of action of this effect is not completely understood, but it is thought that vitamin E phosphate acts as a detergent and forms a barrier that might inhibit the transfer of radicals from one polyunsaturated fatty acid to another. In other words, the detergent barrier acts as a chain terminator of the lipid peroxidation chain reaction. This would be a highly unusual antioxidant mechanism, and more study is needed to determine if this is indeed the antioxidant mechanism of action of vitamin E phosphate.

Incidentally, vitamin E succinate is also known to have detergent-like activity, but in contrast to vitamin E phosphate, vitamin E succinate does not appear to possess an antioxidant effect per se.

Apoptotic activity: Vitamin E phosphate was found to inhibit proliferation and induce apoptosis (programmed cell death) in an MG-63 osteosarcoma cell line and in a THP-1 monocytic leukemia cell line, both in tissue culture. The apoptotic effect was more potent than that obtained with vitamin E succinate and was explained by membrane destabilizing activity due to its action as a detergent. Vitamin E phosphate was found to be more potent than vitamin E succinate in inducing DNA fragmentation and nucleus condensation, two events in the apoptosis process.

The mechanism by which vitamin E phosphate induces apoptosis is not fully understood. It is thought that the apoptotic activity is due, in part, to a detergent-like effect of vitamin E phosphate causing membrane destabilization of the malignant cells.

Cardioprotective activity: In a laboratory study, one group of rats was gavaged with vitamin E phosphate for a period of 30 days while a control group of rats were given water only. After 30 days, the rats were sacrificed and their hearts were excised. Both the treated and control groups were subjected to 30 minutes of global ischemia, followed by two hours of reperfusion.

Myocardial reperfusion injury refers to the damage to myocardial tissue caused when blood returns to the tissue after a period of ischemia.

The vitamin E phosphate-fed rats exhibited significant cardioprotection as evidenced by improved ventricular performance and reduced myocardial infarct size and apoptosis of the cardiomyocytes. Supplementation of vitamin E phosphate appeared to convert the mitogen activated protein (MAP) kinase-induced death signal into a survival signal via enhancing anti-apoptotic p42/44 extracellular signal-regulat-

ed (ERK) kinase and p38 MAPKbeta and reducing pro-apoptotic proteins p38 MAPKalpha and c-JUN N-terminal kinases (JNK). In concert, the phosphorylation of pro-apoptotic cellular sarcoma-inducing gene (c-Src) was also reduced. Vitamin E phosphate increased the DNA binding of the redox-sensitive transcription factor, nuclear factor (NF)-kappaB, and potentiated the activation of anti-death protein Bcl-2 and survival signaling protein Akt (protein kinase B). In summation, vitamin E phosphate appeared to ameliorate myocardial ischemia reperfusion injury by converting the ischemia/reperfusion-mediated death signal into a survival signal via modulating MAP kinase signaling.

Thus, signaling may be the most important feature of vitamin E phosphate. Vitamin E phosphate clearly does not qualify as a storage form of vitamin E, since the amounts found in tissue are so small. Signaling molecules are present in small amounts in tissue. Perhaps this is what the investigators of the 1940s (see Description above) were looking at, but the concepts to explain what they were looking at were not yet invented.

Continued study of this area is needed and warranted. Looking for kinases and phosphatases, major components of signaling systems, should be high priority. And, the next time this type of experiment is performed with vitamin E phosphate, vitamin E succinate, vitamin E acetate and alpha-tocopherol should be used as additional controls.

Protection against ultraviolet B-induced damage to skin: Cultured mouse skin that is exposed to ultraviolet B (UVB) rays undergoes photodamage manifested as sunburn cell formation, DNA degradation and lipid peroxidation. Alpha-tocopherol-6-O-phosphate was found to significantly protect against UVB photodamage when the mouse skin was pretreated with a solution of the vitamin. The protection was found to be greater than that seen with alpha-tocopherol acetate, a common form of vitamin E used in commercial skin care products.

UVB damage to skin is mediated mainly via oxidative stress. The effect of alpha-tocopherol-6-O-phosphate is probably via its antioxidant activity. It was found, however, that the difference in UVB protection of vitamin E phosphate when compared with vitamin E acetate may be explained by the greater conversion of vitamin E phosphate to alpha-tocopherol. In that case, vitamin E phosphate serves as a better delivery form of alpha-tocopherol to the skin than vitamin E succinate, and the protective effect has to do with the antioxidant activity of alpha-tocopherol, not vitamin E phosphate per se.

Transdermal delivery form for insulin: It has been reported that vitamin E phosphate can penetrate the skin nine times more than alpha-tocopherol. Vitamin E phosphate is presently being studied in a transdermal delivery form system for insulin. In this regard, vitamin E phosphate can be considered to be a penetration enhancer. Again, this may be due, at least in part, to its detergent-like activity.

PHARMACOKINETICS

There is very little known on the pharmacokinetics of vitamin E phosphate.

Esterified forms of vitamin E—vitamin E acetate and vitamin E succinate—undergo hydrolysis via esterases secreted by the pancreas. The alpha-tocopherol produced via esterase action is emulsified together with dietary lipids. Bile acids and salts secreted by the liver aid in the emulsification process. Lipolysis and emulsification of the formed lipid droplets lead to the spontaneous formation of mixed micelles. The micelles containing vitamin E are absorbed at the brush border of the intestinal mucosa in the enterocytes. Vitamin E is secreted by the enterocytes into the lymphatics in the form of chylomicrons. (See Vitamin E for a more complete discussion of the pharmacokinetics of vitamin E).

There are animal studies suggesting that vitamin E phosphate, or at least a fraction of it that enters the small intestine, is not hydrolyzed by esterases or phosphatases, but is absorbed intact and reaches the circulatory system, which carries it to various organs. A recent *in vitro* study found that vitamin E phosphate is transported across cell membranes via an organic anion transporter (OAT) mechanism.

Much more study is needed on the absorption, distribution, metabolism and excretion of vitamin E phosphate.

INDICATIONS AND USAGE

Though efforts have been made recently to market vitamin E phosphate as the most important biological form of vitamin E and/or as something "new," there is little support for these marketing claims. Research on vitamin E phosphate dates back to at least the 1940s. There is some very preliminary nonclinical evidence that vitamin E phosphate may have some anticancer and cardioprotective effects, related in part to reported antioxidant, apoptotic and signaling activities. Some very dated research has suggested a possible favorable effect on muscle metabolism. In nonsupplement form, vitamin E might be a useful sun blocker and, possibly, a vehicle for transdermal insulin delivery, according to more preliminary research.

RESEARCH SUMMARY

In a study of rat liver microsomes, vitamin E phosphate was said to be a more effective inhibitor of lipid peroxidation than some other vitamin E-related compounds. It was also said to be superior to those other compounds in its ability to conserve its oxidative potential. And reportedly acting as a detergent capable of forming a barrier that might be able to inhibit the transfer of radicals from one fatty acid to another, vitamin E phosphate was said by this group of researchers to possibly constitute a new antioxidant class. The validity and significance of these findings needs further clarification and research.

There is some *in vitro* evidence that vitamin E phosphate may have some ability to favorably modulate signaling cascades and gene expression in macrophages and smooth muscle cells, inhibiting some important atherogenic events in the process. In a study of rabbits fed a high cholesterol diet, vitamin E phosphate was more effective than vitamin E acetate in inhibiting atherosclerotic progression, as measured by aortic plaque formation. In a study of rats fed 5mg/kg body weight of vitamin E phosphate daily for 30 days, significant cardioprotection was demonstrated (compared with controls that received no supplement). After sacrifice, hearts were removed and subjected to an ischemia/reperfusion challenge. Protection was demonstrated in terms of improved ventricular performance, reduced myocardial infarct size and cardiomyocyte apoptosis. Further research is warranted.

One study demonstrated that vitamin E phosphate has apoptotic effects in an osteosarcoma cell line. This effect was attributed to the substance's detergent-like activity. Again, more research is indicated.

Two papers from the same laboratory in the 1940s reported some favorable vitamin E phosphate *in vitro* effects on muscle metabolism. Reported results are so preliminary and equivocal that no useful conclusion can be drawn concerning a role for this substance in muscle health. Similarly, far more research will be needed to confirm suggestions that vitamin E phosphate might be an effective sun blocker and that it might be a useful vehicle for transdermal delivery of insulin.

CONTRAINDICATIONS, PRECAUTIONS, ADVERSE REACTIONS

CONTRAINDICATIONS

Vitamin E phosphate is contraindicated in those with known hypersensitivity to any component of a vitamin E phosphate-containing product.

PRECAUTIONS

Vitamin E phosphate possesses anticoagulant and antithrombotic activities. Those taking warfarin should avoid vitamin E phosphate. Likewise, individuals with vitamin K deficiencies, such as those with liver failure, should avoid vitamin E phosphate. Vitamin E phosphate should be avoided by those with lesions that have a propensity to bleed (eg, bleeding peptic ulcers), a history of hemorrhagic stroke or inherited bleeding disorders (eg, hemophilia). Vitamin E phosphate should be avoided by pregnant women and nursing mothers.

Vitamin E phosphate supplementation should be stopped about two to four weeks before surgical procedures, including dental procedures, and may be resumed following recovery from the procedure.

ADVERSE REACTIONS
None known.

INTERACTIONS
DRUGS
Antiplatelet drugs (eg, aspirin, dipyridamole, clopidogrel, ticlopidine, tirofiban, abciximab and eptifibatide): Vitamin E phosphate may potentiate the effects of these antiplatelet drugs.

Anticoagulants (eg, warfarin and heparin): Vitamin E phosphate may potentiate the effects of these anticoagulant drugs.

NUTRITIONAL SUPPLEMENTS
Fish oils possess antiplatelet activity. Vitamin E phosphate may potentiate the antiplatelet activity of fish oils.

HERBS
Some herbal products, including garlic, ginkgo, ginseng and curcuminoids, possess antithrombotic activity. Vitamin E phosphate used at the same time as these herbs may enhance their antithrombotic activity.

OVERDOSAGE
There are no reports of overdosage with vitamin E phosphate.

DOSAGE AND ADMINISTRATION
Vitamin E phosphate is available in 400 IU capsules. Doses higher than 400 IU daily are not recommended.

LITERATURE
Devlin HB, Mattill, HA. The chemical determination of tocopherols in muscle tissue. *J Biol Chem* 1942;146:123-130.

Eppstein SH, Morgulis S. Factors Influencing the Onset and Cure of Nutritional Muscular Dystrophy. *J Nut* 1942;23:473-482.

Gianello R, Hall WC, Kennepohl E, et al. Subchronic oral toxicity study of mixed tocopheryl phosphates in rats. *Int J Toxicol.* September-October 2007;26(5):475-490.

Gianello R, Libinaki R, Azzi A, et al. Alpha-tocopheryl phosphate: a novel, natural form of vitamin E. *Free Radic Biol Med.* October 2005;39(7):970-976.

Houchin OB. The In Vitro Effect of alpha-Tocopherol and its Phosphate Derivative on Oxidation in Muscle Tissue. *J. Biol Chem* 1942;146:313-321.

Houchin OB, Mattill HA. The influence of parenteral administration of alpha-tocopheryl phosphate on the metabolic processes in dystrophic muscles. *J Biol Chem.* 1942;146:309-312.

Hummel JP, Basinski DH. The In Vitro Effect of Tocopherol Phosphate on the Respiration of Muscle from Normal and Dystrophic Rabbits. *J Biol Chem.* 1948;172:417-420.

Karrer P. Bussmann G. d, l-alpha-tocopherol-phosphorsäure-ester. *Helv Chim Acta.* 1940;23:1137-1138.

Libinaki R, Ogru E, Gianello R, et al. Evaluation of the safety of mixed tocopheryl phosphates (MTP) – a formulation of alpha-tocopheryl phosphate plus alpha-di-tocopheryl phosphate. *Food Chem Toxicol.* July 2006;44(7):916-932.

Lowenthal J, Fisher LM. The inhibition of blood clotting by phosphate esters of vitamins K and E. *Can J Biochem Physiol* 1959;37:501-505.

Mukherjee S, Vaishnava S, Hooper LV. Multi-layered regulation of intestinal antimicrobial defense. *Cell Mol Life Sci.* 2008;65(19):3019-3027.

Munteanu A, Zingg JM, Ogru E, et al. Modulation of cell proliferation and gene expression by alpha-tocopheryl phosphates: relevance to atherosclerosis and inflammation. *Biochem Biophys Res Commun.* 2004;318(1):311-316.

Negis Y, Aytan N, Ozer N, et al. The effect of tocopheryl phosphates on atherosclerosis progression in rabbits fed with a high cholesterol diet. *Arch Biochem Biophys.* 2006;450(1):63-66.

Negis Y, Meydani M, Zingg JM, et al. Molecular mechanism of alpha-tocopheryl-phosphate transport across the cell membrane. *Biochem Biophys Res Commun.* 2007;359(2):348-353.

Negis Y, Zingg JM, Ogru E, et al. On the existence of cellular tocopheryl phosphate, its synthesis, degradation and cellular roles: a hypothesis. *IUBMB Life.* 2005;57(1):23-25.

Ogru E, Libinaki R, Gianello R, et al. Modulation of cell proliferation and gene expression by alpha-tocopheryl phosphates: relevance to atherosclerosis and inflammation. *Ann N Y Acad Sci.* 2004;1031:405-411.

Rezk BM, Haenen GR, Van Der Vijgh WJ, et al. The extraordinary antioxidant activity of vitamin E phosphate. *Biochim Biophys Acta.* 2004;1683(1-3):16-21.

Rezk BM, van der Vijgh WJ, Bast A, et al. Alpha-tocopheryl phosphate is a novel apoptotic agent. *Front Biosci.* 2007;12:2013-2019.

West SM, Kanner D. Transdermal transport of compounds. U.S. Patent Application 20050089495, April 28, 2005.

Williams MJ, Clapp MP. Action of alpha-tocopherol phosphate on hemolysis in paroxysmal nocturnal hemoglobinuria. *Blood.* 1953;8(4):336-341.

Ziierler KL, Andres R, Levy RI, Anderson HM, et al. On the mechanism of action of alpha-tocopheryl phosphate, with special reference to carbohydrate metabolism of striated muscle. II. Effect on the capacity of rat diaphragm to dissimilate hexose phosphates. *Bull Johns Hopkins Hosp.* 1953;92(1):32-39.

Ziierler KL, Folk BP, Lilienthal JL Jr. On the mechanism of action of alpha-tocopheryl phosphate, with special reference to carbohydrate metabolism of striated muscle. I. Modification of epinephrine effect, hyperlactacidemia, by alpha-tocopheryl phosphate in the rat. *Bull Johns Hopkins Hosp.* 1953;92(1):26-30.

Ziierler KL, Levy RI, Lilienthal JL Jr. On the mechanism of action of alpha-tocopheryl phosphate, with special reference to carbohydrate metabolism of striated muscle. III. Inhibition of insulin-induced glycogenesis in isolated rat diaphragm. *Bull Johns Hopkins Hosp.* 1953;92(1):41-46.

Vitamin K

DESCRIPTION

Vitamin K is a generic term for a group of substances which contain the 2-methyl-1, 4-naphthoquinone ring structure and which possess hemostatic activity. Substances with vitamin K activity were originally identified in green leafy vegetables, hemp seeds, liver and fish meal. These substances were found to have antihemorrhagic activity and their collective name was derived from koagulation, the German word for clotting. In addition to its essential role in hemostasis, vitamin K is involved in bone metabolism, among other processes.

Vitamin K_1 or phylloquinone is the principal dietary source of vitamin K and its predominant circulating form. Green leafy vegetables are rich in vitamin K_1 and contribute 40%-50% of total dietary intake of the vitamin. The next largest contributors to dietary vitamin K intake are the vegetable oils olive oil, canola oil, soybean oil and cottonseed oil. These vegetable oils also contain vitamin K_1. Vitamin K_1 is a fat-soluble substance. Vitamin K_2, which is also fat soluble, is the collective term for a number of substances known as menaquinones. Vitamin K_2 is found in chicken egg yolk, butter, cow liver, certain cheeses and fermented soybean products such as natto. This form of vitamin K is also produced by certain bacteria, including some of the bacteria that comprise the microflora of the intestine. The dietary contribution of vitamin K_2 is much less than that of vitamin K_1. The amount of vitamin K contributed to the body by the intestinal microflora remains unclear. Vitamin K_3 or menadione is a fat-soluble synthetic compound which is used in animal feed and dog and cat food. It is metabolized to vitamin K_2.

Vitamin K is involved as a cofactor in the posttranslational gamma-carboxylation of glutamic acid residues of certain proteins in the body. These proteins include the vitamin K-dependent coagulation factors II (prothrombin), VII (proconvertin), IX (Christmas factor), X (Stuart factor), protein C, protein S, protein Zv and a growth-arrest-specific factor (Gas6). In contrast to the other vitamin K-dependent proteins in the blood coagulation cascade, protein C and protein X serve anticoagulant roles. The two vitamin K-dependent proteins found in bone are osteocalcin, also known as bone G1a (gamma-carboxyglutamate) protein or BGP, and the matrix G1a protein or MGP. Gamma-carboxylation is catalyzed by the vitamin K-dependent gamma-carboxylases. The reduced form of vitamin K, vitamin K hydroquinone, is the actual cofactor for the gamma-carboxylases. Proteins containing gamma-carboxyglutamate are called G1a proteins.

Vitamin K deficiency can occur under certain conditions. These include, inadequate dietary intake, malabsorption syndromes (cystic fibrosis, Crohn's disease, ulcerative colitis, Whipple's disease, celiac sprue, short bowel syndrome) and loss of storage sites due to hepatocellular disease. Vitamin K deficiency frequently occurs in those with chronic liver disease, such as primary biliary cirrhosis. Coumarin anticoagulants, such as warfarin, induce a state analogous to vitamin K deficiency by inhibiting the reduction and recycling of vitamin K, and certain cephalosporin antibiotics (see Interactions) may also induce a vitamin K deficiency state by inhibiting the reduction and recycling of the vitamin. Recently, it has been found that space flight may impair vitamin K metabolism and also induce a state of vitamin K deficiency. Symptoms of vitamin K deficiency include easy bruisability, epistaxis, gastrointestinal bleeding, menorrhagia and hematuria. Chronic vitamin K deficiency may also result in osteoporosis and increased risk of fractures. There is some evidence that chronic warfarin use may also cause osteoporosis.

Vitamin K_1, in addition to being known as phylloquinone, is also known as phytonadione and 2-methyl-3-phytyl-1, 4-naphthoquinone. The lipophilic side chain is located at position 3 of the naphthoquinone ring. Its molecular formula is $C_{31}H_{46}O_2$ and its molecular weight is 450.71 daltons. The structural formula is:

Vitamin K_1

Vitamin K_2 is the collective term for a group of vitamin K compounds called menaquinones. The menaquinone homolgues are characterized by the number of isoprene residues comprising the side chain. The side chain is located at position 3 of the naphthoquinone ring. The group chemical name of the menaquinones is 2-methyl-3-all-*trans*-polyprenyl-1, 4-naphthoquinones. Menaquinones with side chains of up to 15 isoprene units have been described. Menaquinones of from two to 13 isoprene units have been found in human and animal tissues. Menaquinones are designated by the name menaquinone followed by a number. The number refers to the number of isoprene residues in the structure. Thus, menaquinone-4, abbreviated MK-4, possesses four isoprene residues in the side chain. Menaquinone-7 possesses seven isoprene units in the side chain. The menaquinones may also be designated by the number of carbons in the side chain. An isoprene residue contains five carbons. Thus, menaquinone-4 is also called vitamin K_2 (20) and menaquinone-7 is also called vitamin K_2 (35). Menaquinone-4 is also known as menatetrenone. The fermented soybean product natto is rich in menaquinone-7. Menaquinone-4 is the predominant form of vitamin K in the rat brain.

Vitamin K_3 or menadione is a synthetic naphthoquinone derivative. It is also known as 2-methyl-1, 4-naphthoquinone. Its molecular formula is $C_{11}H_8O_2$ and its molecular weight is 172.18 daltons. Vitamin K_3 does not possess a lipophilic side chain.

The nutritional supplement forms of vitamin K are vitamin K_1 and vitamin K_2.

ACTIONS AND PHARMACOLOGY
ACTIONS
Vitamin K has hemostatic activity and may have anti-osteoporotic, antioxidant and anticarcinogenic activities.

MECHANISM OF ACTION
The hemostatic activity of vitamin K is well known. Vitamin K is used to treat anticoagulant-induced prothrombin deficiency caused by warfarin, hypoprothrombinemia secondary to antibiotic therapy and hypoprothrombinemia secondary to vitamin C deficiency from various causes, including malabsorption syndromes. The pharmacological action of vitamin K in the treatment of hypoprothrombinemia is related to the normal physiological function of the vitamin. Vitamin K is an essential cofactor for the gamma-carboxylase enzymes which catalyze the posttranslational gamma-carboxylation of glutamic acid residues in inactive hepatic precursors of coagulation factors II, VII, IX and X. Gamma-carboxylation converts these inactive precursors into active coagulation factors which are secreted by hepatocytes into the blood. Supplement vitamin K has no hemostatic activity in those who are not vitamin K-deficient.

The mechanism of the possible anti-osteoporotic activity of vitamin K is not completely understood. Two vitamin K-dependent proteins are found in bone: osteocalcin or bone Gla protein (BGP) and the matrix Gla protein or MGP. Osteocalcin appears to be the most abundant non-collagenous protein in the bone. Most of the osteocalcin synthesized by the osteoblasts during bone matrix formation is incorporated into bone. This is due to the high specificity of the gamma-carboxyglutamyl residues for the calcium ions of hydroxyapatite. A small amount of osteocalcin is released into the circulation. Osteocalcin appears to act as a regulator of bone mineralization. High levels of circulating undercarboxylated (under-gamma-carboxylated) osteocalcin have been associated with low bone mineral density and increased risk of hip fractures. The serum level of undercarboxylated osteocalcin may be a more sensitive marker of vitamin K status than blood coagulation tests. High levels of undercarboxylated osteocalcin are frequently found in the context of normal blood coagulation tests.

In vivo and *in vitro* studies have shown that vitamin K may directly act on bone metabolism. *In vitro* studies have demonstrated that vitamin K_2 inhibits bone resorption by, in part, inhibiting the production of bone resorbing substances such as prostaglandin E_2 and interleukin-6. Vitamin K_2 has been reported to enhance human osteoblast-induced mineralization *in vitro* and to inhibit bone loss in steroid-treated rats and ovariecomized rats.

The reduced form of vitamin K, vitamin K-hydroquinone, is the active cofactor for the gamma-carboxylase enzymes. Vitamin K hydroquinone is produced in the vitamin K cycle. In the vitamin K cycle, vitamin K-hydroquinone is continuously regenerated. Vitamin K-hydroquinone is a potent reactive oxygen species scavenger. Vitamin K-hydroquinone has been found to inhibit lipid peroxidation.

Certain naphthoquinones, in particular the synthetic vitamin K menadione, have been found to have antitumor activity *in vitro* and *in vivo*. Vitamin K_2 has been found to induce the in vitro differentiation of myeloid leukemic cell lines. The mechanism of the possible anticarcinogenic activity of vitamin K is not well understood. Menadione is an oxidative stress inducer and its possible anticarcinogenic activity may, in part, be explained by induction of apoptotic cell death. One study suggested that the induction of apoptosis by menadione is mediated by the Fas/Fas ligand system. Another study reported that menadione induces cell cycle arrest and cell death by inhibiting Cda 25 phosphatase.

PHARMACOKINETICS
Vitamin K, mainly in the form of vitamin K_1, is principally absorbed from the jejunum and ileum. The efficiency of absorption is variable and ranges from 10% to 80%. Vitamin K is delivered to the enterocytes in micelles formed from bile salts and other substances. Vitamin K is secreted by enterocytes into the lymphatics in the form of chylomicrons. It enters the circulation via the thoracic duct and is carried in the circulation to various tissues including hepatic, bone and spleen, in the form of chylomicron remnants. In the liver, some vitamin K is stored, some is oxidized to inactive end products and some secreted with VLDL (very low-density

lipoprotein). Approximately 50% of vitamin K is carried in the plasma in the form of VLDL, about 25% in LDL (low-density lipoprotein) and about 25% in HDL (high-density lipoprotein). Vitamin K undergoes some oxidative metabolism. Excretion of vitamin K and its metabolites is mainly via the feces. Some urinary excretion of vitamin K also occurs.

INDICATIONS AND USAGE

Vitamin K is indicated in those with vitamin K deficiency, in some cases of hemorrhagic disease of the newborn, in some malabsorption syndromes and in some on long-term total parenteral nutrition. There is emerging evidence that adequate vitamin K intake may help protect against osteoporosis generally. There is the suggestion in early research that vitamin K may also have some anti-atherosclerotic effects. Claims that vitamin K is an anti-cancer agent derive from very preliminary work utilizing, primarily, vitamin K_3 or menadione. There is little or no reliable data yet available to support further claims that vitamin K inhibits platelet aggregation, that it has favorable effects on insulin and glucose, that it is helpful in Alzheimer's disease and that it favorably modulates immunity and has anti-inflammatory effects.

RESEARCH SUMMARY

Though primary vitamin K deficiency is uncommon, deficiencies secondary to disease or drug therapy arise more often. The most significant instance of acquired vitamin K deficiency manifests as hemorrhagic disease of the newborn (HDN). Causes of HDN are varied and include exclusive breast feeding (vitamin K is in short supply in breast milk) and liver dysfunction. Vitamin K prophylaxis, via oral and intramuscular administration at birth, has been widely used for decades with apparent efficacy. Intramuscular administration is considerably more effective but has been less used in recent years following publication of an epidemiological study suggesting an association between this treatment and a reported doubling of cancer risk in later life. Whether this association is genuinely causal has yet to be confirmed. No such association is seen with oral administration.

A number of drug therapies, including vitamin A and E in pharmacologic doses, some broad-spectrum antibiotics, the 4-hydroxycoumarins and salicylates, antagonize the action of vitamin K and, in some instances, result in deficiencies requiring additional vitamin K intake under a physician's supervision. TPN is frequently another indication for supplemental vitamin K, as are some malabsorption syndromes and gastrointestinal disorders. Those with parenchymal liver disease often have vitamin K deficiency. Recently vitamin K deficiency was found to be significant in many with cystic fibrosis.

Over the past decade, some very important vitamin K roles in bone metabolism have begun to be elucidated. Vitamin K has been demonstrated to promote the gamma-carboxylation of glutamyl residues on many bone proteins. This carboxylation is associated with increased bone mineral density, while undercarboxylation results in diminished bone mineral density and increased risk of bone fracture.

In a prospective analysis, the diets of 72,327 women 38-63 years of age were assessed and the incidence of hip fractures monitored over a ten-year period. A significant association was found between low dietary vitamin K intake and increased risk of hip fracture. This study looked at several specific dietary components and found a significant protective effect from lettuce, a source rich in vitamin K. Women who consumed lettuce (iceberg and romaine) one or more times daily had a significant 45% lower risk of hip fracture than did women who ate lettuce once a week or less.

In another study, gammacarboxyglutamate (Gla) proteins, the formation of which, as noted above, are promoted by vitamin K activity, were observed to play regulatory roles in calcification processes in both bone tissue and atherosclerotic vessel wall. This research suggested that reduced vitamin K status increases vessel wall calcification and reduces bone calcification and that increased vitamin K status might do the opposite.

A recent review of vitamin K research foresees the use of vitamin K in dietary supplements and in functional foods "for healthy individuals to prevent bone and vascular disease, as well as for patients on oral anticoagulant treatment to offer them protection against coumarin-induced side effects," which may include, among other things, accelerated bone loss. Long-term use of oral anticoagulants is a risk factor for developing osteoporosis and arterial calcification. A recent animal study demonstrated that high vitamin K intake is capable not only of preventing this calcification to some degree but also of inducing regression of pre-formed arterial calcifications. Trials are planned to further investigate this early finding. Another recent study associated high dietary vitamin K intake with reduced coronary calcification and concluded that adequate intake "could therefore be important to prevent cardiovascular disease." The vitamin K_2 menaquinone was the ester thus associated; the vitamin K_1 ester phylloquinone did not have this positive association.

In a recent prospective cohort study, vitamin K dietary intake was inversely and weakly associated with incidence of prostate cancer. The association noted was between menaquinones and not phylloquinones.

CONTRAINDICATIONS, PRECAUTIONS, ADVERSE REACTIONS

CONTRAINDICATIONS

Vitamin K is contraindicated in those hypersensitive to any component of a vitamin K-containing product.

PRECAUTIONS

Those taking warfarin should avoid supplementation with vitamin K unless specifically prescribed by their physicians.

Pregnant women and nursing mothers should avoid supplemental intakes of vitamin K greater than RDA amounts (65 micrograms daily) unless higher amounts are prescribed by their physicians.

Use of vitamin K for the treatment of vitamin K deficiency must be done under medical supervision.

ADVERSE REACTIONS

The supplemental forms of vitamin K, vitamin K_1 and vitamin K_2 are well tolerated. In one study, doses of 90 milligrams daily of vitamin K_2 were given for 24 weeks. Few adverse effects were noted. Reversible elevations of some liver tests were noted in a few subjects in the study. Menadione (vitamin K_3), which is not used as a nutritional supplemental form of vitamin K for humans, has been reported to cause adverse reactions, including hemolytic anemia.

INTERACTIONS

DRUGS

Broad-Spectrum Antibiotics: Broad-spectrum antibiotics may sterilize the bowel and decrease the vitamin K contribution to the body by the intestinal microflora.

Cephalosporins: Cephalosporins containing side chains of N-methylthiotetrazole (cefmenoxime, cefoperazone, cefotetan, cefamandole, latamoxef) or methylthiadiazole (cefazolin) can cause vitamin K deficiency and hypoprothrombinemia. These cephalosporins are inhibitors of hepatic vitamin K epoxide reductase.

Cholestyramine: Concomitant intake of cholestyramine and vitamin K may reduce the absorption of vitamin K.

Colestipol: Concomitant intake of colestipol and vitamin K may reduce the absorption of vitamin K.

Mineral Oil: Concomitant intake of mineral oil and vitamin K may reduce the absorption of vitamin K.

Orlistat: Orlistat may decrease the absorption of vitamin K.

Salicylates: Salicylates in large doses may inhibit vitamin K epoxide reductase resulting in vitamin K deficiency.

Warfarin: Vitamin K can antagonize the effect of warfarin.

NUTRITIONAL SUPPLEMENTS

Medium Chain Triglycerides: Concomitant intake of medium-chain triglycerides and vitamin K may enhance the absorption of vitamin K.

Squalene: Concomitant intake of squalene and vitamin K may decrease the absorption of vitamin K.

Vitamin A: Intake of high doses of vitamin A may decrease the absorption of vitamin K.

Vitamin E: Intake of very large doses of vitamin E may result in vitamin K deficiency. A vitamin E metabolite, vitamin E quinone, can inhibit vitamin K-dependent gamma-glutamyl carboxylase activity.

FOODS

Olestra: The fat substitute olestra inhibits the absorption of vitamin K as well as the other fat-soluble vitamins A, D and E. These vitamins are added to olestra. Olestra contains 8 micrograms of vitamin K per gram.

DOSAGE AND ADMINISTRATION

There is no typical dosage for vitamin K. Some multivitamin preparations contain vitamin K as vitamin K_1 (phylloquinone or phytonadione) or vitamin K_2 (menaquinones) at doses of 25 to 100 micrograms. The amount of vitamin K in these products is stated as the percentage of the daily value (DV) for vitamin K. The DV is the highest RDA for the vitamin, or 80 micrograms. Vitamin K_1 is also available in 10 milligram doses. In Japan, vitamin K, usually in the form of vitamin K_2, is used for the management of osteoporosis. The fermented soybean product natto is rich in menaquinone-7 or vitamin $K_{2\ (35)}$. The bacteria that is used in the preparation of natto, *Bacillus natto*, is also used in Japan as a dietary supplement source of vitamin K_2.

The Food and Nutrition Board of the U.S. National Academy of Sciences has indicated the following Dietary Reference Intakes (DRIs) for vitamin K:

Category	Age (Years)	AI (adequate intake) (micrograms/day)
Infants	0 through 6 months	2.0
	7 through 12 months	2.5
Children	1 through 3 years	30
	4 through 8 years	55
	9 through 13 years	60

Males	14 through 18 years	75
	19 through 30 years	120
	31 through 50 years	120
	51 through 70 years	120
	Older than 70 years	120
Females	14 through 18 years	75
	19 through 30 years	90
	31 through 50 years	90
	51 through 70 years	90
	Older than 70 years	90
Pregnant	18 years or younger	75
	19 through 50 years	90
Lactating	18 years or younger	75
	19 through 50 years	90

The DV (Daily Value) for vitamin K, which is used for determining percentage of nutrient daily values on nutritional supplement and food labels, is 80 micrograms. This is based on the U.S. RDA for vitamin K.

LITERATURE

Beulens JW, Bots ML, Atsma F, et al. High dietary menaquinone intake is associated with reduced coronary calcification. *Atherosclerosis.* Epub: 2008 Jul 19.

Blackwell GJ, Radkomski M, Moncada S. Inhibition of human platelet aggregation by vitamin K. *Throm Res.* 1985;37:103-114.

Booth SL, Al Rajabi A. Determinants of vitamin K status in humans. *Vitam Horm.* 2008;78:1-22.

Booth SL, Dallal G, Shea MK, et al. Effect of vitamin K supplementation on bone loss in elderly men and women. *J Clin Endocrinol Metab.* 2008;93(4):1217-1223.

Booth SL, Mayer J. Warfarin and fracture risk. *Nutr Rev.* 2000;58:20-22.

Booth SL, O'Brien-Morse ME, Dallal GE, et al. Response of vitamin K status to different intakes and sources of phylloquinone-rich food: comparison of younger and older adults. *Am J Clin Nutr.* 1999;70:368-377.

Booth SL, Suttie JW. Dietary intake and adequacy of vitamin K. *J Nutr.* 1998;128:785-788.

Booth SL, Tucker KL, Chen H, et al. Dietary vitamin K intakes are associated with hip fracture but not with bone mineral density in elderly men and women. *Am J Clin Nutr.* 2000;71:1201-1208.

Bügel S. Vitamin K and bone health in adult humans. *Vitam Horm.* 2008;78:393-416.

Caillot-Augusseau A, Vico L, Herr M, et al. Space flight is associated with rapid decreases of under carboxylated osteocalcin and increases of markers of bone resorption without changes in their circadian variation: observations in two cosmonauts. *Clin Chem.* 2000;46:1136-1143.

Caricchio R, Kovalenko D, Kaufmann WK, et al. Apoptosis provoked by the oxidative stress inducer menadione (vitamin K3) is mediated by the Fas/Fas ligand system. *Clin Immunol.* 1999;93:65-74.

Chlebowski RT, Akman SA, Block JB. Vitamin K in the treatment of cancer. *Cancer Treatment Rev.* 1985;12:49-63.

Craciun AM, Wolf J, Knapen MH, et al. Improved bone metabolism in female elite athletes after vitamin K supplementation. *Int J Sports Med.* 1998;19:479-484.

Cranenburg EC, Schurgers LJ, Vermeer C. Vitamin K: the coagulation vitamin that became omnipotent. *Thromb Haemost.* 2007 Jul;98(1):120-125.

Feskanich D, Weber P, Willett WC, et al. Vitamin K intake and hip fractures in women: a prospective study. *Am J Clin Nutr.* 1999;69:74-79.

Hirao M, Hashimoto J, Ando W, et al. Response of serum carboxylated and undercarboxylated osteocalcin to alendronate monotherapy and combined therapy with vitamin K2 in postmenopausal women. *J Bone Miner Metab.* 2008;26(3):260-264.

Institute of Medicine, Food and Nutrition Board. Dietary Reference Intakes for vitamin A, vitamin K, arsenic, boron, chromium, copper, iodine, iron, manganese, molybdenum, nickel, silicon, vanadium, and zinc. Washington, DC: National Academy Press, 2001.

Jamal SA, Browner WS, Bauer D, Cummings SR. Warfarin use and risk for osteoporosis in elderly women. Study of Osteoporotic Fractures Research Group. *Ann Intern Med.* 1998;128:829-832.

Jie K-SG, Bots ML, Vermeer C, et al. Vitamin K status and bone mass in women with and without aortic atherosclerosis: a population-based study. *Calcif Tissue Int.* 1996;59:352-356.

Kawashima H, Nakajima Y, Matubara Y, et al. Effects of vitamin K2 (menatetrenone) on atherosclerosis and blood coagulation in hypercholesterolemic rabbits. *Jpn J Pharmacol.* 1997;75:135-143.

Lipsky JJ. Nutritional sources of vitamin K. *Mayo Clin Proc.* 1994;69:462-466.

Macdonald HM, McGuigan FE, Lanham-New SA, et al. Vitamin K1 intake is associated with higher bone mineral density and reduced bone resorption in early postmenopausal Scottish women: no evidence of gene-nutrient interaction with apolipoprotein E polymorphisms. *Am J Clin Nutr.* 2008;87(5):1513-1520.

Nimptsch K, Rohrmann S, Linseisen J. Dietary intake of vitamin K and risk of prostate cancer in the Heidelberg cohort of the European Prospective Investigation into Cancer and Nutrition (EPIC-Heidelberg). *Am J Clin Nutr.* 2008;87(4):985-992.

Oldenburg J, Marinova M, Müller-Reible C, et al. The vitamin K cycle. *Vitam Horm.* 2008;78:35-62.

Olson RE. Osteoporosis and vitamin K intake (editorial). *Am J Clin Nutr.* 2000;71:1031-1032.

Olson RE. Vitamin K. In: Shils ME, Olson JA, Shike M, Ross AC, eds. *Modern Nutrition in Health and Disease*. 9th ed. Baltimore, MD: Williams and Wilkins; 1999:363-380.

Pearson DA. Bone health and osteoporosis: the role of vitamin K and potential antagonism by anticoagulants. *Nutr Clin Pract*. 2007;22(5):517-544.

Philip WJ, Martin JC, Richardson JM, et al. Decreased axial and peripheral bone density in patients taking long-term warfarin. *QJM*. 1995;88:635-640.

Rashid M, Durie P, Andrew M, et al. Prevalence of vitamin K deficiency in cystic fibrosis. *Am J Clin Nutr*. 1999;70:378-382.

Sakagami H, Satoh K, Hakeda Y, et al. Apoptosis-inducing activity of vitamin C and vitamin K. *Cell Mol Biol* (*Noisy-le-Grand, France*). 2000;46:129-143.

Sakamoto N, Wakabayashi I, Sakamoto K. Low vitamin K intake effects on glucose tolerance in rats. *Int J Vitam Nutr Res*. 1999;69:27-31.

Sano M, Fujita H, Morita I, et al. Vitamin K_2 (menatetrenone) induces iNOS in bovine vascular smooth muscle cells: no relationship between nitric oxide production and gamma-carboxylation. *J Nutr Sci Vitaminol*. (*Tokyo*). 1999;45:711-723.

Shearer MJ. Vitamin K. *Lancet*. 1995;345:229-234.

Takami A, Nakao S, Ontachi Y, et al. Successful therapy of myelodysplastic syndrome with menatetrenone, a vitamin K_2 analog. *Int J Hematol*. 1999;69:24-26.

Tsaioun KI. Vitamin K-dependent proteins in the developing and aging nervous system. *Nutr Rev*. 1999;57:231-240.

Vermeer C, Jie KS, Knapen MH. Role of vitamin K in bone metabolism. *Annu Rev Nutr*. 1995;15:1-22.

Vervoort LM, Ronden FE, Thijssen HH. The potent antioxidant activity of the vitamin K cycle in microsomal lipid peroxidation. *Biochem Pharmacol*. 1997;54:871-876.

Wu FY, Sun TP. Vitamin K_3 induces cell cycle arrest and cell death by inhibiting Cdc25 phosphatase. *Eur J Cancer*. 1999;35:1388-1393.

Yoshida M, Jacques PF, Meigs JB, et al. Effect of vitamin K supplementation on insulin resistance in older men and women. *Diabetes Care*. Epub: 2008 Aug 12.

Wheat Grass/Barley Grass

DESCRIPTION

Cereal grass is the young green plant that grows to produce the cereal grain. Grasses belong to the *Gramineae* family that provides all the world's cereals and most of the world's sugar. Wheat grass and barley grass are popular nutritional supplements. These cereal grasses, along with spirulina (see Spirulina), chlorella (see Chlorella), oat grass and alfalfa are sometimes referred to as "green foods." Wheat grass and barley grass are rich sources of chlorophyll (see Chlorophyll/ Chlorophyllin), which is believed to have some health-promoting activities.

ACTIONS AND PHARMACOLOGY

ACTIONS

Wheat grass and barley grass have putative anticarcinogenic activity.

MECHANISM OF ACTION

Wheat sprout extracts have demonstrated antimutagenic activity *in vitro*. The mechanism of the antimutagenic effect is unclear. Wheat sprouts and wheat grass are rich in chlorophyll, and the antimutagenic activity of wheat sprouts may be accounted for by the presence of this substance, which is known to have antimutagenic and anticarcinogenic activities (see Chlorophyll/Chlorophyllin). Other substances, including flavonoids, may also play a role in these possible activities. Barley grass extracts have been found to protect human fibroblasts against carcinogenic agents. Again, chlorophyll may, in part, account for this effect. Barley grass contains several substances other than chlorophyll that have antioxidant activity and that may contribute to its possible antimutagenic and anticarcinogenic activities.

PHARMACOKINETICS

The proteins, lipids and carbohydrates in wheat grass and barley grass are digested, absorbed and metabolized by normal physiological processes.

INDICATIONS AND USAGE

Wheat grass/barley grass supplements are promoted for multiple uses. Claims have been made that they help prevent and fight cancer, lower cholesterol, detoxify many pollutants, protect against solar and other forms of radiation, boost energy and immunity, enhance wound healing, help with digestion, fight tooth decay and bad breath, promote healthy skin, reverse graying of hair and lower blood pressure, among other things. There is no credible evidence to support any of these claims at this time.

RESEARCH SUMMARY

Research is lacking on the possible effects of wheat grass and barley grass. Given that they contain chlorophyll, it is possible that they might have some of the activities exhibited by that substance, including antimutagenic and anticarcinogenic activities. See Chlorophyll/Chlorophyllin.

CONTRAINDICATIONS, PRECAUTIONS, ADVERSE REACTIONS

CONTRAINDICATIONS

Wheat grass and barley grass are contraindicated in those who are hypersensitive to any component of a wheat grass- or barley grass-containing supplement.

PRECAUTIONS

Pregnant women and nursing mothers should avoid wheat grass- or barley grass-containing supplements.

Wheat grass supplements may contain high amounts of vitamin K. Those on warfarin should exercise caution in the use of wheat grass supplements.

ADVERSE REACTIONS
No reports of adverse reactions.

INTERACTIONS
Some wheat grass supplements may be rich in vitamin K and may affect the INR of those on warfarin.

DOSAGE AND ADMINISTRATION
There are various forms of wheat grass and barley grass supplements. Both are available as a powder, in tablets and as a juice. It is also available as a juice. Wheat grass and barley grass are also found in combination "green food" products with spirulina, chlorella, oat grass and alfalfa. Those who use wheat grass typically take 3.5 grams daily. The typical dose of barley grass is also about 3.5 grams daily.

LITERATURE
Lai C-N. Chlorophyll: the active factor in wheat sprout extract inhibiting the metabolic activation of carcinogens in vitro. *Nutr Cancer.* 1979; 1:19-21.

Lai C-N, Dabney BJ, Shaw CR. Inhibition of in vitro metabolic activation of carcinogens by wheat sprout extracts. *Nutr Cancer.* 1978; 1:27-30.

Peryt B, Miloszewska J, Tudek B, et al. Antimutagenic effects of several subfractions of extract from wheat sprout toward benzo[a]pyrene-induced mutagenicity in strain TA98 of *Salmonella typhimurium. Mutat Res.* 1988; 206:221-225.

Peryt B, Szymczyk T, Lesca P. Mechanism of antimutagenicity of wheat sprout extracts. *Mutat Res.* 1992; 269:201-215.

Tudek B, Peryt B, Miloszewska J, et al. The effect of wheat sprout extract on benzo(a)pyrene and 7,2-dimethylbenz(a)anthracene activity. *Neoplasma.* 1998; 35:515-523.

Whey Proteins

DESCRIPTION
Whey proteins comprise one of the two major protein groups of bovine milk, the other group being the caseins. Caseins account for about 80% of the total protein in bovine milk, while whey proteins account for the remaining approximately 20%. Whey is derived as a natural byproduct of the cheese-making process. In addition to proteins, the raw form contains fat, lactose and other substances. The raw form is processed to produce protein-rich whey protein concentrates (WPC) and whey protein isolates (WPI), among other things.

Whey proteins are comprised of high-biological-value proteins and proteins that have different functions. The main whey proteins are beta-lactoglobulin and alpha-lactoglobulin, two small globular proteins that account for about 70 to 80% of total whey protein. Proteins present in lesser amounts include the immunoglobulins IgG, IgA and IgM, but especially IgG, glycomacropeptides, bovine serum albumin, lactoferrin, lactoperoxidase and lysozyme. Whey proteins also contain smaller peptides derived from various proteins which are called biopeptides.

A few different types of whey proteins are marketed. Whey protein concentrates are rich in whey proteins and also contain fat and lactose. Some whey protein concentrates contain higher amounts of immunoglobulins than others. Whey protein isolates are low in fat and lactose.

There are various processes for preparing whey protein isolates. Ion-exchange whey protein isolates are high in protein but low in glycomacropeptides, lactoferrin, lactoperoxidase and some bioactive peptides. Microfiltration/ultrafiltration whey protein isolates have higher amounts of glycomacropeptides, lactoferrin, lactoperoxidase and the bioactive peptides, but are lower in bovine serum albumin. Interestingly, bovine serum albumin, along with beta-lactoglobulin and IgG1, are proteins with abundant glutamylcysteine sequences. Glutamylcysteine is the precursor to glutathione. Cross-flow microfiltration gives a whey protein isolate which is greater than 90% in protein that is undenatured and that retains all important sub-fractions in natural ratios, with no fat or lactose.

ACTIONS AND PHARMACOLOGY
ACTIONS
Whey proteins may have antimicrobial and immunomodulatory actions. They may also have antioxidant activity.

MECHANISM OF ACTION
The mechanism of the possible antimicrobial actions of whey proteins may be accounted for by examining the activities of some of the whey proteins. Lactoferrin binds iron very tightly. Iron is a nutrient essential to support microbial growth, especially the growth of pathogenic bacteria. Lactoferrin may also inhibit the adsorption and/or penetration of bacteria and viruses in the intestinal wall. Lactoperoxidase may inactivate or kill microorganisms via an enzymatic activity producing reactive oxygen species. The immunoglobulins may also play a passive immunity role.

The possible immunomodulatory activity of whey proteins may also be due, in part, to the immunoglobulins playing a role in passive immunity. Whey proteins are rich in L-cysteine and L-glutamate, two amino acids that are precursors to the tripeptide glutathione. Some are also abundant in the dipeptide sequence of glutamylcysteine. This dipeptide is also a precursor to glutathione. There is some indication that intake of whey proteins enhance monocyte glutathione levels. Enhanced glutathione levels may also contribute to a possible immunomodulatory role of whey proteins, as well as to the possible antioxidant activity of these proteins. In addition, lactoferrin may modulate immune function.

PHARMACOKINETICS

The pharmacokinetics of whey proteins should be similar to those for dietary proteins. There is indication that lactoferrin and some of the immunoglobulins in whey proteins may be more resistant to proteolytic degradation than are other types of proteins. Some proteins may be digested to peptides that may be absorbed and may have various activities (bioactive peptides). Some (e.g., bovine serum albumin, beta-lactoglobulin) may yield glutamylcysteine during their digestion, which may be absorbed and serve as a precursor to glutathione in some tissues.

INDICATIONS AND USAGE

Whey proteins may be useful in the nutrition of some infants and others, and there is some very preliminary evidence that they may have some immune-modulating and anticancer effects. There is no credible evidence that they build muscle faster than other protein sources.

RESEARCH SUMMARY

Whey proteins have been used as the sole proteins in some infant formulas, and this has reportedly resulted in fewer allergies in these infants. In one study, the use of a whey protein formula in the first six months of life significantly reduced atopic disease up to one year of age. In another study, infants receiving a whey protein-hydrolysate formula during the first six months of life had a lower incidence of cow's milk protein sensitivity at age six months, less eczema during the first year of life and less diarrhea of non-infectitious origin during the first half-year of life.

There are several animal studies in which whey and whey factors are said to exert some positive effects on immunity and cancer. Observed immuno-enhancing properties are believed by some researchers to be related only partially to whey's nutritional effects. Enhancement of host humoral immune response has been associated, in some of these studies, with whey's role in increasing glutathione levels in the body.

In animal studies, whey proteins were found to be protective against colon cancer, relative to red meat and some other protein sources. A whey protein diet significantly decreased tumor burden and extended life in mice with colon cancer, compared to mice with colon cancer fed-standard diet.

Whey protein concentrate was administered to five patients with metastatic cancers (30 grams daily for six months). Two of these patients exhibited some evidence of tumor regres-

sion, normalization of hemoglobin and peripheral lympho-cyte counts. In two other patients, there was stabilization of tumor growth and increased hemoglobin levels. More research is needed.

CONTRAINDICATIONS, PRECAUTIONS, ADVERSE REACTIONS

CONTRAINDICATIONS

Whey proteins are contraindicated in those who are hyper-sensitive to milk proteins.

PRECAUTIONS

See Contraindications.

ADVERSE REACTIONS

No reports. However, those who are hypersensitive to milk products are expected to experience allergy symptoms, including possible serious ones, if they use whey protein products.

INTERACTIONS

No known interactions with drugs, nutritional supplements, food or herbs.

DOSAGE AND ADMINISTRATION

There are several types of whey protein supplements available, including whey protein concentrates, ion exchange whey protein isolates, microfiltration/ultrafiltration whey protein isolates and whey protein hydrolysates. Some preparations contain mixtures of these various forms, and some are enriched with other substances, including branched-chain amino acids and L-glutamine. Dosages are variable. Some (athletes, for example) use whey proteins as a protein supplement and take 10 to 25 grams daily and, in some cases, higher doses.

LITERATURE

Barth CA, Behnke U. [Nutritional physiology of whey and whey components.] [Article in German.] *Nahrung.* 1997; 41:2-12.

Bell S J. Whey protein concentrates with and without immunoglobulins: a review. *J med Food.* 2000; 3:1-13.

Bounous G, Batist G, Gold P. Immunoenhancing property of a dietary whey protein in mice: role of glutathione. *Clin Invest Med.* 1989; 12:154-161.

Bounous G, Batist G, Gold P. Whey proteins in cancer prevention. *Cancer Left.* 1991; 57:91-94.

Bounous G, Gervais F, Amer V, et al. The influence of dietary whey protein on tissue glutathione and the diseases of aging. *Clin Invest Med.* 1989; 12:343-349.

Kennedy RS, Konok GP, Bounous G, et al. The use of a whey protein concentrate in the treatment of patients with metastatic carcinoma: a phase I-II clinical study. *Anticancer Res.* 1995; 15(6B):2643-2649.

Kinsella JE, Whitehead DM. Proteins in whey: chemical, physical, and functional properties. *Adv Food Nutr Res.* 1989; 33:343-438.

Papenburg R, Bounous G, Fleiszner D, Gold P. Dietary milk proteins inhibit the development of dimethylhydrazine-induced malignancy. *Tumor Biol.* 1990; 11:129-136.

Tong LM, Sasaki S, McClements DJ, Decker EA. Mechanisms of the antioxidant activity of a high molecular weight fraction of whey. *J Agric Food Chem.* 2000; 48:1473-1478.

Vandenplas Y, Hauser B, Van den Borre C, et al. Effect of a whey hydrolysate prophylaxis of atopic disease. *Ann Allergy.* 1992; 68:419-424.

Wong CW, Watson DL. Immunomodulatory effects of dietary whey proteins in mice. *J Dairy Res.* 1995; 62:359-368.

Xanthohumol

DESCRIPTION

Beer is a fermented aqueous drink based on starch and flavored with hops. Hops provide the characteristic bitterness of the beer and contribute to its aroma and foam stability.

The hop plant (*Humulus lupulus* L.) is a dioecious plant, meaning that there are separate male and female hop plants. Only the female hop plant produces the flowers, or, more specifically, the strobiles that are used for brewing or possible medicinal purposes. Male plants have no commercial value but are used to pollinate the female plants. Pollination stimulates higher yields by increasing cone size and seed set, but because brewers prefer seedless hops, males are only grown with otherwise poor-yielding female varieties. Hop seed from a pollinated female is only planted when a cross between the male and female is desired to obtain a new variety.

The term 'hop' in a strict sense refers to the hop plant, and the term 'hops' refers to the flower cones ("hop cones" or "hops"). However, both terms are commonly used interchangeably. The flowers in a female hop plant are arranged in characteristic clusters on stems. The flower cluster is called an inflorescence. The female inflorescences are rich in polyphenolic compounds and acyl phloroglucides that are widely used to preserve beer and give beer its characteristic flavor and aroma.

The hop cones are green, built like pine cones and vary in size. At the base of the leaves (bracts, also called scales) of the cones, are collections of small, yellow spheres called the lupulin glands. The lupulin glands are little sacs of bitter and aromatic acids and oils. In the lupulin glands can be found the alpha-acids and their derivatives, including the iso-alpha-acids and the rho-iso-alpha acids, the beta acids and xanthohumol, among several other compounds. The iso-alpha-acids, including isohumulone, account for the bitter

taste of beer. The oils in the hops are mainly responsible for the aroma of beer.

In addition to their role in beer, hops extracts have been used for medicinal reasons. The traditional use of hops as a mild sedative has its origin in the observation that the transfer of hop resin from the hands of hop-pickers to their mouths appeared to cause sleepiness and fatigue in the workers. In Germany, the use of hops is approved for the treatment of restlessness, anxiety and sleep disorders. However, high-quality clinical studies supporting the use of hops as a sedative are few and far between. Thus, the effectiveness of the use of hops for the treatment of sleep disorders is uncertain.

Recently, there has been great interest in studying certain phytochemicals found in hops for their possible anti-inflammatory, anticancer, chemopreventive and estrogenic activities. Two of the phytochemicals found in hops that have been receiving a great deal of attention are xanthohumol for its possible anticancer activity and 8-prenylnaringenin for its phytoestrogenic activity (see 8-Prenylnaringenin).

Xanthohumol is a prenylated chalcone derived from hops. In hops, the yellow compound is found in high amounts in the lupulin glands of the female inflorescence.

Xanthohumol is secreted as part of the hop resin (lupulin) by glandular trichomes found on the adaxial surfaces of cone bracts. It is also found in the trichomes on the underside of young leaves. The chalcone is found in small amounts in the Chinese traditional medicine plant, *Sophora flavescens*, extracts of which are used in the treatment a number of diseases, including certain cancers and viral diseases. A chalcone is an aromatic ketone that forms the central core for a variety of biological compounds. Chalcones are the immediate precursors in the biosynthesis of flavonoids, and their structures differ from that of other flavonoids by the inclusion of an open C-ring. (Chalcones are sometimes referred to as open C-ring flavonoids.) Xanthohumol is usually referred to as a prenylflavonoid. It is the precursor of the flavonoid, isoxanthohumol, which belongs to the flavanone subclass of flavonoids. Xanthohumol possesses a free 2'-hydroxy group and can therefore readily isomerize to isoxanthohumol.

Xanthohumol has been found to have broad-spectrum anticancer activity.

However, in contrast to some other phytochemicals in hops, especially 8-prenylnaringenin, xanthohumol per se does not possess phytoestrogenic activity.

Xanthohumol's empirical formula is $C_{21}H_{22}O_5$, its molecular weight is 354.396, and its CAS Registry Number is 6754-58-1. Xanthohumol is described chemically as (*E*)-1-[2,4-dihydroxy-6-methoxy-3-(3-methylbut-2-enyl)phenyl]-3-(4-hydroxyphenyl)prop-2-en-1-one. It is also known as (3'-[3,3-dimethylallyl]-2',4',4-trihydroxy-6'-methoxychalcone).

In addition to being classified as a prenylated chalcone or prenylchalcone and a prenylflavonoid, xanthohumol can be classified as a terpenophenol and a polyphenol.

Xanthohumol is represented by the following chemical formula:

Xanthohumol

Xanthohumol is a plant secondary metabolite and has broad-spectrum activity against bacteria, viruses and fungi, all of which can cause damage to the plant. The amount of xanthohumol in beer is low (about 0.1 milligram per liter). This is due to the thermal conversion of xanthohumol to isoxanthohumol during the brewing process. Xanthohumol does impart some bitter taste to beer and helps to stabilize the foam.

ACTIONS AND PHARMACOLOGY

ACTIONS

Xanthohumol has antioxidant activity. It may also have anticancer/chemopreventive, anti-inflammatory, antimicrobial, antiobesity, antiosteoporosis, and triglyceride-lowering activities.

MECHANISM OF ACTION

Antioxidant activity: Xanthohumol has a number of antioxidant activities. It has been demonstrated to scavenge hydroxyl, peroxyl and superoxide anion radicals. Xanthohumol was also found to inhibit superoxide anion radical formation by 12-O-tetradecanoylphorbol-13-acetate stimulation of differentiated HL-60 human promyelocytic leukemia cells. It is reported to inhibit nitric oxide formation. Xanthohumol was demonstrated to inhibit the oxidation of LDL (low density lipoprotein) *in vitro*. Oxidized LDL is thought to be a major factor in the pathogenesis of atherosclerosis. It was also shown to decrease conjugated diene formation, a measure of lipid peroxidation, and to inhibit liver microsomal lipid peroxidation induced by ferrous ascorbate, ferric-ADP/NADPH or *tert*-butyl hydroperoxide.

Anticancer activity: Xanthohumol appears to be a broad-spectrum anticancer/chemopreventive agent, acting by multiple mechanisms in the initiation, promotion and progression phase.

Xanthohumol was demonstrated to induce apoptosis and inhibit NF-kappaB activation in two different prostate epithelial lines: human benign prostate hyperplasia epithelial cells (BPH-1) and malignant androgen-independent prostate cancer epithelial cells (PC-3), representing both non-tumorigenic hyperplasia and malignant prostate cancer. It was suggested by the authors of this study that xanthohumol may be potentially useful as a chemopreventive agent during prostate hyperplasia and prostate carcinogenesis.

Xanthohumol was reported to kill B-chronic lymphocytic leukemia (B-CLL) cells via an apoptotic mechanism. Cell death was associated with poly (ADP-ribose) polymerase cleavage and annexin V positivity, indicative of an apoptotic mechanism.

Xanthohumol was shown to inhibit the growth of the vascular tumor line KS-IMM, a spontaneously immortalized iatrogenic Kaposi's sarcoma cell line obtained from a biopsy. Histopathology and *in vivo* angiogenesis assays revealed that tumor angiogenesis was involved and that xanthohumol inhibited the growth of the cells via an antiangiogenic mechanism. Xanthohumol was demonstrated to repress both the NF-kappaB and Akt pathways in human umbilical vein endothelial cells (HUVEC), a commonly used endothelial cell line. This finding suggests that components of the two pathways are major targets in the molecular mechanism of xanthohumol. Further, using *in vitro* analysis, it was shown that xanthohumol interferes with several points in the angiogenic process, including inhibition of endothelial cell invasion and migration, growth, and formation of a network of tubular-like structures. The authors of this study suggest that xanthohumol may be useful as an antiangiogenic chemopreventive substance and that its potential in cancer prevention and treatment should be evaluated.

Another study reported that xanthohumol inhibited cell proliferation of both acute myelogenous leukemia (AML) and chronic myelogenous leukemia (CML) cell lines. Inhibition of cell proliferation was associated with induction of apoptosis, reduced vascular endothelial growth factor (VEGF) secretion, decreased cell invasion, decreased metalloprotease production and decreased adhesion to endothelial cells. The authors of this study had previously shown that xanthohumol has antiangiogenic properties both *in vitro* and *in vivo* associated with inhibition of Akt/NF-kappaB activation. They concluded that as endothelial cells and hematopoietic cells are mutually correlated in their development and growth, targeting both tumor cells and endothelial cells with an agent such as xanthohumol, which possesses both cytotoxic and antiangiogenic activities, may lead to synergistic antitumor effects, interrupting a reciprocal stimulatory loop between leukemia and endothelial cells. In short, xanthohumol appears to show potential as a double-edge anticancer agent.

In a recent study, xanthohumol was reported to inhibit MCF7 cell proliferation dose-dependently. (MCF7 is a human breast cancer cell line.) Oral administration of xanthohumol to nude mice inoculated with MCF7 cells (breast cancer xenografts) resulted in central necrosis within tumors, reduced inflammatory cell number, increased percentage of apoptotic cells and decreased microvessel density. Antiangiogenic effects of xanthohumol were appropriately confirmed. A significant reduction in a number of inflammatory factors, including NF-kappaB, was demonstrated. The findings of this study again suggested the double-edge anticancer activity of xanthohumol. Xanthohumol targeted both breast cancer cells and host cells, namely inflammatory and endothelial cells.

The mechanism of action of the anticancer activities of xanthohumol are far from being completely understood. Continued research in this promising area is needed and warranted.

Anti-inflammatory activity: Xanthohumol has been shown to inhibit cyclooxygenase-1 (COX-1) and cyclooxygenase-2 (COX-2). It was also found to downregulate the proinflammatory transcription factor NF-kappaB in human benign prostate hyperplasia epithelial cells (BPH-1). Xanthohumol was demonstrated to repress both the NF-kappaB and Akt (protein kinase B) inflammatory pathways.

Xanthohumol was reported to reduce the expression of the lipopolysaccharide (LPS) receptor components, such as the toll-like receptor 4 (TLR4) and MD2, resulting in the suppression of NF-kappaB activation in lipopolysaccharide (LPS)-activated RAW264.7 cells (a mouse monocytic cell line). In interferon gamma (IFN-gamma)-stimulated RAW264.7 cells, the binding activity of signal transducer and activator of transcription-1 alpha (STAT-1alpha) and that of interferon regulatory factor-1 (IRF-1) was inhibited by xanthohumol. These results suggest that depending on the stimuli, differential signaling pathways are used by xanthohumol for the inhibition of excess inflammatory mediators in macrophages. Further research is needed and warranted in order to fully understand the mechanism of action of the various anti-inflammatory activities of xanthohumol.

Antimicrobial/antiplasmodial activity: Xanthohumol is a plant secondary metabolite and has broad antibacterial, antiviral and antifungal activity against organisms that can do damage to the hop plant. Xanthohumol was also found to prevent the cytopathogenic effects of the human immunodeficiency virus (HIV) and was demonstrated to inhibit the proliferation of the malarial pathogen *Plasmodium falciparum*. The mechanism of action of these effects is unclear.

Antiobesity activity: The effects of xanthohumol and hinokiol, a lignan isolated from *Magnolia officinalis*, on apoptotic signaling in mouse 3T3-L1 adipocytes were studied alone and in combination.

It was found that although xanthohumol and hinokiol showed little or no effect as individual compounds, xanthohumol in combination with hinokiol demonstrated enhanced activity in inducing apoptosis in the 3T3L1 adipocytes via the cytochrome c/caspase-3/PARP and PTEN/Akt pathways. What these results have to do with an antiobesity effect in humans is entirely unclear. However, they do suggest that a clinical study may be worthwhile to see if this combination might have some effect in humans.

Antiosteoporosis activity: In one study, xanthohumol was reported to prevent bone resorption in a model system. The mechanism of this activity is not clear and further investigation is needed and warranted.

Triglyceride-lowering activity: Xanthohumol was demonstrated to inhibit the activity of diacylglycerol acyltransferase (DGAT), an enzyme that catalyzes the acyl residue transfer from acyl-CoA to diacylglycerol to form triglycerides (triacylglycerols, TAGs). Accumulation of TAGs is linked to a number of potentially serious conditions, including nonalcoholic steatohepatitis (NASH), obesity and elevated plasma triglyceride levels (hypertriglyceridemia) associated with diabetes, the metabolic syndrome and atherosclerosis. However, this experiment did not provide any insights into how xanthohumol and DGAT inhibition might regulate hepatic apolipoprotein B (apoB) secretion. Triglyceride availability is known to be a major factor in the regulation of apoB secretion.

A later study examined the role of xanthohumol on apolipoprotein B (apoB) and triglyceride synthesis and secretion, using HepG2 cells. (The HepG2 cell line is a human hepatoma cell line.) Apolipoprotein B is the primary lipoprotein of LDL-cholesterol. Xanthohumol was demonstrated to decrease apoB dose-dependently. The decrease in apoB was associated with increased cellular apoB degradation. Xanthohumol also inhibited the synthesis of triglycerides in the microsomal membrane and the transfer of the newly synthesized triglycerides to the microsomal lumen. This indicated that triglyceride availability is a determining factor in the regulation of apoB secretion under the experimental conditions. The inhibition of triglyceride synthesis was caused by a reduction in DGAT (see above study), which corresponded to a decrease in DGAT-1 messenger RNA expression, but not DGAT-2 expression. Xanthohumol also decreased microsomal triglyceride transfer protein

(MTP) activity dose-dependently. MTP might also control the rate of triglyceride transfer from the microsomal membrane to the active luminal pool. In conclusion, xanthohumol appears to be a potent inhibitor of apoB secretion.

PHARMACOKINETICS

There is little data on the pharmacokinetics (PK) of xanthohumol in humans. Some animal and tissue culture studies are available. Absorption, metabolism and excretion of xanthohumol have been studied in rats. The efficiency of absorption of xanthohumol from the small intestine following oral administration was low. Xanthohumol was detected in the plasma mainly in the form of two mono-glucuronides whose maximum concentration was reached after four hours. The cumulative amounts of both xanthohumol glucuronides excreted in the urine reached a plateau at 12 hours after oral administration and accounted for 0.3% and 0.05% of the oral dose. The recovery of unchanged xanthohumol from the urine was 0.2%.

The metabolism of xanthohumol was investigated *in vitro* using human liver microsomes. Hydroxylation of a prenyl methyl group was the primary route of oxidative metabolism forming the trans isomer of xanthohumol. The double bond on the prenyl group formed an epoxide, which was opened by an intramolecular reaction with the neighboring hydroxyl group. Some xanthohumol can be converted to isoxanthohumol via acid-catalyzed cyclization in the stomach. And, isoxanthohumol can be converted by the microflora of the large intestine to the potent phytoestrogen prenylnaringenin.

Another metabolic study of xanthohumol examined *in vitro* metabolism of the prenylchalcone by human UDP-glucuronosyltransferases and sulfotransferases. Three monoglucuronides as well as three monosulfates were identified. It was concluded that the findings of the study suggested a prominent role for the glucuronidation and sulfation of xanthohumol in the liver as well as in the gastrointestinal tract.

Xanthohumol can be converted to isoxanthohumol via acid-catalyzed cyclization in the stomach. And, isoxanthohumol can be converted by the microflora of the large intestine to the potent phytoestrogen prenylnaringenin (see 8-prenylnaringenin)

PK studies on xanthohumol in humans are needed to in order to fill in all the details on its ADME (absorption, distribution, metabolism and excretion).

INDICATIONS AND USAGE

There is preliminary experimental evidence that xanthohumol, a prenylated chalcone of the hop plant that is an ingredient of beer, may have anti-inflammatory, anticancer, antiatherogenic and anti-infective/immunoprotective potential. Though hops show significant estrogenic activity, xanthohumol itself does not.

RESEARCH SUMMARY

In a review of some of the relevant literature, one group of researchers concluded that xanthohumol appears to be a broad-spectrum cancer chemopreventive agent. They cite *in vitro* studies showing that it can inhibit metabolic activation of procarcinogens, induce carcinogen-detoxifying enzymes and inhibit tumor growth at early stages. In one study, the chalcone demonstrated both antioxidant and anti-inflammatory activity, modulated enzymes involved in carcinogen metabolism and detoxification and significantly prevented carcinogen-induced preneoplastic lesions in mouse mammary gland organ tissues. In a number of *in vitro* and some *in vivo* animal studies, xanthohumol has also demonstrated notable tumor antiangiogenic activity. Male nude mice were injected with a Kaposi sarcoma cell line that forms highly angiogenic tumors. Mice receiving xanthohumol enjoyed significantly reduced tumor growth, compared with controls. The research suggested that the flavonoid may exert this favorable effect through, among other actions, inhibition of nuclear factor-kappaB (NF-kB) activity involved in inflammation and angiogenesis. Xanthohumol was found to again inhibit NF-kB activation and to impede prostate hyperplasia and prostate carcinogenesis *in vitro* in a dose-dependent manner in another study. Still other *in vitro* studies with this prenylchalcone have demonstrated some efficacy against hematologic malignancies, melanoma and other cancers.

While finding these results provocative and promising, most researchers have been careful to point out that levels of this chalcone sufficient to replicate the results seen in their studies cannot be achieved through consumption of beer alone. The concentration of xanthohumol in beer is low and it would take huge amounts of beer to achieve any of the above possible anticancer effects. Some have begun developing xanthohumol-enriched beers. Others believe xanthohumol supplements are the better option. In any case, further research into the anticancer properties of this chalcone, extending the inquiry into the clinical domain, is indicated.

There is *in vitro* evidence that xanthohumol, through its antioxidant activity, may be able to prevent lipid peroxidation and thus have cardioprotective effects. In a series of *in vitro* assays, xanthohumol proved more potent than a number of other recognized antioxidants in its ability to scavenge hydroxyl and peroxyl radicals, as well as superoxide anion radicals. Xanthohumol has shown some preliminary ability to inhibit LDL-cholesterol oxidation. In another *in vitro* study, xanthohumol decreased apolipoprotein B secretion as well as triglyceride synthesis and secretion. In combination with honokiol, a lignan isolated from *Magnolia officinalis*, xanthohumol induced apoptosis in mature adipocytes *in vitro*. Neither agent, when tested alone, was similarly effective. Whether xanthohumol might play a role in the prevention or treatment of obesity is unknown, and far more research will be required to determine whether it can be effective in cardiovascular health generally.

Through some demonstrated immunoprotective effects modulated through its anti-inflammatory activity, xanthohumol may be able to protect against some infections. In one study it helped preserve macrophage function in an inflammatory environment. In a review of the literature, it demonstrated broad-spectrum anti-infective effects, showing some activity against various bacteria, viruses, fungi and malarial protozoa. Among the viruses affected were cytomegalovirus, herpes simplex viruses type 1 and 2 and human immunodeficiency virus 1. Its reported activity against the malaria agent *Plasmodium falciparum* was associated with its inhibition of glutathione-mediated degradation and detoxification of hemin, a by-product of the parasitic digestion of hemoglobin. Animal and clinical investigation of this anti-infective potential is clearly warranted.

Finally, estrogenic effects of hops have been documented for some time. Xanthohumol itself, however, has shown either no or very weak estrogenic activity, and there is no likely role for this substance in the prevention or treatment of perimenopausal symptoms.

CONTRAINDICATIONS, PRECAUTIONS, ADVERSE REACTIONS

CONTRAINDICATIONS

Xanthohumol-containing dietary supplements are contraindicated in those hypersensitive to any component of a xanthohumol-containing product. Hypersensitivity to xanthohumol is probably very rare.

PRECAUTIONS

Those who wish to use xanthohumol supplements for a health condition should first discuss this with his or her physician.

Because of the lack of long-term studies on the safety of xanthohumol-containing dietary supplements, pregnant females and nursing mothers should avoid their use.

ADVERSE REACTIONS

No reports.

INTERACTIONS

DRUGS

Xanthohumol inhibits cytochrome p450, and although there are no known reports of any interactions with drugs and xanthohumol, those using drugs that are metabolized via the cytochrome p450 system, for example, the statin atorvastatin, should be cautious in the use of xanthohumol supplements.

NUTRITIONAL SUPPLEMENTS

None known.

HERBS

None known.

FOOD

None known.

OVERDOSAGE

There are no reports of overdosage.

DOSAGE AND ADMINISTRATION

The optimal dosage of xanthohumol is unknown.

A few xanthohumol-containing dietary supplements are available. Doses higher than those recommended on the label should generally not be exceeded.

The only dietary source of xanthohumol is beer. However, the concentration of xanthohumol in beer is very low, about 0.1 mg per liter.

LITERATURE

Albini A, Dell'Eva R, Vené R, et al. Mechanisms of the antiangiogenic activity by the hop flavonoid xanthohumol: NF-kappaB and Akt as targets. *FASEB J.* 2006;20(3):527-529.

Allen PC. Anticoccidial effects of xanthohumol. *Avian Dis.* 2007;51(1):21-26.

Casaschi A, Maiyoh GK, Rubio BK, et al. The chalcone xanthohumol inhibits triglyceride and apolipoprotein B secretion in HepG2 cells. *J Nutr.* 2004;134(6):1340-1346.

Cho YC, Kim HJ, Kim YJ, et al. Differential anti-inflammatory pathway by xanthohumol in IFN-gamma and LPS-activated macrophages. *Int Immunopharmacol.* 2008;8(4):567-573.

Colgate EC, Miranda CL, Stevens JF, et al. Xanthohumol, a prenylflavonoid derived from hops induces apoptosis and inhibits NF-kappaB activation in prostate epithelial cells. *Cancer Lett.* 2007;246(1-2):201-209.

Dell'Eva R, Ambrosini C, Vannini N. AKT/NF-kappaB inhibitor xanthohumol targets cell growth and angiogenesis in hematologic malignancies. *Cancer.* 2007;110(9):2007-2011.

Dietz BM, Kang YH, Liu G, et al. Xanthohumol isolated from Humulus lupulus Inhibits menadione-induced DNA damage through induction of quinone reductase. *Chem Res Toxicol.* 2005;18(8):1296-1305.

Frölich S, Schubert C, Bienzle U, et al. In vitro antiplasmodial activity of prenylated chalcone derivatives of hops (Humulus lupulus) and their interaction with haemin. *J Antimicrob Chemother.* 2005;55(6):883-887.

Gerhauser C, Alt A, Heiss E, et al. Cancer chemopreventive activity of Xanthohumol, a natural product derived from hop. *Mol Cancer Ther.* 2002;1(11):959-969.

Gerhäuser C. Broad spectrum anti-infective potential of xanthohumol from hop (Humulus lupulus L.) in comparison with activities of other hop constituents and xanthohumol metabolites. *Mol Nutr Food Res.* 2005;49(9):827-831.

Goto K, Asai T, Hara S, et al. Enhanced antitumor activity of xanthohumol, a diacylglycerol acyltransferase inhibitor, under hypoxia. *Cancer Lett.* 2005;219(2):215-222.

Herath W, Ferreira D, Khan SI, et al. Identification and biological activity of microbial metabolites of xanthohumol. *Chem Pharm Bull* (Tokyo). 2003;51(11):1237-1240.

Herath WH, Ferreira D, Khan IA. Microbial transformation of xanthohumol. *Phytochemistry.* 2003;62(5):673-677.

Kac J, Plazar J, Mlinaric A, et al. Antimutagenicity of hops (Humulus lupulus L.): bioassay-directed fractionation and isolation of xanthohumol. *Phytomedicine.* 2008;15(3):216-220.

Kim HJ, Lee IS. Microbial metabolism of the prenylated chalcone xanthohumol. *J Nat Prod.* 2006;69(10):1522-1524.

Koo JH, Kim HT, Yoon HY, et al. Effect of xanthohumol on melanogenesis in B16 melanoma cells. *Exp Mol Med.* 2008;40(3):313-319.

Lee SH, Kim HJ, Lee JS, et al. Inhibition of topoisomerase I activity and efflux drug transporters' expression by xanthohumol. from hops. *Arch Pharm Res.* 2007;30(11):1435-1439.

Meissner O, Häberlein H. Influence of xanthohumol on the binding behavior of GABAA receptors and their lateral mobility at hippocampal neurons. *Planta Med.* 2006;72(7):656-658.

Monteiro R, Calhau C, Silva AO, et al. Xanthohumol inhibits inflammatory factor production and angiogenesis in breast cancer xenografts. *J Cell Biochem.* 2008;104(5):1699-1707.

Nikolic D, Li Y, Chadwick LR, et al. Metabolism of xanthohumol and isoxanthohumol, prenylated flavonoids from hops (Humulus lupulus L.), by human liver microsomes. *J Mass Spectrom.* 2005;40(3):289-299.

Nozawa H. Xanthohumol, the chalcone from beer hops (Humulus lupulus L.), is the ligand for farnesoid X receptor and ameliorates lipid and glucose metabolism in KK-A(y) mice. *Biochem Biophys Res Commun.* 2005;336(3):754-761.

Pan L, Becker H, Gerhäuser C. Xanthohumol induces apoptosis in cultured 40-16 human colon cancer cells by activation of the death receptor- and mitochondrial pathway. *Mol Nutr Food Res.* 2005;49(9):837-843.

Plazar J, Filipic M, Groothuis GM. Antigenotoxic effect of Xanthohumol in rat liver slices. *Toxicol In Vitro.* 2008;22(2):318-327.

Plazar J, Zegura B, Lah TT, et al. Protective effects of xanthohumol against the genotoxicity of benzo(a)pyrene (BaP), 2-amino-3-methylimidazo[4,5-f]quinoline (IQ) and tert-butyl hydroperoxide (t-BOOH) in HepG2 human hepatoma cells. *Mutat Res.* 2007;632(1-2):1-8.

Possemiers S, Bolca S, Grootaert C, et al. The prenylflavonoid isoxanthohumol from hops (Humulus lupulus L.) is activated into the potent phytoestrogen 8-prenylnaringenin in vitro and in the human intestine. *J Nutr.* 2006;136(7):1862-1867.

Radovi B, Schmutzler C, Köhrle J. Xanthohumol stimulates iodide uptake in rat thyroid-derived FRTL-5 cells. *Mol Nutr Food Res.* 2005;49(9):832-836.

Ruefer CE, Gerhäuser C, Frank N, et al. In vitro phase II metabolism of xanthohumol by human UDP-glucuronosyltransferases and sulfotransferases. *Mol Nutr Food Res.* 2005;49(9):851-856.

Vogel S, Ohmayer S, Brunner G, et al. Natural and non-natural prenylated chalcones: synthesis, cytotoxicity and anti-oxidative activity. *Bioorg Med Chem.* 2008;16(8):4286-4293.

Wang Q, Ding ZH, Liu JK, et al. Xanthohumol, a novel anti-HIV-1 agent purified from Hops Humulus lupulus. *Antiviral Res.* 2004;64(3):189-194.

Yang JY, Della-Fera MA, Rayalam S, et al. Enhanced effects of xanthohumol plus honokiol on apoptosis in 3T3-L1 adipocytes. *Obesity* (Silver Spring). 2008;16(6):1232-1238.

Yang JY, Della-Fera MA, Rayalam S, et al. Effect of xanthohumol and isoxanthohumol on 3T3-L1 cell apoptosis and adipogenesis. *Apoptosis.* 2007;12(11):1953-1963.

Yilmazer M, Stevens JF, Buhler DR. In vitro glucuronidation of xanthohumol, a flavonoid in hop and beer, by rat and human liver microsomes. *FEBS Lett.* 2001;491(3):252-256.

Yilmazer M, Stevens JF, Deinzer ML, et al. In vitro biotransformation of xanthohumol, a flavonoid from hops (Humulus lupulus), by rat liver microsomes. *Drug Metab Dispos.* 2001;29(3):223-231.

Zanoli P, Zavatti M. Pharmacognostic and pharmacological profile of Humulus lupulus L. *J Ethnopharmacol.* 2008;116(3):383-396.

Xylitol

DESCRIPTION

Xylitol is classified as a "sugar alcohol." It has similar sweetness to sucrose, but in a strict chemical sense it is not really a sugar; it is a polyhydroxy alcohol. A sugar is defined chemically as a polyhydroxy aldehyde (eg, glucose) or a polyhydroxy ketone (eg, fructose). However, since "sugar alcohol" is the term commonly used, including by the FDA, for xylitol and other polyhydroxy alcohols, that is the term that will be used in this monograph. Xylitol is a five-carbon acyclic polyhydroxy alcohol, or polyol (pentitol), named for its corresponding aldose, the sugar xylose. Xylitol is found naturally in small quantities in fruits and vegetables, including plums, strawberries, raspberries and rowan berries. It is also found in corn husks, mushrooms and oats. Xylitol was first derived from the complex carbohydrate xylan from birch trees in Finland, where it was called birch sugar, or koivusokeri. About 5 to 10 grams of xylitol are made daily in the human body, from its corresponding aldose xylose and from its corresponding ketose xylulose.

Xylitol was first popularized in Europe as a safe sweetener for diabetics. It is now widely used as a low-calorie sweetener and for several health conditions. These include caries, middle ear infections (otitis media), and sinus infections, among other health concerns. Currently, most of the world supply of xylitol is derived from corn sources and reportedly comes mainly from China.

Xylitol is also known as *xylo*-pentane-1,2,3,4,5-pentol, (2*R*,3*R*,4*S*)-pentane-1,2,3,4,5-pentanol, 1,2,3,4,5-pentahydroxypentane, xylite, and birch sugar (see above). Its molecular formula is $C_5H_{12}O_5$, its molecular weight is 152.15, and its CAS registration number is 87-99-0. Xylitol is written without an L or a D prefix owing to the symmetry of the molecule. Xylitol is represented by the following chemical structure.

$$CH_2OH$$
$$H{-}OH$$
$$HO{-}H$$
$$H{-}OH$$
$$CH_2OH$$

Xylitol

When chewed in the form of gum, xylitol has a cooling effect in the mouth, which is accounted for by the endothermic reaction that occurs when xylitol is dissolved. Sportswear is available that uses xylitol infused into the fabric in order to absorb the heat coming from perspiration. The energy content of xylitol is 2.4 kcal per gram. In comparison, the energy content of sucrose is 4 kcal per gram.

The FDA allows the claim to be made that the noncariogenic carbohydrate sweetener xylitol present in the food does not promote tooth decay, and may reduce the risk of tooth decay. Other "sugar alcohols" considered noncariogenic include sorbitol, mannitol, lactitol, isomalt (a disaccharide composed of the sugar glucose and the sugar alcohol mannitol), erythritol, and hydrogenated starch hydrolysates (a mixture of several sugar alcohols). Also, the claim is allowed for the sugars tagatose (a monosaccharide) and isomaltulose (a disaccharide that is a natural constituent of honey). This is because the FDA was convinced that isomaltulose and tagatose were not fermented by oral bacteria to an extent sufficient to lower dental plaque pH to levels that would contribute to the erosion of dental enamel.

ACTIONS AND PHARMACOLOGY

ACTIONS

Xylitol is a low-calorie sweetener, suitable for use by diabetics. Xylitol has anticariogenic activity and may have antimicrobial activity against middle ear infections (otitis media), nasal and sinus infections, and pulmonary infections. It also may have antiosteoporotic activity. Xylitol may have some benefits for the treatment of the inborn errors of metabolism, such as myoadenylate deaminase deficiency and glucose-6-phosphate dehydrogenase deficiency.

MECHANISM OF ACTION

Anticariogenic activity: Dental caries are the localized destruction of susceptible dental hard tissues by acidic by-products from bacterial fermentation of dietary carbohydrates. The disease process starts within the bacterial biofilm also known as dental plaque. The bacteria that comprise the biofilm are mainly *Streptococcus mutans*, *Streptococcus sobrinus* and *Lactobacillus* spp.

These bacteria ferment sugars such as sucrose, producing lactic acid. Lactic acid causes local pH to fall, resulting in the demineralization of tooth tissues. If the diffusion of calcium, carbonate and phosphate out of the tooth is allowed to continue, caries will eventually form. This process can be reversed in its early stages through uptake of calcium, phosphate and fluoride. Fluoride works by causing diffusion of calcium and phosphate into the tooth, which remineralizes the crystalline structure of the lesion. The rebuilt crystalline surfaces are composed of fluoridated hydroxyapatite and fluorapatite, which is much more resistant to acid attack than is the original structure.

Administration of xylitol is another way of preventing dental decay. There are now many human studies, beginning in 1970 in Finland, testing the effect of xylitol on the growth of dental plaque and the formation of dental caries. In the early studies, diets containing xylitol were compared with diets containing sucrose or fructose. In later studies, xylitol was presented to the subjects in the form of chewing gum. In most cases, xylitol was demonstrated to decrease the formation of dental caries. *Streptococcus mutans*, the major cariogenic bacterium in the mouth, is able to transport xylitol into the cell. It does this via the fructose phosphotransferase system. Once inside, xylitol is phosphorylated to xylitol-5-phosphate. *S. mutans* cannot ferment the five carbon structure of xylitol to form lactic acid as it can six- and 12 carbon sugars. *S. mutans* has to expel xylitol-5-phosphate in order to survive. This futile energy-consuming xylitol cycle is thought to be responsible for the inhibition of the growth of the cariogenic bacteria, both *in vitro* and *in vivo*. Xylitol was also thought to prevent the adhesion of the biofilm to the teeth.

Antiosteoporotic: Animal studies found that xylitol prevents experimental osteoporosis and improves the properties of bones and collagen. The mechanism of these effects is unclear, and more research is warranted. There is some evidence that xylitol increases calcium absorption independent of the effect of vitamin D.

Low-calorie sweetener: The energy content of xylitol is 2.4 kcal per gram. In comparison, the energy content of sucrose is 4 kcal per gram. Xylitol and sucrose have equal levels of sweetness and there is no after taste with xylitol, which is to say that, in addition to its reduced calories, xylitol has excellent organoleptic ("mouth feel") qualities for a sugar substitute. Xylitol has been an excellent sugar substitute for diabetics. Following its ingestion, there is little change in plasma glucose and insulin levels.

Nasal and sinus infections: Preliminary studies with xylitol suggest that it also may have some utility against nasal and sinus infections. More research is required to establish this effect. The mechanism of action of such an effect should be similar to that described for xylitol and otitis media (see below).

Otitis media: Xylitol has been found to be effective in preventing acute otitis media (middle ear infection) by up to 42% when administered either in the form of chewing gum or as a syrup. Otitis media develops when bacteria from the nasopharynx—usually *Streptococcus pneumoniae,* whose growth is known to be inhibited by xylitol—enter the middle ear through the Eustachian tube. The mechanism of the inhibitory effect is not completely known. Possibilities include: Xylitol is known to have anti-adhesive effects on both *S. pneumoniae* and *Haemophilus influenzae,* which are mediated by its effect on the cell wall of the bacteria; xylitol is an unsuitable source of energy for these bacteria (see: Anticariogenic activity, above); xylitol causes a marked reduction in the intracellular redox state due to the rapid production of NADH and NADPH in the polyol dehydrogenase reaction. This could improve the oxidative burst in polymorphonuclear leukocytes with consequent bacterial killing via reactive oxygen species.

Pulmonary infections: A study reported in the Proceedings of the National Academy of Sciences (PNAS) has introduced still another way of accounting for the antimicrobial effect of xylitol. It appears that the surface of the airways is covered by a thin layer of liquid. This liquid contains a number of antimicrobial substances, including lysozyme, lactoferrin, secretory leukoproteinase inhibitor, human beta defensins 1 and 2, secretory phospholipase A2 and cathelicidin LL-37. These substances form part of the pulmonary defense system, killing the small numbers of bacteria that are constantly being deposited on the pulmonary airway surface. Importantly, the antibacterial activity of most of these substances is salt sensitive. An increase of the salt concentration in the liquid layer inhibits the antibacterial activity of most of the above agents. The study suggested that xylitol delivered to the airway surface appears to lower the salt concentration, thus enhancing the innate antibacterial de-fense system. Further study is needed to test this interesting hypothesis.

Xylitol and myoadenylate deaminase deficiency: Myoadenylate deaminase (muscle AMP deaminase) deficiency is an inborn error of metabolism disorder that is manifested by muscle weakness and cramping after exercise, decreased muscle mass, hypotonia and generalized weakness in some cases. The diagnostic test is based on the lack of an exertional increase in plasma ammonia in patients and was based on the fact that AMP (adenosine phosphate) deaminase is the major ammonia-producing enzyme in skeletal muscles. AMP is comprised of adenine, ribose and phosphate. Ribose is essential in the synthesis of DNA, RNA and ATP, among many other important biological molecules. In myoadenylate deaminase deficiency, some ribose is effectively lost from the metabolic pool and may create a storage deficiency of this crucial metabolite. It was reported that when oral ribose was administered before and after exercise to a patient with this disorder, exercise-related symptoms diminished.

Xylitol can be converted metabolically to ribose, and there is a report that xylitol was beneficial to one patient when administered orally at 15 grams to 20 grams daily.

Xylitol and glucose-6-phosphate dehydrogenase deficiency: Red blood cell glucose-6-phosphate dehydrogenase deficiency (G6PD) is a widespread genetic disorder. Hemolytic anemia is the most serious feature of this disease. The disease is characterized biochemically by a low or almost absent G6PD and an abnormally low red blood cell reduced glutathione (GSH) level. This is because a normal glucose-6-phosphate dehydrogenase is necessary for the production of NADPH, which in turn maintains glutathione in its reduced state. GSH is the major intracellular buffer against oxidative stress, and a deficiency of red blood cell GSH makes the cell very vulnerable to any oxidative threat. In G6PD, the production of NADPH is impaired.

It turns out that the NADP-linked xylitol dehydrogenase is found in red blood cells and that its enzyme activity is normal in most G6PD-deficient red blood cells. Xylitol was demonstrated to preserve GSH levels *in vitro* (rabbit red blood cells) and *in vivo* (rabbits with deficient GSH) and to prevent hemolysis of the red blood cells. Further research in this promising area is certainly warranted.

PHARMACOKINETICS

Many details of the pharmacokinetics of xylitol are still missing. After ingestion, xylitol is absorbed slowly from the small intestine and a portion passes into the large intestine where it is fermented by the microflora of the gut to the short-chain fatty acids, acetate, propionate and butyrate, and the gases hydrogen, hydrogen sulfide, carbon dioxide and methane. The portion that is absorbed from the small intestine is distributed to several tissues in the body, but mainly to the liver. In the liver, xylitol is converted to xylitol-5-phospate. Xylitol-5-phosphate is converted to xylulose-5-phosphate via a polyol dehydrogenase reaction; this metabolite enters the pentose phosphate cycle to be further metabolized.

INDICATIONS AND USAGE

Some, though not all, studies indicate that xylitol, a sugar alcohol found in a number of fruits and vegetables, is an effective anticaries agent. There is some support for claims that xylitol has significant antimicrobial effects and may be useful in treating and preventing otitis media and some lung and nasopharyngeal infections. Scant preliminary *in vitro* and animal data suggest possible contributions to bone, skin and colon health.

RESEARCH SUMMARY

Xylitol has been promoted for some time as an effective anticaries agent and is sold in the form of gum and other products advertised to protect dental health. Evidence that xylitol gums are any better than gums sweetened with sorbitol or other sugar alcohol is inconsistently demonstrated in clinical trials that have sought to assess the effects of these gums on tooth decay. One review of the literature found that the claimed superiority of xylitol was not demonstrated in two out of four clinical trials comparing the anticaries potential of xylitol with that of sorbitol-sweetened gums. These reviewers, in fact, concluded that, to the extent any positive effect was observed, it was more likely due to the stimulation of salivary flow, which was roughly equal irrespective of the type of gum chewed. They did not, however, entirely rule out the possibility of a relevant xylitol-related antimicrobial effect. Some studies have found that xylitol does, indeed, significantly suppress some oral bacteria, specifically *Streptococcus mutans,* but it has not been conclusively demonstrated that this effect significantly impedes the formation of dental caries. One can say, however, that xylitol is highly unlikely to promote caries, as certain sugars are known to do. More research will be required to definitively determine whether xylitol is superior to sorbitol as an anticaries agent.

A number of recent studies suggest that xylitol may have significant antimicrobial effects that could be clinically beneficial in a number of circumstances. One of these studies, performed double-blind and placebo-controlled, demonstrated that xylitol, whether administered in a gum or in a syrup, was significantly superior to xylitol-devoid chewing gum and xylitol-devoid syrup in preventing acute otitis media (AOM) in healthy children. The study continued for three months, during which time the experimental subjects received 8.4 to 10 grams of xylitol daily. Whereas

41% of the children who received control syrup experienced at least one incident of AOM, only 29% of those receiving xylitol syrup were similarly affected. Occurrence of AOM decreased by even more among those taking the xylitol gum versus those using the non-xylitol gum. Given the apparent efficacy of xylitol in this study and the high economic costs of AOM, further research is needed and warranted.

Numerous animal studies have demonstrated additional antimicrobial effects. In a recent trial, xylitol-supplemented nutrition was found to enhance bacterial killing and prolong survival of rats in experimental pneumococcal sepsis. A finding of the study was enhanced neutrophilic leukocyte function. A previous report had demonstrated that parenteral administration of xylitol could significantly improve survival of rats suffering intestinal sepsis. A study in which xylitol was shown to enhance bacterial killing in the rabbit maxillary sinus led the researchers to conclude that xylitol might be useful in some cases of human sinusitis. Far more study will be required to establish this.

In one double-blind, placebo-controlled clinical trial, xylitol was sprayed for four days into each nostril of volunteers. Compared with saline-administered controls, the experimental subjects receiving the xylitol spray exhibited significantly decreased numbers of nasal coagulase-negative *Staphylococcus.* This research further revealed some evidence suggesting that xylitol might be of benefit in cystic fibrosis through positive effects in the human airway. Again, more research is needed and warranted.

In a study utilizing an *in vitro* colon simulator, another group of researchers reported positive effects of xylitol on the metabolic activity and patterns of colon microbes, suggesting that the sugar alcohol might have some benefit on colonic health. Other, similarly very preliminary *in vitro* and animal research has pointed toward possible positive effects of xylitol on bone and skin. One study showed that dietary xylitol helped protect against weakening of bone biomechanical properties in an experimental model of postmenopausal osteoporosis. The same group subsequently demonstrated improved bone biomechanical properties in xylitol-fed, aged male rats. Clinical trials are needed to see whether xylitol can have any bone-strengthening effects in humans. Similarly, a finding that long-term dietary xylitol supplementation increases the synthesis of collagen in the skin of aging rats needs further exploration and extension into clinical inquiry.

CONTRAINDICATIONS, PRECAUTIONS, ADVERSE REACTIONS
CONTRAINDICATIONS
Xylitol is contraindicated in those who are hypersensitive to any component of a xylitol-containing product.

PRECAUTIONS

Those who develop gastrointestinal symptoms (flatus, bloating, diarrhea) with the use of xylitol should start with lower doses and slowly go up in dose. Those receiving whole body radiation or radiation to the gastrointestinal tract should avoid xylitol until they have completed their course of radiation. Those with diarrhea-prominent irritable bowel syndrome should begin the use of xylitol at low doses and increase the dose as tolerated.

ADVERSE REACTIONS

Doses of xylitol up to 30 to 60 grams daily are usually well tolerated. Higher doses may cause gastrointestinal symptoms, such as flatulence, bloating and diarrhea, in an unadapted user. Adapted users have gone up to 400 grams daily without any side effects. The most common side effect is flatulence. Some may have side effects at lower doses, eg, a person with diarrhea-prominent irritable bowel syndrome.

There are a couple of reports of dogs having serious adverse events after ingesting xylitol. In one report, eight adult dogs were evaluated for treatment of lethargy, vomiting, widespread petechial, ecchymotic, or gastrointestinal hemorrhages, hyperglycemia, hyperbirubinemia and thrombocytopenia. Three dogs were euthanized, two dogs died, two dogs made a complete recovery, and one dog was recovering, but was lost to follow-up. In another report, a 9-month old Labrador retriever developed hypoglycemia nad seizures after ingesting a large quantity of gum swetened with xylitol. There have been other reports of dogs becoming hypoglycemic after consuming xylitol. There are no such reports for humans.

INTERACTIONS

DRUGS

No known interactions.

FOODS

No known interactions.

NUTRITIONAL SUPPLEMENTS

Arginine-containing mints have been found to have anticariogenic activity secondary to their ability to buffer the acid produced by cariogenic bacteria. Mints containing a combination of xylitol and arginine may give better anticariogenic effects that the use of either alone.

OTHER

The combination of xylitol and the use of fluoride toothpastes may give better anticariogenic effects than the use of either alone.

OVERDOSAGE

No reports.

DOSAGE AND ADMINISTRATION

Xylitol is available as chewing gum, as a nasal wash, in bulk as a sugar substitute and as mints. For dental benefits, 4 to 12 grams of xylitol daily are used. The chewing gum and mints typically contain about 1 gram of xylitol in each piece. One can start by chewing one piece four times a day for a total of 4 grams and work up from there to a total of 12 to 15 grams daily. For prevention of otitis media, 8.5 to 10 grams of chewing gum or syrup was used taken in five divided doses over a course of two months a study.

LITERATURE

Alanen P. Does chewing explain the caries-preventive results with xylitol? *J Dent Res.* 2001;80(7):1600-1601.

Amaechi BT, Higham SM, Edgar WM. Caries inhibiting and remineralizing effect of xylitol in vitro. *J Oral Sci.* 1999;41(2):71-76.

Brown CL, Graham SM, Cable BB, et al. Xylitol enhances bacterial killing in the rabbit maxillary sinus. *Laryngoscope.* 2004;114(11):2021-2024.

Caglar E, Kavaloglu SC, Kuscu OO, et al. Effect of chewing gums containing xylitol or probiotic bacteria on salivary mutans streptococci and lactobacilli. *Clin Oral Investig.* 2007;11(4):425-429.

Chunmuang S, Jitpukdeebodintra S, Chuenarrom C, et al. Effect of xylitol and fluoride on enamel erosion in vitro. *J Oral Sci.* 2007;49(4):293-297.

Granström TB, Izumori K, Leisola M. A rare sugar xylitol. Part II: biotechnological production and future applications of xylitol. *Appl Microbiol Biotechnol.* 2007;74(2):273-276.

Granström TB, Izumori K, Leisola M. A rare sugar xylitol. Part I: the biochemistry and biosynthesis of xylitol. *Appl Microbiol Biotechnol.* 2007;74(2):277-281.

Grillaud M, Bandon D, Nancy J, et al. [The polyols in pediatric dentistry: advantages of xylitol] [Article in French.] *Arch Pediatr.* 2005;12(7):1180-1186.

Hildebrandt GH, Sparks BS. Maintaining mutans streptococci suppression with xylitol chewing gum. *J Am Dent Assoc.* 2000;131(7):909-916.

Kontiokari T, Uhari M, Koskela M. Effect of xylitol on growth of nasopharyngeal bacteria in vitro. *Antimicrob Agents Chemother.* 1995;39(8):1820-1823.

Maguire A, Rugg-Gunn AJ. Xylitol and caries prevention–is it a magic bullet? *Br Dent J.* 2003;194(8):429-436.

Makinen KK. Xylitol: the sugar that does not cause tooth decay. *Refuat Hapeh Vehashinayim.* 1978;27(2):36-37.

Makinen KK. Xylitol—a therapeutic and caries inhibitory natural carbohydrate. *N M Dent J.* 1976;26(4):13,20-21.

Mattila P, Knuuttila M, Kovanen V, et al. Improved bone biomechanical properties in rats after oral xylitol administration. *Calcif Tissue Int.* 1999;64(4):340-344.

Mattila PT, Knuuttila ML, Svanberg MJ. Dietary xylitol supplementation prevents osteoporotic changes in streptozotocin-diabetic rats. *Metabolism*. 1998;47(5):578-583.

Mattila P, Svanberg M, Knuuttila M. Diminished bone resorption in rats after oral xylitol administration: a dose-response study. *Calcif Tissue Int*. 1995;56(3):232-235.

Mattila PT, Svanberg MJ, Jämsä T, et al. Improved bone biomechanical properties in xylitol-fed aged rats. *Metabolism*. 2002;51(1):92-96.

Mattila PT, Svanberg MJ, Knuuttila ML. Increased bone volume and bone mineral content in xylitol-fed aged rats. *Gerontology*. 2001;47(6):300-305.

Mattila PT, Svanberg MJ, Pökkä P, et al. Dietary xylitol protects against weakening of bone biomechanical properties in ovariectomized rats. *J Nutr*. 1998;128(10):1811-1814.

Mattila PT, Pelkonen P, Knuuttila ML. Effects of a long-term dietary xylitol supplementation on collagen content and fluorescence of the skin in aged rats. *Gerontology*. 2005;51(3):166-169.

Renko M, Valkonen P, Tapiainen T, et al. Xylitol-supplemented nutrition enhances bacterial killing and prolongs survival of rats in experimental pneumococcal sepsis. *BMC Microbiol*. 2008;8:45.

Tapiainen T, Kontiokari T, Sammalkivi L, et al. Effect of xylitol on growth of Streptococcus pneumoniae in the presence of fructose and sorbitol. *Antimicrob Agents Chemother*. 2001;45(1):166-169.

Uhari M, Kontiokari T, Koskela M, et al. Xylitol chewing gum in prevention of acute otitis media: double blind randomised trial. *BMJ*. 1996;313(7066):1180-1184.

Uhari M, Kontiokari T, Niemelä M. A novel use of xylitol sugar in preventing acute otitis media. *Pediatrics*. 1998;102(4 Pt 1):879-884.

Uhari M, Tapiainen T, Kontiokari T. Xylitol in preventing acute otitis media. *Vaccine*. 2000;19 Suppl 1:S144-147.

Van Loveren C. Sugar alcohols: what is the evidence for caries-preventive and caries-therapeutic effects? *Caries Res*. 2004;38(3):286-293.

Yeast Beta-D-Glucan

DESCRIPTION

Beta-D-glucans are nondigestible polysaccharides widely found in nature in such sources as cereal grains, including oats and barley, as well as in yeast, bacteria, algae and mushrooms. Beta-D-glucans are primarily located in the cell walls. Yeast beta-D-glucan is marketed as a nutritional supplement. The yeast beta-D-glucan in the supplement is a polyglucose polysaccharide derived from the cell walls of baker's yeast or *Saccharomyces cerevisiae*.

Yeast beta-D-glucan, usually referred to as yeast beta-glucan, consists of straight-chain and branched polymers. The straight-chain structures are (1/3)-beta-D-linked glucose polymers and (1/6)-beta-D-linked glucose polymers. The branched polymers consist of a (1/3)-beta-D-linked backbone containing varying degrees of (1-6)-beta branches. Yeast beta-glucan is sometimes designated as beta 1, 3/1, 6 glucan.

Yeast beta-glucan appears to have immunomodulatory properties. It can bind to various cells of the non-specific immune system, such as macrophages and neutrophils. PGG-glucan or poly- [1, 6]-beta-D-glucopyranosyl- [1,3]-beta-D-glucopyranose is a genetically modified *Saccharomyces cerevisiae* beta-glucan. It is being evaluated in clinical studies as an immunomodulatory agent and a biological response modifier.

Zymosan is the name of a cell wall preparation derived from *Saccharomyces cerevisiae*, which contains beta (1/3)-glucan, beta (1/6)-glucan and other components of the cell wall, such as chitin and mannoprotein. Zymosan's immunological effects are mainly attributed to the beta-glucans.

ACTIONS AND PHARMACOLOGY

ACTIONS

Yeast beta-glucan may have immunomodulatory and lipid-lowering activity.

MECHANISM OF ACTION

Most of the studies done with yeast beta-glucan have been performed in tissue culture, in animals and with PGG-glucan, which is administered parenterally. Yeast beta-glucan can bind to a beta-glucan receptor in macrophages and stimulate the production of such cytokines as TNF (tumor necrosis factor)-alpha and IL (interleukin)-I beta. Binding to the beta-glucan receptor may also induce the release of such reactive oxygen species as superoxide anions and hydrogen peroxide. Yeast beta-glucan may also stimulate such cells as neutrophils NK (natural killer cells) and LAK (lymphokine-activated killer) cells. All of the above stimulation effects may result in antimicrobial and tumoricidal activities.

Research on PGG-glucan indicates that it interacts with receptors on monocytes and neutrophils. It is thought that this interaction primes these cells for production of cytokines and other immune-modulating substances when they are needed. In this sense, yeast beta-glucan may be considered an immune system primer.

The possible immunomodulatory effects of oral yeast beta-glucan remain unclear. Yeast beta-glucan is an indigestible polysaccharide and very little hydrolysis of it takes place in the stomach or small intestine. There is some digestion of yeast beta-glucan that does take place in the large intestine via bacterial beta-glucosidases, and some remnants of this digestion, oligosaccharides with molecular weights of up to 20,000 daltons, have been detected in the serum of animals, as well as of humans, following ingestion of yeast beta-glucan. However, it is not known if these absorbed oligosaccharides have any immunological or other biological activity. Oral yeast beta-glucan may have immunological activity by virtue of its interaction with gut-associated lymphoid tissue (GALT). Immune cells associated with GALT may be activated via their contact with yeast beta-glucan in the gut and migrate to other tissues where they may exert immunomodulatory effects.

Yeast beta-glucan has been found to lower total cholesterol levels as well as to increase levels of HDL-cholesterol. The mechanism of the HDL-elevation activity is unknown. Also, it is not well understood how beta-glucans, including oat beta-glucans, lower total cholesterol levels. It is thought that the cholesterol-lowering effect of oat beta-glucan may be accounted for, in large part, by its promotion of the excretion of bile acids. Yeast beta-glucan may also promote the excretion of bile acids.

PHARMACOKINETICS

Following ingestion, there is virtually no digestion of yeast beta-glucan in the small intestine. The glycosidic linkages of yeast beta-glucan are of the beta type, and there are no beta-glucosidases among the digestive enzymes. Some digestion of yeast beta-glucan does take place in the large intestine via the action of bacterial beta-glucosidases. Some oligosaccharides up to molecular weight of 20,000 daltons that are produced via the bacterial beta-glucosidases may get absorbed. A large percentage of the ingested yeast beta-glucan is excreted in the feces.

INDICATIONS AND USAGE

Yeast beta-glucan appears to be a non-specific immune enhancer via its ability, among other possible mechanisms, to activate macrophages. It may have some anticarcinogenic, antiatherosclerotic and anti-inflammatory effects, may enhance wound healing and promote skin health in some circumstances.

RESEARCH SUMMARY

Yeast beta-glucan has been demonstrated to have non-specific immune-enhancing effects in *in vitro* and some animal and human studies. This substance binds to an activating receptor site on macrophages in humans, as well as in many animal species. In some of these experiments, yeast beta-glucan has exhibited antibacterial, antifungal and antiviral effects.

A genetically modified yeast beta-glucan enhanced the ability of monocytes and neutrophils to kill microbes in healthy volunteers. Subsequently, high-risk surgical patients were given placebo or this yeast beta-glucan in a double-blind, randomized trial. Those receiving the beta-glucan had significantly fewer postoperative infections than did controls. They also had decreased antibiotic requirement and shorter length of stay in intensive care.

Macrophage activation may be one of the mechanisms that also accounts for some of the anti-inflammatory and anticarcinogenic activities associated with yeast beta-glucan in preliminary experimental work. This substance has shown some activity against human melanoma and basal cell carcinoma *in vitro*. Tumor growth inhibition and increased survival times have been observed in animals with transplanted melanoma, adenocarcinoma, mammary carcinoma and lymphocytic leukemia.

Used in combination with some antimicrobial and anticancer drugs, yeast beta-glucan appears to have beneficial synergistic effects in some circumstances. Synergy has been reported with respect to ampicillin, gentamicin, amphotericin B and 5-fluorouracil, among others, in certain situations.

Yeast beta-glucan has been shown to be radioprotective in some circumstances when administered either pre- or post-radiation. This largely *in vitro* and animal work needs clinical followup.

Given that the oat beta-glucan (see Oat Beta-Glucan) has established hypocholesterolemic effects, research has been conducted to see if yeast beta-glucan also has this activity. Recently, obese hypercholesterolemic men given 15 grams of yeast beta-glucan fiber daily for eight weeks had significantly reduced plasma total cholesterol. They had a non-significant decline in LDL-cholesterol. A significant increase in HDL-cholesterol levels was noted four weeks after cessation of fiber administration.

Lipid effects of yeast beta-glucan were said to be similar to those seen with the use of oat beta-glucan with respect to total cholesterol and superior with respect to HDL-cholesterol. This superiority, however, might be due to the use in this study of significantly higher doses of fiber than were used in the oat studies.

The ability of yeast beta-glucan to activate the macrophagic activity of the Langerhans cells of the skin may account for some of the reported significant wound healing properties of this substance. Yeast beta-glucan has also been reported to improve skin dryness and elasticity, and has thus been promoted for cosmetic uses.

There is one study that suggests this substance can have some revitalizing effects on aging skin. Among 150 female volunteers, aged 35 to 60, those given a cosmetic preparation containing yeast beta-glucan were said to have significantly reduced number, depth and length of wrinkles, compared with controls. Dryness and elasticity of skin were also improved. Further research is needed to confirm or refute these findings.

CONTRAINDICATIONS, PRECAUTIONS, ADVERSE REACTIONS

CONTRAINDICATIONS

Yeast beta-glucan is contraindicated in those who are hypersensitive to any component of a yeast beta-glucan containing product.

PRECAUTIONS

Pregnant women and nursing mothers should avoid yeast beta-glucan supplementation.

INTERACTIONS

DRUGS

Antibiotics, antifungal agents, cancer chemotherapeutic agents: Animal studies have shown some synergistic effects when these substances were used concomitantly with yeast beta-glucan.

OVERDOSAGE

There are no reports of overdosage.

DOSAGE AND ADMINISTRATION

The introduction of yeast beta-glucan supplements has been recent. There are no typical doses.

LITERATURE

Babineau TJ, Hackford A, Kenler A, et al. A phase II multicenter, double-blind, randomized, placebo-controlled study of three dosages of an immunomodulator (PGG-glucan) in high-risk surgical patients. *Arch Surg.* 1994; 129:1204-1210.

Babineau TJ, Marcello P, Swails W, et al. Randomized phase I/II trial of a macrophage-specific immunomodulator (PGG-glucan) in high risk surgical patients. *Ann Surg.* 1994; 220:601-609.

Bell S, Goldman VM, Bistrian BR, et al. Effect of beta-glucan from oats and yeast on serum lipids. *Crit Rev Food Sci Nutr.* 1999; 39:189-202.

Nicolosi R, Bell SJ, Bistrian BR, et al. Plasma lipid changes after supplementation with beta-glucan fiber from yeast. *Am J Clin Nutr.* 1999; 70:208-212.

Williams DL, Mueller A, Browder W. Glucan-based macrophage stimulators: a review of their anti-infective potential. *Clin Immunother.* 1996; 5:392-399.

Yogurt

DESCRIPTION

Yogurt is a coagulated milk product that results from the fermentation of milk by the bacteria *Lactobacillus bulgaricus* and *Streptococcus thermophilus*. In addition to *L. bulgaricus* and *S. thermophilus*, other members of the *Lactobacillus* genus, such as *L. acidophilus* and other lactic acid-bacteria, can be used in the process of producing yogurt. Collectively, the bacteria used to make yogurt are called lactic acid bacteria (LAB). All of the LAB produce lactic acid. The acid fermentation curdles the milk and preserves it from putrefaction and spoilage. For centuries, many have believed that fermented milk products such as yogurt are beneficial for health. Elie Metchnikoff, the father of modern immunology, wrote in his book, *The Prolongation of Life: Optimistic Studies*, that yogurt was beneficial for gastrointestinal health, as well as for the promotion of longevity. Some recent research on yogurt suggests that it may have immunostimulatory effects, as well as other benefits.

ACTIONS AND PHARMACOLOGY

ACTIONS

Yogurt may have immunostimulatory and other immunomodulatory activities. It may also have hypocholesterolemic activity.

MECHANISM OF ACTION

The possible immunostimulatory activity of yogurt is probably due to the presence of lactic acid bacteria, as well as nonbacterial components of yogurt. The cell wall of lactic acid bacteria is composed of peptidoglycans, teichoic acid and polysaccharides. The peptidoglycans may induce adjuvant activity at the mucosal surface. Muramyl dipeptide, a lower-molecular-weight breakdown product of the peptidoglycans, may stimulate cytokine production by macrophages, monocytes and lymphocytes. Teichoic acid may also stimulate the production of certain cytokines by monocytes. The lactic acid bacteria may increase secretory IgA activity in the gastrointestinal tract, as well.

Nonbacterial components of yogurt may also contribute to the possible immunostimulatory activity of yogurt. Oligopeptides produced via the fermentation process may enhance phagocytic activity. Some bioactive peptides resulting from the fermentation process may stimulate the proliferation and maturation of T lymphocytes and natural killer (NK) cells for defense against pathogenic enteric bacteria.

Yogurt may have a higher concentration of conjugated linoleic acid (CLA) than nonfermented milk. CLA may have immunomodulatory and anticarcinogenic activity, among other possible health benefits (see Conjugated Linoleic Acid). Whey proteins found in yogurt may be another nonbacterial contributor to yogurt's possible immunostimulatory and other beneficial activities. Whey proteins (see Whey Proteins) are especially high in L-cysteine, a key precursor in the biosynthesis of the tripeptide glutathione. Glutathione has antioxidant activity and is involved in the detoxification of many xenobiotics, including some carcinogens. Whey proteins, in addition to their involvement in the synthesis of glutathione, may have immunomodulatory activities.

The mechanism of the possible anti-allergic activity of yogurt is unclear. It is speculated that yogurt may stimulate interferon-gamma production, which in turn may modulate T cell function by downregulating the Th-2 response.

Some studies have suggested a possible hypocholesterolemic activity of yogurt. Again, the mechanism of this possible effect is unclear. It has been speculated that hydroxymethylglutarate in yogurt may inhibit hydroxymethylglutarate coenzyme A (HMG CoA) reductase activity.

PHARMACOKINETICS

The proteins, peptides and amino acids in yogurt are digested, absorbed and metabolized by normal physiological processes. The same is true for the carbohydrates and lipids in yogurt. Most of the lactic acid bacteria in yogurt adhere only temporarily to the mucosa of the colon. Some, *Lactobacillus acidophilus* for example, persist longer. Most of the lactic acid bacteria do not survive stomach acid. Again, some, such as *L. acidophilus*, are more resistant to stomach acid.

INDICATIONS AND USAGE

Yogurt may have a variety of positive immunologic effects and may help fight certain infections. Yogurt may be anticarcinogenic and antiatherogenic in some circumstances. It may also be useful in some gastrointestinal disorders and in some with allergies and asthma. See also Prebiotics, Probiotics and Symbiotics.

RESEARCH SUMMARY

In vitro, animal and a few human studies indicate that yogurt has a number of favorable immunologic effects. These studies have shown that yogurt consumption increases antibody production, cytokine production, phagocyte activity, natural killer cell activity and T cell function. Both bacterial and non-bacterial components in yogurt have been hypothesized to play roles in these effects on immune function.

In a recent study of long-term yogurt consumption among two different age groups (young adults 20 to 40 years of age and seniors 55 to 70), intake of live-culture yogurt, more than pasteurized yogurt, was associated with decreased allergic symptoms in both age groups. Seniors consuming 200 grams of yogurt daily for one year had consistently lower levels of total immunoglobulin than did control seniors who did not consume yogurt.

Some other studies have also shown that yogurt may be effective in reducing IgE-mediated disorders such as asthma. Results, however, have been mixed, and further research is needed.

Some years ago, a small study suggested that a cup of yogurt daily could significantly reduce the incidence of recurrent vaginitis. The study involved women who had at least five occurrences of vaginitis due to candidal infections annually. The yogurt used in the study was confirmed to contain *Lactobacillus acidophilus*. A three-fold reduction in vaginitis was reported in the women who received yogurt daily for six months.

Various yogurt preparations have been shown to inhibit the growth of several cancers in animal studies. Several of the bacterial components of yogurt have been shown to inhibit tumorigenesis, possibly by reducing nitrite concentrations, through immune-modulation and other mechanisms.

Epidemiological data are somewhat conflicting with respect to yogurt intake and cancer incidence. A significantly lower consumption of fermented milk products (primarily yogurt and buttermilk) was seen among breast-cancer patients in one case-control study. But, in another study, greater yogurt consumption was associated with a higher incidence of ovarian cancer. Further research is needed.

There is some evidence that the bacterial components of yogurt can protect against some gastrointestinal tract infections. Some studies have shown that yogurt products can enhance recovery from some forms of diarrhea. Yogurt has also been used with some success to help restore intestinal microflora diminished by antibiotic treatment. Yogurt is also helpful in some with lactose intolerance.

Several studies spanning many years have concluded that yogurt has hypocholesterolemic effects. In one study, animals were fed high-cholesterol diets. Some were supplemented with yogurt and some were not. The supplemented animals had reduced serum cholesterol and reduced low-density lipoproteins. No effects were noted on serum triglycerides.

Recently, a fermented milk product produced a small but statistically significant reduction in total cholesterol and LDL-cholesterol levels in a double-blind, placebo-controlled, crossover study.

For more information, see Prebiotics, Probiotics and Symbiotics.

CONTRAINDICATIONS, PRECAUTIONS, ADVERSE REACTIONS

CONTRAINDICATIONS

Yogurt is contraindicated in those who are hypersensitive to any component of a yogurt-containing preparation.

PRECAUTIONS

Although yogurt contains much less lactose than nonfermented milk, some with lactase-deficiency may still not be able to tolerate yogurt. Generally, however, it is much better tolerated by those with lactase-deficiency than nonfermented milk.

ADVERSE REACTIONS

There are some reports of flatulence and diarrhea in some with lactase-deficiency.

OVERDOSAGE

None known.

DOSAGE AND ADMINISTRATION

Yogurt is available in many different preparations. Yogurt may be considered a functional food. In some yogurt preparations, the lactic acid bacteria have been killed during the processing of the product via pasteurization. Yogurt preparations in which the lactic acid bacteria have been killed may still confer some, but probably not all, of the possible health benefits.

Intake of yogurt is variable. One study showing a possible anti-allergy effect of yogurt used 200 grams daily for one year. Unpasteurized yogurt was found to be more effective than pasteurized yogurt in this study.

LITERATURE

Bertolami MC, Faludi AA, Batlouni M. Evaluation of the effects of a new fermented milk product (G$_{910}$) on primary hypercholesterolemia. *Eur J Clin Nutr.* 1999; 53:97-101.

Danielson AD, Peo ER Jr, Shahani KM, et al. Anticholesterolemic property of Lactobacillus acidophilus yogurt fed to mature boars. *J Anim Sci.* 1989; 67:966-974.

Hepner G, Fried R, St Jeor S, et al. Hypocholesterolemic effect of yogurt and milk. *Am J Clin Nutr.* 1979; 32:19-24.

Hitchins AD, McDonough FE. Prophylactic and therapeutic aspects of fermented milk. *Am J Clin Nutr.* 1989; 49:675-684.

Kolars JC, Levitt MD, Aouji M, Savaiano DA. Yogurt—an autodigesting source of lactose. *N Engl J Med.* 1984; 310:1-3.

Mann GV. A factor in yogurt which lowers cholesterolemia in man. *Atherosclerosis.* 1977; 28:335-340.

Metchnikoff E. *The Prolongation of Life: Optimistic Studies.* The English translation. Mitchell PC, ed. 1908; GP Putnam's Sons: New York.

Meydani SN, Ha W-K. Immunologic effects of yogurt. *Am Clin Nutr.* 2000; 71:861-872.

Van de Water J, Keen CL, Gershwin ME. The influence of chronic yogurt consumption on immunity. *J Nutr.* 1999; 129:1492S-1495S.

Zinc

DESCRIPTION

Zinc is an essential element in human and animal nutrition with a wide range of biological roles. Zinc plays catalytic, structural or regulatory roles in the more than 200 zinc metalloenzymes that have been identified in biological systems. These enzymes are involved in nucleic acid and protein metabolism and the production of energy, among other things. Zinc plays a structural role in the formation of the so-called zinc fingers. Zinc fingers are exploited by transcription factors for interacting with DNA and regulating the activity of genes. Another structural role of zinc is in the maintenance of the integrity of biological membranes resulting in their protection against oxidative injury, among other things.

Zinc is a metallic element with atomic number 30 and an atomic weight of 65.37 daltons. Its atomic symbol is Zn. Zinc exists under physiological conditions in the divalent state. The adult body contains about 1.5 to 2.5 grams of zinc. It is present in all organs, tissues, fluids and secretions. Approximately 90% of total body zinc is found in skeletal muscle and bone. Over 95% of total body zinc is bound to proteins within cells and cell membranes. Plasma contains only 0.1% of total body zinc. Most of the zinc (75% to 88%) in blood is found in the red blood cell zinc metalloenzyme carbonic anhydrase. In the plasma, approximately 18% of zinc is bound to alpha-2-macroglobulin, 80% to albumin and 2% to such proteins as transferrin and ceruloplasmin.

Physiologically, zinc is vital for growth and development, sexual maturation and reproduction, dark vision adaptation, olfactory and gustatory activity, insulin storage and release and for a variety of host immune defenses, among other things. Zinc deficiency can result in growth retardation, immune dysfunction, increased incidence of infections, hypogonadism, oligospermia, anorexia, diarrhea, weight loss, delayed wound healing, neural tube defects of the fetus, increased risk for abortion, alopecia, mental lethargy and skin changes.

Moderate to severe zinc deficiency is rare in industrialized countries. However, it is highly prevalent in developing countries. Many, however, are at risk for mild zinc deficiency in industrialized countries. Several diseases and situations predispose to zinc deficiency, including the autosomal recessive disease acrodermatitis enteropathica, alcoholism, malabsorption, thermal burns, total parenteral nutrition (TPN) without zinc supplementation and certain drugs, such as diuretics, penicillamine, sodium valproate and ethambutol. Zinc intake in many of the elderly may be suboptimal and, if compounded with certain drugs and diseases, can lead to mild or even moderate zinc deficiency.

Zinc acetate is an FDA-approved orphan drug for the treatment of the copper-overload disorder Wilson's disease.

ACTIONS AND PHARMACOLOGY

ACTIONS

Zinc may have immunomodulatory activity. It may also have antioxidant activity. Zinc has putative antiviral, fertility-enhancing and retinoprotective activities.

MECHANISM OF ACTION

Zinc is required for a number of immune functions, including T-lymphocyte activity. Zinc deficiency results in thymic involution, depressed delayed hypersensitivity, decreased peripheral T-lymphocyte count, decreased proliferative T-lymphocyte response to phytohemagglutinin (PHA), decreased cytotoxic T-lymphocyte activity, depressed T helper lymphocyte function, depressed natural killer cell activity, depressed macrophage function (phagocytosis), depressed neutrophil functions (respiratory burst, chemotaxis) and depressed antibody production. Zinc supplementation can restore impaired immune function in those with zinc deficiency, as found in malabsorption syndromes and acrodermatitis enteropathica.

There is little evidence that zinc supplementation will enhance immune responses in those who are not zinc deficient. High doses of zinc may even be immunosuppressive. Zinc supplementation may improve immune function in healthy elderly individuals who are marginally zinc deficient.

The mechanism underlying the immune effects of zinc is not fully understood. Some of these effects may be accounted for by zinc's membrane-stabilization effect. This could affect signaling processes involved in cell-mediated immunity. Zinc is known to be involved in such signaling processes. Zinc may also influence gene expression by structural stabilization of different immunological transcription factors. Zinc ions can induce blast formation of human peripheral blood monocytes (PBMCs). In PBMCs, zinc induces cytokines, including interleukin (IL)-1, IL-6 and tumor necrosis factor (TNF)-alpha. Cytokine induction by zinc is caused by a direct interaction of zinc with monocytes. The stimulation by zinc of T-lymphocytes appears to occur via monocyte released IL-1 and cell-cell contact. High zinc concentrations inhibit T-lymphocyte proliferation by blocking the IL-1 type 1 receptor-associated kinase. T-lymphocyte activation appears to be delicately regulated by zinc concentrations.

Zinc may have secondary antioxidant activity. Zinc does not have redox activity under physiological conditions. Zinc may influence membrane structure by its ability to stabilize thiol groups and phospholipids. It may also occupy sites that might otherwise contain redox active metals such as iron. These effects may protect membranes against oxidative damage. Zinc also comprises the structure of copper/zinc-superoxide dismutase (Cu/Zn-SOD). Zinc plays a structural role in Cu/Zn-SOD. Zinc may also have antioxidant activity via its association with the copper-binding protein metallothionein.

The role of zinc gluconate in the management of the common cold remains controversial (see Research Summary). The mechanisms proposed for zinc's effects on the duration of colds are inhibition by zinc of the replication of rhinoviruses and/or inhibition of virus entry into cells. Zinc ions, however, have only modest nonselective inhibitory effects for rhinoviruses *in vitro*.

Zinc is involved in sperm formation and testosterone metabolism. Zinc deficiency results in oligospermia. There is little evidence that zinc supplementation affects sperm production in those who are not zinc deficient.

The mechanism of the putative effect of zinc in age-related macular degeneration (ARMD) is unknown.

PHARMACOKINETICS

The efficiency of absorption (fractional absorption) of a zinc salt on an empty stomach ranges from 40% to 90%. The fractional absorption of zinc with food appears to be lower. Zinc-histidine, zinc-methionine and zinc-cysteine complexes appear to be more efficiently absorbed than other zinc supplementary forms. Zinc is absorbed all along the small intestine. Most ingested zinc appears to be absorbed from the jejunum. Zinc uptake across the brush border appears to occur by both a saturable barrier-mediated mechanism and a nonsaturable nonmediated mechanism. The exact mechanism of zinc transport into the enterocytes remains unclear. Zinc transporters have been identified in animal models. Once zinc is within the enterocyte, it can be used for zinc-dependent processes, become bound to metallothionein and held within the enterocyte or pass through the cell. Transport of zinc across the serosal membrane is carrier mediated and energy dependent.

Zinc is transported to the liver via the portal circulation. A fraction of zinc is extracted by the hepatocytes, and the remaining zinc is transported to the various cells of the body via the systemic circulation. Zinc is transported in the plasma bound to albumin (about 80%), alpha-2-macroglobulin (about 18%) and to such proteins as transferrin and ceruloplasmin (about 2%). The major route of zinc excretion is via the gastrointestinal tract. Fecal zinc excretion is comprised of unabsorbed zinc and zinc derived from biliary, pancreatic, and gastrointestinal secretions and zinc from sloughing of mucosal cells.

Much of the pharmacokinetics of zinc in humans is unknown. Research is ongoing.

INDICATIONS AND USAGE

Even borderline zinc deficiency or disturbances in zinc metabolism can have profound adverse health effects. Those at greatest risk of such deficiencies and disturbances include infants, children, the elderly and pregnant women. Due to conditions that can limit the bioavailability of zinc, even when there is adequate zinc intake, zinc deficiency may affect still larger populations.

Among diseases and conditions associated with zinc deficiency are alcoholism, malabsorption syndromes, acrodermatitis enteropathica, anorexia nervosa, thermal burns and total parenteral nutrition (TPN) without zinc supplementation. Supplemental zinc may be helpful in some of the foregoing, in some conditions of immune impairment, in some complications of pregnancy, in the prevention of some cases of fetal neural tube defects, diarrhea, oligospermia, delayed wound healing and some cognitive disorders. It may also help protect against some inflammatory conditions.

Some claim that zinc is neuroprotective, others that it is neurotoxic in some circumstances. Some have suggested it might be useful in depression, and some others have proposed that it might be used as an antiaging substance. Mixed results are reported in the use of zinc in childhood pneumonia.

Widely publicized claims that zinc is efficacious in preventing and ameliorating symptoms of the common cold are supported by some studies but not by others. There is the suggestion in some experimental research that zinc might have some anticarcinogenic effects. There is little evidence that zinc is helpful in diabetes. Topical zinc is useful in treating some skin conditions. Claims that it can prevent or reverse baldness are unsubstantiated except in some cases of severe zinc deficiency. It has no effect on typical male pattern baldness. It may be useful in dysgeusia (taste disorder) in those who are zinc deficient. There is growing evidence that zinc might be helpful in preventing age-related macular degeneration.

RESEARCH SUMMARY

Zinc deficiency has been shown to impair immunity in many ways. It decreases T- and B-lymphocyte function and diminishes proliferative responses to mitogens. It also reduces the biological activity of many cytokines. Zinc deficiency has been shown to impair placental transport of antibodies from mother to fetus. Even mild zinc deficiency has been shown to produce an imbalance between cell-mediated and humoral immunity. Zinc supplementation has reversed many of these and other immune deficits in several *in vitro*, animal and human studies.

Supplementation with zinc reduced the incidence of childhood pneumonia by 41% and incidence of diarrhea in children by 25%, according to the findings of a review of ten randomized, controlled studies in the developing world. Zinc was found, in this review analysis, to be more effective than any other treatment for childhood pneumonia and was said to equal most other effective interventives for diarrhea in these populations. The diarrheas studied were related to diminished immune competence and high rates of exposure to infectious diseases. The significance of these findings is underscored by the fact that respiratory infections, and pneumonia in particular, are the cause of approximately one-third of all deaths among children in developing countries.

Many healthy elderly individuals and even more unhealthy elderly have marginal zinc deficiencies. There is both clinical and experimental evidence of impaired T-lymphocyte function, with associated increases in morbidity and mortality due to infectious diseases, among the elderly. Zinc deficiency has been shown to play a key role in this situation. Zinc supplementation in the elderly has produced mixed results with respect to immune restoration. Many researchers agree, however, that some of the negative results are probably due to the heterogeneity of elderly populations with respect to immune response, and most call for better-designed studies to bring hitherto ambiguous data into sharper focus.

Disturbances in metabolism, as well as zinc deficiency, have been associated with some inflammatory conditions, including some inflammatory bowel diseases and rheumatoid arthritis. The use of supplemental zinc in gastrointestinal inflammation, however, is highly experimental and is not without peril since inappropriate or uncontrolled administration can exacerbate, rather than ameliorate, some of these conditions. In some circumstances, however, supplemental zinc has enhanced the mucosal capacity of the small bowel to absorb water and electrolytes, thus easing inflammation. There is also some experimental evidence that zinc can stimulate tissue repair in some ulcer conditions.

There is some preliminary clinical evidence that supplemental zinc can produce benefit in some with rheumatoid arthritis. Diminished plasma zinc has been reported in some with this disease. Zinc has demonstrated an ability to inhibit mixed lymphocyte reaction in some of these subjects. Some researchers have suggested that further research is warranted to see if zinc might be a useful new therapy in T-cell-mediated auto-immune and graft-versus-host diseases.

One review author has presented evidence that zinc can be neurotoxic in some experimental circumstances and neuroprotective in others. The author warned that "there is a large and growing body of evidence showing that after CNS injury, large quantities of free zinc can be released, not just from pre-synaptic vesicles but also from metalloproteins and from mitochondrial zinc pools, resulting in neuronal damage and death." Some *in vitro* work has shown neurotoxic zinc effects, and some *in vivo* studies have shown free zinc accumulation reportedly leading directly to neuronal death after ischemia, traumatic brain injury and seizure. And there is some, albeit inconsistent, data suggesting that zinc chelators may protect neurons after injury. At the same time, there is data indicating that following traumatic brain injury, the risk for moderate-to-severe zinc deficiency increases significantly in humans. Hence the reviewer stated that "while these data make it clear that systemic zinc deficiency after CNS injury should be avoided, our understanding of the role of free zinc in neuronal death raises the question of whether clinicians should be treating brain-injured patients with supplemental zinc."

This issue was tested in a rat model of traumatic brain injury. Dietary supplementation with zinc subsequent to the induced brain trauma did not have deleterious effects, but the researchers cautioned that in patients with severe traumatic brain injury zinc supplementation would necessarily be administered parenterally with, potentially, significantly different effects. Another study provided at least some reassurance in this context: brain injured human adults received intravenous zinc for 15 days beginning within 72 hours of injury; three weeks after treatment began no adverse effects were observed, and, in fact, within two weeks after injury, those receiving zinc compared to those who did not receive it had improved recovery scores on the Glasgow Coma Scale. In another study, however, zinc chloride administered intraperitoneally 30 minutes prior to embolization of the middle cerebral artery in adult male rats resulted in increased infarct size and diminished behavioral outcomes, compared with other agents tested. Both studies used the same zinc form and dose. But the methods used to induce transient ischemia and reperfusion were different. Clearly more research needs to be done to try to further clarify the issues raised in these conflicting studies.

A group of reviewers examined data they said might indicate a role for zinc in treating depression. They presented evidence indicating that zinc deprivation influences brain homeostasis, mental function and susceptibility to epileptic convulsions. They also pointed to recent rat studies showing that chronic treatment with antidepressants and electroconvulsive shock therapy induces increased brain concentrations of zinc. Zinc supplementation has produced antidepressant-like effects in various animal depression models. The activity of some antidepressants was said to be enhanced when used in combination with zinc. There have been some reports that depression in humans is associated with lower serum zinc concentrations. At least one such inquiry, however, failed to find such an association. A preliminary clinical trial found

some benefit from zinc supplementation in depressed individuals. More research is needed and warranted.

Another group of researchers, surveying a broad range of zinc data, recently concluded that zinc may have general antiaging properties: "An overall estimation of all experimental and clinical observations on the biological role of zinc seems to lead us to the conclusion that zinc supply may be useful in reducing infection relapse and in restoring immune efficiency in ageing and in preventing age-related degenerative disease." However, they cautioned that it is far from being the ideal antiaging substance since there is also the potential for "acute and chronic zinc poisoning."

Diminished zinc status has been associated with HIV disease and higher incidence of opportunistic infections. Zinc supplementation has produced higher CD4+ lymphocyte cell counts and reduced incidence of bacterial infections among patients with HIV disease in one study.

In a double-blind study, subjects were randomized to receive zinc lozenges containing 13.3 milligrams of zinc every two hours while awake for as long as they had symptoms of the common cold. Subjects enrolled within 24 hours of first reporting cold symptoms. Median time to complete resolution of cold symptoms was 4.4 days in those supplemented with zinc, compared with 7.6 days in those receiving placebo. Patients dissolved the lozenges in their mouths, rather than immediately swallowing them.

A recent review of studies found findings similar to those reported above in three additional studies. Four other studies, however, found no benefit from zinc in shortening duration of cold symptoms. In one of the other positive studies, zinc supplementation reduced duration of symptoms by 42%, compared with placebo, when initiated on the first day of symptoms. When withheld until the second day, zinc reduced cold duration by 26%, compared with placebo.

Some have challenged the validity of the four studies that found no zinc effect on the basis of poor bioavailability of the zinc lozenge preparations, either due to a proposed failure of the lozenge formulations to provide adequate amounts of free zinc ions to the saliva and oral tissues or due to doses of zinc in the lozenge that were below a possible therapeutic threshold. On the other hand, some have also argued that there were significant methodological flaws in some of the positive studies. A recent review of the zinc/cold data evaluated 14 randomized, placebo-controlled studies. Half reported positive effects; half reported no effect. Of the four studies the review authors considered the most rigorous and best-designed, three found no effect, and one reported a positive effect—but it used a nasal gel as the delivery form. Whether zinc is truly effective against colds remains an unresolved issue.

A group of researchers has recently concluded that supplemental zinc has been shown to reduce the incidence of childhood pneumonia. Some studies in which it has been used as an adjunct to antibiotic therapy have yielded mixed results. A recent trial suggested that supplemental zinc might actually be detrimental in some cases of childhood pneumonia. Again, the picture is unclear, and more research is required.

Zinc supplementation has reversed some of the signs of anorexia nervosa, including weight loss, in some women. Weight has increased in some zinc-supplemented women with this condition, and menstruation has been restored in some supplemented with zinc.

Zinc supplementation has overcome some forms of both female and male infertility in those who are zinc deficient. Zinc is essential for proper formation and maturation of spermatozoa.

Zinc plays many roles in pregnancy, and disturbances in zinc metabolism, as well as zinc deficiency, can have serious adverse effects on the course of pregnancy and upon the growth of the fetus and newborn. Zinc deficiency can be teratogenic, producing neural tube defects. Zinc is also very important to the newborn when breast milk may be its only source of zinc (during the first few months of life). Premature infants may be at even greater risk of zinc deficiency. Impaired disease resistance and diminished vaccine efficacy in infants may result from zinc deficiency at this stage. Some studies have shown that giving 15 milligrams of zinc daily to breast-feeding mothers produced more weight gain in their babies than in the babies of unsupplemented mothers. Zinc supplementation in infants not breast fed has also shown benefits. Zinc supplementation has also shown benefit in regulating and promoting proper growth in some groups of young children with non-organic failure to thrive.

There is some evidence that zinc can promote and accelerate wound healing in some circumstances. There is very preliminary experimental evidence that it may have some protective effects against prostate cancer and some equally preliminary data suggesting that it might enhance neuropsychological performance in children, most likely those with zinc deficiencies.

There was an early report that 100 milligrams of zinc twice a day with meals significantly reduced visual loss in subjects with macular degeneration. Subsequently, in a much larger study organized by the National Eye Institute, a combination of zinc, vitamin E, beta-carotene and vitamin C reportedly reduced the risk of developing age-related macular degeneration and prevented blindness in a high-risk group of elderly subjects. Mortality was also increased in the supplemented group.

CONTRAINDICATIONS, PRECAUTIONS, ADVERSE REACTIONS

CONTRAINDICATIONS

Zinc is contraindicated in those who are hypersensitive to any component of a zinc-containing supplement.

PRECAUTIONS

Pregnant women and nursing mothers should avoid zinc doses higher than RDA amounts (15 milligrams/day for pregnant women, 19 mg/day for lactating women during the first six months and 16 mg/day for lactating women during the second six months).

ADVERSE REACTIONS

Doses of zinc up to 30 milligrams daily are generally well tolerated. Higher doses may cause adverse reactions. The most common adverse reactions are gastrointestinal and include nausea, vomiting and gastrointestinal discomfort. Other adverse reactions include a metallic taste, headache and drowsiness. There are some reports of decreased HDL-cholesterol in those taking high doses of zinc. Chronic intake of high doses of zinc can lead to copper deficiency and hypochromic, microcytic anemia secondary to zinc-induced copper deficiency.

High doses of zinc may be immunosuppressive.

INTERACTIONS

DRUGS

Bisphosphonates (alendronate, etidronate, risedronate): Concomitant intake of a bisphosphonate and zinc may decrease the absorption of both the bisphosphonate and zinc.

Quinolones (ciprofloxacin, gatifloxacin, levofloxacin, lomefloxacin, moxifloxacin, norfloxacin, ofloxacin, sparfloxacin, trovafloxacin): Concomitant intake of a quinolone and zinc may decrease the absorption of both the quinolone and zinc.

Penicillamine: Concomitant intake of penicillamine and zinc may depress absorption of zinc.

Tetracyclines (doxycycline, monocycline, tetracycline): Concomitant intake of a tetracycline and zinc may decrease the absorption of both the tetracycline and zinc.

NUTRITIONAL SUPPLEMENTS

Calcium: Concomitant intake of calcium and zinc may depress zinc absorption in postmenopausal women.

Copper: Concomitant intake of copper and zinc may depress the absorption of copper. Intake of large doses of zinc can negatively affect the copper status of the body. This is the basis for the use of high doses of zinc for the treatment of Wilson's disease. It is thought that high intakes of zinc induce synthesis of the copper-binding protein metallothionine in the gastrointestinal mucosal cells. Metallothionine can sequester copper. This makes copper unavailable for copper absorption.

L-cysteine: Concomitant intake of L-cysteine and zinc may enhance the absorption of zinc.

L-histidine: Concomitant intake of L-histidine and zinc may enhance the absorption of zinc.

Inositol Hexaphosphate: Concomitant intake of inositol hexaphosphate and zinc may depress the absorption of zinc.

Iron: Concomitant intake of iron and zinc may depress the absorption of both iron and zinc.

L-methionine: Concomitant intake of L-methionine and zinc may enhance the absorption of zinc.

N-acetyl-L-cysteine (NAC): Concomitant intake of NAC and zinc may enhance the absorption of zinc.

Phosphate Salts: Concomitant administration of zinc and phosphate salts may decrease the absorption of zinc.

FOODS

Caffeine: Concomitant intake of coffee, caffeinated beverages or caffeine and zinc may depress the absorption of zinc.

Cysteine-containing Proteins: Foods rich in cysteine-containing proteins (e.g., animal muscle tissue) may increase the absorption of zinc if ingested concomitantly.

Oxalic Acid: Concomitant intake of zinc with foods rich in oxalic acid (spinach, sweet potatoes, rhubarb and beans) may depress the absorption of zinc.

Phytic Acid: Concomitant intake of zinc with foods rich in phytic acid (unleavened bread, raw beans, seeds, nuts and grains and soy isolates) may depress the absorption of zinc.

Tea: Concomitant intake of tea (tannins) and zinc may cause decreased absorption of zinc.

OVERDOSAGE

There are no reports of overdosage from use of zinc supplements.

DOSAGE AND ADMINISTRATION

There are several zinc supplementary forms. These include zinc gluconate, zinc oxide, zinc aspartate, zinc picolinate, zinc citrate, zinc monomethionine and zinc histidine. Zinc supplements are available in stand-alone or in combination products. A typical dose of zinc is about 15 milligrams (as elemental zinc) daily.

The Food and Nutrition Board of the Institute of Medicine of the National Academy of Sciences has recommended the following Dietary Reference Intakes (DRI) for zinc:

	Recommended Daily Allowance (RDA)
0-6 months	2 mg/day (AI, adequate intake)
7-12 months	3 mg/day
Children	Recommended Daily Allowance (RDA)
1-3 years	3 mg/day
4-8 years	5 mg/day
Boys	
9-13 years	8 mg/day
14-18 years	11 mg/day
Girls	
9-13 years	8 mg/day
14-18 years	9 mg/day
Men	
19-30 years	11 mg/day
31-50 years	11 mg/day
51-70 years	11 mg/day
Older than 70 years	11 mg/day
Women	
19-30 years	8 mg/day
31-50 years	8 mg/day
51-70 years	8 mg/day
Older than 70 years	8 mg/day
Pregnancy	
14-18 years	12 mg/day
19-30 years	11 mg/day
31-50 years	11 mg/day
Lactation	
14-18 years	13 mg/day
19-30 years	12 mg/day
31-50 years	12 mg/day

The following summarizes the Tolerable Upper Intake Level (UL) for various age groups and conditions:

Infants	
0-6 months	4 mg/day
7-12 months	5 mg/day
Children	(UL)
1-3 years	7 mg/day
4-8 years	12 mg/day
9-13 years	23 mg/day
Adolescents	
14-18 years	34 mg/day

Adults
19 years and older .... 40 mg/day

Pregnancy
14-18 years .... 34 mg/day
19 years and older .... 40 mg/day

Lactation
14-18 years .... 34 mg/day
19 years and older .... 40 mg/day

The DV (Daily Value) for zinc, which is used for determining percentage of nutrient daily values on nutritional supplement and food labels, is 15 mg. The basis for the DV for zinc is the 1973 U.S. RDA.

LITERATURE

Anon. Zinc lozenges reduce cold symptoms. *Nutr Rev.* 1997;55:82-88.

Arnold LE, DiSilvestro RA. Zinc in attention-deficit/hyperactivity disorder. *J Child Adolesc Psychopharmacol.* 2005;15(4):619-627.

Beletate V, El Dib RP, Atallah AN. Zinc supplementation for the prevention of type 2 diabetes mellitus. *Cochrane Database Syst Rev.* 2007;(1):CD005525.

Berg JM, Shi Y. The galvanization of biology: a growing appreciation for the roles of zinc. *Science.* 1996;271:1081-1085.

Bhutta ZA, Black RE, Brown KH, et al. Prevention of diarrhea and pneumonia by zinc supplementation in children in developing countries: Pooled analysis of randomized controlled trials. *J Pediatr.* 1999;135:689-697.

Caruso TJ, Prober CG, Gwaltney JM Jr. Treatment of naturally acquired common colds with zinc: a structured review. *Clin Infect Dis.* 2007;45(5):569-574.

Chandra RK. Excessive intake of zinc impairs immune response. *JAMA.* 1984;252:1443-1446.

Cuajungco MP, Lees GJ. Zinc metabolism in the brain; relevance to human neurodegenerative disorders. *Neurobiol Dis.* 1997;4:137-169.

Cuevas LE, Koyanagi A. Zinc and infection: a review. *Ann Trop Paediatr.* 2005;25(3):149-160.

Duchateau J, Delepesse G, Vrijens R, et al. Beneficial effects of oral zinc duration on the immune response of old people. *Am J Med.* 1981;70:1001-1004.

Fabris N, Mocchegiani E. Zinc, human diseases and aging. *Aging Clin Exp Res.* 1995;7:77-93.

Fong LY, Zhang L, Jiang Y, et al. Dietary zinc modulation of COX-2 expression and lingual and esophageal carcinogenesis in rats. *J Natl Cancer Inst.* 2005;97(1):40-50.

Grahn BH, Paterson PG, Gottschall-Pass KT, et al. Zinc and the eye. *J Am Coll Nutr.* 2001;20(2 Suppl):106-118.

Grüngreiff K, Grüngreiff S, Reinhold D. Zinc deficiency and hepatic encephalopathy: results of a long-term follow-up on zinc supplementation. *J Trace Elem Exp Med.* 2000;13:21-31.

Hambridge M. Human zinc deficiency. *J Nutr.* 2000;130:1344S-1349S.

Herbein G, Varin A, Fulop T. NF-kappaB, AP-1, Zinc-deficiency and aging. *Biogerontology.* 2006;7(5-6):409-419.

Heyland DK, Jones N, Cvijanovich NZ, et al. Zinc supplementation in critically ill patients: a key pharmaconutrient? *JPEN J Parenter Enteral Nutr.* 2008;32(5):509-519.

Hughes S, Samman S. The effect of zinc supplementation in humans on plasma lipids, antioxidant status and thrombogenesis. *J Am Coll Nutr.* 2006;25(4):285-291.

Hulisz D. Efficacy of zinc against common cold viruses: an overview. *J Am Pharm Assoc* (2003). 2004;44(5):594-603.

Institute of Medicine, Food and Nutrition Board. Dietary Reference Intakes for vitamin A, vitamin K, arsenic, boron, chromium, copper, iodine, iron, manganese, molybdenum, nickel, silicon, vanadium, and zinc. Washington, DC: National Academy Press, 2001.

Jackson JL, Peterson C, Lesho E. A meta-analysis of zinc salts, lozenges and the common cold. *Arch Intern Med.* 1997;157:2373-2376.

King JC, Keen CL. Zinc. In: Shils ME, Olson JA, Shike M, Ross AC, eds. Modern *Nutrition in Health and Disease.* Baltimore, MD: Williams and Wilkins; 1999:223-239.

Klug A, Rhodes D. "Zinc fingers": a novel protein motif for nucleic acid recognition. *Trends Biochem Sci.* 1987;5:464-469.

Levenson CW. Zinc supplementation: neuroprotective or neurotoxic? *Nutr Rev.* 2005;63(4):122-125.

Lonnerdal B. Dietary factors influencing zinc absorption. *J Nutr.* 2000;130(5S Suppl):1378S-1383S.

Macknin ML. Zinc lozenges for the common cold. *Cleveland Clin J Med.* 1999;66:27-31.

Macknin ML, Piedmonte M, Calendine C, et al. Zinc gluconate lozenges for treating the common cold in children. A randomized controlled trial. *JAMA.* 1998;279:1962-1967.

Mares-Perlman JA, Klein R, Klein BE, et al. Association of zinc and antioxidant nutrients with age-related maculopathy. *Arch Opthalmol.* 1996;114:991-997.

Maret W, Sandstead HH. Zinc requirements and the risks and benefits of zinc supplementation. *J Trace Elem Med Biol.* 2006;20(1):3-18.

McMahon RJ, Cousins RJ. Mammalian zinc transporters. *J Nutr.* 1998;128:667-670.

McMahon RJ, Cousins RJ. Regulation of the zinc transporter ZnT-1 by dietary zinc. *Proc Natl Acad Sci USA.* 1998;95:4841-4846.

Mocchegiani E; Zincage Consortium. Zinc, metallothioneins, longevity: effect of zinc supplementation on antioxidant response: a Zincage study. *Rejuvenation Res.* 2008;11(2):419-423.

Mossad SB, Macknin ML, Medendorp SV, Mason PM. Zinc gluconate lozenges for treating the common cold. *Ann Intern Med.* 1996;125:81-88.

Natchu UC, Fataki MR, Fawzi WW. Zinc as an adjunct for childhood pneumonia—interpreting early results. *Nutr Rev.* 2008;66(7):398-405.

Newsome DA, Swartz M, Leone NC. Oral zinc in macular degeneration. *Arch Opthalmol.* 1988;106:192-198.

Noseworthy MD, Bray TM. Zinc deficiency exacerbates loss of blood-brain barrier integrity induced by hyperoxia measured by dynamic MRI. *Proc Soc Exp Biol Med.* 2000;223:175-182.

Nowak G, Szewczyk B, Pilc A. Zinc and depression. An update. *Pharmacol Rep.* 2005;57(6):713-718.

O'Dell BL. Role of zinc in plasma membrane function. *J Nutr.* 2000;130:1432S-1436S.

Olsen RJ, Olsen P. Zinc as a treatment for age related macular degeneration (review). *J Trace Elem Exp Med.* 1998;11:137-145.

Patro B, Golicki D, Szajewska H. Meta-analysis: zinc supplementation for acute gastroenteritis in children. *Aliment Pharmacol Ther.* Epub: 2008 Jul 1.

Prasad AS. Discovery of human zinc deficiency and studies in an experimental human model. *Am J Clin Nutr.* 1991;53:403-412.

Prasad AS. Zinc deficiency in women, infants and children. *J Am Coll Nutr.* 1996;15:113-120.

Prasad AS. Zinc in human health: effect of zinc on immune cells. *Mol Med.* 2008;14(5-6):353-357.

Prasad AS. Zinc: mechanisms of host defense. *J Nutr.* 2007;137(5):1345-1349.

Prasad AS. Zinc: the biology and therapeutics of an ion. *Ann Intern Med.* 1996;125:142-144.

Salgueiro MJ, Zubillaga M, Lysionek AK, et al. Zinc an essential micronutrient: a review. *Nutr Rev.* 2000;20:737-755.

Sandstead HH, Frederickson CJ, Penland JG. History of zinc as related to brain function. *J Nutr.* 2000;130:496S-502S.

Sazawal S, Black RE, Bhan MK, et al. Zinc supplementation in young children with acute diarrhea in India. *N Engl J Med.* 1995;333:839-844.

Schwartz JR, Marsh RG, Draelos ZD. Zinc and skin health: overview of physiology and pharmacology. *Dermatol Surg.* 2005;31(7 Pt 2):837-47; discussion 847.

Solomons NW. Mild human zinc deficiency produces an imbalance between cell-mediated and humoral immunity. *Nutr Rev.* 1998;56:27-28.

Stefanidou M, Maravelias C, Dona A, Spiliopoulou C. Zinc: a multipurpose trace element. *Arch Toxicol.* 2006;80(1):1-9.

Sturniolo GC, Di Leo V, Barollo M, et al. The many functions of zinc in inflammatory conditions of the gastrointestinal tract. *J Trace Elem Exp Med.* 2000;13:33-39.

Temple VJ, Masta A. Zinc in human health. *P N G Med J.* 2004;47(3-4):146-158.

Tubek S. Zinc supplementation or regulation of its homeostasis: advantages and threats. *Biol Trace Elem Res.* 2007;119(1):1-9.

Umeta M, West CE, Haidar J, et al. Zinc supplementation and stunted infants in Ethiopia: a randomized controlled trial. *Lancet.* 2000;355:2021-2026.

Zinc L-Carnosine

DESCRIPTION

Zinc L-carnosine is a chelate of divalent zinc and the dipeptide L-carnosine. L-carnosine (see Carnosine) is comprised of the nonprotein amino acid beta-alanine (see Beta-alanine) and the protein amino acid L-histidine.

Zinc L-carnosine was synthesized by the Japanese in the late 1980s. It was first known as Z-103 and later on as polaprezinc. The idea for the synthesis of zinc L-carnosine came from the knowledge that L-carnosine was reported to increase granulation tissue and accelerate gastric healing in rats, and that zinc had been reported to have protective action against various experimental gastric lesions and also had been reported to possess antiulcer action in clinical studies. The thinking was that the combination of the beneficial effects of zinc and L-carnosine under the chemical roof of one molecule would make for a novel and potent antiulcer agent. Japanese researchers found that the zinc L-carnosine complex did exhibit marked antiulcer activity against various experimental models of gastric ulcers and duodenal ulcers by acting directly on the gastric and intestinal mucosa. However, even during the early days of zinc L-carnosine research, it was already demonstrated to have other activities, such as inhibition of bone resorption in experimental animals. Recently, zinc L-carnosine entered the dietary supplement marketplace in the United States.

Zinc L-carnosine is described chemically as 2-[(3-azanidyl-1-oxidopropylidene)amino]-3-(3*H*-imidazol-4-yl)propanoate. It is also known as polaprezinc, zinc carnosine, β-alanyl-L-histidinato zinc, *N*-(3-aminopropionyl)-L-histidinato zinc, [*N*-β-alanyl-L-histidinato(2-)-*N*,*N*^{N}, O$^\alpha$]zinc, and catena-(*S*)-[lm-[*N*$^\alpha$-(3-aminopropionyl)-L-histidinato (2-)-*N*^{1},N^2,O:*N*$^\tau$]-zinc]. Originally known as Z-103, zinc L-carnosine was demonstrated to be much more active against gastric ulceration in rats than various other Zn(II) complexes. Zinc D-carnosine was found to have little or no activity. Spectroscopic data indicated that the zinc ions coordinate with L-carnosine to form a quadridentate 1:1 complex of polymeric nature in order to maintain low strain of the chelate rings. Small amounts of zinc L-carnosine may be found in muscle and nervous tissue. (Carnosine in muscle and nervous tissue may form chelates with zinc, copper and iron.)

Zinc L-carnosine's empirical formula is $(C_9H_{12}N_4O_3Zn)_n$, its molecular weight is 288.62, and its CAS Registry Number is 107667-60-7. It is insoluble in water and common organic solvents, but does dissolve in acid, including stomach acid.

Zinc L-carnosine is represented by the following chemical structure.

Zinc L-carnosine

ACTIONS AND PHARMACOLOGY

ACTIONS

Zinc L-carnosine has antiulcer, antigastritis and mucosal protective activities. It may also have bone-protective and hepatoprotective activities.

MECHANISM OF ACTION

Antiulcer activity: In an early study of zinc L-carnosine and peptic ulcer disease, it was found that the agent prevented ethanol-induced gastric mucosal damage in rats through increases in the activities of the gastric mucosal antioxidant enzymes superoxide dismutase (SOD) and glutathione peroxidase (GSH-px). Zinc L-carnosine also inhibited the increase in thiobarbituric acid reactive substances (TBARS) in gastric mucosa injured by the ethanol. (TBARS is a measure of oxidative stress.) The study authors concluded that the protective mechanism of zinc L-carnosine against gastric ulceration was due, at least in part, to the scavenging of oxygen-derived free radicals via increases in the synthesis of SOD and GSH-px in the gastric mucosa, induced by zinc L-carnosine.

The antiulcer pharmacological effects of zinc L-carnosine on indomethacin-induced gastric lesions and acetic acid-induced gastric ulcers, were found to be significantly greater than those of either of its components, L-carnosine and divalent zinc, or than a mixture of the two. In a study with rats, it was determined that zinc L-carnosine, which acts directly in

mucosal lesions, was retained in the stomach much longer and adhered to the ulcerous sites more strongly than did divalent zinc or L-carnosine. The characteristics of the compound were thought to arise from its much lower solubility when compared to the high solubility of divalent zinc forms, such as zinc sulfate or L-carnosine.

In a study with primary monolayer cultures of rat gastric fundic mucosa, it was demonstrated that zinc L-carnosine protected gastric cells from oxidative stress caused by hydrogen peroxide and ethanol *in vitro*, that ethanol-induced cytotoxicity was linked with superoxide anion radical production from cells, and that zinc L-carnosine-induced protection against ethanol seemed to be due, at least in part, to the scavenging of reactive oxygen species (ROS). The authors of the study concluded that zinc L-carnosine worked via an antioxidant mechanism and directly protected gastric mucosal cells from noxious agents via its antioxidant properties *in vitro*, independently of microcirculatory and neural or hormonal factors.

The antiulcer and mucocytoprotective effects of zinc L-carnosine may be explained, in part, by its antioxidant properties, as well as its stimulative effect on mucus secretion and its membrane-stabilizing effect. However, this does not completely explain the mechanism of action of its antiulcer activity. In a study using gastric epithelial cells (MKN28, a cell line derived from moderately differentiated gastric carcinoma), it was reported that zinc L-carnosine suppressed interleukin-8 (IL-8) secretion induced by tumor necrosis factor-alpha (TNF-alpha) or interleukin-1beta (IL-1beta) dose-dependently. IL-8 messenger RNA expression was also inhibited by zinc L-carnosine. Proinflammatory cytokine nuclear factor-kappaB (NF-kappaB) activation in response to TNF-alpha, IL-1beta, phorbol ester, and hydrogen peroxide, was downregulated by zinc L-carnosine. Further, Western blot analysis revealed inhibition of TNF-alpha-induced IkappaB-alpha phosphorylation in the presence of zinc L-carnosine.

Thus, an anti-inflammatory action, specifically the downregulation of proinflammatory cytokine-induced NF-kappaB activation and IL-8 expression in gastric epithelial cells, can be added to the list of zinc L-carnosine's antiulcer mechanisms of action.

To add yet another mechanistic possibility, zinc L-carnosine was shown to inhibit indomethacin-induced apoptosis in the rat gastric epithelial cell line RGM1, a diploid and non-transformed epithelial cell line isolated from normal Wistar rat gastric mucosa. Pretreatment of the cells with zinc L-carnosine suppressed caspase-3 activation and subsequent apoptosis in the cells exposed to indomethacin, dose-dependently. Treatment of the cells with indomethacin did produce

ROS, but zinc L-carnosine did not scavenge ROS in the indomethacin-treated cells, ruling out an antioxidant mechanism of action. Thus, in this case, zinc L-carnosine inhibited apoptosis via inhibition of caspase-3 activation, not by antioxidant activity.

Zinc L-carnosine was reported to help in the healing of acute gastric lesions in diabetic rats. In this case, enhancement of mucosal insulin-like growth factor-1 (IGF-1) messenger RNA expression was thought to contribute to the effect.

The effect of zinc L-carnosine on cellular proliferation was studied in human umbilical vein endothelial cells (HUVEC), human foreskin fibroblasts and guinea pig gastric mucosal cells. Zinc L-carnosine stimulated cellular proliferation in the HUVEC and the human foreskin fibroblasts, but did not stimulate proliferation in the guinea pig gastric mucosal cells. Stimulation of cellular proliferation was accompanied by increased IGF-1 messenger RNA levels. The authors of the study concluded that their results suggested that the promotion of wound healing by zinc L-carnosine was related to a proliferative effect on nonparenchymal cells, with zinc and IGF-1 being important for the action. Although divalent zinc in the form of zinc sulfate also demonstrated a proliferative effect, its action was much weaker than that of zinc L-carnosine.

The effects of the roles of inflammatory cytokines, neutrophil accumulation and lipid peroxidation in the protective effect of zinc L-carnosine against aspirin-induced gastric mucosal injury was examined in rats. Zinc L-carnosine dose-dependently inhibited the total gastric erosive area following aspirin administration, inhibited increases in thiobarbituric acid-reactive substances (TBARS), an index of lipid peroxidation, and inhibited tissue-associated myeloperoxidase activity. TBARS and myeloperoxidase activity are both markers of oxidative stress. In addition, zinc L-carnosine dose-dependently inhibited the aspirin-induced rise in the inflammatory cytokine tumor necrosis factor-alpha (TNF-alpha). This study suggested that the protective effects of zinc L-carnosine on aspirin-induced gastric mucosal injury may be attributed to its antioxidative and anti-inflammatory activities.

Helicobacter pylori is a common cause of chronic gastritis and peptic ulcer disease. In *H. pylori*-colonized gastric mucosa, activated neutrophils generate superoxide anion radicals and hydrogen peroxide. Myeloperoxidase in neutrophils catalyzes the oxidation of chloride by hydrogen peroxide to produce hypochlorous acid. The hypochlorous acid reacts with ammonia generated by *H. pylori* to produce monochloramine, which is reactive, toxic and causes gastric mucosal cell injury via damage to DNA. Zinc L-carnosine has been reported to inhibit *H. pylori*-induced gastritis and

DNA damage in Mongolian gerbils through its scavenging action against monochloramine.

The treatment of *H. pylori* is a course of triple therapy, usually with the two antibiotics—amoxicillin and clarithromycin—and a proton pump inhibitor. In a clinical study, a seven-day course of triple therapy with amoxicillin, clarithromycin and lansoprazole was found to be effective in *H. pylori* eradication, but the regimen was significantly improved by the addition of zinc L-carnosine.

Zinc L-carnosine has also been found to protect against colonic mucosal injury. A study investigated the effects of zinc L-carnosine on acetic acid-induced colonic mucosal injury in rats *in vivo*. Zinc L-carnosine inhibited visible damage in the rat colonic mucosa and this was accompanied by a significant increase in the expression of heat shock protein 72 (HSP72) and suppression of nuclear factor-kappaB (NF-kappaB) activation in the colonic mucosa. Heat shock proteins protect cells against heat stress as well as other stressors. The authors of the study suggested that, based on the findings, zinc L-carnosine may be a novel treatment for inflammatory bowel disease. The mechanism of action of this effect is not completely understood, but continued research in this area is needed and warranted.

Bone-protective activity: Zinc L-carnosine has been reported to have possible antiosteoporosis and bone-sparing activities. However, the mechanism of action of these effects is unclear. In one study, prolonged administration of zinc L-carnosine to ovariectomized rats was found to prevent bone loss. In another study, using mouse marrow cultures, an inhibitory effect of zinc L-carnosine on parathyroid hormone (PTH)-stimulated osteoclast-like cell formation was reported. It was speculated that the zinc L-carnosine inhibition of the PTH-stimulated osteoclast-like cell formation was mediated via calcium-dependent activation of protein kinase C.

A small clinical pilot study of postmenopausal women with rheumatoid arthritis reported that zinc L-carnosine improved periarticular osteoporosis, probably through an increase in bone formation.

Zinc L-carnosine has been found to promote the differentiation of osteoblasts, to suppress the formation of osteoclasts and to prevent the progression of osteoporosis. These findings, if they can be verified, could have powerful applications to promote new bone formation, including periodontal bone regeneration. High quality randomized, double-blind, placebo-controlled clinical trials are very much needed and warranted in order to learn if zinc L-carnosine has any role to play in bone regeneration.

Hepatoprotective activity: Non-alcoholic steatohepatitis (NASH) is an increasingly common disorder, which may have serious consequences. This has only recently been recognized. In some cases, it may lead to liver fibrosis, cirrhosis and even hepatocellular carcinoma. The pathogenesis of NASH is unclear. Although a similar condition can occur in people who abuse alcohol, NASH occurs in those who drink little or no alcohol.

The effects of zinc L-carnosine on the development of NASH was investigated in a mouse model of the disease. Zinc L-carnosine was demonstrated to reduce lipid peroxidation, to suppress messenger RNA expression of proinflammatory cytokines and to suppress the activation of hepatic stellate cells. (Stellate cell activation is the central event in hepatic fibrosis.) The results suggested that zinc L-carnosine attenuated fibrosis in NASH by reducing lipid peroxidation and inflammation, and, during a later phase, promoting fibrinolysis by inhibiting tissue inhibitors of metalloproteinase expression.

In a small clinical trial of patients with early liver cirrhosis, it was reported that those patients who received zinc L-carnosine demonstrated reduction in the activity of tissue inhibitors of metalloproteinase-1 as well as decreased levels of type IV collagen, a marker of fibrosis.

Further research in this area is needed and warranted.

A few studies on the effects of zinc L-carnosine have also been performed in patients with chronic hepatitis C infection. In one study, it was reported that zinc L-carnosine administration resulted in reduced hepatocyte injury as measured by the increase in serum transaminase enzyme levels in patients with hepatitis C who were on therapy with pegylated interferon alpha-2b and ribavirin. The mechanism of this effect was not clear. However, the authors of the study speculated that the effect of zinc L-carnosine had to do with its possible antioxidant activity.

In another study of patients with chronic hepatitis C infection, it was reported that those patients receiving zinc L-carnosine had reduced iron overload as determined by serum ferritin levels. Again, the mechanism of this effect was unclear.

PHARMACOKINETICS
There is very little on the pharmacokinetics (PK) of zinc L-carnosine in humans. Studies of the PK of zinc L-carnosine in rats show that, following ingestion, zinc L-carnosine slowly dissociates into its components, L-carnosine and divalent zinc. Zinc L-carnosine, which acts directly in mucosal lesions, is retained in the stomach much longer than other forms of divalent zinc and adheres to the mucosal lesions and ulcerous sites much more than do divalent zinc and L-carnosine themselves. The characteristics of the compound may arise from its much lower solubility when compared to the high solubility of divalent zinc, for example, in the form of zinc sulfate, and L-carnosine. One can think of zinc L-carnosine in this regard as a slow-release form of divalent zinc and L-carnosine.

In the rat studies, zinc was found to be efficiently absorbed from the small intestine. However, it is unclear how much zinc L-carnosine, if any, is transported into the body. It is known that following absorption, zinc is mainly bound to albumin and transported from the intestine to the liver via the portal system. Zinc was found mainly excreted in the feces; a small amount was found excreted in the urine. (See Zinc and L-carnosine for further information on the PK of zinc and of L-carnosine.)

INDICATIONS AND USAGE
Zinc L-carnosine is a one-to-one complex of a synthetic derivative of carnosine and zinc. It is marketed as a zinc supplement with claimed benefits for gastric health. It may help protect the liver against hepatitis C infection and other stressors. It could have some radioprotective effects.

RESEARCH SUMMARY
Polaprezinc (zinc L-carnosine), an anti-ulcer drug which is a chelate compound consisting of zinc and L-carnosine, has been used in a number of studies in which it demonstrates an ability to protect against gastric mucosal injury. It inhibited indomethacin-induced apoptosis in a rat gastric mucosal cell line in a dose-dependent manner, apparently by suppressing activation of caspase-3, which plays a role in cell death by cleaving cellular protein substrates. An antioxidant mode of action was not observed in this study, and the zinc, rather than the L-carnosine, was thought to be responsible for the caspase-3 inhibition. In another study, polaprezinc was shown to inhibit *Helicobacter pylori*-associated gastritis in gerbils. The authors believe the agent scavenged monochloramine, which has been associated with *H. pylori*-associated gastric mucosal injury. Rats administered zinc L-carnosine were protected against acetic-acid induced colonic mucosal injury in another study. The effect was attributed to induction of heat shock protein 72 and suppression of nuclear factor kappa B (NF-kB). The heat shock proteins are thought to have cytoprotective functions in the presence of various stressors. NF-kB is involved in inflammation. These authors concluded that zinc L-carnosine may have significant potential as a new therapeutic drug for inflammatory bowel disease.

More recently, a number of studies have suggested a possible role for zinc L-carnosine in the treatment of chronic hepatitis C infection. Human subjects with this disease were randomly administered 150 mg of polaprezinc daily for 48 weeks in combination with the drugs interferon and ribavirin and 300 mg of vitamin E and 600 mg of vitamin C daily or, in the case of the controls, the same regimen devoid of the zinc L-carnosine supplement. Increase in transaminase was significantly prevented in those receiving the zinc L-carnosine, compared with controls. The authors of this study concluded that the zinc L-carnosine supplementation thus reduced hepatocyte injury during the treatment period and attributed this favorable effect to an antioxidative action.

In another recent study of 14 patients with hepatitis C-related chronic liver disease, subjects were given polaprezinc 225 mg/day for six months along with other medications. The zinc L-carnosine supplement was credited in this study with a significant decrease in iron overload, thought to have resulted from the supplement's anti-inflammatory activity in the liver. The authors recommend zinc L-carnosine as a complementary therapy for hepatitis C-related chronic liver disease.

Also recently, another group of researchers has shown that polaprezinc attenuates liver fibrosis in a mouse model of non-alcoholic steatohepatitis. An inhibition of inflammation and lipid peroxidation was reported. Oral supplementation with polaprezinc for 24 weeks resulted in benefit to patients with early cirrhosis, again primarily due to hepatitis C infection, compared with controls.

The extent to which zinc L-carnosine supplementation can be liver-protective in healthy individuals is unknown. More research is needed and warranted.

Noting that polaprezinc has exhibited various antiapoptotic effects in the gut, researchers have recently examined the effects of this substance on radiation-induced apoptosis in rat jejunal crypt cells. Pretreatment with the agent significantly reduced the number of apoptotic cells. Whether this could be of benefit in ameliorating damage related, for example, to radiotherapy for pelvic malignancies demands further study.

CONTRAINDICATIONS, PRECAUTIONS, ADVERSE REACTIONS

CONTRAINDICATIONS

Zinc L-carnosine dietary supplements are contraindicated in those who are hypersensitive to any component of a zinc L-carnosine-containing supplement.

PRECAUTIONS

Those who wish to try a zinc L-carnosine supplement for a health condition should first discuss its use with his or her physician.

Because of the lack of long-term safety studies on zinc L-carnosine dietary supplements, pregnant women and nursing mothers should avoid their use.

ADVERSE REACTIONS

No reports.

INTERACTIONS

DRUGS

H2 blockers (cimetidine, ranitidine, famotidine): The combination of an H2 blocker and zinc L-carnosine may be more effective than when each agent is used alone.

Sucralfate: The combination of the cytoprotectant sucralfate and zinc L-carnosine may be more effective than when each agent is used alone.

NUTRITIONAL SUPPLEMENTS

No known interactions.

FOOD

No known interactions.

HERBS

No known interactions.

OVERDOSAGE

There are no reports of overdosage from use of zinc L-carnosine supplements.

DOSAGE AND ADMINISTRATION

Zinc L-carnosine supplements are available in strengths of 37.5 milligrams and 75 milligrams. Amounts used in most gastric ulcer studies were 75 milligrams twice daily. Doses higher than those recommended on the supplement label should not be exceeded.

LITERATURE

Fuji Y, Matsura T, Kai M, et al. Protection by polaprezinc, an anti-ulcer drug, against indomethacin-induced apoptosis in rat gastric mucosal cells. *Jpn J Pharmacol.* 2000;84(1):63-70.

Furuta S, Toyama S, Miwa M, et al. Residence time of polaprezinc (zinc L-carnosine complex) in the rat stomach and adhesiveness to ulcerous sites. *Jpn J Pharmacol.* 1995;67(4):271-278.

Hamano H, Yoshinaga K, Eta R, et al. Effect of polaprezinc on taste disorders in zinc-deficient rats. *Biofactors.* 2006;28(3-4):185-193.

Handa O, Yoshida N, Tanaka Y, et al. Inhibitory effect of polaprezinc on the inflammatory response to Helicobacter pylori. *Can J Gastroenterol.* 2002;16(11):785-789.

Hiraishi H, Sasai T, Oinuma T, et al. Polaprezinc protects gastric mucosal cells from noxious agents through antioxidant properties in vitro. *Aliment Pharmacol Ther.* 1999;13(2):261-269.

Ishihara R, Iishi H, Sakai N, et al. Polaprezinc attenuates Helicobacter pylori-associated gastritis in Mongolian gerbils. *Helicobacter.* 2002;7(6):384-389.

Ito M, Shii D, Segami T, et al. Preventive actions of N-(3-aminopropionyl)-L-histidinato zinc (Z-103) through increases in the activities of oxygen-derived free radical scavenging enzymes in the gastric mucosa on ethanol-induced gastric mucosal damage in rats. *Jpn J Pharmacol.* 1992;59(3):267-274.

Kishi S, Segawa Y, Yamaguchi M. Histomorphological confirmation of the preventive effect of beta-alanyl-L-histidinato zinc on bone loss in ovariectomized rats. *Biol Pharm Bull.* 1994;17(6):862-865.

Korolkiewicz RP, Fujita A, Seto K, et al. Polaprezinc exerts a salutary effect on impaired healing of acute gastric lesions in diabetic rats. *Dig Dis Sci.* 2000;45(6):1200-1209.

Maeno M, Ito-Kato E, Suzuki N, et al. Effect of beta-alanyl-L-histidinato zinc on the differentiation pathway of human periodontal ligament cells. Life Sci. 2004;74(20):2493-2504.

Mahmood A, FitzGerald AJ, Marchbank T, et al. Zinc carnosine, a health food supplement that stabilizes small bowel integrity and stimulates gut repair processes. *Gut.* 2007;56(2):168-175.

Matsukura T, Tanaka H. Applicability of zinc complex of L-carnosine for medical use. *Biochemistry* (Mosc). 2000;65(7):817-823.

Matsuu-Matsuyama M, Shichijo K, Okaichi K, et al. Protection by Polaprezinc Against Radiation-Induced Apoptosis in Rat Jejunal Crypt Cells. *J Radiat Res* (Tokyo). 2008; 49:341-347.

Miller DJ, O'Dowd A. Vascular smooth muscle actions of carnosine as its zinc complex are mediated by histamine H(1) and H(2) receptors. *Biochemistry* (Mosc). 2000;65(7):798-806.

Naito Y, Yoshikawa T, Yagi N, et al. Effects of polaprezinc on lipid peroxidation, neutrophil accumulation, and TNF-alpha expression in rats with aspirin-induced gastric mucosal injury. *Dig Dis Sci.* 2001;46(4):845-851.

Odashima M, Otaka M, Jin M, et al. Zinc L-carnosine protects colonic mucosal injury through induction of heat shock protein 72 and suppression of NF-kappaB activation. *Life Sci.* 2006;79(24):2245-2250.

Odashima M, Otaka M, Jin M, et al. Induction of a 72-kDa heat-shock protein in cultured rat gastric mucosal cells and rat gastric mucosa by zinc L-carnosine. *Dig Dis Sci.* 2002;47(12):2799-2804.

Ohkawara T, Nishihira J, Nagashima R, et al. Polaprezinc protects human colon cells from oxidative injury induced by hydrogen peroxide: relevant to cytoprotective heat shock proteins. *World J Gastroenterol.* 2006;12(38):6178-6181.

Segawa Y, Tsuzuike N, Itokazu Y, et al. Effect of beta-alanyl-L-histidinato zinc on bone metabolism in rats with adjuvant arthritis. *Biol Pharm Bull.* 1993;16(7):656-659.

Sugino H, Kumagai N, Watanabe S, et al. Polaprezinc attenuates liver fibrosis in a mouse model of non-alcoholic steatohepatitis. *J Gastroenterol Hepatol.* pub: 2008 Apr 19. Epub: 2008 Apr 19.

Suzuki H, Mori M, Seto K, et al. Polaprezinc attenuates the Helicobacter pylori-induced gastric mucosal leucocyte activation in Mongolian gerbils–a study using intravital videomicroscopy. *Aliment Pharmacol Ther.* 2001;15(5):715-725.

Takada T, Suzuki N, Ito-Kato E, Noguchi Y, Ito M, Maeno M, Otsuka K. Effect of beta-alanyl-L-histidinato zinc on the differentiation of C2C12 cells. *Life Sci.* 2004;76(5):509-520.

Tameyasu T, Yamada M, Tanaka M, et al. Effect of zinc-carnosine chelate compound on muscle function in mdx mouse. *Jpn J Physiol.* 2002;52(1):111-120.

Yamaguchi M, Hashizume M. Effect of beta-alanyl-L-histidinato zinc on protein components in osteoblastic MC3T3-El cells: increase in osteocalcin, insulin-like growth factor-I and transforming growth factor-beta. *Mol Cell Biochem.* 1994;136(2):163-169.

Yamaguchi M, Kishi S. Effect of zinc-chelating dipeptide on bone metabolism in weanling rats: comparison with beta-alanyl-L-histidinato zinc-related compounds. *Peptides.* 1994;15(4):671-673.

Yamaguchi M, Kishi S. Prolonged administration of beta-alanyl-L-histidinato zinc prevents bone loss in ovariectomized rats. *Jpn J Pharmacol.* 1993;63(2):203-207.

Yoshikawa T, Naito Y, Tanigawa T, et al. The antioxidant properties of a novel zinc-carnosine chelate compound, N-(3-aminopropionyl)-L-histidinato zinc. Biochim *Biophys Acta.* 1991;1115(1):15-22.

Supplement Product Tables

On the following pages you'll find a series of tables designed to provide you with an at-a-glance comparison of related multi-ingredient products. Both prescription and over-the-counter supplements are included. The tables cover five product types:

■ Calcium Combination Products
■ Iron Combination Products
■ Multivitamin Products
■ Multivitamin and Mineral Products
■ Vitamin B Complex Products

Entries in the Calcium Combination Products table have been organized in order of the amount of calcium, from highest to lowest. Entries in the other tables are listed alphabetically.

Secondary ingredients—nutrients found only in selected products—are covered in the "Other" column at the right of each table. In the table of Multivitamin and Mineral Products, many of which include a substantial number of trace elements and other nutrients, this column simply indicates whether or not other ingredients appear in the formulation. For a complete list of the extra ingredients found in each product, check the alphabetical product listings immediately following the table.

The following acronyms are used in various tables: FDA=Food and Drug Administration, Rx=requires a prescription, OTC=available over the counter, IU=international units, mg=milligram(s), and PABA=para-aminobenzoic acid.

Calcium Combination Products

NOTE: Products are listed according to the amount of calcium per tablet or capsule, from highest to lowest.

Product (Manufacturer)	Calcium (mg)	Vitamin D (IU)	Calcium Form	Other
Liquid Calcium Soft gels (Carlson Laboratories)	1,000	1,000	Calcium carbonate	Phosphorus 774 mg, Protein 0.8 g per 3 capsules
Calcium/Magnesium/Zinc Tablets (Rexall Naturalist)	1,000			Magnesium 500 mg, Zinc 50 mg
Vita-Calcium Wafers (Vitaline)	1,000 per 3 wafers	400 per 3 wafers	Calcium carbonate	
Cal-600 W/D (PDK Labs)	600	200	Calcium carbonate	
Goldline Calcarb 600 With Vitamin D Tablets (Teva Pharmaceuticals)	600	200	Calcium carbonate	
Caltrate 600 + D + Minerals Tablets (Wyeth Consumer Healthcare)	600	400	Calcium carbonate	Magnesium 50 mg, Zinc 7.5 mg, Copper 1 mg, Manganese 1.8 mg, Boron 250 mcg
Calcium Carbonate/Vitamin D (TriMarc Labs)	600	400	Calcium carbonate	
Nature's Blend Calcium Carbonate with D (National Vitamin Company)	600	400	Calcium carbonate	
Nature's Blend Liquid Calcium Softgel Capsules (National Vitamin Company)	600	200	Calcium carbonate	
Calcium 600/Vitamin D (Cardinal Health)	600	200	Calcium carbonate	
Calcium 600 + Vitamin D Tablets (Perrigo)	600	200	Calcium carbonate	
Calcium-600 W/D (American Pharmacal)	600	200	Calcium carbonate	
Caltrate 600 + D Tablets (Wyeth Consumer Healthcare)	600	400	Calcium carbonate	
Liqua-Cal Capsules (The Key Company)	600	200	Calcium carbonate	
Liquid Calcium 1200 Plus Vitamin D Capsules (Mason Vitamins)	600	200	Calcium carbonate	
Super Calcium w/Vitamin D Tablets (Mason Vitamins)	600	400	Calcium carbonate	
Calcium 600 mg with Vitamin D Tablets (Cypress Pharmaceuticals)	600	200	Calcium carbonate	
Calcium Carbonate with Vitamin D Tablets (Amneal Pharmaceuticals)	600	200	Calcium carbonate	
Calcium 600 + Vitamin D with Soy Isoflavones (Nature's Bounty)	600	200	Calcium carbonate	Soy isoflavones 30 mg
Calcium 600-D (Rugby Laboratories)	600	400	Calcium carbonate	
Calcium 600/Vitamin D Tablets (Basic Vitamins)	600	200	Calcium carbonate	
Calcium 600 Plus Vitamin D Tablets (Amerisource Bergen Corporation)	600	200	Calcium carbonate	
Calcium 600 Plus Vitamin D Tablets (Nature's Bounty)	600	400	Calcium carbonate	
Calcium Carbonate/Vitamin D Tablets (Major Pharmaceuticals)	600	200	Calcium carbonate	
Nature's Blend Calcium Carbonate with Vitamin D Tablets (National Vitamin Company)	600	125	Calcium carbonate	
Calcium Carbonate/Vitamin D Tablets (PD-Rx Pharmaceuticals)	600	125	Calcium carbonate	
Calcium 1200 w/Vit D (Rexall Naturalist)	600	100	Calcium carbonate	
Os-Cal Ultra (GlaxoSmithKline)	600	200	Calcium carbonate	Vitamin C 60 mg, Magnesium 20 mg, Zinc 7.5 mg, Copper 1 mg, Boron 0.25 mg, Manganese 1 mg, Vitamin E 15 IU
Calcium 200 mg Liquid Softgels (Major Pharmaceuticals)	600	180	Calcium carbonate	Vitamin A 825 IU
Chewable Calcium 600 with D Chewable Tablets (Mason Vitamins)	600	400	Calcium carbonate	
Chewable Calcium + D Wafers (Nature's Bounty)	560 per 4 wafers	400 per 4 wafers	Calcium carbonate, Dicalcium phosphate	
Cal-Cyum Wafers (Bio-Tech Pharmacal)	519	150	Calcium carbonate	
AdvaCal Ultra Fast Release Capsules (Lane Labs)	500 per 3 capsules		Calcium hydroxide, Calcium oxide	Amino acids <1 mg per 3 capsules
Calcium 500 mg with Vitamin D Tablets (Nature's Bounty)	500	125	Calcium carbonate	
Oyster Shell Calcium/Vitamin D Tablets (Reese Pharmaceutical Company)	500	200	Calcium carbonate	
Os-Cal 500 + D Tablets (GlaxoSmithKline)	500	200	Calcium carbonate	
Os-Cal 500 + Extra D Caplets (GlaxoSmithKline)	500	400	Calcium carbonate	
Os-Cal 500 + Extra D Chewable (GlaxoSmithKline)	500	400	Calcium carbonate	
Oyster Shell Calcium/Vitamin D Tablets (McKesson Drug Company)	500	200	Calcium carbonate	
Oyster Shell Calcium/Vitamin D Tablets (Perrigo)	500	200	Calcium carbonate	

Product (Manufacturer)	Calcium (mg)	Vitamin D (IU)	Calcium Form	Other
Oyster Shell Calcium Natural/Vitamin D Tablets (Cardinal Health)	500	200	Calcium carbonate	
Calcium 500 w/Vitamin D Tablets (Basic Vitamins)	500	125	Calcium carbonate	
Calcium 500 w/Vitamin D Tablets (Rexall Naturalist)	500	125	Calcium carbonate	
Oysco 500 + D Tablets (Rugby Laboratories)	500	200	Oyster shell calcium	
Goldline Oyst-Cal-D 500 Tablets (Teva Pharmaceuticals)	500	200	Oyster shell calcium	
Oyster Shell Calcium/Vitamin D Tablets (Major Pharmaceuticals)	500	200	Oyster shell calcium	
Oyster Shell Calcium/Vitamin D Tablets (Mason Vitamins)	500	400	Oyster shell calcium	
Nature's Blend Oyster Shell Calcium/Vitamin D Tablets (National Vitamin Company)	500	125	Oyster shell calcium	
Oystercal-D 500 Tablets (Nature's Bounty)	500	400	Oyster shell calcium	
Oyster Shell Calcium/Vitamin D (Basic Vitamins)	500	200	Oyster shell calcium	
Vivactiv Calcium Softchew Tablets (McNeil Consumer Health)	500	200	Calcium carbonate	Vitamin K 0.04 mg
Parva-Cal 500 Tablets (Freeda Vitamins)	500	200	Elemental calcium	
Goldline Calcium and Magnesium Tablets (Teva Pharmaceuticals)	500		Oyster shell calcium carbonate, Calcium gluconate	Magnesium 250 mg
AdvaCal Chewable Wafers (Lane Labs)	400 per 2 wafers		Calcium hydroxide, Calcium oxide	Stevia leaf 700 mcg per 2 wafers, heat-treated Hijiki seaweed extract 320 mcg per 2 wafers
Liquid Calcium-Magnesium Softgel Capsules (Carlson Laboratories)	400	1,000	Calcium carbonate	Magnesium 200 mg, protein 600 mg per 2 softgels
Florical Capsules (Mericon Industries)	364		Calcium carbonate	Sodium fluoride 8.3 mg
Florical Tablets (Mericon Industries)	364		Calcium carbonate	Sodium fluoride 8.3 mg
Calcium, Magnesium & Zinc Tablets (Mason Vitamins)	334		Calcium carbonate	Magnesium 134 mg, Zinc 5 mg
Chew-Cal Wafers (The Key Company)	333	40	Calcium carbonate	
Calcium/Magnesium/Zinc Tablets (Cardinal Health)	333		Calcium carbonate	Magnesium 133 mg, Zinc 5 mg
Calcium Citrate 1500 with Vitamin D Caplets (Mason Vitamins)	315	200	Calcium citrate	
Citracal Caplets + D (Bayer Healthcare)	315	200	Calcium citrate	
Calcium Citrate + D Tablets (Cardinal Health)	315	200	Calcium citrate	
Calcium Citrate + D Tablets (Family Pharmacy)	315	200	Calcium citrate	
Calcium 900 w/Vitamin D Capsules (Rexall Naturalist)	300	100	Calcium carbonate	
AdvaCal Ready to Drink Calcium Powder (Lane Labs)	300		Calcium hydroxide, Calcium oxide	Hijiki seaweed extract 1 mg
Oysco D Tablets (Rugby Laboratories)	250	125	Calcium carbonate	
Goldline Oyst-Cal-D Tablets (Teva Pharmaceuticals)	250	200	Oyster shell calcium	
Oyster Shell Calcium/Vitamin D Tablets (Major Pharmaceuticals)	250	125	Oyster shell calcium	
Oyster Shell Calcium/Vitamin D Tablets (McKesson Drug Company)	250	125	Oyster shell calcium	
Nature's Blend Oyster Shell Calcium/Vitamin D Tablets (National Vitamin Company)	250	250	Oyster shell calcium	
Oyster Shell Calcium/Vitamin D Tablets (Rexall Naturalist)	250	125	Calcium carbonate	
Magnebind 300 Tablets (Nephro-Tech)	250		Calcium carbonate	Magnesium carbonate 300 mg
Monocal Tablets (Mericon Industries)	625		Calcium carbonate	Sodium Monoflurophosphate 22.75 mg
Citracal 250 mg+D tablets (Bayer Healthcare)	250	200	Calcium citrate	
Parva-Cal 250 Tablets (Freeda Vitamins)	250	100	Elemental calcium	
Cal-Citrate Plus Vitamin D Tablets (Freeda Vitamins)	250	100	Calcium citrate	
Cal-Citrate Plus Magnesium Tablets (Freeda Vitamins)	250		Calcium citrate	Magnesium 100 mg
Coral Calcium 1500 Plus D & Magnesium Capsules (Mason Vitamins)	250	200	Coral calcium	
Cal-K (Key Company)	225	40	Calcium carbonate, Calcium gluconate	
Cal-Co3 Capsules (Bio-Tech Pharmacal)	200		Calcium carbonate	
Citracal Petites with Vitamin D Tablets (Bayer Healthcare)	200	200	Calcium citrate	
Citrus Calcium + D Tablets (Rugby Laboratories)	200	200	Calcium citrate	
Magnebind 400 Rx Tablets (Nephro-Tech)	200		Calcium carbonate	Folic acid 1 mg, Magnesium carbonate 400 mg

Product (Manufacturer)	Calcium (mg)	Vitamin D (IU)	Calcium Form	Other
Cal/Mag Chewable Tablets (Freeda Vitamins)	200		Calcium carbonate	Magnesium 100 mg
Chelated Calcium & Magnesium Tablets (Carlson Laboratories)	400		Calcium glycinate chelate	Magnesium 200 mg per 2 tablets
Calcium & Magnesium Chelate Capsules (The Key Company)	180		Calcium carbonate, Calcium amino acid chelate	Magnesium 90 mg
Magnebind 200 Tablets (Nephro-Tech)	160		Calcium carbonate	Magnesium 57 mg
Advacal Capsules (Lane Labs)	150		Calcium hydroxide, Calcium oxide	Amino acids <1 mg per 3 capsules
Calcet Tablets (Mission Pharmacal)	150	100	Calcium carbonate, Calcium gluconate, Calcium lactate	
Mag-SR with Calcium Tablets (Cypress Pharmaceutical)	106		Calcium carbonate	Magnesium chloride 64 mg
Calvite P&D Tablets (Cypress Pharmaceutical)	105	120	Dicalcium phosphate	Phosphorus 81 mg
Cal/Mag Chelated Tablets (Freeda Vitamins)	100		Calcium chelate	Magnesium chelate

IU = international units; mg = milligrams.

Iron Combination Products

Product/Form (Manufacturer)	FDA Class	Iron Sulfate (mg)	Iron Fumarate (mg)	Iron Carbonyl (mg)	Iron (mg)	Polysaccharide Iron Complex (mg)	A (IU)	D (IU)	E (IU)	C (mg)	B1 (mg)	B2 (mg)	Niacin/Niacinamide (B3) (mg)	Calcium Pantothenate (B5) (mg)	B6 (mg)	B12 (mg)	Folic Acid (mg)	Other
Animal Shapes Plus Iron Chewable Tablet Vitamins (Major Pharmaceuticals)	OTC		15				2,500	400	15	60	1.05	1.2	13.5		1.05	0.0045	0.3	
Children's Chewable Vite Tablets with Iron (Rugby Laboratories)	OTC		15				2,500	400	15	60	1.05	1.2	13.5		1.05	0.0045	0.3	Sodium 9 mg
Chromagen Caplets (Ther-Rx Corp)	Rx				70					152						0.01		Succinic acid 75 mg, Stomach, desiccated 50 mg
Chromagen FA Caplets (Ther-Rx Corp)	Rx				70					152						0.01	1	Succinic acid 75 mg
Chromagen Forte Caplets (Ther-Rx Corp)	Rx		151							60.8						0.01	1	Ferrous asparto glycinate 50 mg, Succinic acid 50 mg
Conison Capsules (Ethex Corporation)	Rx		110							75						0.015	0.5	Intrinsic factor 240 mg
Daily Multiple Vitamins with Iron Tablets (Sundown)	OTC		18				5,000	400	30	60	1.5	1.7	20	10	2	0.006	0.4	
Daily-Vite with Iron and Beta-Carotene Tablets (Rugby Laboratories)	OTC		18				5,000	400	30	60	1.5	1.7	20	10	2	0.006	0.4	
Ed Cyte F Tablets (Edwards Pharmaceuticals)	Rx		325														1	Docusate sodium 50 mg
Fe C Tab Plus Tablets (Boca Pharmacal)	Rx				100					250						0.025	1	
Fe C Tab Tablets (Boca Pharmacal)	OTC				100					250								
Ferocon Capsules (Breckenridge Pharmaceutical)	Rx		110							75						0.015	0.5	Intrinsic factor 240 mg
Fero-Folic 500 Extended Release Tablets (Abbott Pharmaceutical)	Rx	525								500							0.8	
Fero-Grad-500 Extended Release Tablets (Abbott Pharmaceutical)	OTC	105								500								
Ferotrinsic Capsules (Contract Pharmacal Corporation)	Rx		110							75						0.015	0.5	Intrinsic factor 240 mg
Ferralet 90 (Mission Pharmacal)	Rx			90						120						0.012	1	Docusate sodium 50 mg
Ferrex 150 Forte Capsules (Breckenridge Pharmaceutical)	Rx					150										0.025	1	
Ferrocite Plus Tablets (Breckenridge Pharmaceutical)	Rx		325							200	10	6	30	10	5	0.015	1	Zinc 18.2 mg, Magnesium 6.9 mg, Manganese 1.3 mg

Product (Manufacturer)															Other
FerroGels Forte Liquid Filled Capsules (Cypress Pharmaceuticals)	Rx	151											0.01	1	
Ferro-Sequels Extended Release Tablets (Inverness Medical)	OTC	150													Docusate sodium 100 mg
Ferrous Fumarate DS Extended Release Capsules (Vita-Rx Corp)	OTC	150													Docusate sodium 100 mg
Ferrous Sulfate-Docusate Sodium Film Coated Caplets (Time-Cap Laboratories)	Rx	150													Docusate sodium 100 mg
Fetrin Extended Release Capsules (Lunsco)	Rx	200											0.005		
Flintstones with Iron Chewable Tablets (Bayer Healthcare)	OTC		15	2,500	400	60	1.05	1.2	13.5	15		1.05	0.0045	0.3	Sodium 10 mg
Folitab 500 Extended Release Tablets (Rising Pharmaceuticals)	Rx	525				500								0.8	
Foltrin Capsules (Sandoz)	Rx	110				75							0.015	0.5	Intrinsic factor 240 mg
Fumatinic Extended Release Capsules (Laser Pharmaceuticals)	Rx	200				60							0.005		
Goldline Baby Vitamin Drops with Iron (Teva Pharmaceuticals) *per mL*	OTC		10	1,500	400	35	0.5	0.6	8	5		0.4			
Goldline One Tablet Daily W/Iron Tablets (Teva Pharmaceuticals)	OTC		18	5,000	400	60	1.5	1.7	20	30	10	2	0.006	0.4	
Hemantic with Folic Acid Tablets (Cypress Pharmaceuticals)	Rx	325												1	
Hemocyte Plus Capsules (U.S. Pharmaceutical Corp)	Rx	325				200	10	6	30		10	5	0.015	1	Zinc 18.2 mg, Magnesium 6.9 mg, Manganese 1.3 mg, Copper 0.8 mg
Hemocyte-F Tablets (U.S. Pharmaceutical Corp)	Rx	325												1	
Hemoplex F Tablets (Contract Pharmacal)	Rx	106												1	
Icar-C Plus SR Capsules (Hawthorn Pharmaceuticals)	Rx		100			320							0.025	1	
Icar-C Plus Tablets (Hawthorn Pharmaceuticals)	Rx		100			250							0.025	1	
Icar-C Tablets (Hawthorn Pharmaceuticals)	OTC		100			250									
Iferex 150 Forte Capsules (Nnodum Corporation)	Rx		150										0.025	1	
Iroon-FA Tablets (PharmaDerm)	OTC	250												0.8	
Iron Advanced Tablets (Rexall Naturalist)	OTC	28	25												Calcium 58.5 mg
Iron-Folic Tablets (Major Pharmaceuticals)	OTC	500				500	6	6	30			5	0.025	0.8	Calcium 105 mg, Sodium 65 mg
Little Animals Children's Chewable Tablets with Iron (Mason Vitamins)	OTC		15	2,500	400	60	1.05	1.2	13.5	15		1.05	0.004	0.3	Sodium 5 mg
Martinic Capsules (Marlop Pharmaceuticals)	Rx	110				75							0.015	0.5	Intrinsic factor 240 mg
Maxaron Forte Capsules (Centrix Pharmaceutical)	Rx		150 (elemental)			60							0.025	1	

Product/Form (Manufacturer)	FDA Class	Iron Sulfate (mg)	Iron Fumarate (mg)	Iron Carbonyl (mg)	Iron (mg)	Polysaccharide Iron Complex (mg)	A (IU)	D (IU)	E (IU)	C (mg)	B1 (mg)	B2 (mg)	Niacin/Niacinamide (B3) (mg)	Calcium Pantothenate (B5) (mg)	B6 (mg)	B12 (mg)	Folic Acid (mg)	Other
Multi-Delyn with Iron Liquid (Silarx Pharmaceuticals) per 5 mL	OTC				10		2,500	400	15	60	1.05	1.2	13.5	10	1.05	0.0045		
Multiret Folic-500 Extended Release Tablets (Actavis Pharmaceuticals)	Rx	105								500	6	6	30	10	5	0.025	0.8	
Multivitamin With Iron Chewable Tablets (Akyma Pharmaceuticals)	OTC				15 (ferric phosphate)		2,500	400	15	60	1.05	1.2	13.5		1.05	0.0045	0.3	Sodium 5 mg
Multivitamin with Iron Tablets (Basic Vitamins)	OTC		18				5,000	400	30	60	1.5	1.7	20		2	0.006	0.4	
Multivitamins W/Iron Children's Chewable Tablets (Cardinal Health)	OTC				15		2,500	400	15	60	1.05	1.2	13.5		1.05	0.0045	0.3	
Myferon 150 Forte Capsules (Me Pharmaceuticals)	Rx					150										0.025	1	
Nature's Blend Daily Vite Plus Iron Tablets (National Vitamin Company)	OTC		15				5,000	400		500	1.5	1.7	20		2	0.006		
Nature's Blend Stress with Iron Tablets (National Vitamin Company)	OTC				20				30	500	10	10	100	20	5	0.012	0.4	Biotin 0.045 mg
Nephron FA Tablets (Nephro-Tech)	Rx		200							40	1.5	1.7	20	10	10	0.006	1	Biotin 0.3 mg, Docusate sodium 75 mg
Niferex 150 Capsules (Ther-Rx Corp)	Rx				150 (elemental)					50								Succinic acid 50 mg
Niferex Gold Tablets (Ther-Rx Corp)	Rx					150				60.8						0.025	1	Ferrous bis-glycinate chelate 50 mg, Succinic acid 50 mg, Zinc 10mg, Docusate sodium 50 mg
Niferex-150 Forte Capsules (Ther-Rx Corp)	Rx					100				60.8						0.025	1	Ferrous asparto glycinate 50 mg, Succinic acid 50 mg
Poly Iron 150 Forte Capsules (Contract Pharmacal Corporation)	Rx					150										0.025	1	
Poly Vitamin Drops with Iron (Hi-Tech Pharmacal) per mL	OTC				10		1,500	400	5	35	0.5	0.6	8		0.4	0.002		
Poly Vitamin Drops with Iron & 0.25 mg Fluoride (Hi-Tech Pharmacal) per mL	Rx				10		1,500	400	5	35	0.5	0.6	8		0.4	0.002		Fluoride 0.25 mg
Poly Vitamin Drops with Iron & Fluoride 0.5 mg (Hi-Tech Pharmacal) per mL	Rx				10		1,500	400	5	35	0.5	0.6	8		0.4	0.002		Fluoride 0.5 mg
Poly-Iron 150 Forte Capsules (Cypress Pharmaceuticals)	Rx					150										0.025	1	
Poly-Vi-Sol W/Iron Drops (Mead Johnson) per mL	OTC				10 (elemental)		1,500	400	5	35	0.5	0.6	8		0.4			

Product	Rx/OTC	Iron (mg)		Vit A	Vit D	Vit E	Vit C	B1	B2	Niacin	B5	B6	B12	Folic Acid	Other
Poly-Vitamin with Iron & 0.25 mg Fluoride Drops (Silarx) per mL	Rx	10		1,500	400	5	35	0.5	0.6	8		0.4			Fluoride 0.25 mg
Poly-Vitamin with Iron Drops (Silarx Pharmaceuticals) per mL	OTC	10		1,500	400	5	35	0.5	0.6	8		0.4			
Proferrin Forte (Colorado Biolabs)	Rx	12												1	
Promar Capsules (Marlop Pharmaceuticals)	Rx	115					150						0.015	1	Intrinsic factor 75 mg
Re Kar C Plus SR Capsules (River's Edge Pharmaceuticals)	Rx	100					320						0.025	1	
Repliva 21/7 Tablets (Ther-Rx Corp)	Rx	81 (elemental)					140						0.01	1	Ferrous asparto glycinate (elemental) 70 mg, Succinic acid 150 mg, Calcium ascorbate 60 mg, Calcium threonate 0.8 mg
Slow FE W/Folic Acid Extended Release Tablets (Novartis Consumer Health)	OTC	50												0.4	
Stress Formula + Iron Tablets (Cardinal Health)	OTC	18				30	500	10	10	100	20	5	0.012	0.4	Biotin 0.045 mg
Stress Formula with Iron Tablets (Basic Vitamins)	OTC	4				30	300	10	10	100	20	5	0.012	0.4	Biotin 0.045 mg, Calcium 20 mg, L-taurine 75 mg, L-glutamine 20 mg, L-carnitine 5 mg, Green tea 50% Polyphenols 5 mg
Stress Formula with Iron Tablets (Major Pharmaceuticals)	OTC	18				30	500	10	10	100	20	5	0.012	0.4	Biotin 0.045 mg, Calcium 65 mg
Tandem Capsules (U.S. Pharmaceutical Corporation)	OTC	162	115.2												
Tandem DHA Capsules (U.S. Pharmaceutical Corporation)	Rx	15	15				20					25		1	Omega-3 fatty acids 310.1 mg, Docosahexaenoic acid 215.12 mg, Eicosapentaenoic acid 53.46 mg
Tandem F Capsules (U.S. Pharmaceutical Corporation)	Rx	162	115.2											1	
Tandem OB Capsules (U.S. Pharmaceutical Corporation)	Rx	162	115.2				200	10	6	30		5	0.015	1	Zinc 18.2 mg, Magnesium 6.9 mg, Manganese 1.3 mg, Copper 0.8 mg
Tandem Plus Capsules (U.S. Pharmaceutical Corporation)	Rx	162	115.2				200	10	6	30		5	0.015	1	Zinc 18.2 mg, Manganese 1.3 mg, Copper 0.8 mg
Tri-Vi-Sol W/Iron Drops (Mead Johnson & Company) per mL	OTC	50 (10 mg elemental iron)		1,500	400		35								
Tri-Vitamin Drops with Iron & Fluoride (Hi-Tech Pharmacal) per mL	Rx	10		1,500	400		35								Fluoride 0.25 mg
Vita Drops with Iron (Major Pharm) per mL	OTC	10		1,500	400	5	35	0.5	0.6	8		0.4			
Vitamins W/Iron Children's Chewable Tablets (Marlex Pharmaceuticals)	OTC	15		2,500	400	15	60	1.05	1.2	13.5		1.05	0.0045	0.3	
Vitron-C Tablets (Heritage Brand/Insight Pharm)	OTC	200					125								
Vitron-C Tablets (Heritage Brand/Insight Pharm)	OTC	66					125								

FDA = Food and Drug Administration. Rx = requires a prescription; OTC = available over the counter.

IU = international units; mg = milligram(s).

Multivitamin Products

Product/Form (Manufacturer)	FDA Class	A (IU)	B1 (mg)	B2 (mg)	Niacin (B3) (mg)	Niacinamide (B3) (mg)	Calcium Pantothenate (B5) (mg)	B6 (mg)	B12 (mg)	C (mg)	D (IU)	E (IU)	K (mg)	Biotin (mg)	Folic acid (mg)	Other
ACES Soft Gel Capsules (Carlson Laboratories)	OTC	5,000								500		200				Selenium 0.5 mg
Animal Shape Chewable Tablet Vitamins (Major Pharmaceuticals)	OTC	2,500	1.05	1.2	13.5			1.05	0.0045	60	400	15			0.3	
Animal Shapes Plus Iron Chewable Tablet Vitamins (Major Pharmaceuticals)	OTC	2,500	1.05	1.2		13.5		1.05	0.0045	60	400	15			0.3	Iron (Ferrous fumarate) 15 mg
Bee Zee Tablets (Rugby Laboratories)	OTC		15	10.2		100	25	10	0.006	600		45		0.3	0.4	Zinc 22.5 mg
Cardiotek Rx Tablets (SJ Pharmaceuticals)	Rx							50	0.5						2	Black pepper extract 5 mg, L-arginine 500 mg
Cardiotek Tablets (SJ Pharmaceuticals)	OTC							50	0.5	100		200			0.8	Black pepper extract 5 mg, L-arginine 75 mg
Children's Chewable Animal Chews with Calcium Tablets (Vitamin World)	OTC	2,500	0.75	0.85		10	5	1	0.003	60	200	15		0.05	0.2	Calcium 125 mg
Children's Chewable Vite Tablets (Rugby Laboratories)	OTC	2,500	1.05	1.2		13.5		1.05	0.0045	80	400	15			0.3	Sodium 10 mg
Children's Chewable Vite Tablets with Iron (Rugby Laboratories)	OTC	2,500	1.05	1.2	13.5			1.05	0.0045	60	400	15			0.3	Iron (Ferrous fumarate) 15 mg, Sodium 9 mg
Children's Multivitamin Chewable Tablets (Akyma Pharmaceuticals)	OTC	2,500	1.05	1.2		13.5		1.05	0.0045	60	400	15			0.3	
Children's Multivitamin Chewable Tablets (Basic Vitamins)	OTC	2,500	1.05	1.2	13.5			1.05	0.005	250	400	15			0.3	Sodium 15 mg
Compete Tablets (Mission Pharmacal Company)	OTC	5,000	2	2.6	30			20	0.009	90	400	43			0.4	Iron 27 mg, Zinc 25 mg
Cran Plus Capsules (The Key Company) *per 6 capsules*	OTC	12,000	24	24		24	24		0.048	150		30				Zinc 24 mg
Daily Multiple Vitamin Tablets (Mason Vitamins)	OTC	5,000	1.5	1.7	20		10	2	0.006	60	400	30			0.4	
Daily Multiple Vitamins Tablets (Marlex Pharmaceuticals)	OTC	5,000	2	2.5	20		1	1	0.001	50	800					
Daily Multiple Vitamins with Iron Tablets (Sundown)	OTC	5,000	1.5	1.7		20	10	2	0.006	60	400	30		0.03	0.4	Iron (Ferrous fumarate) 18 mg
Daily Multivitamin Tablets (Basic Vitamins)	OTC	5,000	1.5	1.7	20		10	2	0.006	60	400	30			0.4	
Daily Value Multi-Vitamin Tablets (Freeda Vitamins)	OTC	5,000	1.5	1.7	20		10	2	0.006	60	400	30		0.3	0.4	

Product/Form (Manufacturer)	FDA Class	A (IU)	B1 (mg)	B2 (mg)	Niacin (B3) (mg)	Niacinamide (B3) (mg)	Calcium Pantothenate (B5) (mg)	B6 (mg)	B12 (mg)	C (mg)	D (IU)	E (IU)	K (mg)	Biotin (mg)	Folic acid (mg)	Other
Daily Vitamins Supplement Liquid (Rugby Laboratories) *per 5 mL*	OTC	2,500	1.05	1.2 per	13.5			1.05	0.0045	60	400	15				
Daily-Vite Tablets (Rugby Laboratories)	OTC	3,000	1.5	1.7	20		10	2	0.006	60	400	30			0.4	Calcium 23 mg
Daily-Vite with Iron and Beta-Carotene Tablets (Rugby Laboratories)	OTC	5,000	1.5	1.7	20		10	2	0.006	60	400	30			0.4	Iron (Ferrous fumarate) 18 mg
Dino Life Chewable Multivitamins with Iron & Zinc Tablets (National Vitamin Company)	OTC	2,500	0.75	0.85		5		1	0.003	30	200	15			0.2	Iron 4.5 mg, Zinc 3.75 mg
Ex-L Tablets (The Key Company)	OTC							50		100		30				Potassium alginate 75 mg, Lemon bioflavonoid complex 100 mg, Lemon pectin complex 50 mg, DL-methionine 15 mg, L-lysine 15 mg, L-cysteine 50 mg
Extress Super Tablets (The Key Company)	OTC		50	50		50	50	50	0.05					0.05	0.4	Calcium 25 mg, Choline 50 mg, Inositol 50 mg, PABA (Para-Aminobenzoic Acid) 50 mg
Extress Tablets (The Key Company)	OTC		10	10		100	10	10	0.025	200				0.01	0.1	PABA 30 mg, Choline bitartrate 20 mg, Inositol 20 mg
Flintstones Plus Calcium Chewable Tablets (Bayer Consumer Healthcare)	OTC	2,500	1.05	1.2	13.5			1.05	0.0045	60	400	15			0.3	Calcium (elemental) 200 mg, Sodium 10 mg
Flintstones Chewable Tablets with Extra Vitamin C (Bayer Consumer Healthcare)	OTC	2,500	1.05	1.2	13.5			1.05	0.0045	250	400	15			0.3	Sodium 25 mg
Flintstones Gummies (Bayer Consumer Healthcare) *per 2 gummies*	OTC	2,000					5	1	0.005	30	200	20		0.075	0.2	Iodine 0.04 mg, Zinc 2.5 mg, Choline 38 mg, Inositol 0.02 mg, Sugars 3 g
Flintstones Gummies Vita Packs (Bayer Consumer Healthcare) *per 6 gummies*	OTC	2,000					5	1	0.005	20	200	20		0.075	0.2	Iodine 0.04 mg, Zinc 2.5 mg, Choline 38 mg, Inositol 0.020 mg, Protein <1 g; Sugars 6 g
Flintstones Sour Gummies (Bayer Consumer Healthcare) *per 2 gummies*	OTC	2,000					5	1	0.005	30	200	20		0.075	0.2	Iodine 0.04 mg, Zinc 2.5 mg, Choline 38 mg, Inositol 0.02 mg, Sugars 3 g
Flintstones with Iron Chewable Tablets (Bayer Consumer Healthcare)	OTC	2,500	1.05	1.2	13.5			1.05	0.0045	60	400	15			0.3	Iron 15 mg, Sodium 10 mg
Folgard OS Tablets (Upsher Smith Laboratories)	Rx							12.5	0.25		300				1.1	Calcium 500 mg, Magnesium 100 mg, Boron 1.5 mg
Folgard Rx Tablets (Upsher Smith Laboratories)	Rx							25	1						2.2	

Product/Form (Manufacturer)	FDA Class	A (IU)	B1 (mg)	B2 (mg)	Niacin (B3) (mg)	Niacinamide (B3) (mg)	Calcium Pantothenate (B5) (mg)	B6 (mg)	B12 (mg)	C (mg)	D (IU)	E (IU)	K (mg)	Biotin (mg)	Folic acid (mg)	Other
Folgard Tablets (Upsher Smith Laboratories)	OTC							10	0.115						0.8	
Folpace Rx Tablets (Alaven Pharmaceuticals)	Rx							25	0.425	100		100			2.05	Magnesium 100 mg
Fosfree Tablets (Mission Pharmacal Company) per 2 tablets	OTC	3,000	9	4	21		2	5	0.004	100	300					Calcium 351 mg, Iron 29 mg
Goldline Baby Vitamin Drops (Teva Pharmaceuticals) per mL	OTC	1,500	0.5	0.6	8			0.4	0.002	35	400	5				
Goldline Baby Vitamin Drops with Iron (Teva Pharmaceuticals) per mL	OTC	1,500	0.5	0.6	8			0.4		35	400	5				Iron 10 mg
Goldline One Tablet Daily (Teva Pharmaceuticals)	OTC	5,000	1.5	1.7	20		10	2	0.006	60	400	30			0.4	
Gummy Fruits (The Coromega Company) per 2 gummies	OTC	2,500				7	4	1.05	0.003	20	120	15	0.15		0.2	Calcium 6 mg, Iodine 0.049 mg, Zinc 8 mg
Hexavitamin Tablets (Upsher-Smith Laboratories)	OTC	5,000	2	3		20				75	400					Calcium carbonate 50 mg
Infuvite Adult (Baxter Healthcare Corporation) per 5 mL	Rx	3,300	6	3.6		40		6	0.005	200	200	10	0.15	0.06	0.6	Dexopanthenol 15 mg
Infuvite Pediatric (Baxter Healthcare Corporation) per 4 mL	Rx	2,300	1.2	1.4		17		1	0.001	80	400	7	0.2	0.02	0.14	Dexopanthenol 5 mg
Little Animals Chewables (Mason Vitamins)	OTC	2,500	1.05							60	400	15			0.3	
Little Animals Chewables with Iron (Mason Vitamins)	OTC	2,500	1.05	1.2		13.5		1.05	0.004	60	400	15			0.3	Iron 15 mg, Sodium 5 mg
M.V.I.-12 (without Vitamin K) (Hospira) per 10 mL	Rx	3,300	6	3.6		40		6	0.005	200	200	10				Dexopanthenol 15 mg
M.V.I. Adult (Hospira) per 10 mL	Rx	3,300	6	3.6		40			0.005	200	200	10	0.15	0.06	0.600	Dexopanthenol 15 mg
M.V.I. Pediatric (Hospira) per 5 mL	Rx	2,300	1.2	1.4		17		1	0.001	80	400	7	0.2	0.02	0.14	Dexopanthenol 5 mg
Mega Vita Liquid (Puritan's Pride) per 15 mL	OTC	5,000	21	25		150	150	45	0.05	250	400	125		0.05	0.4	PABA (Para-Aminobenzoic Acid) 25 mg, Choline bitartrate 200 mg, Inositol 100 mg
Mission Prenatal F.A. Tablets (Mission Pharmacal Company)	OTC	4,000	4.7	2	10		1	10	0.002	100	400				0.8	Calcium 50 mg, Iron 29.5 mg, Zinc 15 mg

Product/Form (Manufacturer)	FDA Class	A (IU)	B1 (mg)	B2 (mg)	Niacin (B3) (mg)	Niacinamide (B3) (mg)	Calcium Pantothenate (B5) (mg)	B6 (mg)	B12 (mg)	C (mg)	D (IU)	E (IU)	K (mg)	Biotin (mg)	Folic acid (mg)	Other
Mission Prenatal H.P. Tablets (Mission Pharmacal Company)	OTC	4,000	4	2	10		1	20	0.002	100	400				0.8	Calcium 50 mg, Iron 29.5 mg
Mission Prenatal Tablets (Mission Pharmacal Company)	OTC	4,000	4.7	2	10		1	2.8	0.002	100	400				0.4	Calcium 50 mg, Iron 29.5 mg
Multi-Day Plus Iron Tablets (Nature's Bounty)	OTC	5,000	1.5	1.7		20	10	2	0.006	60	400	30			0.4	Iron (Ferrous fumarate) 18 mg
Multi-Day Tablets (Puritan's Pride)	OTC	5,000	1.5	1.7		20	10	2	0.006	60	400	10			0.4	
Multi-Day Tablets (Nature's Bounty)	OTC	5,000	1.5	1.7		20	10	2	0.006	60	400	10			0.4	
Multi-Delyn Liquid (Silarx Pharmaceuticals) *per 5 mL*	OTC	2,250	0.842	1.08	12.2			0.945	0.00405	54	360	13.5				
Multi-Delyn with Iron Liquid (Silarx Pharmaceuticals) *per 5 mL*	OTC	2,500	1.05	1.2	13.5			1.05	0.0045	60	400	15				Iron 10 mg
Multiret Folic 500 Extended Release Tablets (Actavis Group)	Rx		6	6		30	10	5	0.025	500					0.8	Iron (Ferrous sulfate) 525 mg
Multivitamin Capsules (Numark Laboratories)	OTC	5,000	2.5	2.5		20	5	0.5	0.002	60	400	10				
Multivitamin With Iron Chewable Tablets (Amneal Pharmaceuticals)	OTC	2,500	1.05	1.2		13.5		1.05	0.0045	60	400	15			0.3	Iron 15 mg, Sodium 5 mg
Multivitamin with Iron Tablets (Basic Vitamins)	OTC	5,000	1.5	1.7		20	10	2	0.006	60	400	30			0.4	Iron (Ferrous fumarate) 18 mg
Multi-Vitamins Supplement Tablets (Rugby Laboratories, Inc)	OTC	5,000	1.5	2		20	1	0.1		37.5	400					Calcium 28.5 mg
Natachew Chewable Tablets (Warner Chilcott)	Rx	1,000	2	3		20		10	0.012	120	400	11			1	Iron (Ferrous fumarate) 29 mg
Natafort Tablets (Warner Chilcott)	Rx	1,000	2	3		20		10	0.012	120	400	11			1	
Nature's Blend Children's Multivitamin Chewable Tablets (National Vitamin Company)	OTC	2,500	1.05	1.2		13.5		1.05	0.0045	60	400	15			0.3	
Nature's Blend Daily Vite Plus Iron Tablets (National Vitamin Company)	OTC	5,000	1.5	1.7		20		2	0.006	50	400	11			1	Iron (Ferrous fumarate) 15 mg
Nature's Blend Stress with Iron Tablets (National Vitamin Company)	OTC		10	10		100	20	5	0.012	500		30		0.045	0.4	Iron 27 mg
Nephron FA Tablets (Nephro-Tech)	Rx		1.5	1.7		20	10	10	0.006	40				0.3	1	Iron (Ferrous fumarate) 200 mg, Docusate 75 mg
Nutrinate Chewable Tablets (Ethex Corporation)	Rx	1,000	2	3		20		10	0.012	120	400	11			1	Iron 29 mg

Product/Form (Manufacturer)	FDA Class	A (IU)	B1 (mg)	B2 (mg)	Niacin (B3) (mg)	Niacinamide (B3) (mg)	Calcium Pantothenate (B5) (mg)	B6 (mg)	B12 (mg)	C (mg)	D (IU)	E (IU)	K (mg)	Biotin (mg)	Folic acid (mg)	Other
Ocuvite DF Tablets (Bausch & Lomb)	OTC		0.75			10		1		100		100				Alpha lipoic acid 140 mg, Genistein 25 mg
Once Daily Tablets (Prime Marketing)	OTC	5,000	2	2.5		20	1	1	0.001	50	400					
Oncovite Tablets (Mission Pharmacal Company)	OTC	9,000	0.34	0.5	5		2.3	25	0.0016	500	400	100			0.4	Zinc 7.5 mg
One A Day Essential Tablets (Bayer Consumer Healthcare)	OTC	3,000	1.5	1.7	20		10	2	0.006	60	400	30			0.4	Calcium 45 mg (elemental)
One A Day Scooby Doo Gummies (Bayer Consumer Healthcare) per 2 gummies	OTC	2,000					5	1	0.005	30	200	20		0.075	0.2	Iodine 0.04 mg, Zinc 2.5 mg, Choline 0.03 mg, Inositol 0.02 mg, Sugars 3 g
One Daily Multiple Vitamin Tablets (Amneal Pharmaceuticals)	OTC	5,000	1.5	1.7		20		2	0.006	60	400	15			0.4	
Poly Vi Sol Liquid (Mead Johnson & Company) per mL	OTC	1,500	0.5	0.6	8			0.4	0.002	35	400	5				
Poly Vitamin Chewable Tablets (Rugby Laboratories)	OTC	2,500	1.05	1.2	13.5			1.05	0.0045	60	400	15			0.3	
Poly Vitamin Drops (Hi-Tech Pharmacal Co) per mL	OTC	1,500	0.5	0.6	8			0.4	0.002	35	400	5				
Poly Vitamin Drops with 0.25 mg Fluoride (Hi-Tech Pharmacal Co) per mL	Rx	1,500	0.5	0.6	8			0.4	0.002	35	400	5				Fluoride 0.25 mg
Poly Vitamin Drops with 0.50 mg Fluoride (Hi-Tech Pharmacal Co) per mL	Rx	1500	0.5	0.6	8			0.4	0.002	35	400	5				Fluoride 0.50 mg
Poly Vitamin Drops with Iron & Fluoride 0.25 mg (Hi-Tech Pharmacal Co) per mL	Rx	1,500	0.5	0.6	8			0.4	0.002	35	400	5				Iron 10 mg, Fluoride 0.25 mg
Poly Vitamin Drops with Iron & Fluoride 0.5 mg (Hi-Tech Pharmacal Co) per mL	Rx	1500	0.5	0.6	8			0.4	0.002	35	400	5				Iron 10 mg, Fluoride 0.5 mg
Poly-Vi-Sol W/Iron Drops (Mead Johnson & Company) per mL	OTC	1,500	0.5	0.6	8			0.4	0.002	35	400	5				Iron 10 mg
Poly-Vitamin Drops (Silarx Pharmaceuticals) per mL	OTC	1,500	0.5	0.6	8			0.4	0.002	35	400	5				
Poly-Vitamin Drops with Iron (Hi-Tech Pharmacal Co.) per mL	OTC	1500	0.5	0.6	8			0.4	0.002	35	400	5				Iron 10 mg
Poly-Vitamin with 0.25 mg Fluoride Drops (Silarx Pharmaceuticals) per mL	Rx	1,500	0.5	0.6	8			0.4	0.002	35	400	5				Fluoride 0.25 mg

Product/Form (Manufacturer)	FDA Class	A (IU)	B1 (mg)	B2 (mg)	Niacin (B3) (mg)	Niacinamide (B3) (mg)	Calcium Pantothenate (B5) (mg)	B6 (mg)	B12 (mg)	C (mg)	D (IU)	E (IU)	K (mg)	Biotin (mg)	Folic acid (mg)	Other
Poly-Vitamin with 0.5 mg Fluoride Drops (Silarx Pharmaceuticals) *per mL*	Rx	1,500	0.5	0.6	8			0.4	0.002	35	400	5				Fluoride 0.5 mg
Poly-Vitamin with Iron & 0.25 mg Fluoride Drops (Silarx Pharmaceuticals) *per mL*	Rx	1,500	0.5	0.6	8			0.4		35	400	5				Iron 10 mg, Fluoride 0.25 mg
Poly-Vitamin with Iron Drops (Silarx Pharmaceuticals) *per mL*	OTC	1,500	0.5	0.6	8			0.4		35	400	5				Iron 10 mg
Prenatal Vitamin Tablets (Puritan's Pride)	OTC	4,000	1.84	1.7		18		2.6	0.004	100	400	11			0.8	Calcium 200 mg, Iron (Ferrous fumarate) 27 mg, Zinc 25 mg
Prenatal Vitamins (Vitamin World)	OTC	4,000	1.84	1.7		18		2.6	0.004	100	400	11			0.8	Calcium 200 mg, Iron (Ferrous fumarate) 27 mg, Zinc 25 mg
Prenavite Protein Coated Tablets (Rugby Laboratories)	OTC	8,000	1.7	2		20		4	0.008	60	400	30			0.8	Calcium sulfate 200 mg, Iron (Ferrous fumarate) 28 mg, Iodine 0.15 mg, Magnesium 100 mg
Prevent Softgel Capsules (A.G. Marin Pharmaceuticals)	OTC	5,000						6	0.4	500		400			0.4	Selenium 0.05 mg, L-glutathione 30 mg
Quintabs (Freeda Vitamins)	OTC	5,000	30	30		100	30	30	0.03	300	400	50		0.03	0.4	
Rhino Gummy Bear Vitamins (Nutrition Now) *per 2 gummy bears*	OTC	2,500					5	0.7	0.004	18	60	15		0.06	0.24	Iodine 0.037 mg, Zinc 2.2 mg, Inositol 0.01 mg, Sugars 3 g
Sigtab Tablets (Lee Pharmaceuticals)	OTC	5,000	10.3	10	100		20	6	0.018	333	400	15			0.4	
SourceCF Chewable Tablets (SourceCF)	OTC	9,000	1.5	1.7		10	12	1.9	0.006	100	800	200		0.1	0.2	Vitamin K 0.6 mg, Zinc 10 mg
SourceCF Pediatric Drops (SourceCF) *per mL*	OTC	3,170	0.5	0.6			3	0.7	0.004	45	400	50		0.015		Vitamin K 0.3 mg, Zinc 5 mg
SourceCF Softgel Capsules (SourceCF)	OTC	9,000	1.5	1.7		20	12	1.9	0.006	100	400	200		0.1	0.2	Vitamin K 0.5 mg, Zinc 10 mg
Stress Formula Tablets (Upsher-Smith Laboratories)	OTC		10	10		100	20	5	0.012	500		30		0.045	0.4	Calcium 67 mg
Stress Formula Tablets (Nature's Bounty)	OTC		10	10		100	20	5	0.012	500		30		0.045	0.4	
Stress Formula with Zinc Tablets (Basic Vitamins)	OTC		10	10		100	20	5	0.012	250		30		0.045	0.4	Calcium 70 mg, Phosphorus 34 mg, Magnesium 25 mg, Zinc 24 mg, Copper 3 mg
Super Antioxidant Formula Softgel Capsules (Nature's Bounty)	OTC	25,000								500		400				Selenium 0.05 mg
Super Antioxidant Formula Softgels (Vitamin World)	OTC	25,000								500		400				Selenium 0.05 mg
Surbex T Tablets (Abbott Laboratories)	OTC		12.4	9	90.7		16.6	3.7	0.009	450						Sodium 65 mg

Product/Form (Manufacturer)	FDA Class	A (IU)	B1 (mg)	B2 (mg)	Niacin (B3) (mg)	Niacinamide (B3) (mg)	Calcium Pantothenate (B5) (mg)	B6 (mg)	B12 (mg)	C (mg)	D (IU)	E (IU)	K (mg)	Biotin (mg)	Folic acid (mg)	Other
Surbex with C Tablets (Abbott Laboratories)	OTC		4.96	5.4	27.2		8.28	1.85	0.0045	225						Sodium 35 mg
Tab A Vite + Iron Tablets (Major Pharmaceuticals)	OTC	5,000	1.5	1.7		20	10	2	0.006	60	400	30			0.4	Iron 18 mg
Thera Multi-Vitamin Liquid (Major Pharmaceuticals) *per 5 mL*	OTC	5,000	10	10	100		21.4	4.1	0.005	200	400					
Thera Tablets (Major Pharmaceuticals)	OTC	5,000	3	3.4	20		10		0.009	90	400	30		0.03	0.4	Calcium 66 mg
Thera Tablets (Amneal Pharmaceuticals)	OTC	5,000	3	3.4		20	10	3	0.009	90	400	30		30	0.4	
Therapeutic Multivitamin Tablets (Upsher-Smith Laboratories)	OTC	5,000	3	3.4		30	10	3	0.009	120	400	30		0.015	0.4	Calcium 150 mg
Thera-Plus Liquid (Hi-Tech Pharmacal Co) *per 5 mL*	OTC	5,000	10	10	100		21.4	4.1	0.005	200	400	30				
Therems (Rugby Laboratories)	OTC	5,000	3	3.4		20	10	3	0.009	90	400	30		0.03	0.4	
Tri-Vi-Sol W/ Iron Drops (Mead Johnson & Company) *per mL*	OTC	1,500								35	400					Iron 10 mg
Tri-Vitamin Drops (Hi-Tech Pharmacal Co) *per mL*	OTC	1,500								35	400					
Tri-Vitamin Drops with Fluoride (Hi-Tech Pharmacal Co)	Rx	1,500								35	400					Fluoride 0.25 mg
Tri-Vitamin Drops with Fluoride (Hi-Tech Pharmacal Co) *per mL*	Rx	1,500								35	400					Fluoride 0.5 mg
Tri-Vitamin Drops with Iron & Fluoride (Hi-Tech Pharmacal Co)	Rx	1,500								35	400					Iron 10 mg, Fluoride 0.25 mg
Tri-Vitamin with Fluoride 0.25 mg Drops (Silarx Pharmaceuticals) *per mL*	Rx	1,500								35	400					Fluoride 0.25 mg
Uni-Daily Plus Iron Tablets (United Research Laboratories)	OTC	5,000	2	2.5	20		1	1	0.001	50	400				0.4	Iron (Ferrous sulfate) 15 mg
Uni-Daily Tablets (United Research Laboratories)	OTC	5,000	1.5	1.7	20			2	0.006	60	400				0.4	
Viactiv Multivitamin Chews (McNeil Nutritionals)	OTC	2,500	1.5	1.7	15		10	2	0.006	60	400	33		0.03	0.4	Calcium 200 mg, Sodium 25 mg
Vimar Syrup (Marlop Pharmaceuticals) *per 5 mL*	OTC	2,500	1.05	1.2	13.5			1.05	0.0045	60	400	15				

Product/Form (Manufacturer)	FDA Class	A (IU)	B1 (mg)	B2 (mg)	Niacin (B3) (mg)	Niacinamide (B3) (mg)	Calcium Pantothenate (B5) (mg)	B6 (mg)	B12 (mg)	C (mg)	D (IU)	E (IU)	K (mg)	Biotin (mg)	Folic acid (mg)	Other
Vimar Syrup with Iron (Marlop Pharmaceuticals) *per 5 mL*	OTC	2,500	1.05	1.2	13.5			1.05	0.0045		400	15				Iron 10 mg
Vita Drops Liquid (Major Pharmaceuticals) *per mL*	OTC	1,500	0.5	0.6	8			0.4	0.002	35	400	5				
Vita Drops with Iron (Major Pharmaceuticals) *per mL*	OTC	1,500	0.5	0.6	8			0.4		35	400	5				Iron 10 mg
Vita Zinc Tablets (Major Pharmaceuticals)	OTC		15	10.2		100	25	10	0.006	600		45				Zinc 22.5 mg
Vital D Tablets (Nephro-Tech)	Rx		1.5	1.7		20	10	10	0.006	60	1750			0.3	1	Zinc 12.5 mg
Vitamin Children's Chewable Tablets (Prime Marketing)	OTC	2,500	1.05	1.2	13.5			1.05	0.0045	60	400	15			0.3	
Yummi Bears (Hero Nutritional Products) *per 3 gummy bears*	OTC	2,500							60			15				Choline 0.015 mg, Inositol 0.015 mg, Sugars 3 g

FDA = Food and Drug Administration. Rx = requires a prescription; OTC = available over the counter.

IU = international units; mg = milligram(s); PABA = para-aminobenzoic acid.

Multivitamin and Mineral Products

Product/Form (Manufacturer)	FDA Class	A (IU)	D (IU)	E (IU)	B1 (mg)	B2 (mg)	B6 (mg)	B12 (mg)	C (mg)	Folic acid (mg)	Zinc (mg)	Selenium (mg)	Copper (mg)	Calcium (mg)	Biotin (mg)	Chromium (mg)	Manganese (mg)	Calcium Pantothenate B5 (mg)	Niacinamide B3 (mg)	Niacin B3 (mg)	Other
ABC Plus Senior Tablets (Nature's Bounty)	OTC	3,500	400	45	1.5	1.7	3	0.025	60	0.4	15	0.02	2	200	0.03	0.15	2	10	20		Yes
ABC Plus Senior Tablets (Puritan's Pride)	OTC	3,500	400	45	1.5	1.7	3	0.025	60	0.4	15	0.02	2	200	0.03	0.15	2	10	20		Yes
ABC Plus Tablets (Nature's Bounty)	OTC	3,500	400	30	1.5	1.7	2	0.006	60	0.4	15	0.02	2	166	0.03	0.12	2	10	20		Yes
ABC Plus Tablets (Puritan's Pride)	OTC	3,500	400	30	1.5	1.7	2	0.006	60	0.4	15	0.02	2	162	0.03	0.12	2	10	20		Yes
ACES Gold Tablets (Carlson Laboratories)	OTC	5,000		200					500		3.75	0.05	0.5	50			1				Yes
ACES Plus Zinc Liquid Filled Capsules (Carlson Laboratories)	OTC	5,000		200					250		7.5	0.05		25							
Actical Softgel Capsules (A.G. Marin Pharmaceuticals)	OTC		100							0.8				500							Yes
Adult Chewable Multivitamin Tablets (Puritan's Pride)	OTC	5,000	400	100	15	15	15	0.015	150	0.4	0.325		0.05	10 (carbonate)	0.02		0.017	20	25		Yes
Adult Chewable Pineapple Flavor Tablets (Vitamin World)	OTC	5,000	400	100	15	15	15	0.015	150	0.4	0.325		0.05	10 (carbonate)	0.02		0.017	20	25		Yes
Advanced Natalcare Tablets (Ethex)	Rx	2,700	400	30	3	3.4	20	0.012	120	1	25		2	200 (carbonate)				20	20		Yes
Advanced Prenatal Tablets (Hillestad Pharmaceuticals USA) per 3 tabs	OTC	2,700	400	45	3	3.4	3	0.012	120	0.8	25	0.0875	2	125 (citrate)	0.3	0.12	5	10	25		Yes
Advanced RF Natalcare Tablets (Ethex)	Rx		400	30	3	3.4	20	0.012	120	1	25		2	200 (carbonate)				20	20		Yes
Advanced Therabasic M Tablets (Basic Vitamins)	OTC	5,000	400	60	6	3.4	6	0.012	90	0.4	15	0.07	2	40	0.03	0.05	2	10	20	20	Yes
A-Free Prenatal Tablets (Freeda Vitamins) per 3 tabs	OTC		400	30	6	6	3	0.006	100	0.8	22.5		0.3	1,000	0.03	0.2	0.3	15	30		Yes
Alpha Betic Caplets (Abkit)	OTC	2,500	400	60	1.5	1.7	2	0.006	120	0.4	15	0.07		100 (carbonate)	0.3	0.2	5	10	20		Yes
Androvite Tablets (Optimox) per 6 tabs	OTC	25,000	400	400	50		100	0.125	1,000	0.4	50	0.2	2		0.125	0.2	10	100	50		Yes
Antioxidant 4,000 Capsules (Nature's Bounty)	OTC	10,000		125					200			0.025									Yes
Apetimar with Iron Solution (Marlop Pharmaceuticals) per 5 mL	OTC				10		5	0.025													Yes
Aquadeks Pediatric Liquid (Axcan Pharma) per mL	OTC	5,751	400	65	0.6	0.6		45		5	0.01		0.015				3	6			Yes

Product/Form (Manufacturer)	FDA class	A (IU)	D (IU)	E (IU)	B1 (mg)	B2 (mg)	B6 (mg)	B12 (mg)	C (mg)	Folic acid (mg)	Zinc (mg)	Selenium (mg)	Copper (mg)	Calcium (mg)	Biotin (mg)	Chromium (mg)	Manganese (mg)	Calcium Pantothenate B5 (mg)	Niacinamide B3 (mg)	Niacin B3 (mg)	Other
Aquadeks Soft Gel Capsules (Axcan Pharma)	OTC	18,167	800	150	1.5	1.7	1.9	0.012	75	0.2	10	0.075			0.1			12	20		Yes
Bacmin Tablets (Marnel Pharmaceuticals)	Rx	5,000		30	20	20	25	0.05	500	1	22.5	0.05	3		0.15	0.1	5	25		100	Yes
Body, Hair, Skin, and Nails Formula Capsules (Mason Vitamins) *per 3 caps*	OTC	6,000		30	1.5	1.7	2	0.006	60	0.4	5		2	400	0.6		10	15		20	Yes
Bounty Buddies Plus Extra C Chewable Tablets (Nature's Bounty)	OTC	2,500	400	15	1.05	1.2	1.05	0.005	250	0.3									13.5		Yes
Calafol Rx Tablets (Alaven Pharmaceutical)	Rx		400	30			25	0.425		1.6				600 (carbonate)							Yes
Calcet Plus Tablets (Mission Pharmacal)	OTC	5,000	400	30	2.25	2.55	3	0.009	500	0.8	15		2	160				15		30	Yes
Calcifol DT Wafers (Everett Laboratories)	Rx		300				10	0.125		1				1,342 (carbonate)							Yes
Calcifol Wafers (Everett Laboratories)	Rx		200				10	0.025		1.6				1,342 (carbonate)							Yes
Calna Tablets (The Key Company)	OTC	1,000	100	10	5	2	5	0.01	50	0.4	10	0.03	0.5	250	0.15	0.04	2	5	15		Yes
Cal-Nate Tablets (Ethex)	Rx		400	30	3	3.4	20	0.006	120	1	25		2	125 (citrate)					20		Yes
Cardenz Tablets (Miller Pharmacal Group)	OTC	2,000	100	5			1.5	0.001	25										20		Yes
CareNatal DHA Tablets (Ethex)	Rx	3,000	400	30	1.8	4	25	0.012	120	1	25		2	200 (carbonate)					20		Yes
Carlson for Kids Chewable Vitamin and Mineral Tablets (Carlson Laboratories)	OTC	5,000	400	60	1.5	1.7	2	0.006	120	0.4	7.5	0.035	1	50	0.15	0.06	1.75	10	5		Yes
Cenogen Ultra Tablets (US Pharmaceuticals)	Rx	2,500		30	10	6	5	0.015	200	1			0.8				1.3	10	30		Yes
Centamin Liquid (Silarx Pharmaceuticals) *per 15 mL*	OTC	2,500	400	30	1.5	1.7	2	0.006	60		3				0.3			10		20	Yes
Centrum Cardio Tablets (Wyeth Consumer Healthcare)	OTC	1,750	200	15	0.75	0.85	2.5	0.1	30	0.2	3.75	0.01	0.35	54	0.015	0.06	1	5		10	Yes
Centrum Chewable Tablets (Wyeth Consumer Healthcare)	OTC	3,500	400	30	1.5	1.7	2	0.006	60	0.4	15		2	108	0.045	0.02	1	10		20	Yes
Centrum Kids Complete Dora the Explorer Chewable Vitamin Tablets (Wyeth Consumer Healthcare)	OTC	3,500	400	30	1.5	1.7	2	0.006	60	0.4	15		2	108	0.045	0.02	1	10		20	Yes
Centrum Kids Complete Rugrats Chewable Vitamin Tablets (Wyeth Consumer Healthcare)	OTC	3,500	400	30	1.5	1.7	2	0.006	60	0.4	15		2	108	0.045	0.02	1	10		20	Yes
Centrum Kids Complete Sponge Bob Square Pants Chewable Vitamin Tablets (Wyeth Consumer Healthcare)	OTC	3,500	400	30	1.5	1.7	2	0.006	60	0.4	15		2	108	0.045	0.02	1	10		20	Yes

Product (Manufacturer)	Status																			
Centrum Liquid (Wyeth Consumer Healthcare) *per 15 mL*	OTC	1,300	400	30	1.5	1.7	2	0.006	60	0.4	3				0.3	0.025	2	10	20	Yes
Centrum Performance Tablets (Wyeth Consumer Healthcare)	OTC	3,500	400	60	4.5	5.1	6	0.018	120	0.5	11	0.07	0.9	100	0.05	0.12	4	12	40	Yes
Centrum Silver Chewable Tablets (Wyeth Consumer Healthcare)	OTC	4,000	400	70	2.2	2.7	7	0.025	75	0.5	15	0.0225	2	200	0.045	0.1	4.5	10	12	Yes
Centrum Silver Tablets (Wyeth Consumer Healthcare)	OTC	2,500	500	50	1.5	1.7	3	0.025	90	0.5	11	0.055	0.9	220	0.03	0.045	2.3	10	20	Yes
Centrum Tablets (Wyeth Consumer Healthcare)	OTC	3,500	400	30	1.5	1.7	2	0.006	90	0.5	11	0.055	0.9	200	0.03	0.035	2.3	10	20	Yes
Cerovite Advanced Formula Tablets (Rugby Laboratories)	OTC	3,500	400	30	1.5	1.7	2	0.006	90	0.5	11	0.055	0.9	200	0.03	0.035	2.3	10	20	Yes
Cerovite Jr. Chewable Tablets (Rugby Laboratories)	OTC	3,500	400	30	1.5	1.7	2	0.006	60	0.4	15		2	108	0.045	0.02	1	10	20	Yes
Cerovite Liquid Advanced Formula (Rugby Laboratories) *per 15 mL*	OTC	1,300	400	30	1.5	1.7	2	0.006	60	0.4	3				0.3	0.025	2	10	20	Yes
Cerovite Senior Tablets (Rugby Laboratories)	OTC	2,500	500	50	1.5	1.7	3	0.025	90	0.5	11	0.055	0.9	220	0.03	0.045	2.3	10	20	Yes
CertaVite Liquid (Major Pharmaceuticals) *per 15 mL*	OTC	2,500	400	30	1.5	1.7	2	0.006	60		3				0.3	0.025	2.5	10	20	Yes
CertaVite Performance Tablets (Major Pharmaceuticals)	OTC	5,000	400	60	4.5	5.1	6	0.018	120	0.4	15	0.07	2	100	0.04	0.12	4	10	40	Yes
CertaVite Senior with Lutein Tablets (Major Pharmaceuticals)	OTC	5,000	400	45	1.5	1.7	3	0.025	60	0.4	15	0.02	2	200	0.03	0.15	2	10	20	Yes
Certavite with Lutein Tablets (Major Pharmaceuticals)	OTC	5,000	400	30	1.5	1.7	2	0.006	60	0.4	15	0.02	2	162	0.03	0.12	2	10	20	Yes
Chew-12 Chewable Tablets (The Key Company)	OTC	1,250	200	5	0.35	0.4	0.35	1.5	20	0.1	15				0.075		2.5		4.5	
Children's Chewable Layered Tablets (Hillestad Pharmaceuticals USA) *per 2 tabs*	OTC	2,500	200	10	0.4	0.5	0.6	0.003	46	0.2	2	0.005	0.08	40	0.075	0.008	2	6	5	Yes
Children's Multi Gummies (Vitamin World) *per 2 gummies*	OTC	1,500	200	15			0.5	0.003	15	0.2	2				0.045			2.5		Yes
CitraNatal 90 DHA Capsules (Mission Pharmacal)	Rx	400		30	3	3.4	20	0.015	120	1	25	0.075	2	200					20	Yes
CitraNatal DHA Capsules (Mission Pharmacal)	Rx	400		30	3	3.4	20	0.006	120	1	25		2	125					20	Yes
CitraNatal Rx Capsules (Mission Pharmacal)	Rx	400		30	3	3.4	20	0.006	120	1	25		2	125					20	Yes
Clusimar Liquid (Marlop Pharmaceuticals) *per 5 mL*	OTC	2,500	400		1	1	0.6	0.002		0.5	0.5						0.5	2.5	5	Yes
Complere Tablets (Miller Pharmacal Group)	OTC	10,000	400	60	15	15	15	0.015	200	0.075	30	0.075	1	450	0.015	0.075	2	15	50	Yes
Daily Multi Caplets (Sundown)	OTC	2,500	400	30	1.5	1.7	2	0.006	60	0.4	15	0.02	2	162	0.03	0.065	3.5	10	20	Yes
Daily Prenatal Tablets (Freeda Vitamins)	OTC	2,000	400	15	2	3	3	0.01	100	0.8	15		2	200	0.1		2	10	20	Yes

Product/Form (Manufacturer)	FDA Class	A (IU)	D (IU)	E (IU)	B1 (mg)	B2 (mg)	B6 (mg)	B12 (mg)	C (mg)	Folic acid (mg)	Zinc (mg)	Selenium (mg)	Copper (mg)	Calcium (mg)	Biotin (mg)	Chromium (mg)	Manganese (mg)	Calcium Pantothenate B5 (mg)	Niacinamide B3 (mg)	Niacin B3 (mg)	Other
Daily Vitamins with Calcium & Extra Iron for Women Tablets (Basic Vitamins)	OTC	2,500	400	30	1.5	1.7	2	0.006	60	0.4	15			450 (carbonate)				5	10		Yes
DermaVite Tablets (Stiefel Laboratories)	OTC	3,500		60		8.5	10		120	0.4	45	0.05	2	2	0.6	0.2	5				Yes
Diabetic Support Formula Tablets (Vitamin World)	OTC			30	20	2.5	12.5	0.045	100	0.15	7.5	0.07	0.75	50	0.35	0.5	2		15		Yes
Diabetiks Tablets (The Green Turtle Bay Vitamin Company) per 2 tabs	OTC	500		50					150		7.5	0.0175			0.125	0.15	2.5				Yes
Diasense Multivitamin Tablets (Blaine Pharmaceuticals)	OTC	5,000	400	100	1.5	1.7	10	0.03	120	0.4	15	0.07	2		0.3	0.2	2	10	20		Yes
Diatx Zn Tablets (Pamlab)	Rx				1.5	1.5	50	2	60	5	25		1.5		0.3			10	20		
Duet Chewable Tablets (Xanodyne Pharmaceuticals)	Rx	3,000	400	30	1.8	4	25	0.012	120	1	25		2	100					20		Yes
Duet DHA Enteric Coated Soft Gel Capsules (Xanodyne Pharmaceuticals)	Rx	3,000	400	3	1.8	4	25	0.012	120	1	25		2	200 (carbonate)					20		Yes
Duet DHA Tablets (Xanodyne Pharmaceuticals)	Rx	3,000	400	30	1.8	4	25	0.012	120	1	25		2	200 (carbonate)					20		Yes
Duet Tablets (Xanodyne Pharmaceuticals)	Rx	3,000	400	30	1.8	4	25	0.012	120	1	25		2	200					20		Yes
Encora Tablets (Ther-Rx) per daily dose	Rx		800	50			37.5		50	2.5				1,000							Yes
Enfamil Kindercal Liquid (Mead Johnson & Company) per 8 fl oz	OTC	970	125	8.8	0.4	0.5	0.5	0.0014	58	0.038	3	0.0075	0.3	240	0.038	0.0125	0.5	3.1		4.9	Yes
Enfamil Kindercal Liquid with Fiber (Mead Johnson & Company) per 8 fl oz	OTC	970	125	8.8	0.4	0.5	0.5	0.0014	58	0.038	3	0.0075	0.3	240	0.038	0.0125	0.5	3.1		4.9	Yes
Extress-30 Extended Release Capsules (The Key Company)	OTC				30	30	30	0.03	30	0.2	15				0.1			2.5	30		Yes
Fem Cal Citrate Tablets (Freeda Vitamins) per 5 tabs	OTC		400											1,000 (citrate)			20				Yes
Fem Cal Plus Tablets (Freeda Vitamins) per 3 tabs	OTC		400											1,000 (carbonate)			2				Yes
Fem Cal Tablets (Freeda Vitamins) per 4 tabs	OTC		400											1,000 (carbonate)			20				Yes
Femtabs (Azur Pharma)	Rx	5,000		30	3	3.4	40	0.012	120	1	15	0.05			0.6						Yes
Ferrocite Plus Tablets (Breckenridge Pharmaceuticals)	Rx				10	6	5	0.015	200	1	18.2		0.8				1.3	10	30		Yes
Ferrotate Junior Capsules (The Key Company)	OTC							0.05	100	0.4			1				2				Yes

Product																					
Flintstones Complete Chewable Tablets (Bayer Consumer Healthcare)	OTC	3,000	400	30	1.5	1.7	2	0.006	60	0.4	12		2	100 (elemental)	0.04			10		15	Yes
Folbee Plus Tablets (Breckenridge Pharmaceuticals)	Rx				1.5	1.5	50	1	60	5					0.3			10	10	20	
Foltabs Prenatal + DHA Tablets (Midlothian Laboratories)	Rx		400	30	3	3.4	20		120	1	25		2	125 (citrate)			6.1		20		Yes
Foltabs Prenatal Tablets (Midlothian Laboratories)	Rx		400	30	3	3.4	20		120	1	25		2	125 (citrate)			5		20		Yes
Formula 100 Tablets (Puritan's Pride)	OTC	10,000	400	150	100	100	100	0.1	250	0.4	15	0.025	0.5	100 (carbonate)	0.1	0.2		100	100		Yes
Formula B Plus Tablets (Major Pharmaceuticals)	Rx	5,000	400	30	20	20	25	0.05	500	0.8	22.5		3		0.15	0.1		25	100		Yes
Freedavite Tablets (Freeda Vitamins)	OTC	5,000	400	30	1.5	1.7	2	0.006	60	0.4	1.5	0.035	0.1	20	0.03	0.625		10	20		Yes
Geriaton Liquid (Silarx Pharmaceuticals) *per 30 mL*	OTC				5	2.5	1	0.001			2						2	2	50		Yes
Geri-Freeda Tablets (Freeda Vitamins)	OTC	5,000	400	15	15	15	15	0.015	150	0.4	7.5	0.035	0.5	50	0.015	0.06	1	15	50		Yes
Geritol Complete Tablets (GlaxoSmithKline Consumer Healthcare)	OTC	6,100	400	30	1.5	1.7	2	0.0067	57	0.38	13.5	0.001	1.8	148	0.044	0.012	2.4	13	20	20	Yes
Geritol Extend Tablets (GlaxoSmithKline Consumer Healthcare)	OTC	3,333	200	13	1.2	1.3	2	0.0025	55	0.2	14	0.035	2							15	Yes
Geritol Tonic Liquid (GlaxoSmithKline Consumer Healthcare) *per 15 mL*	OTC				2.5	2.5	0.5											2		50	Yes
Glutofac-MX Caplets (Pharmaderm) *per dose*	Rx							0.01	100	0.8	40	0.07	5	500	0.3	0.2	5	25	500		Yes
Glutofac-ZX Caplets (Pharmaderm)	Rx	5,000	400	30	20	20	25	0.05	500	0.8	40	0.05	5	50	0.2	0.2	5	25	50		Yes
Glutofac-ZX Caplets (Pharmaderm)	Rx	5,000	400	100	20	20	25	2.5	200	2.8	15	0.1	2.5		0.2	0.2	2.5	10	100		Yes
GNC Kid's MultiBite Minerals and Calcium Chewable Tablets (General Nutrition Centers) *per 2 tabs*	OTC	5,000	400	30	5	5	5	0.01	90	0.4	3		0.2	200	0.1		0.12	15	20		Yes
GNC Kid's MultiBite plus Minerals Chewable Tablets (General Nutrition Centers)	OTC	5,000	400	30	5	5	5	0.01	90	0.4	3		0.2	30	0.1			15	20		
GNC Maximum Greens Ultra Mega Green without Iron Caplets (General Nutrition Centers) *per 2 caps*	OTC	5,000	600	30	25	25	25	0.25	500	0.4	15	0.2	2		0.05	0.12	0.12	25	25		Yes
GNC Multi-Gel Multivitamin Capsules (General Nutrition Centers) *per 2 caps*	OTC	10,000	400	300	50	50	50	0.05	300	0.4	15	0.05	2	200	0.05			50	200		Yes
GNC Multi-Gel without Iron Capsules (General Nutrition Centers) *per 2 caps*	OTC	10,000	400	300	50	50	50	0.05	300	0.4	15	0.05	2	200	0.05		10	50	200		Yes
GNC Soloday Multivitamin Tablets (General Nutrition Centers)	OTC	3,500	400	30	1.5	1.7	2	0.006	60	0.4	15	0.02	2	162	0.03	0.12	2	10	20		Yes

Product/Form (Manufacturer)	FDA Class	A (IU)	D (IU)	E (IU)	B1 (mg)	B2 (mg)	B6 (mg)	B12 (mg)	C (mg)	Folic acid (mg)	Zinc (mg)	Selenium (mg)	Copper (mg)	Calcium (mg)	Biotin (mg)	Chromium (mg)	Manganese (mg)	Calcium pantothenate B5 (mg)	Niacinamide B3 (mg)	Niacin B3 (mg)	Other
GNC Solotron Chewable Wafers (General Nutrition Centers) per 2 wafers	OTC	5,000	400	100	15	15	15	0.015	150	0.1					0.02		1.7	20	25		Yes
GNC Solotron Multivitamin Caplets (General Nutrition Centers)	OTC	10,000	400	30	30	30	30	0.03	200	0.4	30	0.025	0.5	60 (carbonate)	0.03	0.025	5	30	30		Yes
GNC Solotron Platinum Multivitamin Tablets (General Nutrition Centers)	OTC	15,000	400	100	35	35	35	0.03	250	0.4	15	0.025	2	200 (carbonate)	0.03	0.1	3	20		35	Yes
GNC Solotron without Iron Multivitamin Caplets (General Nutrition Centers)	OTC	10,000	400	30	30	30	30	0.03	200	0.4	30	0.025	0.5	60 (carbonate)	0.03	0.025	5	30	30		Yes
GNC Ultra Mega Multivitamin Caplets (General Nutrition Centers)	OTC	10,000	400	100	75	75	75	0.075	200	0.4	15	0.01	0.25	100 (carbonate)	0.075	0.01	0.006	75	75		Yes
Goldline Certagen Tablets (Teva Pharmaceuticals)	OTC	5,000	400	30	1.5	1.7	2	0.006	60	0.4	15	0.02	2	162	0.03	0.065	3.5	10	20		Yes
Goldline Prenatal S Tablets (Teva Pharmaceuticals)	OTC	4,000	400	11	1.84	1.7	2.6	0.004	100	0.8	25			200 (carbonate)					18		Yes
Green Source Tablets (Nature's Bounty) per 3 tabs	OTC	15,000	400	250	25	25	25	0.025	1,000	0.4	15	0.025	0.5	250	0.05	0.1	4	25		25	Yes
Gynovite Plus Tablets (Optimox) per 6 tabs	OTC	5,000	400	400	10	10	20	0.125	180	0.4	15	0.2	2	500	0.125	0.2	10	10	20		Yes
Hair, Skin & Nails Formula Tablets (Nature's Bounty) per 3 tabs	OTC	5,000	100	15	5	5	5	0.008	120	0.2	7.5	0.0125		834	3		5	15	25		Yes
Hematinic Plus Vitamins and Minerals (Cypress Pharmaceuticals)	Rx				10	6	5	0.015	200	1	18.2		0.8				1.3	10	30		Yes
Hemocyte Plus Capsules (US Pharmaceutical)	Rx				10	6	5	0.015	200	1	18.2		0.8				1.3	10	30		Yes
Hep-Forte Soft Gel Capsules (Marlyn Nutraceuticals)	OTC	1,200		10	1	1	0.5	0.001	10	0.06	2				0.0033			2	10		Yes
Hi-Kovite Tablets (Freeda Vitamins)	OTC	5,000	400	30	10	10	10	0.01	200	0.4	7.5	0.0175	0.5	120 (carbonate)	0.03		1	10	100		Yes
Hyalex Tablets (Miller Pharmacal Group)	OTC	1,500	100	3	3	3.4	10	0.002	30		0.7							5			Yes
Icar Prenatal Tablets (Hawthorn Pharmaceuticals)	Rx	4,000	200	30	3	2	20	0.012	120	1	15	0.075	2		0.03	0.1	2	5	20		Yes
Ironmin-G Tablets (Mission Pharmacal)	OTC	4,000	400		4.8			0.002	100	0.8				57				1		10	Yes
Keytab Tablets (The Key Company) per 6 tabs	OTC	10,000	100	400	100	50	100	0.1	1,200	0.8	30	0.2	2	650 (carbonate)	0.3	0.2	10	500	150	50	Yes
Keytab Tablets w/o Glandulars (The Key Company) per 6 tabs	OTC	10,000	100	400	100	50	100	0.1	1,200	0.8	30	0.2	2	650 (carbonate)	0.3	0.2	10	500	150	50	Yes
Keytab Tablets w/o Iron, Copper, or Glandulars (The Key Company) per 6 tabs	OTC	10,000	100	400	100	50	100	0.1	1,200	0.8	30	0.2		650 (carbonate)	0.3	0.2	10	500	150	50	Yes

Product	Rx/OTC																			
KPN Prenatal Tablets (Freeda Vitamins) *per 3 tabs*	OTC	2,000	400	30	6	6	3	0.006	100	0.8	22.5		0.3	1,000	0.03			15	30	Yes
LYC Capsules (The Key Company)	OTC								310					50 (carbonate)						Yes
LYC-2,000 Powder for Suspension (The Key Company) *per 5 mL*	OTC								1,410					270 (carbonate)						Yes
Manly Machovites Tablets (Neurovites)	OTC	1,041	16.67	16.67	4.17	4.17	50	0.017	250	0.07	4.17	0.017	0.08	20.83	0.017	0.017	1.67	4.17	4.17	Yes
Maple Melts Chewable Tablets (The Green Turtle Bay Vitamin Company)	OTC	1,250	50	25	1.5	1.5	2.5	0.025	100	0.2	2.5	0.01	0.2	25	0.0375		1.5	6	10	Yes
Maximum Blue Tablets (Integrative Therapeutics) *per 2 tabs*	OTC	5,000	33	133	16	16	33	0.033	400	0.266	10	0.066	0.1	166	0.066	0.666	10	133	63	Yes
Mega Vita Gel Iron Free Softgels (Puritan's Pride) *per 2 softgels*	OTC	10,000	400	300	50	50	50	0.05	300	0.4	15	0.025	0.05	200	0.003	0.003	10	50	50	Yes
Mega Vita Gel Softgels (Vitamin World) *per 2 softgels*	OTC	10,000	400	300	50	50	50	0.05	300	0.4	15	0.025	0.05	200	0.003	0.003	10	50	50	Yes
Mega Vita Min for Seniors Tablets (Vitamin World)	OTC	8,000	400	150	4.5	5.1	50	0.018	250	0.4	1.4	0.025	0.045	200 (carbonate)	0.025	0.012	2	10	20	Yes
Mega Vita Min for Teen Tablets (Puritan's Pride) *per 3 tabs*	OTC	5,000	30	30	4.5	5.1	6	0.018	350	0.4	15	0.005	0.045	100	0.02	2	2	10	20	Yes
Mega Vita Min for Teens Tablets (Vitamin World) *per 3 tabs*	OTC	5,000	30	30	4.5	5.1	6	0.018	350	0.4	15	0.005	0.045	100	0.02	2	2	10	20	Yes
Mega Vita-Min Tablets (Puritan's Pride)	OTC	8,000	125	125	80	80	80	0.08	250	0.4	15	0.025	0.08	15	0.025	0.12		80	80	Yes
Mega Vita-Min Time Release Tablets (Vitamin World)	OTC	8,000	125	125	80	80	80	0.08	250	0.4	1.4	0.025	0.08	8 (carbonate)	0.025	0.12		80	80	Yes
Mega Vitamins for the Hair Tablets (Puritan's Pride) *per 3 tabs*	OTC	10,000		84	100	81	0.1	1,000	0.4	5		2			2			100		Yes
Mega Vitamins for the Hair Tablets (Vitamin World) *per 3 tabs*	OTC	10,000		100	100	100	0.1	1,000	0.4	5		2			2			100		Yes
Mega VM-80 Tablets (Nature's Bounty)	OTC	8,000	125	80	80	80	0.08	250	0.4	1.4	0.025	0.07	19	0.025	0.12		80		80	Yes
Mega-Multi Capsules (Innovative Health Products)	OTC	10,000	200	100	10	12.5	4.5	0.006	250	0.2	3.75	0.05	0.15	20	0.2	0.5	45	7		Yes
Men's Multivitamin Health Formula Tablets (Basic Vitamins)	OTC	3,500	400	45	1.2	1.7	3	0.018	90	0.4	15	0.105	0.03	210	0.12	2	5			Yes
Men's Daily Formula Capsules (Mason Vitamins)	OTC	3,500	400	45	1.2	1.7	3	0.018	90	0.4	15	0.105	0.03	210	0.12	2	5			Yes
Mini-Multi Tablets (Carlson Laboratories)	OTC	5,000	60	60	1.5	1.7	2	0.006	120	0.4	15	0.025	0.03	20	0.025	2	10	20		Yes
Mini-Prenatal Tablets (Freeda Vitamins)	OTC	2,000	15	15	2	3	3	0.01	100	0.8	15		0.1	200		2	10	20		Yes
Monocaps Tablets (Freeda Vitamins)	OTC	5,000	15	15	15	15	15	0.015	120	0.4	3.75	0.035	0.015	50	0.1	1	15	40		Yes
Multi-Day Plus Minerals Tablets (Nature's Bounty)	OTC	2,500	400	30	1.5	1.7	2	0.006	60	0.4			0.03	162	0.03	2	10	20		Yes

Product/Form (Manufacturer)	FDA class	A (IU)	D (IU)	E (IU)	B1 (mg)	B2 (mg)	B6 (mg)	B12 (mg)	C (mg)	Folic acid (mg)	Zinc (mg)	Selenium (mg)	Copper (mg)	Calcium (mg)	Biotin (mg)	Chromium (mg)	Manganese (mg)	Calcium Pantothenate B5 (mg)	Niacinamide B3 (mg)	Niacin B3 (mg)	Other
Multi-Day Women's with Calcium and Iron Tablets (Nature's Bounty)	OTC	2,500	400	30	1.5	1.7	2	0.006	60	0.4	15			450				5		10	Yes
Multifol Plus Tablets (Breckenridge Pharmaceuticals)	Rx	2,700	400	30	1.6	1.8	2.5	0.012	70	1	25		2	100						18	Yes
Multi-Gel Liquid Filled Capsules (Carlson Laboratories) per 6 caps	OTC	6,000	1,200	400	50	50	50	0.1	1,000	0.6	15	0.105	2	1,000	0.3	0.18	2	50	50		Yes
Multilex Film Coated Tablets (Rugby Laboratories)	OTC	10,000	400	5.5	10	5	1.7	0.003	100		1.5		1				1	10	30		
Multilex T&M Tablets (Rugby Laboratories)	OTC	10,000	400	5.5	15	10	2	0.0075	150		1.5		1				1	10	100		Yes
M-Vit Caplets (R.A. McNeil)	Rx	2,000		30	20	20	25	0.05	500	1	22.5	0.05	3		0.15	0.1	5	25	100		Yes
Myadec Multivitamin-Multimineral Supplement Tablets (J&J Consumer Products)	OTC	5,000	400	30	1.7	2	3	0.006	60	0.4	15	0.025	2	162	0.03	0.025	2.5	10		20	Yes
NanoVM Packets (Solace Nutrition) per 2 packets	OTC	1,000	200	9	0.5	0.5	0.5	0.009	15	0.15	3	0.02	0.34	500	0.008	0.011	1.2	2		6	Yes
NataCaps Capsules (Ethex)	Rx				10	6	5	0.015	200	1			0.8				1.3	10	30		Yes
NatalCare GlossTabs (Ethex)	Rx	2,700	400	10	3	3.4	20	0.012	120	1	15		2	200 (carbonate)	0.03			6	20		Yes
NatalCare PIC Forte Tablets (Ethex)	Rx	5,000	400	30	3	3.4	4	0.012	80	1	25		2	250 (carbonate)					20		Yes
NatalCare PIC Tablets (Ethex)	Rx	4,000	400	22	2.43	3	1.64	0.003	50	1	18			125 (carbonate)					10		Yes
NatalCare Plus Tablets (Ethex)	Rx	4,000	400	22	1.84	3	10	0.012	120	1	25		2	200					20		Yes
NatalCare Rx Tablets (Ethex) per 2 tabs	Rx	4,000	400	15	1.5	1.6	4	0.0025	80	1	25		3	200 (carbonate)	0.03			7	17		Yes
NatalCare Three Tablets (Ethex)	Rx	3,000	400	22	1.8	4	25	0.012	120	1	25		2	200 (carbonate)					20		Yes
NataTab C Fe Tablets (Ethex)	Rx	4,000	400	30	3	3	3	0.008	120	1	15			200 (carbonate)					20		Yes
NataTab FA Tablets (Ethex)	Rx	4,000	400	30	3	3	3	0.008	120	1	15			200 (carbonate)					20		Yes
NataTab Rx Tablets (Ethex)	Rx	4,000	400	30	3	3	3	0.008	120	1	15		3	200 (carbonate)	0.03			7	20		Yes
Natelle C Tablets (Azur Pharma)	Rx	2,000	400	25	3	3	50	0.012	150	1	15		2		0.03			6	18		Yes
Natelle EZ Tablets (Azur Pharma)	Rx	2,700	400	20	3	3.5	30	0.012	120	1	15	0.05	2	100	0.03			8	20		Yes
Natelle Plus w/ DHA Tablets (Azur Pharma)	Rx	2,600	420	20	3	3.5	30	0.012	120	1	15	0.05	2	100	0.03			8	20		Yes

Product (Manufacturer)	Rx/OTC	1	2	3	4	5	6	7	8	9	10	11	12	13	14	15	16	17	18	19
Natelle Prefer Tablets (Azur Pharma)	Rx	3,000	400	30	3	3.5	50	0.012	120	1	15		2.5	150	0.03			8	20	Yes
Natelle Tablets (Azur Pharma)	Rx	3,000	400	30	3	3.5	30	0.012	120	1	15		2.5	150 (carbonate)	0.03			8	20	Yes
Nature's Blend Mega Multivitamin with Minerals Tablets (National Vitamin)	OTC	4,800	400	100	50	50	50	0.2	250	0.4	10		2	150			5	50	50	Yes
Nature's Blend Multi-Vitamin with Minerals Soft Gel Capsules (National Vitamin)	OTC	10,000	400	2	5	2.5	1	0.002	75	0.2	0.5			75			0.5	4	40	Yes*
Nature's Blend Multi-Vitamin with Minerals Tablets (National Vitamin)	OTC	5,000	400	15	2.5	2.5	1	0.001	60	0.4	1.5			100				5	15	Yes
Nature's Blend Prenatal and Iron Tablets (National Vitamin)	OTC	4,000	400	30	1.8	1.7	2.6	0.008	120	0.8	25			200 (carbonate)					20	Yes
Nature's Blend Stress with Zinc Tablets (National Vitamin)	OTC			30	10	10	5	0.012	500	0.4	23.9		3		0.045			20	100	
Nature's Blend Super Theravite M Tablets (National Vitamin)	OTC	5,000	400	30	3	3.4	3	0.009	90	0.4	15	0.01	2	40	0.03	0.015		10	20	Yes
Nature's Blend Theratrum Complete 50 Plus Tablets (National Vitamin)	OTC	5,000	400	45	1.5	1.7	3	0.025	60	0.4	15	0.02	2	200	0.03	0.15	2	10	20	Yes
Nature's Blend Theratrum Complete Tablets (National Vitamin)	OTC	5,000	400	30	1.5	1.7	2	0.006	60	0.4	15	0.02	2	162	0.03	0.12	2	10	20	Yes
Neevo Caplets (Pamlab)	Rx		400	30	3	3.4	2.6	0.5	80	0.4	15		2	200 (carbonate)	0.03			7	20	Yes
NovaNatal Tablets (Azur Pharma)	Rx		400	30	3	3	3	0.008	120	1	15		2	200 (carbonate)					20	Yes
NovaStart Tablets (Azur Pharma)	Rx	4,000	400	30	3	3	3	0.008	120	1	15		2	200 (carbonate)					20	Yes
Nutri-100 Gold Tablets (Vitamin World)	OTC	10,000	400	150	100	100	100	0.1	250	0.4	15	0.025	0.5	100 (carbonate)	0.1	0.2	6.1	100	100	Yes
Nutrimin-Plus Tablets (The Key Company)	OTC	5,000	400	30	15	15	30	0.05	75	0.4	15	0.02	1	100	0.05		10	25	20	Yes
Nutrision Capsules (Westlake Laboratories)	Rx	8,000								15	15		1		3					
NutriSpire Tablets (Ethex)	Rx		400	30	3	3	3	0.008	120	1	15		2	200 (carbonate)					20	Yes
Nutrivit (Llorens Pharmaceutical International Division) *per 15 mL*	OTC			15	15	3	2	0.025	10	1	10								100	Yes
O-Cal FA Tablets (Pharmics)	Rx	2,500	400	30	3	3	4	0.012	90	1	15		2	200 (carbonate)					20	Yes
O-Cal Prenatal Tablets (Pharmics)	Rx	2,500	400	30	3	3	4	0.012	90	1	15		2	200 (carbonate)					20	Yes
Ocuvite Adult 50+ Soft Gel Capsules (Bausch & Lomb)	OTC			30					150		9		1							Yes
Ocuvite Extra Tablets (Bausch & Lomb)	OTC	1,000	100	40	3				300		40	0.055	2				5		40	Yes
Ocuvite Lutein Capsules (Bausch & Lomb)	OTC		30	15					60		15		2							Yes
Ocuvite Tablets (Bausch & Lomb)	OTC	1,000	60	40					200		40	0.055	2							Yes

Product/Form (Manufacturer)	FDA class	A (IU)	D (IU)	E (IU)	B1 (mg)	B2 (mg)	B6 (mg)	B12 (mg)	C (mg)	Folic acid (mg)	Zinc (mg)	Selenium (mg)	Copper (mg)	Calcium (mg)	Biotin (mg)	Chromium (mg)	Manganese (mg)	Calcium Pantothenate B5 (mg)	Niacinamide B3 (mg)	Niacin B3 (mg)	Other
One A Day Active Tablets (Bayer Consumer Healthcare)	OTC	5,000	400	60	4.5	5.1	6	0.018	120	0.4	15	0.045	2	110 (elemental)	0.04	0.1	2	10		40	Yes
One A Day Kids Bugs Bunny & Friends Complete Chewable Tablets (Bayer Consumer Healthcare)	OTC	3,000	400	30	1.5	1.7	2	0.006	60	0.4	12		2	100 (elemental)	0.04			10		15	Yes
One A Day Kids Scooby Doo Complete Chewable Tablets (Bayer Consumer Healthcare)	OTC	3,000	400	30	1.5	1.7	2	0.006	60	0.4	12		2	100 (elemental)	0.04			10		15	Yes
One A Day Kids Scooby Doo Plus Calcium Chewable Tablets (Bayer Consumer Healthcare)	OTC	2,500	400	15	1.05	1.2	1.05	0.0045	60	0.3				200 (elemental)						13.5	Yes
One A Day Maximum Tablets (Bayer Consumer Healthcare)	OTC	2,500	400	30	1.5	1.7	2	0.006	60	0.4	15	0.02	2	162	0.03	0.065	3.5	10		20	Yes
One A Day Men's 50+ Advantage Tablets (Bayer Consumer Healthcare)	OTC	2,500	400	33	4.5	3.4	6	0.025	120	0.4	22.5	0.105	2	120 (elemental)	0.03	0.18	4	15		20	Yes
One A Day Men's Health Formula Tablets (Bayer Consumer Healthcare)	OTC	3,500	400	45	1.2	1.7	3	0.018	90	0.4	15	0.105	2	210	0.03	0.12	2	5		16	Yes
One A Day Weight Smart Advanced Tablets (Bayer Consumer Healthcare)	OTC	2,500	400	30	1.9	2.1	2.5	0.0075	60	0.4	15	0.07	2	200		0.2	2	12.5		25	Yes
One A Day Women's 50+ Advantage Tablets (Bayer Consumer Healthcare)	OTC	2,500	800	33	4.5	3.4	6	0.025	60	0.4	22.5	0.02	2	405	0.03	0.18	4	15		20	Yes
One A Day Women's Prenatal Tablets (Bayer Consumer Healthcare)	OTC	4,000	400	30	1.7	2	2.5	0.008	60	0.8	15		2	300	0.3			10		20	Yes
One A Day Women's Tablets (Bayer Consumer Healthcare)	OTC	2,500	800	30	1.5	1.7	2	0.006	60	0.4	15	0.02	2	450	0.03	0.12	2	5		10	Yes
One Daily Maximum Vitamin Tablets (Basic Vitamins)	OTC	5,000	400	30	1.5	1.7	2	0.006	60	0.4	15	0.02	2		0.03	0.065	3.5	10		20	Yes
Opti-C Tablets (The Key Company)	OTC								250		15										Yes
OptiNate Tablets (Sciele Pharma)	Rx		400	10	3		20	0.012	120	1	15		2	200	0.03			6	20		Yes
Opti-Plus Capsules (The Key Company)	OTC			50					25		15	0.025	1			1.25			20		Yes
Optisource Chewable Tablets (Novartis Nutrition)	OTC	1,875	100		0.375	0.425	0.5	0.125	15	0.2	7.5	0.0175	0.5	250	0.075	0.03	0.5	2.5		5	Yes
Optivite P.M.T. Tablets (Optimox) per 6 tabs	OTC	12,500	100	100	25	25	300	0.06	1,500	0.2	25	0.1	1	125	0.06	0.1	10	25	25		Yes
OsCal Ultra Tablets (GlaxoSmithKline Consumer Healthcare)	OTC		200	15					60		7.5		1	600			1				Yes

Product (Manufacturer)	Type	Vit A (IU)	Vit D (IU)	Vit E (IU)	Vit C (mg)	Thiamine (mg)	Riboflavin (mg)	Niacin (mg)	Folic Acid (mg)	Calcium (mg)	Sugar Free
Parvlex Tablets (Freeda Vitamins)	OTC	—	—	—	60	20	20	10	0.4	—	Yes
PMS Formula Tablets (Neurovites)	OTC	1,041	16.67	16.67	250	4.17	4.17	50	0.07	20.83	Yes
Poly Vitamin w/Iron Chewable Tablets (Rugby Laboratories)	OTC	2,500	400	15	60	1.05	1.2	1.05	0.3	—	Yes
Potent 75 Super VM Tablets (Puritan's Pride)	OTC	10,000	400	150	250	60.8	75	61.5	0.4	50	Yes
Powermate Tablets (The Green Turtle Bay Vitamin Company)	OTC	5,000	—	100	250	—	—	—	—	—	Yes
PowerVites Tablets (The Green Turtle Bay Vitamin Company) per 2 tabs	OTC	5,000	300	25	250	12.5	12.5	25	0.3	165	Yes
PreCare Chewables (Ther-Rx)	Rx	—	6 mcg	3.5	50	—	—	2	1	250 (carbonate)	Yes
PreCare Conceive Tablets (Ther-Rx)	Rx	—	—	30	60	—	3.4	50	1	200	Yes
PreCare Premier Tablets (Ther-Rx)	Rx	—	6 mcg	3.5	50	—	3.4	50	1	250 (carbonate)	Yes
PreferaOB Tablets (Alaven Pharmaceuticals)	Rx	—	400	10	—	1.5	1.6	50	1	—	Yes
Premesis Rx Tablets (Ther-Rx)	Rx	—	—	—	75	—	—	75	—	200	Yes
Prenafirst Tablets (Cypress Pharmaceuticals)	Rx	4,000	400	30	120	3	3	3	1	200 (carbonate)	Yes
Prenatabs FA Tablets (Cypress Pharmaceuticals)	Rx	4,000	400	30	120	3	3	3	1	200	Yes
Prenatabs Rx Tablets (Cypress Pharmaceuticals)	Rx	4,000	400	30	120	3	3	3	1	200 (carbonate)	Yes
Prenatal 1 + 1 Tablets (Amneal Pharmaceuticals)	Rx	4,000	400	11	120	1.84	3	10	0.8	200	Yes
Prenatal 19 Chewable Tablets (Cypress Pharmaceuticals)	Rx	1,000	400	30	100	3	3	20	1	200 (carbonate)	Yes
Prenatal 19 Tablets (Cypress Pharmaceuticals)	Rx	1,000	400	30	100	3	3	20	1	200	Yes
Prenatal AD Tablets (Cypress Pharmaceticals)	Rx	2,700	400	30	120	3	3.4	20	1	200 (carbonate)	Yes
Pre-Natal Complex Capsules (Puritan's Pride) per 4 caps	OTC	8,000	400	30	60	1.7	2	2.5	0.8	1300	Yes
Pre-Natal Complex Capsules (Vitamin World) per 4 caps	OTC	8,000	400	30	60	1.7	2	2.5	0.8	1300	Yes
Prenatal MR 90 Fe Tablets (Ethex)	Rx	4,000	400	30	120	3	3.4	20	1	250 (carbonate)	Yes
Prenatal MTR with Selenium Tablets (Ethex)	Rx	5,000	400	30	120	1.5	1.6	4	1	200	Yes
Prenatal Plus Tablets (Amneal Pharmaceuticals)	Rx	4,000	400	22	120	1.84	3	10	1	200 (carbonate)	Yes
Prenatal Rx 1 Tablets (Ethex)	Rx	4,000	400	15	80	1.5	1.6	4	1	200	Yes
Prenatal Tablets (Major Pharmaceuticals)	OTC	4,000	400	11	100	1.84	1.7	2.6	0.8	200 (carbonate)	Yes
PreNATAL Tablets (Carlson Laboratories) per 4 tablets	OTC	8,000	400	150	300	6.8	8	10	0.3	1,000 (carbonate)	Yes
Prenatal U Capsules (Cypress Pharmaceuticals)	Rx	—	—	—	200	10	6	5	1	—	Yes

Product/Form (Manufacturer)	FDA class	A (IU)	D (IU)	E (IU)	B1 (mg)	B2 (mg)	B6 (mg)	B12 (mg)	C (mg)	Folic acid (mg)	Zinc (mg)	Selenium (mg)	Copper (mg)	Calcium (mg)	Biotin (mg)	Chromium (mg)	Manganese (mg)	Calcium Pantothenate B5 (mg)	Niacinamide B3 (mg)	Niacin B3 (mg)	Other
Prenatal Vitamins (Nature's Bounty)	OTC	4,000	400	30	1.8	1.7	2.6	0.008	120	0.8	25			200 (carbonate)					20		Yes
Prenatal Vitamins (Basic Vitamins)	OTC	4,000	400	30	1.8	1.7	2.6	0.008	120	0.8	25			200 (carbonate)					20		Yes
Prenatal Z Advanced Formula Tablets (Ethex)	Rx	3,000	400	10	1.5	1.6	2.2	0.0022	70	1	15			200 (carbonate)					17		Yes
Prenate DHA Tablets (Sciele Pharma)	Rx		200	10			25	0.012	85	1	15			150 (carbonate)							
Prenate Elite Tablets (Sciele Pharma)	Rx		400	10	3	3.4	20	0.012	120	1	15		2	200 (carbonate)	0.03			6	20		Yes
Prenavite Tablets (Rugby Laboratories)	OTC	4,000	400	30	1.8	1.7	2.6	0.008	120	0.8	25		2						20		Yes
Prescriptive Formulas Men's Optimal Vitamin Packets (Nature's Bounty)	OTC	3,500	400	430	6.5	6.7	3	0.007	560	0.4	15	0.02	2	188	0.03	0.12	2	14.6	60		Yes
Prescriptive Formulas Women's Optimal Vitamin Packets (Nature's Bounty)	OTC	2,500	525	30	7	7	3.5	0.0085	560	0.4	15	0.07	2	975		0.4	2	17	60		Yes
PreserVision AREDS Soft Gel Capsules (Bausch & Lomb)	OTC	14,320		200					226		34.8		0.8								Yes
PreserVision Lutein Soft Gel Capsules (Bausch & Lomb)	OTC			200					226		34.8		0.8								Yes
PrimaCare (Ther-Rx) *per daily dose*	Rx		400	30	3	3.4	50	0.012	100	1	11	0.075	1.3	400	0.035	0.045		7	20		Yes
PrimaCare One Capsules (Ther-Rx)	Rx		170	30			25		25	1				150							Yes
Prosight Lutein Tablets (Major Pharmaceuticals)	OTC			30					60		15		2	22							Yes
Prosight Tablets (Major Pharmaceuticals)	OTC	5,000		30		25			60	0.4	40	0.04	2	44							
Puritan's Pride Complete One Tablets (Puritan's Pride)	OTC	10,000	400	30	25	25	50	0.05	250	0.4	15	0.025	2	54	0.05	0.1	5	50	50		Yes
Q.S. Tablets (McGuff) *per 6 tabs*	OTC	10,000	200	400	100	50	25	0.15	1,200	0.8	25	0.2	2	500		0.2	25	350	150	50	Yes
Quench Capsules (Bio-Tech Pharmacal) *per 4 caps*	OTC			80	5	37		1	1,500		50	0.2	1			0.2	4		60		Yes
Quintabs-M Tablets (Freeda Vitamins)	OTC	5,000	400	50	30	30	30	0.03	300	0.4	7.5	0.035	0.2	30	0.03		2	30	100		Yes
Quintabs-M Tablets-Iron Free (Freeda Vitamins)	OTC	5,000	400	50	30	30	30	0.03	300	0.4	7.5	0.035	0.2	30	0.03		2	30	100		Yes
Ragus Tablets (Miller Pharmacal Group)	OTC	5,000	400	10	20	3	5	0.009	100		2		1	580			2	5	80		Yes
Recover Tablets (The Key Company)	OTC				5	5	8	0.005	200	0.4	25	0.4						50		50	

Product	Form																			
Renatabs (Hawthorn Pharmaceuticals)	Rx			5	1.5	1.7	10	0.006	60	1	5				0.3			10	20	
Renatabs with Iron (Hawthorn Pharmaceuticals)	Rx			5	1.5	1.7	10	0.006	60	1	5				0.3			10	20	
Replace Liquid Filled Capsules (The Key Company)	OTC	2,250	500	20	12.5	12.5	12.5	0.025	50	0.2	5	0.025	0.05	45	0.01	0.025	1.25	37.5	20	Yes
Replace Liquid Filled Capsules w/o Iron (The Key Company)	OTC	2,250	500	20	12.5	12.5	12.5	0.025	50	0.2	5	0.025	0.05	45	0.01	0.025	1.25	37.5	20	Yes
Savision Tablets (Mason Vitamins) *per 2 tabs*	OTC	14,320		200					226		34.8		0.8							
Sclerex Tablets (Miller Pharmacal Group)	OTC	2,500	200	100	5	5	5	0.005	100	0.1	9		1				2	7.5	30	Yes
Select OB Caplets (Everett Laboratories)	Rx	1,700	400	30	1.6	1.8	2.5	0.005	60	1	15		1						15	Yes
Senior Eye Vision Capsules (Vitamin World) *per 4 caps*	OTC	16,250		200	10	12.5	15	0.024	250	0.4	15	0.1	1.5	50 (carbonate)				50		Yes
Siderol Tablets (A.G. Marin Pharmaceuticals)	Rx				15	15	15	0.06	250	0.8			8				3	25	20	Yes
Sterling Layered Tablets (Hillestad Pharmaceuticals USA) *per 3 tabs*	OTC	21,000	698	75	8.4	17.5	18.9	0.0168	210	0.2814	15.6	34.8	1.5	701	0.210	0.07	4.2	71.4	72.2	Yes
Stress Formula Vitamin Tablets (Major Pharmaceuticals)	OTC			30	10	10	5	0.012	500	0.4				69	0.045			20	100	
Stress Formula with Iron Tablets (Basic Vitamins)	OTC			30	10	10	5	0.012	300	0.4				20	0.045			20	100	Yes
Stress Formula with Iron Tablets (Major Pharmaceuticals)	OTC			30	10	10	5	0.012	500	0.4	23.9		3	65	0.045			20	100	
Stress Formula with Zinc Tablets (Nature's Bounty)	OTC			30	10	10	5	0.012	500	0.4	23.9		3		0.045			20	100	Yes
Stress Formula with Zinc Tablets (Upsher-Smith Laboratories)	OTC			30	10	10	5	0.012	500	0.4	23.9		3	59	0.045			20		
Strovite Advance Caplets (Everett Laboratories)	Rx	3,000	400	100	20	5	25	0.05	300	1	25	0.1	1.5		0.1	0.5	1.5	15	25	Yes
Strovite Forte Tablets (Everett Laboratories)	Rx	4,000	600	60	20	20	25	0.05	500	0.8	15	0.05	3		0.15	0.1	3	25	100	Yes
Stuart Prenatal Tablets (Xanodyne Pharmaceuticals)	OTC	4,000	400	30	1.8	1.7	2.6	0.008	120	0.8	25		0.8	200					20	Yes
Summit Gold Junior Tablets (Hillestad Pharmaceuticals USA) *per 3 tabs*	OTC	7,500	250	37.5	3	3.75	6.75	0.006	75	0.1005	5.6	0.0125	0.5	250.5	0.075	0.025	1.5	0.0255	25.8	Yes
Summit Gold Layered Tablets (Hillestad Pharmaceuticals USA) *per 3 tabs*	OTC	15,000	500	75	6	7.5	13.5	0.012	150	0.201	11.3	0.025	1	501	0.15	0.05	3	51	51.6	Yes
Summit Gold Special Formula Tablets (Hillestad Pharmaceuticals USA) *per 3 tabs*	OTC	15,000	500	75	6	7.5	13.5	0.012	150	0.201	11.3	0.025	1	501	0.15	0.05	3	51	51.6	Yes
Summit Max Layered Tablets (Hillestad Pharmaceuticals USA) *per 3 tabs*	OTC	10,000	500	75	6	7.5	13.5	0.012	150	0.201	11.3	0.035	1	501	0.15	0.06	3	51	51.6	Yes

Product/Form (Manufacturer)	FDA Class	A (IU)	D (IU)	E (IU)	B1 (mg)	B2 (mg)	B6 (mg)	B12 (mg)	C (mg)	Folic acid (mg)	Zinc (mg)	Selenium (mg)	Copper (mg)	Calcium (mg)	Biotin (mg)	Chromium (mg)	Manganese (mg)	Calcium Pantothenate B5 (mg)	Niacinamide B3 (mg)	Niacin B3 (mg)	Other
Sundown Spiderman Complete Children's Multiple Vitamin Chewable Tablets (Sundown)	OTC	5,000	400	30	1.5	1.7	2	0.006	60	0.4	15		2	100	0.04			10		20	Yes
Sunnie Tablets (The Green Turtle Bay Vitamin Company) per 4 tabs					10	10	10	0.1	500	0.4	10		0.5		0.05		20		25		
Sunvite Platinum Tablets (Rexall Naturalist)	OTC	6,000	400	45	1.5	1.7	3	0.0025	60	0.2	15	0.025	2	200	0.03	0.025	2.5	10	10		Yes
Sunvite Tablets (Rexall Naturalist)	OTC	5,000	400	30	1.5	1.7	2	0.006	60	0.4	15	0.025	2	162	0.03	0.025	2.5	10	20	20	Yes
Super 1 Daily Tablets (Carlson Laboratories)	OTC	10,000	400	200	25	25	25	0.1	250	0.4	15	0.105	1	50	0.025	0.12	3	25	25		Yes
Super 2 Daily Liquid Filled Capsules (Carlson Laboratories)	OTC	10,000	600	400	25	25	25	0.1	500	0.8	15	0.2	2	50	0.3	0.2	3	25	25		Yes
Super 75 Tablets (Carlson Laboratories)	OTC	10,000	400	200	75	75	75	0.075	250	0.4	10	0.025		35	0.075	0.025	5	75	75		Yes
Super High Vitamins & Minerals Tablets (Rugby Laboratories)	OTC	10,000	400	150	75	75	75	0.075	250	0.4	1.5	0.01	0.025	10	0.075	0.025	0.61	75	75		Yes
Supermins Tablets (The Key Company)	OTC			200					250			0.025									Yes
Support Liquid (A.G.Marin Pharmaceutical) per 5 mL	OTC	1,500	100		8	2	2	0.01		0.8	2.86							10	30		Yes
Support-500 Softgel Capsules (A.G. Marin Pharmaceuticals)	Rx	5,000	100	400	20	20	20	0.025	500	0.4	28	0.05					1.3	18	25		Yes
Surbex 750 with Zinc Tablets (Abbott Laboratories)	OTC			27	12	13.5	4.5	0.018	750	0.36	20.3										Yes
Tab A Vite Essential Tablets (Major Pharmaceuticals)	OTC	5,000		30					60			0.04	2	44							
Tab A Vite Maximum Tablets (Major Pharmaceuticals)	OTC	5,000	400	30	1.5	1.7	2	0.006	60	0.4	40	0.01	2	130	0.03	0.01	2.5	10	20		Yes
Tab A Vite Women's Formula Tablets (Major Pharmaceuticals)	OTC	5,000	400	30	1.5	1.7	2	0.006	60	0.4	15			450 (carbonate)				10	20		Yes
Tandem DHA Capsules (US Pharmaceuticals)	Rx						25		20	1	15										Yes
Tandem OB Capsules (US Pharmaceuticals)	Rx				10	6	5	0.015	200	1	18.2		0.8				1.3	10	30		Yes
Tandem Plus Capsules (US Pharmaceuticals)	Rx				10	6	5	0.015	200	1	18.2		0.8				1.3	10	30		Yes
Thera M Tablets (Amneal Pharmaceuticals)	OTC	5,500	400	30	3	3.4	3	0.009	120	0.4	15	0.01	2	40	0.015	0.015	5	10	30		Yes
Theradex M (Mason Vitamins)	OTC	5,500	400	30	3	3.4	3	0.009	120	0.4	15	0.01	2	40	0.015	0.015	5	10	30	30	Yes

Product (Manufacturer)	Rx/OTC	(1)	(2)	(3)	(4)	(5)	(6)	(7)	(8)	(9)	(10)	(11)	(12)	(13)	(14)	(15)	(16)	(17)	(18)	(19)	(20)
Thera-M Enhanced Tablets (Major Pharmaceuticals)	OTC	5,000	400	60	3	3.4	6	0.012	90	0.4	15	0.07	2	40	0.03	0.05	2	10	10	20	Yes
Thera-M w/Mineral Tablets (Prime Marketing)	OTC	5,000	400	30	3	3.4	3	0.009	90	0.4	15	0.021	2	40	0.03	0.026	3.5	10	10	20	Yes
Theramill Forte Capsules (Miller Pharmacal Group) *per 6 caps*	OTC	21,000	200	400	100	75	100	0.1	1,000	0.4	15	0.2	400	400	0.3	0.2	10	100	160	40	Yes
Theramill Plus Capsules (Miller Pharmacal Group) *per 6 caps*	OTC	21,000	200	400	75	38	75	0.1	1,000	0.4	15	0.2	1,200	400	0.3	0.2	10	100	160	40	Yes
Theramill Plus Liquid Filled Capsules (Miller Pharmacal Group)	OTC	21,000	200	400	75	38	75	0.1	1,000	0.4	15	0.2	1.2	400	0.3	0.2	10	100	160	40	Yes
Therapeutic Multivitamin with Mineral Tablets (Upsher-Smith Laboratories)	OTC	5,000	400	30	3	3.4	3	0.009	120	0.4	15	0.01	2	40	0.015	0.015	5	10	30		Yes
Theravim-M Tablets (Nature's Bounty)	OTC	5,000	400	60	3	3.4	6	0.012	90	0.4	15	0.07	2	35	0.03	0.05	2	10	20		Yes
Theravim-M Tablets (Puritan's Pride)	OTC	5,000	400	30	3	3.4	3	0.009	90	0.4	15	0.01	2	40	0.03	0.015	5	10	20		Yes
Therems-H Tablets (Rugby Laboratories)	OTC	1,400	140	5	3.3	3.3	3.3	0.05	100	0.33	15		0.67	130				11.7	33.3		Yes
Therems-M Tablets (Rugby Laboratories)	OTC	5,000	400	60	3	3.4	6	0.012	90	0.4	15	0.07	2	40	0.03	0.05	2	10	20		Yes
Therobec Plus Tablets (Qualitest Products)	Rx	5,000	30	30	20	20	25	0.05	500	0.8	22.5	0.025	3		0.15	0.1	5	25		100	Yes
Time Release Mega Vita-Min Iron Free Tablets (Puritan's Pride)	OTC	8,000	125	80	80	80	80	0.08	250	0.4	1.4	0.025	0.07	18	0.08	0.025	0.12	80	80		Yes
Total Formula 3 Tablets (Integrative Therapeutics)	OTC	10,000	400	30	15	15	25	0.025	100	0.4	30	0.025	2	100	0.3	0.2	2	25	25		Yes
Triamin Tablets (The Key Company)	OTC		30								125			125							Yes
T-Vites Tablets (Freeda Vitamins)	OTC		400		25	25	25	0.03	100	0.4	3.75	0.1	2		0.03		0.5	25	150		Yes
Ultra Freeda A Free Tablets (Freeda Vitamins) *per 3 tabs*	OTC	400	200	50	50	50	50	0.1	1,000	0.8	22.5	0.1	250	250	0.3	0.2	10	100	100		Yes
Ultra Freeda, Iron Free Tablets (Freeda Vitamins) *per 3 tabs*	OTC	400	200	50	50	50	50	0.1	1,000	0.8	22.5	0.1	250	250	0.3	0.2	10	100	100		Yes
Ultra Freeda, With Iron Tablets (Freeda Vitamins) *per 3 tabs*	OTC	400	200	50	50	50	50	0.1	1,000	0.8	22.5	0.1	250	250	0.3	0.2	10	100	100		Yes
Ultra NatalCare Tablets (Ethex)	Rx	2,700	400	30	3	3.4	20	0.012	120	1	25	0.035	2	200 (citrate)	0.001	0.00235	0.76	12.5	20	20	Yes
Ultra Vita-Min Iron Free Tablets (Puritan's Pride)	OTC	10,000	400	12.5	24	25	14	0.05	150	0.4	0.72	0.01	0.035	60	0.001	0.00235	0.76	12.5	50	50	Yes
Ultra Vita-Min Tablets (Nature's Bounty)	OTC	10,000	400	12.5	25	25	15	0.05	150	0.4	0.66	0.01	0.035	60	0.001	0.00235	1	12.5	50	50	Yes
Unicomplex-M Tablets (Rugby Laboratories)	OTC	5,000	30	30	1.5	1.7	2	0.006	60	0.4	15	0.006	2	60	0.006		2	10		20	Yes
Uni-Thera M Advanced Tablets (United Research Laboratories)	OTC	5,000	60	60	3	3.4	6	0.012	90	0.4	15	0.07	2	40	0.03	0.05	2	10	20	90	Yes
V-C Forte Capsules (Breckenridge Pharmaceuticals)	Rx	8,000	50	50	10	5	2	0.01	150	1	80							10		25	Yes
Vicap Forte Capsules (Major Pharmaceuticals)	Rx	8,000	50	50	10	5	2	0.01	150		80							10		25	

Product/Form (Manufacturer)	FDA Class	A (IU)	D (IU)	E (IU)	B1 (mg)	B2 (mg)	B6 (mg)	B12 (mg)	C (mg)	Folic acid (mg)	Zinc (mg)	Selenium (mg)	Copper (mg)	Calcium (mg)	Biotin (mg)	Chromium (mg)	Manganese (mg)	Calcium Pantothenate B5 (mg)	Niacinamide B3 (mg)	Niacin B3 (mg)	Other
Vicon C Capsules (UCB)	OTC				17.9	10	4		300		15.9							22	95		Yes
Vigomar Forte Tablets (Marlop Pharmaceuticals)	OTC	10,000	400	15	10	10	5	0.005	200	1	1.5		2				1	20	100		Yes
Vinate AZ Extra Tablets (Breckenridge Pharmaceuticals)	Rx	3,000	400	30	3	3.5	60	0.012	120	1	15				0.03			8	20		Yes
Vinate AZ Tablets (Breckenridge Pharmaceuticals)	Rx	3,000	400	30	3	3.5	30	0.012	120	1	15		2.5	160 (carbonate)	0.03			8	20		Yes
Vinate GT Tablets (Breckenridge Pharmaceuticals)	Rx	2,700	400	10	3	3.4	20	0.012	120	1	15		2	200 (carbonate)	0.3			6	20		Yes
Vinate II Tablets (Breckenridge Pharmaceuticals)	Rx	3,000	400	30	1.8	4	25	0.012	120	1	25		2	200 (carbonate)					20		Yes
Vinate M Tablets (Breckenridge Pharmaceuticals)	Rx	5,000	400	30	3	3.4	10	0.012	120	1	25	0.02	2	200 (carbonate)	0.03	0.025	5	10	20		Yes
Vision Vitamin Tablets (Mason Vitamins)	OTC	5,000		30					60		40	0.04	2	44							
Vision Vitamin Tablets Plus Lutein (Mason Vitamins)	OTC	1,000		60					200		40	0.055	2								Yes
Vita S Forte Tablets (Rising Pharmaceuticals)	Rx	4,000	400	60	20	20	25	0.05	500	1	15	0.05	3		0.15	0.05		25	100		Yes
Vita Zinc Tablets (Major Pharmaceuticals)	OTC			45	15	10.2	10	0.006	600	0.4	22.5							25		100	Yes
Vitabasic Active Tablets (Basic Vitamins)	OTC	5,000	400	60	4.5	5.1	6	0.018	120	0.4	15	0.07	2	100	0.04	0.12	4	10		40	Yes
Vitabasic Complete Tablets (Basic Vitamins)	OTC	3,500	400	30	1.5	1.7	2	0.006	60	0.4	15	0.02	2	162	0.03	0.12	2	10		20	Yes
Vitabasic Senior Tablets (Basic Vitamins)	OTC	3,500	400	45	1.5	1.7	3	0.025	60		15	0.02	2	200	0.03	0.15	2	10		20	Yes
Vitadec Tablets (Major Pharmaceuticals)	OTC	5,000	400	30	1.7	2	3	0.006	60	0.4	15	0.025	2	162	0.03	0.025	2.5	10		20	Yes
Vitafol OB +DHA Caplets (Everett Laboratories)	Rx	2,700	400	30	1.6	1.8	2.5	0.012	70	1	25		2	100 (carbonate)					18		Yes
Vitafol OB Caplets (Everett Laboratories)	Rx	2,700	400	30	1.6	1.8	2.5	0.012	70	1	25		2	100					18		Yes
Vitalets Children's Chewable Tablets (Freeda Vitamins)	OTC	2,500	200	15	0.75	0.85	1	0.003	40	0.2	0.8			80	0.15		0.1	5	10		Yes
Vita-Min Capsules (Bio-Tech Pharmacal)	OTC	7,500	333	100	25	25	13	0.2	193	0.8	10	0.067	0.05	47	0.5	0.2	0.2	25	25	12.5	Yes
Vitamin Tonic for Seniors (Major Pharmaceuticals) per 15 mL	OTC				1.5	1.7		0.006			15		2				2	10		20	Yes
Vitamins for Hair Tablets (Basic Vitamins)	OTC	5,000		30	2	4	2	0.006		0.4	15			80	0.3		2	50	25	35	Yes

Product (manufacturer)	FDA																			
Vitamins for the Hair Tablets (Vitamin World)	OTC								0.4	15						5	100	35	Yes
Vitamins for the Hair Tablets (Puritan's Pride)	OTC						0.006		0.4	15						5	100	35	Yes
VitaTRUM Chewable Tablets (Mason Vitamins)	OTC	3,500	400	60	1.5	1.7	2	0.006	60	0.4	15	0.02	2	108	0.045	0.02	1	10	20	Yes
VitaTRUM Complete Multivitamin/Multimineral tablets (Mason Vitamins)	OTC	3,500	400	30	1.5	1.7	2	0.006	60	0.4	15	0.02	2	162	0.03	0.12	2	10	20	Yes
Vitrum Senior Complete Multivitamin/Multimineral tablets (Mason Vitamins)	OTC	3,500	400	45	1.5	1.7	3	0.025	60	0.4	15	0.02	2	200	0.03	0.15	2	10	20	Yes
Women's Exclusive Formula Tablets (Puritan's Pride) *per 2 tabs*	OTC	5,000	400	30	30	30	30	0.13	60	0.4	15	0.025	0.5	500	0.03	0.025	5	30	30	Yes
Women's Exclusive Formula Tablets (Vitamin World) *per 2 tabs*	OTC	5,000	400	30	30	30	30	0.13	60	0.4	15	0.025	0.5	500	0.03	0.025	5	30	30	Yes
Women's One Daily Caplets (Sundown)	OTC	2,500	400	30	1.5	1.7	2	0.006	60	0.4	15		2	450				5	10	Yes
Women's Ultra Mega Active Caplets (General Nutrition Centers) *per 2 caps*	OTC	5,000	600	30	50	50	50	0.05	200	0.4	15	0.02	2	500	0.3	0.12	2	50	35	Yes
Xtramins Tablets (The Key Company)	OTC	1,000	100	10	5	2	5	0.01	50	0.4	10	0.03	0.5	250	0.03	0.04	2	5	15	Yes
Yelets Tablets (Freeda Vitamins)	OTC	5,000	400	30	10	10	10	0.01	100	0.4	7.5	0.0175		60	0.03	0.06	1	10	25	Yes
Yummi Bears Chewables (Hero Nutritional Products)	OTC	2,500	200	15			1	0.003	30	0.2	7.5			9.2 (Calcium citrate)	0.15			5	10	Yes
Yummi Bears Multivitamin and Mineral (Hero Nutritionals) *per 3 gummy bears*	OTC	2,500	200	15			1	0.003	30	200	7.5			9.2 (Calcium citrate)	0.15			5	10	Yes

FDA = Food and Drug Administration. Rx = requires a prescription; OTC = available over the counter.
IU = international units; mg = milligram(s).

OTHER INGREDIENTS:

ABC Plus Senior Tablets (Nature's Bounty)
Vitamin K 0.01 mg, Phosphorus 48 mg, Iodine 0.15 mg, Magnesium 100 mg, Molybdenum 0.075 mg, Chloride 72 mg, Potassium 80 mg, Boron 0.15 mg, Nickel 0.005 mg, Silica 2 mg, Vanadium 0.01 mg, Lycopene 0.3 mg, Lutein 0.25 mg

ABC Plus Senior Tablets (Puritan's Pride)
Vitamin K 0.01 mg, Phosphorus 51 mg, Iodine 0.15 mg, Magnesium 100 mg, Molybdenum 0.075 mg, Chloride 72 mg, Potassium 80 mg, Boron 0.15 mg, Nickel 0.005 mg, Silica 2 mg, Vanadium 0.01 mg, Lycopene 0.3 mg, Lutein 0.25 mg

ABC Plus Tablets (Nature's Bounty)
Vitamin K 0.025 mg, Ferrous fumarate 18 mg, Phosphorus 113 mg, Iodine 0.15 mg, Magnesium 100 mg, Molybdenum 0.075 mg, Chloride 72 mg, Potassium 80 mg, Boron 0.15 mg, Nickel 0.005 mg, Silica 2 mg, Tin 0.01 mg, Vanadium 0.01 mg, Lutein 0.25 mg, Lycopene 0.3 mg

ABC Plus Tablets (Puritan's Pride)
Vitamin K 0.025 mg, Iron (Ferrous fumarate) 18 mg, Phosphorus 109 mg, Iodine 0.15 mg, Magnesium 100 mg, Molybdenum 0.075 mg, Chloride 72 mg, Potassium 80 mg, Boron 0.15 mg, Nickel 0.005 mg, Silica 2 mg, Tin 0.01 mg, Vanadium 0.01 mg, Lutein 0.25 mg, Lycopene 0.3 mg

ACES Gold Tablets
Coenzyme Q10 7.5 mg, Glutathione 1.5 mg, N-Acetyl Cysteine 25 mg, Alpha-lipoic acid 3 mg, Citrus bioflavonoids 50 mg, Quercetin bioflavonoid 15 mg, Garlic (odorless) 50 mg, Grape seed extract 5 mg, Green tea 1.5 mg, Lutein 0.5 mg

Actical Softgel Capsules
Vitamin K 0.04 mg, Magnesium 45 mg

Adult Chewable Multivitamin Tablets
Iron (Ferrous fumarate) 5 mg, Iodine 0.1 mg, Magnesium 0.145 mg, Soy lecithin 25 mg, Choline bitartrate 5 mg, Hesperidin complex 5 mg, Betaine HCl 5 mg, Rutin 2.5 mg, Citrus bioflavonoids 2.5 mg, PABA (Para-Aminobenzoic Acid) 2.5 mg, Inositol 2.5 mg

Adult Chewable Pineapple Flavor Tablets
Iron (Ferrous fumarate) 5 mg, Iodine 0.1 mg, Magnesium 0.145 mg, Soy lecithin 25 mg, Choline bitartrate 5 mg, Hesperidin complex 5 mg, Betaine HCl 5 mg, Rutin 2.5 mg, Citrus bioflavonoids 2.5 mg, PABA (Para-Aminobenzoic Acid) 2.5 mg, Inositol 2.5 mg

Advanced Natalcare Tablets
Iron 90 mg, Magnesium 30 mg, Docusate sodium 50 mg

Advanced Prenatal Tablets
Magnesium 125 mg, Iodine 0.075 mg, Iron (Ferrous fumarate) 30 mg, Potassium 25 mg, Inositol 25 mg, PABA (Para-Aminobenzoic Acid) 25 mg, Bioflavonoids complex 135 mg, Choline bitartrate 150 mg, Pancreatin 8X 37.5 mg, Betaine HCl 30 mg, DHA (Docosahexanoic Acid) 100 mg

Advanced RF Natalcare Tablets
Iron 90 mg, Magnesium 30 mg, Docusate sodium 50 mg

Advanced Therabasic M Tablets
Vitamin K 0.028 mg, Iron 9 mg, Phosphorus 31 mg, Iodine 0.15 mg, Magnesium 100 mg, Molybdenum 0.075 mg, Chloride 7 mg, Potassium 7.5 mg, Boron 0.15 mg, Tin 0.01 mg, Vanadium 0.01 mg, Nickel 0.005 mg, Silica 2 mg

A-Free Prenatal Tablets
Iron (Ferrous fumarate) 27 mg, Magnesium 100 mg, Natural base (contains Bioflavonoids and Hesperidin) 66 mg

Alpha Betic Caplets
Iodine 0.15 mg, Magnesium 200 mg, Potassium 100 mg, Alpha-lipoic acid 100 mg, Lutein 1.5 mg, Vanadium 0.1 mg

Androvite Tablets
Iron 18 mg, Iodine 0.15 mg, Magnesium 500 mg, PABA (Para-Aminobenzoic Acid) 25 mg, Betaine HCl 100 mg, Pancreatin 4X 75 mg, Inositol 36 mg, Hesperidin 35 mg, Rutin 25 mg, Boron 3 mg

Antioxidant 4,000 Capsules
Proprietary blend (Carrot powder, Broccoli powder, Spinach powder) 3 mg

Apetimar with Iron Solution
Iron 15 mg, L-lysine 150 mg

Aquadeks Pediatric Liquid
Vitamin K 0.4 mg, Beta carotene 3 mg, Coenzyme Q10 3 mg

Aquadeks Soft Gel Capsules
Vitamin K 0.7 mg, Beta carotene 10 mg, Coenzyme Q10 10 mg

Bacmin Tablets
Bioflavonoids 50 mg, Iron 27 mg, Magnesium 50 mg

Body, Hair, Skin, and Nails Formula Capsules
Iron (Ferrous fumarate) 9 mg, Phosphorus 200 mg, Iodine 0.15 mg, Magnesium 100 mg, Choline bitartrate 500 mg, Gelatin 250 mg, Inositol 100 mg, PABA (Para-Aminobenzoic Acid) 60 mg

Bounty Buddies Plus Extra C Chewable Tablets
Sodium 15 mg

Calafol Rx Tablets
Policosanol 5 mg

Calcet Plus Tablets
Iron 18 mg

Calcifol DT Wafers
Magnesium 50 mg, Boron 0.25 mg

Calcifol Wafers
Magnesium 60 mg, Boron 1 mg

Calna Tablets
Iron 10 mg, Iodine 0.15 mg, Magnesium 20 mg, Boron 1 mg, PABA (Para-Aminobenzoic Acid) 5 mg, Potassium 45 mg

Cal-Nate Tablets
Iron 27 mg, Iodine 0.15 mg, Docusate sodium 50 mg

Cardenz Tablets (Miller Pharmacal Group)
Inositol 30 mg, PABA (Para-Aminobenzoic Acid) 9 mg, Potassium 8 mg, Iodine 0.05 mg, Magnesium 23 mg

CareNatal DHA Tablets
Iron 29 mg, Magnesium 25 mg

Carlson for Kids Chewable Vitamin and Mineral Tablets
Vitamin K 0.04 mg, Iron 9 mg, Phosphorus 22 mg, Iodine 0.075 mg, Magnesium 25 mg, Molybdenum 0.038 mg, Potassium 2.5 mg, Lemon bioflavonoids 10 mg

Cenogen Ultra Tablets
Iron (Ferrous fumarate) 324 mg

Centamin Liquid
Iron 9 mg, Iodine 0.15 mg

Centrum Cardio Tablets
Vitamin K 0.0125 mg, Iron 3 mg, Phosphorus 40 mg, Iodine 0.075 mg, Magnesium 20 mg, Molybdenum 0.0375 mg, Chloride 29 mg, Potassium 32 mg, Boron 0.016 mg, Nickel 0.0025 mg, Silicon 1 mg, Tin 0.005 mg, Vanadium 0.005 mg, Phytosterols 400 mg

Centrum Chewable Tablets
Vitamin K 0.01 mg, Iron 18 mg, Phosphorus 50 mg, Iodine 0.15 mg, Magnesium 40 mg, Molybdenum 0.02 mg

Centrum Kids Complete Dora the Explorer Chewable Vitamin Tablets
Vitamin K 0.01 mg, Iron 18 mg, Phosphorus 50 mg, Iodine 0.15 mg, Magnesium 40 mg, Molybdenum 0.02 mg

Centrum Kids Complete Rugrats Chewable Vitamin Tablets

Vitamin K 0.01 mg, Iron 18 mg, Phosphorus 50 mg, Iodine 0.15 mg, Magnesium 40 mg, Molybdenum 0.02 mg

Centrum Kids Complete Sponge Bob Square Pants Chewable Vitamin Tablets

Vitamin K 0.01 mg, Iron 18 mg, Phosphorus 50 mg, Iodine 0.15 mg, Magnesium 40 mg, Molybdenum 0.02 mg

Centrum Liquid

Iron 9 mg, Iodine 0.15 mg, Molybdenum 0.025 mg

Centrum Performance Tablets

Vitamin K 0.025 mg, Iron 18 mg, Phosphorus 48 mg, Iodine 0.15 mg, Magnesium 40 mg, Molybdenum 0.075 mg, Chloride 72 mg, Potassium 80 mg, Ginseng root 50 mg, Ginkgo biloba 60 mg, Boron 0.06 mg, Nickel 0.005 mg, Silicon 4 mg, Tin 0.01 mg, Vanadium 0.01 mg

Centrum Silver Chewable Tablets

Phosphorus 125 mg, Iodine 0.1 mg, Magnesium 50 mg, Molybdenum 0.025 mg, Nickel 0.005 mg, Silicon 4 mg, Tin 0.01 mg, Vanadium 0.01 mg, Lutein 0.25 mg

Centrum Silver Tablets

Vitamin K 0.03 mg, Phosphorus 110 mg, Iodine 0.15 mg, Magnesium 50 mg, Molybdenum 0.045 mg, Chloride 72 mg, Potassium 80 mg, Boron 0.15 mg, Nickel 0.005 mg, Silicon 2 mg, Vanadium 0.01 mg, Lutein 0.25 mg, Lycopene 0.3 mg

Centrum Tablets

Vitamin K 0.025 mg, Iron 18 mg, Phosphorus 109 mg, Iodine 0.15 mg, Magnesium 100 mg, Molybdenum 0.045 mg, Chloride 72 mg, Potassium 80 mg, Boron 0.15 mg, Nickel 0.005 mg, Silicon 2 mg, Tin 0.01 mg, Vanadium 0.01 mg, Lutein 0.25 mg, Lycopene 0.3 mg

Cerovite Advanced Formula Tablets

Vitamin K 30 IU; Iron (Ferrous fumarate) 18 mg, Phosphorus 109 mg, Iodine 0.15 mg, Magnesium 100 mg, Molybdenum 0.045 mg, Chloride 72 mg, Potassium 80 mg, Boron 0.15 mg, Nickel 0.005 mg, Tin 0.01 mg, Silicon 2 mg, Vanadium 0.01 mg, Lutein 0.25 mg, Lycopene 0.3 mg

Cerovite Jr. Chewable Tablets

Vitamin K 0.01 mg, Iron (Ferrous fumarate) 18 mg, Phosphorus 50 mg, Iodine 0.15 mg, Magnesium 40 mg, Molybdenum 0.02 mg

Cerovite Liquid Advanced Formula

Iron (Ferrous gluconate) 9 mg, Iodine 0.15 mg, Molybdenum 0.025 mg

Cerovite Senior Tablets

Vitamin K 0.03 mg, Phosphorus 110 mg, Iodine 0.15 mg, Magnesium 50 mg, Molybdenum 0.045 mg, Chloride 72 mg, Potassium 80 mg, Boron 0.15 mg, Nickel 0.005 mg, Silica 2 mg, Vanadium 0.01 mg, Lutein 0.25 mg, Lycopene 0.3 mg

CertaVite Liquid

Iodine 0.15 mg, Iron 9 mg, Molybdenum 0.025 mg

CertaVite Performance Tablets

Boron 0.60 mg, Chloride 72 mg, Ginkgo biloba extract 60 mg, Iodine 0.15 mg, Korean ginseng extract 50 mg, Magnesium 40 mg, Molybdenum 0.075 mg, Nickel 0.005 mg, Phosphorus 48 mg, Potassium 80 mg, Silica 4 mg, Tin 0.01 mg, Vanadium 0.01 mg, Vitamin K 0.025 mg

CertaVite Senior with Lutein Tablets

Boron 0.150 mg, Chloride 72 mg, Iodine 0.15 mg, Lutein 0.25 mg, Magnesium 100 mg, Molybdenum 0.075 mg, Nickel 0.005 mg, Phosphorus 48 mg, Potassium 80 mg, Silica 2 mg, Vanadium 0.01 mg, Vitamin K 0.01 mg

Certavite with Lutein Tablets

Boron 0.150 mg, Chloride 72 mg, Iodine 0.150 mg, Lutein 0.250 mg, Magnesium 100 mg, Molybdenum 0.075 mg, Nickel 0.005 mg, Phosphorus 109 mg, Potassium 80 mg, Silica 2 mg, Vanadium 0.01 mg, Vitamin K 0.025 mg

Children's Chewable Layered Tablets

Iron (Ferrous fumarate) 4 mg, Iodine 0.075 mg, Magnesium 10 mg, Molybdenum 0.003 mg, Potassium 4 mg

Children's Multi Gummies

Iodine 0.03 mg, Magnesium 2 mg, Sodium 10 mg, Inositol 0.01 mg, Sugars 3 g

CitraNatal 90 DHA Capsules

Iron 90 mg, Iodine 0.15 mg, Docusate sodium 50 mg, Docosahexaenoic acid (DHA) 250 mg

CitraNatal DHA Capsules

Iron 27 mg, Iodine 0.15 mg, Docusate sodium 50 mg, Docosahexaenoic acid (DHA) 250 mg

CitraNatal Rx Capsules

Iron 27 mg, Iodine 0.15 mg, Docusate sodium 50 mg

Clusimar Liquid

Panthenol 3 mg, Magnesium 3 mg

Complere Tablets (Miller Pharmacal Group)

Iron 15 mg, Phosphorus 345 mg, Iodine 0.1 mg, Magnesium 80 mg, Potassium 30 mg, L-lysine monohydrochloride 30 mg, DL-Methionine 30 mg

Daily Multi Caplets

Vitamin K 0.025 mg, Iron 18 mg, Iodine 0.15 mg, Magnesium 100 mg, Molybdenum 0.16 mg, Chloride 72 mg, Potassium 80 mg, Boron 0.15 mg, Tin 0.01 mg, Vanadium 0.01 mg, Nickel 0.005 mg, Silica 2 mg

Daily Prenatal Tablets

Iron (Ferrous fumarate) 27 mg, Magnesium 60 mg

Daily Vitamins with Calcium & Extra Iron for Women Tablets

Iron (Ferrous fumarate) 18 mg, Magnesium 50 mg

DermaVite Tablets

Lycopene 5 mg, Silicon 20 mg

Diabetic Support Formula Tablets

Magnesium 250 mg, Alpha-lipoic acid 30 mg, Vanadyl sulfate 10 mg, Ginkgo biloba 20 mg, Coenzyme Q10 5 mg, Taurine 50 mg, L-carnitine 125 mg

Diabetiks Tablets

Magnesium 150 mg, Molybdenum 0.0125 mg, Bilberry extract 50 mg, Citrus bioflavonoids 12.5 mg, Ginkgo biloba 10 mg, Green tea extract 20 mg, Huckleberry leaf 100 mg, Pine bark extract-OPC-85% 1 mg, L-carnitine-L-tartrate 7.5 mg, N-acetyl-L-cysteine 50 mg, Taurine 375 mg, Coenzyme Q10 1 mg, Lipoic acid 5 mg

Diasense Multivitamin Tablets

Iodine 0.15 mg, Magnesium 200 mg, Potassium 100 mg, Alpha-lipoic acid 60 mg, Coenzyme Q10 5 mg, Lutein 0.5 mg, Vanadium 0.1 mg

Duet Chewable Tablets

Iron 29 mg, Magnesium 25 mg

Duet DHA Enteric Coated Soft Gel Capsules

Iron 29 mg, Magnesium 25 mg

Duet DHA Tablets

Iron 29 mg, Magnesium 25 mg

Duet Tablets

Iron 29 mg, Magnesium 25 mg

Encora Tablets

Essential Fatty Acids (omega-3) 650 mg, DHA and EPA 550 mg, Alpha-linolenic acid (ALA) 100 mg, Linoleic acid (LA) 10 mg

Enfamil Kindercal Liquid

Vitamin K 0.0075 mg, Choline 63 mg, Inositol 20 mg, L-carnitine 15 mg, Taurine 15 mg, Phosphorus 200 mg,

Magnesium 50 mg, Iron 2.5 mg, Iodine 0.03 mg, Sodium 88 mg, Potassium 310 mg, Chloride 175 mg, Molybdenum 0.0125 mg

Enfamil Kindercal Liquid with Fiber
Vitamin K 0.0075 mg, Choline 63 mg, Inositol 20 mg, L-carnitine 15 mg, Taurine 15 mg, Phosphorus 200 mg, Magnesium 50 mg, Iron 2.5 mg, Iodine 0.03 mg, Sodium 88 mg, Potassium 310 mg, Chloride 175 mg, Molybdenum 0.0125 mg, Fiber 1.5 g

Extress-30 Extended Release Capsules
Magnesium 15 mg

Fem Cal Citrate Tablets
Magnesium 400 mg, Boron 2 mg, Silica 10 mg

Fem Cal Plus Tablets
Magnesium 400 mg, Boron 2 mg, Silica 10 mg

Fem Cal Tablets
Magnesium 400 mg, Boron 2 mg, Silica 10 mg

Femtabs Tablets
Magnesium 80 mg

Ferrocite Plus Tablets
Iron (Ferrous fumarate) 324 mg, Magnesium 6.9 mg

Ferrotate Junior Capsules
Iron 25 mg, Magnesium 50 mg

Flintstones Complete Chewable Tablets
Iron 18 mg, Phosphorus 100 mg, Iodine 0.15 mg, Magnesium 20 mg, Sodium 10 mg, Choline 38 mg

Foltabs Prenatal + DHA Tablets
Iron 27 mg, Iodine 0.15 mg; Docusate sodium 50 mg, Docosahexaenoic Acid (DHA) 250 mg

Foltabs Prenatal Tablets
Iron 27 mg, Iodine 0.15 mg, Docusate sodium 50 mg

Formula 100 Tablets
Iron (Ferrous fumarate) 18 mg, Iodine 0.15 mg, Magnesium 50 mg, Potassium 10 mg, PABA (Para-Aminobenzoic Acid) 100 mg, Choline bitartrate 100 mg, Inositol 100 mg, Rutin 25 mg, Lemon bioflavonoids 50 mg, Hesperidin 12.5 mg, Betaine HCl 30 mg, Octacosanol 0.05 mg, Proprietary blend (Alfalfa leaf, Watercress, Parsley leaf, Rice bran and Soy lecithin) 5 mg

Formula B Plus Tablets
Iron (Ferrous fumarate) 27 mg, Magnesium 50 mg

Freedavite Tablets
Iron (Ferrous fumarate) 8 mg, Iodine 0.075 mg, Magnesium 8 mg

Geriaton Liquid
Iron 15 mg, Iodine 0.1 mg, Magnesium 2 mg, Choline 100 mg

Geri-Freeda Tablets
Iodine 0.15 mg, Magnesium 25 mg, Betaine HCl 10 mg, Choline 10 mg, Hesperidin 10 mg, Inositol 25 mg, L-lysine 25 mg, PABA (Para-Aminobenzoic Acid) 10 mg

Geritol Complete Tablets
Vitamin K 0.024 mg, Iron 16 mg, Iodine 0.12 mg, Magnesium 86 mg, Phosphorus 118 mg, Potassium 36 mg, Chloride 20 mg, Molybdenum 0.001 mg

Geritol Extend Tablets
Vitamin K 0.08 mg, Iron 9.5 mg, Iodine 0.13mg: Magnesium 32 mg, Calcium 120 mg, Phosphorus 98 mg

Geritol Tonic Liquid
Methionine 25 mg, Choline bitartrate 50 mg, Iron 18 mg

Glutofac-MX Caplets
Iron 82 mg, Magnesium 300 mg, Iodine 0.15 mg, Molybdenum 0.075 mg, Phosphorus 130 mg, Dioctyl sodium sulfosuccinate 50 mg, Nickel 0.005 mg, Tin 0.01 mg, Vanadium 0.01 mg, Boron 0.15 mg

Glutofac-ZX Caplets
Magnesium 50 mg

Glutofac-ZX Caplets
Lutein 0.5 mg, Lycopene 0.5 mg, Magnesium 100 mg

GNC Kid's MultiBite plus Minerals and Calcium Chewable Tablets
Iron 12 mg, Phosphorus 45 mg, Iodine 0.1 mg, Magnesium 100 mg, Citrus bioflavonoids complex 6 mg, Inositol 5 mg, Choline bitartrate 1 mg

GNC Kid's Multibite plus Minerals Chewable Tablets
Iron (Ferrous fumarate) 12 mg, Phosphorus 15 mg, Iodine 0.11 mg, Magnesium 15 mg, Choline bitartrate 1 mg, Inositol 5 mg, PABA (Para-Aminobenzoic Acid) 1 mg, Citrus bioflavonoids complex 6 mg

GNC Multi-Gel Multivitamin Capsules
Iron (Ferrous fumarate) 18 mg, Phosphorus 50 mg, Iodine 0.15 mg, Magnesium 50 mg, Potassium 30 mg, Soybean oil 442 mg, Lecithin 80 mg, Inositol 50 mg, PABA (Para-Aminobenzoic Acid) 50 mg, Choline bitartrate 50 mg

GNC Multi-Gel without Iron Capsules
Phosphorus 50 mg, Iodine 0.15 mg, Magnesium 50 mg, Potassium 30 mg, Soybean oil 442 mg, Lecithin 80 mg, Inositol 0.05 mg, PABA (Para-Aminobenzoic Acid) 50 mg, Choline bitartrate 50 mg

GNC Soloday Multivitamin Tablets
Vitamin K 0.025 mg, Iron (Ferrous fumarate) 18 mg, Phosphorus 109 mg, Iodine 0.15 mg, Magnesium 100 mg, Molybdenum 0.075 mg, Chloride 72 mg, Potassium 80 mg, Boron 0.15 mg, Silica 2 mg, Lycopene 0.3 mg, Lutein 0.25 mg, Tin 0.01 mg, Vanadium 0.01 mg, Nickel 0.005 mg

GNC Solotron Chewable Wafers
Iron (Ferrous gluconate) 5 mg, Iodine 0.076 mg, Lecithin 25 mg, Hesperidin complex 5 mg, Betaine HCl 5 mg, Rutin 2.5 mg, Citrus bioflavonoids complex 2.5 mg, PABA (Para-Aminobenzoic Acid) 2.5 mg, Inositol 2.5 mg, Choline bitartrate 5 mg

GNC Solotron Multivitamin Caplets
Vitamin K 0.025 mg, Iron (Ferrous fumarate) 18 mg, Iodine 0.15 mg, Magnesium 30 mg, Molybdenum 0.025 mg, Potassium 30 mg, Choline bitartrate 14 mg, PABA (Para-Aminobenzoic Acid) 30 mg, Citrus bioflavonoids complex 25 mg, Green tea leaves extract 5 mg, N-acetyl-L-cysteine (NAC) 0.5 mg, Lutein 0.3 mg, Boron 0.1 mg, Inositol 0.03 mg, Vanadium 0.01 mg, Silicon 0.01 mg

GNC Solotron Platinum Multivitamin Tablets
Iron 10 mg, Phosphorus 35 mg, Iodine 0.03 mg, Magnesium 100 mg, Molybdenum 0.025 mg, Chloride 72 mg, Potassium 80 mg, Silica 0.01 mg, Nickel 0.005 mg, Inositol 0.05 mg, Choline bitartrate 0.05 mg, PABA (Para-Aminobenzoic Acid) 0.05 mg, Citrus bioflavonoids complex 50 mg, Coenzyme Q10 0.075 mg, Lecithin powder 50 mg, Lupinus albus & Triticum vulgare 0.3 mg

GNC Solotron without Iron Multivitamin Caplets
Vitamin K 0.025 mg, Iodine 0.15 mg, Magnesium 30 mg, Molybdenum 0.025 mg, Potassium 30 mg, Choline bitartrate 30 mg, PABA (Para-Aminobenzoic Acid) 25 mg, Citrus bioflavonoids complex 10 mg, Green tea leaves extract 5 mg, N-acetyl-L-cysteine (NAC) 0.5 mg, Lutein 0.3 mg, Boron 0.1 mg, Inositol 0.03 mg, Vanadium 0.01 mg, Silica 0.01 mg

GNC Maximum Greens Ultra Mega Green without Iron Caplets
Iodine 0.15 mg, Molybdenum 0.075 mg

GNC Ultra Mega Multivitamin Caplets
Iron (Ferrous fumarate) 18 mg, Iodine 0.15 mg, Potassium 10 mg, Boron 0.1 mg, Silica 0.01 mg, Choline bitartrate 35 mg, Inositol 0.075 mg, PABA (Para-Aminobenzoic Acid) 75 mg, Trimethylglycine (TMG) 10 mg, Rutin powder 25 mg, Citrus bioflavonoids complex 25 mg, Hesperidin complex 5 mg, N-acetyl-L-cysteine (NAC) 0.5 mg, Alpha-lipoic acid 1 mg, Green tea leaves extract 5 mg

Goldline Certagen Tablets
Vitamin K 0.025 mg, Ferrous fumarate 18 mg, phosphorus 109 mg, Iodine 0.15 mg, Magnesium 10 mg, Molybdenum 0.16 mg, Chloride 72 mg, Potassium 80 mg, Boron 0.15 mg, Nickel 0.005 mg, Silica 2 mg, Tin 0.01 mg, Vanadium 0.01 mg

Goldline Prenatal S Tablets
Iron (Ferrous fumarate) 27 mg

Green Source Tablets
Iron 15 mg, Iodine 0.15 mg, Magnesium 125 mg, Molybdenum 0.05 mg, Potassium 50 mg, Boron 1 mg, Choline bitartrate 50 mg, Inositol 25 mg, PABA (Para-Aminobenzoic Acid) 25 mg, Citrus bioflavonoids complex 100 mg, Quercetin 25 mg, Rutin 25 mg, Hesperidin complex 10 mg, Bromelain 20 mg, Betaine HCl 20 mg, Papain 20 mg, Amylase 5 mg, Lipase 5 mg, Protease 1 mg, Cellulase 2.5 mg, Propietary lactobacillus blend (L.acidophilus, L.bifidus, L. bulgaricus) 25 mg, Oat bran 25mg, Pectin 25 mg, RNA 35 mg, DNA 10 mg, Carotenoids 10 mg, Chlorophyll 4 mg, Vegetable oil 100 mg, L-glutathione 5 mg, Spirulina 1,000 mg, Wheat grass 100 mg, Barley juice concentrate 100 mg, Flaxseed oil 100 mg, Chinese chlorella 100 mg, Bee pollen 100 mg, Korean ginseng 50 mg, Dehydrated garlic 10 mg, Proprietary herbal blend (Echinacea, Milk thistle, Goldenseal; Ginger root; Ginkgo biloba; Cayenne pepper) 60 mg

Gynovite Plus Tablets
Iron 18 mg, Iodine 0.15 mg, Magnesium 600 mg, PABA (Para-Aminobenzoic Acid) 25 mg, Betaine HCl 100 mg, Pancreatin 4X 93 mg, Inositol 50 mg, Hesperidin 35 mg, Rutin 25 mg, Boron 3 mg

Hair, Skin & Nails Formula Tablets
Iron (Ferrous gluconate) 3 mg, Phosphorus 150 mg, Iodine 112.5 mg, Magnesium 100 mg, Sodium 10 mg, PABA (Para-Aminobenzoic Acid) 25 mg, Choline bitartrate 75 mg, Inositol 30 mg, Ribonucleic acid (RNA) 30 mg, Citrus bioflavonoids 25 mg, Rutin 12.5 mg, Horsetail extract 3 mg, Betaine HCl 25 mg

Hematinic Plus Vitamins and Minerals
Magnesium 6.9 mg, Iron (Ferrous fumarate) 324 mg

Hemocyte Plus Capsules
Iron (Ferrous fumarate) 324 mg, Magnesium 6.9 mg

Hep-Forte Soft Gel Capsules
Choline 10 mg, Liver defatted 194 mg, Liver concentrate 65 mg, Liver fraction #2 65 mg, Yeast dried 65 mg, Melatonin 10 mg, Inositol 10 mg

Hi-Kovite Tablets
Iron (Ferrous fumarate) 9 mg, Iodine 0.075 mg, PABA (Para-Aminobenzoic Acid) 60 mg, Potassium 35 mg, phosphorus 10 mg, Bioflavonoids 10 mg, L-lysine 10 mg, Inositol 10 mg

Hyalex Tablets (Miller Pharmacal Group)
Magnesium oxide 5 mg, Magnesium salicylate 260 mg, Magnesium p-aminobenzoate 163 mg

Icar Prenatal Tablets
Iodine 0.15 mg, Iron 29 mg, Magnesium 225 mg, Vitamin K 0.065mg: Molybdenum 0.075 mg, Boron 1 mg

Iromin-G Tablets
Iron 29.5 mg

Keytab Tablets
Beta carotene 15,000; Inositol 100 mg, PABA (Para-Aminobenzoic Acid) 50 mg, Bioflavonoids 200 mg, Choline 100 mg, L-cysteine HCl 250 mg, DL-Methionine 62.5 mg, Magnesium 325 mg, Potassium 99 mg, Iron 20 mg, Molybdenum 0.1 mg, Iodine 0.244 mg, Boron 1 mg, Raw gland (thymus, spleen, liver, adrenal) (2:2:2:1)180 mg

Keytab Tablets w/o Glandulars
Beta carotene 15,000 IU; Inositol 100 mg, PABA (Para-Aminobenzoic Acid) 50 mg, Bioflavonoids 200 mg, Choline 100 mg, L-cysteine HCl 250 mg, DL-Methionine 62.5 mg, Magnesium 325 mg, Potassium 99 mg, Iron 20 mg, Molybdenum 0.1 mg, Iodine 0.244 mg, Boron 1 mg

Keytab Tablets w/o Iron, Copper, or Glandulars
Beta carotene 15,000; Inositol 100 mg, PABA (Para-Aminobenzoic Acid) 50 mg, Bioflavonoids 200 mg, Choline 100 mg, L-cysteine HCl 250 mg, DL-Methionine 62.5 mg, Magnesium 325 mg, Potassium 99 mg, Molybdenum 0.1 mg, Iodine 0.244 mg, Boron 1 mg

KPN Prenatal Tablets
Iron (Ferrous fumarate) 27 mg, Magnesium 100 mg, Natural base (contains Bioflavonoids and Hesperidin) 66 mg

LYC Capsules
Magnesium 33 mg, Potassium 13 mg, L-lysine 440 mg

LYC-2,000 Powder for Suspension
Magnesium 150 mg, Potassium 60 mg, L-lysine 2,000 mg

Manly Machovites Tablets
Betaine 16.67 mg, Bioflavonoids 41.67 mg, Choline 52.08 mg, Inositol 4.17 mg, Iodine 0.013 mg, Iron 2.5 mg, Magnesium 41.67 mg, PABA 4.17 mg, Pancreatin GX 16.67 mg, Potassium 7.92 mg, Rutin 4.17 mg

Maple Melts Chewable Tablets
Iodine 0.001 mg, Magnesium 12.5 mg, Molybdenum 0.005 mg, Potassium 5 mg, Inositol 5 mg, Lactoferrin 1 mg, N-Acetyl-D-Glucosamine 1 mg, Pantethine 0.5 mg, Boron 0.011 mg, Vanadium 0.002 mg, Soy extracts 2.5 mg

Maximum Blue Tablets
Iodine 0.05 mg, Magnesium 166 mg, Molybdenum 0.016 mg, Sodium 5 mg, Potassium 35 mg, Lysine 200 mg, Choline bitartrate 66 mg, Inositol 33 mg, Mixed bioflavonoids 33 mg, PABA (Para-Aminobenzoic Acid) 16 mg, Silicon 0.8 mg, Boron 0.666 mg, Vanadium 0.008 mg

Mega Vita Gel Iron Free Softgels
Phosphorus 50 mg, Iodine 0.15 mg, Magnesium 50 mg, Potassium 30 mg, Boron 1 mg, Rutin 10 mg, Citrus bioflavonoids 30 mg, PABA (Para-Aminobenzoic Acid) 50 mg, Royal Jelly 5 mg, Choline bitartrate 50 mg, Inositol 0.05 mg, Garlic oil 135 mg, Soy lecithin 80 mg, Octacosanol 0.01 mg, RNA 2 mg, DNA 2 mg, Coenzyme Q10 0.1 mg

Mega Vita Gel Softgels
Iron (Ferrous fumarate) 15 mg, Phosphorus 50 mg, Iodine 0.15 mg, Magnesium 50 mg, Potassium 30 mg, Boron 1 mg, Rutin 10 mg, Citrus bioflavonoid 30 mg, PABA (Para-Aminobenzoic Acid) 50 mg, Royal Jelly 5 mg, Choline bitartrate 50 mg, Inositol 0.05 mg, Garlic oil 135 mg, Soy lecithin 80 mg, Octacosanol 0.01 mg, RNA 2mg, DNA 2 mg, Coenzyme Q10 0.1 mg

Mega Vita Min for Seniors Tablets
Vitamin K 0.01 mg, Iodine 0.15 mg, Magnesium 15 mg, Molybdenum 0.025 mg, Potassium 1.67 mg, Boron 0.5 mg, Choline bitartrate 100 mg, Inositol 50 mg, PABA (Para-Aminobenzoic Acid) 50 mg, Rutin 30 mg, Citrus bioflavonoid complex 25 mg, Hesperidin complex 5 mg, Betaine HCl 25 mg, Coenzyme Q10 0.5 mg, Deodorized garlic 1 mg, Korean ginseng 1mg, Pine bark extract 0.5 mg, Natural alpha carotene 0.375 mg, Other carotenoids (Lutein, Cryptoxanthin, Zeaxanthin) 1.4 mg, Ginkgo biloba extract 10 mg, Alpha-lipoic acid 5 mg

Mega Vita Min for Teens Tablets (Puritan's Pride)
Vitamin K 0.01 mg, Iron (Ferrous fumarate) 18 mg, Phosphorus 20 mg, Iodine 0.15 mg, Magnesium 50 mg, Molybdenum 0.02 mg, Choline bitartrate 0.05 mg, Inositol 0.05 mg

Mega Vita Min for Teens Tablets (Vitamin World)
Vitamin K 0.01 mg, Iron (Ferrous fumarate) 18 mg, Phosphorus 20 mg, Iodine 0.15 mg, Magnesium 50 mg, Molybdenum 0.02 mg, Sodium 5 mg, Choline bitartrate 0.050 mg, Inositol 0.05 mg

Mega Vita-Min Tablets
Iron (Ferrous gluconate) 2 mg, Iodine 0.15 mg, Magnesium 6 mg, Molybdenum 0.025 mg, Sodium 5 mg, Potassium 1.6 mg, Boron 0.5 mg, Choline bitartrate 80 mg, Inositol 80 mg, PABA (Para-Aminobenzoic Acid) 80 mg, Rutin 30 mg, Citrus bioflavonoid complex 25 mg, Hesperidin complex 5 mg, Betaine HCl 25 mg, Coenzyme Q10 0.5 mg, Deodorized garlic 1 mg, Korean ginseng 1 mg, Natural food base 4 mg, Pinus pinaster 0.5 mg

Mega Vita-Min Time Release Tablets
Iron (Ferrous gluconate) 2 mg, Iodine 0.15 mg, Magnesium 6 mg, Molybdenum 0.025; Potassium 1.6 mg, Boron 0.5 mg, Choline bitartrate 80 mg, Inositol 80 mg, PABA (Para-Aminobenzoic Acid) 80 mg, Rutin 30 mg, Citrus bioflavonoids 25 mg, Hesperidin 5 mg, Betaine HCl 25 mg, Coenzyme Q10 0.5 mg, Deodorized garlic 1 mg, Korean ginseng 1 mg, Pycnogenol 0.5 mg, Proprietary blend (Alfalfa leaf, Watercress, Parsley leaf, Rice bran and Lecithin) 4 mg

Mega Vitamins for the Hair Tablets (Puritan's Pride)
Choline bitartrate 500 mg, Inositol 500 mg, PABA (Para-Aminobenzoic Acid) 100 mg, L-cysteine 334 mg

Mega Vitamins for the Hair Tablets (Vitamin World)
Choline bitartrate 500 mg, Inositol 500 mg, PABA (Para-Aminobenzoic Acid) 100 mg, L-cysteine 334 mg

Mega VM-80 Tablets
Ferrous gluconate 2 mg, Iodine 0.15 mg, Magnesium 6 mg, Molybdenum 0.025 mg, Potassium 1.67 mg, Boron 0.5 mg, Choline bitartrate 80 mg, Inositol 80 mg, PABA (Para-Aminobenzoic Acid) 80 mg, Rutin 30 mg, Citrus bioflavonoid complex 25 mg, Hesperidin complex 5 mg, Betaine HCl 25 mg, Coenzyme Q10 0.5 mg, Deodorized garlic 1 mg, Korean ginseng 1 mg, Natural food base (Alfalfa leaf powder, Watercress powder, Parsley powder, Rice bran powder, Soy lecithin) 4 mg, Pinus maritima 0.5 mg

Mega-Multi Capsules
Iodine 0.038 mg, Iron 4.5 mg, Magnesium 30 mg, Phosphorus 15 mg, Potassium 100 mg

Men's Multivitamin Health Formula Tablets
Vitamin K 0.02 mg, Potassium 100 mg, Magnesium 120 mg, Lycopene 0.6 mg

Men's Daily Formula Capsules
Vitamin K 0.02 mg, Magnesium 120 mg, Potassium 100 mg, Lycopene 0.6 mg

Mini-Multi Tablets
Iodine 0.075 mg, Magnesium 40 mg

Mini-Prenatal Tablets
Iron (Ferrous fumarate) 27 mg, Magnesium 60 mg

Monocaps Tablets
Iron (Ferrous fumarate) 14 mg, Iodine 0.15 mg, Magnesium 30 mg, L-lysine 10 mg, Lecithin 10 mg, PABA (Para-Aminobenzoic Acid) 10 mg

Multi-Day Plus Minerals Tablets
Vitamin K 0.025 mg

Multi-Day Women's with Calcium and Iron Tablets
Iron (Ferrous fumarate) 18 mg, Magnesium 50 mg

Multifol Plus Tablets
Iron (elemental) 65 mg, Magnesium 25 mg

Multi-Gel Liquid Filled Capsules
Vitamin K 0.04 mg, Iron 18 mg, Iodine 0.15 mg, Magnesium 400 mg, Lutein 0.6 mg, Coenzyme Q10 12 mg, Alpha-lipoic acid 12 mg, Bioflavonoids 60 mg, Rutin 60 mg, Papaya concentrate 60 mg, Lecithin 60 mg, Phosphatidyl choline 107mg, Phosphatidyl inositol 7 mg

Multilex Film Coated Tablets
Iron (Ferrous sulfate) 15 mg, Iodine 0.15 mg, Magnesium 5 mg

Multilex T&M Tablets
Iron (Ferrous fumarate) 15 mg, Iodine 0.15 mg, Magnesium 5 mg

M-Vit Caplets
Lemon bioflavonoids 50 mg, Iron (Ferrous fumarate) 27 mg, Magnesium 50 mg

Myadec Multivitamin-Multimineral Supplement Tablets
Vitamin K 0.025 mg, Iron 18 mg, Phosphorus 125 mg, Iodine 0.15 mg, Magnesium 100 mg, Molybdenum 0.025 mg, Chloride 36 mg, Potassium 40 mg, Nickel 0.005 mg, Tin 0.01 mg, Silicon 0.01 mg, Vanadium 0.01 mg, Boron 0.15 mg

NanoVM Packets
Vitamin K 0.03 mg, Phosphorus 460 mg, Iron 7 mg, Magnesium 65 mg, Iodine 0.09 mg, Molybdenum 0.017 mg, Potassium 575 mg

NataCaps Capsules
Iron (Ferrous fumarate) 324 mg

NatalCare GlossTabs
Iron 90 mg, Magnesium 30 mg, Docusate sodium 50 mg

NatalCare PIC Forte Tablets
Iron 60 mg, Iodine 0.2 mg, Magnesium 10 mg

NatalCare PIC Tablets
Iron 60 mg

NatalCare Plus Tablets
Iron (Ferrous fumarate) 27 mg

NatalCare Rx Tablets
Iron (Ferrous fumarate) 54 mg, Magnesium 100 mg

NatalCare Three Tablets
Iron (Ferrous fumarate) 28 mg, Magnesium 25 mg

NataTab C Fe Tablets
Iron 50 mg, Iodine 0.15 mg

NataTab FA Tablets
Iron (Ferrous fumarate) 29 mg, Iodine 0.15 mg

NataTab Rx Tablets
Iron 29 mg, Iodine 0.15 mg, Magnesium 100 mg

Natelle C Tablets
Magnesium 40 mg, Choline 90 mg, Iron 28 mg

Natelle EZ Tablets
Iron 25 mg, Magnesium 50 mg, Choline bitartrate 55 mg

Natelle Plus w/DHA Tablets
Iron 26 mg, Magnesium 50 mg, Choline 60 mg, Docosahexaenoic Acid (DHA) 200 mg

Natelle Prefer Tablets
Iron 29 mg, Magnesium 75 mg

Natelle Tablets
Iron 27 mg, Magnesium 75 mg

Nature's Blend Mega Multivitamin with Minerals Tablets
Iron 18 mg, Iodine 0.225 mg, Magnesium 100 mg

Nature's Blend Multi-Vitamin with Minerals Soft Gel Capsules
Iron 27 mg, Phosphorus 58 mg, Iodine 0.15 mg, Potassium 2 mg, Choline bitartrate 14.9 mg, Inositol 15 mg,

Nature's Blend Multi-Vitamin with Minerals Tablets
Iron 7.5 mg, Phosphorus 80 mg, Iodine 0.075 mg, Magnesium 0.5 mg

Nature's Blend Prenatal and Iron Tablets
Iron (Ferrous fumarate) 20 mg

Nature's Blend Super Theravite M Tablets
Iron (Ferrous fumarate) 27 mg, Phosphorus 31 mg, Iodine 0.15 mg, Magnesium 100 mg, Molybdenum 0.015 mg, Chloride 5 mg, Potassium 10 mg

Nature's Blend Theratrum Complete 50 Plus Tablets
Vitamin K 0.01 mg, Phosphorus 48 mg, Iodine 0.15 mg, Magnesium 100 mg, Molybdenum 0.075 mg, Chloride 72 mg, Potassium 80 mg, Boron 0.15 mg, Nickel 0.005 mg, Silicon 2 mg, Vanadium 0.01 mg, Lutein 0.25 mg

Nature's Blend Theratrum Complete Tablets
Vitamin K 0.025 mg, Iron (Ferrous fumarate) 18 mg, Phosphorus 109 mg, Iodine 0.15 mg, Magnesium 100 mg, Molybdenum 0.075 mg, Chloride 72 mg, Potassium 80 mg, Silicon 2 mg, Lutein 0.25 mg, Boron 0.15 mg, Vanadium 0.01 mg, Tin 0.01 mg, Nickel 0.005 mg

Neevo Caplets
L-methylfolate 1 mg, Iron 29 mg, Magnesium 40 mg

NovaNatal Tablets
Iodine 0.15 mg, Iron 29 mg

NovaStart Tablets
Iodine 0.15 mg, Iron (Ferrous fumarate) 17 mg

Nutri-100 Gold Tablets
Iron (Ferrous fumarate) 18 mg, Iodine 0.15 mg, Magnesium 50 mg, Potassium 10 mg, PABA (Para-Aminobenzoic Acid) 100 mg, Choline bitartrate 100 mg, Inositol 100 mg, Rutin 25 mg, Lemon bioflavonoids 50 mg, Hesperidin 12.5 mg, Betaine HCl 30 mg, Octacosanol 0.05 mg, Proprietary blend (Alfalfa leaf, Watercress, Parsley leaf, Rice bran and Soy lecithin) 5 mg

Nutrimin-Plus Tablets
Iron 18 mg, Phosphorus 0.05 mg, Iodine 0.15 mg, Magnesium 25 mg, Chrominin 1 mg

NutriSpire Tablets
Iron 29 mg, Iodine 0.15 mg

Nutrivit
L-lysine HCl 800 mg, Panthenol 15 mg, Iron 15 mg

O-Cal FA Tablets
Iron (Ferrous fumarate) 27 mg, Iodine 0.15 mg, Magnesium 100 mg, Fluoride 0.5 mg

O-Cal Prenatal Tablets
Iron (Ferrous fumarate) 27 mg, Iodine 0.15 mg, Magnesium 100 mg, Fluoride 0.5 mg

Ocuvite Adult 50+ Soft Gel Capsules
Lutein 6 mg, Omega-3 150 mg

Ocuvite Extra Tablets
L-glutathione 5 mg, Lutein 2 mg

Ocuvite Lutein Capsules
Lutein 6 mg

Ocuvite Tablets
Lutein 2 mg

One A Day Active Tablets
Vitamin K 0.025 mg, Iron 9 mg, Phosphorus 48 mg, Iodine 0.15 mg, Magnesium 40 mg, Molybdenum 0.025 mg, Chloride 180 mg, Potassium 200 mg, Nickel 0.005 mg, Tin 0.01 mg, Silicon 6 mg, Vanadium 0.01 mg, Boron 0.15 mg, American ginseng standardized extract 55 mg

One A Day Kids Bugs Bunny & Friends Complete Chewable Tablets
Iron 18 mg, Phosphorus 100 mg, Iodine 0.15 mg, Magnesium 20 mg, Sodium 10 mg

One A Day Kids Scooby Doo Complete Chewable Tablets
Iron 18 mg, Phosphorus 100 mg, Iodine 0.15 mg, Magnesium 20 mg, Sodium 10 mg

One A Day Kids Scooby Doo Plus Calcium Chewable Tablets
Sodium 10 mg

One A Day Maximum Tablets
Vitamin K 0.025 mg, Iron 18 mg, Phosphorus 109 mg, Iodine 0.15 mg, Magnesium 100 mg, Molybdenum 0.16 mg, Chloride 72 mg, Potassium 80 mg, Nickel 0.005 mg, Tin 0.01 mg, Silicon 2 mg, Vanadium 0.01 mg, Boron 0.15 mg

One A Day Men's 50+ Advantage Tablets
Vitamin K 0.02 mg, Iodine 0.15 mg, Magnesium 100 mg, Molybdenum 0.09 mg, Potassium 40 mg, Ginkgo biloba extract 120 mg, Lycopene 0.6 mg

One A Day Men's Health Formula Tablets
Vitamin K 0.02 mg, Magnesium 120 mg, Potassium 100 mg

One A Day Weight Smart Advanced Tablets
Vitamin K 0.08 mg, Iron 18 mg, Magnesium 50 mg, Guarana blend: Guarana seed (powder & extract), Caffeine 180 mg, Green tea/Cayenne blend: Green tea powder (leaf), Cayenne pepper powder (fruit) 10 mg

One A Day Women's 50+ Advantage Tablets
Vitamin K 0.02 mg, Iodine 0.15 mg, Magnesium 50 mg, Molybdenum 0.090 mg, Ginkgo biloba extract 120 mg

One A Day Women's Prenatal Tablets
Iron 28 mg, Iodine 0.15 mg, Magnesium 50 mg

One A Day Women's Tablets
Vitamin K 0.025 mg, Iron 18 mg, Magnesium 50 mg

One Daily Maximum Vitamin Tablets
Vitamin K 0.025 mg, Iron 18 mg, Phosphorus 109 mg, Iodine 0.15 mg, Magnesium 100 mg, Molybdenum 0.16 mg, Chloride 72 mg, Potassium 80 mg, Boron 0.15 mg, Tin 0.01 mg, Vanadium 0.01 mg, Nickel 0.005 mg, Silica 2 mg

Opti-C Tablets
Magnesium 20 mg, Beta carotene 5,000 IU

OptiNate Tablets
Iron 90 mg: Magnesium 30 mg, Docusate sodium 50 mg, Docosahexaenoic Acid (DHA) 250 mg

Opti-Plus Capsules
Beta carotene 1,000 IU; Lutein 10 mg, L-glutathione 2.5 mg, Zeaxanthin 10 mg, Bilberry 150 mg, L-taurine 20 mg

Optisource Chewable Tablets
Vitamin K 0.04 mg, Iron 7.5 mg, Phosphorus 50 mg, Iodine 0.0375 mg, Magnesium 100 mg, Molybdenum 0.01875 mg, Sodium 5 mg

Optivite P.M.T. Tablets
Iron 15 mg, Iodine 0.075 mg, Magnesium 250 mg, Potassium 48 mg, Choline 313 mg, Citrus bioflavonoids 250 mg, Betaine HCl 100 mg, Pancreatin 4X 93 mg, Inositol 24 mg, PABA (Para-Aminobenzoic Acid) 25 mg, Rutin 25 mg

OsCal Ultra Tablets
Magnesium 20 mg, Boron 0.25 mg

Parvlex Tablets
Iron (Ferrous fumarate) 29 mg

PMS Formula Tablets
Betaine 16.67 mg, Bioflavonoids 41.67 mg, Choline 52.08 mg, Inositol 4.17 mg, Iodine 0.013 mg, Iron 2.5 mg, Magnesium 41.67 mg, PABA (Para-Aminobenzoic Acid) 4.17 mg, Pancreatin GX 16.67 mg, Potassium 7.92 mg, Rutin 4.17 mg

Poly Vitamin w/Iron Chewable Tablets
Iron 12 mg

Potent 75 Super VM Tablets
Iron 10 mg, Iodine 0.15 mg, Magnesium 25 mg, Potassium 10 mg, PABA (Para-Aminobenzoic Acid) 75 mg, Choline bitartrate 75 mg, Inositol 75 mg, Rutin 25 mg, Citrus bioflavonoids 25 mg, Hesperidin 5 mg, Betaine HCl 25 mg, L-glutamic acid 25 mg, Proprietary blend (Alfalfa, Watercress, Parsley) 3 mg

Powermate Tablets
Ginkgo biloba 5 mg, Green tea extract 100 mg, Pine bark extract-OPC-85% 50 mg, Echinacea 50 mg, Golden seal root 20 mg, N-acetyl-L-cysteine 25 mg, Glutathione 5 mg, Coenzyme Q10 2 mg

PowerVites Tablets
PABA (Para-Aminobenzoic Acid) 12.5 mg, Inositol 12.5 mg, Choline bitartrate 25 mg, Magnesium 120 mg, Potassium 25 mg, Boron 1 mg, Citrus bioflavonoids 25 mg, Rutin 5 mg, Hesperidin 5 mg, Bee pollen 250 mg, Betaine HCl 10 mg

PreCare Chewables
Iron 40 mg, Magnesium 50 mg

PreCare Conceive Tablets
Iron (Ferrous fumarate) 30 mg, Magnesium 100 mg

PreCare Premier Tablets
Iron 30 mg, Magnesium 25 mg, Docusate sodium 50 mg, Succinic acid 35 mg

PreferaOB Tablets
Iron 28 mg, Iodine 0.175 mg

Prenafirst Tablets
Iron (Ferrous fumarate) 17 mg, Iodine 0.15 mg

Prenatabs FA Tablets
Iron (Ferrous fumarate) 29 mg, Iodine 0.15 mg

Prenatabs Rx Tablets
Iron (carbonyl) 29 mg, Magnesium 100 mg, Iodine 0.15 mg

Prenatal 1 + 1 Tablets
Iron (Ferrous fumarate) 65 mg

Prenatal 19 Chewable Tablets
Docusate sodium 25 mg, Iron (Ferrous fumarate) 29 mg

Prenatal AD Tablets
Magnesium 30 mg, Docusate sodium 50 mg, Iron (carbonyl) 90 mg

Pre-Natal Complex Capsules
Iron (Ferrous fumarate) 18 mg, Iodine 0.15 mg, Magnesium 450 mg, Molybdenum 0.075 mg, Potassium 10 mg, Sodium 5 mg, Cranberry fruit powder 60 mg, Choline bitartrate 20 mg, Ginger root 20 mg, Inositol 20 mg, Peppermint oil 20 mg, PABA (Para-Aminobenzoic Acid) 2 mg

Pre-Natal Complex Capsules
Iron (Ferrous fumarate) 18 mg, Iodine 0.15 mg, Magnesium 450 mg, Molybdenum 0.075 mg, Potassium 10 mg, Sodium 5 mg, Cranberry fruit 60 mg, Choline bitartrate 20 mg, Ginger root 20 mg, Inositol 20 mg, Peppermint oil 20 mg, PABA (Para-Aminobenzoic Acid) 2 mg

Prenatal MR 90 Fe Tablets
Iron 90 mg, Docusate sodium 50 mg

Prenatal MTR with Selenium Tablets
Iron (Ferrous fumarate) 27 mg, Iodine 0.15 mg, Magnesium 25 mg, Molybdenum 0.025 mg

Prenatal Plus Tablets
Iron (Ferrous fumarate) 27 mg

Prenatal Rx 1 Tablets
Iron (Ferrous fumarate) 60 mg, Magnesium 100 mg

Prenatal Tablets
Iron 27 mg

PreNATAL Tablets
Iron 36 mg, Iodine 0.15 mg, Magnesium 450 mg, Grape seed extract 10 mg, Citrus bioflavonoids complex 100 mg

Prenatal U Capsules
Iron (Ferrous fumarate) 106.5 mg

Prenatal Vitamins (Nature's Bounty)
Iron (Ferrous fumarate) 28 mg

Prenatal Vitamins (Basic Vitamins)
Iron (Ferrous fumarate) 28 mg

Prenatal Z Advanced Formula Tablets
Iron (Ferrous fumarate) 65 mg, Iodine 0.175 mg, Magnesium 100 mg

Prenate DHA Tablets
Iron (Ferrous fumarate) 27 mg, Magnesium 50 mg, Docosahexaenoic Acid (DHA) 300 mg, Calcium docusate ≤50 mg

Prenate Elite Tablets
Iron 90 mg, Magnesium 30 mg, Docusate sodium 50 mg

Prenavite Tablets
Calcium carbonate 200 mg, Iron (Ferrous fumarate) 28 mg

Prescriptive Formulas Men's Optimal Vitamin Packets
Vitamin K 0.025 mg, Biotin 0.03 mg, Iron (Ferrous fumarate) 18 mg, Phosphorus 129 mg, Iodine 0.15 mg, Magnesium 100 mg, Molybdenum 0.075 mg, Chloride 72 mg, Sodium 10 mg, Potassium 80 mg, Fish oil 1,000 mg, Omega-3 340 mg, Omega-6 20 mg, Desicated liver 100 mg, Brewer's yeast 50 mg, Citrus bioflavonoids 25 mg, Choline bitartrate 20 mg, Rose hips 14 mg, Inositol 10 mg, Saw palmetto extract 160 mg, Silica 2 mg, Lycopene 0.3 mg, Lutein 0.25 mg, Boron 0.15 mg, Vanadium 0.01 mg, Nickel 0.01 mg, Tin 0.01 mg

Prescriptive Formulas Women's Optimal Vitamin Packets
Vitamin K 0.08 mg, Iron (Ferrous fumarate) 18 mg, Phosphorus 58 mg, Magnesium 50 mg, Sodium 15 mg, Fish oil 1,000 mg, Omega-3 340 mg, Omega-6 20 mg, Desicated liver 100 mg, Brewer's yeast 50 mg, Green tea extract 32 mg, Citrus bioflavonoids 25 mg, Choline bitartrate 20 mg, Rose hips 14 mg, Inositol 10 mg

PreserVision Lutein Soft Gel Capsules
Lutein 5 mg

PrimaCare
Omega-3 fatty acids 330 mg, Docosahexaenoic Acid (DHA) 260 mg, Eicosapentaenoic Acid (EPA) 40 mg, Alpha-linolenic acid (ALA) 30 mg, Linoleic acid 30 mg, Vitamin K 0.09 mg, Iron 30 mg, Molybdenum 0.05 mg, Docusate sodium 50 mg, Succinic acid 30 mg

PrimaCare One Capsules
Omega-3 fatty acids 330 mg, Docosahexaenoic Acid (DHA) 260 mg, Eicosapentaenoic Acid (EPA) 40 mg, Alpha-linolenic acid (ALA) 30 mg, Linoleic acid 30 mg, Iron 27 mg

Prosight Lutein Tablets
Lutein 6 mg

Puritan's Pride Complete One Tablets
Iron (Ferrous fumarate) 54 mg, Phosphorus 23 mg, Iodine 0.15 mg, Magnesium 100 mg, Molybdenum 0.015 mg, Chloride 1 mg, Potassium 1 mg, PABA (Para-Aminobenzoic Acid) 50 mg, Inositol 15 mg, Choline bitartrate 15 mg

Q.S. Tablets
Choline 100 mg, Inositol 100 mg, PABA (Para-Aminobenzoic Acid) 100 mg, Citrus bioflavonoids 150 mg, Magnesium 500 mg, Potassium 99 mg, Iron (Ferrous fumarate) 20 mg, Molybdenum 0.1 mg, Iodine 0.2 mg, Boron 1 mg, Vanadium 0.03 mg

Quench Capsules
Vitamin K$_1$ 1 mg, Reduced l-Glutathione 40 mg, N-acetyl-L-cysteine 300 mg, Alpha-lipoic acid (ALA) 100 mg, Coenzyme Q10 15 mg, Natural beta carotene 15 mg, Lycopene 8 mg, Super oxide dismutase 2,000 units; Catalase 1,000 units; Citrus bioflavonoid complex 400 mg, Deodorized garlic 3:1 Conc. 100 mg, Melatonin 0.25 mg

Quintabs-M Tablets
Iron (Ferrous fumarate) 10 mg, Iodine 0.15 mg, Magnesium 15 mg, PABA (Para-Aminobenzoic Acid) 10 mg

Quintabs-M Tablets- Iron Free
Iodine 0.15 mg, Magnesium 15 mg, PABA (Para-Aminobenzoic Acid) 10 mg

Ragus Tablets
Phosphorus 450 mg, Magnesium 27 mg, L-lysine 25 mg, DL-Methionine 50 mg, Iron (gluconate) 20 mg, Potassium 10 mg, Iodine 0.1 mg

Replace Liquid Filled Capsules
Potassium 10 mg, Iron 5 mg, Iodine 0.1125 mg, Magnesium 45 mg, Molybdenum 0.01 mg, Boron 2.5 mg, Lycopene 2.5 mg, Citrus bioflavonoid complex 25 mg

Replace Liquid Filled Capsules w/o Iron
Potassium 10 mg, Iodine 0.1125 mg, Magnesium 45 mg, Molybdenum 0.01 mg, Boron 2.5 mg, Lycopene 2.5 mg, Citrus bioflavonoid complex 25 mg

Sclerex Tablets
Succinate 25 mg, Inositol 2 g, Magnesium 34 mg, Iron (gluconate) 10 mg, Iodine 0.1 mg

Select OB Caplets
Iron 29 mg, Magnesium 25 mg

Senior Eye Vision Capsules
Magnesium 125 mg, Lutein 5 mg, N-acetyl cysteine 125 mg, Bilberry 20 mg, Ginkgo biloba extract 30 mg, Quercetin 150 mg, L-taurine 250 mg, L-methionine 100 mg, L-glutamic acid 25 mg, L-glycine 25 mg

Siderol Tablets
Iron 150 mg, Desiccated stomach substance 100 mg, Desiccated liver 50 mg, Vegetable fiber 40 mg

Sterling Layered Tablets
Iron 12.6 mg, Iodine 0.105 mg, Magnesium 280 mg, Molybdenum 0.0318 mg, Choline 105 mg, Inositol 105 mg, DL Methionine 45 mg, Aloe vera gel concentrate equivalent to 900 mg, Pancreatin 3X 34.8 mg, PABA (Para-Aminobenzoic acid) 6 mg

Stress Formula with Iron Tablets (Basic Vitamins)
Iron (Ferrous fumarate) 4 mg, L-taurine 75 mg, L-glutamin 20 mg, L-carnitine 5 mg, Green tea 50% Polyphenols 5 mg

Stress Formula with Iron Tablets (Major Pharmaceuticals)
Iron (Ferrous Fumarate) 18 mg

Strovite Advance Caplets
Magnesium 50 mg, Alpha-lipoic acid 15 mg, Lutein 5 mg

Strovite Forte Tablets
Iron 10 mg, Magnesium 50 mg, Molybdenum 25 mg

Stuart Prenatal Tablets
Iron 28 mg

Summit Gold Junior Tablets
Iron (Ferrous fumarate) 4.5 mg, Phosphorus 60 mg, Iodine 0.0375 mg, Magnesium 100 mg, Molybdenum 0.00375 mg, Potassium 7.5 mg, Choline 37.5 mg, Inositol 37.5 mg

Summit Gold Layered Tablets
Iron (Ferrous fumarate) 9 mg, Phosphorus 120 mg, Iodine 0.075 mg, Magnesium 200 mg, Molybdenum 0.0075 mg, Potassium 15 mg, Choline 75 mg

Summit Gold Special Formula Tablets
Phosphorus 120 mg, Iodine 0.075 mg, Magnesium 200 mg, Molybdenum 0.0075 mg, Potassium 15 mg, Choline 75 mg, Inositol 75 mg

Summit Max Layered Tablets
Iron (Ferrous fumarate) 9 mg, Phosphorus 120 mg, Iodine 0.075 mg, Magnesium 200 mg, Molybdenum 0.0375 mg, Potassium 15 mg, Choline 75 mg, Inositol 75 mg, Coenzyme Q10 5 mg, Lycopene 1.5 mg

Sundown Spiderman Complete Children's Multiple Vitamin Chewable Tablets
Iron (Ferrous sulfate) 18 mg, Iodine 0.15 mg, Magnesium 20 mg

Sunnie Tablets
d-Cal pantothenate 50 mg, PABA (Para-Aminobenzoic Acid) 10 mg, L-cystine 25 mg, Choline bitartrate 25 mg, Magnesium 50 mg, L-glutamine 150 mg, Ginkgo biloba 10 mg, St. John's wort 900 mg, Betaine TMG 500 mg

Sunvite Platinum Tablets
Chloride 72 mg, Iodine 0.15 mg, Iron 9 mg, Magnesium 100 mg, Molybdenum 0.025 mg, Nickel 0.005 mg, Phosphorus 48 mg, Potassium 80 mg, Silicon 0.01 mg, Vanadium 0.01 mg, Vitamin K 0.01 mg

Sunvite Tablets
Boron 0.15 mg, Chloride 36.3 mg, Iodine 0.15 mg, Magnesium 100 mg, Molybdenum 0.025 mg, Nickel 0.005 mg, Phosphorus 125 mg, Potassium 40 mg, Silicon 2 mg, Tin 0.01 mg, Urib 18 mg, Vanadium 0.01 mg, Vitamin K 0.025 mg

Super 1 Daily Tablets
Vitamin K 0.04 mg, Iron 9 mg, Iodine 0.15 mg, Magnesium 50 mg, Potassium 45 mg, Lutein 0.5 mg, Lemon bioflavonoids complex 25 mg, Lecithin 25 mg, Inositol 25 mg, Choline 25 mg, Betaine HCl 25 mg

Super 2 Daily Liquid Filled Capsules
Iodine 0.15 mg, Magnesium 100 mg, Lutein 0.5 mg, Lemon bioflavonoids complex 25 mg, Lecithin 60 mg, Phosphatidyl choline 50 mg, Phosphatidyl inositol 3mg, Phosphatidyl ethanolamine 10 mg, Fish oil concentrate 770 mg, EPA (EicosaPentaenoic Acid) 130 mg, DHA (DocosaHexaenoic Acid) 90 mg

Super 75 Tablets
Iron 9 mg, Iodine 0.15 mg, Magnesium 15 mg, Potassium 10 mg, Choline 75 mg, Inositol 75 mg, PABA (Para-Aminobenzoic Acid) 75 mg, Lemon bioflavonoids complex 25 mg, Betaine HCl 10 mg

Super High Vitamins & Minerals Tablets
Iron (Ferrous fumarate) 1 mg, Iodine 0.15 mg, Magnesium 1.44 mg, Potassium 2 mg, Choline 75 mg, Inositol 75 mg, PABA (Para-Aminobenzoic Acid) 75 mg, Citrus bioflavonoid complex 25 mg, Rutin 25 mg, Hesperidin complex 5 mg, Betaine 25 mg, Glutamic acid 25 mg

Supermins Tablets
Beta carotene 12,500 IU; Magnesium 40 mg, Potassium complex 49.5 mg

Support Liquid
Magnesium 0.069 mg, Lysine 275 mg

Support-500 Softgel Capsules
Magnesium 100 mg, L-glutathione 30 mg

Surbex 750 with Zinc Tablets
Sodium 100 mg

Tab A Vite Maximum Tablets
Iodine 0.15 mg, Iron (Ferrous fumarate) 18 mg, Magnesium 100 mg, Molybdenum 0.01 mg, Phosphorus 100 mg, Potassium 40 mg

Tab A Vite Women's Formula Tablets
Iron (Ferrous fumarate) 27 mg

Tandem DHA Capsules
Iron (Ferrous fumarate) 15 mg, Polysaccharide iron complex 15 mg, Omega 3 fatty acids 310.1 mg, Docosahexaenoic Acid (DHA) 215.12 mg, Eicosapentaenoic Acid (EPA) 53.46 mg

Tandem OB Capsules
Iron (Ferrous fumarate) 162 mg, Polysaccharide iron complex 115.2 mg, Magnesium 6.9 mg

Tandem Plus Capsules
Iron (Ferrous fumarate) 162 mg, Polysaccharide iron complex 115.2 mg

Thera M Tablets
Iron (Ferrous fumarate) 18 mg, Phosphorus 31 mg, Iodine 0.15 mg, Magnesium 100 mg, Molybdenum 0.015 mg, Potassium 7.5 mg

Theradex M
Iron 27 mg, Iodine 0.15 mg, Magnesium 100 mg, Molybdenum 0.015 mg, Potassium 0.01 mg

Thera-M Enhanced Tablets
Boron 0.15 mg, Iodine 0.15 mg, Iron 9 mg, Magnesium 100 mg, Molybdenum 0.075 mg, Nickel 0.005 mg, Phosphorus 31 mg, Potassium 7.5 mg, Silica 2 mg, Tin 0.01 mg, Vanadium 0.01 mg

Thera-M w/Mineral Tablets
Chloride 7.5 mg, Iodine 0.15 mg, Iron 18 mg, Magnesium 100 mg, Molybdenum 0.032 mg, Phosphorus 31 mg, Potassium 7.5 mg, Vitamin K 0.028 mg

Theramill Forte Capsules
Pyridoxal 5 phosphate 25 mg, Pantothine 25 mg, Choline bitartrate 75 mg, Inositol 75 mg, PABA (Para-Aminobenzoic Acid) 50 mg, Potassium 99 mg, Iodine 0.2 mg, Molybdenum 0.05 mg, Vanadium 0.02 mg, Bioflavonoids 100 mg, Boron 1.5 mg, Magnesium 400 mg

Theramill Plus Capsules
Iron 15 mg, Iodine 0.2 mg, Magnesium 100 mg, Molybdenum 0.05 mg, Potassium 99 mg, Pyridoxyl 5 phosphate 25 mg, Pantethine 25 mg, Choline bitartrate 75 mg, Inositol 75 mg, Vanadium 0.02 mg, Bioflavonoids 100 mg, Boron 1.5 mg

Theramill Plus Liquid Filled Capsules
Pyridoxal 5 Phosphate 25 mg, Pantothine 25 mg, Choline bitartrate 75 mg, Inositol 75 mg, PABA (Para-Aminobenzoic Acid) 50 mg, Potassium 99 mg, Iodine 0.2 mg, Molybdenum 0.05 mg, Vanadium 0.02 mg, Iron 15 mg, Bioflavonoids 100 mg, Boron 1.5 mg, Magnesium 400 mg

Therapeutic Multivitamin with Mineral Tablets
Iron (Ferrous fumarate) 27 mg, Iodine 0.15 mg, Magnesium 100 mg, Molybdenum 0.015 mg

Theravim-M Tablets (Nature's Bounty)
Vitamin K 0.028 mg, Iron (Ferrous fumarate) 9 mg, Phosphorus 27 mg, Iodine 0.15 mg, Magnesium 100 mg, Molybdenum 0.075 mg, Chloride 7 mg, Potassium 7.5 mg, Boron 0.15 mg, Tin 0.01 mg, Vanadium 0.01 mg, Nickel 0.005 mg, Silica 2 mg

Theravim-M Tablets (Puritan's Pride)
Iron (Ferrous fumarate) 27 mg, Phosphorus 31 mg, Iodine 0.15 mg, Magnesium 100 mg, Molybdenum 0.015 mg, Potassium 7.5 mg

Therems-H Tablets
Iron (Ferrous fumarate) 27 mg, Magnesium 41.7 mg, Sodium 12 mg

Therems-M Tablets
Vitamin K 0.028 mg, Iron (Ferrous fumarate) 9 mg, Phosphorus 31 mg, Iodine 0.15 mg, Magnesium 100 mg, Molybdenum 0.075 mg, Chloride 7.5 mg, Potassium 7.5 mg, Boron 0.15 mg, Nickel 0.005 mg, Silica 2 mg, Tin 0.01 mg, Vanadium 0.01 mg

Therobec Plus Tablets
Iron 27 mg, Magnesium 50 mg

Time Release Mega Vita-Min Iron Free Tablets
Iodine 0.15 mg, Magnesium 6 mg, Molybdenum 0.025 mg, Potassium 1.6 mg, Boron 0.5 mg, Choline bitartrate 80 mg, Inositol 80 mg, PABA (Para-Aminobenzoic Acid) 80 mg, Rutin 30 mg, Citrus bioflavonoids 25 mg, Hesperidin Complex 5 mg, Natural food base 4 mg, Betaine HCl 25 mg, Coenzyme Q10 0.5 mg, Deodorized garlic 1 mg, Korean ginseng 1 mg, Pinus pinaster 0.5 mg

Total Formula 3 Tablets
Vitamin K 0.07 mg, Iodine 0.1 mg, Magnesium 100 mg, Molybdenum 100 mg, Potassium 25 mg, Choline bitartrate 10 mg, Citrus bioflavonoids complex 10 mg, Hesperidin complex 10 mg, Inositol 10 mg, Rutin 10 mg, PABA (Para-Aminobenzoic acid) 8 mg, Silicon 2.4 mg, Boron 1 mg, Vanadium 0.025 mg

Triamin Tablets
Magnesium 62.5 mg, Potassium 49.5 mg

T-Vites Tablets
Magnesium 100 mg, Potassium 35 mg

Ultra Freeda A Free Tablets
Iron (Ferrous fumarate) 18 mg, Iodine 0.15 mg, Magnesium 100 mg, Molybdenum 0.0125 mg, Potassium 35 mg, Base (Choline, Inositol, PABA) 100 mg

Ultra Freeda, Iron Free Tablets
Iodine 0.15 mg, Magnesium 100 mg, Molybdenum 0.0125 mg, Potassium 35 mg, Bioflavonoids 100 mg, Base (Choline, Inositol, PABA) 100 mg

Ultra Freeda, With Iron Tablets
Iron (Ferrous fumarate) 18 mg, Iodine 0.15 mg, Magnesium 100 mg, Molybdenum 0.0125 mg, Potassium 35 mg, Bioflavonoids 100 mg, Base (Choline, Inositol, PABA) 100 mg

Ultra NatalCare Tablets
Iron 90 mg, Iodine 0.15 mg, Docusate sodium 50 mg

Ultra Vita-Min Iron Free Tablets
Phosphorus 24.3 mg, Iodine 0.1 mg, Magnesium 0.42 mg, Molybdenum 0.01 mg, Potassium 0.5 mg, PABA (Para-Aminobenzoic Acid) 15 mg, Choline bitartrate 25 mg, Inositol 25 mg, Boron 0.5mg, Betaine HCl 25 mg, Rose hips 10 mg, Rutin 5 mg, Citrus bioflavonoids complex 15 mg, Royal jelly 5 mg, Bee propolis 5 mg, Coenzyme Q10 0.03 mg, Octacosanol 0.05 mg, Deodorized garlic 10 mg, Korean ginseng 15 mg, RNA 2 mg, DNA 2 mg

Ultra Vita-Min Tablets
Iron (Ferrous gluconate) 5.79 mg, Phosphorus 24.3 mg, Iodine 0.1 mg, Magnesium 0.39 mg, Molybdenum 0.01 mg, Potassium 0.5 mg, PABA (Para-Aminobenzoic Acid) 15 mg, Choline bitartrate 25 mg, Inositol 25 mg, Boron 0.5 mg, Betaine HCl 25 mg, Rose hips 10 mg, Rutin 5 mg, Citrus bioflavonoid complex 15 mg, Royal jelly 5 mg, Bee propolis 5 mg, Coenzyme Q10 0.03 mg, Octacosanol 0.05 mg, Deodorized garlic 10 mg, Korean ginseng 15 mg, RNA 2 mg, DNA 2 mg

Unicomplex-M Tablets
Iron (Ferrous fumarate) 18 mg, Phosphorus 45 mg, Iodine 0.15 mg, Potassium 5 mg

Uni-Thera M Advanced Tablets
Vitamin K 0.028 mg, Iron (Ferrous fumarate) 9 mg, Phosphorus 31 mg, Iodine 0.15 mg, Magnesium 100 mg, Molybdenum 0.075 mg, Chloride 7 mg, Potassium 7.5 mg, Boron 0.15 mg, Tin 0.01 mg, Vanadium 0.01 mg, Nickel 0.005 mg, Silica 2 mg

V-C Forte Capsules
Magnesium sulfate 70 mg, Magnesium chloride 4 mg

Vicon C Capsules
Magnesium 6.4 mg

Vigomar Forte Tablets
Iodine 0.15 mg, Iron (Ferrous fumarate) 12 mg, Magnesium 65 mg

Vitrum Senior Complete Multivitamin/Multimineral Tablets

Vitamin K 0.01 mg, Phosphorus 48 mg, Iodine 0.15 mg, Magnesium 100 mg, Molybdenum 0.075 mg, Chloride 72 mg, Potassium 0.08 mg, Silicon 2 mg, Boron 0.150 mg, Vanadium 0.01 mg, Nickel 0.005 mg, Lycopene 0.300 mg, Lutein 0.250 mg

Women's Exclusive Formula Tablets (Puritan's Pride)

Iron (Ferrous gluconate) 15 mg, Phosphorus 30 mg, Iodine 0.15 mg, Magnesium 250 mg, Molybdenum 0.025 mg, Sodium 5 mg, Potassium 30 mg, Inositol 30 mg, Choline bitartrate 30 mg, PABA (Para-Aminobenzoic Acid) 30 mg, Citrus bioflavonoids 25 mg, Betaine HCl 25 mg, L-cysteine 50 mg, Dong quai 50 mg

Women's Exclusive Formula Tablets (Vitamin World)

Iron (Ferrous gluconate) 15 mg, Phosphorus 30 mg, Iodine 0.15 mg, Magnesium 250 mg, Molybdenum 0.025 mg, Sodium 5 mg, Potassium 30 mg, Inositol 30 mg, Choline bitartrate 30 mg, PABA (Para-Aminobenzoic Acid) 30 mg, Citrus bioflavonoids 25 mg, Betaine HCl 25 mg, L-cysteine 50 mg, Dong quai 50 mg

Women's One Daily Caplets

Iron 18 mg, Magnesium 50 mg

Women's Ultra Mega Active Caplets

Vitamin K 0.08 mg, Iron (Ferrous fumarate) 18 mg, Iodine 0.15 mg, Magnesium 100 mg, Molybdenum 0.075 mg, Chloride 72 mg, Potassium 80 mg, Proprietary performance blend (Panax ginseng root extract, Gingko biloba leaf extract, Green tea leaf extract, L-valine, L-leucine, L-isoleucine) 100 mg, Alpha-lipoic acid 25 mg, Choline bitartrate 10 mg, Inositol 10 mg, Cranberry concentrate 10 mg, Silica 4 mg, Lutein 0.95 mg, Lycopene 0.95 mg, Boron 0.06 mg, Astaxanthin 0.05 mg, Zeaxanthin 0.05 mg, Vanadium 0.01 mg

Xtramins Tablets

Potassium 45 mg, Iron 10 mg, Iodine 0.15 mg, Magnesium 20 mg, PABA (Para-Aminobenzoic Acid) 5 mg, Boron 1 mg

Yelets Tablets

Iron (Ferrous fumarate) 18 mg, Iodine 0.15 mg, Magnesium 20 mg, L-lysine 10 mg

Yummi Bears Chewables

Iodine 0.075 mg, Magnesium 8 mg, Vitamin K 0.04 mg

Yummi Bears Multivitamin and Mineral

Iodine 0.075 mg, Magnesium 8 mg, Sugars 3 g

Vitafol OB +DHA Caplets

Iron (Ferrous fumarate) 65 mg, Magnesium 25 mg, Dexahexaenoic Acid (DHA) 250 mg

Vitafol OB Caplets

Iron (Ferrous fumarate) 65 mg, Magnesium 25 mg

Vitalets Children's Chewable Tablets

Iron (Ferrous fumarate) 10 mg, Phosphorus 60 mg, Magnesium 20 mg

Vita-Min Capsules

Vitamin K1 0.3 mg, Phosphorus 4 mg, Iodine 0.1 mg, Magnesium 28 mg: Molybdenum 0.25 mg, Potassium 20 mg, Mixed mineral aspartates, Orotates, & Amino phosphate complex (AEP) Natural mixed cartenoids 52.5 mg, Inositol 2.5mg, Choline 25 mg, PABA (Para-Aminobenzoic Acid) 25 mg, Atlantic kelp 40 mg, Lemon bioflavonoid complex 13 mg, Alpha-lipoic acid 10 mg, Bromelain 10 mg, Hesperidin 6 mg, Boron 0.5 mg, Vanadium 0.25 mg

Vitamin Tonic for Seniors

Magnesium 15 mg

Vitamins for Hair Tablets (Basic Vitamins)

Iron 4.5 mg, Phosphorus 60 mg, Iodine 0.15 mg, Choline bitartrate 200 mg, Inositol 125 mg, PABA (Para-Aminobenzoic Acid) 35 mg, Glycin 12 mg, Silica 10.5 mg, Gelatin 13 mg

Vitamins for the Hair Tablets (Vitamin World)

Iron (Ferrous sulfate) 15 mg, Iodine 0.15 mg, Sodium 5 mg, PABA (Para-Aminobenzoic Acid) 30 mg, Choline bitartrate 125 mg, Inositol 50 mg, Isolated soy protein 100 mg, Brewer's yeast 5 mg

Vitamins for the Hair Tablets (Puritan's Pride)

Iron (Ferrous sulfate) 15 mg, Iodine 0.15 mg, Sodium 5 mg, PABA (Para-Aminobenzoic Acid) 30 mg, Choline bitartrate 125 mg, Inositol 50 mg, Isolated soy protein 100 mg, Brewer's yeast 5 mg

VitaTRUM Chewable Tablets

Vitamin K 10 IU; Iron 18 mg, Phosphorus 50 mg, Iodine 0.150 mg, Magnesium 40 mg, Molybdenum 20 mg

VitaTRUM Complete Multivitamin/Multimineral Tablets

Vitamin K 0.025 mg, Iron 18 mg, Phosphorus 109 mg, Iodine 0.15; Magnesium 100 mg, Molybdenum 0.075 mg, Chloride 72 mg, Potassium 0.08 mg, Silicon 2 mg, Boron 0.150 mg, Tin 0.15 mg, Vanadium 0.01 mg, Nickel 0.005 mg, Lycopene 0.300 mg, Lutein 0.250 mg

Vinate AZ Extra Tablets

Iron 29 mg, Magnesium 75 mg

Vinate AZ Tablets

Iron 27 mg, Magnesium 75 mg

Vinate GT Tablets

Elemental iron (Carbonyl iron) 90 mg, Magnesium 30 mg, Docusate 50 mg

Vinate II Tablets

Iron 29 mg, Magnesium 25 mg

Vinate M Tablets

Iodine 0.15 mg, Iron (Ferrous fumarate) 27 mg, Magnesium 25 mg, Molybdenum 0.025 mg

Vision Vitamin Tablets Plus Lutein

Lutein 2 mg

Vita S Forte Tablets

Iron (Ferrous fumarate) 10 mg, Magnesium 50 mg, Molybdenum 0.02 mg

Vitabasic Active Tablets

Vitamin K 0.025 mg, Potassium 80 mg, Phosphorus 48 mg, Iodine 0.15 mg, Magnesium 40 mg, Molybdenum 0.075 mg, Chloride 72 mg, Iron 18 mg, Boron 0.06 mg, Ginkgo biloba 0.06 mg, Vanadium 0.01 mg, Nickel 0.005 mg, Silica 4 mg, Tin 0.01 mg, Panax ginseng ex 0.25 mg

Vitabasic Complete Tablets

Vitamin K 0.025 mg, Potassium 80 mg, Phosphorus 109 mg, Iodine 0.15 mg, Magnesium 100 mg, Molybdenum 0.075 mg, Chloride 72 mg, Iron 18 mg, Boron 0.15 mg, Lycopene 0.3 mg, Vanadium 0.01 mg, Nickel 0.005 mg, Silica 2 mg, Tin 0.01 mg, Lutein 0.25 mg

Vitabasic Senior Tablets

Vitamin K 0.01 mg, Potassium 80 mg, Phosphorus 48 mg, Iodine 0.15 mg, Magnesium 100 mg, Molybdenum 0.075 mg, Chloride 72 mg, Lutein 0.25 mg, Boron 0.15 mg, Lycopene 0.3 mg, Vanadium 0.01 mg, Nickel 0.005 mg, Silica 2 mg

Vitadec Tablets

Boron 0.15 mg, Chloride 37.5 mg, Iodine 0.15 mg, Iron 18 mg, Magnesium 100 mg, Molybdenum 0.025 mg, Nickel 0.005 mg, Phosphorus 125 mg, Potassium 40 mg, Silica 0.01 mg, Tin 0.01 mg, Vanadium 0.01 mg, Vitamin K 0.025 mg

Vitamin B Complex Products

PRODUCT (Manufacturer)	FDA Class	B1 (mg)	B2 (mg)	B3 (mg)	Niacin-amide (mg)	B5 (mg)	B6 (mg)	B12 (mg)	Biotin (mg)	C (mg)	Folic Acid (mg)	Other
Animi-3 (PBM Pharmaceuticals)	Rx						12.5	500			0.5	Omega-3 fatty acids 1 mg
B-100 Complex (Rexall)	OTC	100	100		100	100	100	0.1	0.1		0.4	
B-100 ULTRA B-Complex (Nature's Bounty)	OTC	100	100		100	0.1	100	0.1	0.1		0.1	Inositol, PABA, Choline Bitartrate, Proprietary Blend
Balance B100 (National Vitamin)	OTC	100	100		100	100	100	0.1	0.1		0.2	Aminobenzoic Acid 100 mg, Choline 100 mg, Yeast, Dried 100 mg
Biotin (Nature's Bounty)	OTC	0.3										
B-plex Tablets (Contract Pharmacal)	Rx	15	15		100	18	4	0.005		500	0.5	
Cerefolin (PamLab)	Rx		50				5	5.635				L-methylfolate 1 mg
Dialyvite (Hillestad Pharmaceuticals)	Rx	1.5	1.7	20		10	10	0.006	0.3	100	1	
Diatx Zn (Pan American Laboratories)	Rx	1.5	1.5	20		10	50	2		60	5	Zinc 25 mg, Copper 1.5 mg
Folgard (Upsher-Smith Laboratories)	OTC						10	0.115			0.8	
Folic Acid Injection (Pharma Labs)	Rx							15/Ml			15/Ml	Sodium hydroxide, Hydrochloric acid
Folic Acid XTRA (Rexall)	OTC										0.8	
Formula B plus Tablets (Major Pharmaceuticals)	Rx	20	20		100	25	25	0.05	0.15	500	0.8	Chromium 0.1 mg, Manganese 5 mg, Zinc Oxide 22.5 mg, Iron 27 mg, Vitamin A 5,000 IU, Vitamin E 30 IU, Magnesium Oxide 50 mg, Copper 3 mg
Iberet-Folic-500 (Abbott Laboratories)	OTC	6	6		30	10	5	0.025		500	0.08	Ferrous sulfate 525 mg
Mega B (Arco Pharma)	OTC	100	100		100	100	100	0.1	0.06	60	0.1	Choline bitartrate 100 mg, Inositol 100 mg, PABA 100 mg
Nephplex Rx (Nephro-Tech, Inc)	Rx	1.5	1.7	20		10	10	6	0.3	60	1	
Nephrocaps (Fleming)	Rx	1.5	1.7	20		5	10	0.006	0.3	100	1	
Nephro-vite Rx (Watson)	Rx	1.5	1.7		20	10	10	0.006	0.3	60	1	
Neurofolic (Medical Products Panamericana)	OTC						125	1			0.8	
Niacin (Nature's Bounty)	OTC			100								

PRODUCT (Manufacturer)	FDA Class	B1 (mg)	B2 (mg)	B3 (mg)	Niacin-amide (mg)	B5 (mg)	B6 (mg)	B12 (mg)	Biotin (mg)	C (mg)	Folic Acid (mg)	Other
Strovite Rx (Everett)	Rx	20	20		100	25	25	0.005			0.8	Chromium 0.1 mg, Magnesium 5 mg, 3 mg, Zinc oxide 22.5 mg, Iron 27 mg, Vitamin A 500 IU, Vitamin E 30 IU, Copper 3 mg
Therobic (Qualitest)	Rx	15	15		100	18	4	0.005		500	0.5	
Thiamine Hydrochloride, Injection (APP Pharma)	Rx	100 per mL										Chlorobutanol 0.5%, Monothioglycerol 0.5%, Sodium hydroxide
Vita-Bee with C Tablets (Rugby Labs)	OTC	15	10.2		50	10	5			300		
Vitamin B Complex 100 (Bioniche Pharma)	Rx	100	2		100	2						
Vitamin B Complex Capsules (Rugby Labs)	OTC	3	3	20		5	0.5	0.001				Brewer's yeast 60 mg, desiccated liver 60 mg
Vitamin B12 Sl Jr (Carlson Laboratories)	OTC							1				
Vitamin B6 (Mason Vitamins)	OTC						50					
Vitaplex (Actavis)	Rx	15	15		100	18	4	0.005		500	0.5	

FDA = Food and Drug Administration classification. Rx = requires a prescription; OTC = available over the counter.

IU = international units; mg = milligram(s); PABA = para-aminobenzoic acid.